HERZOG'S
CCU BOOK

Eyal Herzog, MD

Director
Cardiac Care Unit
Director
Echocardiography Laboratories
Mount Sinai St. Luke's Hospital
Associate Professor of Medicine
Icahn School of Medicine at Mount Sinai
New York, New York

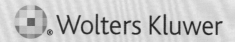

Philadelphia • Baltimore • New York • London
Buenos Aires • Hong Kong • Sydney • Tokyo

Senior Acquisitions Editor: Sharon Zinner
Editorial Coordinator: Lauren Pecarich
Production Project Manager: Linda Van Pelt
Design Coordinator: Holly McLaughlin
Manufacturing Coordinator: Beth Welsh
Marketing Manager: Rachel Mante Leung
Prepress Vendor: S4Carlisle Publishing Services

9 8 7 6 5 4 3 2 1

Printed in China

Library of Congress Cataloging-in-Publication Data
Names: Herzog, Eyal, editor.
Title: Herzog's CCU book / [edited by] Eyal Herzog.
Other titles: CCU book | Cardiac care unit book
Description: Philadelphia: Wolters Kluwer Health, [2018] | Includes
   bibliographical references and index.
Identifiers: LCCN 2017044559 | ISBN 9781496362612 (paperback)
Subjects: | MESH: Heart Diseases | Critical Care
Classification: LCC RC682 | NLM WG 210 | DDC 616.1/2—dc23 LC record
available at https://lccn.loc.gov/2017044559

LWW.com

To my family, patients, colleagues, and trainees
who have taught me so much over the years
Eyal Herzog

Contributors

Eric Adler, MD
Medical Director
Cardiac Transplant
Clinical Professor of Medicine
University of California San Diego
La Jolla, California

Jeanine Albu, MD, FACP
Chief
Division of Endocrinology, Diabetes and Nutrition
Mount Sinai St. Luke's and Mount Sinai West Hospitals
Professor of Medicine
Icahn School of Medicine at Mount Sinai
New York, New York

Diana Anca, MD
Cardiothoracic Anesthesiologist
Assistant Clinical Professor of Anesthesiology
Icahn School of Medicine at Mount Sinai
Mount Sinai St. Luke's Hospital
New York, New York

Edgar Argulian, MD, MPH, FACC, FASE
Assistant Professor of Medicine
Co-Director Echocardiography Laboratory
Mount Sinai St. Luke's Hospital
Mount Sinai Heart Institute
Icahn School of Medicine at Mount Sinai
New York, New York

Emad F. Aziz, DO, MBCHB, FACC, FHRS
Director Cardiovascular Research
Associate Director of Cardiovascular Fellowship
Associate Professor of Medicine
Icahn School of Medicine at Mount Sinai
New York, New York

Joshua Aziz, BMEs
Rutgers University
New Brunswick, New Jersey

May Bakir, MD
Department of Cardiology
Mount Sinai St. Luke's Hospital
New York, New York

Sandhya K. Balaram, MD, PhD
Associate Professor of Surgery
Department of Cardiovascular Surgery
Icahn School of Medicine at Mount Sinai
Mount Sinai St. Luke's Hospital
New York, New York

Gabriela Bambrick-Santoyo, MD
Director of Simulation
Associate Program Director
Internal Medicine Residency Program
Hackensack University Medical Center
Mountainside Hospital
Montclair, New Jersey

Chirag Bavishi, MD, MPH
Fellow
Cardiovascular Diseases
Mount Sinai St. Luke's and Mount Sinai West Hospitals
Icahn School of Medicine at Mount Sinai
New York, New York

Louis Brusco, MD, FCCM
Chief Medical Officer
Morristown Medical Center
Morristown, New Jersey

Sujata B. Chakravarti, MD
Medical Director
Congenital Cardiovascular Care Unit
Hassenfeld Children's Hospital at NYU Langone Health
Assistant Professor of Pediatrics
Division of Pediatric Cardiology
New York University School of Medicine
New York, New York

Patricia Chavez, MD
Cardiology Fellow
Mount Sinai St. Luke's and Mount Sinai West Hospitals
New York, New York

Joanna Chikwe, MD

The Eugene and Carol Chen Chair of
    Cardiothoracic Surgery
Professor and Chief
Cardiothoracic Surgery
Co-Director of the Heart Institute
Stony Brook University Hospital
Professor
Department of Cardiovascular Surgery
Icahn School of Medicine at Mount Sinai
New York, New York

Ankit Chothani, MD

Chief Fellow in Cardiovascular Medicine
Mount Sinai St. Luke's and Mount Sinai West Hospitals
New York, New York

Randy Cohen, MD

Attending Physician
Crystal Run Healthcare
West Nyack, New York

Johanna Contreras, MD, MSc, FACC, FAHA, FASE, FHFSA

Assistant Professor
Advanced Heart Failure and Transplant Cardiology
Director Heart Failure
Mount Sinai St. Luke's and Mount Sinai West Hospitals
Icahn School of Medicine at Mount Sinai
New York, New York

Ashish Correa, MD

Chief Resident
Internal Medicine
Mount Sinai St. Luke's and Mount Sinai
    West Hospitals
Icahn School of Medicine at Mount Sinai
New York, New York

Jacqueline Danik, MD, DrPH

Cardiology Division
Massachusetts General Hospital
Boston, Massachusetts

Asaf Danon, MD, MSc

Consultant
Electrophysiology Unit
Carmel Medical Center
Haifa, Israel

Seyed Hamed Hosseini Dehkordi, MD

Resident Physician
Mount Sinai St. Luke's and Mount Sinai West Hospitals
Icahn School of Medicine at Mount Sinai
New York, New York

Ernest G. DePuey, MD

Director of Nuclear Medicine
Mount Sinai St. Luke's and Mount Sinai West Hospitals
Clinical Professor of Radiology
Icahn School of Medicine at Mount Sinai
New York, New York

Matthew Durst, MD

House Staff
Icahn School of Medicine at Mount Sinai
New York, New York

Aeshita Dwivedi, MD

Fellow in Cardiovascular Diseases
The Leon H. Charney Division of Cardiology
New York University Medical School of Medicine
New York, New York

Karim El Hachem, MD

Attending Physician
Assistant Professor of Medicine
Icahn School of Medicine at Mount Sinai
Mount Sinai St. Luke's and Mount Sinai West Hospitals
New York, New York

Moshe Flugelman, MD

Director
Department of Cardiology
Lady Davis Carmel Medical Center
Faculty of Medicine
Technion – Israel Institute of Technology
Haifa, Israel

Diandra Fortune, BS

Research Assistant
Mount Sinai St. Luke's Hospital
New York, New York

Elissa K. Fory, MD

Attending Neurologist
Mount Sinai St. Luke's Hospital
Assistant Professor of Neurology
Icahn School of Medicine at Mount Sinai
New York, New York

Rodolfo J. Galindo, MD

Assistant Professor of Medicine
Emory University School of Medicine
Investigator
Center for Diabetes and Metabolism Research
Division of Endocrinology, Diabetes and Lipids
Medical Chair
Hospital Diabetes Taskforce
Emory Healthcare System
Atlanta, Georgia

Carly E. Glick, MD

Gastroenterology Fellow
Mount Sinai Beth Israel, Mount Sinai St. Luke's, and
    Mount Sinai West Hospitals
New York, New York

Jacob Goldstein, MD, FESC

Cardiology Department
Lady Davis Carmel Medical Center
Haifa, Israel

Gustavo S. Guandalini, MD

Cardiovascular Disease Fellow
The Leon H. Charney Division of Cardiology
New York University School of Medicine
New York, New York

Dan G. Halpern, MD

Director
Adult Congenital Heart Disease Program
Assistant Professor of Medicine
The Leon H. Charney Division of Cardiology
New York University School of Medicine
New York, New York

Harvey Hecht, MD, FACC, FSCCT

Director of Cardiovascular Computed Tomography
Mount Sinai St. Luke's and Mount Sinai West Hospitals
Professor of Medicine
Icahn School of Medicine at Mount Sinai
New York, New York

Yaron Hellman, MD

Cardiology Department
Rambam Health Care Campus
Haifa, Israel

Eyal Herzog, MD

Director
Cardiac Care Unit
Director
Echocardiography Laboratories
Mount Sinai St. Luke's Hospital
Associate Professor of Medicine
Icahn School of Medicine at Mount Sinai
New York, New York

Lee Herzog

Icahn School of Medicine at Mount Sinai
New York, New York

Andrew Higgins, MD

Fellow in Cardiovascular Disease
Cleveland Clinic Lerner College of Medicine
Case Western Reserve University
Cleveland Clinic
Cleveland, Ohio

Chetan Huded, MD

Fellow in Cardiovascular Disease
Cleveland Clinic Lerner College of Medicine
Case Western Reserve University
Cleveland Clinic
Cleveland, Ohio

Ronen Jaffe, MD

Director of Interventional Cardiology
Carmel Medical Center
Assistant Professor of Medicine
Rappaport School of Medicine
Technion – Israel Institute of Technology
Haifa, Israel

James Jones, MD[†]

Division of Nephrology
Mount Sinai St. Luke's and Mount Sinai West Hospitals
New York, New York

Karen Kan, MD

Fellow
Cardiovascular Disease
NYU Langone Medical Center
New York, New York

Samir Kapadia, MD

Professor of Medicine
Section Head
Interventional Cardiology
Director
Cardiac Catheterization Laboratory
Cleveland Clinic
Cleveland, Ohio

Basheer Karkabi, MD

Senior Cardiologist
Cardiology Division
Lady Davis Carmel Hospital
Haifa, Israel

Bette Kim, MD

Director
Cardiomyopathy Program
Director
Mount Sinai West Echocardiography Laboratory
Assistant Professor of Clinical Medicine
Mount Sinai West Hospital
Icahn School of Medicine at Mount Sinai
New York, New York

Todd Kobrinski, DO, MD

Clinical Cardiac Electrophysiology Fellow
Icahn School of Medicine at Mount Sinai
Mount Sinai Heart
Mount Sinai St. Luke's Hospital
New York, New York

Donald P. Kotler, MD

Chief
Division of Gastroenterology
Jacobi Medical Center
Bronx, New York

Ismini Kourouni, MD

Senior Fellow
Pulmonary and Critical Care Medicine
Mount Sinai St. Luke's and Mount Sinai West Hospitals
Icahn School of Medicine at Mount Sinai
New York, New York

[†] Deceased. His untimely passing at the end of 2016 has left a void in our hearts and minds.

Itzhak Kronzon, MD

Professor in Cardiology
Hofstra University School of Medicine
Lenox Hill Hospital—Northwell Health
Department of Cardiology
New York, New York

Nina Kukar, MD

Director
Women's Heart NY
Director
Cardiac MRI Mount Sinai West and Mount Sinai
    St. Luke's Hospitals
Assistant Professor of Medicine
Icahn School of Medicine at Mount Sinai
New York, New York

Marrick L. Kukin, MD, FACC, FAHA, FHFSA

Professor of Medicine
Mount Sinai St. Luke's Hospital
Icahn School of Medicine at Mount Sinai
New York, New York

Gina LaRocca, MD

Associate Director
Adult Congenital Heart Disease
Assistant Professor of Medicine in Cardiology
Icahn School of Medicine at Mount Sinai
New York, New York

Shawn Lee, MD

Medical Resident
Mount Sinai St. Luke's Hospital
New York, New York

Steven B. Levy, PharmD

Assistant Director of Clinical Pharmacy
Department of Pharmacy
Mount Sinai St. Luke's Hospital
New York
Clinical Associate Professor
Long Island University
LIU Pharmacy
Brooklyn, New York
Adjunct Assistant Professor
University of Connecticut School of Pharmacy
Storrs, Connecticut

Pavan K. Mankal, MD

Division of Gastroenterology
Department of Medicine
Mount Sinai St. Luke's and Mount Sinai West Hospitals
New York, New York

Petra Zubin Maslov, MD

Medical Resident
Internal Medicine
Mount Sinai St. Luke's and Mount Sinai
    West Hospitals
New York, New York

Joseph P. Mathew, MD, FACP, FCCP

Co-Director
Critical Care Ultrasonography Program
Medical Director
Center for Advanced Medical Simulation (CAMS)
Division of Pulmonary, Critical Care, and Sleep Medicine
Mount Sinai St. Luke's and Mount Sinai West Hospitals
Associate Professor of Medicine
Icahn School of Medicine at Mount Sinai
New York, New York

Stephan A. Mayer, MD, FCCM

Director
Neurocritical Care
Mount Sinai Health System
Professor of Neurology and Neurosurgery
Icahn School of Medicine at Mount Sinai
New York, New York

Davendra Mehta, MD

Director
Cardiac Electrophysiology Cardiology
Mount Sinai St. Luke's Hospital
New York, New York

Ira Meisels, MD

Chief
Division of Nephrology
Mount Sinai St. Luke's and Mount Sinai West Hospitals
Associate Professor of Medicine
Icahn School of Medicine at Mount Sinai
New York, New York

Venu Menon, MD, FACC, FAHA

Director
CICU
Director
Cardiovascular Fellowship
Associate Director
Professor of Medicine
Cleveland Clinic Lerner College of Medicine
Case Western Reserve University
Cleveland, Ohio

Arie Militianu, MD

Director
Arrhythmia Service
Lady Davis Carmel Medical Center
Technion – Israel Institute of Technology
Haifa, Israel

Ahmadreza Moradi, MD

Internal Medicine Resident
Mount Sinai St. Luke's and Mount Sinai West Hospitals
Icahn School of Medicine at Mount Sinai
New York, New York

Noah Moss, MD

Medical Director of Mechanical Circulatory Support
Mount Sinai Hospital
Assistant Professor of Medicine
Icahn School of Medicine at Mount Sinai
New York, New York

Gopal Narayanswami, MD, FCCP

Associate Director
Medical Intensive Care Unit
Mount Sinai St. Luke's Hospital
Assistant Professor of Medicine
Icahn School of Medicine at Mount Sinai
New York, New York

Mary O'Sullivan, MD

Director of Margarita Camche Smoking Cessation Clinic
Mount Sinai St. Luke's Hospital
Associate Professor of Medicine
Icahn School of Medicine at Mount Sinai
New York, New York

Angela Palazzo, MD, FACC

Associate Chief Cardiology
Clinical Operations
Mount Sinai St. Luke's Hospital
Assistant Professor of Medicine
Icahn School of Medicine at Mount Sinai
New York, New York

Yuvrajsinh J. Parmar, MD

Fellow
Department of Cardiology
Hofstra University School of Medicine
Lenox Hill Hospital – Northwell Health
New York, New York

Vishal P. Patel, DO

Attending Physician
Naples Community Hospital
Naples, Florida

Sean P. Pinney, MD

Director
Heart Failure and Transplantation
Mount Sinai Health System
Professor of Medicine
Icahn School of Medicine at Mount Sinai
New York, New York

Hooman Poor, MD

Assistant Professor of Medicine
Director of Pulmonary Vascular Disease
Mount Sinai–National Jewish Health Respiratory Institute
Associate Program Director
Fellowship Training Program
Division of Pulmonary, Critical Care and Sleep Medicine
Zena and Michael A. Wiener Cardiovascular Institute
Icahn School of Medicine at Mount Sinai
New York, New York

Jonathan Price, MD

Department of Surgery
Mount Sinai St. Luke's Hospital
New York, New York

Olga Reynbakh, MD

Medical Resident
Mount Sinai St. Luke's Hospital
New York, New York

Mario Rodriguez Rivera, MD

Resident
Internal Medicine
Mount Sinai St. Luke's and Mount Sinai West Hospitals
New York, New York

Richard Ro, MD

Clinical Cardiologist
Division of Cardiovascular Diseases
Assistant Professor of Medicine
Columbia University Medical Center
Mount Sinai Medical Center
Miami, Florida

Alan Rozanski, MD

Director
Cardiovascular Fellowship Training Program
Director
Nuclear Cardiology and Cardiac Stress Testing
Professor of Medicine
Icahn School of Medicine at Mount Sinai
New York, New York

Ronen Rubinshtein, MD, FACC, FESC

Director
Cardiovascular Imaging
Lady Davis Carmel Medical Center
Clinical Associate Professor of Medicine
Technion – Israel Institute of Technology
Haifa, Israel

Manpreet Sabharwal, MBBS

Cardiologist
United Heart and Vascular Clinic
St. Paul, Minnesota

Javier Sanz, MD, FACC

Director
Cardiac CT/MR
Zena and Michael A. Wiener Cardiovascular Institute and
    Marie-Josée and Henry R. Kravis Center for Cardiovascular
    Health
Associate Professor of Medicine/Cardiology & Radiology
Icahn School of Medicine at Mount Sinai
New York, New York

Muhamed Saric, MD, PhD

Associate Professor
Director
Noninvasive Cardiology
The Leon H. Charney Division of Cardiology
New York University
New York, New York

Kimberly M. Sarosky, MS, PharmD

Clinical Pharmacy Specialist
Critical Care/Infectious Disease
Department of Pharmacy
Mount Sinai St. Luke's Hospital
Clinical Associate Professor
Long Island University
LIU Pharmacy
Brooklyn, New York

Jorge E. Schliamser, MD

Director
Cardiac Electrophysiology Laboratory
Department of Cardiovascular Medicine
Lady Davis Carmel Medical Center
Haifa, Israel

Allison Selby, DO

Cardiology Fellow
Mount Sinai St. Luke's and Mount Sinai West Hospitals
New York, New York

Ziad Sergie, MD, MBA, FACC

Monmouth Cardiology Associates, LLC
Director
Cardiovascular MRI
Jersey Shore University Medical Center
Eatontown, New Jersey

Arpit Shah, MD

Interventional Cardiology Fellow
Mount Sinai St. Luke's Hospital
New York, New York

Janet M. Shapiro, MD, FCCP

Director
Medical Intensive Care Unit
Mount Sinai St. Luke's Hospital
Associate Professor of Medicine
Icahn School of Medicine at Mount Sinai
New York, New York

Avinoam Shiran, MD

Director
Echocardiography
Lady Davis Carmel Medical Center
Clinical Associate Professor
The Ruth and Bruce Rappaport Faculty of Medicine
Technion – Israel Institute of Technology
Haifa, Israel

Nektarios Souvaliotis, MD

Clinical Cardiac Electrophysiology Fellow
Mount Sinai St. Luke's Hospital
New York, New York

Karan Sud, MD

Resident Physician
Department of Internal Medicine
Icahn School of Medicine at Mount Sinai
Mount Sinai St. Luke's and Mount Sinai West Hospitals
New York, New York

Jacqueline E. Tamis-Holland, MD, FACC, FSCAI, FAHA

Associate Director
Cardiac Catheterization Laboratory
Mount Sinai St. Luke's Hospital
Assistant Professor of Medicine
Icahn School of Medicine at Mount Sinai
New York, New York

Henry Tannous, MD

Associate Professor of Cardiovascular Surgery
Icahn School of Medicine at Mount Sinai
Associate Professor of Cardiothoracic Surgery
Stony Brook University Medical Center
New York, New York

Seth Uretsky, MD

Medical Director
Cardiovascular Imaging
Atlantic Health System
Associate Professor of Medicine
Sidney Kimmel Medical College
Thomas Jefferson University
Morristown, New Jersey

Alan F. Vainrib, MD

Clinical Instructor
The Leon H. Charney Division of Cardiology
New York University
New York, New York

Indra Warren, MD, FRCPC

Staff Cardiologist
Assistant Clinical Professor (Adjunct)
McMaster University
Joseph Brant Hospital
Burlington, Canada

Barak Zafrir, MD, FESC, FACC

Director
Cardiac Prevention and Rehabilitation Service
Department of Cardiovascular Medicine
Lady Davis Carmel Medical Center
Haifa, Israel

Preface

Heart disease is the leading cause of death in the world. Advances in the treatment of heart disease are considered among the greatest achievements of modern medicine. Physicians, nurses, and all health care providers who care for patients with heart disease consider the cardiac care unit (CCU) the most exciting place in the hospital.

The *CCU Book* is essentially two books combined into one. Most chapters have two sections: the first is for physicians and other health care providers, and the second is for patients and their families.

The first section of each chapter is aimed toward physicians (interns, residents, fellows, and attendings), medical students, nurses, physician assistants, and other health care providers who rotate or practice in the CCU. It is organized such that readers will not need to consult any textbooks regarding the topics discussed and will be able to understand the simplified pathophysiology and management of the disease. This includes diagnostic modalities, initial critical care management in the CCU, follow-up care in a step-down unit, and plans for discharge. Algorithms and pathways for management are provided for easy implementation in any health care system.

The second part of each chapter covers the same topics previously discussed but is directed toward the patients and their families. The language and the medical terminology are simpler and geared toward the general public.

It is my hope that this book will serve as a teaching tool to save the lives of patients with heart disease in the CCU.

Eyal Herzog

Acknowledgments

I would like to acknowledge the extraordinary work of LaToya Selby and Candice Francis from my office at Mount Sinai St. Luke's Hospital in New York; they are my right hand in assisting my trainees and patients in the hospital and are also the editing coordinators for this book.

Thank you,
Eyal Herzog

Contents

Section III

ARRHYTHMIA IN THE CCU

Section IV

AORTIC, PERICARDIAL, AND VALVULAR DISEASE IN THE CCU

ACUTE CORONARY SYNDROME

Eyal Herzog
Jacqueline E. Tamis-Holland
Emad F. Aziz

1

Pathway for the Management of Acute Coronary Syndrome

The practice of medicine is changing at unprecedented speed. Today's reasonable assumption is outlined by tomorrow's evidence. We face a deluge of data as we confront the onslaught of acute coronary syndrome (ACS). ACS subsumes a spectrum of clinical entities, ranging from unstable angina (UA) to ST-elevation myocardial infarction (STEMI). The management of ACS is deservedly scrutinized because it accounts for about 2 million hospitalizations and a remarkable 30% of all deaths in the United States each year. Clinical guidelines on the management of ACS, which are based on clinical trials, have been updated and published.[1–3]

In this chapter, we describe a novel pathway for the management of ACS in our health care system.[4,5]

The pathway has been designated with the acronym PAIN (*P*riority risk, *A*dvanced risk, *I*ntermediate risk, and *N*egative/Low risk), which reflects the patient's most immediate risk stratification upon admission (**Figure 1.1**). This risk stratification reflects the patient's 30-day risks for death and myocardial infarction (MI) following the initial ACS event.

The pathway is color coded with the "PAIN" acronym (P—red, A—yellow, I—yellow, N—green), which guides patient management according to the patient's risk stratification. These colors—similar to the traffic light code—have been chosen as an easy reference for the provider about the sequential risk level of patients with ACS.[6]

In comparison with the North American and European guidelines for ACS,[1–3] in the proposed PAIN algorithm, P (priority) is equivalent to STEMI or STE (ST-elevation)-ACS; A (advanced) and I (intermediate) are equivalent to non–STE-ACS; and N (negative) means that there is no evidence of ACS.

INITIAL ASSESSMENT OF PATIENTS WITH CHEST PAIN OR CHEST PAIN EQUIVALENT

Patients who present to emergency departments with chest pain or chest pain equivalent will be enrolled into this pathway.

Figure 1.2 shows the chest pain equivalent symptoms. The initial assessment is seen in **Figure 1.3**. All patients should have an electrocardiogram (ECG) performed within 10 minutes as well as a detailed history and physical examination.

Non-ACS chest pain should be excluded urgently. These conditions include aortic dissection, pericarditis and pericardial effusion, pulmonary emboli, aortic stenosis, and hypertrophic cardiomyopathy. If any of these emergency conditions is suspected, we recommend immediately obtaining an echocardiogram or a computed tomography (CT) scan and treating accordingly.

Our recommended initial laboratory tests include complete blood count, basic metabolic panel, cardiac markers (to include creatine phosphokinase [CPK], CPK-muscle and brain [CPK-MB], and troponin), brain natriuretic peptide (BNP), prothrombin time, partial thromboplastin time, international normalized ratio, magnesium level, and a lipid profile.

INITIAL MANAGEMENT OF PRIORITY PATIENTS

Priority patients are those with symptoms of chest pain or chest pain equivalent lasting longer than 30 minutes with one of the following ECG criteria for acute MI:

1. Group (1): New ST-elevation at the J point in at least two contiguous leads: ≥ 2 mm (0.2 mV) in men or ≥ 1.5 mm (0.15 mV) in women in leads V2–V3 and/or ≥ 1 mm (0.1 mV) in other contiguous chest leads or the limb leads
2. Group (2): New left bundle branch block (LBBB) or
3. Group (3): Acute posterior wall MI (ST-segment depression in leads V1–V3)

The initial treatment of these patients includes obtaining an intravenous line; providing oxygen; treating patients with oral aspirin (chewable 325 mg stat) and a loading dose of one of the following agents: ticagrelor (180 mg), clopidogrel (600 mg), or prasugrel (60 mg); and giving high-dose statin (atorvastatin 80 mg po). We also recommend considering a bolus of IV heparin (1 mg/kg to a maximum dose of 4000 units) and nitroglycerin if it will not delay the transfer of the patient to the Cardiac Catheterization Laboratory (**Figure 1.4**).

The key question for further management of these patients is the duration of the patients' symptoms. For patients whose symptoms exceed 12 hours, presence of persistent or residual chest pain determines the next strategy. If there is no evidence of continued symptoms, these patients will generally be treated as though they had been risk stratified with the advanced risk group.

For patients whose symptoms are less than 12 hours or with ongoing chest pain, the decision for further management is

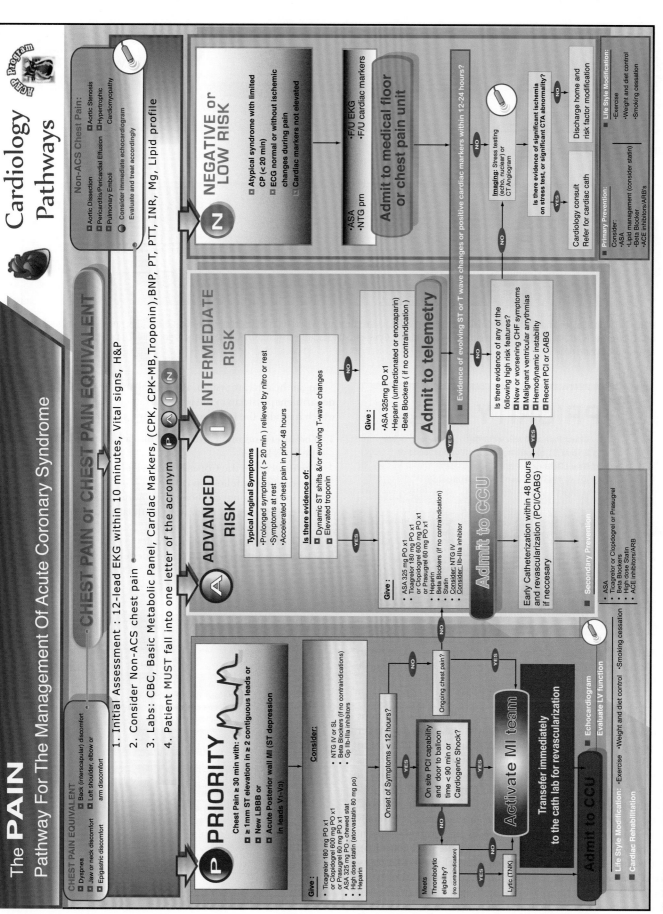

FIGURE 1.1 The PAIN pathway for the management of acute coronary syndrome. ACE, angiotensin converting enzyme; ACS, acute coronary syndrome; ARB, angiotensin receptor blocker; BNP, brain natriuretic peptide; CABG, coronary artery bypass surgery; CHF, congestive heart failure; CCU, coronary care unit; CPK, creatine phosphokinase; CPK-MB, CPK-muscle and brain; ECG, electrocardiogram; INR, international normalized ratio; LBBB, left bundle branch block; MI, myocardial infarction; PCI, percutaneous coronary intervention; PT, prothrombin time; PTT, partial thromboplastin time.

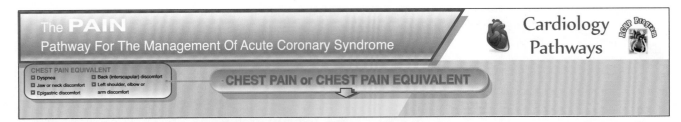

FIGURE 1.2 Chest pain and chest pain equivalent symptoms.

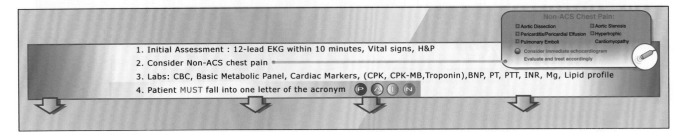

FIGURE 1.3 Initial assessment of patients with chest pain. ACS, acute coronary syndrome; CBC, complete blood count; CPK, creatine phosphokinase; CPK-MB, CPK-muscle and brain; BNP, brain natriuretic peptide; ECG, electrocardiogram; INR, international normalized ratio; PT, prothrombin time; PTT, partial thromboplastin time.

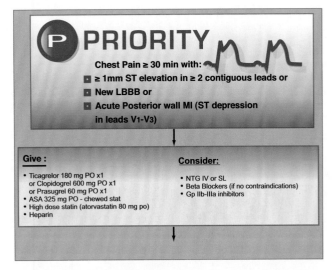

FIGURE 1.4 The initial management of priority patients (those with ST-elevation myocardial infarction). LBBB, left bundle branch block; MI, myocardial infarction.

In our health care system, a single call made by the emergency department physician to the page operator activates the MI team, which includes the following healthcare providers:

1. The interventional cardiologist on call (who is considered the team leader
2. The director of the Coronary Care Unit (CCU)
3. The cardiology fellow on call
4. The interventional cardiology fellow on call
5. The catheterization laboratory (cath lab) nurse on call
6. The cath lab technologist on call
7. The CCU nursing manager on call
8. The senior internal medicine resident on call

based on the availability of on-site angioplasty (percutaneous coronary intervention [PCI]) capability or the ability to transfer the patient to a PCI-capable hospital for immediate PCI within 120 minutes, and the clinical condition of the patient. Patients presenting to a PCI-capable hospital or patients presenting to a non–PCI-capable hospital but who can be transferred to a PCI-capable hospital with an expected "first door to balloon" time of less than 120 minutes should be transferred immediately to the cardiac catheterization laboratory for revascularization. The MI team is activated for this group of patients (**Figure 1.5**). Furthermore, patients with cardiogenic shock should be transferred immediately to the cardiac catheterization laboratory even if they present to a non–PCI-capable hospital and anticipated time to transfer is more than 120 minutes.

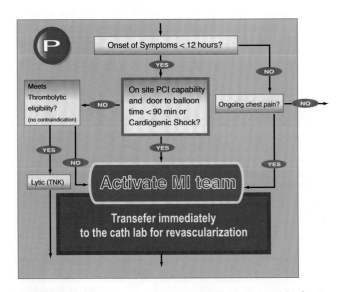

FIGURE 1.5 Advanced management of priority myocardial infarction patients. MI, myocardial infarction; PCI, percutaneous coronary intervention.

Activating these groups of people has been extremely successful in our institution and has reduced markedly our door to balloon time as well as our first medical contact to device time.

For hospitals without PCI capability and with expected first door-balloon time of more than 120 minutes, we recommend thrombolytic therapy if there are no contraindications.

CORONARY CARE UNIT MANAGEMENT AND SECONDARY PREVENTION FOR PATIENTS WITH PRIORITY MYOCARDIAL INFARCTION

Patients with priority MI should be admitted to the CCU (**Figure 1.6**). All patients should have an echocardiogram to evaluate left ventricle systolic and diastolic function and to exclude valvular abnormality and pericardial involvement. We recommend a CCU stay of 24 to 48 hours to exclude arrhythmia or mechanical complications. For patients with no evidence of mechanical complications or significant arrhythmia, secondary prevention drugs should be started, including aspirin, one of the additional antiplatelet drugs (ticagrelor, clopidogrel, or prasugrel) a high-dose statin, a beta-blocker, and an angiotensin converting enzyme (ACE) inhibitor, or an angiotensin receptor blocker (ARB). Aldosterone blocking agents should be considered for patients with diabetes or LV ejection fraction less than 40%.

Most patients can be discharged within 48 hours with recommendation for lifestyle modification, including exercise, weight and diet control, smoking cessation, and cardiac rehabilitation. Secondary prevention drugs should be continued on discharge.

MANAGEMENT OF ADVANCED RISK ACUTE CORONARY SYNDROME

Typical anginal symptoms are required to be present in patients who will be enrolled into the advanced or intermediate risk groups.

These symptoms include the following:

1. Prolonged chest pain (>20 minutes) relieved by nitroglycerine or rest
2. Chest pain at rest or
3. Accelerated chest pain within 48 hours

To qualify for the advanced risk group, patients must have dynamic ST changes on the ECG (>0.5 mm), dynamic ischemic

T-wave changes, or elevated cardiac biomarkers (troponin >0.2 ng/mL) (**Figure 1.7**).

We recommend that patients be admitted to the CCU and be treated with aspirin; ticagrelor or clopidogrel; anticoagulation, including either intravenous heparin or low molecular weight heparin; a beta-blocker; and a statin; consider glycoprotein IIb–IIIa inhibitor or nitroglycerin if there are no contraindications (**Figure 1.8**).

These patients should have early cardiac catheterization within 48 hours and revascularization by PCI or coronary artery bypass surgery (CABG) if there is obstructive coronary artery disease noted on coronary angiography. All patients should have an echocardiogram to evaluate left ventricular (LV) function. Recommendation for secondary prevention medication, lifestyle modification, and cardiac rehabilitation should be provided as in the case of patients in the priority risk group (**Figure 1.6**).

MANAGEMENT OF INTERMEDIATE RISK GROUP

Both the intermediate risk group and the advanced risk patients present to the hospital with typical anginal symptoms. Compared with the advanced risk patients, the immediate risk patients *do not* have evidence of dynamic ST changes or ischemic T-wave changes on the ECG or evidence of positive cardiac markers. These patients should be admitted to the telemetry floor and be given aspirin, heparin, and a beta-blocker if there is no contraindication (**Figure 1.9**). We recommend a minimum telemetry stay of 12 to 24 hours. During this period of time, if there is evidence of dynamic ST changes or ischemic T-wave changes on the ECG or evidence for positive cardiac markers, the patients should be treated as if they had been stratified to the advanced group.

The intermediate risk group patients are assessed again for the following high-risk features:

1. New or worsening heart failure symptoms
2. Malignant ventricular arrhythmias
3. Hemodynamic instability
4. Recent PCI or CABG

If there is evidence of any of these high-risk features, we recommend cardiac catheterization within 48 hours and revascularization by PCI or CABG if necessary. Patients with no evidence

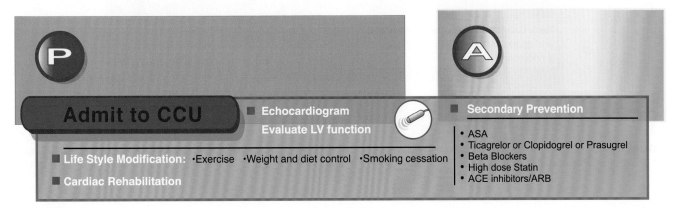

FIGURE 1.6 Coronary care unit management and secondary prevention for patients with priority myocardial infarction. ACE, angiotensin converting enzyme; ARB, angiotensin receptor blocker; CCU, coronary care unit.

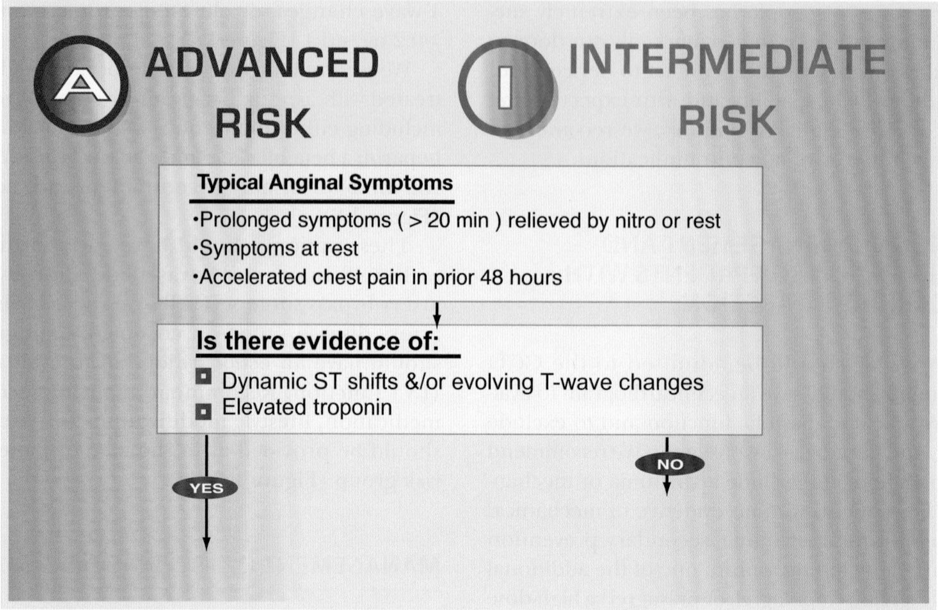

FIGURE 1.7 Risk stratification as advanced risk acute coronary syndrome.

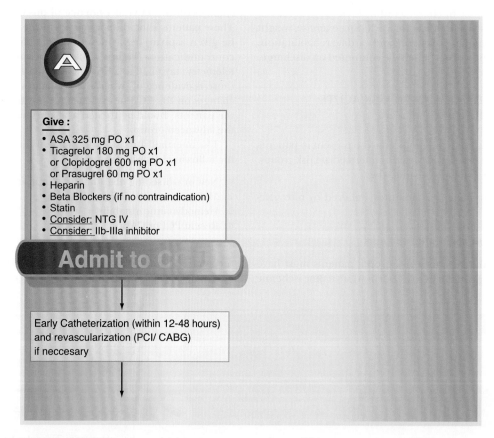

FIGURE 1.8 Management of patients with advanced risk acute coronary syndrome. CCU, coronary care unit; CABG, coronary artery bypass surgery; PCI, percutaneous coronary intervention.

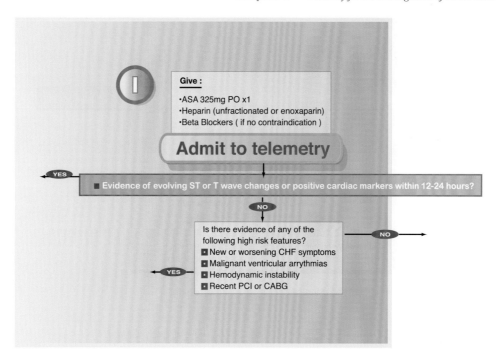

FIGURE 1.9 Management of patients with intermediate risk acute coronary syndrome. CHF, congestive heart failure; CABG, coronary artery bypass surgery; PCI, percutaneous coronary intervention.

of high-risk features should be referred for cardiac imaging and stress testing (stress echocardiography or stress nuclear test) or for CT angiography.

MANAGEMENT OF NEGATIVE- OR LOW-RISK GROUP PATIENTS

These groups of patients have atypical symptoms, do not have significant ischemic ECG changes during pain, and do not have elevated cardiac biomarkers.

These patients should be treated only with aspirin and given sublingual nitroglycerin if needed. If a decision is made to admit them to the hospital, they should be admitted to a chest pain unit or to a regular medical floor. They should be followed up for 12 to 24 hours with repeated ECG and cardiac biomarkers (**Figure 1.10**). If there is evidence of evolving ST changes or ischemic T-wave changes on the ECG or any evidence of positive cardiac markers, the patients should be treated aggressively, as for the advanced risk group patients.

If there are no significant ECG changes and all cardiac markers are negative, we recommend cardiac imaging and stress testing by stress echocardiography or stress nuclear test or a CT angiography (**Figure 1.11**).

Evidence of significant ischemia on any of these stress imaging modalities will be followed by a referral for cardiac catheterization. If there is no evidence of significant ischemia on stress testing, the patients will be discharged home with a recommendation for risk factor modification, to include primary prevention medication and lifestyle modification (**Figure 1.12**).

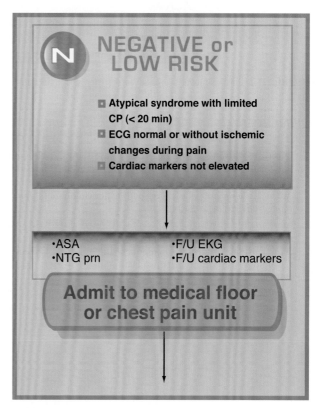

FIGURE 1.10 Initial management of patients with negative- or low-risk acute coronary syndrome; ASA, acetylsalicylic acid; CP, chest pain; ECG, electrocardiogram; NTG, nitroglycerin.

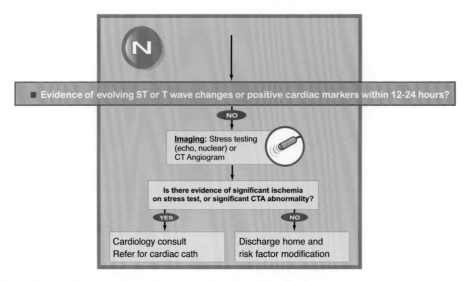

FIGURE 1.11 Risk stratification of low-risk patients by using cardiac imaging stress testing.

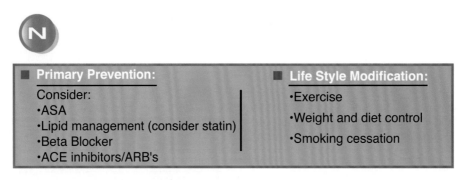

FIGURE 1.12 Primary prevention for low-risk patients. ACE, angiotensin converting enzyme; ARB, angiotensin receptor blocker; ASA, acetylsalicylic acid.

REFERENCES

1. O'Gara PT, Kushner FG, Ascheim DD, et al. 2013 ACC/AHA guideline for the management of ST-elevation myocardial infarction: a report of the American College of Cardiology Foundation/American Heart Association Task Force on Practice Guidelines. *J Am Coll Cardiol.* 2013;61(4):e78-e140.

2. Amsterdam EA, Wenger NK, Brindis RG, et al. 2014 AHA/ACC guideline for the management of patients with non-ST-elevation acute coronary syndromes. A report of the American College of Cardiology/American Heart Association Task Force on Practice Guidelines. *Circulation.* 2014;130:e344-e426.

3. Roffi M, Patrono C, Collet J-P, et al. 2015 ESC guidelines for the management of acute coronary syndromes in patients presenting without persistent ST-segment elevation. *Eur Heart J.* 2016;37(3): 267-315.

4. Herzog E, Saint-Jacques H, Rozanski A. The PAIN pathway as a tool to bridge the gap between evidence and management of acute coronary syndrome critical. *Pathw Cardiol.* 2004;3:20-24.

5. Herzog E, Aziz EF, Hong MK. A novel pathway for the management of acute coronary syndrome. In: Herzog E, Chaudhry F. *Echocardiography in Acute Coronary Syndrome: Diagnosis, Treatment and Prevention.* London, England: Springer; 2009:9-19.

6. Saint-Jacques H, Burroughs VJ, Watowska J, et al. Acute coronary syndrome critical pathway: chest PAIN Caremap: a qualitative research study-provider-level intervention. *Crit Pathw Cardiol.* 2005;4: 145-156.

Chirag Bavishi
Eyal Herzog
Jacqueline E. Tamis-Holland

2

ST-Segment Elevation Myocardial Infarction

INTRODUCTION

ST-segment elevation myocardial infarction (STEMI) represents the most urgent form of acute coronary syndromes (ACS). Pathophysiologically, it is characterized by occlusive intracoronary thrombus formation, resulting in the total cessation of coronary artery blood flow, and the characteristic pattern of ST-segment elevation on the electrocardiogram (ECG), indicative of an acute current of injury from transmural ischemia. Prompt recognition is the key step in the management of such patients to ensure early revascularization, thus limiting the extent of ischemic myocardium and minimizing early and late morbidity and mortality associated with STEMI.

EPIDEMIOLOGY

STEMI remains a major public health problem in both developed and developing nations. In the United States, there are approximately 1 million hospitalizations each year for ACS, and STEMI comprises 25% to 40% of these cases.[1,2] Approximately one-third of the patients with STEMI are women. In the past decade, there has been a marked decline in the incidence of STEMI, presumably as a result of the widespread institution of aggressive preventive therapies. In-hospital mortality for patients with STEMI ranges from 5% to 6%, whereas 1-year mortality is variable and estimated to range from 7% to 18%.[1] However, important age-related, sex-related, and geographic differences exist.

PATHOPHYSIOLOGY

The occlusive intracoronary thrombus is usually the result of rupture, ulceration, or erosion of an atherosclerotic plaque. Plaque rupture accounts for the majority of the cases. This leads to either partial obstruction, which generally causes myocardial ischemia in the absence of ST-segment elevation (non–ST-segment elevation ACS), or complete occlusion and STEMI. The myocardium supplied by the culprit artery loses its contractile ability, which leads to the following abnormal contractile patterns: dyssynchrony, hypokinesis, akinesis, and dyskinesis. The remaining noninfarcted myocardium usually manifests hyperkinesis unless there is underlying coronary artery disease affecting the territory supplied by these arteries. If a large area of myocardium is jeopardized, left ventricular pump function becomes depressed.

Diastolic dysfunction is invariably associated with systolic dysfunction. Severely reduced systolic function leads to a decrease in left ventricular stroke volume, which lowers systemic pressures and coronary perfusion pressure, potentiating myocardial ischemia and leading to a vicious cycle. In extreme cases of severe myocardial damage, this will eventually lead to cardiogenic shock.

CLINICAL DIAGNOSIS AND ASSESSMENT

The diagnosis of STEMI generally requires symptoms suggestive of myocardial ischemia associated with persistent ST-segment elevation on ECG and evidence of myocardial necrosis, which is typically supported by an elevation in cardiac enzymes.

SYMPTOMS

The sudden onset of chest discomfort is the most common presenting symptom. The chest discomfort is usually retrosternal, with a mid- to left-sided predisposition. The pain is usually described as "pressure-like," "crushing," "squeezing," or "compressing." The pain may sometimes radiate to the left arm, left shoulder, neck, or jaw. These symptoms may be associated with shortness of breath, diaphoresis, nausea, or vomiting. These typical clinical symptoms are present in many, but not all, patients with STEMI. Women, elderly patients, and patients with diabetes may present with atypical symptoms. Such symptoms can include epigastric pain, shortness of breath, back pain, or nausea and diaphoresis alone. In some patients, the presentation of STEMI is manifested by symptoms of ventricular tachycardia or symptoms of left ventricular failure. Occasionally, patients with STEMI may present with cardiac arrest. A focused history and physical exam should be performed on all patients with suspected STEMI, to aid in making the diagnosis and identifying high-risk patients.

ELECTROCARDIOGRAM

A 12-lead ECG should be acquired and interpreted promptly (within 10 minutes) in all suspected cases of acute myocardial infarction (MI). In the presence of a strong clinical suspicion, if the initial ECG is nondiagnostic, a repeat ECG should be performed 5 to 10 minutes later to assess for evolving ST elevation. Hyperacute T waves are the earliest ECG manifestations of a STEMI and may precede the characteristic ST-segment elevation. On the other hand, up to 15% of patients with STEMI can have a normal ECG. In these circumstances, the left circumflex artery is often the culprit vessel.

The European Society of Cardiology/ACCF/AHA/World Heart Federation Task Force for the Universal Definition of MI and the ACCF/AHA/SCAI Guidelines for the Management of ST Elevation Myocardial Infarction include the following criteria for the ECG definition of ST elevation infarction[1,3]:

1. New ST elevation at the J point in at least two contiguous leads of ≥2 mm (0.2 mV) in men or ≥1.5 mm (0.15 mV) in women in leads V2–V3 and/or of ≥1 mm (0.1 mV) in other contiguous chest leads or the limb leads.
2. New ST depressions in ≥2 precordial leads (V1–V4) are indicative of a transmural posterior infarction.
3. New or presumably new left bundle branch block (LBBB). (While this may be a STEMI equivalent, the diagnostic accuracy of this finding has recently been questioned.[1] There are algorithms that may help to further differentiate a true STEMI in the setting of LBBB.)

In patients with suspected right ventricular infarction, right precordial leads (V3R and V4R) could further aid in the diagnosis. In addition, in cases of a suspected posterior infarction, recording of posterior leads is strongly recommended (V7 lead should be recorded at the left posterior axillary line, V8 lead should be recorded at the left midscapular line, and V9 lead should be recorded at the left paraspinal border).[3] The presence of "reciprocal changes" in the form of ST-segment depression in the leads that are opposite to the location of the ST elevations is a characteristic finding that greatly increases the specificity of the diagnosis of STEMI. Multilead ST-segment depression with coexistent ST elevation in lead aVR alone has been described in patients with left main or proximal left anterior descending artery occlusion.

It is important to recognize that the ECG changes that are depicted in a patient with suspected STEMI are a dynamic finding. The ST-segment changes will evolve throughout the patient's postinfarction course and will often reflect the extent to which the patient has achieved restoration of myocardial blood flow at the tissue level. **Figure 2.1** outlines the evolution of ECG changes in a patient with a large anterior infarction who received prompt reperfusion therapy.

BIOMARKERS

Serum biomarkers can be detected when they are released from damaged myocardial cells. Because this is a time-bound process, serum biomarkers are not useful for early detection of STEMI

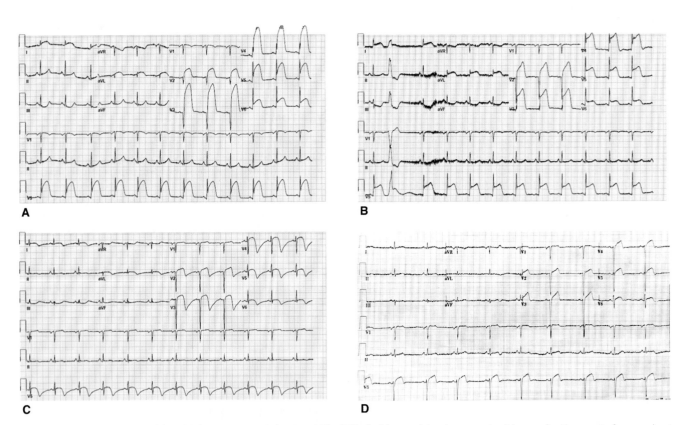

FIGURE 2.1 The evolution of the ECG during an acute infarction. A, The ECG of a 54-year-old male presenting 2 hours after the onset of severe chest pain demonstrating a large anterolateral infarction. B, The ECG in this same patient immediately after reperfusion therapy with primary PCI. Despite restoration of TIMI III flow in the infarct artery and complete relief of chest pain, there remains moderate ST-segment elevation. Note, however, that the ST-segment elevation has been reduced by more than 50% in the lead with the greatest degree of ST elevation on initial ECG. This usually indicates achievement of tissue-level reperfusion. C, The ECG 48 hours after the acute infarction. The patient was asymptomatic at the time the ECG was performed, and his cardiac enzymes were downtrending. Note the marked ST and T wave changes and the prolongation of the QT interval. This finding is not uncommon postinfarction even in patients treated successfully with reperfusion therapy. D, The ECG was performed 2 weeks after the infarction. Note the marked improvement in the ST and T wave abnormalities. ECG, electrocardiogram; PCI, percutaneous coronary intervention; STEMI, ST-segment elevation myocardial infarction; TIMI, thrombolysis in myocardial infarction.

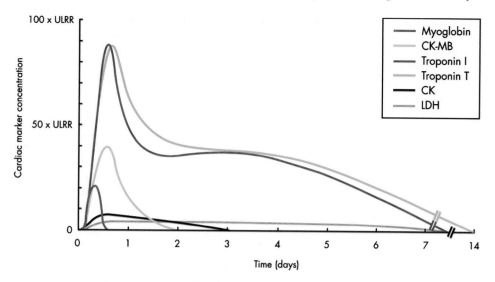

FIGURE 2.2 Cardiac biomarkers in STEMI. These biomarker profiles are schematic and do not differentiate the course of the occlusion (ie, early reperfusion vs persistent occlusion). ST-segment elevation myocardial infarction. CK, creatine kinase; CK-MB, creatine kinase muscle–brain; LDH, lactate dehydrogenase; STEMI, ST-elevation myocardial infarction; URLL, upper limit reference range. (Reproduced from French JK, White HD. Clinical implications of the new definition of myocardial infarction. *Heart.* 2004;90(1):99-106, with permission of the publisher. Copyright 2016, BMJ Publishing Group Ltd & British Cardiovascular Society.)

but can confirm myocardial injury if a patient is presenting late after symptom onset. Established cardiac biomarkers used to detect acute MI are cardiac-specific troponins (troponin I and troponin T), creatine kinase (CK) and CK isoenzymes (CK-MB fraction), and myoglobin. **Figure 2.2** depicts the Kinetic profiles of the various biomarkers used in the diagnosis of acute STEMI. Myoglobin elevations peak early but are not cardiac-specific. Cardiac troponin is the preferred biomarker for the diagnosis of MI because of its high specificity and sensitivity. The biomarkers of myocardial injury, however, do not provide any information on the cause of injury. Elevated levels should always be correlated clinically because it could be secondary to nonischemic insults. In STEMI, clinicians should not wait for the results of cardiac biomarkers to initiate treatment. Clinical presentation and 12-lead ECG should serve as the initial diagnostic tools. CK and CK-MB are the tests of choice to define a recurrent MI in the early days after STEMI.

RISK ASSESSMENT

It is important to perform a risk assessment for all patents with STEMI. This assessment should be done on initial presentation, and repeat assessments should be performed throughout the hospital stay. A risk assessment provides the physician with important estimates of the patient's overall prognosis and guides the health care team on the most appropriate therapies on the basis of this risk. For example, in a post hoc analysis of the DANish trial in Acute Myocardial Infarction-2 (DANAMI-2),[4] primary percutaneous coronary intervention (PCI) was associated with a significant reduction in 3-year mortality compared with fibrinolysis (25% vs 36%) in high-risk patients with a thrombolysis in myocardial infarction (TIMI) risk score ≥5. Risk assessments also allow the physician to provide realistic information to patients and their families regarding a patient's prognosis. A risk assessment is often based on the historical and clinical information that is available to the health care team when the patient first presents to the hospital, and is further modified by the patient's subsequent hospital course.

Scoring systems such as the TIMI risk score[5] or the Global Registry of Acute Coronary Events (GRACE) score[6] are tools that provide a qualitative assessment of risk and the likelihood that the patient will suffer a subsequent ischemic or terminal event in the short term. The TIMI risk score is an easy to use risk score for patients with STEMI. The TIMI score was derived from a dataset of patients enrolled in the TIMI-II trial and validated using information from those patients enrolled in the TIMI-9 trial. The score comprises eight variables, each of which is assigned a certain number of points. The variables include the following: (1) Age: 65 to 74 years = 2 points; and ≥75 years = 3 points; (2) Systolic blood pressure < 100 mm Hg = 3 points; (3) Heart rate > 100 beats/min = 2 points; (4) Kilip class II–IV = 2 points; (5) History of diabetes or hypertension or angina = 1 point; (6) Weight < 67 kg = 1 point; (7) Anterior infarct or LBBB = 1 point; and (8) Time to treatment > 4 hours = 1 point. Across the spectrum of risk, mortality at 30 days varies from less than 1% for low-risk patients (those with a TIMI score of 1) to over 35% for high-risk patient (those with a TIMI score of 8).

The GRACE risk score assesses the likelihood of in-hospital and 6-month mortality among patients with ACS, including STEMI, non–ST-elevation MI, or unstable angina. The score was derived using variables from an unselected population of patients enrolled in the GRACE Registry, an international clinical registry of all patients with ACS admitted to selected hospitals. The GRACE risk score gives a broader range of weighted values for each particular risk factor. Because the GRACE score was derived from an unselected population of patients (rather than data from patients enrolled in clinical trials), it incorporates a larger range of clinical variables than the TIMI risk score. Eight factors are used in this score: (1) Age, (2) Heart rate, (3) Systolic blood pressure, (4) serum creatinine, (5) Cardiac arrest on presentation, (6) ST-segment deviation, (7) Elevated/abnormal cardiac enzymes, and (8) Rales or jugular venous distension versus pulmonary edema versus shock. The GRACE score calculator is available as a web-based tool for easy use (http://www.outcomes-umassmed.org/grace/). The GRACE score was validated using the clinical data of the patients enrolled in the Global Use of Strategies to Open Occluded Arteries IIb (GUSTO IIb) study. The predicted mortality for the patients in the GUSTO IIb study calculated with the GRACE scoring system was strongly correlated with the observed mortality (c-statistic = 0.791), thus emphasizing the strong predictive accuracy of this scoring system.

REPERFUSION THERAPY

The management of STEMI involves an integrated strategy that begins with early recognition of symptoms and diagnosis, contact with emergency medical services, time-efficient practices in emergency departments to shorten door-to-balloon times or door-to-needle times, and a skilled heart team to ensure timely revascularization. To achieve these goals, the American Heart Association recommends that each community develops a STEMI system of care, which includes[1,7]:

1. A process for prehospital identification of STEMI and prehospital activation of the cardiac catheterization laboratory, with destination protocols in place to bypass non-PCI hospitals and direct patients with suspected STEMI diagnosed in the field to PCI-capable hospitals.
2. Protocols enabling the rapid diagnosis and treatment of STEMI at non–PCI-capable hospitals, including the facilitation of transfer of such patients to PCI-capable hospitals and/or the rapid and early use of fibrinolytic therapy for those patients who present to hospitals without PCI capability and who cannot be transferred to PCI-capable hospitals in a timely manner.
3. Ongoing multidisciplinary team meetings (including emergency medical services, non-PCI hospitals, and PCI centers) to evaluate outcomes and quality improvement metrics.

PRIMARY PERCUTANEOUS CORONARY INTERVENTION

Current guidelines recommend that reperfusion with either fibrinolysis or primary PCI be performed as soon as possible after arrival at the hospital.[1] In general, primary PCI is the preferred reperfusion therapy. Several randomized controlled trials (RCTs) and observational studies have shown the superiority of primary PCI compared with fibrinolytic therapy.[8,9] In a meta-analysis of 23 randomized trials, primary PCI was associated with a reduction in short-term and long-term major adverse cardiovascular events, including death, nonfatal Recurrent MI, and stroke.[8] The benefits of PCI over fibrinolytic therapy were seen irrespective of the type of fibrinolytic agent used, and even when reperfusion was delayed because of transfer for primary PCI. Restoration of TIMI-3 flow has a major impact on short- and long-term mortality. Primary PCI can achieve TIMI-3 flow in the infarct artery in >85% of patients,[9,10] compared with only about 60% to 63% of patients using thrombolytic therapy.[11] Conceivably, PCI has been shown to limit infarct size and salvage greater myocardium compared with fibrinolysis.[12] Primary PCI also reduces recurrent ischemia, resulting in fewer revascularization procedures and a shorter length of stay compared with fibrinolysis.[13] Primary PCI should be performed in patients with ischemic symptoms of <12 hours' duration presenting to PCI-capable hospitals, and for patients presenting to non–PCI-capable hospitals only if PCI can be performed within 120 minutes of first hospital arrival (see below). For patients with a delayed presentation of 12 to 24 hours after symptom onset,

PCI can still be considered. Patients who present to hospitals without PCI capabilities should be transferred for primary PCI if they have contraindications to fibrinolytic therapy or cardiogenic shock, irrespective of the time delay from first medical contact.[1]

Transfer for Primary Percutaneous Coronary Intervention

Several trials have shown benefits in transferring patients with STEMI for primary PCI from a non–PCI-capable hospital to a PCI-capable hospital. The DANAMI-2 trial[14] conducted in Denmark was the largest of such studies, involving 1572 patients. The trial found that the transfer of patients with STEMI from a non–PCI-capable hospital to a PCI-capable hospital for primary PCI was superior to the use of fibrinolytic therapy at the referring hospital. The median transfer time was 67 minutes, and average first door-to-device time was approximately 110 minutes. Most of these transfer studies were performed in European centers where transfer times are generally relatively short, and efficient systems with protocols for transport are already in place. Data from the recent AHA Mission: Lifeline Program of 14,518 patients transferred from non–PCI-capable hospitals for primary PCI between 2008 and 2012 in the United States showed that more than one-third of the patients with STEMI who were transferred for primary PCI failed to achieve a first door-to-device time ≤120 minutes, despite estimated transfer times of less than 60 minutes.[15] If the time to treatment with primary PCI falls beyond the window of 120 minutes, it is possible that the relative benefit from primary PCI as compared with fibrinolytic therapy may be lost. These findings suggest that ongoing efforts to optimize STEMI systems across the country are still needed to achieve primary PCI care for transfer patients as mandated by the guidelines.

FIBRINOLYTIC THERAPY

When it is anticipated that primary PCI cannot be performed within 120 minutes of first medical contact and the onset of ischemic symptoms is within 12 hours, then fibrinolytic therapy should be given. As stated earlier, myocardial salvage is a time-dependent process, and successful epicardial perfusion can be achieved if fibrinolytic therapy is administered early after symptom onset. In fact, studies have demonstrated the superiority of fibrinolysis over primary PCI when therapy is administered within 1 to 2 hours of symptom onset (concept of the "golden hour").[16] The efficacy and utility of fibrinolytic agents diminish with time, and their benefit in patients who present >12 hours after symptom onset is uncertain; however, the guidelines still provide a window of use within 12 to 24 hours of symptom onset for large infarct or patients with ongoing symptoms. It is recommended that when fibrinolytic therapy is indicated or chosen as the primary reperfusion strategy, it should be administered within 30 minutes of arrival at the hospital. Unfortunately, not all patients are candidates for fibrinolytic therapy because of possible contraindications, but should instead be considered for transfer for primary PCI.[1] **Table 2.1** outlines the absolute and relative contraindications to fibrinolytic therapy. Major complications of fibrinolytic therapy include bleeding, particularly intracranial hemorrhage (<1%) and other serious bleeding (<2%). Approximately 20% to 25% of patients have failure of reperfusion,[17] and an additional 25% to 30% have reocclusion,[18] which is associated with increased in-hospital mortality and significant impairment in left ventricular function.[19]

TABLE 2.1	Contraindications to Fibrinolytic Therapy
ABSOLUTE	**RELATIVE**
Any prior intracranial hemorrhage	History of chronic, severe poorly controlled hypertension
Known structural cerebral vascular lesion (ie, arteriovenous malformation)	Severe hypertension (systolic blood pressure > 180 mm Hg or diastolic blood pressure > 110 mm Hg)
Malignant cerebral neoplasm (primary or metastatic)	History of prior ischemic stroke >3 mo
Ischemic stroke within 3 mo	Dementia
Active bleeding or bleeding diathesis (excluding menses)	Other known intracranial pathology
Important closed-head or facial trauma within 3 mo	Traumatic or prolonged (>10 min) cardiopulmonary resuscitation
Intracranial or intraspinal surgery within 3 mo	Major surgery (<3 wk)
Severe and uncontrolled hypertension unresponsive to therapies	Recent (within 2–4 wk) internal bleeding
For planned streptokinase use: streptokinase within 6 mo	Noncompressible vascular punctures
	Pregnancy
	Active peptic ulcer

MEDICAL MANAGEMENT

GENERAL MEASURES

Oxygen is provided to treat hypoxia. In a randomized study evaluating the benefits of oxygen therapy administered routinely to patients at 8 L/min (in the absence of clinical hypoxia), oxygen therapy was associated with increased rates of recurrent MI and ventricular arrhythmias and increased infarct size.[20] For this reason, oxygen should be reserved for those patients with signs of hypoxia, including an oxygen saturation of <95% on room air. In patients with severe pulmonary edema compromising the respiratory status, endotracheal intubation and mechanical ventilation may be necessary. Morphine or nitrates should be given to control pain and associated increased sympathetic activity, but these therapies have little effect on overall clinical outcome. Nitrates are contraindicated in patients with suspected right ventricular infarction, hypotension, or recent use of 5′ phosphodiesterase inhibitors.

ANTIPLATELET THERAPY

A cascade of thrombotic processes follow rupture, fissure, or erosion of an atherosclerotic plaque. Circulating platelets become activated on contact with the lipid-filled core, collagen, and other thrombogenic contents. Activated platelets release adenosine diphosphate (ADP) and thromboxane A_2 and cause expression of the glycoprotein IIb/IIIa receptors, which bind to adhesive proteins such as von Willebrand factor and fibrinogen

and amplify the thrombotic process at the ruptured plaque. Of the various receptors involved in the process, the P2Y12 receptors activated by ADP play a key role in platelet activation, adhesion, and aggregation. A thrombus rich in platelets promotes reocclusion after successful fibrinolysis[21] and even after primary PCI.[22] Antiplatelet agents thus play a central role in the treatment of patients with STEMI. **Figure 2.3** illustrates the various receptors seen on the surface of the platelet and the interaction of the platelet receptor inhibitors with these receptors.

Aspirin

Aspirin irreversibly inhibits the cyclooxygenase enzyme, which is the mediator of the initial step in the synthesis of thromboxane A_2 and arachidonic acid. Non–enteric-coated aspirin in doses of 162 to 325 mg should be given to patients to "chew" immediately on initial presentation. After primary PCI or fibrinolysis, the preferred maintenance dose is 81 mg. In the CURRENT-OASIS 7 trial,[23] there were no differences in the efficacy and safety end points between aspirin 325 mg and aspirin 81 mg in patients with ACS undergoing invasive treatment. Observational studies, however, have suggested increased bleeding in follow-up with higher doses of maintenance aspirin,[24] and hence the lower dose is generally advised.

P2Y12 Inhibitors

The P2Y12 inhibitors include oral (clopidogrel, prasugrel, and ticagrelor) and intravenous (cangrelor) agents. These medications block the binding of ADP to the P2Y12 receptor, thus inhibiting the P2Y12 receptor–mediated activation of the glycoprotein IIb/IIIa receptor and subsequent platelet aggregation. Adding P2Y12 inhibitors to aspirin offers added benefit in patients with MI, and benefits have been noted in medically treated patients as well. **Table 2.2** outlines the properties of the currently available oral P2Y12 inhibitors.

Clopidogrel

Clopidogrel, a prodrug, converts to active metabolite and binds irreversibly to the P2Y12 receptor on platelets. Numerous RCTs have demonstrated that pretreatment with clopidogrel reduces cardiovascular mortality and ischemic events post-PCI.[25] Clopidogrel administered at a loading dose of 600 mg (as compared with 300 mg) is associated with a 42% relative reduction in the rates of definite stent thrombosis.[23] The AHA/ACC guidelines recommend a loading dose of 600 mg to be given as early as possible for those patients planned for primary PCI.[1] The Clopidogrel and Metoprolol in Myocardial Infarction Trial/Second Chinese Cardiac Study (COMMIT/CCS-2) study[26] showed that the use of clopidogrel for medically treated STEMI benefited patients through a 9% reduction in the composite end point of death, recurrent MI, and stroke; further, a 7% reduction in all-cause death was noted among patients randomized to clopidogrel treatment. A 300 mg loading dose of clopidogrel is advised for medically treated patients (fibrinolytic-treated patients or patients who did not receive reperfusion therapy), followed by a maintenance dose of 75 mg daily. A loading dose is not recommended for medically treated patients over 75 years old.

Prasugrel

As with clopidogrel, prasugrel is a prodrug that, on converting to active metabolite, irreversibly blocks the P2Y12 receptor.

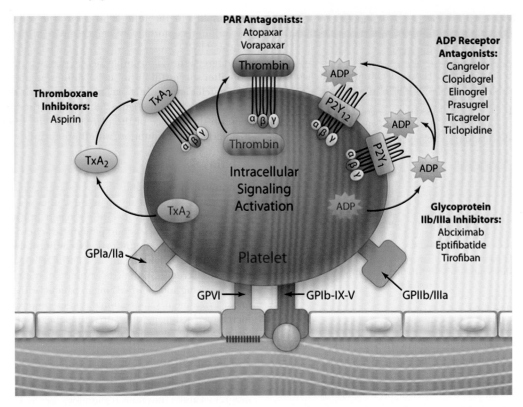

FIGURE 2.3 Schematic diagram of the interplay of platelet receptors and platelet receptor inhibitors. There are various targets of action for antiplatelet therapies. ADP, adenosine diphosphate; GP, glycoprotein; PAR, protease-activated receptor; Tx, Thromboxane. (Reproduced from Bhatt DL, Hulot J-S, Moliterno DJ, et al. Antiplatelet and anticoagulation therapy for acute coronary syndromes. *Circ Res*. 2014;114:1929-1943, with permission of the publisher. Copyright 2016, American Heart Association.)

TABLE 2.2	Comparison of P2Y12 Inhibitors		
P2Y12 INHIBITOR	**CLOPIDOGREL**	**PRASUGREL**	**TICAGRELOR**
Class	Thienopyridine	Thienopyridine	Cyclopentyl-triazolopyrimidine
Prodrug	Yes	Yes	No
Receptor binding	Irreversible	Irreversible	Reversible
Onset of effect	2–4 h	30 min	30 min
Duration of effect	3–10 d	5–10 d	3–4 d
Metabolism	Hepatic	Hepatic	Hepatic
Clearance	Renal 50%, fecal 46%	Renal 68%, fecal 27%	Renal 26%, fecal 58%
Loading dose	300–600 mg	60 mg	180 mg
Maintenance dose	75 mg daily	10 mg daily	90 mg twice daily
Withdrawal before surgery	5 d	7 d	5 d

As compared with clopidogrel, prasugrel achieves faster and more potent platelet inhibition. In a prespecified subgroup analysis of patients with STEMI enrolled in the Trial to Assess Improvement in Therapeutic Outcomes by Optimizing Platelet Inhibition with Prasugrel-TIMI (TRITON-TIMI 38),[27] prasugrel, as compared with clopidogrel, was associated with a 32% reduction in the primary composite end point of cardiovascular death, MI, or stroke without any increase in non–coronary artery bypass graft

(CABG) bleeding. Prasugrel was also associated with a 52% reduction in stent thrombosis in follow-up. It is important to note that despite the absence of an increase in bleeding events in the patients with STEMI enrolled in the TRITON-TIMI 38 trial, a higher rate of non-CABG major bleeding was noted in the overall trial. Therefore, prasugrel should be used with caution in patients who are ≥75 years of age or whose body weight ≤60 kg. Prasugrel is contraindicated in those patients with a history of prior stroke or transient ischemic attack. The recommended loading dose of prasugrel is 60 mg, followed by a maintenance dose of 10 mg daily.

Ticagrelor

Ticagrelor is a direct acting selective antagonist that binds reversibly to the P2Y12 receptor. In a subgroup analysis of patients with STEMI enrolled in the Platelet Inhibition and Patient Outcomes (PLATO) trial,[28] ticagrelor showed a 13% reduction in the combined end point of cardiovascular death, MI, or stroke with no increase in the risk of any bleeding, compared with clopidogrel. Mortality was also significantly reduced with ticagrelor. The recommended loading dose of ticagrelor is 180 mg, and the recommended maintenance dose is 90 mg twice a day. When ticagrelor is used, the maintenance dose of aspirin is 81 mg daily. Dyspnea is one of the frequently reported side effects of ticagrelor, with about 14% of patients reporting dyspnea in the main PLATO trial; however, drug discontinuation caused by dyspnea was less than 1%.[29]

Cangrelor

Cangrelor is an intravenous, nonthienopyridine, direct P2Y12 receptor blocker that has rapid onset and rapid offset (within minutes) of its effects. Pooled analysis of the Cangrelor versus Standard Therapy to Achieve Optimal Management of Platelet Inhibition (CHAMPION) trials[30] showed that cangrelor decreased periprocedural outcomes of all-cause death, MI, ischemia-driven revascularization, or stent thrombosis. An increase in minor bleeding, but not major bleeding, was noted. Although these trials came under scrutiny because of their designs and timing of administration of clopidogrel, the results of the trials collectively support the use of cangrelor in those patients who are "inadequately" pretreated with clopidogrel before PCI.

Glycoprotein IIb/IIIa Receptor Inhibitors

Glycoprotein IIb/IIIa receptor inhibitors (GPI) block the binding of the glycoprotein IIb/IIIa receptors to fibrinogen, thereby inhibiting fibrinogen-platelet bridging. They are potent parenteral platelet inhibitors. Three agents are available—abciximab, eptifibatide, and tirofiban. In the setting of primary PCI, abciximab has been studied the most. Compared with unfractionated heparin (UFH) or low-molecular-weight heparin alone, GPIs are associated with a significant reduction in cardiovascular events, largely driven by a reduction in periprocedural MI.[31] An increased risk for bleeding was also observed in the trials studying GPI use. Studies supporting the use of these agents during PCI were largely performed before the widespread use of dual antiplatelet therapy, and the role of GPI in the current era is less well defined. Furthermore, data on the benefits of these agents in the setting of STEMI have shown variable results.[32,33] Per guidelines, it is reasonable to begin treatment with GPI at the time of primary PCI in selected patients (large thrombus burden or inadequate P2Y12 receptor antagonist loading) with STEMI who are receiving UFH.

ANTICOAGULATION THERAPY

Anticoagulant therapy is used in the acute setting of STEMI in preparation for primary PCI. It is also used in medically treated patients following fibrinolysis, or in those patients who are not otherwise eligible for reperfusion therapy. The choice of anticoagulation depends on the patient's risk of bleeding and the treatment strategy.

Unfractionated Heparin or Bivalirudin in Primary Percutaneous Coronary Intervention

UFH titrated to an appropriate activated clotting time (approximately 250 seconds) and bivalirudin are the most commonly used therapies for primary PCI. UFH can be used with or without planned GPI, whereas bivalirudin is typically administered with provisional use of GPI. Many studies have compared the use of bivalirudin with UFH in patients with STEMI. These studies consistently demonstrated a lower rate of major bleeding with bivalirudin and lower net adverse cardiac events but a higher risk of stent thrombosis. A meta-analysis of randomized trials comparing these two anticoagulants in patients undergoing primary PCI demonstrated a 19% reduction in all-cause mortality, a 32% reduction in cardiac mortality, and a 38% reduction in major bleeding with bivalirudin.[34] Bivalirudin, however, was associated with a 3-fold higher rate of stent thrombosis. Prolonged bivalirudin infusion post-PCI may help to mitigate this early risk of stent thrombosis in patients with STEMI; in those with higher risk for bleeding, bivalirudin is preferred.

Unfractionated Heparin, Enoxaparin, or Fondaparinux with Fibrinolytic Therapy

Patients undergoing fibrinolysis should receive anticoagulant therapy for a minimum of 48 hours, and preferably for the duration of the index hospitalization, or until revascularization is performed.[1] Based on age, weight, and renal function, either UFH, enoxaparin, or fondaparinux can be used. The Enoxaparin and Thrombolysis Reperfusion for Acute Myocardial Infarction Treatment (ExTRACT)- TIMI 25 study[35] demonstrated a 17% reduction in the rates of death or recurrent MI at 30 days with the use of enoxaparin as compared with UFH following fibrinolytic therapy, but a higher rate of major bleeding was observed. Despite the higher rates of major bleeding, net adverse events, including a composite of death, nonfatal recurrent MI, and nonfatal intracerebral hemorrhage, was lower with enoxaparin. If anticoagulation therapy is extended beyond 48 hours, enoxaparin is preferred. In patients undergoing PCI post–fibrinolytic therapy, heparin is a reasonable alternative. Finally limited data have shown some benefit to fondaparinux for medically treated and fibrinolytic-treated patients with STEMI.[36] It should be noted, however, that if PCI is planned, fondaparinux should not be used as the sole anticoagulant to support the PCI because of the risk of catheter-related thrombosis.[36]

β-BLOCKERS

β-Blockers decrease the risk for ventricular arrhythmias, reduce remodeling, improve left ventricular hemodynamics, and may reduce infarct size.[37] Oral β-blockers should be initiated within the first 24 hours in all patients with STEMI, in the absence of any contraindication. Patients with initial contraindications to β-blockers should be reevaluated after 24 hours for β-blocker therapy. Intravenous β-blockers can be given at the time of presentation in patients who are hypertensive or have ongoing ischemia, but the routine use of IV β-Blockers has not been proven beneficial. β-Blockers are contraindicated in patients with signs of heart failure, evidence of a low output state, increased risk for cardiogenic shock, or other contraindications to use (PR interval >0.24 seconds, second- or third-degree heart block, active asthma, or reactive airways disease).

STATIN THERAPY

In stabilized patients, a fasting lipid panel should be obtained, and high-intensity statin therapy (atorvastatin or rosuvastatin) should be initiated or continued if there are no contraindications. Numerous studies have demonstrated that statins lower the risk of future cardiovascular events and the need for coronary revascularization in patients with ACS.[38] Statin therapy is beneficial even in patients with baseline low-density lipoprotein cholesterol levels <70 mg/dL.[39]

ANGIOTENSIN-CONVERTING ENZYME INHIBITORS OR ANGIOTENSIN RECEPTOR BLOCKERS

In a meta-analysis of four RCTs and >98,000 patients in which angiotensin-converting enzyme (ACE) inhibitors were started within 36 hours of MI, compared with placebo, ACE inhibitors significantly reduced 30-day mortality and heart failure.[40] Although data have shown a benefit of ACE inhibitors in all patients with STEMI, the benefits appear most pronounced in patients with large areas of myocardium involved or in patients with congestive heart failure. Therefore, ACE inhibitors should be administered within the first 24 hours to all patients with STEMI with anterior location, heart failure, or ejection fraction ≤40%, unless contraindicated. ACE inhibitors can also be given to otherwise stable and low-risk patients with STEMI as well. The major contraindications of ACE inhibitors/ARBs (angiotensin receptor blockers) are hypotension, worsening renal function, or drug allergy. ARBs are indicated for patients who are ACE inhibitor–intolerant.

ALDOSTERONE ANTAGONISTS

Spironolactone and eplerenone are aldosterone antagonists. The AHA/ACC guidelines recommend initiation of an aldosterone antagonist in patients with STEMI and no contraindications in those who are already receiving an ACE inhibitor and β-blocker and who have an ejection fraction ≤0.40 and either symptomatic congestive heart failure or diabetes mellitus.[1] This recommendation is supported by the results from the Eplerenone Post–Acute Myocardial Infarction Heart Failure Efficacy and Survival trial,[41] which studied the effect of eplerenone in addition to standard therapy in patients with acute MI and an ejection fraction ≤40% and signs of heart failure. Eplerenone resulted in a 15% reduction in total mortality and a 17% reduction in cardiovascular mortality mainly because of a reduction in sudden cardiac death. Aldosterone antagonists should not be given to patients with renal failure (creatinine ≥ 2.5 mg/dL in men and ≥2.0 mg/dL in women) and hyperkalemia (potassium ≥5.0 mEq/L).

ADDITIONAL MANAGEMENT

ECHOCARDIOGRAPHY

An echocardiogram is a simple tool to assess post-MI ejection fraction and can provide useful information regarding a patient's overall prognosis. All patients with STEMI should receive an echocardiogram before hospital discharge and ideally within the first 24 hours of presentation. Echocardiography can also aid in identifying stunned or jeopardized myocardium, evaluate ejection fraction following reperfusion, and can help detect mechanical complications of STEMI such as free wall rupture, acute ventricular septal defect, and mitral regurgitation (see section on Mechanical Complications). Finally, in patients with ST elevation of uncertain etiology, echocardiography performed on initial presentation can help distinguish myocardial ischemia from common nonischemic causes of chest pain such as perimyocarditis, valvular heart disease, pulmonary embolism, or aortic dissection.

CORONARY ANGIOGRAPHY

Although the majority of patients with STEMI will be treated with primary PCI, a substantial minority of patients will present to hospitals without timely access to primary PCI and will therefore be treated with fibrinolytic therapy; these patients should be considered for coronary angiography at some point during the hospital course. In general, patients with severe heart failure or cardiogenic shock should be transferred for immediate coronary angiography following fibrinolytic therapy. It is also recommended that patients who do not demonstrate evidence for restoration of myocardial blood flow following fibrinolytic therapy be considered for immediate transfer for coronary angiography.

Over the last decade, numerous studies have supported a strategy of early coronary angiography (within 3 to 24 hours) following fibrinolytic therapy even in seemingly stable patients.[42,43] The Trial of Routine Angioplasty and Stenting after Fibrinolysis to Enhance Reperfusion in Acute Myocardial Infarction (TRANSFER-AMI) study[42] was the largest of all such trials evaluating the benefit of routine early angiography following fibrinolytic therapy, and reported a 36% reduction in clinical events, including 30-day death, recurrent MI, worsening heart failure, or shock in the group of patients assigned to early catheterization. A meta-analysis of all such trials reported a 64% reduction in the rate of death or recurrent infarction at 30 days with early coronary angiography following fibrinolytic therapy, which was particularly pronounced among the trials enrolling high-risk patients.[43] As a result of these data, routine early coronary angiography (within 3 to 24 hours of fibrinolytic therapy) should be considered for all stable patients. For the remaining patients who may not have been referred for early angiography, the AHA/ACC guidelines give a class I recommendation for coronary angiography in cases of spontaneous or inducible ischemia.[1] In the absence of these findings, routine coronary angiography before hospital discharge (to define the anatomy) may still be considered.

STRESS TESTING

For those medically treated patients who do not undergo initial coronary angiography, noninvasive stress testing should be performed. This allows the clinician to assess for residual ischemia post-MI (both in the infarct-related artery and to assess ischemia in areas remote from the infarct which might be indicative of multivessel disease). After the first 48 to 72 hours, pharmacologic stress testing may be performed and has been shown to be safe and effective. Alternatively, a submaximal exercise stress test might also be considered to help guide recommendations for postdischarge exercise plans but should be followed with a maximal stress test within 6 weeks once the patient is fully recovered.

PERCUTANEOUS CORONARY INTERVENTION OF THE NONCULPRIT ARTERY

In patients with STEMI, approximately 50% will have multivessel disease.[44] There are three options for the treatment of multivessel disease in STEMI. These include: (1) Treatment of the culprit artery only with ischemia-guided management of nonculprit arteries; (2) performing multivessel PCI at the time of primary PCI; or (3) treatment of the culprit artery only during the primary PCI followed by staged PCI of nonculprit arteries at a later date. Several randomized trials evaluating these strategies have reported benefits from PCI of the nonculprit artery (done either at the time of primary PCI or as a staged procedure).[45,46] The Preventive Angioplasty in Acute Myocardial Infarction trial[45] randomized 465 patients to a strategy of multivessel PCI performed at the time of the primary PCI or usual care. This study demonstrated a 65% reduction in major cardiovascular events with multivessel PCI, including a composite of death from cardiac causes, nonfatal MI, and refractory angina. Although the study was not powered to show a reduction in the individual components of the composite end points, the benefits reported in this study were consistent across all of the individual components of the composite end point. In the Third Danish Study of Optimal Acute Treatment of Patients with ST-Segment Elevation Myocardial Infarction (DANAMI 3-PRIMULTI) trial,[46] the patients were randomized to a strategy of fractional flow reserve (FFR)–guided staged PCI or conservative care. In this study of 607 patients, FFR-guided staged PCI was associated with a 44% reduction in the composite of death, nonfatal MI, or ischemia-driven revascularization. This appeared to be entirely driven by a lower rate of ischemia-driven revascularization. It is important to note that all of the trials to date examining PCI strategies for patients with STEMI and multivessel disease have been small or moderate in size and none of the trials were powered to evaluate the individual components of the composite end point. The Complete versus Culprit-only Revascularization to Treat Multi-vessel Disease After Primary PCI for STEMI (COMPLETE) trial[47] will randomize 3900 patients to a strategy of staged multivessel PCI or culprit artery only revascularization and should provide us with important information regarding staged PCI for patients with STEMI and multivessel disease. Until we have a larger data set of results, it is important to remember that the management of multivessel disease in STEMI should be individualized. Factors that might influence the decision to proceed with additional revascularization include patient-related factors (the presence of severe left ventricular dysfunction, recurrent angina, or arrhythmias might favor complete revascularization; on the other hand, older patients or patients with chronic kidney disease might benefit from a more conservative approach to care), coronary anatomy (patients with relatively discrete lesions with a low complexity might be appropriate for multivessel PCI performed at the time of primary PCI), and patient preferences.

COMPLICATIONS ARISING AFTER STEMI

BLEEDING

Bleeding after MI is associated with increased mortality, recurrent MI, longer hospital stay, and increased cost.[48] Major bleeding may occur in up to 5% to 10% of patients undergoing PCI; however, the incidence rates vary depending on patient population, antithrombotic combinations, and bleeding definition.[49] Various definitions and risk scores have been developed to assess the severity and prognosis of bleeding.[50] Access-site bleeding accounts for the majority of bleeding; however, gastrointestinal and intracerebral bleeding may occur (in particular in fibrinolytic-treated patients) and could be life-threatening. Bleeding risk increases with age and is particularly notable in patients with low body weight, female sex, femoral access, or those receiving fibrinolytic therapy or GPI. There is an exponential increase in the risk of bleeding when triple therapy is required during or after hospitalization. Every effort should be made to minimize bleeding complications. Bleeding risk can be mitigated with the use of bivalirudin anticoagulant therapy during PCI or through radial access PCI. In addition, when triple therapy is indicated, careful titration of the international normalized ratio with a narrower goal of 2.0 to 2.5 is recommended.

LEFT VENTRICULAR RUPTURE

Left ventricular rupture is a rare complication of acute MI occurring in 0.17% to 0.31% of cases.[51] Rupture develops after a large STEMI usually at the junction of infarcted and normal myocardium and is often lethal. Rupture typical occurs about 2 to 5 days following acute infarction but has been shown to occur as early as day 1 post-MI. Risk factors for rupture include delayed time to reperfusion, advanced age, and female sex. Rupture can occur at the free wall, resulting in immediate death, or present subacutely with signs of shock because of contained rupture and cardiac tamponade. Frank free wall rupture is often immediately fatal, whereas survival in a contained rupture will depend on the timing to the recognition of the rupture, hemodynamic stabilization and, most importantly, surgical repair. A telltale sign of a contained rupture is the sudden onset of hypotension or shock with clear lungs and elevated jugular venous pressure. Another form of left ventricular wall rupture includes ventricular septal rupture. Anterior infarctions are associated with rupture of the septum in an apical location, whereas ruptures associated with inferior infarctions usual involve the basal septum. In these cases, patients typically present with hemodynamic instability, heart failure, and development of a loud, holosystolic murmur. Echocardiography is instrumental in the diagnosis of any of these forms of rupture. Definitive management for all forms of rupture is surgical repair; however, the feasibility of surgical repair and timing of surgery are controversial and vary with clinical presentation.

ACUTE MITRAL REGURGITATION

Significant mitral regurgitation is noted in approximately 3% of cases of acute MI.[52] The etiology of acute mitral regurgitation includes ischemic papillary muscle displacement/rupture, left ventricular dilatation, or true aneurysm. Papillary muscle rupture, partial or complete, is a life-threatening complication. This usually occurs 2 to 7 days after the infarct. Clinical manifestation includes hypotension, pulmonary edema, and a mid- to late systolic murmur in the mitral area. Diagnosis is confirmed by echocardiography (with color flow Doppler). The management includes prompt diagnosis, afterload reduction with nitrates, diuretics, intra-aortic balloon pump, and emergent surgery. Nevertheless, mortality remains high.

LEFT VENTRICULAR ANEURYSM

True aneurysms consist of a discrete, dyskinetic area of thin left ventricular wall with a broad neck. Rupture of these aneurysms is uncommon. This should be differentiated from a *pseudoaneurysm,* which is a contained ventricular rupture (see above). Aneurysms are most often noted in patients who are not treated with reperfusion therapy or who have lack of evidence of tissue level reperfusion following fibrinolytic therapy or PCI (persistent ST-segment elevation noted on the ECG in the immediate hours and days after treatment). Diagnosis is made by noninvasive imaging modalities. Possible sequelae of left ventricular aneurysm include congestive heart failure, ventricular arrhythmias, and left ventricular thrombus. Because of the risk for mural thrombosis and systemic embolization, oral anticoagulation therapy should be considered in patients with aneurysms, especially in the first 3 months post-MI. Surgical aneurysmectomy is reserved for select cases of patients who are severely symptomatic.

LEFT VENTRICULAR THROMBUS

Although the incidence of left ventricular thrombus has decreased with the use of primary PCI and the use of potent antithrombotic therapies, it is not an uncommon complication after STEMI, occurring in 4% to 8% of cases and usually associated with anterior wall infarctions.[53] Systemic embolization is always a potential risk. High-risk features for embolization on echocardiography include increased mobility, protrusion into the ventricular chamber, and contiguous zones of akinesis and hyperkinesis. Cardiac MRI can also be helpful to aid in diagnosis. Treatment requires anticoagulation with warfarin for at least 3 to 6 months.

ATRIOVENTRICULAR BLOCK

Ischemic injury can produce a variety of conduction blocks. Complete atrioventricular block is more common in inferior than in anterior infarct. It is usually transient and improves with revascularization. Some patients may require temporary pacing, but permanent complete heart block associated with an inferior infarction is generally rare.

VENTRICULAR ARRHYTHMIAS

Ventricular tachycardia and ventricular fibrillation are the most dreaded complications. Nonsustained ventricular tachycardia in the first 24 hours postinfarct is generally benign and not associated with a worse prognosis.[54] Correction of electrolyte abnormalities, including hypokalemia, hypomagnesemia, and institution of β-blockers serve as prophylaxis for occurrence of malignant arrhythmias. Occasionally, postinfarction arrhythmias can indicate reocclusion and may necessitate additional coronary angiography even in the absence of other signs or symptoms of reocclusion. Treatment of unstable ventricular tachycardia/ventricular fibrillation consists of electrical defibrillation, administration of antiarrhythmic agents such as amiodarone or lidocaine, and repeat coronary angiography if clinically warranted. Generally, the presence of sustained ventricular arrhythmias beyond 48 to 72 hours in the absence of evidence of reocclusion is associated with a poor prognosis, and consideration should be given to the placement of a cardiac defibrillator.

CARDIOGENIC SHOCK

Cardiogenic shock is the most common cause of death in patients with STEMI, occurring in 5% to 15% of all acute infarctions.[55] Cardiogenic shock can either be a manifestation of severe pump failure in the setting of a large infarct or a sequela of mechanical complications of MI. It is characterized by a constellation of findings reflecting systemic hypotension, low cardiac output, and evidence of vital organ hypoperfusion (eg clouded sensorium, cool extremities, oliguria, acidosis). The formal diagnostic criteria for cardiogenic shock will vary depending on the dataset examined, but, in general, cardiogenic shock requires refractory (not transient) hypotension in the absence of any other underlying causes with evidence of a low output state. **Table 2.3** outlines the diagnostic criteria for shock taken from the Should We Emergently Revascularize Occluded Coronaries for Cardiogenic Shock (SHOCK) trial.[56] The diagnosis of shock can be confirmed through the use of right heart catheterization measurements; however, the clinical presentation and use of Doppler and 2D echocardiography provide similar information to right heart catheterization, and therefore right heart catheterization is not always indicated. Early revascularization with PCI or CABG is the recommended reperfusion strategy for patients with STEMI and shock, irrespective of the time delay.[56] For patients who are unsuitable candidates for PCI or CABG, fibrinolysis can be given if there are no contraindications. Inotropes and vasopressor agents can be used to maintain hemodynamic stability and organ perfusion. Norepinephrine, dopamine, or dobutamine are used for the initial pharmacologic management. However, in patients with elevated systemic vascular resistance, vasopressor agents and high-dose inotropes may be counterproductive, and these patients should be evaluated for mechanical circulatory support devices.

Intra-aortic balloon pumps (IABP) can be used in patients with cardiogenic shock who do not stabilize with pharmacologic therapies. Although observational data support the use of IABP in patients with cardiogenic shock demonstrating improved

TABLE 2.3	Criteria for Cardiogenic Shock
CLINICAL CRITERIA	
Persistent hypotension (a systolic blood pressure of <90 mm Hg for at least 30 min or the need for supportive measures to maintain a systolic blood pressure of ≥90 mm Hg)	

End-organ hypoperfusion
    Altered mental status
    Cool extremities
    Urine output of <30 mL/h
    Elevated serum lactate levels	

Heart rate of ≥60 beats/min	
HEMODYNAMIC CRITERIA	
Cardiac index (<1.8 L/min/m^2 without support or <2.0 to 2.2 L/min/m^2 with support)	
Adequate or elevated filling pressure (left ventricular end-diastolic pressure >18 mm Hg or right ventricular end-diastolic pressure >10 to 15 mm Hg or pulmonary capillary wedge pressure of ≥15 mm Hg)	

outcomes,[57] the Intra-aortic Balloon Pump in Cardiogenic Shock II (IABP-SHOCK II) trial[58] failed to show any benefit from the use of IABP in patients with acute MI complicated by cardiogenic shock. The study examined patients presenting with acute MI and shock who were planned for early revascularization. The primary end point, 30-day all-cause mortality, was not significantly reduced with the use of IABP in shock. The study, however, did not address the optimal management of patients who develop shock later in the hospital course following revascularization. Fewer data are available to guide the use of IABP in cases of shock that develop after reperfusion, and most physicians would try to support these patients with mechanical circulatory support devices as a bridge to recovery, or as a bridge to additional revascularization and/or surgical repair of complications. Other temporary mechanical circulatory support devices such as Impella 2.5 or Impella CP, Tandem Heart, and percutaneous extracorporeal membrane oxygenator, may be helpful in severe cases of shock, but randomized data are not available. There are advantages and limitations to each of the support devices, and the decision to initiate hemodynamic support should be individualized.

DISCHARGE PLANNING

TIMING OF DISCHARGE

The timing of discharge is highly variable and often influenced by the clinical and Socio-demographic variables of the patient. There are no recommendations as to what constitutes appropriate duration of hospitalization for patients with STEMI. In low-risk patients with single vessel disease, who undergo successful primary PCI and are free of early sustained ventricular tachyarrhythmias, hypotension, heart failure, or any bleeding episodes, discharge home at 48 hours is generally reasonable.

PATIENT EDUCATION AND COUNSELING

One of the critical aspects of discharge planning is education of patients and their families. The plan of care for the patients should include the following domains of care:

1. Review of medications, including the importance of adherence
2. Follow-up appointments and testing
3. Dietary counseling
4. Physical and sexual activities counseling
5. Smoking cessation (if applicable)
6. Secondary prevention
7. Cardiac rehabilitation

CARDIAC REHABILITATION

Cardiac rehab is a medically supervised exercise program that has been shown to improve the cardiovascular health of patients with acute MI. The goals of exercise-based cardiac rehabilitation after STEMI are to increase functional capacity, improve symptoms, decrease potential disability, improve the quality of life, help the patient to modify coronary risk factors and thereby reduce morbidity and mortality.[1,59] Core components include a baseline and follow-up patient assessment, exercise counseling, nutritional counseling, smoking cessation counseling, psychosocial counseling, and management of blood pressure, lipids, and diabetes

mellitus with pharmacologic treatment, as appropriate.[59] In spite of the proven benefits of cardiac rehabilitation, it is underutilized because of several hospital-level factors and insurance issues.[60] Efforts must be concentrated on ensuring timely access to cardiac rehabilitation in patients with STEMI.

FUTURE DIRECTIONS

There remains a strong need to improve public awareness and educate the general population about symptoms of heart attacks and the importance of timely care, to improve the time from symptom onset to presentation for medical evaluation. Multicultural and multilingual efforts should be made, especially in those for whom English is not the first language. Research into newer therapies should continue. Research into treatments to minimize or reverse ventricular remodeling, and novel therapies involving stem cell or bone marrow precursor cells, stent technology, antiplatelets, and anticoagulants are ongoing.

REFERENCES

1. O'Gara PT, Kushner FG, Ascheim DD, et al. 2013 ACCF/AHA guideline for the management of ST-elevation myocardial infarction: a report of the American College of Cardiology Foundation/American Heart Association Task Force on Practice Guidelines. *Circulation.* 2013;127(4):529-555.
2. Mozaffarian D, Benjamin EJ, Go AS, et al; on behalf of the American Heart Association Statistics Committee and Stroke Statistics Subcommittee. Heart disease and stroke statistics—2016 update: a report from the American Heart Association. *Circulation.* 2016;133:e38-e360.
3. Thygesen K, Alpert JS, Jaffe AS, et al; the Writing Group on behalf of the Joint ESC/ACCF/AHA/WHF Task Force for the Universal Definition of Myocardial Infarction. Third universal definition of myocardial infarction. *Circulation.* 2012;126(16):2020-2035.
4. Thune JJ, Hoefsten DE, Lindholm MG, et al. Simple risk stratification at admission to identify patients with reduced mortality from primary angioplasty. *Circulation.* 2005;112(13):2017-2021.
5. Morrow DA, Antman EM, Charlesworth A, et al. TIMI risk score for ST-elevation myocardial infarction: a convenient, bedside, clinical score for risk assessment at presentation: an intravenous nPA for treatment of infarcting myocardium early II trial substudy. *Circulation.* 2000;102(17):2031-2037.
6. Granger CB, Goldberg RJ, Dabbous O, et al. Predictors of hospital mortality in the global registry of acute coronary events. *Arch Intern Med.* 2003;163(19):2345-2353.
7. Jollis JG, Granger CB, Henry TD, et al. Systems of care for ST-segment-elevation myocardial infarction: a report from the American Heart Association's Mission: Lifeline. *Circ Cardiovasc Qual Outcomes.* 2012;5(4):423-428.
8. Keeley EC, Boura JA, Grines CL. Primary angioplasty versus intravenous thrombolytic therapy for acute myocardial infarction: a quantitative review of 23 randomised trials. *Lancet.* 2003;361(9351):13-20.
9. The Global Use of Strategies to Open Occluded Coronary Arteries in Acute Coronary Syndromes (GUSTO IIb) Angioplasty Substudy Investigators. A clinical trial comparing primary coronary angioplasty with tissue plasminogen activator for acute myocardial infarction. *N Engl J Med.* 1997;336(23):1621-1628.
10. Grines CL, Cox DA, Stone GW, et al; for the Stent Primary Angioplasty in Myocardial Infarction Study Group. Coronary angioplasty with or without stent implantation for acute myocardial infarction. *N Engl J Med.* 1999;341(26):1949-1956.

11. Assessment of the Safety and Efficacy of a New Thrombolytic (ASSENT-2) Investigators, Van De Werf F, Adgey J, Ardissino D, et al. Single-bolus tenecteplase compared with front-loaded alteplase in acute myocardial infarction: the ASSENT-2 double-blind randomised trial. *Lancet*. 1999;354(9180):716-722.

12. Kastrati A, Mehilli J, Dirschinger J, et al. Myocardial salvage after coronary stenting plus abciximab versus fibrinolysis plus abciximab in patients with acute myocardial infarction: a randomised trial. *Lancet*. 2002;359(9310):920-925.

13. Machecourt J, Bonnefoy E, Vanzetto G, et al. Primary angioplasty is cost-minimizing compared with pre-hospital thrombolysis for patients within 60 min of a percutaneous coronary intervention center: the Comparison of Angioplasty and Pre-hospital Thrombolysis in Acute Myocardial Infarction (CAPTIM) cost-efficacy sub-study. *J Am Coll Cardiol*. 2005;45(4):515-524.

14. Andersen HR, Nielsen TT, Rasmussen K, et al. A comparison of coronary angioplasty with fibrinolytic therapy in acute myocardial infarction. *N Engl J Med*. 2003;349(8):733-742.

15. Dauerman HL, Bates ER, Kontos MC, et al. Nationwide analysis of patients with ST-segment-elevation myocardial infarction transferred for primary percutaneous intervention: findings from the American Heart Association Mission: Lifeline program. *Circ Cardiovasc Intervent*. 2015;8(5):e002450.

16. Westerhout CM, Bonnefoy E, Welsh RC, Steg PG, Boutitie F, Armstrong PW. The influence of time from symptom onset and reperfusion strategy on 1-year survival in ST-elevation myocardial infarction: a pooled analysis of an early fibrinolytic strategy versus primary percutaneous coronary intervention from CAPTIM and WEST. *Am Heart J*. 2011;161(2):283-290.

17. Anderson JL, Karagounis LA, Califf RM. Meta-analysis of five reported studies on the relation of early coronary patency grades with mortality and outcomes after acute myocardial infarction. *Am J Cardiol*. 1996;78(1):1-8.

18. Armstrong PW, Fu Y, Chang W-C, et al; The GUSTO-IIb Investigators. Acute coronary syndromes in the GUSTO-IIb trial: prognostic insights and impact of recurrent ischemia. *Circulation*. 1998;98(18):1860-1868.

19. Nijland F, Kamp O, Verheugt FW, Veen G, Visser CA. Long-term implications of reocclusion on left ventricular size and function after successful thrombolysis for first anterior myocardial infarction. *Circulation*. 1997;95(1):111-117.

20. Stub D, Smith K, Bernard S, et al. Air versus oxygen in ST-segment-elevation myocardial infarction. *Circulation*. 2015;131(24):2143-2150.

21. Jang IK, Gold HK, Ziskind AA, et al. Differential sensitivity of erythrocyte-rich and platelet-rich arterial thrombi to lysis with recombinant tissue-type plasminogen activator. A possible explanation for resistance to coronary thrombolysis. *Circulation*. 1989;79(4):920-928.

22. Gawaz M, Neumann FJ, Ott I, et al. Platelet function in acute myocardial infarction treated with direct angioplasty. *Circulation*. 1996;93(2):229-237.

23. CURRENT-OASIS 7 Investigators, Mehta SR, Bassand J-P, Chrolavicius S, et al. Dose comparisons of clopidogrel and aspirin in acute coronary syndromes. *N Engl J Med*. 2010;363(10):930-942.

24. Yu J, Mehran R, Dangas GD, et al. Safety and efficacy of high- versus low-dose aspirin after primary percutaneous coronary intervention in ST-segment elevation myocardial infarction: the HORIZONS-AMI (Harmonizing Outcomes With Revascularization and Stents in Acute Myocardial Infarction) trial. *JACC Cardiovasc Interv*. 2012;5(12):1231-1238.

25. Bellemain-Appaix A, O'Connor SA, Silvain J, et al. Association of clopidogrel pretreatment with mortality, cardiovascular events, and major bleeding among patients undergoing percutaneous coronary intervention: a systematic review and meta-analysis. *JAMA*. 2012;308(23):2507-2516.

26. Chen ZM, Jiang LX, Chen YP, et al. Addition of clopidogrel to aspirin in 45,852 patients with acute myocardial infarction: randomised placebo-controlled trial. *Lancet*. 2005;366(9497):1607-1621.

27. Montalescot G, Wiviott SD, Braunwald E, et al. Prasugrel compared with clopidogrel in patients undergoing percutaneous coronary intervention for ST-elevation myocardial infarction (TRITON-TIMI 38): double-blind, randomised controlled trial. *Lancet*. 2009;373(9665):723-731.

28. Steg PG, James S, Harrington RA, et al. Ticagrelor versus clopidogrel in patients with ST-elevation acute coronary syndromes intended for reperfusion with primary percutaneous coronary intervention: a Platelet Inhibition and Patient Outcomes (PLATO) trial subgroup analysis. *Circulation*. 2010;122(21):2131-2141.

29. Storey RF, Becker RC, Harrington RA, et al. Characterization of dyspnoea in PLATO study patients treated with ticagrelor or clopidogrel and its association with clinical outcomes. *Eur Heart J*. 2011;32(23):2945-2953.

30. Steg PG, Bhatt DL, Hamm CW, et al. Effect of cangrelor on periprocedural outcomes in percutaneous coronary interventions: a pooled analysis of patient-level data. *Lancet*. 2013;382(9909):1981-1992.

31. Stone GW, Grines CL, Cox DA, et al. Comparison of angioplasty with stenting, with or without abciximab, in acute myocardial infarction. *N Engl J Med*. 2002;346(13):957-966.

32. Stone GW, Witzenbichler B, Guagliumi G, et al. Bivalirudin during primary PCI in acute myocardial infarction. *N Engl J Med*. 2008;358(21):2218-2230.

33. ten Berg JM, van 't Hof AW, Dill T, et al. Effect of early, pre-hospital initiation of high bolus dose tirofiban in patients with ST-segment elevation myocardial infarction on short- and long-term clinical outcome. *J Am Coll Cardiol*. 2010;55(22):2446-2455.

34. Shah R, Rogers KC, Matin K, et al. An updated comprehensive meta-analysis of bivalirudin vs heparin use in primary percutaneous coronary intervention. *Am Heart J*. 2016;171(1):14-24.

35. Antman EM, Morrow DA, McCabe CH, et al. Enoxaparin versus unfractionated heparin with fibrinolysis for ST-elevation myocardial infarction. *N Engl J Med*. 2006;354(14):1477-1488.

36. Yusuf S, Mehta SR, Chrolavicius S, et al. Effects of fondaparinux on mortality and reinfarction in patients with acute ST-segment elevation myocardial infarction: the OASIS-6 randomized trial. *JAMA*. 2006;295(13):1519-1530.

37. Pizarro G, Fernandez-Friera L, Fuster V, et al. Long-term benefit of early pre-reperfusion metoprolol administration in patients with acute myocardial infarction: results from the METOCARD-CNIC trial (effect of metoprolol in cardioprotection during an acute myocardial infarction). *J Am Coll Cardiol*. 2014;63(22):2356-2362.

38. Cholesterol Treatment Trialists Collaboration, Baigent C, Blackwell L, Emberson J, et al. Efficacy and safety of more intensive lowering of LDL cholesterol: a meta-analysis of data from 170,000 participants in 26 randomised trials. *Lancet*. 2010;376(9753):1670-1681.

39. Lee KH, Jeong MH, Kim HM, et al. Benefit of early statin therapy in patients with acute myocardial infarction who have extremely low low-density lipoprotein cholesterol. *J Am Coll Cardiol*. 2011;58(16):1664-1671.

40. ACE Inhibitor Myocardial Infarction Collaborative Group. Indications for ACE inhibitors in the early treatment of acute myocardial infarction: systematic overview of individual data from 100,000 patients in randomized trials. *Circulation*. 1998;97(22):2202-2212.

41. Pitt B, Remme W, Zannad F, et al. Eplerenone, a selective aldosterone blocker, in patients with left ventricular dysfunction after myocardial infarction. *N Engl J Med*. 2003;348(14):1309-1321.

42. Cantor WJ, Fitchett D, Borgundvaag B, et al. Routine early angioplasty after fibrinolysis for acute myocardial infarction. *N Engl J Med*. 2009;360(26):2705-2718.

43. Borgia F, Goodman SG, Halvorsen S, et al. Early routine percutaneous coronary intervention after fibrinolysis vs. standard therapy in ST-segment elevation myocardial infarction: a meta-analysis. *Eur Heart J.* 2010;31(17):2156-2169.

44. Park DW, Clare RM, Schulte PJ, et al. Extent, location, and clinical significance of non-infarct-related coronary artery disease among patients with ST-elevation myocardial infarction. *JAMA.* 2014;312(19):2019-2027.

45. Wald DS, Morris JK, Wald NJ, et al. Randomized trial of preventive angioplasty in myocardial infarction. *N Engl J Med.* 2013;369(12):1115-1123.

46. Engstrom T, Kelbaek H, Helqvist S, et al. Complete revascularisation versus treatment of the culprit lesion only in patients with ST-segment elevation myocardial infarction and multivessel disease (DANAMI-3-PRIMULTI): an open-label, randomised controlled trial. *Lancet.* 2015;386(9994):665-671.

47. Elgendy IY, Mahmoud AN, Kumbhani DJ, Bhatt DL, Bavry AA. Complete vs culprit-only revascularization to treat multi-vessel disease after primary PCI for STEMI (COMPLETE). *JACC Cardiovasc Interv.* 2017;10(4):315-324. https://clinicaltrials.gov/ct2/show/NCT01740479. Accessed June 16, 2017.

48. Kikkert WJ, Zwinderman AH, Vis MM, et al. Timing of mortality after severe bleeding and recurrent myocardial infarction in patients with ST-segment-elevation myocardial infarction. *Circ Cardiovasc Intervent.* 2013;6(4):391-398.

49. Kwok CS, Rao SV, Myint PK, et al. Major bleeding after percutaneous coronary intervention and risk of subsequent mortality: a systematic review and meta-analysis. *Open Heart.* 2014;1(1):e000021.

50. Mehran R, Rao SV, Bhatt DL, et al. Standardized bleeding definitions for cardiovascular clinical trials: a consensus report from the Bleeding Academic Research Consortium. *Circulation.* 2011;123(23):2736-2747.

51. Jones BM, Kapadia SR, Smedira NG, et al. Ventricular septal rupture complicating acute myocardial infarction: a contemporary review. *Eur Heart J.* 2014;35(31):2060-2068.

52. Pellizzon GG, Grines CL, Cox DA, et al. Importance of mitral regurgitation in-patients undergoing percutaneous coronary intervention for acute myocardial infarction: the Controlled Abciximab and Device Investigation to Lower Late Angioplasty Complications (CADILLAC) trial. *J Am Coll Cardiol.* 2004;43(8):1368-1374.

53. Weinsaft JW, Kim J, Medicherla CB, et al. Echocardiographic algorithm for post-myocardial infarction LV thrombus: a gatekeeper for thrombus evaluation by delayed enhancement CMR. *JACC Cardiovasc Imaging.* 2016;9(5):505-515.

54. Katritsis DG, Zareba W, Camm AJ. Nonsustained ventricular tachycardia. *J Am Coll Cardiol.* 2012;60(20):1993-2004.

55. Thiele H, Ohman EM, Desch S, et al. Management of cardiogenic shock. *Eur Heart J.* 2015;36(20):1223-1230.

56. Hochman JS, Sleeper LA, Webb JG, et al; SHOCK Investigators. Early revascularization in acute myocardial infarction complicated by cardiogenic shock. Should we emergently revascularize occluded coronaries for cardiogenic shock. *N Engl J Med.* 1999;341(9):625-634.

57. Sjauw KD, Engstrom AE, Vis MM, et al. A systematic review and meta-analysis of intra-aortic balloon pump therapy in ST-elevation myocardial infarction: should we change the guidelines? *Eur Heart J.* 2009;30(4):459-468.

58. Thiele H, Zeymer U, Neumann FJ, et al. Intraaortic balloon support for myocardial infarction with cardiogenic shock. *N Engl J Med.* 2012;367(14):1287-1296.

59. Balady GJ, Williams MA, Ades PA, et al. Core components of cardiac rehabilitation/secondary prevention programs: 2007 update: a scientific statement from the American Heart Association Exercise, Cardiac Rehabilitation, and Prevention Committee, the Council on Clinical Cardiology; the Councils on Cardiovascular Nursing, Epidemiology and Prevention, and Nutrition, Physical Activity, and Metabolism; and the American Association of Cardiovascular and Pulmonary Rehabilitation. *Circulation.* 2007;115(20):2675-2682.

60. Aragam KG, Dai D, Neely ML, et al. Gaps in referral to cardiac rehabilitation of patients undergoing percutaneous coronary intervention in the United States. *J Am Coll Cardiol.* 2015;65(19):2079-2088.

Patient and Family Information for: ST-ELEVATION MYOCARDIAL INFARCTION

WHAT IS A STEMI?

ST-elevation myocardial infarction (STEMI) or "heart attack" is a life-threatening emergency condition that occurs when one of the arteries supplying blood to the heart muscle suddenly becomes completely blocked. This is more commonly referred to as a heart attack and is one of the leading causes of death in the United States. A STEMI heart attack is considered an emergency because within a very short period of time, a part of the heart muscle can become permanently damaged because of the absence of blood flow from the blocked artery; therefore, urgent medical attention and treatment is required. Studies have shown that the major delay in treatment of a patient with a STEMI is often related to the patient's ability to recognize the symptoms and call for help. This is why all patients with chest pain or discomfort lasting more than 10 minutes are encouraged to call 911 for immediate evaluation.

WHAT CAUSES A STEMI?

Patients at risk for a heart attack often have mild or intermediate blockages caused by plaque buildup in the arteries of the heart (coronary arteries). Normally, these blockages do not cause any symptoms because the blood flow to the heart muscle is not usually compromised. However, if these plaques rupture (or crack), the blood in the artery is then exposed to the sticky material inside of the plaque, and this will lead to the formation of a large blood clot that will completely block the flow of blood down the artery. Some conditions may increase a patient's risk of developing a heart attack. These are referred to as risk factors. It is important to understand that the presence of risk factors increases a patient's chance of developing a heart attack. However, even if a patient has a lot of risk factors, it does not mean that he or she will definitely have a heart attack. On the contrary, some patients without any risk factors may still have a heart attack. The major risk factors that have been identified to cause coronary artery disease and heart attacks include a family history of heart attacks or coronary artery disease, a history of diabetes, high blood pressure, or high cholesterol levels, smoking cigarettes or other types of tobacco products, being overweight, not being physically active, and male gender. Some of these conditions can be changed or controlled by living a healthier lifestyle and/or taking medications to control the condition.

HOW DO DOCTORS DIAGNOSE A STEMI?

The presentation of heart attacks can be variable, but most commonly patients experience profound chest discomfort or chest pain. Patients may describe this chest pain as a chest "squeezing," "tightness," or "heaviness," and sometimes a patient may have shortness of breath, cold sweats, and nausea. The chest pain is typically located in the center of the chest and often described as radiating to the left shoulder, arm, or jaw. The patient may instead have symptoms of upper belly pain, shoulder or back pain, or shortness of breath in the absence of chest pain. Older patients, female patients, and patients with diabetes are more likely to have these less typical symptoms. When an individual presents with these complaints, medical personnel use a chest pain protocol to allow a rapid evaluation in order to quickly confirm the patient's diagnosis so as to allow for immediate treatment.

The mainstay of diagnosis of a STEMI is the electrocardiogram (ECG). During an ECG, electrodes are attached to the outside of the chest wall with a sticky material, and these electrodes measure the electrical conduction through the heart. If the patient is having a "STEMI" the ECG will have a characteristic appearance, known as ST segment elevation. This characteristic appearance helps to distinguish a STEMI heart attack from other heart conditions or other non–heart-related conditions. It is essential to perform and interpret an ECG early after a patient presents for evaluation. Doctors may also order blood tests called cardiac enzymes (cardiac troponin or creatinine kinase CPK-MB). These enzymes are normally contained within the heart cells; When the heart cells die during a heart attack, the heart cells are destroyed and the enzymes are released into the bloodstream. If the health care team strongly suspects, on the basis of symptoms and the abnormalities seen on ECG, that a patient is having a heart attack, then treatment will be given even before the results of the blood tests are reported.

There are two options doctors may use to reopen blocked arteries. The first treatment is the administration of fibrinolytic medications. These medications dissolve the blood clot in the artery of the heart. The second treatment is a procedure called an angioplasty or stent, commonly referred to as primary percutaneous coronary intervention (PCI). During primary PCI, a balloon and/or stents are used by a cardiologist to physically open up the blocked artery. Extensive research involving multiple studies have shown that primary PCI is the best treatment to restore blood flow for a patient with STEMI. However, not all hospitals have the ability to perform emergency primary PCI. If a patient lives in a region in which there are no nearby hospitals that can provide emergency angioplasty or stent, the doctor may first treat the patient with fibrinolytic medications and later transfer him or her to a hospital for possible angioplasty or stent. Regardless of the type of treatment a patient receives, the goal is to rapidly provide the therapy to open the blocked arteries: Fibrinolytic therapy should be administered within 30 minutes; Primary PCI should be performed within 90 minutes of presentation.

WHAT OTHER TREATMENTS DO PATIENTS WITH STEMI RECEIVE?

Once a patient is diagnosed with a STEMI, doctors will begin therapy with medications that thin the blood and decrease its stickiness. Blood thinners are referred to as anticoagulants.

Agents that decrease the stickiness of the blood are referred to as antiplatelet agents. All patients with a STEMI will also be placed on a cardiac monitor, and their vitals signs (blood pressure, heart rate, and breathing rates) will be closely monitored. The next step for treating patients with STEMI is to open the blocked artery. As previously mentioned, if a patient is admitted to a hospital that offers emergency primary PCI, the blocked artery will be opened by inflating a balloon in the artery and placing a stent. If a patient is admitted to a hospital that does not have the capability of performing emergency stenting, the patient will be transferred to another hospital that can perform primary PCI. If there are no nearby hospitals that have the capability of performing primary PCI, the patient might first receive fibrinolytic therapy and later be transferred to another hospital as needed. On most occasions, when an angioplasty is performed a stent is placed in the coronary artery to prevent reocclusion. The two types of stents that are used are bare-metal stents and drug-eluting stents. Drug-eluting or "coated" stents are less likely to narrow again compared with bare-metal stents, but they require a more prolonged duration of treatment with antiplatelet medications. In some cases, the best way to treat the blocked arteries is open-heart surgery. In addition to antiplatelets therapy, other medications may be given. These include angiotensin-converting enzyme inhibitors and beta-blockers. These medications decrease the work required by the heart, and they help the heart to recover and get stronger after a heart attack. Cholesterol lowering medications, called statins, are an important medication used to treat patients with a heart attack. They help to prevent the occurrence of another heart attack.

PREVENTION AND FOLLOW-UP

There are two types of heart attack prevention. Primary prevention is aimed at decreasing a patient's chance of having a "first" heart attack. The goal of secondary prevention is to prevent the occurrence of another heart attack (a "second heart attack"). In patients with STEMI, the focus is on secondary prevention so that the patient will be less likely to suffer from another heart attack. This requires rigorous efforts and attention to living a good lifestyle and taking medications on a regular basis. It is important that patients eat a heart-healthy diet. Heart-healthy diets are diets that are rich in fruits and vegetables and whole grains, and low in saturated fats, trans fats, sweetened drinks, and processed foods. If possible, patients should begin a regular exercise plan (with a doctor's guidance). Although individual recommendations may vary, the goal is to do at least 30 minutes of moderate-intensity exercise most days of the week. Weight loss, avoidance of excess alcohol, and cessation of smoking are also important components of a healthy lifestyle. It is critical that patients also adhere to taking all of their prescribed medications on a regular basis and discuss any concerns about their medications with their doctor before stopping a prescribed medication. Patients should closely follow up with their cardiologist for regular monitoring to ensure compliance with lifestyle measures and medications so as to prevent the complications from the heart attack and lower the risk of recurrences. From a public health perspective, CPR could save the lives of patients who suffer heart attack and sudden death, and everyone should ideally be certified in CPR.

Ronen Jaffe
Eyal Herzog
Moshe Flugelman

3

Non–ST-Elevation Acute Coronary Syndromes

NON–ST-ELEVATION MYOCARDIAL INFARCTION: DEFINITION AND CLINICAL SPECTRUM

The term non–ST-elevation myocardial infarction (NSTEMI) refers to acute coronary syndrome (ACS) in which myocardial ischemia results in tissue necrosis in the absence of ST-segment elevation on the electrocardiogram (ECG). By definition, NSTEMI is accompanied by elevated levels of cardiac biomarkers, signifying loss of myocardial tissue and differentiating NSTEMI from unstable angina. The clinical spectrum of NSTEMI ranges from mild ischemic insults with preserved left ventricular function to life-threatening ischemic events associated with global myocardial ischemia and hemodynamic compromise as well as cardiac arrest. Detailed practice guidelines have been published by the European Society of Cardiology in 2016,[1] the American Heart Association (AHA), and American Society of Cardiology (ACC) in 2014.[2] A comparison between the two documents has also been published.[3]

PATHOPHYSIOLOGY

Myocardial infarction typically results from formation of a coronary thrombus at the site of an existing atherosclerotic plaque.[4] The degree of coronary stenosis at the culprit site before the acute ischemic event is frequently mild or moderate. Coronary thrombosis is caused by disruption of the fibrous cap that forms a barrier between the blood and procoagulant constituents within the plaque. Postmortem studies as well as intravascular imaging studies indicate that most events are triggered by rupture of a thin-cap fibrous atheroma overlying a lipid-rich necrotic core. Superficial plaque erosions are responsible for most of the remainder of cases. In contrast to ST-elevation myocardial infarction (STEMI), the culprit coronary lesion in most NSTEMI cases is not totally occlusive. Embolization of particulate matter from the thrombus within the epicardial coronary artery to the distal microvasculature, as well as intermittent coronary occlusion, leads to myocardial necrosis in these cases. Rarely, NSTEMI is caused by total occlusion of a major coronary artery without associated elevation of the ST-segment in the ECG.

EPIDEMIOLOGY

Currently, NSTEMI outnumbers STEMI by a ratio of 3:1, with an estimated annual US incidence of around 500,000.[5] Patients with NSTEMI have more comorbidities than those with STEMI. In-hospital mortality is similar for patients with NSTEMI and STEMI (9.5% vs 9.7%); however, 1-year postdischarge mortality is higher in patients with NSTEMI (18.7% vs 11.4%).[6,7]

DIAGNOSIS

HISTORY

Precordial chest pain is a frequent presenting symptom in patients with NSTEMI. Typical angina involves a sensation of retrosternal heaviness or pressure radiating to the left arm. Chest pain may be atypical, may radiate to any anatomic location between the umbilicus and the mandible, and in some cases may be absent. Alternatively, patients may complain of angina equivalents such as dyspnea, palpitations, and generalized weakness. Atypical presentation is more common in females, diabetics, patients with renal failure, and the elderly. Presence of risk factors for atherosclerosis such as diabetes mellitus, hypertension, hyperlipidemia, renal failure, a family history of coronary disease, a history of smoking, advanced age, and a previous diagnosis of coronary or peripheral vascular disease are common in patients with NSTEMI. It is important to document current medications the patient is receiving (which may interact with medications to be administered) and to inquire about use of illicit drugs such as cocaine, which may trigger myocardial ischemia. In a patient with ACS, it is crucial to rule out a history of bleeding before initiating antithrombotic and anticoagulant therapy. Allergy to intravascular contrast media should be ruled out and renal function assessed before referring the patient for cardiac catheterization.

PHYSICAL EXAMINATION

Examination may be normal in patients with NSTEMI. It is important to detect signs of hemodynamic compromise if present (reduced blood pressure, accelerated heart rate, signs of peripheral hypoperfusion, jugular venous distention, pulmonary congestion) because these patients may benefit from intensive care and an early invasive strategy. A hypertensive crisis may trigger myocardial ischemia and should be diagnosed and treated rapidly. A systolic murmur may signify a mechanical complication such as acute ischemic mitral regurgitation. A detailed physical examination is crucial for detecting findings, which may point to an alternative diagnosis such as pericarditis (friction rub and pulsus paradoxus), aortic stenosis (systolic murmur), aortic dissection (differences in blood pressure between limbs), musculoskeletal disorders (sensitivity to palpation of the chest wall), and so on. Irregular heart rhythm may also be present in NSTEMI with premature beats and atrial fibrillation. Rapid rate may play a role in the pathophysiology of NSTEMI and should be documented and referred to in the therapeutic strategy.

ELECTROCARDIOGRAM

The ECG may show a variety of anomalies such as ST-segment depression, transient ST-segment elevation, T wave inversion, as well as tachyarrhythmias and bradyarrhythmias. In more than 30% of patients, the ECG is normal. It is important not to misdiagnose a true posterior-wall STEMI (ST-depression and tall R waves in leads V1–V3) and new-onset left bundle branch block (LBBB), which warrant emergency coronary reperfusion.

CARDIAC BIOMARKERS

Measurement of cardiac troponin (cTn) serum levels using regular assays or high-sensitivity assays (hs-cTn) is an effective quantitative method for identifying myocardial necrosis in patients suspected of having NSTEMI. Many hospitals still use regular troponin assays. cTn is a more sensitive and specific marker for myocardial injury than creatine kinase and its muscle–brain isoenzyme. Whereas elevations up to 3-fold the upper reference limit are a nonspecific finding with limited positive predictive value for diagnosis of acute myocardial infarction (MI), elevations beyond 5-fold the upper reference limit have high (>90%) positive predictive value. High-sensitivity troponin assays detect myocardial necrosis within 1 hour of onset of symptoms and typically remain elevated for several days. A variety of conditions other than MI may be accompanied by troponin elevations including critical illness (e.g. burns), nonischemic cardiac injury (e.g. myocarditis, infiltrative disease), aortic dissection, pulmonary embolism, and renal failure. Renal failure can modify the pathognomonic levels of troponin, but dynamic changes in troponin are indicative of myocardial necrosis.

ANCILLARY TESTING

A variety of functional and anatomic imaging modalities may be used to noninvasively detect and quantify myocardial ischemia, to assess prognosis, and to identify high-risk patients. Chest X-ray may demonstrate noncardiac causes of chest discomfort such as pneumonia, pneumothorax, and rib fracture and should be performed in all patients in whom the diagnosis of an ACS is deemed unlikely. Echocardiography assesses left ventricular ejection fraction, reveals regional wall motion abnormalities suggestive of acute or chronic coronary disease, and is crucial for assessment of patients who are hemodynamically unstable. Echocardiography may assist in diagnosing alternative causes of chest pain such as aortic stenosis, pericarditis (pericardial effusion), pulmonary embolism (pulmonary hypertension and right ventricular dilatation), Takotsubo cardiomyopathy, and aortic dissection. Stress echocardiography (during exercise or administration of dipyridamole or dobutamine) may diagnose and quantify degree of myocardial ischemia and offers superior prognostic information compared with a regular exercise test. Contrast echocardiography may be used to assess myocardial perfusion. Cardiac magnetic resonance may be used to assess myocardial perfusion and wall motion and to diagnose myocardial scar formation (late gadolinium hyperenhancement). Nuclear myocardial perfusion imaging detects myocardial ischemia and may be used to assess myocardial viability and ejection fraction. Multidetector computed tomography enables noninvasive detection of coronary disease; however, efficacy may be limited in patients with severe coronary calcification, prior stent implantation, and irregular and fast heart rhythms.

DIFFERENTIAL DIAGNOSIS

A majority of patients presenting to the emergency department with chest pain have a noncardiac etiology for their complaints. The differential diagnosis of NSTEMI in individuals presenting with chest pain includes STEMI (diagnostic ECG); unstable angina (lack of biomarker elevation); thoracic emergencies such as acute aortic syndromes (e.g. aortic dissection) and pulmonary embolism; infectious or inflammatory conditions such as pneumonia, myocarditis, and pericarditis; gastrointestinal disorders; and musculoskeletal disorders of the chest wall. A detailed history and physical examination are crucial for diagnosing these conditions and should be complemented by judicious use of imaging studies.

DIAGNOSTIC ALGORITHM

In patients presenting with chest pain who are suspected of having an ACS, a key priority is to identify those with indications for emergency coronary reperfusion (eg, STEMI, new-onset LBBB, ongoing ischemia, hemodynamic instability) (**Figure 3.1**). Life-threatening conditions that can mimic NSTEMI such as acute aortic syndromes and pulmonary embolism should be rapidly excluded on the basis of the history, examination, and appropriate imaging studies (e.g. "triple rule out" CT angiography). The remainder should undergo a diagnostic protocol, which is designed to rapidly rule-in or rule-out myocardial ischemia as the underlying cause of their symptoms. cTn assays, preferably hs-cTn assays, are crucial for rapid triage of these patients because serum levels increase rapidly in patients with myocardial damage. A dynamic rise in serum cTn levels above the 99th percentile in patients with a compatible clinical presentation is diagnostic of MI. A typical 0 h/3 h algorithm in patients suspected to have sustained an NSTEMI is based on testing of hs-cTn serum levels on admission to the emergency department. Levels below the upper limit of normal in patients in whom chest pain began more than 6 hours previously effectively rules out the diagnosis. Repeat testing of hs-cTn levels is performed 3 hours later in those who developed chest pain less than 6 hours before presentation, when initial levels were not elevated. Patients in whom hs-cTn levels are not elevated may be discharged or referred for further noninvasive evaluation. In those with elevated hs-cTn levels on admission, a dynamic rise in levels is required to confirm the diagnosis of NSTEMI. Patients with a diagnosis of NSTEMI are referred for invasive management unless contraindicated.

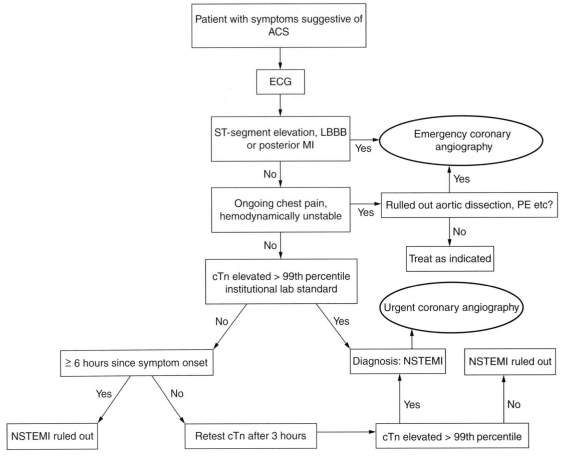

FIGURE 3.1 Diagnostic algorithm in patients with suspected NSTEMI. ACS, acute coronary syndrome; cTn, cardiac troponin; ECG, electrocardiogram; LBBB, left bundle branch block; MI, myocardial infarction; NSTEMI, non–ST-elevation myocardial infarction; PE, pulmonary embolism.

An alternative 0 h/1 h algorithm may be used; however, it is less well validated.

RISK STRATIFICATION

Early triage of patients with NSTEMI is crucial in order to identify individuals who are at high risk for development of further myocardial damage. Ongoing chest pain, dynamic ST-changes on the ECG, and hemodynamic instability suggest need for emergency revascularization. Assessment of the risk for life-threatening cardiac arrhythmias is crucial for selecting the appropriate hospital environment and degree of monitoring required for these patients. Predictors of serious arrhythmias include hemodynamic instability, documented major arrhythmias, ejection fraction ≤40%, untreated significant coronary lesions on angiography, and complications related to coronary intervention. Patients with NSTEMI and risk factors for serious arrhythmias should be kept in cardiac care unit.

Several scores provide quantitative assessment of ischemic risk and prognostication up to 3 years. The thrombolysis in myocardial infarction (TIMI) risk score (online calculator: http://www.timi.org/index.php?page=calculators) uses seven metrics to assess prognosis. The variables included in the risk score are:

age ≥65 years, presence of ≥3 risk factors for coronary disease, known coronary disease, recent aspirin use (within the past week), severe angina (≥2 episodes within the past 24 hours), ST deviation ≥0.5 mm on the ECG, and elevated cardiac biomarkers. The Global Registry of Acute Coronary Events (GRACE) 2.0 risk score (online calculator: http://www.gracescore.org/WebSite/default.aspx?ReturnUrl=%2f) has been shown to provide superior prognostication compared with the TIMI risk score. Variables included in the GRACE 2.0 risk score are: age, blood pressure, heart rate, renal function, cardiac arrest, Killip class, elevated cardiac biomarkers, and ST-segment deviation.

Assessment of risk for bleeding is crucial before administration of anticoagulant and antiplatelet drugs. Current risk scores are relevant mainly for predicting bleeding in patients with NSTEMI undergoing coronary angiography; however, their relevance to patients selected for noninvasive treatment or those receiving oral anticoagulants is unclear. The *C*an *R*apid risk stratification of *U*nstable angina patients *S*uppress *AD*verse outcomes with *E*arly implementation of the ACC/AHA guidelines (CRUSADE) bleeding risk score (online calculator: http://www.crusadebleedingscore.org) uses the following variables: female sex, diabetes, peripheral vascular or cerebrovascular disease, heart rate, blood pressure, heart failure, hematocrit, and creatinine clearance. The Acute Catheterization and Urgent Intervention Triage strategy

(ACUITY) bleeding risk score takes into account the following variables: female sex, advanced age, elevated serum creatinine, white blood cell count, anemia, and presentation as NSTEMI or STEMI. These scores may require updating in view of recent changes in clinical practice, which include increasing use of transradial vascular access, diminishing popularity of glycoprotein IIb/IIIa inhibitors, substitution of clopidogrel for more potent oral antiplatelet drugs, and shift in anticoagulant regimens from heparin to bivalirudin.

MEDICAL TREATMENT

ANTI-ISCHEMIC AGENTS

The objective of medical therapy is to correct the imbalance between myocardial supply and demand and to reduce thrombus-related events (**Figure 3.2**). Some of the research relating to pharmacologic treatment of NSTEMI dates back to the era before the advent of current antiplatelet and anticoagulant medications and preceded modern invasive treatment strategies.

General Measures

Bed rest minimizes physical activity, reduces myocardial oxygen demand, and enables effective patient monitoring. Oxygen should not be administered universally, but only to hypoxic patients with arterial oxygen saturation <90%. Opiates reduce chest pain and anxiety and therefore myocardial oxygen demand; however, they may reduce intestinal absorption of oral antiplatelet medications and may lower blood pressure in hypotensive patients—especially in those given concomitant nitrates. Nitrates may lower blood pressure in hypertensive patients and facilitate regression of ST-segment depression on the ECG. Their role is symptom relief

with no proven impact on patient outcome. Nitrates should be given cautiously to hemodynamically unstable patients and are contraindicated in patients who have received phosphodiesterase type 5 inhibitors (sildenafil, tadalafil) within the past 24 to 48 hours.

β-Adrenergic-Blocking Agents

β-Blockers reduce myocardial oxygen demand (reduced contractility, heart rate, and blood pressure). Early studies found a mortality benefit for administration of β-blockers; however, they should be given cautiously to hypotensive and bradycardic patients because they may increase the incidence of cardiogenic shock. β-Blockers may worsen coronary spasm in patients who have used cocaine.

ANTIPLATELET THERAPY

Combined antiplatelet therapy with aspirin and an inhibitor of the $P2Y_{12}$ receptor decreases the occurrence of recurrent ischemic event and improves clinical outcomes in patients with NSTEMI compared with aspirin monotherapy. Dual therapy also increases the risk of bleeding, especially if ticagrelor or prasugrel is substituted for clopidogrel. This bleeding risk is especially relevant to the estimated 10% of NSTEMI patients who are referred for coronary artery bypass surgery (CABG). Prasugrel administration should be withheld until coronary angiography has been performed and need for CABG has been excluded.

Aspirin

Aspirin suppresses platelet thromboxane A_2 production by irreversibly inactivating cyclooxygenase-1. Pivotal trials of aspirin in ACS, performed before the recognition of the importance of an early invasive strategy, found a reduction in occurrence of MI and death. High-dose (300 to 325 mg/d) and low-dose (75 to 100 mg/d) aspirin are equally effective and should be given following a loading dose of 150 to 300 mg of a nonenteric-coated formulation.

$P2Y_{12}$ Receptor Blockers

Clopidogrel

Clopidogrel irreversibly inactivates platelet $P2Y_{12}$ receptors and inhibits adenosine diphosphate (ADP)-induced platelet aggregation. Clopidogrel is a pro-drug that undergoes hepatic metabolism via the cytochrome p450 to release an active metabolite. In patients with ACS, combined treatment of aspirin and clopidogrel decreases ischemic events. Some patients have inadequate response to clopidogrel and may be at risk for increased ischemic events and stent thrombosis. Individual responsiveness to clopidogrel may be related to gene polymorphisms; however, the role of screening for platelet responsiveness to clopidogrel in clinical practice is unclear. The loading dose of clopidogrel is 300 to 600 mg and maintenance dose is 75 mg/d. In the Clopidogrel and Aspirin Optimal Dose Usage to Reduce Recurrent Events–Seventh Organization to Assess Strategies in Ischemic Syndromes (CURRENT-OASIS7) study, doubling the maintenance dose during the first week reduced the risk of ischemic events.[8]

Prasugrel

Prasugrel irreversibly inactivates platelet $P2Y_{12}$ receptors and inhibits ADP-induced platelet aggregation with faster onset and greater

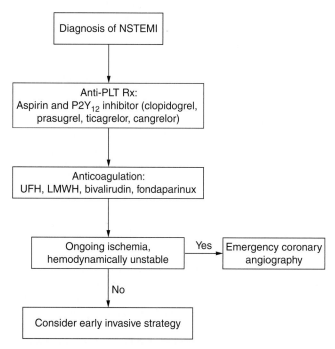

FIGURE 3.2 Treatment algorithm in patients with diagnosis of NSTEMI. Anti-PLT Rx, antiplatelet therapy; LMWH, low-molecular-weight heparin; NSTEMI, non–ST-elevation myocardial infarction; UFH, unfractionated heparin.

inhibitory effect than clopidogrel. In the Trial to Assess Improvement in Therapeutic Outcomes by Optimizing Platelet Inhibition with Prasugrel-TIMI (TRITON-TIMI 38) study, prasugrel reduced the risk of MI and stent thrombosis compared with clopidogrel but increased the risk of bleeding.[9] Prasugrel is contraindicated in patients with known cerebrovascular disease, elderly patients (>75 years old) and those with low body weight (<60 kg). Loading dose is 60 mg and the maintenance dose is 10 mg/d.

Ticagrelor

Ticagrelor reversibly inhibits platelet $P2Y_{12}$ receptors with onset of action and efficacy similar to prasugrel. The half-life of 6 to 12 hours mandates that ticagrelor is taken twice daily. In the Platelet Inhibition and Patient Outcomes (PLATO) study, ticagrelor decreased death, MI, and stroke as well as stent thrombosis compared with clopidogrel but increased the risk of nonfatal bleeding.[10] Side effects include dyspnea. Loading dose is 180 mg, and maintenance does is 90 mg twice daily.

Cangrelor

Cangrelor is administered intravenously and induces short-term (1 to 2 hours) inhibition of platelet $P2Y_{12}$ receptors. Cangrelor reduces thrombotic events and stent thrombosis compared with clopidogrel but increases the risk of bleeding.[11]

Glycoprotein IIb/IIIa Receptor Inhibitors

Glycoprotein IIb/IIIa receptor inhibitors effectively prevent platelet aggregation; however, their use is associated with an increased risk of bleeding. Studies performed before the era of oral $P2Y_{12}$ antagonists suggested a clinical benefit; however, the safety of administering these drugs concomitantly with ticagrelor and prasurel is unknown. Currently, administration of these agents is recommended only in the setting of thrombotic complications of PCI.

ANTICOAGULATION

Anticoagulants target thrombin generation and fibrin formation and act in synergy with antiplatelet agents. A challenge in treating these patients is to achieve the optimal balance between the need to safely and effectively prevent thrombus-related events and the desire to reduce bleeding complications.

Unfractionated Heparin

Unfractionated heparin (UFH) is composed of an assortment of molecules of variable size that generate a conformational change in antithrombin and inactivate factors II (thrombin) and X. UFH is administered intravenously, the dose–response of UFH is unpredictable, the therapeutic window narrow, and the treatment predisposes patients to development of heparin-induced thrombocytopenia (HIT). Anticoagulation can be reversed by administration of protamine sulfate, and the degree of anticoagulation can be assessed by measuring the activated Partial Thromboplastin Time (aPTT).

Low-Molecular-Weight Heparin

Low-molecular-weight heparin (LMWH) is administered subcutaneously and achieves more predictable anticoagulant effect compared with UFH. Protamine achieves partial reversal of LMWH-induced anticoagulation. LMWH causes HIT less often than UFH, and the LMWH dose should be reduced in patients with renal failure.

Fondaparinux

Fondaparinux is a reversible selective inhibitor of factor X. Fondaparinux is administered subcutaneously and does not induce HIT. Fondaparinux lowers rates of bleeding and mortality compared with LMWH without increasing ischemic events; however, UFH should be added during PCI to avoid catheter thrombosis.[12,13]

Bivalirudin

Bivalirudin is an intravenously administered direct thrombin inhibitor. Bivalirudin with bailout administration of glycoprotein IIb/IIIa inhibitors achieves an anti-ischemic effect comparable to UFH or LMWH with routine co-administration of glycoprotein IIb/IIIa inhibitors, but with reduced bleeding complications.

INITIAL CONSERVATIVE VERSUS INITIAL INVASIVE APPROACH

Routine coronary angiography in patients with NSTEMI enables rapid confirmation of the diagnosis of ACS by identification of the culprit lesion in an epicardial coronary artery, risk assessment based on the coronary anatomy and performance of early coronary revascularization. Randomized trials have shown that an invasive strategy achieved superior clinical outcomes (reduced mortality and rehospitalization) compared with a strategy of selective angiography based on positive findings in noninvasive tests.[14,15] Selection of patients for an early invasive strategy should be individualized and should take into consideration the presence of comorbidities, cognitive impairment, renal failure, frailty, etc. An early invasive strategy (angiography with 12 to 48 hours of hospital admission) reduced the risk of adverse cardiac events compared with a delayed invasive strategy, especially in high-risk patients (GRACE risk score > 140).[16] Coronary angiography and intervention via transradial vascular access decreases mortality and vascular complications compared with transfemoral access[17] and complete revascularization is associated with superior clinical outcomes compared with culprit-only revascularization.[18] Revascularization should be performed after demonstration of a hemodynamically significant flow-limiting coronary stenosis. Stenting is generally performed in discrete coronary lesions, whereas patients with diffuse coronary disease (SYNTAX score > 23 to 33) should be considered for CABG.

DISCHARGE PLANNING

Secondary prevention of coronary events is crucial in patients being discharged after hospitalization for NSTEMI. Patients should be educated about the importance of modifying their risk profile and instructed regarding the importance of a healthy lifestyle, smoking cessation, weight reduction, routine aerobic exercise, optimal blood pressure control, and consumption of a Mediterranean diet low in saturated fats and rich in vegetable products. Enrollment in a cardiac rehabilitation program may enhance patient compliance, reduce cardiac mortality and hospital admissions, and improve quality of life.[19]

STATINS

High-intensity statin therapy is recommended to reduce low-density lipoprotein (LDL)-cholesterol levels to below 70 mg/dL or as low as possible, depending on the specific hospital's protocol. Ezetimibe treatment may be considered in patients who are intolerant to high-dose statins and those who fail to reach the desired LDL levels.

BETA BLOCKERS AND ACE INHIBITORS

Beta Blockers and ACE Inhibitors are indicated in patients with a reduced left ventricular ejection fraction (<40%); however, their efficacy in patients with preserved left ventricular ejection fraction in the current era of routine coronary revascularization is unproven.

ANTIPLATELET THERAPY

Dual antiplatelet therapy (DAPT) with aspirin and a $P2Y_{12}$ inhibitor is mandatory after coronary stenting and also in patients who did not undergo coronary revascularization. Tailoring the duration of DAPT involves a tradeoff between reductions in stent thrombosis and MI and increases in major hemorrhage.[20] DAPT should be continued for at least 1 year, and continuation of DAPT beyond that time frame has been suggested to reduce ischemic events[21]; however, duration of DAPT should be individualized according to the estimated patient's risk of future ischemic events as well as bleeding risk.[22]

REFERENCES

1. Roffi M, Patrono C, Collet JP, et al. 2015 ESC guidelines for the management of acute coronary syndromes in patients presenting without persistent ST-segment elevation: task force for the management of acute coronary syndromes in patients presenting without persistent ST-segment elevation of the European Society of Cardiology (ESC). *Eur Heart J.* 2016;37:267-315.

2. Amsterdam EA, Wenger NK, Brindis RG, et al. 2014 AHA/ACC guideline for the management of patients with non-ST-elevation acute coronary syndromes: a report of the American College of Cardiology/American Heart Association task force on practice guidelines. *J Am Coll Cardiol.* 2014;64:e139-e228.

3. Rodriguez F, Mahaffey KW. Management of patients with NSTE-ACS: a comparison of the recent AHA/ACC and ESC guidelines. *J Am Coll Cardiol.* 2016;68:313-321.

4. Libby P. Mechanisms of acute coronary syndromes and their implications for therapy. *N Engl J Med.* 2013;368:2004-2013.

5. Mozaffarian D, Benjamin EJ, Go AS, et al; on behalf of the American Heart Association Statistics Committee and Stroke Statistics Subcommittee. Heart disease and stroke statistics—2016 update: a report from the American Heart Association. *Circulation.* 2016;133:e38-e360.

6. McManus DD, Gore J, Yarzebski J, Spencer F, Lessard D, Goldberg RJ. Recent trends in the incidence, treatment, and outcomes of patients with STEMI and NSTEMI. *Am J Med.* 2011;124:40-47.

7. Vora AN, Wang TY, Hellkamp AS, et al. Differences in short- and long-term outcomes among older patients with ST-elevation versus non-ST-elevation myocardial infarction with angiographically proven coronary artery disease. *Circ Cardiovasc Qual Outcomes.* 2016;9:513-522.

8. Mehta SR, Tanguay JF, Eikelboom JW, et al. Double-dose versus standard-dose clopidogrel and high-dose versus low-dose aspirin in individuals undergoing percutaneous coronary intervention for acute coronary syndromes (CURRENT-OASIS 7): a randomised factorial trial. *Lancet.* 2010;376:1233-1243.

9. Wiviott SD, Braunwald E, McCabe CH, et al. Prasugrel versus clopidogrel in patients with acute coronary syndromes. *N Engl J Med.* 2007;357:2001-2015.

10. Wallentin L, Becker RC, Budaj A, et al. Ticagrelor versus clopidogrel in patients with acute coronary syndromes. *N Engl J Med.* 2009;361:1045-1057.

11. Steg PG, Bhatt DL, Hamm CW, et al. Effect of cangrelor on periprocedural outcomes in percutaneous coronary interventions: a pooled analysis of patient-level data. *Lancet.* 2013;382:1981-1992.

12. Yusuf S, Mehta SR, Chrolavicius S, et al; The Fifth Organization to Assess Strategies in Acute Ischemic Syndromes Investigators. Comparison of fondaparinux and enoxaparin in acute coronary syndromes. *N Engl J Med.* 2006;354:1464-1476.

13. Jolly SS, Faxon DP, Fox KA, et al. Efficacy and safety of fondaparinux versus enoxaparin in patients with acute coronary syndromes treated with glycoprotein IIb/IIIa inhibitors or thienopyridines: results from the OASIS 5 (Fifth Organization to Assess Strategies in Ischemic Syndromes) trial. *J Am Coll Cardiol.* 2009;54:468-476.

14. Fox KA, Clayton TC, Damman P, et al. Long-term outcome of a routine versus selective invasive strategy in patients with non-ST-segment elevation acute coronary syndrome a meta-analysis of individual patient data. *J Am Coll Cardiol.* 2010;55:2435-2445.

15. Fox KA, Poole-Wilson PA, Henderson RA, et al. Interventional versus conservative treatment for patients with unstable angina or non-ST-elevation myocardial infarction: the British Heart Foundation RITA 3 randomised trial. Randomized intervention trial of unstable angina. *Lancet.* 2002;360:743-751.

16. Mehta SR, Granger CB, Boden WE, et al. Early versus delayed invasive intervention in acute coronary syndromes. *N Engl J Med.* 2009;360:2165-2175.

17. Valgimigli M, Gagnor A, Calabro P, et al. Radial versus femoral access in patients with acute coronary syndromes undergoing invasive management: a randomised multicentre trial. *Lancet.* 2015;385: 2465-2476.

18. Genereux P, Palmerini T, Caixeta A, et al. Quantification and impact of untreated coronary artery disease after percutaneous coronary intervention: the residual SYNTAX (Synergy Between PCI with Taxus and Cardiac Surgery) score. *J Am Coll Cardiol.* 2012;59:2165-2174.

19. Anderson L, Oldridge N, Thompson DR, et al. Exercise-based cardiac rehabilitation for coronary heart disease: cochrane systematic review and meta-analysis. *J Am Coll Cardiol.* 2016;67:1-12.

20. Bittl JA, Baber U, Bradley SM, Wijeysundera DN. Duration of dual antiplatelet therapy: a systematic review for the 2016 ACC/AHA guideline focused update on duration of dual antiplatelet therapy in patients with coronary artery disease: a report of the American College of Cardiology/American Heart Association task force on clinical practice guidelines. *J Am Coll Cardiol.* 2016;68:1116-1139.

21. Mauri L, Kereiakes DJ, Yeh RW, et al. Twelve or 30 months of dual antiplatelet therapy after drug-eluting stents. *N Engl J Med.* 2014;371:2155-2166.

22. Levine GN, Bates ER, Bittl JA, et al. 2016 ACC/AHA guideline focused update on duration of dual antiplatelet therapy in the patients with coronary artery disease: a report of the American College of Cardiology/American Heart Association task force on clinical practice guidelines. *J Am Coll Cardiol.* 2016;68:1082-1115.

Patient and Family Information for:
NON–ST-ELEVATION ACUTE CORONARY SYNDROMES

WHAT IS CORONARY ARTERY DISEASE, AND WHAT IS A HEART ATTACK?

Coronary disease results from blockages in the arteries that supply oxygenated blood to the heart muscle. Coronary disease results from atherosclerosis, which is a process in which cholesterol accumulates in cells within the vessel wall. Atherosclerosis is very common in the general population and is linked to several risk factors such as smoking, obesity, high blood pressure, diabetes, and a family history of coronary disease. A heart attack results from sudden development of a blood clot on top of an atherosclerotic plaque, which occludes the coronary artery and prevents blood flow to the heart muscle. Because the pumping heart needs a constant blood supply, occlusion of a coronary artery may cause irreversible damage and replacement of the normal muscle cells with scar tissue. The typical symptom during a heart attack is crushing chest pain radiating to the left arm; however, the presenting symptoms of a heart attack may be atypical, and many other diseases may be associated with symptoms that mimic a heart attack.

HOW IS A HEART ATTACK DIAGNOSED?

Diagnosis of a heart attack is based on assessment of the patient's complaints, physical examination, the ECG, and various blood tests and ancillary tests.

ELECTROCARDIOGRAM

The ECG in a patient with a heart attack may show a finding called ST-elevation, which usually signifies complete blockage of a coronary artery. Heart attack patients with ST-elevation on the ECG are usually referred for emergency coronary catheterization in order to open the blocked artery immediately and prevent further damage to the heart muscle. More often, the ECG in patients with a heart attack does not show ST-elevation. These patients usually do not require emergency catheterization, but are typically referred for catheterization within 1 to 2 days in order to evaluate the patency of the coronary arteries and select the best treatment approach.

BLOOD TESTS

Even minimal damage to the heart muscle may lead to secretion of a protein called troponin into the blood stream. Measurement of blood troponin levels enables accurate diagnosis of a heart attack.

ADDITIONAL TESTS

- Echocardiography uses ultrasound to evaluate the structure and functioning of the heart. This noninvasive test is very useful for detecting damage to the heart muscle following a heart attack.

- Exercise testing: During physical exercise, the workload on the heart increases in order to supply larger volumes of oxygenated blood to the skeletal muscles. This increased cardiac workload means that the heart muscle itself requires increased blood supply through the coronary arteries. Obstruction to blood flow in the coronaries during exercise may cause an imbalance between oxygen supply and demand in the heart muscle, which is called myocardial ischemia. ECG changes during exercise may reflect ischemia and signify that catheterization should be performed in order to accurately analyze the anatomy of the coronary arteries.
- Myocardial perfusion scans measure the uptake of radioactive substances in the heart muscle at rest and during exercise to detect ischemia.
- Cardiac CT is a noninvasive test that enables accurate mapping of the coronary anatomy and detection of blockages within these arteries.

TREATMENT

MEDICATIONS

Various medications have proven benefit in patients with coronary artery disease. Aspirin is a blood thinner, which is used to prevent development of blood clots within the coronaries. In patients with a heart attack, an additional oral blood thinner is usually given to enhance the effect of aspirin. Three commonly used blood thinners are clopidogrel (Plavix), prasugrel (Effient), and ticagrelor (Brilinta). Statins are cholesterol-lowering drugs that may prevent heart attacks and death in patients with coronary disease. β-Blockers are drugs that lower the heart rate and blood pressure and therefore decrease the workload on the heart. Nitrates are drugs that improve blood supply to the heart muscle in patients with coronary disease.

CARDIAC CATHETERIZATION

During catheterization, a thin tube (catheter) is inserted via an artery in the groin or in the wrist to the heart. The procedure is performed in a special room, which is called a catheterization laboratory where X-ray is used to study the heart and coronary arteries. Injection of a fluid called contrast media enables accurate mapping of the course and patency of the coronary arteries and detection of blockages within them.

CORONARY ANGIOPLASTY

Angioplasty is a technique that enables opening of blockages within the coronary arteries through a catheter. A small balloon is used to open the blockages. A stent is a metallic cylinder that is placed within the blockage to keep it open. Modern stents (drug-eluting stents) have special drugs attached to them that prevent renarrowing of the arteries.

CORONARY BYPASS SURGERY

Bypass surgery is open-heart surgery in which alternative blood vessels (bypass grafts) are connected to the diseased coronary arteries beyond the point at which they are blocked. This is done in order to renew blood supply to the heart muscle. Bypass surgery is usually performed in patients with multiple blockages in the coronary arteries who are not considered good candidates for angioplasty, especially in diabetics.

RECOVERY

- Diet: Patients with coronary disease should use a "Mediterranean" diet with a high consumption of vegetables and fruit and low in saturated fats and red meat. Patients should lower their calorie consumption in order to achieve an ideal body weight.

- Exercise: Aerobic exercise has proven benefit in preventing future heart attacks, lowering blood pressure, and achieving weight loss. A typical exercise regimen entails walking an hour a day at a speed of 3 mph.
- Smoking: Continued smoking after a heart attack significantly increases the risk of repeated heart attacks, stroke, and death. Smoking cessation is crucial in patients with coronary disease and may be assisted by special counseling.
- Medications: Patients with coronary disease require life-long aspirin to prevent future heart attacks and statins to lower the blood cholesterol. Patients who have received coronary stents require an additional blood thinner (clopidogrel, prasugrel, ticagrelor) for a period ranging between several months and 1 year. Some patients require additional medications to control high blood pressure and diabetes, to treat heart failure or rhythm disturbances, and to reduce chest pain (angina).

Eyal Herzog
Indra Warren

4

Echocardiography in Acute Coronary Syndrome

INTRODUCTION

The past few decades have witnessed remarkable progress in the understanding of the pathophysiology of acute coronary syndrome (ACS). This, in turn, has led to advances in various imaging techniques for diagnosis and therapeutic options. Developments in the field of echocardiography have paralleled the progress made in ACS. The initial use of echocardiography was to detect pericardial effusions and cardiac tumors. However, the current applications of various forms of echocardiography include an extended list of pathologic and therapeutic indications. Advances in echocardiographic techniques and instrumentation have rivaled those in management of ACS.[1] This chapter is focused on the role of echocardiography in ACS.

ASSESSMENT OF REGIONAL SYSTOLIC FUNCTION IN ACUTE CORONARY SYNDROME

Occlusion of an epicardial coronary artery at the time of ACS may lead to a loss of contractile function in the myocardial segments subtended by that vessel. The magnitude and duration of wall motion abnormalities depend on the severity, extent, and duration of the coronary occlusion.

In unstable angina, left and right ventricular wall motion may be normal unless transthoracic echocardiography happens to be performed during an episode of chest pain.

Non–ST-elevation myocardial infarction (NSTEMI) usually results from an occlusion of a coronary branch vessel often in an elderly patient with pre-existing collateral coronary circulation. Typically, the loss of contractile function is restricted to the subendocardial layer, which is most vulnerable to ischemia. However, on standard echocardiography, the contractility loss may be observed in the entire thickness of the affected myocardial segment. This overestimation of contractile loss is attributed to tethering (an apparent passive loss of contractility in normal segments because of contractile loss in an adjacent area).

ST-elevation myocardial infarction (STEMI) often results from an acute occlusion of a major coronary vessel and tends to occur in a younger age group compared with NSTEMI. If the total session of coronary flow lasts for more than 3 to 6 hours, myocardial necrosis will occur and the myocardium in the affected segments will be replaced with a fibrous tissue over the ensuing weeks.[2]

The magnitude of regional contractile loss in ACS is usually assessed semiquantitatively. It is usually interpreted clinically as follows[2]:

1. Interpretation of wall motion abnormalities:
   Normal: Contractility preserved
   Hypokinesis: Partial loss of contractility
   Akinesis: Complete loss of contractility
   Dyskinesis: Paradoxical movement of the affected segment away from the center of the ventricle during systole
   Aneurysmal: Outward movement of the affected segment during both systole and diastole
2. Extent and location of affected segments
3. Suspected coronary artery distribution (left anterior descending artery [LAD] vs right coronary artery vs left circumflex artery).

ASSESSMENT OF GLOBAL SYSTOLIC FUNCTION IN ACUTE CORONARY SYNDROME

Global ventricular systolic function in ACS is assessed through both wall motion scoring and global ventricular ejection fraction (EF).

Wall Motion Scoring

Wall motion scoring analysis assigns a numeric value to the degree of contractile dysfunction in each segment. The most common scoring criteria are seen in **Table 4.1**.[3]

Once all segments are assigned individual scores, a total score is calculated as a sum of individual scores. A Wall Motion Score Index (WMSI) is then calculated as a ratio between the total score over the number of evaluated segments. The WMSI is a dimensionless index.

A 17-segment model is commonly used to allow for standardized communication within echocardiography and with other imaging modalities. In this 17-segment model, the apex is divided into five segments (septal, anterior, inferior, lateral, and an "apical cap" defined as the myocardium beyond the end of the left ventricular [LV] cavity).[3] For a fully visualized normal ventricle, the total score is 17 (all segments have normal contractility). Because all 17 segments are evaluated, the WMSI of a normal heart is $17/17 = 1$. For abnormal ventricles, the higher the WMSI, the more significant the wall motion abnormally is. A score above 1.7 represents significant wall motion abnormality.

Assessment of Ventricular Ejection Fraction

Numerous studies have consistently shown left ventricular ejection fraction (LVEF) as one of the most powerful predictors of future mortality and morbidity in patients with heart disease.[4] LVEF is the single most powerful predictor of mortality and the risk for developing life-threatening ventricular arrhythmias after myocardial infarction.[5] Furthermore, once the ACS resolves, the residual LVEF is important for treatment options as LVEF cutoff values are built into recommendations for both medical and electrical device therapies. Even with treatment and clinical stabilization of heart failure, there is an inverse, almost linear, relationship between LVEF and survival in patients whose LVEF is less than 45% (**Figure 4.1**).[6]

By definition, LVEF is the percentage of the end-diastolic volume that is ejected with each systole as the stroke volume. Thus, to calculate the LVEF, one needs to estimate the end-systolic and end-diastolic volume of the left ventricle.

For two-dimensional echocardiography, biplane Simpson's rule is routinely used for estimation of the LVEF.[7,8] Most modern ultrasound systems provide a semiautomated software package for the Simpson's rule analysis. Operators are usually only required to trace the LV endocardial border at end-diastolic and end-systolic in the apical four-chamber and two-chamber views; the software package then automatically calculates the LV end-diastolic volume, end-systolic volume, and LVEF (**Figure 4.2**).

With the advent of real-time three-dimensional (RT3D) transthoracic techniques, LV volumes and LVEF can now be calculated with even greater accuracy than is possible with the biplane Simpson's rule (**Figure 4.3**). RT3D-derived LV volume data are now comparable to those obtained by cardiac magnetic resonance imaging, the prior gold standard for such calculations.[8]

Thus, whenever available, LV volumes and LVEF in ACS should be calculated from an RT3D system; the biplane Simpson's rule should be the next best method for such calculations when only a two-dimensional ultrasound system is available.

THE ISCHEMIC CASCADE

The ischemic cascade refers to a sequence of events that occurs in the myocardium after the onset of ischemia.[9] Myocardial perfusion is determined by coronary blood flow and myocardial oxygen consumption. Any imbalance in this supply-and-demand relationship results in myocardial ischemia.[10] The mechanical, electrographic, and clinical events that follow the development of ischemia were formally described in 1985 by Hauser et al.[11] and were later termed the "ischemic cascade."[12]

TABLE 4.1	Left Ventricular Wall Motion Scoring	
		SCORE
Normal or hyperkinetic		1
Hypokinetic (reduced thickening)		2
Akinetic (absent or negligible thickening)		3
Dyskinetic (systolic thinning or stretching, aneurysmal)		4

Wall Motion Score Index = Sum of Individual Segment Scores/Number of Evaluated Segments.

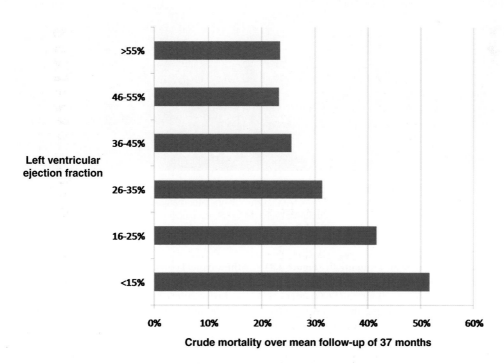

FIGURE 4.1 Relationship between left ventricular ejection fraction and survival. Note the negative, almost linear, relationship between survival and left ejection fractions <45%. (Based on numeric data from Curtis et al.[6])

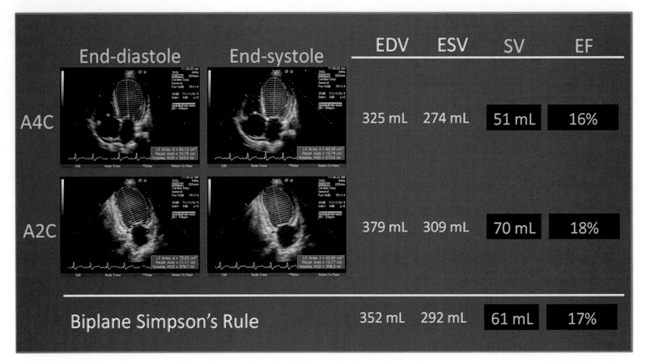

FIGURE 4.2 Calculation of LVEF by biplane Simpson's rule. The operator of an ultrasound system is required to trace the endocardial border of an end-diastolic and an end-systolic frame in the A4C and A2C views. The system then calculates the EDV, ESV, SV, and LVEF. A4C, apical four-chamber; A2C, apical two-chamber; EDV, end-diastolic volume; EF, ejection fraction; ESV, end-systolic volume; LVEF, left ventricular ejection fraction; SV, stroke volume.

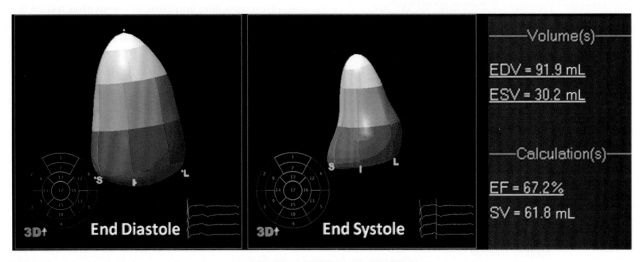

FIGURE 4.3 Calculation of left ventricular volumes and EF by three-dimensional echocardiography. A three-dimensional ultrasound system calculates the EDV, ESV, SV, and LVEF automatically from a three-dimensional data set after an operator manually enters key reference points of the left ventricle. EDV, end-diastolic volume; EF, ejection fraction; ESV, end-systolic volume; LVEF, left ventricular ejection fraction; SV, stroke volume.

Classically, the observable changes occur sequentially (**Figure 4.4**) starting with perfusion abnormalities leading to abnormalities in wall function, then ischemic electrocardiogram (ECG) changes, and finally angina.[13] Echocardiography has the ability to detect these pathophysiologic changes in the myocardium at the most initial stages and therefore is more sensitive than history, physical examination, and ECG for identification of myocardial ischemia.[14] **Figures 4.5** and **4.6** depict echocardiographic views of the left ventricle, demonstrating the LV wall segments and

their typical corresponding coronary distributions.[3] Additionally, the utilization of image-enhancing agents (echocardiographic contrast microbubbles) has improved the detection of even subtle wall motion abnormalities, improving the confidence in the presence or absence of ischemia, and thereby facilitating further management.

Echocardiography for the diagnosis of suspected acute ischemia is most helpful in subjects with a high clinical suspicion but nondiagnostic electrocardiograms, as it allows real-time assessment

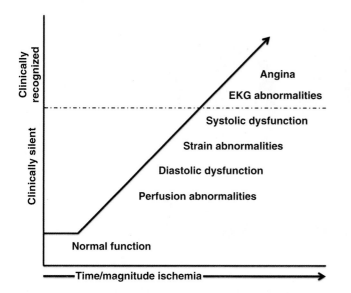

FIGURE 4.4 The ischemic cascade. Myocardial dysfunction occurs in a predictable sequence, which is detectable before clinical symptoms. ECG, electrocardiogram.

of myocardial function. Additionally, through stress modalities, it offers assessment and risk stratification in patients who present to the emergency department with chest pain.

Of note, troponin elevation with chest pain may not be related to an ACS, but rather be secondary to other cardiovascular pathology such as valvular disease (eg, severe aortic stenosis or regurgitation), which can induce ischemia by causing LV wall stress; acute heart failure due to systolic and/or diastolic dysfunction; or even acute pulmonary embolism with right ventricular strain. Echocardiography is a valuable tool to detect and quantify these other abnormalities, regardless of whether the patient is having an ACS.

STRESS ECHOCARDIOGRAPHY

There are different types of stress echocardiography that can be used in the evaluation of patients with coronary artery disease.[15] For patients who are able to exercise, treadmill and supine bicycle stress echocardiograms are the preferred techniques. For patients unable to exercise, pharmacologic stress testing using

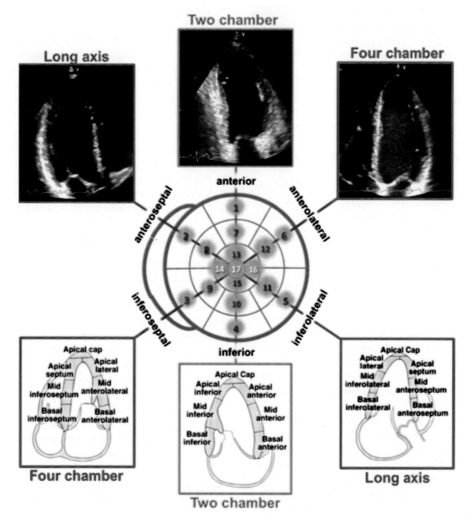

FIGURE 4.5 A4C, A2C, and ALX views in relation to the bull's-eye display of the left ventricular segments (center). Top panels show echocardiographic images and bottom panels depict the left ventricular wall segments visualized in each view. A4C, apical four chamber; A2C, apical two chamber; ALX, apical long axis. (Courtesy of Lang et al.[3])

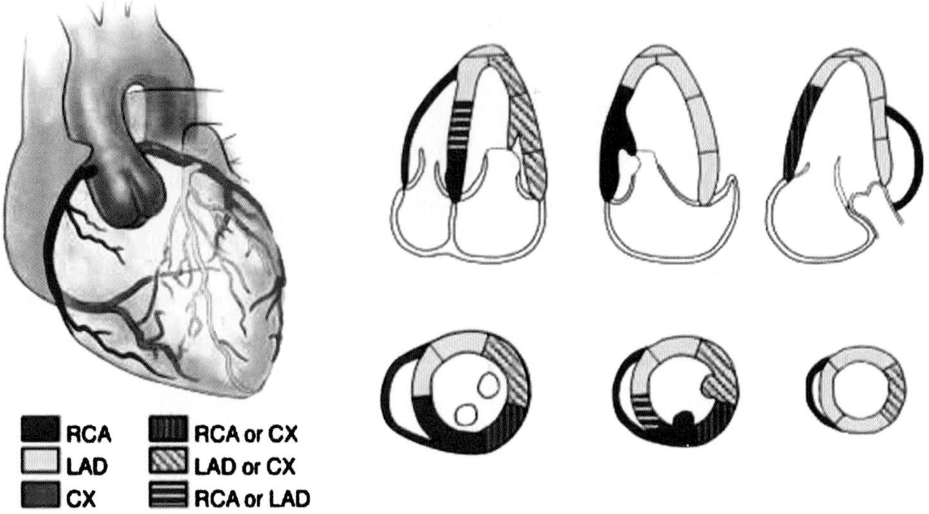

FIGURE 4.6 Distributions of the RCA, LAD, and CX. CX, circumflex coronary artery; LAD, left anterior descending artery; RCA, right coronary artery. (Courtesy of Lang et al.[3])

TABLE 4.2	Methods to Induce Stress
EXERCISE	**PHARMACOLOGIC**
Treadmill	Dobutamine
Supine bicycle	Dipyridamole
Isometric exercise	Adenosine

dobutamine, dipyridamole, or adenosine is an alternative method to provoke ischemia.

Table 4.2 outlines the methods to induce stress. The basic principle of stress echocardiography is the identification of new wall motion abnormalities that occur in the presence of provocable ischemia. This involves the comparison of baseline echocardiographic images obtained under resting conditions with those obtained immediately postexercise in the case of treadmill or during peak exercise in the case of bicycle protocol. Parasternal long and short axes as well as apical two-chamber, three-chamber, and four-chamber views are acquired at baseline and Post-stress testing. The left ventricle is divided into 17 segments as per the recommendation of the American Society of Echocardiography. All images are digitized in a continuous-loop format utilizing a quad-screen format to facilitate the detection of new segmental wall motion abnormalities. The best Post-exercise image is selected and compared with the baseline image by side-by-side comparison in the quad-screen image format.

In the United States, the most commonly used method for provoking ischemia in patients able to exercise is treadmill testing. The sensitivity of exercise testing is strongly dependent upon attaining adequate heart rate and cardiovascular workload. The use of treadmill or bicycle methods of exercise requires the patient to achieve a target heart rate of 85% of the age-predicted maximum heart rate or attain a workload of at least six metabolic equivalents in order to achieve satisfactory sensitivity. In patients who can achieve these workloads, exercise testing is the method of choice to provoke myocardial ischemia.

The most common treadmill protocol used is the Bruce protocol, although other protocols such as the modified Bruce can be used depending upon the level of fitness of the patient. According to standard stress testing protocol, the patient has continuous ECG monitoring with exercise and blood pressure is checked every 3 minutes. With treadmill exercise, the Post-exercise images are obtained ideally within less than 1 minute.

The exercise test should be terminated if any of the following occurs:

1. Severe symptoms such as chest pain or dyspnea
2. Severe ST depressions
3. Hemodynamically significant arrhythmia
4. Severe hypertensive response (BP > 220/120 mm Hg)
5. Hypotension (a decrease of >20 mm Hg)

PHARMACOLOGIC STRESS ECHOCARDIOGRAM

For those patients who cannot exercise, dobutamine or dipyridamole stress echocardiograms can alternatively be performed. By far, dobutamine is the most common pharmacologic agent used to provoke ischemia in stress echocardiograms. Dobutamine is a synthetic catecholamine that binds to β-1 and β-2 receptors. The affinity of dobutamine for β-1 cardiac muscle receptors results in positive inotropic and chronotropic effects. Therefore, dobutamine induces myocardial ischemia in patients with flow-limiting coronary stenosis by increasing LV contractility, heart rate, wall stress, and therefore myocardial oxygen demand. Dobutamine has a short half-life and is rapidly metabolized once the infusion is discontinued. Any adverse side effects or arrhythmias can usually be quickly terminated by discontinuation of the drip or by intravenous β-blockers.[16]

PATHWAY FOR MANAGEMENT OF PATIENTS BASED ON STRESS ECHOCARDIOGRAPHY RESULTS

Risk stratification of patients undergoing stress echocardiography should be based both on peak WMSI (which includes both extent and severity of ischemia/infarction) and on LVEF (resting).

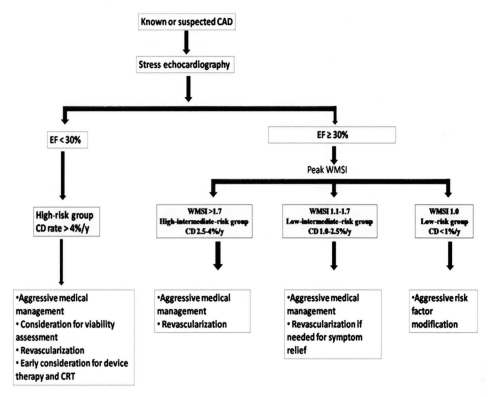

FIGURE 4.7 Schematic for risk stratification of patients undergoing stress echocardiography. CAD, coronary artery disease; CD, cardiac death; CRT, cardiac resynchronization therapy; EF, ejection fraction; WMSI, Wall Motion Score Index.

Figure 4.7 represents a schematic for the risk stratification of patients with known or suspected coronary artery disease referred for stress echocardiography. These data for risk stratification are based on an analysis of 3259 patients (59 ± 13 years; 48% males) followed for up to 4 years.[17]

The first step in the risk stratification process is evaluation of LVEF. Patients with EF <30% are a high-risk group with a cardiac death (CD) rate of >4%/y regardless of the peak WMSI. Such patients should be aggressively managed. These patients may also benefit from viability assessment and consideration for revascularization as deemed necessary. They should also be considered for early device therapy (implantable cardioverter defibrillator/cardiac resynchronization therapy) and for cardiac transplant evaluation.

In patients with EF ≥ 30%, peak WMSI can further risk stratify the patient subgroup into a low-risk group (peak WMSI = 1.0) (CD <1%/y), low-intermediate (peak WMSI 1.1–1.7) (CD 1%–2.5%/y), and a high-intermediate (peak WMSI > 1.7) (CD 2.5%–4.0%/y) risk groups. Patients in the low-risk category will benefit from aggressive risk factor modification. Those in the low-intermediate risk group may benefit from aggressive medical management and consideration of revascularization for symptom relief only. Patients in the high-intermediate risk group may benefit from aggressive medical management and revascularization therapy. Such a risk stratification approach would potentially avoid unnecessary revascularization procedures for low-risk individuals and at the same time provide a framework for the management of intermediate and high-risk subgroups.

REFERENCES

1. Panjrath GS, Herzog E, Chaudhry F. Echocardiography in ACS from prevention to diagnosis and treatment. In: Herzog E, Chaudhry F, eds. *Introduction: Acute Coronary Syndrome and Echocardiography.* New York, NY: Springer-Verlag; 2009:1-4.

2. Saric M. Echocardiography in ACS from prevention to diagnosis and treatment. In: Herzog E, Chaudhry F, eds. *Echo Assessment of Systolic and Diastolic Function in Acute Coronary Syndrome.* New York, NY: Springer-Verlag; 2009:37-57.

3. Lang RM, Badano LP, Mor-Avi V, et al. Recommendations for cardiac chamber quantification by echocardiography in adults: an update from the American Society of Echocardiography and the European Association of Cardiovascular Imaging. *J Am Soc Echocardiogr.* 2015;28:1-39.

4. Multicenter Postinfarction Research Group. Risk stratification and survival after myocardial infarction. *N Engl J Med.* 1983;309(6): 331-336.

5. Carlson MD, Krishen A. Risk assessment for ventricular arrhythmias after extensive myocardial infarction: what should I do? *ACC Curr J Rev.* 2003;12(2):90-93.

6. Curtis JP, Sokol SI, Wang Y, et al. The association of left ventricular ejection fraction, mortality, and cause of death in stable outpatients with heart failure. *J Am Coll Cardiol.* 2003;42(4):736-742.

7. Lang RM, Bierig M, Devereux RB, et al. Recommendations for chamber quantification: a report from the American Society of Echocardiography's Guidelines and Standards Committee and the Chamber Quantification Writing Group, developed in conjunction with the European Association of Echocardiography, a

branch of the European Society of Cardiology. *J Am Soc Echocardiogr.* 2005;18(12):1440-1463.

8. Otterstad JE. Measuring left ventricular volume and ejection fraction with the biplane Simpson's method. *Heart.* 2002;88(6):559-560.

9. Ansari A, Puthumana J. Echocardiography in ACS from prevention to diagnosis and treatment. In: Herzog E, Chaudhry F, eds. *The "Ischemic Cascade".* New York, NY: Springer-Verlag; 2009:149-160.

10. Feigenbaum H, Armstrong WF, Ryan T. *Feigenbaum's Echocardiography.* Philadelphia, PA: Lippincott Williams & Wilkins; 2005.

11. Hauser AM, Vellappillil G, Ramos RG, et al. Sequence of mechanical, electrocardiographic and clinical effects of repeated coronary artery occlusion in human beings: echocardiographic observations during coronary angioplasty. *J Am Coll Cardiol.* 1985;5:193-197.

12. Nesto RW, Kowalchuk MD. The ischemic cascade: temporal sequence of hemodynamic, electrocardiographic and symptomatic expressions of ischemia. *Am J Cardiol.* 1987;57:23C-30C.

13. Harbinson M, Anagnostopoulos CD. Principles of pathophysiology related to noninvasive cardiac imaging. In: Anagnostopoulos C, Nihoyannopoulos P, Bax J, van der Wall E, eds. *Noninvasive Imaging of Myocardial Ischemia.* London, England: Springer; 2006.

14. Lewis WR. Echocardiography in the evaluation of patients in chest pain units. *Cardiol Clin.* 2005;23:531-539.

15. Kim B, Chaudhry FA. Echocardiography in ACS from prevention to diagnosis and treatment. In: Herzog E, Chaudhry F, eds. *How to Perform Stress Echocardiography.* New York, NY: Springer-Verlag; 2009:161-166.

16. Valentini V, Greenfield S, McDermott E, McNeal M, Danao N, Chaudhry FA. Principles and techniques of pharmacologic stress echocardiography. *Video J Echocardiog.* 1993;3:82-89.

17. Bangalore S, Chaudhry FA. Echocardiography in ACS from prevention to diagnosis and treatment. In: Herzog E, Chaudhry F, eds. *Pathway for the Management of Patients Based on Stress Echo Results.* New York, NY: Springer-Verlag; 2009:193-200.

Patient and Family Information for: ECHOCARDIOGRAPHY IN ACUTE CORONARY SYNDROME

INTRODUCTION

The echocardiogram is an ultrasound device that visualizes the heart and surrounding structures in a real-time fashion, which in turn provides important anatomic and physiologic information to the cardiologist. The echocardiogram, like a radar, emits and receives ultrasound waves and constructs an image by employing the differences in the signal properties. At the end of this sophisticated and fast process, an impressive and informative animation of the heart moving in the chest is displayed for further interpretation. In the cardiac care unit (CCU), echocardiography has become an essential tool for real-time bedside diagnosis of heart disease, especially in critical situations. Furthermore, echocardiography lacks any major side effects and is mostly noninvasive.

THE DEVICE STRUCTURE

The echocardiogram itself is made of two major components: the first is the transducer, which is the "radar dish" that relays the ultrasounds waves and is in touch with the patient's body, and the second is a computer console that functions as the "brain" performing the computation. The transducer is filled with multiple crystals (called piezoelectric crystals) that have the natural property of sending and receiving ultrasound waves. Different transducers have different properties. Lower frequency transducers can emit ultrasound waves deeper into the body, but lack the picture quality of the higher frequency ones. When placing the transducer over the chest (this common procedure is referred to as a transthoracic echocardiogram or TTE), a real-time moving image of the heart appears. By rotating and manipulating the transducer over the chest, different areas of the heart are seen; those are referred to as windows. Gel is used to improve the contact between the transducer and the skin, which helps with improving image quality. In TTE, four major areas over the chest are used to create heart images. These include the left chest area between the third and fourth ribs (parasternal), the tip of the heart (apical), under the ribs (subcostal), and above the chest (suprasternal). Several views of the heart are created in each location by rotating the transducer.

THE ECHOCARDIOGRAM ROLE IN THE CCU

In the CCU, echocardiography studies are performed to answer complex clinical questions. Of particular concern in the CCU are the function and integrity of the heart muscle walls (myocardium), the valves, and the heart sac (pericardium). The echocardiogram can provide information such as which chamber of the heart is involved in the disease, the heart's squeezing efficiency, the amount of fluid in the heart's sac, and the presence of clots in the heart chambers.

In the case where there is fluid in the heart sac that compresses the heart (a condition called pericardial tamponade), the echocardiogram can detect this acute life-threatening situation promptly and guide an immediate draining procedure.

"HEART ATTACKS" AND ECHOCARDIOGRAPHY

The majority of disease treated in the CCU is of coronary origin. The coronary arteries are the vessels that feed blood to the heart muscle itself. "Heart attack" or acute myocardial infarction is the condition where a coronary vessel is blocked and thereby prevents oxygenated blood from being delivered to the heart muscle. This in turn causes the heart muscle to start dying, and losing its ability to contract and pump blood. In contrast to a complete blockage, a partial blockage of the coronary artery may result in symptoms such as chest pressure on exertion (referred to as angina), but no impairment in the heart's squeezing function. Interestingly, the patient's symptoms are the last to develop in the cascade of coronary artery blockage. After complete cessation of blood supply to the heart muscle, a sequence of event occurs that is referred to as the ischemic cascade, where the heart muscle wall motion is affected before any ECG changes and before the patient develops symptoms. Therefore, the echocardiogram potentially can detect, in a noninvasive way, heart wall motion contraction impairments in situations where the ECG is nondiagnostic and the patient's symptoms are unclear. During a complete coronary occlusion, the echocardiogram is able to show which wall of heart is not contracting and is thus affected directly by the occlusion. The degree of muscle contraction impairment has a scoring system that provides information about the extent of occlusion and function of the muscle. The walls of the heart are divided into 17 segments. Normal wall motion gets a score of 1; *hypokinesis* is the term used to describe decreased contractility and receives a score of 2; *akinesis* is when no wall motion is seen, with a score of 3; and *dyskinesis* is when the wall motion direction is occurring in the opposite direction, with a score of 4. The sum of the scores of each segment is then divided by 17. A normal score would be 1 (17 divided by the 17 segments) and a score above 1.7 represents significant wall motion abnormality.

There are three major coronary arteries in the heart, and each of them provides blood supply to a certain muscle wall of the heart (with some overlap). The echocardiogram is able to pinpoint the culprit vessel that is occluded. The occluded coronary artery is represented in the echocardiographic study by a specific area of impaired contraction. The assessment of the heart muscle contraction is also assessed as a whole, that is, the heart's overall pumping efficiency. This is referred to as EF. The EF denotes the percentage of blood squeezed from the left ventricle of the heart in one heartbeat to the rest of the body (normal value is 60%). It is known from numerous studies that the lower the EF is, the worse the outcome of the patient.

For example, a patient with an acute myocardial infarction is admitted to the CCU with a LAD occlusion. The LAD supplies blood to the front side of the left heart chamber (main pumping chamber). During the performance of the echocardiogram study, the cardiologist notices that the front portion of the left heart chamber is not squeezing optimally (ie, there is hypokinesis), with an EF of 30%, and there is also some valve leak. Occlusion of an artery can influence the function of a heart valve because the valve's movement relies on muscles attached to the heart wall. The patient is sent thereafter for a cardiac catheterization where the occluded coronary artery is opened. An echocardiogram performed 2 days after the procedure shows some recovery in the wall motion of the front wall with resolution of the valve leakage, as blood supply was restored to the region. The echocardiogram provided up-to-date functional information of various structures of the heart such as the muscle wall and the valves. In contrast, a patient whose echocardiogram shows global LV hypokinesis without any regional wall abnormalities likely had a remote myocardial infarction that initially affected the region of the heart distributed by the occluded coronary artery but progressed to a dilated left ventricle, or had small vessel disease that reduced global perfusion.

MANAGEMENT AFTER THE ACUTE EPISODE

The echocardiogram has a role for diagnosing new or recurrent symptoms during the admission of a patient in the CCU after the primary diagnosis was made. For example, if a patient has recurrent chest pain or shortness of breath, or if the patient's blood pressure is coming down without a reason, the echocardiogram can provide answers. New heart wall motion abnormalities could point to new or recurrent coronary vessel occlusions. A new murmur that is first detected on physical exam with a stethoscope could be the result of a new valve problem (eg leakage), or even a rupture between the heart chambers. These conditions require prompt interventions, and at times may require surgery. The echocardiogram can help in diagnosing dehydration (the main pumping chamber of the heart becomes smaller), fluid overload (due to heart failure or administration of too much fluids), or fluid in the heart sac that compresses the heart (eg pericardial effusion, tamponade).

STRESS TESTING

Some patients who are admitted with chest pain with a high suspicion of a coronary artery disease without an overt heart attack require more testing to confirm the diagnosis. This could be accomplished by performing an echocardiogram while the patient's heart is being "stressed," that is, walking on a treadmill or giving the patient a medication that will make the heart beat faster. Actual stressing or exercising is not performed when the patient is suspected of an evolving heart attack (ACS). Images of the patient's heart muscle contraction are obtained before, during, and after the stress—the muscle could be inspected for wall motion abnormalities that denote probable coronary disease.

TRANSESOPHAGEAL ECHOCARDIOGRAPHY

Some echocardiographic information could be better acquired by using the device in a semi-invasive method called transesophageal echocardiogram—echocardiogram obtained through the esophagus (food pipe). Because there is a short distance between the transducer and the heart while the transducer is positioned in the esophagus, the quality of pictures is better. It is especially useful when imaging cardiac structures that are located at the back part of the heart (eg the left atrium).

LIMITATIONS

There are some limitations in performing an echocardiogram at the bedside as compared with the echocardiography laboratory settings. Usually, the patient is asked to lie on his left side to obtain some of the windows and then to lie on his back for the rest of the images. In the CCU, the patient could be mechanically ventilated, sedated, and might not be able to cooperate. Thus, some of the pictures may be much harder to obtain in order to produce high-quality images.

CONCLUSION

Echocardiography in the CCU provides important anatomic, structural, and clinical information that aids the cardiologist in the diagnosis and treatment of acute heart diseases. It helps to establish a diagnosis in a real-time fashion. It shows the heart muscle function, and this information helps to designate which coronary artery is occluded during heart attacks. It also shows the integrity and function of the heart valves, the amount of fluid in the heart's sac, and the body's fluid balance. Echocardiography aids in managing severely sick patients in the CCU by performing sequential studies. Echocardiography has changed the way cardiologists treat patients in the CCU by having the ability to get live, real-time images of the heart apparatus at the bedside.

Edgar Argulian
Ernest G. DePuey
Seth Uretsky

5

Use of Radionuclide Imaging in Acute Coronary Syndrome

INTRODUCTION

Chest pain is a common complaint and is often the presenting symptom in patients with acute coronary syndrome (ACS). The evaluation of chest pain as a presenting symptom for ACS is complicated by: (1) the numerous etiologies that can cause chest pain, (2) the lack of an "ideal" diagnostic test available at the time of initial evaluation, (3) poor clinical outcomes of patients in whom a diagnosis of ACS is missed, and (4) the medicolegal implications. Because patients with ACS are at a high risk for poor outcomes, the ability to identify these patients rapidly during the initial evaluation is critical. The initial diagnostic workup in patients presenting with symptoms suspicious of ACS include a history, physical examination, electrocardiogram (ECG), and serum cardiac biomarkers (such as cardiac troponins). The ECG is the key diagnostic test used to determine whether the patient has ongoing myocardial ischemia. Unfortunately, the ECG is often nondiagnostic in many patients who present with symptoms suspicious for ACS. Although serum troponin has been shown to be a sensitive test for myocardial damage, there are certain drawbacks to the test, for example, the need for ischemia of sufficient time for myocardial necrosis to take place, and thus the initial serum troponin is often negative in patients with ACS. Patients with unstable angina often do not have significant troponin elevation. Although the newer generation assays ("high-sensitivity troponin") may affect the accuracy and timing of ACS diagnosis significantly, one should bear in mind that troponin elevation (especially mild degrees) is not exclusive to ACS but may happen in other conditions, primarily nonischemic cardiovascular diseases, for example, pulmonary embolism, acute heart failure, and severe sepsis. Based on the pathophysiology of coronary artery plaque rupture as the cause of ACS, one of the earliest signs of ACS is the decrease in blood flow to the myocardium (**Figure 5.1**). This decrease in myocardial blood flow can be evaluated using single photon emission computed tomography (SPECT) myocardial perfusion imaging (MPI), which images the relative amount of myocardial blood flow to all segments of the left ventricle. The use of SPECT MPI in the patient presenting with chest pain has developed over the last several decades to allow for rapid triage in chest pain patients with a view to initiating the necessary medical therapy and revascularization. However, we would also like to identify those patients whose chest pain is not caused by ACS so they are not unnecessarily admitted to the hospital, thus better utilizing health care resources. Stress SPECT MPI can be used for risk stratification in low-risk patients admitted for suspected ACS. It can also identify areas of ischemia in patients with ACS who were not fully revascularized. Finally, radionuclide imaging can assist in assessment of myocardial viability. In this chapter, we will explore the technical, physiologic, and current outcome data of using SPECT MPI in patients with acute chest pain.

OVERVIEW OF SPECT MYOCARDIAL PERFUSION IMAGING

MPI was introduced into clinical practice in the 1970s as a tool to noninvasively assess for myocardial ischemia. In the 1980s, planar imaging gave way to the more robust SPECT imaging most commonly used today. The theory behind SPECT MPI relies on the fact that blood flows preferentially down the path of least resistance, that is, the vessel without coronary occlusion versus the vessel with coronary occlusion (**Figure 5.2**). When comparing myocardial regions with each other, a decrease in tracer uptake in a region is a sign of myocardial hypoperfusion. SPECT MPI utilizes radiotracers whose activity can be detected with a special camera called a scintillation camera. The most commonly used radiopharmaceuticals are Thallium-201 (Tl-201), Technetium-99m (Tc-99m) sestamibi, and Tc-99m tetrofosmin. Radiopharmaceuticals contain atoms that undergo radioactive decay by emitting a particle that can be detected using a SPECT camera. Once injected intravenously, the radiotracer is taken up by the myocardium proportionally to regional coronary blood flow, and the relative "amount" of tracer in each region of the myocardium can be measured and imaged.

SPECT CAMERA

The SPECT camera is designed to detect the radioactivity emitted from a patient after injection of a radiotracer. After injection of the radiotracer, patients are placed in the camera and the images are acquired.

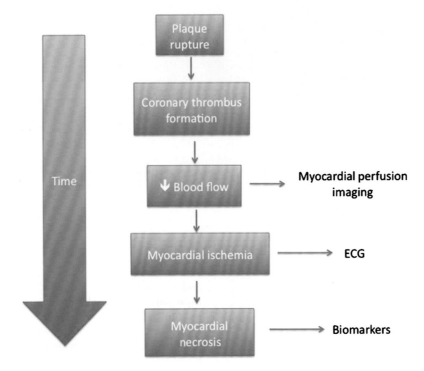

FIGURE 5.1 The ischemic cascade. ECG, electrocardiogram.

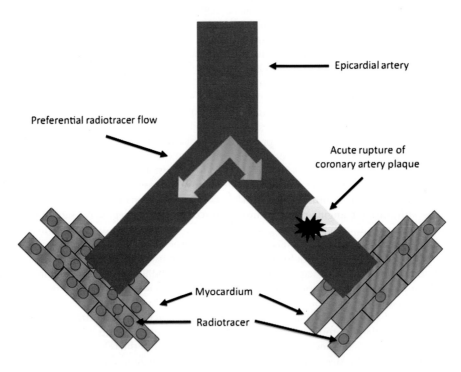

FIGURE 5.2 Differential myocardial radiotracer uptake in myocardium subtended by a normal coronary and a coronary with a ruptured atherosclerotic plaque.

RADIOTRACERS

Radiotracers are tagged molecules that emit radioactivity. The ideal radiotracer has several features:

1. Linear relationship between myocardial uptake and blood flow.
2. High myocardial extraction rate.
3. Low extracardiac uptake.

The most commonly used radiotracers in nuclear cardiology are Tl-201 and Tc-99m. Tc-99m has several advantages over Tl-201, including a shorter half-life, higher energy photons, no redistribution, and availability on site from a Mo-99 generator or in unit doses from a local commercial radiopharmacy. The process whereby Tl-201 decays is called electron capture or isomeric transition (Tl-201 + e$^-$ → Hg-201 + Υ), whereas Tc-99m decays by a process called gamma decay (Tc-99m → Tc-99 + Υ).

RESTING MYOCARDIAL PERFUSION IMAGING

MPI imaging is based on the concept that the injected radiotracer is taken up by the myocardium in proportion to the amount of blood flow that the myocardial region receives. If the blood flow to an area of myocardium is reduced at rest because of coronary occlusion, this area of the myocardium will receive less radiotracer relative to those areas in which blood flow is not reduced (**Figure 5.2**). The resulting SPECT images will have a decrease in tracer activity in the myocardial segments subtended by the diseased coronary artery. In patients with chest pain caused by ACS, there is rupture of coronary plaque, resulting in the formation of intracoronary thrombus and a subsequent decrease in myocardial blood flow to the myocardium supplied by that artery. On the other hand, in patients without coronary occlusion, there will be no decrease in blood flow to the myocardium, and no decrease in tracer activity will be seen.

STRESS MYOCARDIAL PERFUSION IMAGING

In patients with coronary artery disease but with preserved resting blood flow to the myocardium, MPI may appear normal at rest. Stress testing can be used to diagnose physiologically significant coronary artery stenosis in these patients. Stress testing can be performed using exercise or pharmacologic agents. In nuclear cardiology, pharmacologic stress testing is typically performed using a vasodilator agent (such as adenosine, dipyridamole, and regadenoson). During exercise, there is disproportional increase in coronary blood flow to the nondiseased coronary arteries compared with the stenosed coronary arteries. Similarly, during vasodilator pharmacologic stress, coronary vasodilation and increase in blood flow are attenuated in areas supplied by stenosed coronary arteries. As a result, stress testing creates inhomogeneity in myocardial perfusion with decreased regional radiotracer uptake in patients with hemodynamically significant coronary artery disease that can be detected and quantified by MPI.

INTERPRETATION OF SPECT MYOCARDIAL PERFUSION IMAGING

By convention, SPECT images are displayed in three orientations: short axis, vertical long axis, and horizontal long axis (**Figure 5.3**). The left ventricle can be divided into the anterior wall, lateral wall, inferior wall, and septum. While interpreting stress SPECT MPI, images are displayed with the poststress images on the

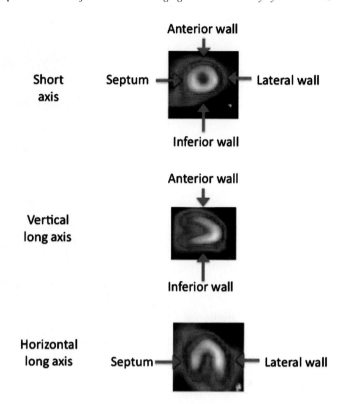

FIGURE 5.3 Short-axis, vertical long-axis, and horizontal long-axis slices with labeled myocardial regions.

top line and the rest images below (**Figure 5.4**). The short axis images are displayed apex to base, followed by the vertical long axis and the horizontal long axis. As previously discussed, SPECT MPI measures relative blood flow to the various segments of the myocardium. When interpreting stress SPECT MPI, one compares the amount of tracer uptake on the stress images with the amount of tracer uptake in the rest images for each myocardial segment. Broadly speaking, if the tracer uptake is homogeneous in both the rest and stress images, there is no decrease in blood flow to the myocardium, that is, no ischemia or scar (**Figure 5.4**). However, if there is a decrease in perfusion on the stress images in a region of normal tracer uptake on the resting images, that is termed a "reversible" defect and may be indicative of ischemia (**Figure 5.5**). If there is a matched in tracer uptake in both the stress and rest images, that is termed a "fixed" defect and may be indicative of myocardial scar (**Figure 5.6**).

VIABILITY ASSESSMENT

In patients with established coronary artery disease and ischemic cardiomyopathy, resting wall motion abnormalities may be present, signifying areas of noncontractile myocardium. However, noncontractile myocardium is not synonymous with scarred and nonviable myocardium. In patients with acute ischemic event, the myocardium can still be viable but stunned (ie regionally decreased contractile function) and may recover contractility over time. In patients with a high-degree coronary stenosis and limited resting blood flow, the myocardium can be in a state of hibernation and can maintain viability. With the restoration of blood flow, the hibernating myocardium can return to its contractile state and improve systolic heart function. SPECT imaging can discern viable myocardial tissue from myocardial

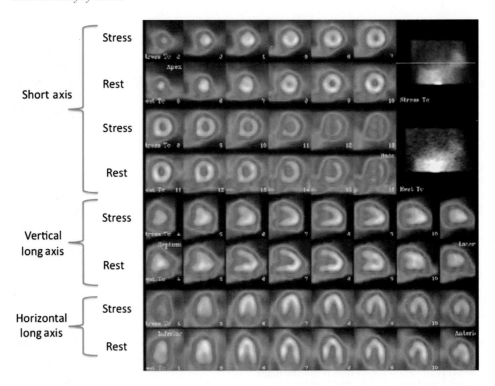

FIGURE 5.4 Normal single photon emission computed tomography myocardial perfusion imaging with homogeneous tracer uptake.

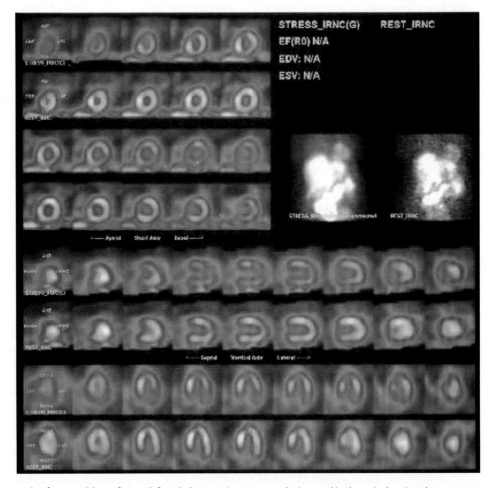

FIGURE 5.5 An example of a reversible perfusion defect. A decrease in tracer uptake is noted in the apical region that reverses on the resting images. This is a reversible perfusion defect and is indicative of ischemia in the distribution of the left anterior descending artery.

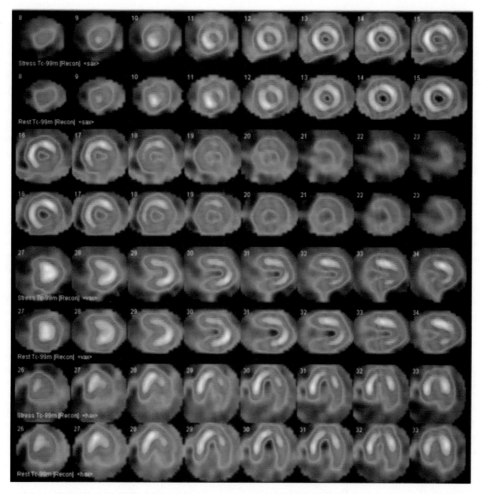

FIGURE 5.6 An example of a fixed perfusion defect. There is a decrease in tracer uptake noted in the lateral and inferior walls at the midventricle and at the base of the stress images. This finding is also noted in the rest images and is termed a fixed defect indicative of myocardial scar.

scar by taking advantage of the redistributive properties of Tl-201. When Tl-201 is injected, it is initially distributed and taken up by the myocardium with good blood flow. Myocardial segments with limited blood flow that are viable and those myocardial segments that are scarred do not take up Tl-201 initially. Over several hours, Tl-201 will redistribute and be taken up by the myocardium that is alive but has limited blood flow, that is, the viable myocardium. Initial defects on imaging study may show reversibility upon redistribution imaging, and the extent of viable myocardium can be assessed.

ROLE OF SPECT MYOCARDIAL PERFUSION IMAGING IN PATIENTS WITH SUSPECTED ACUTE CORONARY SYNDROME

RESTING SPECT MYOCARDIAL PERFUSION IMAGING

The ideal test in patients with suspected ACS enables the clinician to diagnose it early in the course of the disease as well as stratify those patients who are at low risk and can be safely discharged compared with those who are at high risk and need further workup. As previously stated, the combination of history, physical examination, ECG, and serum troponin may be indeterminate

at the time of initial evaluation, and the clinician cannot confidently determine whether the patients are experiencing an ACS. Resting SPECT MPI protocols have been developed and well studied in patients with suspected ACS having active ongoing chest pain. Multiple studies have shown that resting SPECT MPI can identify patients undergoing ACS and also those who can be safely discharged. Heller et al. studied 357 patients who presented with chest pain suspicious for myocardial ischemia and a non-diagnostic EKG. Patients underwent rest SPECT MPI with Tc-99m.[1] Among the 20 patients with myocardial infarction, 18 (90%) had abnormal SPECT images, whereas 2 had normal SPECT images, for a negative predictive value of 99%. In this study, SPECT MPI gave incremental diagnostic value over clinical and ECG variables alone, and an abnormal SPECT was the strongest predictor of myocardial infarction. The Emergency Room Assessment of Sestamibi for Evaluation of Chest Pain (ERASE) trial was a prospective multicenter randomized trial of 2475 patients who presented with chest pain and a normal or nondiagnostic ECG.[2] The patients were randomized to usual care or usual care plus rest SPECT MPI. The authors report that there was no difference in the rate of hospitalization between the study arms among the patients with myocardial infarction. However, among those without ACS, fewer patients were hospitalized in the rest SPECT strategy than in standard care (42% vs 52%).

TRIAGING LOW-RISK PATIENTS HAVING CHEST PAIN WITH SUSPECTED ACUTE CORONARY SYNDROME

Low-risk patients with chest pain evaluated in the acute settings often have nondiagnostic initial ECG and negative cardiac biomarkers. Stress SPECT MPI can be used safely in this patient group for diagnosis and risk stratification. Multiple studies have addressed the role of different imaging modalities in assessing low-risk patients with chest pain in the emergency department and those admitted to the hospital. Most of the studies compared coronary computed tomography (CT) angiography with different stress testing modalities (such as traditional stress SPECT MPI, stress-only SPECT MPI, and stress echocardiography).[3–6] The studies showed largely comparable outcomes among patients assigned to different modalities, and the decision to proceed with a particular test should be determined by patient-specific and institution-specific characteristics. SPECT MPI tests the functionality of the heart (whether occluded coronary arteries cause ischemia of wall segments). In contrast, CTA shows the anatomy of the coronary arteries (whether there is any stenosis) but provides no information about the physiologic significance of the stenosis. Thus, both modalities can be used in complementary ways.[7]

ROLE OF SPECT IN MANAGING PATIENTS POST–MYOCARDIAL INFARCTION

Stress SPECT MPI can also be used in hemodynamically stable patients within 3 months of myocardial infarction to assess for the presence and degree of ischemia and for risk stratification purposes. It can also be used to evaluate for stent thrombosis or restenosis in patients who become symptomatic after revascularization. In general, stress testing is not used in asymptomatic patients if they were fully revascularized, but it can be considered in asymptomatic patients with no or partial revascularization to evaluate for the usefulness of additional revascularization.[8] Myocardial perfusion SPECT using adenosine or dipyridamole infusion can be safely performed 48 hours post–myocardial infarction once the patient is hemodynamically stable.

ROLE OF RADIONUCLIDE IMAGING IN ASSESSING MYOCARDIAL VIABILITY

Thallium-201 SPECT can be used in patients with ischemic cardiomyopathy to assess viability, with the goal of revascularizing viable myocardium. Often, patients admitted to the hospital with heart failure symptoms are found to have new reductions in left ventricular ejection fraction (LVEF) without a known ischemic insult. These patients may have had silent myocardial infarction or may not have presented to the hospital when they had an acute myocardial infarction. Sometimes, patients with newly diagnosed reductions in LVEF may have nonischemic cardiomyopathy caused by long-standing hypertension or myocarditis, in which case revascularization would not be useful. SPECT MPI is useful in differentiating between ischemic and nonischemic cardiomyopathy. Other tests that are used to distinguish viable myocardium from irreversible injury include positron emission tomography, dobutamine echocardiography, and cardiac magnetic resonance.[9] Accumulating evidence is inconclusive about the role of routine viability assessment in patients with ischemic cardiomyopathy, but it can be useful in certain clinical scenarios.[10]

CONCLUSION

Although the cardiac imaging modalities have been rapidly evolving over the past decade, SPECT MPI has been shown to be a useful tool in diagnosing and risk stratifying patients with suspected ACS. It can also be occasionally used in patients post–myocardial infarction and for viability assessment in patients with ischemic cardiomyopathy.

REFERENCES

1. Heller GV, Stowers SA, Hendel RC, et al. Clinical value of acute rest technetium-99m tetrofosmin tomographic myocardial perfusion imaging in patients with acute chest pain and nondiagnostic electrocardiograms. *J Am Coll Cardiol.* 1998;31(5):1011-1017.

2. Udelson JE, Beshansky JR, Ballin DS, et al. Myocardial perfusion imaging for evaluation and triage of patients with suspected acute cardiac ischemia: a randomized controlled trial. *JAMA.* 2002;288(21):2693-2700.

3. Goldstein JA, Chinnaiyan KM, Abidov A, et al. The CT-STAT (Coronary Computed Tomographic Angiography for Systematic Triage of Acute Chest Pain Patients to Treatment) trial. *J Am Coll Cardiol.* 2011;58(14):1414-1422.

4. Hoffmann U, Truong QA, Schoenfeld DA, et al. Coronary CT angiography versus standard evaluation in acute chest pain. *N Engl J Med.* 2012;367(4):299-308.

5. Nabi F, Kassi M, Muhyieddeen K, et al. Optimizing evaluation of patients with low-to-intermediate-risk acute chest pain: a randomized study comparing stress myocardial perfusion tomography incorporating stress-only imaging versus cardiac CT. *J Nucl Med.* 2016;57(3):378-384.

6. Uretsky S, Argulian E, Supariwala A, et al. Comparative effectiveness of coronary CT angiography vs stress cardiac imaging in patients following hospital admission for chest pain work-up: the Prospective First Evaluation in Chest Pain (PERFECT) trial [published online ahead of print on April 5, 2016]. *J Nucl Cardiol.* doi:10.1007/s12350-015-0354-6.

7. Kim HL, Kim YJ, Lee SP, et al. Incremental prognostic value of sequential imaging of single-photon emission computed tomography and coronary computed tomography angiography in patients with suspected coronary artery disease. *Eur Heart J Cardiovasc Imaging.* 2014;15(8):878-885.

8. Hendel RC, Berman DS, Di Carli MF, et al. ACCF/ASNC/ACR/AHA/ASE/SCCT/SCMR/SNM 2009 Appropriate use criteria for cardiac radionuclide imaging: a report of the American College of Cardiology Foundation Appropriate Use Criteria Task Force, the American Society of Nuclear Cardiology, the American College of Radiology, the American Heart Association, the American Society of Echocardiography, the Society of Cardiovascular Computed Tomography, the Society for Cardiovascular Magnetic Resonance, and the Society of Nuclear Medicine Endorsed by the American College of Emergency Physicians. *J Am Coll Cardiol.* 2009;53(23):2201-2229. doi:10.1016/j.jacc.2009.02.013.

9. Anavekar NS, Chareonthaitawee P, Narula J, Gersh BJ. Revascularization in patients with severe left ventricular dysfunction: is the assessment of viability still viable? *J Am Coll Cardiol.* 2016;67(24):2874-2887.

10. Bonow RO, Maurer G, Lee KL, et al. Myocardial viability and survival in ischemic left ventricular dysfunction. *N Engl J Med.* 2011;364(17):1617-1625.

Patient and Family Information for: USE OF RADIONUCLIDE IMAGING IN ACUTE CORONARY SYNDROME

Radionuclide imaging, often called nuclear imaging, has been used since the 1970s to image the heart. Radionuclide imaging uses radiopharmaceuticals that are given via intravenous injection. One component of a radiopharmaceutical is a tracer, a substance that is taken up from the blood by the heart muscle. The amount of the tracer extracted from the blood by the heart muscle is proportional to the amount of the blood flow to the heart muscle. The radiopharmaceutical is a radioactive substance that emits photons that can be captured by a special camera. The information from the camera allows physicians to take pictures of the heart muscle. Essentially, those pictures represent "the map" of blood flow to the heart muscle and identify the areas where the blood flow is compromised because of a blockage in the blood vessels supplying the heart.

Although nuclear imaging employs radioactive substances, the dosage given to an individual patient is relatively small. Mostly, it is in the range of radioactivity comparable to other imaging procedures such as a CT scan and is considered safe. The injection is given by a technician or a doctor. The patient is then imaged by the camera that detects the photons emitted by the radiotracer. This part of the test is crucial: the technician explains to the patient the position they need to maintain and the necessity of staying still while the pictures are obtained. The patient needs to follow the instructions carefully so that high-quality images can be obtained.

Heart attacks are caused by a decrease in the blood flow that nourishes the heart muscle. If blood flow to a part of the heart muscle is blocked, the patient will have a heart attack and the heart muscle can die. In patients who experience chest pain, it is often difficult to determine if the pain is a sign of heart disease. The initial tests for patients with chest pain include an ECG and blood tests. If these tests are inconclusive, the physician may opt to perform radionuclide imaging. Radionuclide imaging maps the blood flow to the heart and is useful in identifying a blood vessel blockage that may signify a heart attack. In patients who have experienced a heart attack, radionuclide imaging enables physicians to determine who will benefit from procedures that restore blood flow to the heart muscle.

The idea behind the stress test is to compare resting images of the heart to those obtained after the stress test. The stress portion can be performed with either exercise or medication. During an exercise stress test, the patient is asked to exercise on a treadmill or a stationary bicycle. If the patient cannot exercise or the physician thinks it is unsafe for the patient to exercise, a medication can be used. The physician or a trained health care professional is always present in the room for the stress test. In general, stress testing is safe and well tolerated, although some patients may experience brief side effects (headache, nausea, chest discomfort) from the medication. Serious events, including heart attacks and heart rhythm disturbances, are rare.

During radionuclide stress testing, two sets of heart images—the rest images and the stress images—are usually obtained as previously described. By comparing the two sets of images, the physician can determine whether there is an impairment of blood flow to the heart. If significant blood flow impairment is identified by the stress test, the patient may be referred for an invasive procedure called cardiac catheterization.

Ronen Rubinshtein
Harvey Hecht

6

Computed Tomographic Angiography in Acute Cardiac Care

INTRODUCTION

Contrast-enhanced multidetector computed tomography (MDCT), which provides high-quality noninvasive images of the heart, great vessels, and coronary vasculature, has been shown to be useful and reliable in the triage of patients with chest pain of possible ischemic origin and specifically in the diagnosis of acute coronary syndrome. Current generation computed tomography (CT) scanners (64-slice and higher) require minimal patient cooperation (short breath hold) and have improved image quality (better spatial and temporal resolution) and high diagnostic accuracy. MDCT can visualize coronary plaques and is also gaining a role in the evaluation of coronary stents and bypass grafts and for evaluation of patients undergoing structural or electrophysiologic cardiac interventions.

TECHNICAL CONSIDERATION

New generation CT scanners allow rapid scanning of the heart by a high gantry rotation speed and wider coverage of the field of view than initial scanners, thus allowing a "freeze" in cardiac motion and overcoming many previously observed breathing artifacts. Some scanners allow a single beat acquisition and very rapid reconstruction of scanned data to be presented to the reader.

However, despite these advancements, it is still recommended to lower the patient heart rate to <65 beats/min to optimize image quality. In the absence of contraindications, it is also recommended to administer sublingual nitroglycerin just prior to scanning to allow coronary vasodilation and improved image quality.

The scan itself is performed using electrocardiogram (ECG) gating to image and reconstruct the heart and the coronary vessels during a certain phase in the cardiac cycle, usually diastole.

About 50 to 100 mL of intravenous contrast media (iodine-based) is typically used to allow opacification of the coronary vessels.

After scanning, the data can be viewed and manipulated on a PC-based or dedicated workstation that utilizes sophisticated software to optimize analysis and overcome artifacts.

CLINICAL USEFULNESS OF CARDIAC CT

NONCONTRAST CALCIUM SCORING

Quantitative assessment of the extent of coronary arterial calcification by electron beam CT had been available for several years before the advent of MDCT. When categorized according to a defined scoring system (eg, the Agatston calcium score), calcification can predict subsequent coronary events in various cohorts. However, calcium scoring is usually performed for screening asymptomatic subjects, especially those with intermediate risk for future cardiovascular adverse events. Those are the patients in whom calcium scoring may identify or rule out definite coronary atherosclerosis (coronary calcifications) and may impact the physician's decision in regard to primary preventive therapies.

CONTRAST-ENHANCED CARDIAC CT APPLICATIONS

Coronary CT angiography (CCTA) is used to diagnose coronary atherosclerosis and coronary narrowing. CCTA is considered the noninvasive test with the highest sensitivity to diagnose coronary stenosis when compared to invasive coronary angiography as the reference standard. This test has a very high negative predictive value (>98%), making it a useful tool to rule out coronary stenosis. On the other hand, because of motion artifacts and coronary calcifications, the positive predictive value is somewhat lower but still very good (85% to 92%).

One of the areas where CCTA has been shown to be especially useful is in the emergency department setting. Patients with acute chest pain but without high-risk features (such as elevated troponin, ECG changes indicative of ischemia, or recurrent/ongoing chest pain) are good candidates for CCTA. A normal or near-normal scan has been shown to be safe and effective in shortening hospital stay (**Figure 6.1**). Infrequently, a "triple rule out" protocol may be used to exclude pulmonary emboli or thoracic aortic dissection in addition to coronary stenosis.

In contrast to conventional invasive coronary angiography, which allows visualization of the coronary lumen but provides only minimal details of the coronary plaque, CCTA can demonstrate the details of coronary plaques (noncalcified/calcified/mixed), and several features that may be demonstrated by CCTA have been suggested to be associated with higher risk of adverse coronary events. Those include low attenuation plaque (<30

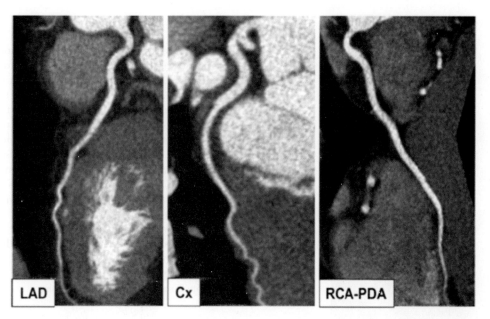

FIGURE 6.1 Normal coronary arteries by coronary computed tomography angiography in a patient with acute chest pain. Cx, circumflex coronary artery; LAD, left anterior descending artery; PDA, posterior descending artery; RCA, right coronary artery.

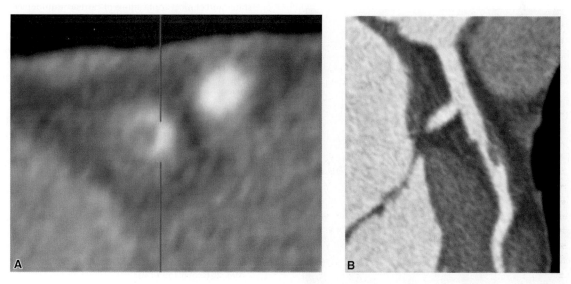

FIGURE 6.2 Cross-section view (A) and long axis (multiplanar reformation) (B) of the left anterior descending coronary artery showing a possible ruptured plaque (napkin ring sign) and stenosis.

Hounsfield units), spotty calcifications (within a non-calcified plaque), and "napkin ring" sign (**Figure 6.2**). Other features shown to be of clinical relevance are plaque eccentricity and positive remodeling.

The presence of nonobstructive coronary atherosclerosis as well as obstructive disease on CCTA has been shown to be of prognostic value. The higher the burden of disease, the higher the likelihood of future cardiovascular events (and vice versa).

Recently, it has been shown that CCTA can also be used to evaluate the physiologic significance of a coronary stenosis (computed tomographic fractional flow reserve) using complex models of computational flow dynamics.

Of note, this may also be shown by using CT for assessment of myocardial perfusion (rest or stress induced), where myocardial hypoenhancement limited to a vessel territory may be indicative of ischemia or infarction.

CCTA is also very useful in the characterization of coronary anomalies or myocardial bridging.

Beyond evaluation of the native coronary vessels, CCTA can evaluate the patency of coronary stents, especially stents ≥3 mm wide, albeit with reduced diagnostic accuracy related to metallic artifacts (**Figure 6.3**). Diagnosis is also possible in patients with coronary bypass grafts (**Figure 6.4**), but again with somewhat reduced accuracy because of the presence of metallic clips in the

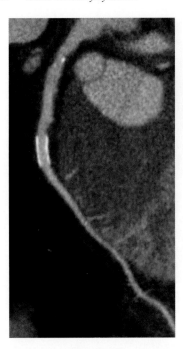

FIGURE 6.3 Patent stent in the left anterior descending coronary artery demonstrated by coronary computed tomography angiography.

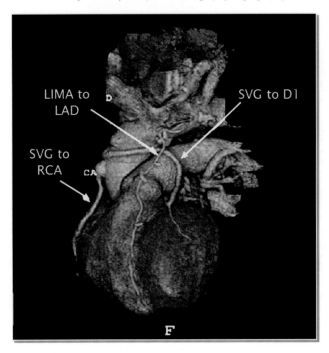

FIGURE 6.4 Volume-rendered image of the heart in a patient with a history of coronary bypass grafting. D1, first diagonal batch; LAD, left anterior descending artery; RCA, right coronary artery; SVG, saphenous vein graft; LIMA, left internal mammary artery.

distal anastomosis and the diffuse nature of calcified coronary atherosclerosis in those patients.

An increasing indication is the evaluation of cardiac structures before interventional cardiac procedures, most importantly for evaluation of the aortic valve and root before transarterial aortic valve replacement or evaluation of the pulmonary veins draining into the left atrium before pulmonary vein isolation (ablation) in patients with atrial fibrillation.

SUMMARY

Cardiac CT is a powerful diagnostic tool, mostly used for the diagnosis of obstructive coronary atherosclerosis in symptomatic patients. Technical advancement in recent years has led to a significant reduction in radiation exposure to patients without compromising image quality. Several future trends in the development of cardiac CT systems may also increase its usefulness for clinical use. Those include the development of dual energy or spectral CT systems that may improve tissue diagnosis and the rapid development in the field of fusion imaging allowing visualization (even in real time) of images derived from two different modalities (eg, two-dimensional angiography and CT or echocardiography and CT).

The exponential increase in the number of structural heart interventions and the increased usefulness that may be derived from combining anatomic and physiologic assessment of the coronary tree are expected to accelerate the use of this imaging modality for cardiovascular diagnosis.

SUGGESTED READINGS

1. Halon DA, Rubinshtein R, Gaspar T, Peled N, Lewis BS. Current status and clinical applications of cardiac multidetector computed tomography. *Cardiology.* 2008;109:73-84.

2. Abbara S, Blanke P, Maroules CD, et al. SCCT guidelines for the performance and acquisition of coronary computed tomographic angiography: a report of the society of Cardiovascular Computed Tomography Guidelines Committee: endorsed by the North American Society for Cardiovascular Imaging (NASCI). *J Cardiovasc Comput Tomogr.* 2016;10:435-449.

3. Hecht HS, Cronin P, Blaha MJ, et al. 2016 SCCT/STR guidelines for coronary artery calcium scoring of noncontrast noncardiac chest CT scans: a report of the Society of Cardiovascular Computed Tomography and Society of Thoracic Radiology. *J Cardiovasc Comput Tomogr.* 2017;11:74–82.

4. Rubinshtein R, Halon DA, Gaspar T, et al. Impact of 64-slice cardiac computed tomographic angiography on clinical decision-making in emergency department patients with chest pain of possible myocardial ischemic origin. *Am J Cardiol.* 2007;100:1522-1526.

5. Litt HI, Gatsonis C, Snyder B, et al. CT angiography for safe discharge of patients with possible acute coronary syndromes. *N Engl J Med.* 2012;366:1393-1403.

6. Taylor AJ, Cerqueira M, Hodgson JM, et al; American College of Cardiology Foundation Appropriate Use Criteria Task Force, Society of Cardiovascular Computed Tomography, American College of Radiology, American Heart Association, American Society of Echocardiography, American Society of Nuclear Cardiology, North American Society for Cardiovascular Imaging, Society for Cardiovascular Angiography and Interventions, Society for Cardiovascular Magnetic Resonance. ACCF/SCCT/ACR/AHA/ASE/ASNC/NASCI/SCAI/SCMR 2010 Appropriate Use Criteria for Cardiac Computed Tomography. A report of the American College of Cardiology Foundation Appropriate Use Criteria Task Force, the Society of Cardiovascular Computed Tomography, the American College of Radiology, the American Heart Association, the American Society of Echocardiography, the American Society of Nuclear Cardiology, the North American Society for Cardiovascular Imaging, the Society for Cardiovascular Angiography and Interventions, and the Society for Cardiovascular Magnetic Resonance. *J Cardiovasc Comput Tomogr.* 2010;4:407.e1-433.e3.

7. Cheruvu C, Precious B, Naoum C, et al. Long term prognostic utility of coronary CT angiography in patients with no modifiable coronary artery disease risk factors: results from the 5 year follow-up of the CONFIRM International Multicenter Registry. *J Cardiovasc Comput Tomogr.* 2016;10:22-27.

8. Motoyama S, Ito H, Sarai M, et al. Plaque characterization by coronary computed tomography angiography and the likelihood of acute coronary events in mid-term follow-up. *J Am Coll Cardiol.* 2015;66:337-346.

9. Min JK, Taylor CA, Achenbach S, et al. Noninvasive fractional flow reserve derived from coronary CT angiography: clinical data and scientific principles. *JACC Cardiovasc Imaging.* 2015;8:1209-1222.

10. Achenbach S, Delgado V, Hausleiter J, et al. SCCT expert consensus document on computed tomography imaging before transcatheter aortic valve implantation (TAVI)/transcatheter aortic valve replacement (TAVR). *J Cardiovasc Comput Tomogr.* 2012;6:366-380.

Patient and Family Information for: COMPUTED TOMOGRAPHIC ANGIOGRAPHY IN ACUTE CARDIAC CARE

Coronary computed tomographic angiography (CTA) is a simple X-ray study involving injection of approximately 6 ounces of contrast containing iodine into an arm vein while the patients hold their breath for 5 seconds. This will be accompanied by a warm sensation throughout the body some patients may find this mildly uncomfortable.

If there is a known allergy to intravenous contrast, premedication with steroids and diphenhydramine will be required. There is no relationship between seafood and contrast allergies. Patients will be able to leave unaccompanied immediately afterward. The X-ray machine is open and does not produce claustrophobia. The CTA provides very detailed pictures of the coronary arteries that are very accurate in determining whether there is narrowing in the arteries. It also produces excellent pictures of the aorta and heart muscle.

Arpit Shah
Angela Palazzo

7

Coronary Angiography and Percutaneous Coronary Intervention

CARDIAC CATHETERIZATION AND ANGIOGRAPHY

Sones and colleagues performed the first coronary arteriography in 1959. Since its advent, cardiac catheterization and coronary angiography have remained the gold standard for diagnosis of coronary artery disease (CAD) as well as structural and valvular heart disease. Although advances in imaging, including cardiac computed tomography and cardiac magnetic resonance imaging, have enhanced the diagnosis of many forms of heart disease, coronary angiography along with advances in percutaneous coronary intervention (PCI) and structural heart disease intervention has revolutionized our ability to manage patients with ischemic, non-ischemic and structural heart disease.

INDICATIONS

The indications for cardiac catheterization and coronary angiography are varied. They include acute coronary syndromes such as ST-elevation myocardial infarction (STEMI) as well as non-ST-elevation myocardial infarction (NSTEMI), unstable coronary syndromes without infarction, heart failure, valvular heart disease, arrhythmia, and sudden cardiac death. In some of these instances, the procedure will be for diagnostic purposes only, but for others, it will be a prelude to intervention.

STABLE ISCHEMIC HEART DISEASE

Coronary angiography is performed in patients with stable ischemic heart disease (SIHD) either as an initial strategy to assess risk or after a workup with noninvasive testing. The 2012 and 2014 multisociety guidelines on diagnosis and management of patients with SIHD have recommended diagnostic angiography based on clinical presentation, symptoms, and findings on noninvasive testing (**Tables 7.1 and 7.2**).[1,2]

REDUCED LEFT VENTRICULAR EJECTION FRACTION

Coronary angiography is considered reasonable when ischemia may be a contributing factor for heart failure to assess the patency of coronary arteries.[3] This may be part of a workup that includes echocardiography, viability studies, and MRI.

SUDDEN CARDIAC DEATH OR VENTRICULAR ARRHYTHMIA

Coronary angiography is an important tool in the assessment of CAD in survivors of cardiac arrest and patients with life-threatening ventricular arrhythmia.[4] If cardiac arrest is associated with ST elevations, coronary angiography should be performed emergently.

PREOPERATIVE CORONARY ANGIOGRAPHY

Routine use of preoperative coronary angiography for noncardiac surgery is not recommended. Indications of coronary angiography are similar to those applied in a nonoperative setting.[5]

For patients who are undergoing cardiac surgery for valvular heart disease, aortic disease, or other structural heart disease, coronary angiography is recommended as part of the preoperative workup for nonemergency indications.

CORONARY ANATOMY

Optimal myocardial function is based on a delicate balance of supply and demand achieved through coronary arterial circulation. Coronary arterial circulation consists of two parts—the conduit vessels formed by large epicardial coronary arteries and resistance vessels formed by medium- and small-sized coronary arterioles. The coronary arterial circulation originates from the aorta as two main branches—the left coronary artery, which consists of the left main coronary artery (LMCA), the left anterior descending and the circumflex artery—and the right coronary artery (RCA). There can be some anatomic variations to this pattern. The left and right coronary arteries arise from the left and right coronary cusps, respectively. Dominance is referred to as right or left, depending on whether the RCA or the left coronary artery supplies the posterior descending artery (PDA). In about 70% of patients, the PDA is a branch of the RCA, and this is referred to as a right dominant circulation. In 20% of individuals, the PDA is codominant or balanced in both the left circumflex artery (LCx) and the RCA, and in 10% of individuals, the PDA arises from the LCx.

In order to correlate angiographic views with coronary anatomy, it is useful to consider the main coronary arteries in two orthogonal planes. The left anterior descending and the

TABLE 7.1	Noninvasive Risk Stratification in Patients With Stable Ischemic Heart Disease[1, 2]

HIGH RISK (>3% ANNUAL DEATH OR MI)

Severe resting LV dysfunction (LVEF<35%) not readily explained by noncoronary causes

Resting perfusion abnormalities ≥10% of the myocardium in patients without prior history or evidence of MI

Stress ECG findings including ≥2 mm of ST-segment depression at low workload or persisting into recovery, exercise-induced ST-segment elevation, or exercise-induced VT/VF

Severe stress-induced LV dysfunction (peak exercise LVEF <45% or drop in LVEF with stress ≥10%)

Stress-induced perfusion abnormalities encumbering ≥10% myocardium or stress segmental scores indicating multiple vascular territories with abnormalities

Inducible wall motion abnormality (involving >2 segments or 2 coronary beds)

Wall motion abnormality developing at low dose of dobutamine (≤10 mg/kg/min) or at a low heart rate<120 beats/min)

CAC score >400 Agatston units

Multivessel obstructive CAD (≥70% stenosis) or left main stenosis ≥50% stenosis) on CCTA

INTERMEDIATE RISK (1-3% ANNUAL DEATH OR MI)

Mild/moderate resting LV dysfunction (LVEF 35% to 49%) not readily explained by noncoronary causes

Resting perfusion abnormalities in 5% to 9.9% of the myocardium in patients without a history or prior evidence of MI

≥1 mm of ST-segment depression occurring with exertional symptoms

Stress-induced perfusion abnormalities encumbering 5% to 9.9% of the myocardium or stress segmental scores (in multiple segments) indicating 1 vascular territory with abnormalities but without LV dilation

Small wall motion abnormality involving 1 to 2 segments and only 1 coronary bed

Coronary Artery Calcium score 100 to 399 Agatston units

One vessel CAD (≥70% stenosis) or moderate CAD stenosis (50% to 69% diameter stenosis) of CCTA in ≥2 arteries on CCTA

LOW RISK (< 1% ANNUAL DEATH OR MI)

Low-risk treadmill score (score ≥5) or no new ST segment changes or exercise-induced chest pain symptoms; when achieving maximal levels of exercise

Normal or small myocardial perfusion defect at rest or with stress encumbering <5% of the myocardium

Normal stress or no change of limited resting wall motion abnormalities during stress

CAC score <100 Agatston units

No coronary stenosis >50% on CCTA

CAC, coronary artery calcium; CAD, coronary artery disease; CCTA, coronary computed tomography angiography; ECG, electrocardiogram; LV, left ventricular; LVEF, left ventricular ejection fraction; MI, myocardial infarction; VF, ventricular fibrillation; VT, ventricular tachycardia.

posterior descending arteries course along the plane of the interventricular septum. The LCx and the RCA run along the plane of the atrioventricular valve perpendicular to the plane of the interventricular septum.

LEFT CORONARY ARTERY

The LMCA is the first portion of the left coronary artery. The LMCA usually bifurcates into the left anterior descending artery (LAD) and the LCx. In some individuals, there may be a trifurcation into a ramus intermedius branch. The LAD artery initially runs along the anterior interventricular groove and terminates at the apex in most individuals. During its course, it gives out septal branches that supply the anterior two-thirds of the interventricular septum, and diagonal branches that supply the anterolateral wall of the left ventricle. The LCx travels along the left atrioventricular groove and gives rise to the obtuse marginal branches. The obtuse marginal branches supply the lateral wall of the left ventricle.

RIGHT CORONARY ARTERY

The RCA runs along the right atrioventricular groove in a mirror fashion to the LCx artery, perpendicular to the long axis of the heart. The first branch arising from the RCA is called the conus artery, which supplies the right ventricular outflow tract. The second branch arising from the RCA is a sinoatrial branch, which supplies the sinus node. It arises out of the RCA in about 60% cases and from the LCx in 40% of individuals. The acute marginal branch arises from the mid-segment of the RCA supplying the right ventricle. The RCA gives off the PDA and at least one posterolateral branch in a right dominant circulation.

POSTERIOR DESCENDING ARTERY

The PDA runs along the posterior interventricular groove parallel to the LAD running in the anterior interventricular groove and meeting the LAD along the apical portion of the interventricular

TABLE 7.2	Indications for Coronary Angiography in Stable Ischemic Heart Disease[1,2]		
INDICATIONS FOR CORONARY ANGIOGRAPHY IN STABLE ISCHEMIC HEART DISEASE			
Class I	*Class IIA*	*Class IIB*	*Class III*
Coronary angiography is useful in patients with presumed SIHD who have unacceptable ischemic symptoms despite GDMT and who are amenable to, and candidates for, coronary revascularization. (Level of Evidence: C)	Coronary angiography is reasonable to further assess risk in patients with SIHD who have depressed LV function (Ejection Fraction <50%) and moderate risk criterion noninvasive testing with demonstrable ischemia. (Level of Evidence: C)	Coronary angiography might be considered in patients with stress test results of acceptable quality that do not suggest the presence of CAD when clinical suspicion of CAD remains high and there is a high likelihood that the findings will result in important changes to therapy. (Level of Evidence: C)	Coronary angiography for risk assessment is not recommended in patients with SIHD who elect not to undergo revascularization or who are not candidates for revascularization because of comorbidities or individual preferences. (Level of Evidence: B)
Patients with SIHD who have survived sudden cardiac death or potentially life-threatening ventricular arrhythmia should undergo coronary angiography to assess cardiac risk. (Level of Evidence: B)	Coronary angiography is reasonable to further assess risk in patients with SIHD and inconclusive prognostic information after noninvasive testing or in patients for whom noninvasive testing is contraindicated or inadequate. (Level of Evidence: C)		Coronary angiography is not recommended to further assess risk in patients with SIHD who have preserved LV function (Ejection Fraction >50%) and low-risk criteria on noninvasive testing. (Level of Evidence: B)
Patients with SIHD who develop symptoms and signs of heart failure should be evaluated to determine whether coronary angiography should be performed for risk assessment. (Level of Evidence: C)	Coronary angiography for risk assessment is reasonable for patients with SIHD who have unsatisfactory quality of life because of angina, have preserved LV function (Ejection Fraction >50%), and have intermediate risk criteria on noninvasive testing. (Level of Evidence: C)		Coronary angiography is not recommended to assess risk in patients who are at low risk according to clinical criteria and who have not undergone noninvasive risk testing. (Level of Evidence: C)
Coronary arteriography is recommended for patients with SIHD whose clinical characteristics and results of noninvasive testing indicate a high likelihood of severe IHD and when the benefits are deemed to exceed risk. (Level of Evidence: C)	Coronary angiography is reasonable to define the extent and severity of CAD in patients with suspected SIHD whose clinical characteristics and results of noninvasive testing (exclusive of stress testing) indicate a high likelihood of severe IHD and who are amenable to, and candidates for, coronary revascularization. (Level of Evidence: C)		Coronary angiography is not recommended to assess risk in asymptomatic patients with no evidence of ischemia on noninvasive testing. (Level of Evidence: C)
	Coronary angiography is reasonable in patients with suspected symptomatic SIHD who cannot undergo diagnostic stress testing or have indeterminate or nondiagnostic stress tests, when there is a high likelihood that the findings will result in important changes to therapy. (Level of Evidence: C)		

CAD, coronary artery disease; GDMT, guideline-directed medical therapy; IHD, ischemic heart disease; LV, left ventricular; SIHD, stable ischemic heart disease.

septum. It supplies the inferoposterior aspects of the left ventricle and gives off septal branches to supply the inferior aspect of the interventricular septum.

POSTEROLATERAL BRANCHES

The posterolateral branches arise as terminal portions of either the RCA after the origin of the PDA or the LCx. They supply the inferior and posterior segments of the left ventricle.

ANGIOGRAPHIC PROJECTIONS

An accurate assessment of coronary arteries requires obtaining multiple angiographic projections to avoid any overlap of vessels. The position of the image intensifier in relation to the patient's body defines the projections. Left anterior oblique (LAO) and right anterior oblique (RAO) describe the position of the image intensifier to the left or right of a patient's chest, respectively. The anteroposterior (AP) views describe the image intensifier directly over the patient. Cranial and caudal projections describe the position of the image intensifier toward the head (cranial) or feet (caudal). The left coronary system requires an AP caudal to assess the LMCA, LAO cranial for the LAD and its branches. The LAO caudal (spider view) is helpful for assessment of the LMCA, proximal LAD, and proximal LCx. The RAO caudal view is useful for the LCx and its obtuse marginal branches, and the RAO cranial view for mid- and distal LAD along with diagonal branches (**Figure 7.1A** and **B**). The RCA should be visualized in LAO cranial, which shows the RCA along with the PDA and

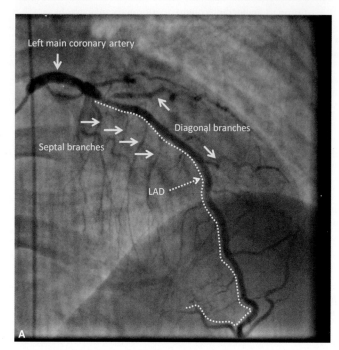 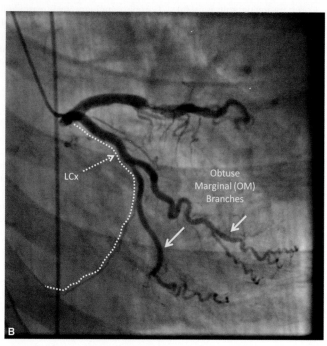

FIGURE 7.1 A, Left anterior descending artery (LAD) and its major branches visualized in a cranially and a slightly rightward angulated view (right anterior oblique [RAO] –9°; cranial +36°). B, Nondominant left circumflex (LCx) artery and its major branches visualized in a caudally and a slightly rightward angulated view (RAO –6°; caudal –21°).

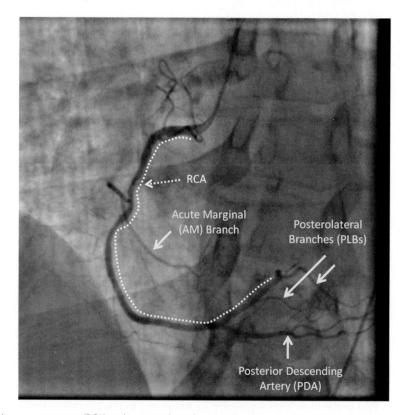

FIGURE 7.2 Dominant right coronary artery (RCA) and its major branches visualized in a slightly cranially angulated left anterior oblique (LAO) view (LAO +28°; cranial +3°).

a RAO projection with cranial angulation for mid-RCA and the entire course of the PDA (**Figure 7.2**). Additional views may be obtained based on the individual patient's coronary anatomy.

PREPROCEDURE PREPARATION

CONSENT

The physician performing the cardiac catheterization should obtain informed consent from the patient. The discussion should include the indication for coronary angiography and PCI if indicated, an overview of the procedure, and risk/benefits of the procedure. The following risks, although not inclusive, should be reviewed with the patient.[6]

Mortality (0.1%)
Myocardial infarction (0.05%)
Cerebrovascular accident (0.07%)
Arrhythmia (0.38%)
Vascular complications and bleeding (0.43%)
Contrast reaction (0.37%)
Hemodynamic complication (0.26%)
Perforation of heart chamber (0.03%)

MEDICATIONS AND ALLERGIES

Complete medication reconciliation along with a review of allergies should be performed before the procedure. Special attention should be given to prior allergies to contrast agents. Mild to moderate reactions can usually be pretreated with diphenhydramine and/or steroids. Careful assessment of risk and benefits along with allergy consultation should be done for more serious reactions. Metformin should be discontinued on the day of the procedure and 48 hours thereafter. Patients on chronic warfarin therapy should have an international normalized ratio < 1.8 for femoral access if anticoagulation can be withheld.[7] Alternatively, radial access can be considered for these patients. The timing of discontinuation for newer oral anticoagulants is guided by the patient's renal function and the particular agent but should be discontinued at least 1 to 2 days prior to the procedure.[7]

PREPROCEDURE WORKUP

A recent laboratory evaluation with baseline renal function, hemoglobin, and coagulation studies (if indicated) should be performed within 30 days in the outpatient setting and within 24 hours in the inpatient setting.[7] Patients with preexisting renal dysfunction or elevated risk scores[8] are at high risk for contrast-induced nephropathy (CIN) and should be considered for adequate hydration with normal saline pre- and periprocedural. The electrocardiogram should be reviewed for all patients because it can help localize the culprit vessel, particularly in the setting of ST-elevation myocardial infarction. Prior angiograms and operative reports for patients with a history of coronary artery bypass grafting (CABG) should also be reviewed if available.

CONSCIOUS SEDATION

A complete assessment of comorbidities and physical examination should be performed before the procedure. Airway assessment

using the Mallampati classification and the American Society of Anesthesiologists Physical Status Classification can help in assessing the patient's eligibility for conscious sedation. Conscious sedation is usually achieved with short-acting agents such as midazolam and fentanyl.

A physical exam should be performed prior to the procedure and include auscultation of the heart for previously undiagnosed murmurs and documentation of neurologic exam, including any pre-existing deficits. A careful assessment of peripheral pulses, including femoral, dorsalis pedis, and posterior tibial, should be recorded in the chart.

ARTERIAL ACCESS

Coronary angiography can be performed using a modified Seldinger technique at three possible sites:

1. Femoral artery
2. Radial artery
3. Brachial artery

FEMORAL ARTERY

The common femoral artery courses medial to the femoral head and bifurcates into the superficial femoral artery and profunda femoris artery distal to the midpoint of the femoral head. The femoral artery should ideally be accessed above the bifurcation and below the inferior epigastric artery. The femoral artery (right or left) is accessed using a modified Seldinger technique with anatomic landmarks and fluoroscopy guidance to locate the midpoint of the femoral head. A 5F or 6F sheath is usually used for diagnostic cardiac catheterization (**Figure 7.3**). There is a risk of retroperitoneal bleeding if the sheath is placed above the inguinal ligament. The risk of a pseudoaneurysm increases if the sheath is placed below the bifurcation of the common femoral artery.

RADIAL ARTERY

Radial artery catheterization has been shown to reduce mortality and major adverse cardiovascular events and reduce major bleeding and vascular complications across the entire spectrum of patients with CAD.[9] Before this procedure, an Allen test is

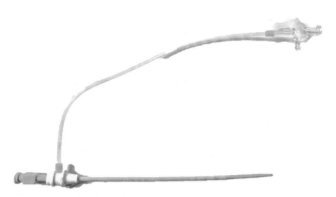

FIGURE 7.3 A 6F arterial sheath is shown here. This serves as the access point for left heart catheterization and coronary angiography.

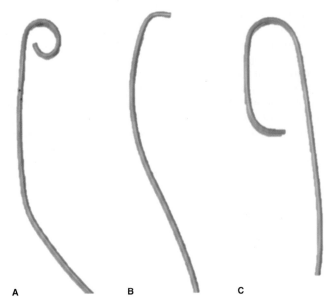

A   **B**   **C**

FIGURE 7.4 Coronary artery catheters used in coronary angiography and left heart catheterization. A, A pigtail catheter is placed across the aortic valve to assess left ventricular function and hemodynamics. B, A Judkins right catheter, shown here, is used to cannulate the right coronary artery. C, A Judkins left catheter, shown here, is used to cannulate the left coronary artery.

performed to assess the patency of ulnar artery flow. The radial artery is accessed using a modified Seldinger technique. Heparin is injected directly into the sheath upon access to prevent thrombosis. Radial artery spasm is prevented by injecting nitroglycerin and Verapamil.

BRACHIAL ARTERY

The brachial artery can also be used for coronary angiography; however, there is a higher risk of compromising the blood supply to the hand in the event of vessel closure.

DIAGNOSTIC CARDIAC CATHETERIZATION

After access has been obtained from any of the sites previously mentioned, coronary angiography and left ventriculography are performed through the sheath. With the help of a J-tipped guidewire, the catheter is advanced through the sheath and into the ascending thoracic aorta under fluoroscopy. The guidewire is removed, and catheters are aspirated followed by a flush with heparinized saline.

CORONARY ANGIOGRAPHY

The LMCA is usually engaged using a Judkins left catheter (**Figure 7.4C**), and the RCA is engaged using a Judkins right catheter through the femoral approach (**Figure 7.4B**). In addition, other catheters are available in cases where Judkins catheters fail to engage the coronary arteries. Similarly, catheters are specially designed to access the coronary arteries from a radial approach. On successful cannulation of coronaries, contrast is injected under fluoroscopy, and various angiographic views are obtained as previously mentioned for each coronary artery.

LEFT VENTRICULOGRAPHY

Left ventriculography is performed with the help of a pigtail catheter in most cases (**Figure 7.4A**). The pigtail catheter is advanced through the aortic valve and positioned in the center of the left ventricle. An RAO projection is obtained as the contrast is injected into the left ventricle. The figure shows left ventriculography performed in an RAO view. This view gives an assessment of the anterolateral wall, inferior wall, and apex. An LAO projection can be performed to visualize the interventricular septum and lateral wall. Left ventriculography can also be used to assess the severity of mitral regurgitation based on the degree of opacification of the left atrium. Left ventriculography should be avoided in patients with underlying chronic kidney disease unless deemed necessary for diagnosis.

SUPRA-AORTIC ANGIOGRAPHY

Positioning the pigtail catheter just above the aortic valve is useful for assessing the ascending aorta as well as evaluating aortic insufficiency.

LEFT HEART HEMODYNAMICS

Intracavitary pressure tracings can be obtained from the pigtail catheter placed in the left ventricle. Left ventricular end-diastolic pressure can be measured from these pressure tracings, which can help in the management of patients presenting with acute coronary syndrome, heart failure, and cardiogenic shock and to guide fluid strategy postprocedure. Aortic stenosis can be assessed from the transvalvular gradient obtained as the pigtail catheter is withdrawn from the left ventricle into the aorta or with simultaneous pressure measurements in the left ventricular (LV) and aorta. Mitral stenosis can be assessed by measurement of gradients between the pulmonary capillary wedge pressure and the LV cavity, and atrial septal defect as well as ventricular septal defect can be evaluated with an oxygen saturation series.

ARTERY BYPASS GRAFTS

It is helpful to know the anatomy of the bypass grafts before cardiac catheterization. Specialized catheters are available to engage the bypass grafts.

POSTPROCEDURE CARE

VASCULAR SITE HEMOSTASIS

After completion of cardiac catheterization, the femoral sheath is removed, and hemostasis is achieved either by manual compression or vascular closure devices. Manual compression can be applied directly at the access site for a minimum of 15 minutes, depending on the size of the sheath. If anticoagulation is given with heparin during the procedure, sheath removal and manual compression can be done if activated clotting time (ACT) is less than 180 seconds. For patients receiving bivalirudin, the sheath can be removed 2 hours after the infusion has stopped. Bed rest of at least 4 hours is advised following manual compression for hemostasis.

A variety of vascular closure devices are available. These achieve hemostasis either with an extravascular plug (Angio-seal/Mynx) or through sutures (Perclose). The Angio-seal vascular closure (St. Jude Medical) device consists of a bioabsorbable intravascular anchor and a collagen extravascular plug to seal the arteriotomy site. Components are absorbed within 60 to 90 days, and the site is available after this time for access. A potential complication is embolization of the intravascular component. Mynx vascular closure (Access closure) uses a bioabsorbable sealant that absorbs blood and expands to seal the arteriotomy site. Perclose (Abbott Laboratories) is a suture-based vascular closure device that functions by percutaneous delivery of sutures. Perclose is also used as a preclosure device when managing a large femoral arteriotomy, as with the use of Impella or Transcatheter Aortic Valve Replacement. Careful assessment of distal pulses is a mandatory part of postprocedure care.

Compared to manual compression, vascular closure devices are noninferior regarding access-site complications but have a higher incidence of infection. They have been shown to have a reduced time to hemostasis and earlier time to mobilization.[10] Careful selection of patients is advised to avoid potential complications.

Radial artery hemostasis is achieved by immediately removing the sheath postprocedure irrespective of anticoagulation status and applying wristband compression devices. Radial artery occlusion is a potential complication. It is important to assess the radial artery flow with pulse oximetry of the corresponding finger by compressing the ulnar artery while using the wristband compression devices. There are no restrictions to ambulation after wristband compression devices, but the patient is advised not to perform strenuous activities using their hand for 2 to 4 hours after the procedure.[7,11]

POSTPROCEDURE MONITORING

Complete bed rest for 2 hours is advised when a vascular closure device has been used in a patient who has not received anticoagulation. Manual compression requires 4 to 6 hours of bed rest. The patient should be recovered in an area with careful monitoring of vital signs and distal pulses to identify early signs of bleeding or vessel closure. Postprocedure labs are recommended in patients undergoing PCI and those with preexisting renal dysfunction. Patients undergoing PCI may be considered for monitoring in a telemetry setting if they are at increased risk for postprocedural adverse cardiac event or CIN or require continuous use of intravenous medications.

COMPLICATIONS

The risk of major adverse cardiac and cerebrovascular events for diagnostic cardiac catheterization occurs in <0.1% of procedures. Vascular site complications include bleeding, retroperitoneal hemorrhage, hematoma, pseudoaneurysm, arteriovenous (AV) fistula formation, dissection, and embolization and are less than 0.5%. Patients with a small pseudoaneurysm (less than 2 cm) can be observed for spontaneous closure. Large pseudoaneurysms (more than 3 cm) require ultrasound-guided compression or, more frequently, ultrasound-guided thrombin injection. Retroperitoneal hemorrhage should be suspected in patients with back or flank pain along with hemodynamic instability. Diagnosis can be confirmed with CT scan without contrast. Management includes close monitoring of vitals and complete blood count in a coronary care unit setting, fluid resuscitation, and transfusion as indicated.

Anticoagulation reversal may be indicated and vascular surgery consultation is advised. AV fistula is a relatively rare complication. Small AV fistulas can be followed serially with ultrasound. Large fistulas associated with swelling, deep vein thrombosis, or high-output failure may require ultrasound-guided compression or surgical closure.

The risk for CIN increases with preexisting renal insufficiency, DM, and with patients with elevated risk scores.[8] The ideal strategy for preventing CIN includes adequate hydration and minimizing the contrast load.[7]

Coronary artery spasm, dissection, and air embolism are infrequent complications. Cardiac perforation is a rare complication after right heart catheterization. Other complications include cardiac arrhythmia, particularly ventricular fibrillation after injecting the RCA, vagal response, heart failure, and rarely infection. Allergic reaction to contrast dye can range from mild to severe anaphylaxis. Patients at high risk should be premedicated as outlined earlier.

PERCUTANEOUS CORONARY INTERVENTION

Andreas Gruentzig ushered in a new era in the management of CAD when he performed the first percutaneous transluminal coronary angioplasty (PTCA) in 1977. PCI has now grown into a complex field of diagnosis and management of CAD. With a marked improvement in safety and efficacy, it is one of the remarkable achievements of modern cardiovascular medicine.

INDICATIONS FOR PERCUTANEOUS CORONARY INTERVENTION

The American College of Cardiology/American Heart Association task force has published guidelines on indications for PCI.[12] In addition, a multisociety committee has developed the appropriate use criteria for nonemergent PCI based on the severity of angina, findings on the noninvasive study, medical therapy, and extent of CAD.[13]

ST-ELEVATION MYOCARDIAL INFARCTION

Coronary angiography and PCI is a Class I indication in STEMI as primary therapy in patients with ischemic symptoms of less than 12 hours' duration or in patients in cardiogenic shock or acute severe heart failure regardless of time to presentation. Delayed PCI of the infarct-related artery in patients who were initially managed either with fibrinolytic or no reperfusion therapy should be performed in the setting of cardiogenic shock, high-risk findings on noninvasive testing, or spontaneous or easily provoked myocardial ischemia. It is not recommended to perform delayed PCI of a totally occluded artery more than 24 hours after STEMI presentation in stable patients (**Tables 7.3** and **7.4**).[14]

NON–ST-ELEVATION ACUTE CORONARY SYNDROME

The management of non-ST-elevation acute coronary syndromes (NSTE-ACS) revolves around two pathways, either an invasive strategy or an ischemia-guided strategy. The invasive strategy is designed to perform coronary angiography initially, with intent to revascularize. In the ischemia-guided strategy, angiography is

TABLE 7.3	Indications for Primary PCI in STEMI[14]

PRIMARY PCI IN STEMI

Class I	Class IIA	Class IIB	Class III
Primary PCI should be performed in patients with STEMI and ischemic symptoms of less than 12 h duration. (Level of Evidence: A)	Primary PCI is reasonable in patients with STEMI if there is clinical and/or ECG evidence of ongoing ischemia between 12 and 24 h after symptom onset. (Level of Evidence: B)	PCI of a noninfarct artery may be considered in selected patients with STEMI and multivessel disease who are hemodynamically stable, either at the time of primary PCI or as a planned staged procedure	
Primary PCI should be performed in patients with STEMI and ischemic symptoms of less than 12 h duration who have contraindications to fibrinolytic therapy, irrespective of the time delay from FMC. (Level of Evidence: B)			
Primary PCI should be performed in patients with STEMI and cardiogenic shock or acute severe HF, irrespective of time delay from MI onset. (Level of Evidence: B)			

ECG, electrocardiogram; FMC, first medical contact; HF, heart failure; MI, myocardial infarction; PCI, percutaneous coronary intervention; STEMI, ST-elevation myocardial infarction.

TABLE 7.4	Coronary Angiography in Patients Who Received Firbrinolytic Therapy or No Reperfusion Therapy

CORONARY ANGIOGRAPHY IN PATIENTS WHO RECEIVED FIBRINOLYTIC THERAPY OR NO REPERFUSION THERAPY

Class I	Class IIA	Class IIB	Class III
Cardiac catheterization and coronary angiography with intent to perform revascularization should be performed after STEMI in patients with any of the following: • Cardiogenic shock or acute severe HF that develops after initial presentation. (Level of Evidence: B) • Intermediate- or high-risk findings on predischarge noninvasive ischemia testing. (Level of Evidence: B) • Myocardial ischemia that is spontaneous or provoked by minimal exertion during hospitalization. (Level of Evidence: C)	Coronary angiography with intent to perform revascularization is reasonable for patients with evidence of failed reperfusion or reocclusion after fibrinolytic therapy. Angiography can be performed as soon as logistically feasible. (Level of Evidence: B)		
	Coronary angiography is reasonable before hospital discharge in stable patients with STEMI after successful fibrinolytic therapy. Angiography can be performed as soon as logistically feasible, and ideally within 24 h, but should not be performed within the first 2–3 h after administration of fibrinolytic therapy. (Level of Evidence: B)		

HF, heart failure; STEMI, ST-elevation myocardial infarction.

performed in patients who do not respond to medical therapy, have high-risk findings on noninvasive testing, or have a high non-ST-elevation acute coronary syndromes or Thrombolysis in Myocardial Infarction (TIMI) score (**Table 7.5**).[15]

CHRONIC STABLE ANGINA

Revascularization in patients with chronic stable angina is recommended on the basis of either improved survival or improved symptoms and is outlined in a document termed the Appropriate Use Criteria. This is a detailed compilation of scenarios based on symptoms, extent of ischemia, and current medications. A full discussion is included in the reference.[13,16]

For patients with complex coronary anatomy, left main disease, or severe LV dysfunction, a "heart team" approach is recommended with input from both cardiac surgery and interventional cardiology with regard to risks and benefits of each approach.

The success of PCI revolves around the following:

- Guiding catheters and guidewires
- Balloon dilatation and coronary stents
- Anticoagulation during PCI
- Lesion modification devices
- Embolic protection devices
- Diagnostic ancillary devices
- Mechanical supportive devices

TABLE 7.5	Management of Patients With NSTE-ACS[15]		
NON--ST-ELEVATION ACUTE CORONARY SYNDROMES			
Class I	*Class IIA*	*Class IIB*	*Class III*
An urgent/immediate invasive strategy (diagnostic angiography with intent to perform revascularization if appropriate based on coronary anatomy) is indicated in patients (men and women) with NSTE-ACS who have refractory angina or hemodynamic or electrical instability (without serious comorbidities or contraindications to such procedures). (Level of Evidence: A)	It is reasonable to choose an early invasive strategy (within 24 h of admission) over a delayed invasive strategy (within 25–72 h) for initially stabilized high-risk patients with NSTE-ACS. For those not at high/intermediate risk, a delayed invasive approach is reasonable. (Level of Evidence: B)	In initially stabilized patients, an ischemia-guided strategy may be considered for patients with NSTE-ACS (without serious comorbidities or contraindications to this approach) who have an elevated risk for clinical events. (Level of Evidence: B)	An early invasive strategy (ie, diagnostic angiography with intent to perform revascularization) is not recommended in patients with: a. Extensive comorbidities (eg, hepatic, renal, pulmonary failure, cancer), in whom the risks of revascularization and comorbid conditions are likely to outweigh the benefits of revascularization. (Level of Evidence: C) b. Acute chest pain and a low likelihood of ACS who are troponin-negative (Level of Evidence: C), especially women (Level of Evidence: B)
An early invasive strategy (diagnostic angiography with intent to perform revascularization if appropriate based on coronary anatomy) is indicated in initially stabilized patients with NSTE-ACS (without serious comorbidities or contraindications to such procedures) who have an elevated risk for clinical events. (Level of Evidence: B)		The decision to implement an ischemia-guided strategy in initially stabilized patients (without serious comorbidities or contraindications to this approach) may be reasonable after considering clinician and patient preference. (Level of Evidence: C)	

GUIDE CATHETERS AND GUIDEWIRES

Appropriate choice of the guide catheter is a key first step in the treatment of a lesion. An ideal catheter should be of sufficient design to deliver equipment, provide adequate support to advance the equipment, and provide monitoring of aortic pressure. Similar to diagnostic angiography, luminal diameter size of guide catheters for PCI is denoted by French size (6F approximately 2 mm). In most cases, a 6F guide catheter will be adequate for percutaneous intervention. However, a large French size guide catheter (7F or 8F) is required for performing complex PCI. Despite the extra support provided by guide catheters, a flexible tip is available to reduce damage to the coronary ostium. Guide catheters also help in monitoring the aortic pressure and alert the operator in case of dampening or ventricularization of the waveform. Dampening of the pressure wave (drop in systolic pressure) is seen when a guide is larger than the coronary ostium or when the guide is deep-seated and pressing against the wall or plaque. In addition to appropriate choice of the guide catheter, additional maneuvers such as a long arterial sheath, guideliner delivery system, or buddy wire techniques may be used to achieve optimal support.

GUIDEWIRES

The next step after the choice of the optimal guide catheter is an appropriate selection of coronary guidewire. An optimal guidewire will cross the lesion without trauma and provide a rail for device delivery. A coronary guidewire consists of an inner core, outer covering, and tip. The choice of guidewire depends on the lesion complexity and type of device delivery. In most cases, "workhorse" wires will suffice for the noncomplex lesion. Complex lesions such as chronic total occlusions may require more advanced techniques and different wires. Soft tip and hydrophilic wires can help navigate tortuous lesions but are more liable to cause dissection and perforation.

BALLOON DILATATION

After the guidewire is advanced distally across the lesion, the next step is to select balloon dilatation catheters. There are two types of balloon dilatation catheter: monorail and over-the-wire. Monorail or rapid-exchange system is designed for a single operator to advance the system while maintaining the distal wire. The over-the-wire system allows delivery to tortuous, calcified vessels and better support for certain devices. Inflation of the balloon is done with a device called an indeflator that measures and controls the amount of pressure. The purpose of predilatation prior to stent implantation includes evaluation of the characteristics and length of the stenosis, determination of the diameter of the stent to be used, and aid in the delivery of the stent. Successful predilatation of the stenosis occurs when both the pressure and the duration of inflation inside the balloon causes the stenotic lesion to yield completely in its entire length. With increasing balloon diameters and higher pressures, inflation can result in an increased risk of vessel injury. On the contrary, lower inflation pressures may not cause sufficient yielding of the stenosis, complicating adequate stent placement.

Compliance of the balloon must be considered while planning PTCA. Compliant balloons can increase in size by >20% when pressure is increased beyond nominal pressure, whereas noncompliant balloons change very little at higher pressures. Noncompliant balloons are better suited for the calcified or fibrotic lesions or for postdilatation of stents. There are many ways to approach balloon inflation, including size, inflation time, and pressures, but the overall concept is to eliminate the "waist" or area of stenosis.

CORONARY STENTS

Before the advent of stents, plain old balloon angioplasty (POBA) was met with the risk of abrupt vessel closure, requiring CABG, in the short term and the risk of restenosis in the long term because of intense smooth muscle proliferation at the site of POBA. These problems were addressed with the introduction of bare metal stents (BMS) and improved upon in the current era of drug-eluting stents (DES). In its basic design, a DES consists of a mesh of metal that is polymer coated with an antiproliferative drug. Despite the reduction in the incidence of abrupt vessel closure with coronary stents, two issues have plagued the use of coronary stents—stent thrombosis and in-stent restenosis (ISR).

Stent thrombosis can be acute (<24 hours), subacute (<30 days), late (30 days to 1 year), and very late (>1 year). Stent thrombosis results from a lack of endothelialization of the stent, resulting in contact between stent struts and platelets. Endothelialization is usually completed within 4 weeks in BMS. This is markedly delayed in DES because of the release of the antiproliferative drug. In addition to the type of stent, several other factors, including lack of stent apposition or malposition/dissection, can increase the risk of stent thrombosis. The use of dual antiplatelet therapy (DAPT) has reduced the incidence of stent thrombosis, but very late thrombosis has been seen rarely after termination of DAPT beyond the 1-year mark. The duration of DAPT has been a matter of intense debate. The recent 2016 AHA/ACC focus update on the duration of DAPT recommends that patients with SIHD who are treated with DES should be treated for at least 6 months and for at least 1 month following BMS (Class I). Treatment beyond the recommended duration may be considered for those patients who can tolerate DAPT without significant bleeding risk (Class IIb). In patients with ACS treated with either BMS or DES, DAPT should be continued for at least 1 year, and continuation beyond that may be reasonable for patients without any bleeding complication or elevated risk for bleeding (Class IIb).[17]

ISR is caused by neointimal hyperplasia. Neointimal hyperplasia refers to smooth muscle proliferation leading to stenosis at the site of stent implantation. The incidence of ISR has significantly decreased with the use of DES. Risks for ISR include stent underexpansion, diabetes, small vessel size, and long lesions. Besides neointimal hyperplasia, de novo neoatherosclerosis caused by chronic inflammation has been proposed as a potential mechanism for late ISR and thrombosis.[18]

ANTICOAGULATION DURING PERCUTANEOUS CORONARY INTERVENTION

Anticoagulation is required during PCI to prevent thrombus formation on the guide catheters, coronary wire, or at the site of any arterial injury.[12] There are several different anticoagulation alternatives for PCI.

UNFRACTIONATED HEPARIN

Unfractionated heparin (UFH) is one of the most commonly used anticoagulants because of ease of use, rapid action availability of the reversal agent, and cost. The degree of anticoagulation with UFH is measured by the ACT using either Hemochron or Hemotec devices. The dosing of heparin is weight-based. UFH should be titrated to achieve an ACT of 200 to 250 seconds if glycoprotein IIb/IIIa receptor inhibitors (GPI) is administered; if no GPI is given, ACT should be targeted toward 250 to 350 seconds (Class I; Level of Evidence C).[12]

BIVALIRUDIN

Bivalirudin is a direct thrombin inhibitor that is used across the entire spectrum of patients undergoing PCI, including STEMI, where it has been shown to reduce cardiac mortality and major bleeding (Class I; Level of Evidence B).[14,19,20] However, recent trials have failed to show a mortality benefit or superiority over heparin.[21,22] Bivalirudin should be the agent of choice for patients with heparin-induced thrombocytopenia. Bivalirudin is given as a bolus of 0.75 mg/kg followed by infusion of 1.75 mg/kg/h for the duration of the procedure. If the patient receives a load of Prasugrel or Brilinta at the time of PCI or is on maintenance therapy with either drug, then bivalirudin can be stopped immediately after PCI. In patients receiving a plavix load at the time of PCI or within 2 hours of PCI, bivalirudin should be continued for at least 2 hours post-PCI until the antiplatelet effect has been achieved.

ENOXAPARIN

Enoxaparin, or low-molecular-weight heparin, can be used in patients with NSTE-ACS undergoing PCI. Enoxaparin may be considered for patients who have not received prior antithrombin therapy or who have received subcutaneous enoxaparin "upstream" for management of NSTE-ACS (Class IIb; Level of Evidence B).[12] An additional dose of enoxaparin is recommended if the patient has received less than 2 doses or if the last dose was received more than 2 hours before PCI (Class I; Level of Evidence B).[12]

FONDAPARINUX

Fondaparinux is an indirect thrombin inhibitor. It is not recommended for use because of an increased risk of catheter thrombosis.[12]

DIAGNOSTIC ANCILLARY DEVICES

Although considered "the gold standard," coronary angiography comes with some limitations. Coronary angiography merely outlines the vessel lumen and provides no information on the anatomic configuration of the vessel wall or functional significance of the lesion. These problems are addressed by recent advances in intravascular ultrasound (IVUS), optical coherence tomography (OCT), and fractional flow reserve (FFR).

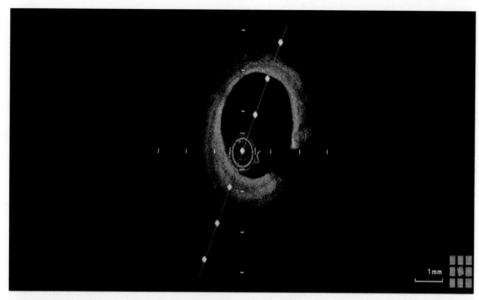

FIGURE 7.5 A cross-sectional optical coherence tomography image of coronary artery.

INTRAVASCULAR ULTRASOUND

IVUS creates a cross-sectional tomographic image of the vessel wall. A standard IVUS image provides a minimal luminal area (MLA, plaque burden, and some characterization of lesion morphology and contents). Criteria for MLA with IVUS have been correlated with FFR. An MLA < 6.0 mm^2 is suggestive of significant hemodynamic lesion in left main, whereas an MLA of <4.00 mm^2 is used as cutoff for non–LMCA. In addition to assessment of lesion severity, IVUS has substantial clinical utility in coronary stenting. IVUS-guided coronary stenting can be useful in assessing vessel size, stent deployment, and proper stent apposition. It can also guide in the identification and management of complications post-stenting such as ISR and coronary dissection.

OPTICAL COHERENCE TOMOGRAPHY

OCT uses scattering and absorption of near infrared emitted from an optical fiber of an imaging catheter. Tomographic images are generated through an automated pullback requiring contrast infusion because OCT cannot image through blood. OCT has far superior resolution compared to IVUS. However, it falls behind in image penetration. OCT can identify thrombus, plaque rupture, stent malapposition, edge dissection, and prolapse of tissue (**Figure 7.5**). A 2014 consensus document of the Society of Cardiovascular Angiography and Interventions gives OCT a "probably beneficial" rating for stent deployment and "possibly beneficial" for plaque morphology.[23]

FRACTIONAL FLOW RESERVE

As compared to the anatomic assessment of lesion severity provided by IVUS and OCT, FFR provides physiologic significance of lesion severity. FFR is the ratio of mean distal coronary pressure after the lesion divided by mean pressure proximal to the lesion during maximal hyperemia achieved with IV adenosine (**Figure 7.6**). Although first validated at a significant level of 0.75, the value was

extended to 0.80 to improve sensitivity. The FAME trial randomized patients with multivessel disease to either FFR-guided PCI or to angiographic-guided PCI. The primary outcome of death, MI, or repeat revascularization was significantly lower in the FFR-guided PCI arm.[24] FAME 2 demonstrated that FFR-guided PCI with optimal medical therapy in patients with stable CAD showed better outcomes than did medical therapy alone.[25] FFR is useful in guiding the management of a patient with SIHD and in assessing the angiographic significance of intermediate lesions (Class IIa; Level of evidence A).[12]

LESION MODIFICATION DEVICES

The procedural success of a calcified lesion depends on the adequate preparation of the vessel. Mild calcification can be managed with routine PTCA followed by stent. Moderate to severe calcification may require the use of the atherectomy devices to both debulk the lesion and modify the architecture of the vessel. Device selection is based on the degree of calcification, operator experience, and clinical presentation of the patient.

Atherectomy devices include rotational atherectomy, orbital atherectomy, excimer laser atherectomy, and cutting balloon atherectomy.

Rotational atherectomy works on the principle of "differential cutting," involving selective ablation of calcium, leaving healthy tissue intact, unlike balloon angioplasty, which causes several intimal tears. Rotational atherectomy ablates plaque using a diamond elliptical burr rotating concentrically on a wire at 140,000 to 160,000 revolutions per minute. It comes in sizes ranging from 1.25 to 2.5 mm. Particulates released from RA can pass through coronary microcirculation and eventually undergo phagocytosis in the body. Occasionally, the microparticles can cause microcirculation obstruction, thereby increasing the risk of slow flow or no-reflow.[26] This can be reduced by gradual burr advancement, short ablation runs, and avoidance of deceleration.[26] Despite its clinical utility, rotational atherectomy has not been shown to improve clinical outcomes. Current guidelines

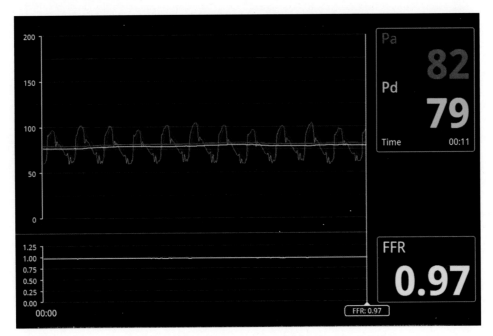

FIGURE 7.6 Normal fractional flow reserve of an indeterminate lesion coronary after IV adenosine infusion.

recommend that rotational atherectomy be used in the setting of severely calcified or fibrotic lesions that are not amenable to adequate balloon dilatation prior to stent implantation (Class IIa; Level of Evidence C).[12]

Diamondback 360 Coronary Orbital Atherectomy System works on the principle of differential sanding and centrifugal force for plaque modification. The system consists of a diamond-coated crown eccentrically mounted on a guidewire. The crown is available in a 1.25-mm size, but the maximum orbit is determined by the rotational speed of the crown. Compared to rotational atherectomy, orbital atherectomy produces microparticles that are smaller in size and allows continuous blood flow.

Excimer laser atherectomy uses laser energy to modify calcified lesions. Similar to rotational atherectomy, guidelines recommend use of excimer laser in fibrotic or moderately calcified lesions that cannot be adequately crossed or dilated with balloon angioplasty (Class IIb; Level of Evidence C).[12]

Cutting balloon atherectomy utilizes a balloon mounted with metallic blades that cut the plaque, allowing balloon dilatation at a lower pressure. Two such devices are available: The Flextome cutting balloon consists of three to four longitudinally directed microsurgical blades on the balloon surface. AngioSculpt consists of a nitinol cage over a balloon that cuts the plaque and also prevents balloon slippage. Cutting balloon atherectomy is frequently used in the setting of ostial lesions and mild- to moderate calcified lesions. Cutting balloon is also recommended to avoid coronary artery trauma caused by balloon slippage during PCI of ISR (Class IIb; Level of Evidence C).[12]

THROMBECTOMY

Thrombectomy devices incorporate removal of complete or partially occluding thrombus in patients with ST-elevation myocardial infarction. In light of recent studies, the 2015 focused update on primary PCI for patients with ST-elevation myocardial infarction has modified the recommendation from Class IIa to Class III for Routine aspiration thrombectomy before primary PCI.[27] Aspiration thrombectomy is performed using a catheter to remove thrombus using negative pressure applied through a syringe with a locking plunger controlled with a three-way stopcock. Angiojet is a rheolytic device based on the Venturi Bernoulli principle. It consists of a flexible catheter, pump, and angiojet console. The console energizes the pump to send pressurized saline to the catheter tip. A vacuum effect is created as the saline jet travels backward in the catheter. The net result is disruption and aspiration of thrombus, which can then be retrieved. Although not routinely recommended, it is extremely useful in patients with heavy clot burden.

EMBOLIC PROTECTION DEVICES

Embolization of atherosclerotic debris into systemic circulation is a complication sometimes encountered during saphenous vein graft intervention. There are two devices currently available for prevention of embolization. The Filterwire EZ uses a distal filter over a fixed wire that is advanced across a saphenous vein graft lesion. The filter prevents embolization of debris but does not compromise the blood flow through the filter pores. The Guardwire uses a balloon mounted on the distal end of the wire. The balloon is inflated distal to the lesion followed by rapid stenting and aspiration of the content of the vessel. Unlike the filter wire, there is the possibility of compromise to blood flow and hemodynamic compromise.

MECHANICAL SUPPORTIVE DEVICES

One of the significant advances in interventional cardiology is the availability of mechanical circulatory support devices.

The purpose of the mechanical support device is to provide end-organ and coronary perfusion and improve myocardial performance in the setting of cardiogenic shock or high-risk PCI.[28] The definition of high-risk PCI has been broad across the literature. It can be defined on the basis of patient-specific, lesion-specific, and clinical-specific variables.[29] Patient-specific characteristics include advanced age, depressed EF <35%, congestive heart failure, chronic kidney disease, diabetes mellitus, severe aortic stenosis, severe mitral regurgitation, or peripheral arterial disease. Lesion-specific characteristics include multivessel disease, left main disease, last patent conduit, bifurcation lesions, or chronic total occlusion. Lastly, clinical presentations include acute coronary syndromes, advanced heart failure, and cardiogenic shock.[29]

Cardiogenic shock and high-risk PCI represent a dynamic patient population group that can have marked hemodynamic and metabolic derangements. It is recommended that a multidisciplinary heart team approach is utilized for prompt identification of these patients. Providing optimal support to these patients may require this team approach and can be accomplished with an array of appropriate mechanical support devices.[30] The 2011 multisociety guidelines for PCI recommend elective insertion of a hemodynamic support device at the time of PCI in carefully selected patient populations as described above (Class IIb; Level of Evidence C).[12] Each device has a particular hemodynamic profile as well as indications and contraindications. It is imperative to carefully consider all clinical parameters before a mechanical support device is selected.

INTRA-AORTIC BALLOON PUMP

The intra-aortic balloon pump (IABP) remains one of the most commonly used support devices. The IABP, which works on the principle of counterpulsation, inflates during diastole to provide diastolic augmentation of pressure and increased coronary perfusion and deflates during systole to reduce afterload and improve cardiac output. The device consists of a balloon catheter and a console. The balloon catheter has a polyethylene balloon attached to its body with two lumens. One lumen is for guidewire insertion and pressure monitoring, and the other lumen is for balloon inflation with helium. The IABP is inserted through the femoral artery and placed in the descending thoracic aorta under fluoroscopic guidance. The position of the balloon should be 1 to 2 cm below the subclavian artery and above the renal artery. A daily chest X-ray should confirm the tip of the IABP between the second and third intercostal spaces. The IABP uses either the electrocardiogram or pressure triggers for timing the balloon cycle. Moderate to severe aortic regurgitation is considered a contraindication for IABP placement, and careful attention is required for patients with severe peripheral arterial and aortic disease. Despite the widespread use of IABP, clinical trials have failed to show a mortality benefit. The Intra-aortic Balloon Pump in Cardiogenic Shock II (IABP-SHOCK II) trail randomized 600 patients with cardiogenic shock complicating acute myocardial infarction into IABP or no IABP. All patients received optimal medical therapy and were expected to undergo revascularization with either PCI or CABG. This trial failed to show a significant reduction in 30-day mortality between the two groups.[31] Despite the lack of evidence, the 2013 guideline for management of ST-elevation myocardial infarction recommends use of IABP for patients with cardiogenic shock who fail to stabilize with pharmacologic therapy (Class IIa; Level of evidence B).[14] Alternate devices for circulatory support may be indicated for patients with refractory cardiogenic shock (Class IIb; Level of Evidence C).[14]

IMPELLA

The Impella device provides a nonpulsatile axial flow of blood from the LV to the ascending aorta. It is available as Impella 2.5 and Impella CP, which can be inserted percutaneously, and as Impella 5.0, which requires a surgical cutdown. The device consists of a pigtail catheter that crosses the aortic valve and is connected to a cannula that contains the pump inlet and outlet.[29] Impella 2.5 can provide an outflow of 2.5 L/min, Impella CP provides support between 3.0 and 4.0 L/min, and Impella 5.0 can provide support of 5.0 L/min. Left ventricular thrombus is an absolute contraindication for the use of Impella. The PROTECT II trial randomized 452 symptomatic patients with complex three-vessel disease or unprotected left main CAD and reduced ejection fraction to intra-aortic balloon or Impella 2.5T support during nonemergent high-risk PCI. The Impella provided superior hemodynamic support compared to IABP, but the 30-day incidence of major adverse events was not statistically significant between the two groups. At 90 days, a trend toward improved outcomes was observed for the Impella 2.5 group.[32]

TANDEM HEART

The Tandem Heart provides extracorporeal circulation up to 5.0 L/min, utilizing a centrifugal pump from the left atrium to the femoral artery. It consists of an inflow cannula inserted into the left atrium through the femoral vein via the transseptal approach and an outflow cannula placed in the femoral artery.

EXTRACORPOREAL MEMBRANE OXYGENATION

Extracorporeal membrane oxygenation (ECMO) can be either Veno-venous ECMO to support oxygenation or veno-arterial ECMO to support both oxygenation and circulation. Veno-arterial is the device of choice for patients with biventricular failure requiring oxygenation and circulatory support.[29] The ECMO system consists of a venous reservoir, external centrifugal pump, membrane oxygenator, and a rewarming heparin-coated circuit.[28] Veno-arterial ECMO can provide circulatory flow up to 6 to 7 L/min, but its use can cause LV distension, and adequate venting with an Impella or IABP may be required.[30]

REFERENCES

1. Fihn SD, Blankenship JC, Alexander KP, et al. 2014 ACC/AHA/AATS/PCNA/SCAI/STS focused update of the guideline for the diagnosis and management of patients with stable ischemic heart disease: a report of the American College of Cardiology/American Heart Association Task Force on Practice Guidelines, and the American Association for Thoracic Surgery, Preventive Cardiovascular Nurses Association, Society for Cardiovascular Angiography and Interventions, and Society of Thoracic Surgeons. *J Am Coll Cardiol.* 2014;64:1929-1949.

2. Fihn SD, Gardin JM, Abrams J, et al. 2012 ACCF/AHA/ACP/AATS/PCNA/SCAI/STS guideline for the diagnosis and management of

patients with stable ischemic heart disease: a report of the American College of Cardiology Foundation/American Heart Association Task Force on Practice Guidelines, and the American College of Physicians, American Association for Thoracic Surgery, Preventive Cardiovascular Nurses Association, Society for Cardiovascular Angiography and Interventions, and Society of Thoracic Surgeons. *Circulation.* 2012;126:e354-e471.

3. Yancy CW, Jessup M, Bozkurt B, et al. 2013 ACCF/AHA guideline for the management of heart failure: a report of the American College of Cardiology Foundation/American Heart Association Task Force on Practice Guidelines. *J Am Coll Cardiol.* 2013;62:e147-e239.

4. Zipes DP, Camm AJ, Borggrefe M, et al. ACC/AHA/ESC 2006 guidelines for management of patients with ventricular arrhythmias and the prevention of sudden cardiac death: a report of the American College of Cardiology/American Heart Association Task Force and the European Society of Cardiology Committee for Practice Guidelines (writing committee to develop guidelines for management of patients with ventricular arrhythmias and the prevention of sudden cardiac death): developed in collaboration with the European Heart Rhythm Association and the Heart Rhythm Society. *Circulation.* 2006;114:e385-e484.

5. Fleisher LA, Fleischmann KE, Auerbach AD, et al. 2014 ACC/AHA guideline on perioperative cardiovascular evaluation and management of patients undergoing noncardiac surgery: a report of the American College of Cardiology/American Heart Association Task Force on Practice Guidelines. *J Am Coll Cardiol* 2014;64:e77-137.

6. Scanlon PJ, Faxon DP, Audet AM, et al. ACC/AHA guidelines for coronary angiography. A report of the American College of Cardiology/American Heart Association Task Force on Practice Guidelines (Committee on Coronary Angiography). Developed in collaboration with the Society for Cardiac Angiography and Interventions. *J Am Coll Cardiol.* 1999;33:1756-1824.

7. Naidu SS, Aronow HD, Box LC, et al. SCAI expert consensus statement: 2016 best practices in the cardiac catheterization laboratory: (Endorsed by the Cardiological Society of India, and Sociedad Latino Americana de Cardiologia Intervencionista; Affirmation of value by the Canadian Association of Interventional Cardiology-Association Canadienne de Cardiologie D'Intervention). *Catheter Cardiovasc Interv.* 2016;88:407-423.

8. Mehran R, Aymong ED, Nikolsky E, et al. A simple risk score for prediction of contrast-induced nephropathy after percutaneous coronary intervention: development and initial validation. *J Am Coll Cardiol.* 2004;44:1393-1399.

9. Ferrante G, Rao SV, Juni P, et al. Radial versus femoral access for coronary interventions across the entire spectrum of patients with coronary artery disease: a meta-analysis of randomized trials. *JACC Cardiovasc Interv.* 2016;9:1419-1434.

10. Schulz-Schupke S, Helde S, Gewalt S, et al. Comparison of vascular closure devices vs manual compression after femoral artery puncture: the ISAR-CLOSURE randomized clinical trial. *JAMA.* 2014;312:1981-1987.

11. Rao SV, Tremmel JA, Gilchrist IC, et al. Best practices for transradial angiography and intervention: a consensus statement from the Society For Cardiovascular Angiography And Intervention's Transradial Working Group. *Catheter Cardiovasc Interv.* 2014;83:228-236.

12. Levine GN, Bates ER, Blankenship JC, et al. 2011 ACCF/AHA/SCAI guideline for percutaneous coronary intervention. A report of the American College of Cardiology Foundation/American Heart Association Task Force on Practice Guidelines and the Society for Cardiovascular Angiography and Interventions. *J Am Coll Cardiol.* 2011;58:e44-e122.

13. Patel MR, Dehmer GJ, Hirshfeld JW, Smith PK, Spertus JA. ACCF/SCAI/STS/AATS/AHA/ASNC/HFSA/SCCT 2012 Appropriate use criteria for coronary revascularization focused update: a report of the American College of Cardiology Foundation Appropriate Use Criteria Task Force, Society for Cardiovascular Angiography and Interventions, Society of Thoracic Surgeons, American Association for Thoracic Surgery, American Heart Association, American Society of Nuclear Cardiology, and the Society of Cardiovascular Computed Tomography. *J Am Coll Cardiol.* 2012;59:857-881.

14. American College of Emergency Physicians, Society for Cardiovascular Angiography and Interventions, and the Society of Thoracic Surgeons. 2013 ACCF/AHA guideline for the management of ST-elevation myocardial infarction: a report of the American College of Cardiology Foundation/American Heart Association Task Force on Practice Guidelines. *J Am Coll Cardiol.* 2013;61:e78-e140.

15. Amsterdam EA, Wenger NK, Brindis RG, et al. 2014 AHA/ACC guideline for the management of patients with non-ST-elevation acute coronary syndromes: a report of the American College of Cardiology/American Heart Association Task Force on Practice Guidelines. *J Am Coll Cardiol.* 2014;64:e139-e228.

16. Patel MR, Dehmer GJ, Hirshfeld JW, Smith PK, Spertus JA. ACCF/SCAI/STS/AATS/AHA/ASNC 2009 Appropriateness criteria for coronary revascularization: a report of the American College of Cardiology Foundation Appropriateness Criteria Task Force, Society for Cardiovascular Angiography and Interventions, Society of Thoracic Surgeons, American Association for Thoracic Surgery, American Heart Association, and the American Society of Nuclear Cardiology: Endorsed by the American Society of Echocardiography, the Heart Failure Society of America, and the Society of Cardiovascular Computed Tomography. *Circulation.* 2009;119:1330-1352.

17. Levine GN, Bates ER, Bittl JA, et al. 2016 ACC/AHA guideline focused update on duration of dual antiplatelet therapy in patients with coronary artery disease: a report of the American College of Cardiology/American Heart Association Task Force on Clinical Practice Guidelines. *J Am Coll Cardiol.* 2016;68:1082-1115.

18. Park SJ, Kang SJ, Virmani R, Nakano M, Ueda Y. In-stent neoatherosclerosis: a final common pathway of late stent failure. *J Am Coll Cardiol.* 2012;59:2051-2057.

19. Stone GW, Witzenbichler B, Guagliumi G, et al. Bivalirudin during primary PCI in acute myocardial infarction. *N Engl J Med.* 2008;358:2218-22130.

20. Stone GW, Clayton T, Deliargyris EN, Prats J, Mehran R, Pocock SJ. Reduction in cardiac mortality with bivalirudin in patients with and without major bleeding: The HORIZONS-AMI trial (Harmonizing Outcomes with Revascularization and Stents in Acute Myocardial Infarction). *J Am Coll Cardiol.* 2014;63:15-20.

21. Shahzad A, Kemp I, Mars C, et al. Unfractionated heparin versus bivalirudin in primary percutaneous coronary intervention (HEAT-PPCI): an open-label, single centre, randomised controlled trial. *Lancet.* 2014;384:1849-1858.

22. Steg PG, van't Hof A, Hamm CW, et al. Bivalirudin started during emergency transport for primary PCI. *N Engl J Med.* 2013;369:2207-2217.

23. Lotfi A, Jeremias A, Fearon WF, et al. Expert consensus statement on the use of fractional flow reserve, intravascular ultrasound, and optical coherence tomography: a consensus statement of the Society of Cardiovascular Angiography and Interventions. *Catheter Cardiovasc Interv.* 2014;83:509-518.

24. Tonino PA, De Bruyne B, Pijls NH, et al. Fractional flow reserve versus angiography for guiding percutaneous coronary intervention. *N Engl J Med.* 2009;360:213-224.

25. De Bruyne B, Pijls NH, Kalesan B, et al. Fractional flow reserve-guided PCI versus medical therapy in stable coronary disease. *N Engl J Med.* 2012;367:991-1001.

26. Tomey MI, Kini AS, Sharma SK. Current status of rotational atherectomy. *JACC Cardiovasc Interv.* 2014;7:345-353.

27. Levine GN, Bates ER, Blankenship JC, et al. 2015 ACC/AHA/SCAI Focused update on primary percutaneous coronary intervention for patients with ST-elevation myocardial infarction: an update of the 2011 ACCF/AHA/SCAI guideline for percutaneous coronary intervention and the 2013 ACCF/AHA guideline for the management of ST-elevation myocardial infarction. *J Am Coll Cardiol.* 2016;67:1235-1250.

28. Myat A, Patel N, Tehrani S, Banning AP, Redwood SR, Bhatt DL. Percutaneous circulatory assist devices for high-risk coronary intervention. *JACC Cardiovasc Interv.* 2015;8:229-244.

29. Rihal CS, Naidu SS, Givertz MM, et al. 2015 SCAI/ACC/HFSA/STS Clinical expert consensus statement on the use of percutaneous mechanical circulatory support devices in cardiovascular care: endorsed by the American Heart Association, the Cardiological Society of India, and Sociedad Latino Americana de Cardiologia Intervencion; affirmation of value by the Canadian Association of Interventional Cardiology-Association Canadienne de Cardiologie d'intervention. *J Am Coll Cardiol.* 2015;65:e7-e26.

30. Atkinson TM, Ohman EM, O'Neill WW, Rab T, Cigarroa JE, Interventional Scientific Council of the American College of Cardiology. A practical approach to mechanical circulatory support in patients undergoing percutaneous coronary intervention: an interventional perspective. *JACC Cardiovasc Interv.* 2016;9:871-883.

31. Thiele H, Zeymer U, Neumann FJ, et al. Intraaortic balloon support for myocardial infarction with cardiogenic shock. *N Engl J Med.* 2012;367:1287-1296.

32. O'Neill WW, Kleiman NS, Moses J, et al. A prospective, randomized clinical trial of hemodynamic support with Impella 2.5 versus intra-aortic balloon pump in patients undergoing high-risk percutaneous coronary intervention: the PROTECT II study. *Circulation.* 2012;126:1717-1727.

Patient and Family Information for: CORONARY ANGIOGRAPHY AND PERCUTANEOUS CORONARY INTERVENTION

CARDIAC CATHETERIZATION AND CORONARY ANGIOGRAPHY

Cardiac catheterization is a procedure that is performed to obtain X-ray pictures of arteries that supply the muscles of the heart. It can also be used to measure the pressures in the right- and left-sided chambers of the heart. This procedure is performed through a blood vessel either in the leg or in the arm or wrist. The doctor may recommend this procedure for a variety of cardiac diseases:

1. CAD: If the doctor is suspecting blockages in coronary arteries, the blood vessels that nourish the heart walls, he/she may recommend cardiac catheterization for identification and assessment of severity of blockages by injecting the coronary arteries with a contrast material that is seen under X-ray.
2. Valvular heart disease: Diseases affecting valves of the heart can be assessed by measuring the pressures in the chambers of the heart and by injecting contrast in the ventricles or the aorta.
3. Congenital heart disease: Some forms of congenital heart disease can be evaluated with cardiac catheterization by pressure measurements and oxygen analysis in the chambers of the heart.

PREPARATION FOR THE PROCEDURE

The patient will most likely be asked not to eat several hours before the procedure, but most medications can be taken with a sip of water. If the patient takes any blood thinners other than aspirin, plavix, prasugrel, ticagrelor, or other antiplatelet drugs, the doctor may discontinue these or modify the doses before the test. For diabetic patients, the doctor may hold or reduce the dose of medications before the procedure.

When the patient arrives in the catheterization laboratory, an intravenous line is started in the arm by the nurse so that medication, including sedation, can be given to the patient during the test. An electrocardiogram and blood tests will be performed before the test. ECG monitoring electrodes will be placed on the chest so that continuous recordings of the heartbeat can be performed throughout the test. To reduce the risk of infection, hair will be shaved from the groin area if the doctor chooses to use the femoral artery in the leg for the insertion of the catheter. The doctor will review the procedure and obtain informed consent from the patient before the procedure.

PROCEDURE

Once the patient is inside the cardiac catheterization room, the doctor will give medications to help relax and relieve any anxiety. The patient will be most likely awake or in a light sleep. The entire body from neck to toe will be covered with a sterile drape. For the catheterization performed through the artery in the leg, the doctor will palpate the femoral artery in the groin. Thereafter, he will inject numbing medication to relieve any pain before inserting a thin plastic sheath into the artery. The doctor may place a similar sheath in the femoral vein that runs next to the femoral artery to measure the pressures in the right-sided chambers of the heart. A similar technique will be used if the catheterization is performed through the wrist of the hand by accessing the radial artery.

LEFT HEART CATHETERIZATION AND CORONARY ANGIOGRAM

After the plastic sheath is placed in the femoral artery, the doctor will pass the catheters through the sheath, which will be advanced under X-ray guidance up to the aorta, the main artery leading to the heart, and reach the left side of the heart. The doctor will then access the coronary arteries and inject "dye" to perform a "coronary angiogram." Digital X-ray pictures will be obtained at the same time to diagnose blockages in coronary arteries. The doctor may also obtain pressures in the left ventricle, which is the main pumping chamber of the heart, by passing a catheter into the left ventricle to perform "left heart catheterization."

RIGHT HEART CATHETERIZATION

After the plastic sheath is placed in the femoral vein, the doctor will pass the catheter under X-ray guidance to the right-sided chambers of the heart. "Right heart catheterization" will be completed by obtaining the pressure measurements of the right-sided chambers of the heart. A combined "right heart catheterization" and "left heart catheterization" will be performed to diagnose the disease of heart valves and muscles of the heart.

POST PROCEDURE

The entire procedure of "left heart catheterization," "coronary angiogram," and "right heart catheterization" will be completed in approximately 30 to 45 minutes if no further procedure is planned. The doctor will then remove the small plastic sheath from the wrist or the leg. If the procedure were performed through the wrist, a small pressure band would be applied and removed in approximately 2 hours. For the procedure performed through the leg, the sheath will be removed, and either manual pressure will be applied for 15 to 20 minutes or a "closure device" will be used. The use of a "closure device" will allow the patient to ambulate earlier compared to the case with manual pressure. The doctor will provide information about postprocedure care required. Typically, the patient is required to stay in bed for about 2 to 4 hours.

After coronary angiogram is performed, the doctor will review the X-ray pictures and decide whether the patient requires an intervention. If the review of X-ray pictures reveals "blockages," the doctor will review the best treatment option for the patient, which can range from medical treatment to PCI or bypass surgery. The choice of treatment option depends on the number of arteries involved and the complexity of the blockages, pumping function of the heart, symptoms of the patient, and presence or absence of diabetes.

The foregoing procedures of "coronary angiogram" and "PCI" may be performed in an elective setting or, in some cases, emergently if the patient presents with symptoms of a heart attack. Two scenarios may occur. In the first scenario, the patient presents with the clinical condition referred to as STEMI. Patients with STEMI have a coronary artery completely blocked by a blood clot known as a thrombus. If the hospital is capable of performing coronary angiogram and PCI, the patient will be rushed to the cardiac catheterization laboratory. If such a capability does not exist, the patient will either be transferred to the nearest hospital and/or given medications to dissolve the clot occluding the artery. In the second scenario, patients may present with a condition referred to as NSTE-ACS, in which, unlike in the case of STEMI, the artery is not completely occluded. Patients presenting with NSTE-ACS are treated with either coronary angiogram and/or PCI within a few hours of presentation if indicated on the basis of clinical presentation, or they may undergo further noninvasive testing to determine the need for a coronary angiogram and/or PCI.

PERCUTANEOUS CORONARY INTERVENTION

We will review different forms of PCI if the doctor decides, on the basis of the coronary angiogram, that there is a need for it. The doctor may perform the PCI immediately after the angiogram or later. The percutaneous intervention is performed through the same small plastic sheath using a different set of catheters and wires.

CORONARY ANGIOPLASTY

This procedure is referred to in medical terminology as PTCA. It is usually performed as a precursor to implantation of stent to prepare the coronary artery. Rarely, it is performed as a "stand alone" procedure, but this is associated with increased risk of repeat blockages because of the formation of scar tissue. The procedure is performed by passing what is known as a guide wire across the coronary artery with "blockages." Once the wire is positioned adequately across the blockage, a flexible catheter with a balloon attached to its distal tip is passed over the wire and placed at the site of the "blockage." The balloon is inflated, compressing the plaque, and is deflated after a few seconds to open the blockage. This may be repeated as necessary to dilate the coronary artery and prepare it for subsequent stent implantation.

CORONARY STENTS

One of the problems with "stand alone" coronary angioplasty, as previously described, was repeat blockage of the coronary artery caused by the formation of scar tissue. This was greatly reduced with the advent of coronary stents. Coronary stents are metallic devices that are placed at the site of the blockage usually after balloon dilatation or sometimes directly. There

are two types of stents: (1) BMS and (2) DES. A DES delivers a drug locally at the site of the blockage and thereby reduces the problem of restenosis. However, the stent itself is considered a foreign material and is at risk for formation of clot because of the interaction of stent material and blood. This risk is greater with DESs because the release of drug prevents cell growth and keeps them "foreign" for a longer time. To prevent this complication of clotting of the stent, the doctor will prescribe two medications, aspirin and another antiplatelet drug such as plavix, prasugrel, or ticagrelor. This form of therapy is called "DAPT." Depending on type of the stent and clinical condition that prompted the stent implantation, the duration of the therapy may last from 1 month to 1 year or even longer. It is essential that the patient consult a doctor before stopping "DAPT."

ROTATIONAL ATHERECTOMY

In some patients, the coronary arteries are severely calcified at the site of the blockage, making the implantation of stent extremely difficult. In those cases, the doctor may decide to perform rotational atherectomy. Rotational atherectomy is performed with a specialized burr mounted on a catheter. The burr rotates at a very rapid speed to pulverize the calcification. This procedure is usually followed by balloon dilatation and stent implantation.

THROMBECTOMY

In patients presenting with STEMI, a blood clot is formed at the site of the blockage. The clot may be aspirated by a catheter with mechanical suction or by devices that generate suction effect by high-pressure saline jets.

INTRAVASCULAR ULTRASOUND

Because coronary angiogram is a two-dimensional image seen on X-ray films, several other devices may be used to determine the severity of blockages in the coronary artery. One such device is called IVUS. This consists of a miniature ultrasound mounted on top of a catheter. The catheter is inserted into the coronary artery and can help visualize the degree of narrowing, calcification, and composition of plaque. It can also help the doctor to guide the implantation of the stent.

OPTICAL COHERENCE TOMOGRAPHY

OCT is a device similar to IVUS to help better understand the severity of the blockage. It is based on fiber optics, and catheters emit near infrared light. The quality of pictures obtained with OCT is far superior to those obtained with IVUS.

FRACTIONAL FLOW RESERVE

FFR is a technique used to assess whether the blockage visualized by coronary angiogram is physiologically limiting the blood supply to heart muscles. A wire is passed across the blockage, and a medication called "adenosine" is given intravenously to simulate maximal blood flow. The wire compares the pressure before and after the blockage to provide a number. If the number is less than 0.80, the doctor will opt to put a stent at the site of the blockage.

MECHANICAL SUPPORT DEVICES

A doctor may insert mechanical support devices in two scenarios: (1) The patient is presenting with a critical condition called "cardiogenic shock," where the patient's blood pressure is extremely low, and the heart is not able to pump sufficient blood to the body despite the use of strong medications. (2) The doctor determines that the blockage is very complex and wants to provide extra support to the heart while the intervention is performed. Several devices are available for use but the most commonly used devices are the IABP and Impella.

Jonathan Price
Sandhya K. Balaram

8

Coronary Artery Bypass Surgery

BACKGROUND

Coronary artery bypass surgery (CABG) is a safe and effective method of treating coronary artery disease.[1-3] Surgical bypass for coronary disease may be performed either in the elective setting or after acute myocardial infarction. The ACC/AHA guidelines for elective CABG in patients with coronary artery disease and emergency CABG after acute myocardial infarction are illustrated in **Tables 8.1** and **8.2**. The principles of surgical technique and postoperative care are similar; however, comorbidities strongly influence outcomes in the intensive care unit (ICU). A standardized approach is useful in the management of these complicated postoperative patients.

BASIC SURGICAL TECHNIQUE AND INTRAOPERATIVE CONSIDERATIONS

CABG is performed under general anesthesia with endotracheal intubation. Patients receive prophylactic antibiotics within 60 minutes prior to incision. Treatment is aimed at normal skin flora; a first-generation cephalosporin is commonly used and redosed in 4 to 6 hours based on clearance during cardiopulmonary bypass (CPB). Vancomycin may be used in regions of high prevalence of methicillin-resistant Staphylococcus species or in those patients with a long preoperative hospital length of stay.[4,5] Continuation of prophylactic antibiotics is not indicated beyond 24 to 48 hours postoperatively.

Intraoperative monitoring is essential in maintaining appropriate physiologic parameters across all body systems. Arterial, central venous, and pulmonary artery (PA) catheterization are used for hemodynamic monitoring. Placement of a PA catheter is not a necessity in those patients with a normal ejection fraction and uncomplicated surgical procedure. Intraoperative transesophageal echocardiograms provide excellent assessment of cardiac function during and after the time of CPB. A bladder catheter with a temperature probe is placed to monitor urine output and core body temperature. Alternatively, a rectal or esophageal temperature probe may be inserted for monitoring during the warming and cooling process of CPB.

Transesophageal echocardiography (TEE) is essential for the intraoperative evaluation of cardiac anatomy, ventricular function, valve anatomy, and pathology. TEE can also be used to confirm placement of intracardiac catheters and devices, evaluate for air or thrombus within the cardiac chambers, and record postrevascularization ventricular function. Epicardial probes may be used by the cardiac surgeon to evaluate the ascending aorta for intraluminal plaque.

CPB and cardioplegic arrest are used in many procedures to provide a motionless and bloodless field during surgical revascularization. CPB uses an extracorporeal circuit to drain the venous system; push the patient's blood through an oxygenator, warmer and filter; and return the blood into arterial circulation. Acting as a gravity siphon, a venous cannula removes blood from the right atrium or inferior vena cava (IVC) and superior vena cava directly into a container called the venous reservoir. A pump then pushes the blood through an oxygenator and a specialized filter to remove particulate matter before returning the blood into arterial circulation. The arterial cannula is most commonly located via the ascending aorta. However, in the case of dense calcification or an aneurysmal ascending aorta, cannulation may be performed in the axillary or femoral vessels. Additional cannulas are placed to infuse cardioplegic solutions and/or vent air from the cardiac chambers. Understanding the location of cannulation sites can be vital to postoperative care in the rare cases that the patient bleeds from one of the suture lines, especially if it is in a location outside of the chest (ie, following axillary or femoral cannulation).

Initiating CPB requires systemic anticoagulation for the patient's entire blood volume will be circulating through an extracorporeal circuit. Intravenous heparin is infused, 300 to 400 units/kg, to achieve an activated clotting time >450 seconds. After CPB has been discontinued, heparin is reversed with intravenous protamine sulfate.[6] Protamine is a naturally occurring protein derived from fish and therefore carries a small risk of anaphylaxis-type reaction with its use. The onset of high pulmonary arterial pressures, systemic hypotension, and acute right heart failure during the administration of protamine is concerning for a protamine reaction. Specific patients at risk include those with known fish allergies, or those who have been previously sensitized (reoperations or diabetics using protamine-containing insulins).[7]

In addition to stopping the heart and substituting circulation and ventilation with CPB, another physiologic change is the systemic cooling of patients to temperatures ranging from 28°C

TABLE 8.1	ACC/AHA Guidelines for CABG in Patients With Coronary Artery Disease

1. ≥50% diameter stenosis in the left main coronary artery

2. ≥70% diameter stenoses in three major coronary arteries, with or without involvement of the proximal LAD artery

3. ≥70% diameter stenosis in the proximal LAD plus one other major coronary artery

4. Survivors of sudden cardiac death with presumed ischemia-mediated ventricular tachycardia caused by significant (≥70% diameter) stenosis in a major coronary artery

5. Patients with one or more significant (≥70% diameter) coronary artery stenoses amenable to revascularization and unacceptable angina despite maximum medical therapy

CABG, coronary artery bypass surgery; LAD, left anterior descending.

TABLE 8.2	Guidelines for Emergency CABG after Myocardial Infarction

1. Patients with acute myocardial infarction (MI) and (a) primary PCI has failed or cannot be performed, (b) coronary anatomy is suitable for CABG, and (c) persistent ischemia of a significant area of myocardium at rest and/or hemodynamic instability refractory to nonsurgical therapy is present

2. Patients undergoing surgical repair of a postinfarction mechanical complication of MI

3. Patients with cardiogenic shock who are suitable for CABG irrespective of the time interval from MI to onset of shock and time from MI to CABG

4. Patients with life-threatening ventricular arrhythmias (believed to be ischemic in origin) in the presence of left main stenosis greater than or equal to 50% and/or 3-vessel CAD

CABG, coronary artery bypass surgery; CAD, coronary artery disease; MI, myocardial infarction; PCI, percutaneous coronary intervention.

to 34°C to reduce cellular metabolism.[6] This provides additional protection to all organ systems. The patient is rewarmed before discontinuing CPB; core temperature is monitored in the immediate postoperative setting to ensure normothermia and prevent abnormal coagulation or an increased risk of infection.[8]

CABG is accomplished by creating a route for blood to travel from a region of good flow (the aorta or subclavian artery), around an occlusive coronary lesion, to an area deprived of adequate flow. Available conduits include the internal mammary arteries, the greater saphenous veins (GSV), and the radial arteries. The internal mammary vessels are most commonly left in situ proximally connected to the subclavian artery and anastomosed distally to the target coronary. When the GSV or radial arteries are used, they are free grafts, requiring anastomosis proximally to the aorta for inflow. Internal mammary arterial patency rates approach 90% at 10 years; GSV patency is reported 70% to 80% at 5 years and 40% to 60% at 10 years.[9] Because of the difference in the native architecture of the venous conduit, there is a higher rate of neointimal hyperplasia and atherosclerosis, leading to earlier stenosis. Radial artery grafts have greater than 80% patency at 5 years.[9]

At the completion of the procedure, the patient is slowly weaned off CPB, and the heart restarts the work of maintaining cardiac output (CO). CPB causes a number of physiologic changes that are evident immediately after its discontinuation and into the postoperative period. Circulating the patient's blood through the extracorporeal circuit activates coagulation, complement, fibrinolytic, and cytokine cascades. This can result in a clinically significant systemic inflammatory response syndrome (SIRS) and/or coagulopathy.[6] The nonpulsatile and relatively hypotensive nature of the CPB circuit leads to activation of the body's natural sympathetic system, which can lead to an increased incidence of postoperative arrhythmias.

CABG can be performed without the use of CPB, thereby decreasing or eliminating the physiologic alterations of the bypass circuit. Off-pump CABG (OPCAB) is performed with special instruments that stabilize the beating heart and allow the surgeon a small area of motionless myocardium to complete the required vascular anastomoses. OPCAB has documented benefits, including decreased hospital costs, length of stay, myocardial dysfunction, stroke, renal dysfunction, transfusion requirements, and gastrointestinal dysfunction.[6,10–14] OPCAB techniques are used mainly by surgeons experienced with this modality. Good candidates are those patients with good cardiac function, no significant valve disease, and good target vessels. Some high-risk patients with many systemic comorbidities may do poorly with the physiologic stresses of CPB and may be candidates for OPCAB.

INITIAL CRITICAL CARE MANAGEMENT

Management of postsurgical patients begins at the time of transfer from the operating room to the ICU. To ensure this safe transit, a team of transporters that includes a member of the surgical team and anesthesia should be present to treat life-threatening situations. Before leaving the operating room, a systematic review of the patient's physiologic status should be performed. Specifically, all monitoring devices are checked, and the patient's vital signs must be appropriate for transport. Significant bleeding, hypothermia, and acidosis should be corrected before leaving the operating room.

The patient is transported with continuous electrocardiogram (ECG) tracings, invasive blood pressure monitoring, and pulse oximetry. The transport team must be equipped with battery-operated infusion pumps to have uninterrupted delivery of the required cardiovascular medications until arrival in the ICU. Sudden changes in cardiac rate, rhythm, and systemic blood pressure can occur quickly, and the transporting team must be prepared to correct them en route. The transporting team must have additional emergency medications readily available. Mechanical breaths are given via bag-mask ventilation from a portable and full oxygen tank.

Upon arrival at the ICU, the team of transporters work together with the accepting ICU staff to provide a seamless transfer of care. The endotracheal tube is immediately connected to the awaiting mechanical ventilator. Cardiovascular medication dosages and rates are confirmed by the ICU staff and, ideally, continued on the same pumps used in transport to avoid any errors. Immediate pump exchange of infusions is made if needed based on pre-transfer communication of medications between the operating room and the ICU nurse. The patient's thoracic drainage tubes are immediately connected to wall suction to evacuate any residual fluid that has collected during transport.

The patient is connected to continuous ECG, invasive and noninvasive blood pressure, pulse oximetry, and the appropriate pulmonary arterial catheter tracings. Immediately after the safe transfer from the operating room to the ICU monitors, a thorough physical examination is performed for vital signs, lateralizing neurologic findings, cardiac murmurs, breath sounds, abdominal distension, quality and quantity of urine and chest tube output, and evidence of extremity malperfusion by examining for color, palpable pulses, and tactile temperature. A 12-lead ECG is obtained upon arrival for postoperative baseline and daily thereafter to evaluate for myocardial ischemia. A portable chest X-ray is checked for placement of the endotracheal tube, the positions of the thoracic drainage tubes, the presence of hemo/

pneumothorax, the width of the mediastinum, and pulmonary vascular congestion. A full set of laboratory values is obtained: arterial blood gas, basic metabolic panel, complete blood count, serum magnesium and phosphorous, serum lactic acid, and a full coagulation profile consisting of prothrombin time, activated thromboplastin time, and international normalized ratio (INR).

Diagnosis and treatment of postoperative abnormalities should involve an algorithmic and systems-based approach. **Figure 8.1** illustrates the algorithm for management of low output state after CABG.

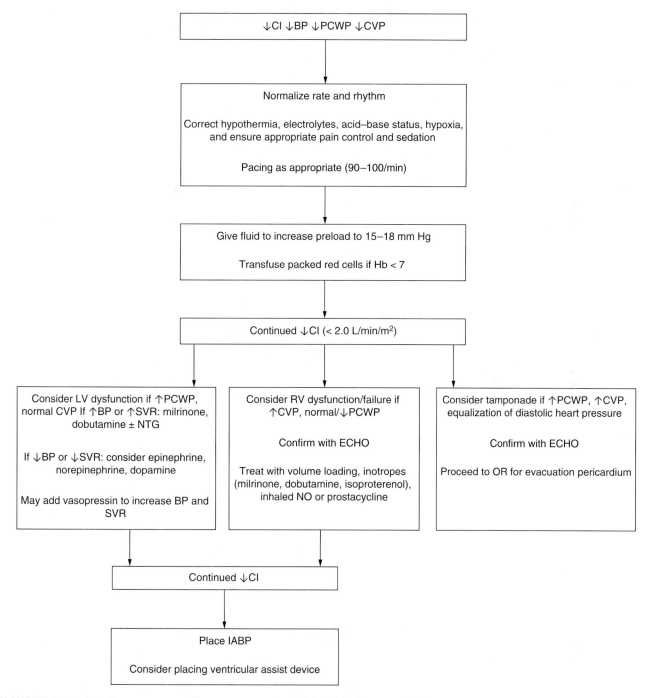

FIGURE 8.1 Algorithm for management of low output state after CABG. BP, blood pressure; CABG, coronary artery bypass surgery; CVP, central venous pressure; ECHO, echocardiogram; Hb, hemoglobin; IABP, intra-aortic balloon pump; LV, left ventricular; PCWP, pulmonary capillary wedge pressure; RV, right ventricle; SVR, systemic vascular resistance.

SYSTEMS MANAGEMENT

CARDIOVASCULAR

Postoperative cardiovascular issues can generally be divided into cardiac rate, rhythm, preload, afterload, contractility, or a combination of these. As discussed earlier, the use of a PA catheter can be omitted in patients with normal preoperative cardiac function; however, its use can provide a significant amount of information and guide management in the intensive care setting. When the PA catheter is not used, non-invasive hemodynamic monitoring, close physical examination, and clinical parameters such as urine output can be used to ensure adequate postoperative end-organ perfusion.

Rate

Rate disturbances are common in the immediate postoperative setting. Tachycardia can be caused by any number of physiologic disturbances such as CPB-induced sympathetic activation, pain, hypothermia, anemia, systemic hypoxemia, or pathologic postoperative conditions such as myocardial ischemia, tamponade, pneumothorax, or postpericardiotomy inflammation. Sinus tachycardia, although not inherently dangerous, contributes significantly to myocardial oxygen demand and should be avoided when possible in the immediate postoperative setting. Treatable causes of tachycardia should be addressed promptly. When secondary to sympathetic activation, atrioventricular (AV) nodal blockade with beta-blockers are considered first-line therapy; however, the use of beta-blockers in the immediate postoperative period is complicated by the depression of myocardial contractility. Postoperative myocardial depression usually dissipates within the first 12 to 24 hours of surgery, and beta-blockers are usually begun on postoperative day 1, with or without the presence of sinus tachycardia.

Asymptomatic bradycardia with or without conduction blockade and without changes to end-organ perfusion may not need to be treated urgently. However, when CO is inadequate, epicardial pacing may be accomplished via temporary ventricular and/or atrial wires placed routinely during the completion of the procedure. Transcutaneous pacing pads can be considered in an expedited fashion when urgent pacing is required in those patients without wires. Transvenous pacing wires can also be placed. When pacing is required, AV sequential pacing for AV nodal blockade or atrial pacing for sinus bradycardia is preferred to ventricular pacing alone to preserve the output of atrial systole, which increases preload and can contribute up to 30% of CO.

Rhythm

Rhythm disturbances, similarly, can be caused by the wide range of etiologies previously discussed, with the addition of electrolyte abnormalities (specifically potassium, magnesium, and calcium), acid–base disturbances, and myocardial irritation from indwelling catheters.

Atrial fibrillation (AF) is the most common post-CABG arrhythmia, occurring in up to 40% of patients. It usually occurs within the first 5 days of surgery but has a peak incidence at postoperative day 2. Risk factors associated with the development of AF include advanced age, history of paroxysmal AF, chronic obstructive pulmonary disease , the use of CPB, and longer intraoperative CPB times.[15,16] Pharmacologic rate control and cardioversion are the two principles of treatment in new-onset AF.

When AF is associated with rapid ventricular response, rate control is employed early to avoid a prolonged increase to myocardial oxygen demand, as is associated with other tachyarrhythmias. Beta-blockers are first-line therapy for acute rate control while corrections of the potential etiologies of the AF are explored.[17,18]

In the absence of an identifiable and treatable cause of the AF in a stable patient, pharmacologic cardioversion may be performed with intravenous amiodarone. Administered as a bolus followed by continuous infusion, amiodarone acts both as a cardioverting agent with its Class III antiarrhythmic properties and as a sympatholytic and AV nodal blocker with its intrinsic beta receptor-blocking properties. Calcium channel blockers and digoxin are not typically used as first-line treatments in this setting.[19] Electrical cardioversion is reserved for patients with AF with rapid ventricular response with associated hemodynamic compromise. With significant hypotension or evidence of end-organ malperfusion associated with the onset of rapid AF, synchronized electrical cardioversion should be performed immediately. When AF persists, systemic anticoagulation with a heparin infusion should be initiated within 48 hours and bridged to therapeutic warfarin therapy with a target INR of 2.0 to 3.0.[18,20]

Preload

Preload is the left ventricular end-diastolic volume (LVEDV), contributing to left ventricular (LV) myocyte stretch just prior to contraction. According to Starling's law, increasing preload is associated with a predictable increase in LV contractility until a critical point is reached where further increases in preload lead to overdistension of the LV and a decrease in contractility. It is therefore necessary to optimize preload to achieve the best CO. The most accurate measure of preload is by direct measurement of the left ventricular end diastolic pressure (LVEDP); this can be accomplished only via transarterial catheterization of the LV. Estimates of LVEDP can be made by measuring pulmonary artery wedge pressure (PAWP), pulmonary arterial diastolic pressure, or central venous pressure (CVP). In general, the further away the measurement from the LV, the less accurate the estimate of the LVEDP. In the postoperative period, however, these measurements can provide easy and rapid estimates of intracardiac volume status.

PAWP is measured after inflating the distally located PA catheter balloon in a segmental PA. This value approximates left atrial pressure, which in turn estimates LV pressure with the open mitral valve. Similarly, pulmonary arterial diastolic pressure, also measured by the PA catheter, estimates transmitted LA pressure. The PA diastolic pressure is, in general, slightly higher than the PAWP; it can be calibrated to the PAWP and trended in real time without having to frequently inflate the PA catheter balloon and risking PA rupture. Both PAWP and PA diastolic pressure are inaccurate in the setting of significant pulmonary hypertension or severe mitral valve disease. CVP provides the least accurate estimate of LVEDP; however, it is readily measured with a central venous catheter. CVP is an inaccurate estimation of LVEDP with right heart dysfunction, pulmonic or tricuspid valve disease. Trends, rather than direct measurements, are the most important aspect of these measurements. Fluctuations in pressure measurements mimic the changes in the LVEDP, and adjustments to postoperative resuscitation can be guided by those values.[6,21]

Preload will be decreased when there is inadequate circulating volume. Active bleeding may be evident via increased chest tube output. More commonly, a postbypass inflammatory state results in a systemic response that includes capillary leakage and third-spacing of intravascular volume. Management is aimed at replacing lost volume, typically with colloid infusions. If there is active bleeding, packed red blood cells may be transfused to maintain adequate tissue oxygenation, as measured by the mixed venous calibration. A thick, stiffened left ventricle typical of patients with long-standing hypertension has poor compliance, and diastolic filling will be compromised. Patients with significant LV hypertrophy may require even higher filling pressures to maintain an adequate preload and normal CO.

Preload can also be compromised in the setting of cardiac tamponade. Postoperative bleeding into the pericardium increases the transmural pressure of the cardiac chambers and compromises venous return to the right heart to restrict filling. Beck Triad (hypotension, distended neck veins, and distant/muffled heart sounds) is the classic finding in tamponade. **Table 8.3** lists the findings in acute tamponade. The diagnosis of tamponade may be subtle, however. The acute or gradual increase in CVP or PA pressures associated with hypotension may be an indication of tamponade without other physical examination findings. One can observe a trend toward equalization of the CVP, right atrial pressure, right ventricular diastolic pressure, PA diastolic pressure, and PAWP. A portable chest X-ray may show increased widening of the mediastinal silhouette, and echocardiography may demonstrate pericardial fluid with compression of the right heart and distension of the IVC. Diagnosis is critical and time-sensitive; treatment should be sought emergently. Evacuation of the pericardial blood is accomplished with resternotomy because this purely mechanical problem will be unresponsive to noninvasive treatments.[6]

Afterload

Afterload is the pressure, or wall tension, generated by the left ventricle to overcome systemic vascular resistance (SVR) to produce adequate ejection of blood; the normal SVR range is 900 to 1200 dynes · seconds/m[5].[6,21] Increased SVR in the postoperative period may occur secondary to increased sympathetic output after CPB, altered baroreceptor activity, hypothermia, pain, or anxiety. Patients with preoperative hypertension, diabetes, peripheral vascular disease, and chronic kidney disease are at higher risk for postoperative hypertension. The goal postoperatively is to achieve a pressure adequate for good organ perfusion, although not placing too much stress on the cardiac and vascular suture lines. This is especially true in older or frail patients with poor tissue strength. Systolic blood pressure is usually maintained

TABLE 8.3	**Findings of Acute Tamponade**

Tachycardia and/or hypotension

Distended neck veins and elevated CVP (only if the patient is not hypovolemic)

Equalization of pressures including CVP, RA mean, RV diastolic, PA diastolic, and PA wedge (usually within 5 mm Hg)

Low voltage ECG tracings or electrical alternans

CXR findings including widening of the mediastinum or cardiac silhouette

TEE findings of RA or RV compression and IVC distension

CVP; central venous pressure; CXR, chest X-ray; ECG, electrocardiogram; IVC, inferior vena cava; PA, pulmonary artery; RA, right atrium; RV, right ventricle; TEE, transesophageal echocardiogram.

between 90 and 130 mm Hg with a mean arterial pressure of less than 90 mm Hg. A higher blood pressure may be needed in patients with significant peripheral arterial disease to maintain end-organ perfusion. Conversely, a high SVR may restrict flow through the systemic microvasculature, thereby decreasing organ perfusion. An elevated SVR places increased stress on the heart by increased LV wall tension and afterload, increasing myocardial oxygen demand and possibly worsening postoperative myocardial function.[6]

Postoperative sedatives such as propofol decrease SVR and blood pressure. Initially after arrival in the ICU, it is important that medications are both rapid onset and quickly cleared in the case of sudden hemodynamic changes.

Sodium nitroprusside lowers both SVR and pulmonary vascular resistance by relaxing arterial smooth muscle and can be used in the setting with an elevated SVR and systemic pressure. Nitroprusside is metabolized to cyanide and may therefore become toxic with prolonged use. Its toxicity is increased with liver dysfunction.

Nitroglycerin is commonly used in the setting of systemic hypertension following CABG. This venodilator increases venous compliance and reduces preload. It should be avoided in states of hypovolemia because it will significantly reduce ventricular filling and may induce a significant reflex tachycardia that will increase myocardial oxygen demand.

Short-acting beta-blockers can also be used for hypertension. However, negative inotropes are generally avoided in the immediate postoperative period. Dihydropyridine calcium channel blocking agents such as nicardipine are almost purely peripheral vasodilators and can be used to treat an elevated SVR. Caution should be exercised because this class of medication has a half-life that is significantly longer than that of nitroprusside and nitroglycerin.

A *low* SVR is also troublesome because it may cause a reflex tachycardia and an increase in CO to maintain peripheral perfusion. Decreased vasomotor tone as a result of SIRS following CPB is the most common cause of a decreased SVR. Other causes include peripheral vasodilation, sepsis, adrenocortical insufficiency, or anaphylaxis. Treatments include maintaining adequate preload, ensuring sufficient CO, and utilizing peripheral vasoconstrictors as needed. Norepinephrine is a first-line agent that may be supplemented with vasopressin or phenylephrine as needed. Epinephrine may also be used in the setting of a patient that requires both vasoconstricting and inotropic effects to maintain perfusion.

Contractility

Myocardial contractility is the intrinsic force of contraction and is generally estimated by left ventricular ejection fraction (LVEF). Patients with poor myocardial contractile function preoperatively have higher risks from surgical intervention. Those with a normal LVEF may also emerge from CABG with depressed myocardial contractility caused by ischemia-reperfusion injury, cardioplegic arrest, myocardial edema, or ischemia.

Intraoperatively, LVEF is recorded with TEE and is compared to the known preoperative values. Postoperatively, contractility may be estimated by measuring the CO using a PA catheter. Utilizing the principle of thermodilution, a small volume of cold saline is injected into the right atrial port, where it mixes with blood. The change in temperature is sensed by a probe at the tip of the catheter located distally in the pulmonary arterial tree.

Cardiac output is estimated by the change in temperature of blood over time between the site of injection of cold saline and the tip of the pulmonary artery catheter. The faster the decrease in temperature, the higher the CO and vice versa. Other less invasive systems exist for estimating CO, including a FloTrac® sensor, which utilizes arterial line pressure measurements and waveforms to estimate the CO based on standardized values of SVR for the patient's height, weight, and age.

Post-CABG myocardial dysfunction is usually transient, especially in patients with normal preoperative function, and usually resolves within 12 to 48 hours. Normal CO is 4.0 to 6.0 L/min, but varies depending on the patient's size. The cardiac index (CI) is a measure of the CO, standardized to the patient's body surface area. The CI, measured in $L/min/m^2$, is a more effective measure of the patient's contractile function. An adequate CI should be greater than $2.0 \ L/min/m^2$. With adequate preload and afterload, a depressed CI requires inotropic medications to augment myocardial contractility.[6]

Epinephrine is a strong alpha and beta-adrenergic agonist and can be simultaneously used as a positive inotrope and vasopressor. Dobutamine is a strong beta agonist and weak alpha agonist. Both exert strong inotropic effects and are titrated to achieve an adequate CO. Their use may be limited because of the intrinsic arrhythmogenic properties of the medications. Higher doses used to achieve an adequate CO may cause tachyarrhythmias that increase myocardial oxygen demand. Epinephrine causes fewer tachyarrhythmias at higher concentrations than does dobutamine, although both are acceptable for use in the immediate postoperative period.

Milrinone is a phosphodiesterase inhibitor that increases myocardial contractility while relaxing peripheral and pulmonary arterial smooth muscle. It is an ideal drug for an adequately volume-loaded patient with depressed myocardial contractility and an elevated SVR or pulmonary hypertension. Milrinone has a significantly longer half-life than epinephrine, and its use can have effects lasting for hours after it has been discontinued.

Other positive inotropes such as dopamine and isoproterenol exist, and their use varies depending on the clinical situation. Any medication used to treat impaired myocardial contractile function must be weighed against other systemic effects that they will induce on the critical care patient. In severe postoperative cardiogenic shock, placement of an intra-aortic balloon pump may be indicated to decrease afterload, increase coronary perfusion, and improve CO.

Although LV dysfunction is more commonly associated with a postoperative decrease in CI, right ventricular dysfunction may play an important role. Preexisting right heart failure, inadequate right ventricular protection during CPB, right ventricular infarction, and pulmonary hypertension may contribute to postoperative right heart dysfunction, which may present as a decreased CO. Common findings include elevated right ventricular filling pressures associated with relatively low or normal LV filling pressure. Echocardiography may demonstrate a hypokinetic and dilated right ventricle and/or new-onset tricuspid regurgitation.

Management of right heart failure is similar to that of left heart failure. The goal is to optimize preload for adequate myocardial stretch, provide inotropic support, and minimize afterload, which in this case is the pulmonary arterial vasculature. Milrinone can provide good inotropic support with pulmonary vasodilation in this setting. Dobutamine, isoproterenol, nitric oxide, prostacyclin, and sildenafil citrate may also be used as adjuncts in the ICU setting to improve RV function and decrease pulmonary hypertension.[22,23]

BLEEDING AND HEMATOLOGIC DISTURBANCES

Bleeding in the immediate postoperative period is not uncommon post-CABG. Multiple reasons for this exist: preoperative antiplatelet agents or anticoagulants, disturbances to the coagulation cascade, hepatic dysfunction, CPB-associated platelet dysfunction, and hypothermia. The volume of hourly bleeding should trend downward from the time of sternal closure. A guideline for acceptable postoperative bleeding is 2 mL/kg for the first 3 hours, followed by 1 mL/kg for the next 3 hours, and then by 0.5 mL/kg up to postoperative hour twelve. We define surgical bleeding mandating re-exploration vs. excessive bleeding with initial conservative measures as illustrated in **Figure 8.2**. Up to 4% of postoperative bleeding in CABG patients requires re-exploration.[24–26] Persistent hemorrhage is quickly communicated to the attending surgeon.

The quality and quantity of chest tube drainage are examined in the bleeding patient. Fresh, bright red blood with brisk flow may indicate arterial surgical bleeding and require re-exploration. Slow draining, dark red blood may be evidence of venous bleeding or oozing from raw surfaces and may be controlled with improved coagulation, warming to normothermia, clotting factors, or watchful waiting.

Frequent laboratory tests of serum hemoglobin, hematocrit, platelet count, prothrombin time, activated partial thromboplastin time (aPTT), and INR are indicated. Although no specific transfusion trigger exists, packed red blood cell transfusions are generally initiated to maintain hemoglobin of at least 7 mg/dL. In patients with relatively more systemic oxygen demand, such as those with a lower threshold for end-organ ischemia, hemoglobin levels are general kept higher, around 8 to 10 mg/dL. In the coagulopathic patient with an elevated INR, fresh frozen plasma (FFP) may be transfused if the INR is greater than 1.5. An elevated aPTT, greater than 1.5 times baseline, may be an indication of residual circulating heparin, and additional protamine may be infused in doses of 50 to 100 mg. Checking the intraoperative anesthesia record is important because the total amount of infused protamine should not exceed 1.3 mg/100 units of heparin given for CPB.[27]

Postoperative platelet dysfunction may be a result of CPB, uremia from chronic kidney disease, or antiplatelet medications. Platelet concentrations should be maintained at 100,000/μL if ongoing coagulopathy and bleeding are present. Desmopressin (DDAVP) may also be used as an adjunct to postoperative bleeding that is thought to originate in platelet dysfunction. It causes a release of von Willebrand factor from vascular endothelium and promotes the adherence of platelets to collagen. Its routine prophylactic use to treat CPB-induced platelet dysfunction is not recommended; it may be used in excessive hemorrhage or when bleeding is secondary to uremia or known von Willebrand disease, type I or II.[26]

Cryoprecipitate, which contains factors VII, VIII, fibrinogen, and von Willebrand factor, may also be used as an adjunct to the bleeding patient receiving packed red blood cells, FFP, and platelets to account for dilution of these factors. When massive volumes of blood product are being transfused, the ratios of packed red blood cell, FFP, and cryoprecipitate should be relatively equal.[26,28]

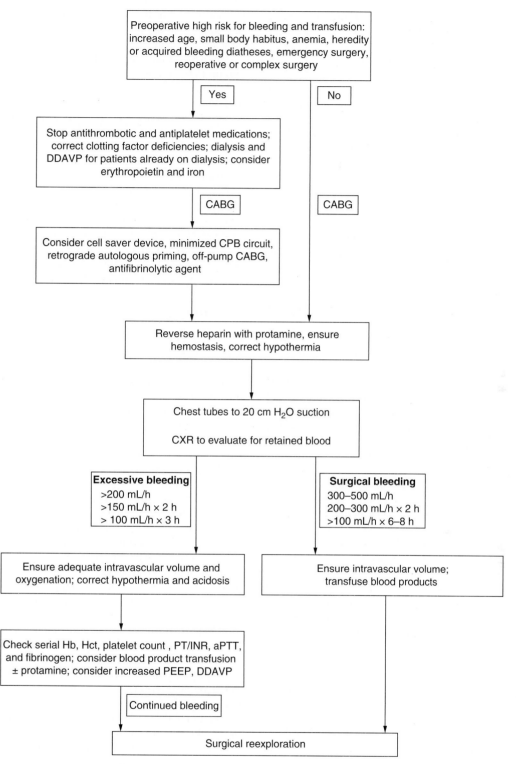

FIGURE 8.2 Algorithm for the management of postoperative bleeding. aPPT, activated partial thromboplastin time; CABG, coronary artery bypass surgery; CPB, cardiopulmonary bypass; CXR, chest X-ray; DDAVP, desmopressin; INR, international normalized ratio; Hb, hemoglobin; Hct, hematocrit; PEEP, positive end-expiratory pressure; PT, prothrombin time.

Increasing intrathoracic pressure may be beneficial by effectively tamponading slowly bleeding surfaces, particularly from the chest wall. This is accomplished by increasing positive end-expiratory pressure (PEEP) on the ventilator, usually from 5 up to 8 to 10 mm Hg. The intravascular fluid status of the patient is important because this increase in PEEP reduces venous return to the heart and may cause hypotension.

Persistent hemorrhage, particularly in the setting of hemodynamic compromise with increased vasopressor requirements and normalized coagulopathy, may be an indication for return to the operating room for re-exploration.

PULMONARY

During transfer to the ICU, patients are manually bag-ventilated on 100% oxygen; they are transitioned to mechanical ventilation immediately after arrival. After arrival, a volume-controlled mode is used to maintain set minute ventilation. This mode of delivery can be programmed via assist-control ventilation or synchronized intermittent mandatory ventilation (SIMV); with the patient fully sedated, SIMV will perform as assist-control mode. The fraction of inspired oxygen is titrated down from 100% to 40% as tolerated by the patient to maintain hemoglobin saturation above 95%. Tidal volumes are set according to the patient's weight, and both tidal volume and respiratory rate should be adjusted as needed to maintain adequate ventilation after examination of the first arterial blood gas.

Most patients will be ready for extubation within 6 hours of arrival in the ICU. Risk factors for prolonged mechanical ventilation include advanced age, tobacco smoking, COPD, female gender, renal failure, emergency surgery, persistent cardiogenic shock, and cerebrovascular accidents (CVA).[29,30]

Hemodynamically stable patients who are fully awake, alert, and following commands can proceed to ventilator weaning. Several protocols exist to ensure safe weaning from mechanical ventilation, and all rely on the patient's ability to breathe spontaneously and ventilate adequately. Initiating a spontaneous breathing trial (SBT) with zero mechanically delivered breaths, a PEEP of 5 cm H_2O, and little pressure support will allow the patient to assume the work of breathing. During the SBT, diaphoresis, agitation, hypoxemia, use of accessory respiratory muscles, or hemodynamic instability are sufficient evidence that the patient is not ready for extubation. After 30 minutes, if the patient does not exhibit signs of physiologic distress, an arterial blood gas is measured to evaluate for adequacy of ventilation and oxygenation. If the pH ≥ 7.32, $Pao_2 \geq 60$ mm Hg, and $Pco_2 \leq 45$ mm Hg, the patient meets the criteria for extubation in the right clinical setting.[6]

The patient is transitioned from mechanical ventilation to supplemental oxygen via facemask delivering humidified air. This should be progressively weaned to nasal cannula as tolerated by the patient to maintain a hemoglobin saturation above 92%. Pulmonary toilet, pain control, and mobilization are critical in the immediate postoperative period to prevent atelectasis and effusions that can delay the patient's progress. Incentive spirometry is taught to each patient and recommended frequently throughout the ICU stay.

If clinically indicated, high-flow oxygen via nasal cannula or continuous positive airway pressure via mask can be used to decrease the work of breathing for the patient and improve oxygenation. This is particularly true in obese patients or those with known preoperative pulmonary dysfunction.

RENAL

Management of fluids following CABG can be divided into two phases: (1) volume loading and (2) diuresis. Initially, maintaining an adequate preload is critical to CO, and infusion of significant volumes of intravenous fluids may be required. A urinary catheter with a temperature probe is inserted before the start of surgery and is left in place for precise hourly measurements of urine output that confirm good organ perfusion. Urine output should be maintained at 0.5 mL/kg/h; oliguria may be evidence of inadequate end-organ perfusion, and addressing problems with preload, afterload, and/or contractile function is mandatory.

Up to 8% of patients will develop acute kidney injury (AKI), and up to 0.7% will require dialysis after CABG. The presence of AKI increases the risk of perioperative mortality to 14%, and that rate is doubled for those requiring dialysis.[27,31]

Within the first 24 to 48 hours, the CPB-associated SIRS response improves, and loss of fluid to the extravascular space secondary to capillary leak will reverse. Oncotic pressure will draw fluid into the intravascular space, and the total body fluid volume will begin to decrease as urine output increases. In some cases, urine output alone is insufficient to remove the excess fluid. CPB can both activate the renin–angiotensin–aldosterone system and stimulate antidiuretic hormone release, both reducing fluid excretion. After the volume loading phase, when managing preload is no longer a concern, typically on the first or second postoperative day, the patient may be started on furosemide or other loop diuretic to aid in volume unloading.

GASTROINTESTINAL

Enteral feeding of the post-CABG patient should be done as soon as it is safe. For patients extubated immediately postoperatively, liquids and then solid food are started on postoperative day 1. For patients who require longer periods of mechanical ventilation, adequate caloric intake is ensured with an orogastric or nasogastric tube placed at the time of surgery. For longer-term enteral nutrition, a soft Dobhoff feeding tube should be inserted.

Gastrointestinal complications occur in 1% to 3% of CABG patients, and, although rare, they increase morbidity and mortality. The most common ones include paralytic ileus (gastric, small bowel, or colonic in origin), upper gastrointestinal bleeding, mesenteric ischemia attributed to diffuse hypoperfusion or acute vascular occlusion, and acute acalculous cholecystitis.

Paralytic ileus of the small bowel or colon may present with abdominal cramping, distension, nausea with bilious emesis, and obstipation. Its cause in the post-CABG patient is usually secondary to the use of opioid analgesics; however, CPB-associated SIRS may play a role. Treatment is largely supportive and requires bowel rest; discontinuation of opioid medications; and maintenance of adequate electrolyte levels, intravenous hydration, and early mobilization. Nasogastric decompression is indicated in the setting of persistent nausea and emesis and should be maintained until evidence of bowel function returns.[32–34]

Upper gastrointestinal bleeding may occur from previously undiagnosed gastroduodenal lesions, stress ulcers, or diffuse gastritis secondary to hypoperfusion. Epigastric pain associated with nausea and bloody or "coffee-ground" emesis should immediately prompt further investigation with esophagogastroduodenoscopy EGD. Other findings include melena and increasing blood urea nitrogen (BUN) with a normal serum creatinine with decreasing serum hemoglobin. In all high-risk patients postoperatively, the use of acid-reducing medications is initiated to reduce the incidence of bleeding caused by stress gastritis.[35–37]

Mesenteric ischemia can be a life-threatening disease that requires urgent work-up. In post-CABG patients, especially those suffering from decreased CO, systemic hypoperfusion may lead to diffuse ischemia. This may be exacerbated in patients with known mesenteric arterial occlusive disease. Presenting symptoms may include vague abdominal pain, abdominal distension, obstipation, or hematochezia, as the endothelium necroses and begins to slough. Acute thrombosis or embolism to a major mesenteric vessel may also produce ischemia. In this case, the onset of pain may be more acute and intense with a patient in more distress than clinical examination would indicate. In both cases, elevations of white blood cell count and serum lactic acid occur as the ischemic bowel transitions to anaerobic metabolism. In a hemodynamically stable patient, a suspicion for mesenteric ischemia should be worked up with computed tomography (CT) angiography. In a rapidly deteriorating patient with a high suspicion for mesenteric ischemia, surgical exploration of the abdomen, possibly with on-table mesenteric angiography and bowel resection, should be planned.

Acalculous cholecystitis is a classic disease of the ICU patient with poor CO and compromised foregut perfusion. Symptoms may include acute onset of right upper quadrant pain with tenderness, fever, rigors, nausea, and emesis. Laboratory studies may be normal or demonstrate a new leukocytosis and hyperbilirubinemia or mild transaminitis. Diagnosis is usually made with right upper quadrant abdominal sonography, specifically looking for thickening of the gallbladder wall, pericholecystic fluid, and usually the absence of gallstones. Patients with acalculous cholecystitis may be treated with antibiotics alone. If the patient begins to clinically deteriorate, and fails nonoperative management, the placement of a percutaneous cholecystostomy tube will usually treat the obstruction without the need for further immediate surgical intervention.[38,39]

NEUROLOGIC

The post-CABG patient is at significant risk for neurologic insults. Clinically significant postoperative CVA following CABG are estimated at 1% to 2%. Risk factors include increasing age, diabetes, previous CVA, carotid artery occlusive disease, significantly calcified aorta, aortic or mitral valve, prolonged CPB time, and AF.[40,41]

CVA can be divided grossly into embolic or hemorrhagic stroke, global hypoperfusion, or hypoxemia. Clinically evident strokes are usually identified after the patient is wakened from anesthesia and a full neurologic examination is completed. Inability to fully regain consciousness once sedation is weaned, hemiplegia or other lateralizing deficits, dysarthria, and visual field abnormalities may be apparent. Immediate noncontrast CT of the head should be obtained in any patient for whom suspicion for CVA exists.

Confusion and agitation are also common neurologic disturbances that occur in the postoperative setting. Although gross agitation is usually clear to all, subtle signs of confusion may be apparent only to a patient's family or nurse who cares for the patient from day to day. A mental status examination should be performed to assess the patient's orientation. If the patient is a threat to himself or others, emergency sedation or 1:1 observation may be indicated.

In all cases, a full assessment of the potential causes of the change in mental status is performed. Etiologies of confusion include narcotic medications, CVA, hypoxemia or hypercapnia, alcohol withdrawal, metabolic derangements such as hypoglycemia, elevated BUN, ammonia or acidosis, and seizure activity. Treatment is aimed at correction of the underlying cause. When none can be reliably identified, noncontrast head CT and/or electroencephalogram may be required. Neurology consultation is always obtained.

REFERENCES

1. Rogers WJ, Coggin CJ, Gersh BJ, et al. Ten-year follow-up of quality of life in patients randomized to receive medical therapy or coronary artery bypass graft surgery. The Coronary Artery Surgery Study (CASS). *Circulation.* 1990;82(5):1647-1658.

2. Takaro T, Hultgren HN, Lipton MJ, et al. The VA cooperative randomized study of surgery for coronary arterial occlusive disease II. Subgroup with significant left main lesions. *Circulation.* 1976;54 (6 suppl):III107-III117.

3. Williams DO, Vasaiwala SC, Boden WE. Is optimal medical therapy "optimal therapy" for multivessel coronary artery disease? Optimal management of multivessel coronary artery disease. *Circulation.* 2010;122(10):943-945.

4. Ariano RE, Zhanel GG. Antimicrobial prophylaxis in coronary bypass surgery: a critical appraisal. *DICP.* 1991;25(5):478-484.

5. Vuorisalo S, Pokela R, Syrjala H. Comparison of vancomycin and cefuroxime for infection prophylaxis in coronary artery bypass surgery. *Infect Control Hosp Epidemiol.* 1998;19(4):234-239.

6. Bojar RM. *Manual of Perioperative Care in Adult Cardiac Surgery.* 5th ed. Malden, MA: Wiley-Blackwell; 2011.

7. Nybo M, Madsen JS. Serious anaphylactic reactions due to protamine sulfate: a systematic literature review. *Basic Clin Pharmacol Toxicol.* 2008;103(2):192-196.

8. Reynolds L, Beckmann J, Kurz A. Perioperative complications of hypothermia. *Best Pract Res Clin Anaesthesiol.* 2008;22(4):645-657.

9. Hillis LD, Smith PK, Anderson JL, et al. 2011 ACCF/AHA guideline for coronary artery bypass graft surgery. A report of the American College of Cardiology Foundation/American Heart Association Task Force on Practice Guidelines. Developed in collaboration with the American Association for Thoracic Surgery, Society of Cardiovascular Anesthesiologists, and Society of Thoracic Surgeons. *J Am Coll Cardiol.* 2011;58(24):e123-e210.

10. Cleveland JC Jr, Shroyer AL, Chen AY, et al. Off-pump coronary artery bypass grafting decreases risk-adjusted mortality and morbidity. *Ann Thorac Surg.* 2001;72(4):1282-1288; discussion 1288-1289.

11. Puskas JD, Edwards FH, Pappas PA, et al. Off-pump techniques benefit men and women and narrow the disparity in mortality after coronary bypass grafting. *Ann Thorac Surg.* 2007;84(5):1447-1454; discussion 1454-1456.

12. Puskas JD, Kilgo PD, Kutner M, Pusca SV, Lattouf O, Guyton RA. Off-pump techniques disproportionately benefit women and narrow the gender disparity in outcomes after coronary artery bypass surgery. *Circulation.* 2007;116(11 suppl):I192-I199.

13. Puskas JD, Thourani VH, Kilgo P, et al. Off-pump coronary artery bypass disproportionately benefits high-risk patients. *Ann Thorac Surg.* 2009;88(4):1142-1147.

14. Raja SG, Dreyfus GD. Current status of off-pump coronary artery bypass surgery. *Asian Cardiovasc Thorac Ann.* 2008;16(2):164-178.

15. Mathew JP, Fontes ML, Tudor IC, et al. A multicenter risk index for atrial fibrillation after cardiac surgery. *JAMA.* 2004;291(14):1720-1729.

16. Zacharias A, Schwann TA, Riordan CJ, Durham SJ, Shah AS, Habib RH. Obesity and risk of new-onset atrial fibrillation after cardiac surgery. *Circulation.* 2005;112(21):3247-3255.

17. Frendl G, Sodickson AC, Chung MK, et al. 2014 AATS guidelines for the prevention and management of perioperative atrial fibrillation and flutter for thoracic surgical procedures. *J Thorac Cardiovasc Surg.* 2014;148(3):e153-e193.

18. January CT, Wann LS, Alpert JS, et al. 2014 AHA/ACC/HRS guideline for the management of patients with atrial fibrillation: a report of the American College of Cardiology/American Heart Association Task Force on Practice Guidelines and the Heart Rhythm Society. *J Am Coll Cardiol.* 2014;64(21):e1-e76.

19. Andrews TC, Reimold SC, Berlin JA, Antman EM. Prevention of supraventricular arrhythmias after coronary artery bypass surgery. A meta-analysis of randomized control trials. *Circulation.* 1991;84 (5 suppl):III236-III244.

20. Dunning J, Nagarajan DV, Amanullah M, Nouraei S. What is the optimal anticoagulation management of patients post-cardiac surgery who go into atrial fibrillation? *Interact Cardiovasc Thorac Surg.* 2004;3(3):503-509.

21. O'Leary JP, Tabuenca A, Capote LR. *The Physiologic Basis of Surgery.* 4th ed. Philadelphia, PA: Wolters Kluwer Health/Lippincott Williams & Wilkins; 2008.

22. De Wet CJ, Affleck DG, Jacobsohn E, et al. Inhaled prostacyclin is safe, effective, and affordable in patients with pulmonary hypertension, right heart dysfunction, and refractory hypoxemia after cardiothoracic surgery. *J Thorac Cardiovasc Surg.* 2004;127(4):1058-1067.

23. Oz MC, Ardehali A. Collective review: perioperative uses of inhaled nitric oxide in adults. *Heart Surg Forum.* 2004;7(6):E584-E589.

24. Karthik S, Grayson AD, McCarron EE, Pullan DM, Desmond MJ. Reexploration for bleeding after coronary artery bypass surgery: risk factors, outcomes, and the effect of time delay. *Ann Thorac Surg.* 2004;78(2):527-534; discussion 534.

25. Sellman M, Intonti MA, Ivert T. Reoperations for bleeding after coronary artery bypass procedures during 25 years. *Eur J Cardiothorac Surg.* 1997;11(3):521-527.

26. Gunter P. Practice guidelines for blood component therapy. *Anesthesiology.* 1996;85(5):1219-1220.

27. Swaminathan M, Shaw AD, Phillips-Bute BG, et al. Trends in acute renal failure associated with coronary artery bypass graft surgery in the United States. *Crit Care Med.* 2007;35(10):2286-2291.

28. Fremes SE, Wong BI, Lee E, et al. Metaanalysis of prophylactic drug treatment in the prevention of postoperative bleeding. *Ann Thorac Surg.* 1994;58(6):1580-1588.

29. Herlihy JP, Koch SM, Jackson R, Nora H. Course of weaning from prolonged mechanical ventilation after cardiac surgery. *Tex Heart Inst J.* 2006;33(2):122-129.

30. Pappalardo F, Franco A, Landoni G, Cardano P, Zangrillo A, Alfieri O. Long-term outcome and quality of life of patients requiring prolonged mechanical ventilation after cardiac surgery. *Eur J Cardiothorac Surg.* 2004;25(4):548-552.

31. Conlon PJ, Stafford-Smith M, White WD, et al. Acute renal failure following cardiac surgery. *Nephrol Dial Transplant.* 1999;14(5):1158-1162.

32. Christenson JT, Schmuziger M, Maurice J, Simonet F, Velebit V. Gastrointestinal complications after coronary artery bypass grafting. *J Thorac Cardiovasc Surg.* 1994;108(5):899-906.

33. Krasna MJ, Flancbaum L, Trooskin SZ, et al. Gastrointestinal complications after cardiac surgery. *Surgery.* 1988;104(4):773-780.

34. Saunders MD. Acute colonic pseudo-obstruction. *Best Pract Res Clin Gastroenterol.* 2007;21(4):671-687.

35. Ali T, Harty RF. Stress-induced ulcer bleeding in critically ill patients. *Gastroenterol Clin North Am.* 2009;38(2):245-265.

36. Norton ID, Pokorny CS, Baird DK, Selby WS. Upper gastrointestinal haemorrhage following coronary artery bypass grafting. *Aust N Z J Med.* 1995;25(4):297-301.

37. Steinberg KP. Stress-related mucosal disease in the critically ill patient: risk factors and strategies to prevent stress-related bleeding in the intensive care unit. *Crit Care Med.* 2002;30(6 suppl):S362-S364.

38. Mastoraki A, Kriaras I, Douka E, Geroulanos S. Complications involving gall bladder and biliary tract in cardiovascular surgery. *Hepatogastroenterology.* 2008;55(85):1233-1237.

39. Rady MY, Kodavatiganti R, Ryan T. Perioperative predictors of acute cholecystitis after cardiovascular surgery. *Chest.* 1998;114(1):76-84.

40. Likosky DS, Leavitt BJ, Marrin CA, et al. Intra- and postoperative predictors of stroke after coronary artery bypass grafting. *Ann Thorac Surg.* 2003;76(2):428-434; discussion 435.

41. Newman MF, Mathew JP, Grocott HP, et al. Central nervous system injury associated with cardiac surgery. *Lancet.* 2006;368(9536):694-703.

Patient and Family Information for: CORONARY ARTERY BYPASS SURGERY

BACKGROUND

CABG is a surgical procedure performed for patients who have blockages in the arteries that deliver oxygenated blood to their heart muscle. These blockages are caused by atherosclerosis, which occurs as a result of risk factors: smoking, hypertension, high cholesterol, diabetes mellitus, and family history.

Not all patients require surgery for these blockages; some can be treated with medications and others with minimally invasive procedures called stents. Surgery is recommended for those patients with a blockage in the main artery to their heart (left main artery) or multiple blockages in a patient with diabetes or decreased heart function. Some complex lesions also require surgical bypass.

Patients can be seen as outpatients to schedule their procedure. Others arrive in the hospital with a small or large heart attack, and it is recommended that they have surgery urgently to prevent complete blockage of the heart arteries that would result in a major heart attack and permanent loss of heart muscle function.

PROCEDURE

CABG surgery is performed with the patient asleep under general anesthesia. Most surgeries require between 3 and 6 hours, depending on the number of grafts that need to be placed. Although there are three main arteries to the heart, the branches of these arteries may be large and supply a significant amount of muscle. For that reason, patients may require between 1 and 6 grafts, depending on the number of specific blockages and their specific anatomy.

The basis of the surgery is to use a vessel, or conduit, to bring new blood supply to the heart. The actual lesion itself is not removed. Rather, blood is rerouted from an area of high blood flow (such as the aorta), past the blockage, to an area of lesser blood flow. This procedure is often performed with the patient on a heart–lung machine, or CPB circuit. This device takes over the work of the heart and lungs while the surgeon is performing the operation. At the completion of the surgery, the patient is weaned off the machine, and the heart resumes beating on its own, pumping blood to the lungs and body.

CRITICAL CARE MANAGEMENT

Most patients are brought straight to the ICU after surgery. The first 48 hours are the most critical time after heart surgery. The patient is monitored closely for any changes in their blood pressure, heart rate, and organ function. Once they are awake after anesthesia and strong enough, they are removed from the ventilator and are able to breathe on their own.

In the ICU, the patients are watched closely for any signs of bleeding, irregular heart rates, and organ dysfunction. They are encouraged to deep breathe and cough to keep their lungs expanded. Pain control is very important for this process, and although they initially receive strong intravenous medications, they are slowly transitioned to oral medications as their pain improves. Respiratory therapists work with the patients immediately after arrival and throughout their hospital stay.

Another important part of recovery is mobilizing the patient after surgery. This helps lung function, bowel function, and overall strength. Deconditioning after heart surgery can be severe, and physical therapy is necessary to prevent this. Physical therapists work with all patients from the first day after surgery and continue to help them as they take a few steps, walk in the hallways, climb stairs, and mobilize on their own.

RECOVERY

Most patients are in the ICU for 24 to 48 hours after CABG surgery, barring any complications. The patient is then moved to a step-down monitored room in preparation for discharge. In uncomplicated cases, families can expect their loved ones to return home within 5 to 7 days after surgery.

Basheer Karkabi
Eyal Herzog
Jacob Goldstein

9

Medications Used in the Management of Acute Coronary Syndrome

The pharmacologic management of an acute coronary syndrome (ACS) has evolved dramatically over the past three decades into a heavily evidence-based discipline. Contemporary treatment strategies have become more targeted, focusing on the unique pathophysiologic underpinnings of this disorder. Additionally, new therapeutic approaches are rigorously tested and proven in large clinical trials before becoming standard therapy. As our armamentarium of new therapeutics continues to grow, our diagnostic and management strategies will necessarily change over time. As such, practitioners caring for patients with ACS must become life-long students of this exciting and dynamic field in order to provide the best care for their patients in the years to come.

Appropriate medical therapy is indicated for all patients presenting with or suspected of having ACS. The goals of initial medical therapy are fourfold: to relieve pain, to halt the progression of disease, to reduce morbidity, and to improve survival. Because the term *ACS* encompasses a spectrum of severity with a common pathophysiology, the difficulty in the pharmacologic management comes in determining where in the spectrum a particular patient falls and balancing the risks and benefits in treating that patient to achieve the desired goals.

Once the diagnosis of ACS is established, the patient should quickly be stratified by risk into one of several treatment strategies. Medical therapy should be immediately started in a rational manner to achieve the initial goals of treatment, namely, to interrupt platelet activation/aggregation and thrombus formation and to relieve pain. Patients diagnosed with an ST-segment elevation myocardial infraction (STEMI) should be emergently stratified to primary percutaneous coronary intervention (PCI) or fibrinolytic therapy, whereas those with unstable angina (UA)/ non–ST-segment elevation myocardial infarction (NSTEMI) should be risk stratified into either an early invasive or an initial conservative approach. Regardless of what treatment strategy is initiated, patients should be continuously evaluated for high-risk features of disease, adverse hemodynamic consequences, and treatment failure. Such features often mandate deviation from the initial management strategy to a more aggressive one. Importantly, as a patient transitions from one treatment strategy to another, the pharmacologic approach can vary substantially.

In general, the pharmacologic approach to managing ACS should be prioritized with an emphasis on rapid treatment with medications known to provide morbidity and mortality benefit. Guidelines for treatment are useful; however, they cannot address every possible nuance experienced in clinical practice. Health care providers must have a thorough understanding of their institutional capabilities and preferences, as well as familiarity with the drugs, doses, indications, and side effects in order to provide patients with optimal benefit and minimal harm.

ANTI-ISCHEMIC AND ANALGESIC THERAPY

β-ADRENERGIC BLOCKERS

Rationale: β-Blockers are used to inhibit the actions of catecholamines on the β_1-adrenergic receptors located in the myocardium. Inhibition of these receptors leads to a reduction in myocardial contractility, atrioventricular (AV) node conduction, sinus node rate, and an overall reduction in systolic blood pressure. The net effect of these actions results in a decrease in cardiac work and myocardial oxygen demand. Additionally, β-blockers increase diastolic pressure-time, which may be important in increasing coronary blood flow. In patients with ACS undergoing PCI, a large meta-analysis showed a significant reduction in mortality at 30 days and 6 months for patients who received β-blocker therapy.[1] However, the COMMIT trial failed to demonstrate a mortality benefit with the early use of β-blockers in patients with myocardial infarction.[2] This finding has been attributed to injudicious use of β-blockers in patients with heart failure or other risk factors for cardiogenic shock and has been instructive in the most recent guidelines involving recommendations for β-blocker usage in ACS. In contrast to the early aggressive use of β-blockers for acute myocardial infraction (MI), the CAPRICORN trial demonstrated a reduction in all-cause mortality, cardiovascular mortality, and nonfatal MI with β-blockers when 1959 patients with acute MI and left ventricular (LV) dysfunction were randomized to receive to low-dose carvedilol versus placebo and treated with a more gradual uptitration strategy.[3]

Indications: ACS (without contraindications), stable angina, compensated chronic heart failure.

Dosing: Multiple preparations available including intravenous (IV) and oral, β_1 selective and nonselective, short and long acting (**Table 9.1**).

TABLE 9.1	β-Blockers Used in ACS		
DRUGS	**SELECTIVITY**	**DOSE**	**COMMENT**
Metoprolol tartrate	β_1	50–200 mg twice daily	Often initiated with 12.5–25 mg every 6–8 h
Metoprolol succinate	β_1	12.5–200 mg daily	Short-acting tartrate preferred for ACS; however, mortality benefit shown for stable patients with CHF
Carvedilol	β_1, β_2, α_1	3.125–25 mg twice daily	Started low and titrate up; mortality benefit for LV dysfunction
Bisoprolol	β_1	1.25–5 mg twice daily	
Atenolol	β_1	25–200 mg daily	
Labetalol	β_1, β_2, α_1	200–600 mg twice daily	
Propranolol	β_1, β_2	20–80 mg twice daily	
Esmolol	β_1	50–300 µg/kg/min	

ACS, acute coronary syndrome; CHF, congestive heart failure; LV, left ventricular.

Side effects: Hypotension, bradycardia, AV block, acute exacerbation of heart failure, bronchospasm, paradoxical hypertension (HTN) in setting of active cocaine use.

Contraindications: High-grade AV block, active bronchoconstriction, hypotension, bradycardia, severe LV dysfunction or heart failure (rales, S3 gallop), or in patients with myocardial infarction at high risk for cardiogenic shock (older age, female sex, relative hypotension, high Killip class, reflexive tachycardia).

Recommendations: The acute use of β-blockers in ACS is recommended in all patients without contraindications, especially in patients with ongoing angina and HTN. Short-acting, β_1 selective agents are typically used to minimize side effects and allow for dose titration. The common practice used to be a regimen of metoprolol 5 mg IV, repeated every 5 minutes, up to a total of 15 mg. Oral therapy can be started at metoprolol 25 to 50 mg every 6 hours, or bisoprolol 1.25 mg every 12 hours, and titrated to achieve the desired heart rate or blood pressure. Frequent heart rate and blood pressure checks, continuous electrocardiography (ECG) monitoring, and routine auscultation for rales and bronchospasm should be performed (preferably in an intensive care unit setting). Once stabilized, patients should receive maintenance doses of up to 100 mg metoprolol twice daily or bisoprolol 2.5 to 5 mg twice daily. In patients with LV dysfunction, β-blockers with proven mortality benefit such as bisoprolol, carvedilol, and metoprolol succinate should be utilized for long-term management.

CALCIUM CHANNEL BLOCKERS

Rationale: Calcium channel blockers (CCBs) inhibit myocardial and vascular smooth muscle contraction by reducing transmembrane inward calcium flux. In ACS, CCBs are useful in decreasing myocardial oxygen demand (by decreasing afterload, contractility, and heart rate) and in coronary vasodilatation. Meta-analyses of UA/NSTEMI trials involving CCBs have suggested no overall benefit in death or nonfatal MI.[4] Retrospective studies of verapamil and diltiazem have shown increased mortality in patients with LV dysfunction.[5,6] Additionally, a trial using nifedipine was stopped early because of concern for harm when taken without concomitant β-blockers.[7]

TABLE 9.2	Calcium Channel Blockers Used in ACS		
DRUG	**DOSE**	**DURATION OF ACTION**	**COMMENT**
Nondihydropyridines			
Diltiazem	Immediate release: 30–90 mg every 6 h	Short	Avoid with known or suspected LV dysfunction
	Slow release: 120–360 mg 3 times daily	Long	
Verapamil	Immediate release: 80–160 mg every 8 h	Short	Avoid with known or suspected LV dysfunction
	Slow release: 120–480 mg daily	Long	
Dihydropyridines			
Amlodipine	5–10 mg daily	Long	
Felodipine	5–10 mg daily	Long	
Nisoldipine	20–40 mg daily	Short	

ACS, acute coronary syndrome; LV, left ventricular.

Indications: In ACS, considered second-line therapy in β-blocker-intolerant patients for relief of angina, blood pressure control, and rate control of supraventricular arrhythmias. CCBs are considered adjuncts to β-blockers and nitrates for the relief of ischemic symptoms. They are generally the preferred treatment for patients with cocaine-induced myocardial ischemia or variant angina.

Dosing: Multiple preparations both IV and oral, short and long acting (**Table 9.2**).

Side effects: Hypotension, bradycardia, myocardial depression (diltiazem and verapamil), flushing, edema, headache.

Contraindications: Hypotension, AV conduction abnormalities, LV dysfunction or congestive heart failure (CHF) (especially diltiazem and verapamil).

TABLE 9.3	Nitrate Preparations Used in ACS		
COMPOUND	**ROUTE**	**DOSE**	**DURATION OF EFFECT**
Nitroglycerin	Sublingual tablets	0.3–0.6 up to 1.5 mg	1 to 7 min
	Spray	0.4 mg as needed	Similar to sublingual tablets, however, has a longer shelf life
	Transdermal	0.2–0.8 mg/h every 12 h	8 to 12 h with intermittent therapy; efficacy improved with 12 h off period
	Intravenous	5–200 µg/min	Tolerance in 7 to 8 h
Isosorbide dinitrate	Oral	5–80 mg, every 8–12 h	Up to 8 h
	Oral, slow release	40 mg, every 12–24 h	Up to 8 h
Isosorbide mononitrate	Oral	20 mg twice daily	12 to 24 h
	Oral, slow release	60–240 mg daily	

ACS, acute coronary syndrome.

Recommendations: In patients with contraindications to β-blockers or in those whom β-blockers and nitrates have failed to achieve relief of ischemia or rate control with supraventricular arrhythmias, CCBs can be used to further reduce blood pressure and chest pain. Caution should be exercised when CCBs and β-blockers are used concomitantly because of depressed AV nodal conduction. Diltiazem and verapamil should be avoided in patients with LV dysfunction. Use of dihydropyridines such as amlodipine and felodipine appear to be safe with LV dysfunction, although their benefit remains undefined in the treatment of ACS; nifedipine should be avoided altogether.

NITRATES

Rationale: Despite a paucity of rigorous clinical trial data, nitrates continue to remain important in the treatment of HTN and chest pain in patients with ACS. Nitrates cause a reduction of myocardial oxygen demand while enhancing myocardial oxygen delivery and affect both peripheral and coronary vascular beds. Nitroglycerin (NTG) increases venous capacitance, thereby decreasing preload and reducing ventricular wall tension. Furthermore, NTG promotes the dilation of the coronary arteries, and possibly has a mild inhibitory effect on platelet aggregation (although the clinical significance of this is not known).

Indications: Angina, HTN, CHF, variant angina.

Dosing: NTG is available in multiple preparations including sublingual tablets and spray, transdermal, and intravenously (**Table 9.3**).

Side effects: Headaches, hypotension, and tachyphylaxis are common with NTG usage.

Contraindications: NTG is contraindicated after the use of phosphodiesterase inhibitors used for the treatment of erectile dysfunction such as sildenafil, tadalafil, and vardenafil as concomitant use can induce profound hypotension. Additionally, nitrates should be avoided in patients suspected of having a right ventricular infarct because its usage can result in severe hypotension even with low doses.

Recommendations: NTG use is typically initiated with three 0.4-mg sublingual NTG tablets taken 5 minutes apart with the concomitant administration of either an oral or IV β-blocker. For patients with ongoing chest pain, HTN, or decompensated heart failure, it is appropriate to switch to IV NTG. This is given at 10 µg/min through continuous infusion via nonabsorbing tubing and can be up titrated by 10 µg/min every 3 to 5 minutes to achieve symptomatic relief or desired blood pressure response. Although there is no published maximal ceiling dose, 200 µg/min is typically used because there is unlikely to be measurable clinical benefit beyond this rate. For blood pressure titrations, NTG should be titrated to less than 110 mm Hg in previously normotensive patients or to greater than 25% lower than the starting Mean Arterial Pressure (MAP) in hypertensive patients. NTG should generally be avoided in patients with starting systolic blood pressures of less than 90 mm Hg, in patients with marked bradycardia or tachycardia, or in patients who present with systolic blood pressures 30 mm Hg or more below their baseline. After a patient has been stable or chest pain free for 12 to 24 hours, it is prudent to attempt weaning IV NTG or transitioning to an oral preparation if still indicated.

MORPHINE

Rationale: Although there is a lack of randomized clinical trials, morphine sulfate provides analgesic and anxiolytic effects that might partially counteract the adrenergic drive associated with ACS. Additionally, it causes mild venodilation, a modest reduction in heart rate via increased vagal tone, and decreased blood pressure, which lowers myocardial oxygen demand.

Dosing: Morphine sulfate 1 to 5 mg IV PRN.

Side effects: Nausea, vomiting, respiratory depression, hypotension.

Recommendations: Morphine should be considered for anginal relief in patients not sufficiently controlled with nitrates, β-blockers, or CCBs and is often given in preparation for further invasive testing.

ANCILLARY THERAPIES

ANGIOTENSIN-CONVERTING ENZYME INHIBITORS AND ANGIOTENSIN II RECEPTOR BLOCKERS

Rationale: Inhibition of the renin–angiotensin–aldosterone system has salutary effects on blood pressure, afterload reduction, and LV remodeling associated with myocardial infarction

(MI)-induced LV dysfunction. Angiotensin-converting-enzyme (ACE) inhibitors have a proven track record in multiple clinical trials for decreasing mortality, particularly when started within 24 hours to 16 days after myocardial infarction in patients with depressed ejection fractions, heart failure, and diabetes mellitus.[8–12] Patients with higher risk gained greater benefit. Additionally, the VALIANT trial demonstrated that valsartan was as effective as captopril in the reduction of death following MI in patients with demonstrable LV dysfunction or clinical heart failure.[13] Therefore, in addition to their proven clinical role in stable CHF, angiotensin receptor blockers (ARBs) appear to also offer benefit in the ACS setting.

Indications: ACS with concurrent pulmonary congestion or LVEF ≤ 40%, in absence of contraindications. ARBs should be given to patients intolerant of ACE inhibitors.

Dosing: Multiple preparations both short and long acting. IV forms are not recommended for ACS (**Table 9.4**).

Side effects: Hypotension, hyperkalemia, angioedema and cough (ACE inhibitors).

Contraindications: Hemodynamic instability, renal failure, hyperkalemia.

Recommendations: Typically initiated early, within the first 24 hours of hospital stay, in patients without contraindications. Use of short-acting formulations (ie, captopril 6.25 mg q8h) allows for dose titration. Once stable, once-daily dosing can be initiated. IV ACE inhibitors should be avoided in the management of ACS.

ALDOSTERONE RECEPTOR ANTAGONISTS

Rationale: Aldosterone receptor antagonists have been shown to prevent deleterious ventricular remodeling after acute MI, decrease the rate of death, and reduce hospitalizations in patients with chronic severe heart failure. The EPHESUS trial further expanded the beneficial role in renin–angiotensin–aldosterone blockade by demonstrating a reduction in morbidity and mortality for patients presenting with acute MI complicated by heart failure and LV dysfunction (LVEF ≤ 40%) when treated with eplerenone.[14]

Indications: ACS with concurrent pulmonary congestion or LVEF ≤ 40%, in absence of contraindications.

Dosing: Eplerenone 25 mg daily with gradual uptitration to a maximum of 50 mg daily. Frequent monitoring of electrolytes, especially potassium and creatinine, is essential.

Side effects: Hypotension, hyperkalemia, renal dysfunction.

Contraindications: Hemodynamic instability, renal failure, hyperkalemia.

Recommendations: Given the totality of evidence to date, ACE inhibitors and ARBs remain preferred first-line therapy agents for renin–angiotensin–aldosterone blockade for patients with

TABLE 9.4	ACE Inhibitors and ARBs Used in ACS			
ACE INHIBITORS				
Drug	*Starting dose*	*Typical dose*	*Maximum dose*	*Comments*
Benazepril	10 mg	20–40 mg	80 mg	May use bid dosing
Captopril	6.25–12 mg bid–tid	25–50 mg bid–tid	450 mg daily	Target dose in HF: 50 mg tid
Enalapril	2.5–5 mg daily–bid	10–40 mg	40 mg	Target dose in HF: 10 mg bid
Fosinopril	10 mg	20–40 mg	80 mg	
Lisinopril	2.5–5 mg	10–40 mg	80 mg	Target dose in HF: 20 mg daily
Moexipril	7.5 mg	7.5–30 mg	30 mg	
Perindopril	4 mg	4–8 mg	16 mg	
Quinapril	10 mg	20–80 mg	80 mg	Target dose in HF: 20 mg daily
Ramipril	2.5 mg	2.5–20 mg	20 mg	
Trandolapril	1 mg	2–4 mg	8 mg	Reduce dose in hepatic dysfunction
ARBs				
Candesartan	8–16 mg	16–32 mg	32 mg	
Eprosartan	600 mg	600–800 mg	800 mg	
Irbesartan	75–150 mg	150–300 mg	300 mg	
Losartan	25–50 mg	50–100 mg	100 mg	Reduce dose in hepatic dysfunction
Valsartan	20 mg	160 mg	320 mg	
Olmesartan	20 mg	20–40 mg	40 mg	
Telmisartan	20–40 mg	40–80 mg	80 mg	

ACE, angiotensin-converting-enzyme; ACS, acute coronary syndrome; ARBs, angiotensin receptor blocker; HF, heart failure.

ACS and concurrent LV dysfunction. However, the addition of an aldosterone receptor blocker such as eplerenone may be considered in patients already receiving optimal medical treatment in the absence of contraindications.

HMG-COA REDUCTASE INHIBITORS (STATINS)

Rationale: Statins have been widely studied both in primary and secondary prevention for chronic coronary artery disease (CAD). The "pleiotropic" effects of statins include not only their well-established ability to lower the levels of low-density lipoprotein (LDL), but also their anti-inflammatory, antioxidant, and antithrombotic properties. The first clinical trial to demonstrate benefit of statins given early (24 to 96 hours) after ACS was MIRACL study—compared with placebo, atorvastatin given for 16 weeks reduced the composite end point of death, nonfatal MI, cardiac arrest with resuscitation, or recurrent symptomatic myocardial ischemia with objective evidence and requiring emergency rehospitalization by 16% (95% CI: 0.7 to 1.0, $P = 0.048$).[15] Also in the setting of ACS, PROVE IT-TIMI 22 showed a significant 16% reduction in the hazard ratio for death, MI, UA, revascularization and stroke in patients treated with intensive lipid-lowering therapy (atorvastatin 80 mg) compared with standard therapy (pravastatin 40 mg) and followed for 18 to 36 months.[16]

Indications: STEMI and UA/NSTEMI.

Dosing: Multiple agents; however, atorvastatin was the most studied for ACS. They are typically given at 40 to 80 mg po daily (**Table 9.5**).

Side effects: Dyspepsia, rash/pruritis, myalgias, hepatotoxicity, rhabdomyolysis (rare).

Contraindications: Caution should be exercised when used with cytochrome P450 inhibitors and in the setting of elevated transaminases.

Recommendations: Statins at high doses should be considered early in the course of patients presenting with ACS, irrespective of the baseline LDL-cholesterol levels. Statins should be considered standard therapy for secondary prevention in the absence of contraindications.

ANTIPLATELET MEDICATIONS

ASPIRIN (ASA)

Rationale: Aspirin is a potent, irreversible platelet COX-1 inhibitor that inhibits the production of thromboxane A_2 and results in

TABLE 9.5	Statins Used in ACS
DRUG	**DOSE**
Atorvastatin	10–80 mg daily
Fluvastatin	20–80 mg daily
Lovastatin	10–80 mg daily
Pravastatin	10–80 mg daily
Rosuvastatin	5–40 mg daily
Simvastatin	10–80 mg daily

decreased platelet aggregation at the site of intimal injury and thrombus formation. Although it is a relatively weak inhibitor of overall platelet aggregation, ASA confers a significant reduction in mortality.[17–21]

Indications: ACS (diagnosed or suspected), chronic CAD.

Dosing: Initial dosing should be 162 to 325 mg given orally as a nonenteric coated, chewable tablet to allow for rapid buccal absorption. If active nausea or vomiting, a 300-mg rectal suppository should be promptly administered. The maintenance dose of ASA is conventionally the lowest available dose, which ranges from 75 to 100 mg/d in different countries (81 mg/d in North America).

Side effects: Nausea, vomiting, dyspepsia, gastrointestinal (GI)/genitourinary (GU) bleeding.

Contraindications: The only contraindication is patients with true ASA allergy (anaphylaxis, hives, nasal polyps, bronchospasm). Such patients should be given a thienopyridine such as clopidogrel, with strong consideration given for ASA desensitization treatment.

Recommendations: Aspirin 325 mg should be administered to all persons as soon as ACS is diagnosed or suspected, typically in the ambulance or the emergency department. In general, therapy with ASA should be continued indefinitely after the first presentation with ACS at a low dose of 75 to 81 mg daily.

P2Y$_{12}$ ADENOSINE DIPHOSPHATE RECEPTOR INHIBITORS

P2Y$_{12}$ inhibitors are inhibitors of adenosine diphosphate (ADP)-induced platelet aggregation and dual antiplatelet therapy (DAPT) of P2Y$_{12}$ inhibitors (thienopyridines and nonthienopyridines) along with ASA have become a cornerstone in the pharmacologic management of patients with ACSs and after coronary stent placement. The first thienopyridine introduced and used after coronary stenting was ticlopidine. Since the introduction of other agents of this group, ticlopidine use has been largely decreased mainly due to unfavorable side-effect profile including GI effects, neutropenia, and thrombotic thrombocytopenic purpura (TTP) in addition to long onset of action and frequent dosing. Therefore, ticlopidine is no longer recommended in the treatment of ACS. During the last two decades, another three oral P2Y$_{12}$ inhibitors have received the Food and Drug Administration (FDA) approval in the United States for use in ACS: clopidogrel, prasugrel, ticagrelor, and another IV agent introduced recently, cangrelor. Each of these drugs work by inhibiting the P2Y$_{12}$ ADP receptor on platelets, with ticagrelor being the only oral drug with reversible inhibition. They differ importantly with respect to their onset of action, side-effect profile, and overall potency. Evidence for the beneficial use of P2Y$_{12}$ inhibitors comes from multiple, large-scale randomized trials. Because DAPT with P2Y$_{12}$ inhibitors exert more robust platelet inhibition than ASA alone, the risk of subsequent bleeding is higher and therefore appropriate P2Y$_{12}$ inhibitors selection should be tailored to a patient's individual bleeding risk.

Clopidogrel

Rationale: Clopidogrel is an irreversible P2Y$_{12}$ receptor inhibitor, the most studied thienopyridine, and the most used until the introduction of ticagrelor. As the maximal therapeutic platelet inhibition of clopidogrel takes 3 to 7 days to reach, the administration of a loading dose of 300 to 600 mg, resulting in substantial inhibition within approximately 2 hours, has been used in ACS studies. In the CURE trial, patients with UA or NSTEMI were found to have a lower rate of cardiovascular death, nonfatal MI, or stroke when treated with ASA and clopidogrel than ASA alone (9.3% vs 11.4%, $P < 0.001$); however, this came at the expense of major bleeding, particularly in patients who subsequently underwent coronary artery bypass graft (CABG).[22] In STEMI patients, the COMMIT-CCS-2 study demonstrated a significant reduction in the composite end point of death, reinfarction, and stroke (9.2% clopidogrel vs 10.1% placebo, $P = 0.002$) in 45,852 patients treated with clopidogrel, 93% of whom had ST elevation.[23] The addition of clopidogrel to fibrinolytic therapy was proven beneficial in the CLARITY-TIMI 28 trial where 3491 patients with STEMI had a significant reduction in occluded infarct artery on angiography, death, or recurrent MI when treated with clopidogrel (15% clopidogrel vs 21.7% placebo, $P < 0.001$).[24] This was felt to be driven by the prevention of infarct-related reocclusion. Randomized controlled trials of clopidogrel versus placebo, added to ASA, in primary PCI for patients with STEMI has not been conducted and its efficacy in that setting has been assumed on the basis of the results of studies of patients with ACS undergoing elective PCI and patients with STEMI treated with fibrinolysis before PCI. On this background, the HORIZONS-AMI trial evaluated two loading doses, 600 versus 300 mg, of clopidogrel in STEMI patients undergoing primary PCI. The higher loading dose resulted in 28% reduction of 30 days' composite of mortality, reinfarction, and stent thrombosis without significantly increasing the rate of major bleeding.[25] The larger CURRENT-OASIS 7 trial has evaluated high dose of clopidogrel, 600 mg loading and 150 mg daily for a week with regular 75-mg daily dose thereafter, to regular loading and maintenance dose among 25,086 patients with ACS. A prespecified analysis of 17,263 individuals who underwent PCI revealed a reduction of cardiovascular events at 30 days, especially to be noticed a 46% reduction in the occurrence definite stent thrombosis with the high-dose regimen of clopidogrel compared with the regular dose.[26]

Indications: STEMI, UA/NSTEMI, alternative to ASA in patients with true ASA intolerance.

Dosing: Loading dose 300 to 600 mg followed by 75 mg daily. When combined with fibrinolytics, a 300-mg loading dose should be used for patients under 75 years of age and no loading dose for patients over 75 years of age.

Side effects: Bleeding, GI intolerance, rash, TTP (rare).

Contraindications: High risk for intracranial/GI/GU bleeding, anticipated CABG within 5 days, high suspicion for diminished clopidogrel response (eg, CYP2C19 variant, stent thrombosis).

Special note on clopidogrel responsiveness: It has become increasingly recognized that there is considerable interindividual variability in platelet inhibition from clopidogrel, often leading to adverse clinical events. This is thought to be primarily related to genetic polymorphisms involving the metabolism of clopidogrel and other drugs by the hepatic CYP450 system, specifically the CYP2C19 isoenzyme, and has led to an FDA warning for the use of clopidogrel. Although genetic and platelet function testing are available, routine use is not specifically recommended at this time. However, patients deemed to be at moderate to high risk (previous history of stent thrombosis, recurrent ischemic events, planned complex interventions) should be considered for platelet function testing or alternative antiplatelet strategies including prasugrel or ticagrelor, two agents that do not appear to have these limitations.

Recommendations: Clopidogrel with loading dose of 300 to 600 mg followed by 75 mg daily alongside with ASA is indicated early in the treatment of UA/NSTEMI (both early invasive and initial conservative strategy), although it is reasonable to use ticagrelor in preference to clopidogrel in patients who are treated with an early invasive strategy. Clopidogrel should be continued for up to 12 months, with treatment beyond that time considered in specific patients. Halting clopidogrel and DAPT may be required in some clinical circumstances earlier than 12 months after the index event, such as with the occurrence of bleeding, the need for noncardiac surgery or if anticoagulant therapy for atrial fibrillation becomes indicated. With no clear answers from randomized controlled trials, it is important to utilize clinical judgment as to the length of DAPT duration for the scenarios mentioned here, taking into consideration the bleeding risk on the one hand and the risk of stent thrombosis on the other (based on clinical and anatomic findings of each patient and the stent type).

Because of the increased bleeding associated with CABG, clopidogrel should be held for at least 5 days and up to 7 days before elective CABG. In patients with a high likelihood of needing bypass, some centers opt to delay clopidogrel loading until coronary anatomy has been defined if angiography can be done in a timely manner. If a loading dose is given and a patient is subsequently found to need urgent surgical revascularization, centers with experienced surgeons can often operate with an acceptable incremental bleeding risk.

For patients with STEMI, when fibrinolysis is planned, clopidogrel alongside with ASA is recommended with a 300-mg loading dose for patients <75 years. However, no loading dose is currently recommended for patients ≥75 years. For patients planned for primary PCI, a loading dose of 600 mg with 75 mg daily thereafter is recommended, but it is reasonable to use ticagrelor or prasugrel in preference to clopidogrel in this setting.

Prasugrel

Rationale: Prasugrel is a newer irreversible $P2Y_{12}$ ADP receptor inhibitor that offers distinct advantages over clopidogrel. Like clopidogrel, prasugrel is a pro-drug that requires hepatic metabolism to its active metabolite. However, its metabolism is not affected by the CYP2C19 allele and does not appear to have the same interpatient variability found with clopidogrel. Additionally, its pharmacodynamic properties result in more rapid and consistent platelet inhibition when compared with clopidogrel. The TRITON-TIMI 38 study is the largest trial to date for prasugrel evaluation, comparing it to clopidogrel in patients with ACS scheduled to undergo PCI. Prasugrel was found to significantly reduce the combined rates of death, nonfatal MI, and stroke when compared with clopidogrel (9.9% prasugrel vs 12.1% clopidogrel, $P < 0.001$). Additionally, significant reductions in MI, urgent target vessel revascularization, and stent thrombosis were shown. However, the benefit of prasugrel came at the expense of significantly increased major bleeding, including fatal bleeding.[27] Patients with prior stroke or transient ischemic attack (TIA) had worse outcome with prasugrel, and bleeding rates were noted to be particularly high in patients with body weight <60 kg or age >75 years.

Indications: STEMI when fibrinolysis is not planned and UA/NSTEMI.

Dosing: Loading dose of 60 mg followed by 10 mg daily.

Side effects: Bleeding.

Contraindications: Age ≥75 years, body weight <60 kg (or use maintenance dose of 5 mg daily), history of stroke/TIA, high risk for intracranial/GI/GU bleeding, active bleeding, CABG planned within 5 to 7 days.

Recommendations: Prasugrel is currently recommended for the treatment of STEMI in patients undergoing primary PCI. For patients undergoing nonprimary PCI, prasugrel should not be given if the patient has received a fibrinolytic. For UA/NSTEMI, prasugrel is a reasonable alternative thienopyridine in patients without the aforementioned contraindications and in whom clopidogrel would otherwise be indicated, especially after coronary stent placement. It must be noted that in TRITON-TIMI 38, patients with UA/NSTEMI treated with prasugrel were given the loading dose only *after* coronary anatomy was defined. Injudicious upstream loading in patients at high risk for surgical disease before knowledge of coronary anatomy may lead to excessive bleeding. This drawback and the introduction of ticagrelor have turned prasugrel to be less preferred in the setting of UA/NSTEMI. Additionally, prasugrel has not been studied in the early conservative management strategy.

Ticagrelor

Rationale: Ticagrelor is a nonthienopyridine reversible $P2Y_{12}$ ADP receptor inhibitor. Like prasugrel, it offers several potential advantages over clopidogrel, namely, it provides more rapid and consistent platelet inhibition. Additionally, because it is a reversible inhibitor, its antiplatelet effects dissipate more rapidly than other thienopyridines. The PLATO trial compared ticagrelor with clopidogrel in the treatment of patients presenting with ACS both with and without STEMI ($n = 18,624$). Ticagrelor was associated with a significant reduction in the primary composite end point of death, MI, and stroke compared with clopidogrel (9.8% vs 11.7%, $P < 0.001$). There was no significant difference in the rates of major bleeding between the two groups; however, the ticagrelor group did have a higher incidence of major bleeding not related to CABG, including more intracranial bleeding.[28] A substudy of PLATO trial including only patients planned for invasive strategy has reached the same results.[29] The PEGASUS-TIMI 54 trial examined the benefit and safety of extended treatment with ticagrelor among patients with previous MI. Comparing two doses of ticagrelor, 90 mg twice daily and 60 mg twice daily, with placebo for a median follow-up of 33 months revealed a significant reduction in the composite end point of cardiovascular death, MI, or stroke with the expense of increased risk of bleeding.[30]

Indications: STEMI when fibrinolysis is not planned and UA/NSTEMI (both early invasive or initial conservative strategy).

Dosing: Initial loading dose of 180 mg followed by 90 mg twice daily.

Side effects: Bleeding, dyspnea, ventricular pauses.

Contraindications: High risk for intracranial/GI/GU bleeding, active bleeding.

Recommendations: Ticagrelor is indicated in STEMI when percutaneous intervention is planned. As it has not been studied in conjunction with fibrinolytic agents, ticagrelor is not indicated when these agents are planned to be given or immediately after being given as in rescue PCI—in these circumstance clopidogrel is more appropriate. Ticagrelor is indicated for the treatment of UA/NSTEMI whether they planned for invasive strategy or

conservative/medical management. Particularly advantageous is ticagrelor's reversible pharmacokinetic properties and short half-life, which make upstream loading possible irrespective of the patient's risk for surgical CAD.

Cangrelor

Rationale: Cangrelor is an IV nonthienopyridine blocker of the ADP activated $P2Y_{12}$ receptor. The rapid onset of action and the rapid return of platelets function after cessation of its infusion are thought to be its clinical advantage. The CHAMPION PHOENIX trial of 11,145 patients compared bolus and infusion of cangrelor to clopidogrel 300 or 600 mg in patients undergoing elective or urgent PCI. Cangrelor reduced the occurrence of primary end point (composite of death, MI, ischemia-driven revascularization, and stent thrombosis at 48 hours) by 22% to 4.7% in the cangrelor group versus 5.9% in the clopidogrel (95% CI: 0.66 to 0.93, $P = 0.005$). To be noted, the secondary end point of stent thrombosis at 48 hours was reduced to 0.8% with cangrelor in comparison with 1.4% with clopidogrel (95% CI: 0.43 to 0.90, $P = 0.01$).[31]

Indications: As adjunct to PCI in patients who have not been treated with $P2Y_{12}$ receptor inhibitors and who are not being given a glycoprotein IIb/IIIa inhibitors (GIPs).

Dosing: Cangrelor is given as 30 µg/kg bolus followed by 4 µg/kg/min infusion at the time of PCI for 2 hours up to a maximum of 4 hours.

Side effects: Bleeding, worsening renal function, hypersensitivity.

Contraindications: Significant active bleeding, hypersensitivity reaction.

Recommendations: Cangrelor is recommended as adjunct to PCI in patients who have not been treated with oral $P2Y_{12}$ receptor inhibitors at the time of PCI and who are not being given a GIP.

PLATELET GP IIB/IIIA RECEPTOR ANTAGONISTS

GPIs decrease platelet aggregation and thrombus formation by inhibiting the ability of fibrinogen to cross-link platelets. Three GPI medications that are currently approved for use in the United States include abciximab, eptifibatide, and tirofiban. The benefit of GPI medications seems to be predominantly in patients managed invasively with PCI and with high-risk clinical features (positive troponins, diabetics). However, in the modern era of DAPT with aspirin plus a $P2Y_{12}$ inhibitor, the benefit of upstream use before PCI in the ACS population has become less apparent. For UA/NSTEMI patients, the *EARLY-ACS* trial compared routine upstream use of eptifibatide in addition to standard DAPT versus delayed use at the time of angiography. No significant reduction in ischemic complications was observed with early upstream use of GPI, even though eptifibatide was used in only approximately 25% of patients in the "delayed" arm.[32] Similarly, the *ACUITY Timing* trial failed to show benefit of the strategy of upstream GPI inhibitors when compared with provisional use at the time of PCI. For patients treated with upstream use, increased major bleeding was observed at 30 days.[33] As such, the routine *upstream* use of GPI is not recommended in NSTEMI.[34] Accordingly, in NSTEMI, guidelines recommend DAPT with aspirin plus *either* a $P2Y_{12}$ inhibitor or GPI, but not *routine* triple antiplatelet therapy with all three class of agents. GPIs should be used in addition to aspirin, especially at the time of PCI if there was no adequate pretreatment with ADP receptor blockers. If adequate pretreatment with an ADP receptor blockers was given, the administration of GPI at the time of PCI is according to class 2a recommendation.

For patients with STEMI, the FINESSE and BRAVE-3 studies showed no benefit with regard to infarct size or ischemic events in patients treated upstream with abciximab, as compared with administering GPI during primary PCI.[35,36] According to STEMI 2012 European guidelines.[37] in primary PCI patients:

1. GPIs should be considered for bailout therapy if there is angiographic evidence of massive thrombus, slow or no-reflow, or a thrombotic complication as a class 2a recommendation.
2. Routine use of a GP IIb/IIIa inhibitor as an adjunct to primary PCI performed with unfractionated heparin (UFH) may be considered in patients without contraindications as a class 2b recommendation.
3. Upstream use of a GPI (vs in-lab use) may be considered in high-risk patients undergoing transfer for primary PCI as a class 2b recommendation.

Additionally, the 2013 STEMI guidelines of ACC/AHA[38] emphasizes the following points:

1. It is reasonable to administer GPI at the time of primary PCI in the cath-lab in selected STEMI patients treated with UFH irrespective of the pretreatment of ADP receptor blockers—a 2a recommendation. It is possible to consider intracoronary abciximab—a 2b recommendation.
2. Upstream administration of GPI in planed primary PCI—as a class 2b recommendation.

Many of these trials predated the routine use of P2Y12 inhibitors. Although the relative efficacy of prasugrel and ticagrelor in the trials appeared consistent among patients receiving and not receiving GIPs, the efficacy and safety of GPIs on top of these P2Y12 inhibitors have not been prospectively addressed.[27,28] In patients treated with prasugrel or ticagrelor, GPIs should be limited to bail out situations *or* thrombotic complications during PCI. All GPIs should be used in conjunction with ASA and heparin or enoxaparin. Benefit must be weighed against increased incidence of bleeding, especially in patients at a higher risk for this adverse outcome such as elderly patients.

Abciximab

Rationale. Abciximab is a Fab fragment of a humanized murine antibody that inhibits the GP IIb/IIIa receptor, endothelial cell vitronectin receptors, and leukocyte MAC-1 receptors. Although it has a short half-life, its binding to GP IIb/IIIa receptors can persist for weeks although platelet aggregation gradually returns to normal 24 to 48 hours after discontinuation of the infusion. The role of abciximab in ACS was first established with the EPIC trial, which demonstrated a significant reduction in the rate of death, MI, or emergent revascularization in the group treated with a bolus and infusion of the drug before undergoing PCI.[39] In the contemporary era, the ISAR-REACT 2 trial demonstrated a significant reduction in death, MI, or urgent revascularization in high-risk (troponin positive) UA/NSTEMI patients treated with abciximab who underwent PCI (8.9% abciximab vs 11.9% placebo, *P* = 0.03).[40] However, for UA/NSTEMI patients who are risk-stratified to the early

conservative strategy, the GUSTO IV-ACS trial showed abciximab to be of no additional benefit.[41]

Indications. UA/NSTEMI as adjunct to PCI in bailout situations or thrombotic complications during PCI, STEMI during primary PCI.

Dosing. 0.25 mg/kg 10 to 60 minutes before PCI followed by 0.125 μg/kg/min for 12 hours (maximum rate 10 μg/min).

Side effects. Bleeding, thrombocytopenia, hypersensitivity reactions.

Contraindications. Prior hypersensitivity, high risk for intracranial/GI/GU bleeding.

Recommendations. Abciximab should not be used in the treatment of UA/NSTEMI when PCI is not planned. For STEMI, it should be initiated at the time of primary PCI.

Eptifibatide

Rationale. A heptapeptide antagonist that reversibly inhibits GP IIb/IIIa. In the PURSUIT trial, patients with UA/NSTEMI treated with eptifibatide in addition to ASA and heparin had reduced rates of death and nonfatal MI at 96 hours and 6 months, particularly in those who underwent PCI.[42]

Indication. UA/NSTEMI treated with PCI with high-risk features. STEMI during primary PCI.

Dosing. Upstream ACS: Loading dose 180 μg/kg bolus followed by 2 μg/kg/min for 96 hours. If CrCl ≤ 50 mL/min, dose should be reduced to 1 μg/kg/min.

Primary PCI: Loading dose of 180 μg/kg bolus twice, separated by 10 minutes, followed by 2 μg/kg/min for 18 to 24 hours. If CrCl ≤ 50 mL/min, dose should be reduced to 1 μg/kg/min.

Side effects. Bleeding, thrombocytopenia (rarely severe).

Contraindications. Renal dialysis, severe thrombocytopenia, high risk for intracranial/GI/GU bleeding.

Recommendations. Eptifibatide use is acceptable in the management of UA/NSTEMI for patients as adjunct to PCI in bailout situations or thrombotic complications during PCI, or in addition to other standard antiplatelet medications for patients with high-risk features or recurrent ischemia. Daily monitoring of hemoglobin and platelets is recommended. For STEMI, eptifibatide should be initiated at the time of primary PCI.

Tirofiban

Rationale. Tirofiban is a nonpeptide antagonist that reversibly inhibits GP IIb/IIIa receptor. When combined with UFH, it has been shown to reduce death, MI, and refractory ischemia up to 30 days in patients with high-risk presentations (ischemic ECG features, elevated cardiac biomarkers).[43]

Dosing. High dose—25 μg/kg bolus, followed by 0.15 μg/kg/min infusion for 18 to 24 hours; standard dose—0.4 μg/kg/min for 30 minutes, then 0.1 μg/kg/min for 96 hours. Dose should be reduced by half for patients with CrCl < 30 mL/min.

Side effects. Bleeding, thrombocytopenia (rarely severe).

Contraindications. High risk for intracranial/GI/GU bleeding, severe thrombocytopenia.

Recommendations. Typically, its addition to other standard antiplatelet medications is reserved for patients with high-risk features or recurrent ischemia. Most contemporary trials utilize the high-dose regimen for patients undergoing PCI due to more robust platelet inhibition. Daily monitoring of hemoglobin and platelets is recommended.

ANTICOAGULANTS

UNFRACTIONATED HEPARIN

Rationale: Heparin accelerates the action of circulating antithrombin, which leads to inactivation of factor IIa (thrombin), factor IXa, and factor Xa. Ultimately, this prevents further clot propagation but not lysis of existing thrombus. A meta-analysis involving six trials showed a nonsignificant relative risk reduction of 33% ($P = 0.06$) in death or MI when combined with ASA.[44]

Indications: ACS (both STEMI and UA/NSTEMI).

Dosing: Weight-based nomogram preferred to fixed-dose regimens. Bolus: 60 U/kg (max 4000 U) with initial infusion at 12 U/kg/h (max 1000 U/h). The activated partial thromboplastin time (aPTT) should be monitored q6h until dosing is therapeutic (aPTT 50 to 70).

Side effects: Mild thrombocytopenia, bleeding, heparin-induced thrombocytopenia (HIT).

Contraindications: Severe thrombocytopenia, previously documented HIT.

Recommendations: UFH is recommended early in the management of STEMI and UA/NSTEMI (for both conservative and early invasive strategies) and during PCI. A weight-based dosing regimen should be utilized with frequent monitoring of aPTT, hemoglobin, and platelets. For conservative management strategy, UFH should be continued for at least 48 hours or until discharge (up to 8 days). For CABG or PCI, it should be continued up until the time of procedure (holding according to institutional practices).

LOW-MOLECULAR-WEIGHT HEPARIN: ENOXAPARIN

Rationale: Enoxaparin is a low-molecular-weight heparin (LMWH) that is more selective than UFH at inhibition of factor Xa. When compared with UFH, LMWHs have decreased binding to plasma proteins and endothelial cells, dose-independent clearance, a longer half-life, and more sustained and predictable anticoagulation. Multiple clinical trials have shown a reduction in death, MI, and recurrent angina up to 40 days when compared with UFH.[45–47] For patients with STEMI treated with fibrinolysis, the ExTRACT TIMI 25 study showed that enoxaparin was superior to UFH with regard to death, nonfatal reinfarction, and urgent revascularization but with increased rates of major bleeding.[48]

Advantages over UFH: More predictable anticoagulation, more cost-effective (less monitoring), less occurrence of HIT, twice-daily subcutaneous (SC) dosing, better reduction of nonfatal MI, death, or recurrent angina.

Disadvantages compared with UFH: Unable to give in setting of severe renal impairment, not reversible with protamine, increased major bleeding,[49] inability to reliably monitor ACT (Activated Clotting Time) during PCI.

Indications: UA/NSTEMI and STEMI.

Dosing: Enoxaparin 30 mg IV × 1 may be given early and then 1 mg/kg q12h for 2 to 8 days. It should be avoided in patients with CrCl < 30 (or reduction to q24h should be considered). Unclear dosing strategy for morbidly obese patients; however, often an anti-Xa level is measured, with a commonly accepted therapeutic target of 0.5 to 1.0 anti-Xa units/mL. For patients >75 years, no IV bolus should be given and dose at 0.75 mg/kg q12h.

Side effects: Bleeding, HIT (rare), injection-site complications.

Contraindications: CrCl < 30 mL/min.

Recommendations: In patients with UA/NSTEMI, use of enoxaparin is considered an acceptable alternative to UFH, especially in those being managed conservatively. Duration of treatment is at least 48 hours and typically until discharge (up to 8 days). If CABG is pursued, enoxaparin should be discontinued 12 to 24 hours prior and bridged with UFH according to institutional practice. Although there are limited data for the use of dalteparin for this indication, enoxaparin remains the preferred LMWH. For STEMI patients treated with fibrinolysis, enoxaparin has proven efficacy, albeit at increased risk for bleeding, and can be used throughout the index hospitalization up to 8 days.

DIRECT THROMBIN INHIBITORS: BIVALIRUDIN

Rationale: Direct thrombin inhibitors (DTIs) bind reversibly to thrombin and inhibit clot-bound thrombin more effectively than does UFH. Bivalirudin is a synthetic derivative of hirudin (older DTI no longer used clinically) with a shorter half-life. The ACUITY trial studied UA/NSTEMI patients undergoing PCI and showed noninferiority of bivalirudin monotherapy as compared with UFH or LMWH plus GPI with respect to ischemia (9% vs 8%, $P = 0.45$), but importantly a significant reduction in major bleeding (4% vs 7%, $P < 0.0001$).[50] The HORIZONS-AMI trial showed that STEMI patients undergoing primary PCI treated with bivalirudin alone compared with UFH plus GPI had significantly reduced 30-day rates of death from cardiac causes (1.8% vs 2.9%, $P = 0.03$) and a lower rate of major bleeding (4.9% vs 8.3%, $P < 0.001$).[51] When followed out to 1 year, patients classified as high risk had a decreased mortality (8.4% vs 15.9%, $P = 0.01$) and a decreased rate of recurrent MI (3.6% vs 7.9%, $P = 0.04$).[52] Yet, a recently published meta-analysis of 13 randomized controlled trials, involving 24,605 patients with ACS treated with PCI revealed a significant reduction in the rate of major bleeding with bivalirudin compared with UFH with routine use of GPIs, but not when provisional use of GPIs with UFH was attempted. Additionally, there was a significant increase in the rate of 30 days' definite stent thrombosis largely driven by a 4-fold increase in acute (<24 hours) stent thrombosis regardless of routine or provisional use of GPIs with UFH.[53]

Indications: UA/NSTEMI (early invasive strategy only); STEMI undergoing primary PCI.

Dosing: Bolus 0.75 mg/kg followed by infusion of 1.75 mg/kg/h up to 4 hours. Then it should be decreased to 0.2 mg/kg/h for up to 20 hours.

Side effects: Bleeding.

Contraindications: Dosing adjustments for renal impairment.

Recommendations: Bivalirudin is an acceptable alternative for treatment of UA/NSTEMI in patients undergoing early invasive strategy when used with P2Y$_{12}$ inhibitor given upstream of PCI. It is not recommended for UA/NSTEMI patients being treated with an initial conservative strategy. For STEMI, bivalirudin can be used during primary PCI with or without prior treatment with UFH.

FACTOR XA INHIBITORS: FONDAPARINUX

Rationale: Fondaparinux is a synthetic pentasaccharide that selectively binds to and potentiates antithrombin thereby promoting factor Xa inhibition. Its dose-independent clearance and long half-life allow for once-daily administration and predictable and sustained anticoagulation effects. The OASIS 5 study compared fondaparinux with enoxaparin in the treatment of UA/NSTEMI. Patients treated with fondaparinux had similar rates of death, MI, and refractory ischemia at 9 days, but significantly less major bleeding. At 180 days, fondaparinux was associated with a significant reduction in all major end points.[54] However, there was an increased incidence of catheter-associated thrombus formation during PCI, which led to the open-labeled use of UFH. The OASIS 6 study found that patients with STEMI treated with fondaparinux and fibrinolysis had reduced mortality and reduced rates of reinfarction without increased bleeding or strokes,[55] although again there was evidence of increased thrombotic complications during coronary intervention. These adverse events have turned fondaparinux to be contraindicated as a sole anticoagulant to support PCI in ACS.[38]

Indications: UA/NSTEMI and STEMI.

Dosing: Initial dose of 2.5 mg IV followed by 2.5 mg SC injection daily (maximum antifactor Xa activity is reached in 3 hours).

Side effects: Bleeding, rash/pruritus at injection site, mild elevation of aminotransferases, thrombocytopenia.

Contraindications: CrCl < 30 mL/min, caution if body weight < 50 kg.

Recommendations: Fondaparinux is an alternative anticoagulant for the treatment of UA/NSTEMI patients being managed conservatively and should be continued for up to 8 days. Its use is preferred in the treatment of those with an increased bleeding risk. In the event of PCI, co-administration of UFH or bivalirudin is recommended to decrease the incidence of catheter-associated thrombosis. Fondaparinux should be avoided in patients with planned CABG within 24 hours owing to its long half-life. For STEMI, fondaparinux is an acceptable alternative to UFH in patients undergoing fibrinolysis and should be continued for up to 8 days. The incidence of catheter-associated thrombosis has limited its use for primary PCI and therefore fondaparinux should not be used in this setting.

WARFARIN

Rationale: Warfarin exerts its anticoagulant effect by inhibiting the hepatic synthesis of the vitamin K–dependent coagulation factors II, VII, IX, and X as well as the anticoagulant proteins C and S. Although older, small studies found limited benefit when used in the post-MI setting, the role of warfarin for ACS in the modern era is primarily relegated to the treatment of LV thrombus, atrial fibrillation, or mechanical heart valves. Given the role of DAPT for ACS, the addition of warfarin ("triple antithrombotic therapy") for other indications introduces a greater overall risk of bleeding and can often be challenging to manage in clinical practice.

Indications: Atrial fibrillation, LV thrombus, mechanical heart valve, venous thromboembolism (VTE).

Dosing: 2 to 5 mg po daily should be started and adjusted according to international normalized ratio (INR). Standard nomograms or genotype-specific dosing strategies are available. Starting lower dose in elderly or debilitated patients should be considered. Target INR varies with indication.

Side effects: Bleeding, hypersensitivity reactions, skin/tissue necrosis (rarely).

Contraindications: Active bleeding or unacceptable bleeding risk, unsupervised patient with high nonadherence risk, pregnancy.

Recommendations: The use of warfarin during or after ACS is predominately guided by expert opinion with limited evidence in the current literature. Warfarin should generally be started or continued in high-risk patients with a clear indication for its use (atrial fibrillation, LV thrombus, mechanical heart valve, or VTE). When used in combination with aspirin and a thienopyridine, the benefit of warfarin should outweigh the incremental risk of bleeding, and it should be given for the minimal time necessary to achieve the desired protection. Patients on triple antithrombotic therapy should be closely monitored for bleeding with strict attention paid to maintaining a therapeutic INR.

NEW ORAL ANTICOAGULANTS

During the last decade, the oral DTI Dabigatran and the direct factor Xa inhibitors Rivaroxaban, Apixaban, and Edoxaban have gained widespread use to reduce the thromboembolic risk in nonvalvular atrial fibrillation (NVAF) and in VTE with superior efficacy and safety profile, as a group, over warfarin.[56] Therefore, they are used in patients with ACS mainly for above-mentioned indications, NVAF, and VTE. As with warfarin, the addition of one of these agents to DAPT after coronary syndrome and PCI is associated with increased risk of bleeding. For the meantime, no large randomized clinical trials to examine different protocols and combinations of these agents have been completed. Therefore, as with warfarin, triple antithrombotic therapy should be given for the minimal time necessary, with reduced dosage of new oral anticoagulants (NOACs) and with addition of proton pump inhibitors. Additionally, when triple therapy is needed, it is a common practice to prefer clopidogrel to ticagrelor and prasugrel.[57] As the clearance of these agents is partly renal, they are not given with severe impairment of renal function (CrCl < 15 mL/min).

Except for their common use in NVAF and VTE, clinical trials have shown some reduction in ischemic events when NOACs were given to patients after ACS but with the expense of increased bleeding events.[58]

Indications: NVAF, VTE.

Dosing: Dabigatran 110 to 150 twice daily, rivaroxaban 20 mg once daily (15 mg for CrCl 15 to 49 mL/min) (15 mg twice daily for 21 days as a loading dose for VTE), apixaban 5 mg twice daily (2.5 mg twice daily when two of the following exists: Serum Creatinine > 1.5 mg%, age > 80, weight < 60 kg).

Side effects: Bleeding.

Contraindications: Active bleeding or unacceptable bleeding risk, advanced renal failure, pregnancy.

Recommendations: NVAF, VTE.

FIBRINOLYTICS

All fibrinolytic agents are plasminogen activators and work by catalyzing the cleavage of endogenous plasminogen to generate plasmin. Their thrombolytic action is derived from the ability of plasmin to degrade the fibrin matrix of the thrombus. Although contemporary practice favors the use of a catheter-based reperfusion strategy when available, fibrinolytic reperfusion still remains an important component in the treatment of STEMI in the United States and worldwide. The mortality benefit of fibrinolytic therapy is well proven and, when compared with control, fibrinolysis has been estimated to confer a significant 18% relative reduction in 35-day mortality.[59] Similar to primary PCI, fibrinolytic reperfusion offers the greatest benefit when given early, ideally within the 30 minutes of diagnosis. As a thrombus becomes more organized over time, the efficacy of fibrinolytic therapy decreases. Patients at higher risk for adverse consequences (anterior MI, diabetes, hypotension, left bundle branch block) seem to derive the most benefit when pharmacologic reperfusion is initiated early in the course.

Fibrinolytic agents differ substantially with regard to their antigenicity, specificity for clot-bound fibrin, dosing, and cost. There is no preferred fibrinolytic agent currently recommended by ACC/AHA guidelines. Instead, the choice of fibrinolytic agent should be selected on the basis of physician familiarity, timely availability, and, in the case of streptokinase, past exposure. The most feared and catastrophic adverse consequence of fibrinolytic therapy is intracranial hemorrhage, which is estimated to occur in 0.5% to 0.7% of patients. As such, the absolute contraindications for fibrinolytic therapy include patients with increased risk for intracerebral hemorrhage (ICH) (prior hemorrhagic stroke, prior ischemic stroke within 3 months, intracranial neoplasm or vascular lesions, or closed-head injury within 3 months). Fibrinolytic reperfusion is contraindicated in the treatment of UA/NSTEMI.

Concominant use of anticoagulants in patients treated with fibrinolytics: All patients receiving fibrinolytic reperfusion should receive anticoagulant therapy for a minimum of 48 hours and preferably for the duration of the hospitalization, up to 8 days. UFH, enoxaparin, and fondaparinux have established efficacy when used with fibrinolytics and are the recommended anticoagulants. UFH should be dosed according to recommended ACS weight-based dosing guidelines. However, use for greater than 48 hours is discouraged due to the increased risk of developing HIT and therefore should be changed to enoxaparin or fondaparinux. Enoxaparin should be dosed with specific attention to age, weight, and CrCl. In patients <75 years with normal creatinine, an initial 30-mg IV bolus is given followed by 1-mg/kg SC every 12 hours. If ≥75 years, the IV bolus is eliminated and 0.75 mg/kg SC every 12 hours is given. For all patients with CrCl < 30 mL/min, 1 mg/kg SC daily should be given. Fondaparinux is dosed with an initial 2.5-mg IV followed by 2.5-mg SC daily. It should be avoided in patients with creatinine less than 3.0 mg/dL.

STREPTOKINASE

Rationale: Streptokinase (SK) is a first-generation non–fibrin-specific lytic that exerts its effects both on clot-bound and circulating plasminogen. Although inexpensive by comparison, SK is limited by the possible development of neutralizing antibody titers in previously treated patients. Additionally, SK results in systemic fibrinolysis.

Indication: STEMI.

Dosing: 1.5 million IU over 60 minutes.

Side effects: Bleeding, bronchospasm, anaphylaxis, hypotension, angioedema, periorbital swelling, fever, urticaria.

Contraindications: See **Table 9.6**.

ALTEPLASE (RTPA)

Rationale: A second-generation fibrinolytic considered to be more specific for clot-bound fibrin. Compared with SK, alteplase was shown to confer a significant 30-day mortality reduction (15%) when administered with UFH.[60] However, alteplase is associated with a slightly higher risk of ICH than SK.

Indications: STEMI.

Dosing: Accelerated protocol—(for patients > 67 kg) 15 mg IV bolus, then 50 mg over 30 minutes, then 35 mg over 60 minutes

TABLE 9.6	Contraindications for the Use of Fibrinolytic Agents in STEMI

ABSOLUTE CONTRAINDICATIONS

Any prior ICH
Known intracranial neoplasm or cerebral vascular lesion
Ischemic stroke within 3 mo (EXCEPT acute ischemic stroke within 3 h)
Suspected aortic dissection
Active bleeding or bleeding diathesis (excluding menopause) such as active peptic ulcer
Significant closed-head or facial trauma within 3 mo

RELATIVE CONTRAINDICATIONS

Severe, uncontrolled HTN on presentation (SBP > 180 mm Hg or DBP > 110 mm Hg)
History of ischemic stroke > 3 months, dementia, or intracranial pathology not specified above
Traumatic or prolonged (>10 min) CPR
Noncompressible vascular punctures
Pregnancy
Recent (2–4 wk) internal bleeding
Major surgery within past 3 weeks

Adapted from Antman EM, Anbe DT, Armstrong PW, et al. ACC/AHA guidelines for the management of the patients with ST-elevation myocardial infarction: a report of the American College of Cardiology/American Heart Association Task Force on Practice Guidelines (Committee to Revise the 1999 Guidelines for the Management of Patients with Acute Myocardial Infarction). *J Am Coll Cardiol.* 2004;44:E1-E211.

CPR, cardiopulmonary resuscitation; DPB, diastolic blood pressure; ICH, intracerebral hemorrhage; HTN, hypertension; SBP, systolic blood pressure; STEMI, ST-elevation myocardial infarction.

(total dose = 100 mg). For patients ≤ 67 kg, 15 mg IV bolus, then 0.75 mg/kg (50 mg maximum) over 30 minutes, then 0.5 mg/kg (35 mg maximum) over 60 minutes (total dose < 100 mg).

Side effects: Bleeding, hypotension, nausea/vomiting.

Contraindications: See **Table 9.6**.

RETEPLASE (RPA)

Rationale: rPA is a third-generation fibrinolytic similar to alteplase but with less high-affinity fibrin binding and increased potency. Although no increased mortality was shown over alteplase in GUSTO III, its ability to be given as a double bolus may confer a theoretical advantage related to it by timely administration and less dosing errors.

Indications: STEMI.

Dosing: 10 units IV bolus followed by a second 10 units IV bolus in 30 minutes.

Side effects: Bleeding.

Contraindications: See **Table 9.6**.

TENECTEPLASE (TNK)

Rationale: TNK is a third-generation fibrinolytic that, compared with alteplase, has increased fibrin specificity, decreased clearance, and decreased inhibition from plasminogen activator 1. The ASSENT 2 trial showed similar 30-day mortality rates when compared with alteplase, however fewer mild-to-moderate systemic bleeding complications and need for blood transfusions.[61]

Indications: STEMI.

Dosing: Single 30-to-50-mg IV bolus given over 5 seconds, dosed by weight. For <60 kg, 30 mg should be given; for 60 to 70 kg, 35 mg; for 70 to 80 kg, 40 mg; for 80 to 90 kg, 45 mg; for ≥ 90 kg, 50 mg.

Side effects: Bleeding, hypotension.

Contraindications: See **Table 9.6**.

REFERENCES

1. Ellis K, Tcheng JE, Sapp S, Topol EJ, Lincoff MA. Mortality benefit of beta blockade in patients with acute coronary syndromes undergoing coronary intervention: pooled results from the Epic, Epilog, Epistent, Capture and Rapport trials. *J Interv Cardiol*. 2003;16(4):299-305.

2. Chen ZM, Pan HC, Chen YP, et al. Early intravenous then oral metoprolol in 45,852 patients with acute myocardial infarction: randomised placebo-controlled trial. *Lancet*. 2005;366(9497):1622-1632.

3. Dargie HJ. Effect of carvedilol on outcome after myocardial infarction in patients with left-ventricular dysfunction: the CAPRICORN randomised trial. *Lancet*. 2001;357(9266):1385-1390.

4. Held PH, Yusuf S, Furberg CD. Calcium channel blockers in acute myocardial infarction and unstable angina: an overview. *BMJ*. 1989;299(6709):1187-1192.

5. Hansen JF, Hagerup L, Sigurd B, et al. Cardiac event rates after acute myocardial infarction in patients treated with verapamil and trandolapril versus trandolapril alone. Danish Verapamil Infarction Trial (DAVIT) Study Group. *Am J Cardiol*. 1997;79(6):738-741.

6. Gibson RS, Boden WE, Theroux P, et al. Diltiazem and reinfarction in patients with non-Q-wave myocardial infarction. Results of a double-blind, randomized, multicenter trial. *N Engl J Med*. 1986;315(7):423-429.

7. Lubsen J, Tijssen JG. Efficacy of nifedipine and metoprolol in the early treatment of unstable angina in the coronary care unit: findings from the Holland Interuniversity Nifedipine/Metoprolol Trial (HINT). *Am J Cardiol*. 1987;60(2):18A-25A.

8. Yusuf S, Pepine CJ, Garces C, et al. Effect of enalapril on myocardial infarction and unstable angina in patients with low ejection fractions. *Lancet*. 1992;340(8829):1173-1178.

9. Rutherford JD, Pfeffer MA, Moye LA, et al. Effects of captopril on ischemic events after myocardial infarction. Results of the Survival and Ventricular Enlargement trial. SAVE Investigators. *Circulation*. 1994;90(4):1731-1738.

10. ACE Inhibitor Myocardial Infarction Collaborative Group. Indications for ACE inhibitors in the early treatment of acute myocardial infarction: systematic overview of individual data from 100,000 patients in randomized trials. *Circulation*. 1998;97(22):2202-2212.

11. Gustafsson I, Torp-Pedersen C, Køber L, Gustafsson F, Hildebrandt P, Trace Study Group. Effect of the angiotensin-converting enzyme inhibitor trandolapril on mortality and morbidity in diabetic patients with left ventricular dysfunction after acute myocardial infarction. Trace Study Group. *J Am Coll Cardiol*. 1999;34(1):83-89.

12. Buch P, Rasmussen S, Abildstrom SZ, Køber L, Carlsen J, Torp-Pedersen C. The long-term impact of the angiotensin-converting enzyme inhibitor trandolapril on mortality and hospital admissions in patients with left ventricular dysfunction after a myocardial infarction: follow-up to 12 years. *Eur Heart J*. 2005;26(2):145-152.

13. Pfeffer MA, McMurray JJ, Velazquez EJ, et al. Valsartan, captopril, or both in myocardial infarction complicated by heart failure, left ventricular dysfunction, or both. *N Engl J Med*. 2003;349(20):1893-1906.

14. Pitt B, Remme W, Zannad F, et al. Eplerenone, a selective aldosterone blocker, in patients with left ventricular dysfunction after myocardial infarction. *N Eng J Med*. 2003;348(14):1309-1321.

15. Schwartz G, Olsson AG, Ezekowitz MD, et al. Effects of atorvastatin on early recurrent ischemic events in acute coronary syndromes. The MIRACL study: a randomized controlled trial. *JAMA*. 2001;285(13):1711-1718.

16. Cannon CP, Braunwald E, McCabe CH, et al. Intensive versus moderate lipid lowering with statins after acute coronary syndromes. *N Engl J Med*. 2004;350(15):1495-1504.

17. Antiplatelet Trialists' Collaboration. Collaborative overview of randomized trials of antiplatelet therapy—I: prevention of death, myocardial infarction, and stroke by prolonged antiplatelet therapy in various categories of patients. *BMJ*. 1994;308(6921):81-106.

18. Lewis HD Jr, Davis JW, Archibald DG, et al. Protective effects of aspirin against acute myocardial infarction and death in men with unstable angina. Results of a Veterans Administration Cooperative Study. *N Engl J Med*. 1983;309(7):396-403.

19. Cairns JA, Gent M, Singer J, et al. Aspirin, sulfinpyrazone, or both in unstable angina. Results of a Canadian multicenter trial. *N Engl J Med*. 1985;313(22):1369-1375.

20. Theroux P, Ouimet H, McCans J, et al. Aspirin, heparin, or both to treat acute unstable angina. *N Engl J Med*. 1988;319(17):1105-1111.

21. The RISC Group. Risk of myocardial infarction and death during treatment with low dose aspirin and intravenous heparin in men with unstable coronary artery disease. *Lancet*. 1990;336(8719):827-830.

22. Yusuf S, Fox KAA, Tognoni G, et al. Effects of clopidogrel in addition to aspirin in patients with acute coronary syndromes without ST-segment elevation. *N Engl J Med*. 2001;345(7):494-502.

23. Chen ZM, Jiang LX, Chen YP, et al. Addition of clopidogrel to aspirin in 45,852 patients with acute myocardial infarction: randomised placebo-controlled trial. *Lancet*. 2005;366(9497):1607-1621.

24. Scirica BM, Sabatine MS, Morrow DA, et al. The role of clopidogrel in early and sustained arterial patency after fibrinolysis for ST-segment elevation myocardial infarction: the ECG CLARITY-TIMI 28 Study. *J Am Coll Cardiol*. 2006;48(1):37-42.

25. Dangas G, Mehran R, Guagliumi G, et al. Role of clopidogrel loading dose in patients with ST-segment elevation myocardial infarction undergoing primary angioplasty: results from the HORIZONS-AMI (harmonizing outcomes with revascularization and stents in acute myocardial infarction) trial. *J Am Coll Cardiol*. 2009;54(15):1438-1446.

26. The CURRENT-OASIS 7 Investigators. Dose comparisons of clopidogrel and aspirin in acute coronary syndromes. *N Engl J Med*. 2010;363(10):930-942.

27. Wiviott SD, Braunwald E, McCabe CH, et al. Prasugrel versus clopidogrel in patients with acute coronary syndromes. *N Engl J Med*. 2007;357(20):2001-2015.

28. Wallentin L, Becker RC, Budaj A, et al. Ticagrelor versus clopidogrel in patients with acute coronary syndromes. *N Engl J Med*. 2009;361(11):1045-1057.

29. Cannon C, Harrington RA, James S, et al. Comparison of ticagrelor with clopidogrel in patients with a planned invasive strategy for acute coronary syndromes (PLATO): a randomised double-blind study. *Lancet*. 2010;375(9711):283-293.

30. Bonaca M, Bhatt DL, Cohen M, et al. Long-term use of ticagrelor in patients with prior myocardial infarction. *N Engl J Med*. 2015;372(19):1791-1800.

31. Bhatt D, Stone GW, Mahaffey KW, et al. Effect of platelet inhibition with cangrelor during PCI on ischemic events. *N Engl J Med*. 2013;368(14):1303-1313.

32. Giuliano RP, White JA, Bode C, et al. Early versus delayed, provisional eptifibatide in acute coronary syndromes. *N Engl J Med*. 2009;360(21):2176-2190.

33. Stone GW, Bertrand ME, Moses JW, et al. Routine upstream initiation vs deferred selective use of glycoprotein IIb/IIIa inhibitors in acute coronary syndromes. *JAMA*. 2007;355(6):2203-2216.

34. Amsterdam EA, Wenger NK, Brindis RG, et al. 2014 ACC/AHA Guidelines for the management of patients with non-ST elevation acute coronary syndromes. *J Am Coll Cardiol.* 2014;64(24):e139-e228.

35. Ellis S, Tendera M, De Belder MA, et al. Facilitated PCI in patients with ST-elevation myocardial infarction. *N Engl J Med.* 2008;358(21):2205-2217.

36. Mehilli J, Kastrati A, Schulz S, et al. Abciximab in patients with acute ST-segment-elevation myocardial infarction undergoing primary percutaneous coronary intervention after clopidogrel loading: a randomized double-blind trial. *Circulation.* 2009;119(14):1933-1940.

37. Steg PG, James SK, Atar D, et al. ESC guidelines for the management of acute myocardial infarction in patients presenting with ST-segment elevation. *Eur Heart J.* 2012;33:2569-2619.

38. O'Gara P, Kushner FG, Ascheim DD, et al. 2013 ACCF/AHA guidelines for the management of ST-Elevation Myocardial Infarction: executive summary. *Circulation.* 2013;127:1-51.

39. The EPIC Investigators. Use of a monoclonal antibody directed against the platelet glycoprotein IIb/IIIa receptor in high-risk coronary angioplasty. *N Engl J Med.* 1994;330(14):956-961.

40. Kastrati A, Mehilli J, Neumann FJ, et al. Abciximab in patients with acute coronary syndromes undergoing percutaneous coronary intervention after clopidogrel pretreatment: the ISAR-REACT 2 randomized trial. *JAMA.* 2006;295(13):1531-1538.

41. Simoons ML. Effect of glycoprotein IIb/IIIa receptor blocker abciximab on outcome in patients with acute coronary syndromes without early coronary revascularisation: the GUSTO IV-ACS randomised trial. *Lancet.* 2001;357(9272):1915-1924.

42. The PURSUIT Trial Investigators. Inhibition of platelet glycoprotein IIb/IIIa with eptifibatide in patients with acute coronary syndromes. *N Engl J Med.* 1998;339(7):436-443.

43. (PRISM-PLUS) Study Investigators. Inhibition of the platelet glycoprotein IIb/IIIa receptor with tirofiban in unstable angina and non-Q-wave myocardial infarction. *N Engl J Med.* 1998;338(21):1488-1497.

44. Oler A, Whooley MA, Oler J, Grady D. Adding heparin to aspirin reduces the incidence of myocardial infarction and death in patients with unstable angina. A meta-analysis. *JAMA.* 1996;276(10):811-815.

45. FRISC Study Group. Low-molecular-weight heparin during instability in coronary artery disease, fragmin during instability in coronary artery disease. *Lancet.* 1996;347(9001):561-568.

46. Antman EM, McCabe CH, Gurfinkel EP, et al. Enoxaparin prevents death and cardiac ischemic events in unstable angina/non-Q-wave myocardial infarction. Results of the thrombolysis in myocardial infarction (TIMI) 11B trial. *Circulation.* 1999;100(15):1593-1601.

47. Cohen M, Demers C, Gurfinkel EP, et al. A comparison of low-molecular-weight heparin with unfractionated heparin for unstable coronary artery disease. Efficacy and Safety of Subcutaneous Enoxaparin in Non-Q-Wave Coronary Events Study Group. *N Engl J Med.* 1997;337(7):447-452.

48. Antman EM, Morrow DA, McCabe CH, et al. Enoxaparin versus unfractionated heparin with fibrinolysis for ST-elevation myocardial infarction. *N Engl J Med.* 2006;354(14):1477-1488.

49. Ferguson JJ, Califf RM, Antman EM, et al. Enoxaparin vs unfractionated heparin in high-risk patients with non-ST-segment elevation acute coronary syndromes managed with an intended early invasive strategy: primary results of the SYNERGY randomized trial. *JAMA.* 2004;292(1):45-54.

50. Stone GW, McLaurin BT, Cox DA, et al. Bivalirudin for patients with acute coronary syndromes. *N Engl J Med.* 2006;355(21):2203-2216.

51. Stone GW, Witzenbichler B, Guagliumi G, et al. Bivalirudin during primary PCI in acute myocardial infarction. *N Engl J Med.* 2008;358(21):2218-2230.

52. Parodi G, Antoniucci D, Nikolsky E, et al. Impact of bivalirudin therapy in high-risk patients with acute myocardial infarction: 1-year results from the HORIZONS-AMI trial. *JACC Cardiovasc Interv.* 2010;3(8):796-802.

53. Navarese EP, Schulze V, Andreotti F, et al. Comprehensive meta-analysis of safety and efficacy of bivalirudin versus heparin with or without routine glycoprotein IIb/IIIa inhibitors in patients with acute coronary syndrome. *J Am Coll Cardiol.* 2015;8:201-213.

54. Yusuf S, Mehta SR, Bassand JP, et al. Comparison of fondaparinux and enoxaparin in acute coronary syndromes: the OASIS-5 trial. *N Engl J Med.* 2006;354(14):1464-1476.

55. Yusuf S, Mehta SR, Chrolavicius S, et al. Effects of fondaparinux on mortality and reinfarction in patients with acute ST-segment elevation myocardial infarction: the OASIS-6 randomized trial. *JAMA.* 2006;295(13):1519-1530.

56. Dentali F, Riva N, Crowther M, Turpie AG, Lip GY, Ageno W. Efficacy and safety of the novel oral anticoagulants in atrial fibrillation clinical perspective—a systematic review and meta-analysis of the literature. *Circulation.* 2012;126:2381-2391.

57. Kirchhof P, Benussi S, Kotecha D, et al. 2016 ESC guidelines for the management of atrial fibrillation developed in collaboration with EACTS. *Eur Heart J.* 2016;37:2893-2962.

58. Mega J, Braunwald E, Wiviott SD, et al. Rivaroxaban in patients with a recent acute coronary syndrome: the ATLAS ACS 2—TIMI 51 trial. *N Engl J Med.* 2012;366(1):9-19.

59. Fibrinolytic Therapy Trialists' (FTT) Collaborative Group. Indications for fibrinolytic therapy in suspected acute myocardial infarction: collaborative overview of early mortality and major morbidity results from all randomised trials of more than 1000 patients. *Lancet.* 1994;343(8893):311-322.

60. The GUSTO investigators. An international randomized trial comparing four thrombolytic strategies for acute myocardial infarction. *N Engl J Med.* 1993;329(10):673-682.

61. Van De Werf F, Adgey J, Ardissino D, et al. Single-bolus tenecteplase compared with front-loaded alteplase in acute myocardial infarction: the ASSENT-2 double-blind randomised trial. *Lancet.* 1999;354(9180):716-722.

Patient and Family Information for: MEDICATIONS USED IN THE MANAGEMENT OF ACS

The medicines used to treat heart attacks in the modern-era stem from decades of laboratory and clinical trial research. As more and more is learned about CAD, the drugs used to treat heart attack victims will hopefully become even more safe and effective. Today, medical therapy forms the cornerstone of heart attack care. Early after diagnosis, much emphasis is placed on controlling chest pain, interrupting further heart damage, and maintaining a safe blood pressure and heart rate. Powerful blood thinners, pain medications, blood pressure– and cholesterol-lowering drugs, catheterization procedures, and sometimes even bypass surgery are used to varying degrees in the early treatment of heart attacks. Alongside these therapies, other medicines may be added to treat cardiac arrhythmias, CHF, diabetes, or tobacco addiction. The decisions underlying which medicines are used to treat a specific patient are complex and often change depending on one's age, cardiac risk factors, medical history, and type of heart attack encountered.

The following sections are divided into various classes and types of medications routinely used in the treatment of heart attacks. Many of the medicines described are also used to treat other conditions, both related and unrelated to the heart. The rationale behind each medication's use, both generic and commonly used trade names, potential side effects, and important details are provided. It is important to emphasize that the following pages should be used only as a general guide. Specific details about each drug, doses, and potential interactions with other medications should always be discussed with a physician and pharmacist.

TREATING THE PAIN OF A HEART ATTACK

A heart attack results from the interruption of blood flow to the muscle of the heart, most commonly by a small blood clot known as a thrombus. As heart muscle is dependent on the oxygen and nutrients carried by the blood, it quickly becomes starved in a process known as ischemia. Ischemia in most patients results in chest pain or angina. It is classically described as a chest pressure or tightness, often moving to the shoulder, neck, jaw, or arms. Other symptoms may include nausea, vomiting, or shortness of breath. For patients who have experienced chest pain or pressure in the past, the discomfort associated with a heart attack is usually more intense, more frequent, and even occurring at rest. In some patients, particularly diabetics and the elderly, symptoms may be more subtle and present only as mild stomach pain or indigestion, occasional palpitations, or even no symptoms at all. The onset of chest pain is often the first sign of a heart attack, and it provides warning that the heart muscle is threatened. While the primary goal in treating all heart attacks is to restore blood flow within the jeopardized coronary artery, the adequate treatment of pain is of paramount importance to all patients.

Medications used to specifically treat the pain of a heart attack are called "antianginals" and include nitrates, β-blockers,

and CCBs. For pain unrelieved with these classes of drugs, various forms of narcotic medications, known as opioids, are commonly used.

NITRATES

Names: NTG (*Minitran, Nitro-Bid, Nitro-Dur, Nitro-Time, Nitrolingual, NitroQuick, Nitrostat*)

Related medications: Isosorbide mononitrate (*Imdur, Ismo, Monoket*), isosorbide dinitrate (*Isordil, Dilatrate-SR, Isochron*)

NTG is one of the most commonly used medicines for the treatment of chest pain. It is a "vasodilator" and primarily works by dilating, or expanding, the size of coronary arteries. The net effect is that more blood can get to the heart muscle. Even in patients with a completely blocked coronary artery, NTG is useful because it recruits blood flow to other, less diseased arteries. NTG lowers blood pressure, a property that is helpful in relieving pain and decreasing the amount of strain placed on the heart. NTG can be administered in a variety of forms, a feature that makes it particularly useful when treating someone with ongoing nausea and vomiting. When given as permanent medication, people treated with nitrates develop a situation called "tolerance," which means that the influence of nitrates decreases by time. On the other hand, when kept for only s.o.s. use as in heart attacks, nitrates retain their above-mentioned benefits.

Preparations: Sublingual (dissolved under the tongue), translingual (sprayed into the mouth), oral, transcutaneous (absorbed through the skin), and IV.

Side effects: Headache (most common), flushing, dizziness, lightheadedness, nausea, vomiting, blurred vision, swelling.

Important information: The patients who use medications to treat erectile dysfunction such as sildenafil (*Viagra*), tadalafil (*Cialis*), or vardenafil (*Levitra*) should not use NTG because combined use may result in a severe, rapid reduction in blood pressure or even death. The prior or ongoing use of any of these medications should immediately be reported to a physician.

β-BLOCKERS

Names: Metoprolol (*Lopressor, Toprol-XL*), carvedilol (*Coreg*), bisoprolol (*Zebeta*), atenolol (*Tenormin*), labetalol (*Trandate*), propranolol (*Inderal*), esmolol (*Brevibloc*)

β-Blockers are a class of blood pressure medications commonly used in the treatment of heart attacks, abnormal heart rhythms, and CHF. They work to relieve angina by both lowering blood pressure and reducing the heart rate. When the heart is forced to pump blood against a high blood pressure or beat at a fast rate, it requires greater amounts of oxygen and thus greater coronary blood flow. During exercise and especially during a heart attack, blood flow to the heart muscle is jeopardized and unable to meet the demands required. By lowering both the blood pressure and heart rate, β-blockers are useful at reducing this strain on the heart and often result in reduced levels of chest pain.

Preparations: Oral, IV.

Side effects: Dizziness, fatigue, lightheadedness, change in sexual ability or desire, depression, diarrhea, slow heartbeat.

Important information: Some patients with asthma, emphysema, bronchitis, or related diseases of the lungs may experience excessive wheezing or shortness of breath while taking β-blockers. Such reactions should be reported to a physician. Additionally, abruptly discontinuing β-blockers has been reported sometimes to result in worsening of chest pain.

CALCIUM CHANNEL BLOCKERS

Names: Diltiazem (*Cardizem, Cartia, Dilacor, Dilt, Diltia, Diltzac, Taztia, Tiazac*), verapamil (*Calan, Covera, Isoptin, Verelan*), amlodipine (*Norvasc*), felodipine (*Plendil*), nisoldipine (*Sular*), lercanidipine (*Zanidep*)

CCBs, a class of blood pressure medications, are also used to treat angina and abnormal heart rhythms. CCB have various effects, with part of them working similar to β-blockers, reducing the heart rate and blood pressure, thus reducing strain on the heart. Yet, it is a common practice to avoid this group of medications in heart attacks because they can result in significant decrease in heart contractility and may aggravate heart failure. On the other side, patients with a combination of heart attack and elevated blood pressure may gain benefit from CCB treatment.

Preparations: Oral, IV.

Side effects: Dizziness, lightheadedness, headache, nausea or vomiting, constipation, swelling, slow heartbeat.

NARCOTICS (OPIOIDS)

Names: Morphine (*Avinza, MS Contin, Roxanol*), fentanyl (*Sublimaze*), oxycodone (*OxyContin, OxyFast, Percocet, Endocet, Magnacet*), hydrocodone (*Lortab, Norco, Vicodin, Zydone*), hydromorphone (*Dilaudid*), meperidine (*Demerol*)

Narcotics such as morphine do not specifically treat angina. Rather, they act more generally to block pain signals in the body from reaching the brain. Narcotics are often prescribed for heart attack patients when other antianginal medications have failed to completely control pain. Additionally, they have several beneficial side effects, one of which is to help slow the heart rate. Like β-blockers and CCBs, this helps to reduce the work load exerted on the heart thereby reducing strain on the heart. Narcotics come in many different preparations, but in the context of heart attacks narcotics are used mainly intravenously; by this route, they provide the most rapid relief of symptoms needed at the initial phase of management.

Preparations: Oral, IV, transdermal (through the skin).

Side effects: Nausea, vomiting, constipation, dizziness, flushing, slow heartbeat, shallow breathing.

ANTIPLATELET MEDICATIONS

Platelets are specialized blood cells that constantly survey the body for areas of injury. In blood vessels, and in the coronary arteries in particular, platelets are responsible for identifying damaged areas of vessel wall and then sealing off these areas before further harm ensues. Unfortunately, other adverse processes, such as cholesterol deposits and thickening of arterial wall, may cause activation of platelets as these small cells recognize these arterial wall changes as damage to be sealed. When this occurs, platelets quickly change their shape, become sticky, and along with other platelets form a small blood clot—thrombus. Unfortunately, this small blood clot may often grow large enough to completely or incompletely impede flow through the entire artery. This, most simply, is the cause of a heart attack. Antiplatelet drugs are special medications that interfere with the ability of platelets to form clots, particularly large obstructive clots. Antiplatelet medications work particularly well at reducing heart attacks caused by blood clots in the coronary arteries. However, because they block the natural actions of platelets throughout the body, they can also increase the risk of unintended bleeding.

ASPIRIN

Names: Aspirin (*Bayer Aspirin, Ecotrin, Anacin*)

Aspirin is one of the oldest, most widely used, cheap, and effective antiplatelet medicines around. Even today, it remains an essential component in the treatment of heart attacks both during hospitalization and after discharge. With very few exceptions, aspirin therapy should be taken for life in individuals who suffer a heart attack.

Preparations: Oral, rectal.

Side effects: Upset stomach, heartburn, stomach bleeding, easy bruising.

Important information: Because aspirin remains such an important medicine in the treatment and prevention of heart attacks, patients should take it daily. This is especially important if a stent is used in the treatment of one's heart disease. Although a true aspirin allergy exists, fortunately, it is rare and most side effects from aspirin can be overcome with the use of coated formulations and certain medicines to reduce stomach acid. Consultation with a cardiologist is recommended before stopping aspirin, even temporarily, for situations such as elective surgery.

P2Y$_{12}$ INHIBITOR

Names: Clopidogrel (*Plavix*), prasugrel (*Effient*), ticagrelor (*Brilinta*)

These medications each work as potent antiplatelet medications, most commonly taken in addition to aspirin, and work to greatly reduce the body's ability to form blood clots in the coronary arteries and elsewhere. Studies of patients with heart attacks have consistently proven that these drugs, when added to aspirin, help reduce the incidence of future heart attacks and prolong one's lifespan. In addition to their role in the treatment of heart attacks, they are critically important in patients who have been treated with coronary stents.

Preparations: Oral.

Side effects: Easy bruising or bleeding, nausea, dizziness.

Important information: Like with aspirin, patients prescribed medications from this class should strive to take them exactly as requested by a physician. In patients with coronary stents, this becomes of even greater importance because the abrupt discontinuation can result in new blood clots forming within the stent itself. Although such events are rare, they often lead to a second heart attack and can be fatal. As with aspirin, consultation with a cardiologist is recommended prior to electively stopping these medications for upcoming surgeries. Patients should avoid missing doses or running out before a prescription can be renewed.

PLATELET GLYCOPROTEIN IIB/IIIA RECEPTOR ANTAGONISTS

Names: Abciximab (*Reopro*), eptifibatide (*Integrilin*), tirofiban (*Aggrastat*)

Glycoprotein IIb/IIIa receptor antagonists are molecules named for the specific platelet receptor they bind. As with other antiplatelet medications, they work to decrease the ability of platelets to form clots within the coronary arteries. However, this class of medications is only given intravenously. Although these drugs are often used in addition to aspirin for the early treatment of heart attacks, they are most commonly used during coronary intervention during catheterization, including stent placements. Their highly potent platelet-blocking effects make them particularly well suited to prevent clot formation within stents, thereby increasing stent durability. Like with other antiplatelet medications, drugs from this class have been proven in thousands of patients who had heart attack to prolong life and reduce future heart attacks.

Preparation: IV.

Side effects: Easy bruising or bleeding, nausea, stomach aches.

ANTICOAGULANTS

A blood clot, or thrombus, is not only formed by platelets. Within the circulating blood exists a multitude of microscopic proteins that work alongside platelets to assist in the formation of blood clots at sites of vessel injury. When damage is detected, these proteins form long, thin threads call fibrin. In turn, these fibrin threads create a mesh-like plug that helps to stabilize blood clots. Whereas antiplatelet medications block the actions of platelets, anticoagulants block the body's ability to form fibrin. Because they work to prevent blood clot formation, they too are often referred to as "blood thinners."

HEPARIN AND RELATED MEDICATIONS

Names: Heparin

Related medications: Enoxaparin (*Lovenox*), bivalirudin (*Angiomax*), fondaparinux (*Arixtra*), dalteparin (*Fragmin*)

Heparin and its related medicines comprise a central role in the treatment of heart attacks. They are given early in the course of a heart attack and sometimes continued throughout the duration of a hospital stay. In addition to preventing blood clots associated with heart attacks, heparin or similar drugs are routinely used in the prevention of clots associated with other disorders. Typical uses may include the prevention of blood clots in the legs (deep vein thrombosis), those associated with mechanical heart valves, and those that may form with certain abnormal heart rhythms.

Preparations: IV, SC (under the skin) injections.

Side effects: Easy bruising or bleeding, pain at injection site, abnormal blood counts (especially platelets), rash.

Important information: A rare condition known as HIT can occur in some patients who have had previous exposure to heparin. This condition causes a dramatic drop in platelets and can lead to both excessive bleeding and clotting. Patients with a history of HIT should promptly notify their physicians during any hospital admission or office visit.

WARFARIN

Names: Warfarin (*Coumadin, Jantoven*)

Related medications: Dabigatran (*Pradaxa*)

Warfarin is an orally given blood thinner that has been used for decades to treat a multitude of conditions associated with blood clotting. Inherited clotting disorders, mechanical heart valves, abnormal heart rhythms, and prior blood clots in the legs or lungs are all common reasons for warfarin to be prescribed. Although it is rarely used to specifically treat or prevent heart attacks, warfarin deserves special mention because it is often used in addition to the antiplatelet and anticoagulant medications commonly prescribed for patients who had heart attack. A unique and often frustrating feature of warfarin is that it requires frequent blood tests to monitor its activity.

Preparations: Oral.

Side effects: Easy bruising or bleeding, nausea, vomiting, altered sense of taste.

Important information: Each blood thinner added to a patient's list of medications introduces an incremental risk of unintended bleeding. In properly selected patients, these drug combinations can be safely followed but often require more aggressive monitoring and physician visits. It is not uncommon for warfarin dosing, even if stable for years, to need adjusting after the initiation of new medications. Patients should pay close attention to early signs of bleeding, especially bleeding related to the stomach or intestines, and report these to their physician.

NEW ORAL ANTICOAGULANTS (NOACs)

Names: Dabigatran (*Pradaxa*), Rivaroxaban (*Xarelto*), Apixaban (*Eliquis*)

This class of orally taken blood thinners was introduced during the last decade to treat several conditions that, until then, were treated by warfarin. There is no need to continuously monitor their activity by blood tests, and they have additional benefit in efficacy and safety over warfarin. Still, as blood thinners, they may increase the risk of unintended bleeding especially when taken with antiplatelet agents as in patients after heart attacks.

Preparations: Oral.

Side effects: Bleeding.

FIBRINOLYTICS OR "CLOT BUSTERS"

Names: Streptokinase (*Streptase*), alteplase (*Activase*), reteplase (*Retavase*), Tenecteplase (*TNKase*)

Fibrinolytics, also called "thrombolytics" or "clot busters," are a class of medications used to treat a specific type of heart attack where blood flow through a coronary artery is completely obstructed. Unlike antiplatelet and anticoagulant drugs, which prevent blood clots from forming or expanding, fibrinolytics actually target and destroy clots that have already formed. These extremely potent medications work best when given very early in the course of a heart attack and typically are used in areas where a cardiac catheterization laboratory is not immediately available. Unfortunately, they have not proven to be useful in treating heart attacks caused by only partially obstructive clots.

Preparations: IV.

Side effects: Easy bruising or bleeding, stroke (rare).

OTHER IMPORTANT MEDICATIONS USED IN TREATING HEART ATTACKS

The immediate control of chest pain, addition of antiplatelet and anticoagulant medications, and often cardiac catheterization or use of fibrinolytics are crucially important during the early stages of a heart attack. These therapies are largely targeted at aborting further damage and salvaging heart muscle from permanent damage. Aggressive and early control of blood pressure, fluid volume, and cholesterol levels are equally important in achieving these goals. In many cases, additional blood pressure medications may be added to more closely control one's HTN. In other cases, they may be added simply for the unique and beneficial properties they provide to patients with heart disease.

ACE INHIBITORS AND ARBs

Names: **ACE inhibitors**—benazepril (*Lotensin*), captopril (*Capoten*), enalapril (*Vasotec*), fosinopril (*Monopril*), lisinopril (*Prinivil, Zestril*), moexipril (*Univasc*), perindopril (*Aceon*), quinapril (*Accupril*), ramipril (*Altace*), trandolapril (*Mavik*); **ARBs**—cadesartan (*Atacand*), eprosartan (*Teveten*), irbesartan (*Avapro*), losartan (*Cozaar*), olmesartan (*Benicar*), valsartan (*Diovan*), telmisartan (*Micardis*)

Medications from these two classes of blood pressure drugs are commonly used alongside other therapies to treat specific consequences of heart attacks, such as CHF, that is, a weakened heart muscle. Apart from being blood pressure–lowering drugs, these medications have shown to be beneficial in prolonging life, reducing the incidence of CHF, and protecting the kidneys in diabetic patients.

Preparations: Oral.

Side effects: Dizziness, lightheadedness, cough (ACE inhibitors), abnormal electrolyte levels, swelling.

DIURETICS

Names: furosemide (*Lasix*), bumetanide (*Bumex*), torsemide (*Demadex*), hydrochlorothiazide (*Esidrix, Microzide*), chlorothiazide (*Diuril*), metolazone (*Zaroxolyn*), amiloride (*Midamor*), triamterene (*Dyrenium*), spironolactone (*Aldactone*), eplerenone (*Inspra*).

Diuretics, commonly referred to as "water pills," are routinely used in the care of patients who had heart attack and who suffer from CHF or any condition characterized by increased fluid in the body, most often in the lower extremities or lungs. They work to remove excess fluid by stimulating urine production in the kidneys. Furosemide (*Lasix*) remains the most prescribed drug used in the hospital for this purpose. Some weaker diuretics are often added for their blood pressure–lowering properties, whereas others such as spironolactone (*Aldactone*) and eplerenone (*Inspra*) may be added in special circumstances characterized by severe CHF.

Preparations: Oral, IV.

Side effects: Dizziness, lightheadedness, dry mouth, thirst, hearing difficulty, abnormal electrolyte levels, and kidney function.

CHOLESTEROL-LOWERING MEDICATIONS

Names: atorvastatin (*Lipitor*), fluvastatin (*Lescol*), lovastatin (*Mevacor, Altoprev*), pravastatin (*Pravachol*), rosuvastatin (*Crestor*), simvastatin (*Zocor*)

Related medications: niacin (*Niaspan, Niacor*), gemfibrozil (*Lopid*), fenofibrate (*Tricor*), cholestyramine (*Questran*), colestipol (*Colestid*), colesevelam (*Welchol*), ezetimibe (*Zetia*)

Cholesterol-lowering medications, most notably the statins, have emerged as some of the most important drugs used in the treatment CAD in the past three decades. Stringent cholesterol control helps prevent both future heart attacks and strokes. Additionally, clinical trials have shown the benefits of statins, especially powerful agents as atorvastatin (*Lipitor*), simvastatin (*Zocor*), or rosuvastatin (*Crestor*), when given during the early phase of heart attack management. The related medications listed above are sometimes added to better control certain types of cholesterol or triglycerides abnormalities, most often in addition to statins.

Preparations: Oral.

Side effects: Muscle aches or pains, nausea, stomach aches, flushing or itching (niacin), insomnia (niacin), gas, diarrhea.

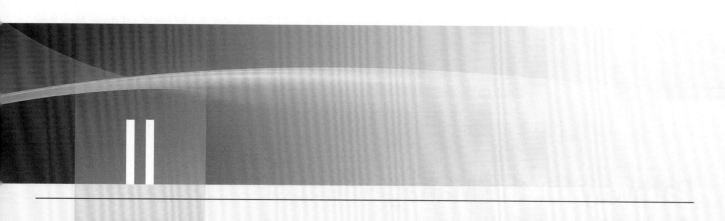

HEART FAILURE

Edgar Argulian
Marrick L. Kukin
Emad F. Aziz
Eyal Herzog

10

Pathway for the Management of Acute Heart Failure

EPIDEMIOLOGY AND IMPACT

Heart failure is a common and growing problem in the developed nations owing to an aging population. If the overall prevalence of heart failure among adults is 1% to 2%, it exceeds 10% in the elderly (over 70 years old).[1] Moreover, acute decompensated heart failure is among the most common causes of hospitalization among elderly patients. Besides being common and costly, heart failure hospitalization has important prognostic implications: it carries subsequent 1-year mortality risk close to 30%.[1] The current chapter is intended to outline a simple yet comprehensive approach to diagnosis and management of acute decompensated heart failure by synthesizing the evidence from multiple studies and major cardiology society recommendations.[1,2] It is based on the initial acute heart failure management pathway published by our heart failure team (**Figure 10.1**).[3]

DEFINITIONS

Acute decompensated heart failure refers to the acute onset of symptoms (predominantly dyspnea, congestion, and fatigue) due to elevated cardiac filling pressures and/or decreased cardiac output. It can be newly diagnosed heart failure or exacerbation of preexisting chronic heart failure condition. Despite major advances in confirmatory laboratory and diagnostic modalities, heart failure remains a clinical diagnosis of a constellation of signs and symptoms. Careful history taking and focused physical examination are the cornerstones of the diagnosis. The diagnosis is established by the combination of symptoms of heart failure (such as dyspnea and orthopnea), signs of fluid overload (such as jugular venous distention, pulmonary crackles, and peripheral edema), signs of hypoperfusion (such as cold extremities, confusion, and narrow pulse pressure), and objective evidence of structural heart disease (such as third heart sounds, cardiac murmurs, and echocardiographic findings). Acute decompensated heart failure is a continuum of clinical presentations ranging from mild dyspnea to florid pulmonary edema to cardiogenic shock; therefore, urgent evaluation and triage of suspected acute decompensated heart failure are warranted.

Although initially described for patients with myocardial infarction, the Forrester classification can be applied to all patients with acute decompensated heart failure to guide the management.[4] It assigns patients to groups on the basis of bedside estimation of fluid overload status ("wet," meaning apparent signs of congestion) and perfusion state ("cold," meaning low perfusion state). "Wet" signs include pulmonary congestion, jugular venous distention, congestive hepatomegaly, and peripheral edema. "Cold" signs include cold extremities, confusion, narrow pulse pressure, and oliguria. Most but not all patients in the "cold" category are hypotensive. Most patients with acute decompensated heart failure fall into the "wet" and "warm" category: They have evidence of pulmonary congestion/pulmonary edema with normal or high blood pressure. Patients with pulmonary edema and hypoperfusion are in or at risk for cardiogenic shock, which typically signifies bad prognosis unless a reversible cause is rapidly identified and corrected (eg, reperfusion therapy in a patient with acute myocardial infarction or a corrective surgery in a patient with acute valvular dysfunction). Sometimes patients with cardiogenic shock ("cold" state) have no evidence of pulmonary congestion and systemic hypoperfusion dominates the clinical picture. Patients with acute right ventricular infarction are a classic example in this category.

ETIOLOGY AND PRECIPITATING FACTORS

There is a long list of possible heart failure etiologies, but in reality a few causes account for the majority of cases. From long-term heart failure management perspective, the causes can be broadly divided into heart failure with reduced left ventricular ejection fraction (LVEF) and heart failure with preserved LVEF. Recently, a new category of heart failure with mid-range ejection fraction of 40% to 49% has been proposed, which represents a "gray zone" between the traditional categories.[1,2] Coronary artery disease is the most common cause of heart failure with reduced LVEF. Less common causes include myocardial diseases resulting in dilated cardiomyopathy that can be idiopathic, genetic, or associated with other conditions (such as infections, toxins, immune-mediated condition, peripartum, and so on). The prevalence of heart failure with preserved LVEF increases with age and overall accounts for approximately 50% of heart failure cases. The etiology of heart failure with preserved ejection fraction is complex and relates to important cardiovascular risk factors such as hypertension.

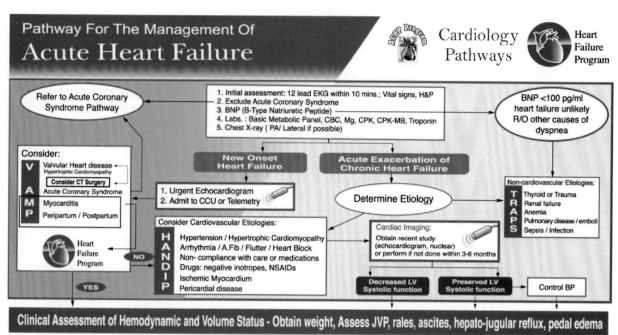

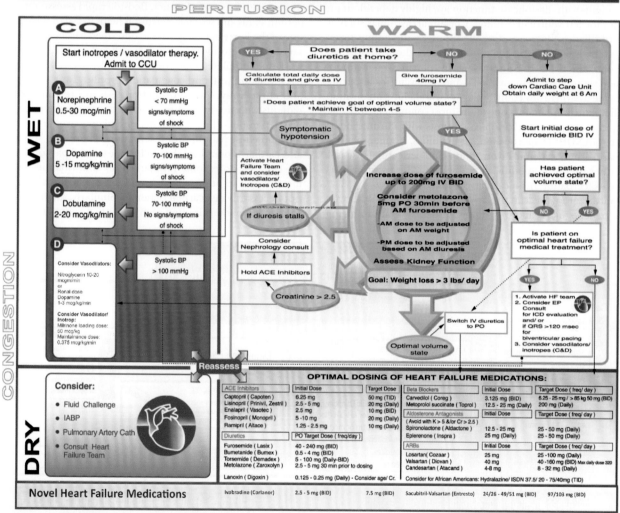

FIGURE 10.1 Pathway for the evaluation and management of acute decompensated heart failure. ACE, angiotensin converting enzyme; ARB, angiotensin receptor blocker; BNP, B-type natriuretic peptides; BP, blood pressure; CBC, complete blood count; CCU, coronary care unit; CPK, creatine phosphokinase; CPK-MB, CPK-muscle and brain; CT, computed tomography; EKG, electrocardiogram; HANDIP, hypertension, arrhythmias, noncompliance with care, drugs, ischemic myocardium, and pericardial disease; IABP, intra-aortic balloon pump; IV, intravenous; JVP, jugular venous pressure; LV, left ventricular; NSAIDs, nonsteroidal anti-inflammatory drugs; PA, pulmonary artery; TRAPS, thyroid, renal failure, anemia, pulmonary disease, and sepsis; VAMP, valvular disease, acute coronary syndromes, myocarditis, and peripartum/postpartum cardiomyopathy.

Some valvular diseases (such as aortic stenosis and mitral regurgitation), hypertrophic cardiomyopathy, and restrictive cardiomyopathy also present as heart failure with preserved LVEF.

In any patient who presents with new-onset acute decompensated heart failure or chronic heart failure exacerbation, the precipitating cause should be identified and adequately addressed. Myocardial ischemia is a common precipitating factor and should be considered in the differential diagnosis. Valvular pathology can cause acute heart failure if it develops suddenly: Typical examples include flail mitral valve with chordal rupture or aortic valve perforation in infective endocarditis. Similarly, mechanical complication of myocardial infarction (such as papillary muscle rupture and ventricular septal rupture) can cause sudden profound hemodynamic deterioration. Myocarditis and postpartum cardiomyopathy can present as acute heart failure. VAMP (valvular disease, acute coronary syndromes, myocarditis, and peripartum/postpartum cardiomyopathy) is a useful mnemonic in evaluating a patient with new-onset acute heart failure (**Figure 10.2**).[3] Severe hypertension is another common condition that is typically associated with preserved LVEF and better in-hospital outcomes. Both supraventricular and ventricular arrhythmias can precipitate heart failure. It is important to know that patients with diastolic dysfunction are highly dependent on preload for left ventricular filling. Certain arrhythmias such as atrial fibrillation decrease diastolic filling by increasing heart rate and eliminating atria kick, and therefore they can provoke florid heart failure in an otherwise stable patient. Interestingly, frequent ventricular premature beats and right ventricular pacing can create dyssynchrony contributing to heart failure. Medication and diet noncompliance is one of the most common factors that precipitate acute exacerbation in patients with chronic heart failure. HANDIP (hypertension, arrhythmias, noncompliance with care, drugs, ischemic myocardium, and pericardial disease) is another useful mnemonic in evaluating patients with heart failure exacerbation from cardiac causes (**Figure 10.2**).[3]

Noncardiac factors can precipitate heart failure in otherwise stable patients by creating high oxygen demand and inducing tachycardia (such as anemia, thyroid diseases, drugs, fever and infection, and pulmonary emboli), causing fluid overload (in-hospital intravenous fluid administration, renal failure, and nonsteroidal anti-inflammatory agents), or decreasing myocardial contractility (negative inotropes such as verapamil). TRAPS (thyroid, renal failure, anemia, pulmonary disease, and sepsis) is a mnemonic to help categorize noncardiac precipitants of heart failure exacerbation (**Figure 10.2**).[3]

DIAGNOSIS AND WORKUP

Once the history and physical examination findings consistent with heart failure are ascertained, further work-up is directed toward confirming the diagnosis, establishing the cause of the heart failure, addressing the precipitating factor(s), and identifying prognostic indicators. Physical examination should specifically focus on the degree of respiratory failure (tachypnea, accessory respiratory muscle use), vital signs, signs of fluid overload (pulmonary crackles, jugular venous distension and peripheral edema), and signs of hypoperfusion (cold extremities, confusion, feeble pulses). Cardiac assessment may provide important clues to the diagnosis (eg, a new murmur). Bedside rapid assessment of congestion status and systemic perfusion helps to assign the patient to one of the Forrester categories as described earlier. The essential set of initial tests includes electrocardiogram (ECG), laboratory work-up (complete blood count, electrolytes, renal function and liver function test, and coagulation profile), cardiac troponins, and chest X-ray. Thyroid function tests are recommended in patients with newly diagnosed acute decompensated heart failure. Up to one-third of patients with acute coronary syndrome have no chest pain upon presentation. Therefore, serial ECGs and cardiac biomarkers should be an essential part of the initial work-up. Of note, some repolarization abnormalities and QTc interval prolongation can be caused by acute heart failure per se, not necessarily myocardial ischemia. Similarly, small increase in cardiac biomarkers is often seen in acute decompensated heart

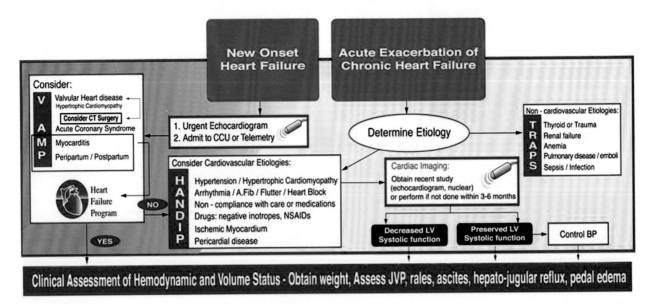

FIGURE 10.2 Differential diagnosis between new-onset heart failure and acute exacerbation of chronic heart failure, with timing of imaging and consideration of precipitating pathophysiology. BP, blood pressure; CCU, coronary care unit; CT, computed tomography; HANDIP, hypertension, arrhythmias, noncompliance with care, drugs, ischemic myocardium, and pericardial disease; JVP, jugular venous pressure; LV, left ventricular; NSAIDs, nonsteroidal anti-inflammatory drugs; TRAPS, thyroid, renal failure, anemia, pulmonary disease, and sepsis; VAMP, valvular disease, acute coronary syndromes, myocarditis, and peripartum/postpartum cardiomyopathy.

failure. Other important findings on ECG include arrhythmias, conduction delays, and hypertrophy. Chest X-ray can confirm pulmonary congestion and can demonstrate some other relevant pathology (large pleural effusion, infiltrates, and cardiomegaly). Arterial blood gases provide information about oxygenation, ventilation, and acid–base status; arterial blood gases should be considered in all patients with significant respiratory distress as well as low perfusion ("cold") state.

B-type natriuretic peptides (BNP and pro-BNP) are released from myocardial cells in response to increase in the wall stress. Their levels are elevated in both heart failure with preserved LVEF and that with reduced LVEF, but on average they are lower in patients with heart failure with preserved LVEF. Measuring BNP level can supplement the evaluation of patients with suspected acute decompensated heart failure if used in the appropriate clinical context.[5] Low BNP levels (<100 pg/mL) have a high negative predictive value that makes the diagnosis of heart failure unlikely in a patient who presents to the emergency department with dyspnea. Values > 400 pg/mL are consistent with heart failure, whereas intermediate values (100 to 400 pg/mL) are in the gray zone. Studies showed linear correlation between the admission BNP levels in patients with acute decompensated heart failure and in-hospital mortality.[6] Of note, obese patients with heart failure have lower BNP levels, which should be factored in during clinical decision making. Sudden, "flash" pulmonary edema can sometimes be associated with falsely low BNP levels. At the same time, the positive predictive value of elevated BNP levels (especially gray-zone values) is not very high because they can be elevated in patients with atrial fibrillation, left ventricular hypertrophy, pulmonary hypertension, sepsis, renal dysfunction, and liver disease. For example, in a septic patient with persistent atrial fibrillation and possible heart failure, elevated BNP levels add little information to the clinical judgment. In the patients with preexisting chronic heart failure who come with acute exacerbation, one-time elevated BNP level conveys little information.

Echocardiography is an essential tool in evaluating patients with acute decompensated heart failure. The urgency of getting echocardiogram is determined by the clinical presentation. For example, in a patient suspected to have acute valvular pathology or an acute mechanical complication of myocardial infarction, a bedside echocardiogram can immediately confirm the diagnosis, whereas in a patient with known chronic heart failure, subacute symptoms, and medication noncompliance, the immediate test would add little information. In the acute settings, an echocardiogram helps to assess the presence and degree of systolic dysfunction, right ventricular size and function, and valvular and pericardial pathology. It can assess the diastolic dysfunction and give the estimate of right-sided pressures as well as left-sided filling pressures. Regional wall motion abnormalities and dyssynchrony can provide clues to the possible causes of the symptoms. Determination of LVEF (heart failure with reduced LVEF vs preserved LVEF) is fundamental in long-term management of heart failure patients.

The routine insertion of a pulmonary artery catheter in patients with acute decompensated heart failure is *not* recommended because it has not been shown to improve major clinical outcomes.[7] It can be considered under specific circumstances to estimate left-sided filling pressures and cardiac output. Possible scenarios include complex patients with cardiac and pulmonary disease, persistent hypotension, worsening renal function, and so forth. The benefits of getting important hemodynamic information should

be weighed in each individual patient against the complications of the invasive monitoring and limitations of the technique.

Coronary angiography is indicated in patients with acute decompensated heart failure believed to be precipitated by myocardial ischemia. Successful reperfusion in these settings has been shown to improve survival.

Comprehensive assessment of patients admitted for acute decompensated heart failure includes identification of prognostic indicators. The indicators of poor prognosis include clinical variables (age, poor functional status at baseline, low admission blood pressure, etc), Laboratory factors and ECG changes (wide QRS complex, certain arrhythmias, hyponatremia, positive cardiac biomarkers, marked elevation of BNP, etc), and imaging findings (low LVEF, restrictive mitral inflow pattern, abnormal RV function, etc).[1]

MANAGEMENT

The management of acute decompensated heart failure should be approached in systematic manner and tailored to each individual patient. **Figure 10.1** outlines the general approach to the management of acute decompensated heart failure. The following components of the therapy should be addressed: (1) oxygenation, (2) hemodynamics, (3) fluid overload, and (4) precipitating factors.

OXYGENATION

The range of respiratory distress varies along the spectrum of presentations in acute decompensated heart failure. Rapid assessment of oxygenation and respiratory status is an important initial step. Mild respiratory distress might require oxygen supplementation via nasal cannula or a mask, with the goal of keeping the patient comfortable and maintaining oxygen saturation above 90% to 92%. Caution should be exercised in chronic CO_2 retainers because high-flow oxygen delivery in these patients can result in acute CO_2 retention and respiratory acidosis. Patients with significant respiratory distress need arterial blood gas analysis to assess oxygenation, ventilation, and acid–base status. Patients with pulmonary edema have been shown to benefit from noninvasive positive pressure ventilation, provided they do not have contraindications (eg, impaired level of consciousness, agitation, inability to protect airways, high risk of aspiration, etc). The benefits of noninvasive positive pressure ventilation result from improved V/Q mismatch and decreased cardiac preload. Meta-analyses of randomized clinical trials in patients with pulmonary edema suggest a decrease in the need of intubation and improvement in respiratory signs and symptoms.[8] Mortality benefit from noninvasive positive pressure ventilation in those patients has not been consistently demonstrated. Patients in significant respiratory distress and those who have contraindications to noninvasive positive pressure ventilation should be intubated and mechanical ventilation should be initiated.

HEMODYNAMICS

Rapid bedside assessment of hemodynamics as described earlier is important in initial management of acute decompensated heart failure. Most heart failure patients are in "warm" and "wet" category and need treatment with diuretics and vasodilators. Patients with borderline or low blood pressure, poor perfusion, and pulmonary edema ("cold" and "wet") are in/at risk of cardiogenic shock and generally carry poor prognosis. Rapid correction of precipitating factors may improve their condition (eg, revascularization in acute coronary syndrome). Patients with borderline and low systolic blood pressure and poor perfusion (cold and clammy) and patients who are resistant to diuretic therapy experience symptomatic improvement from inotropic agents. Dobutamine, which is a β-adrenergic agonist, can be used in these settings. Phosphodiesterase inhibitors (such as milrinone) are potent inotropes and can also provide significant symptomatic relief. It is important to remember that inotropic agents should be used only as temporary measure and withdrawn as early as possible once adequate perfusion is restored and congestion has been relieved. Symptomatic relief provided by those agents comes at the expense of increased risk of ischemia, arrhythmias, and myocardial damage. They have been shown to increase short-term and long-term mortality in patients with congestive heart failure.[1] Their use should be restricted to patients with known severe systolic left ventricular dysfunction. In addition, vasodilator effect of inotropic agents may cause hypotension. Vasopressor agents (preferably norepinephrine) can be used in these settings to maintain blood pressure. Finally, patients with hypotension and no signs of significant pulmonary congestion ("cold" and "dry" state) can receive a fluid challenge, if volume depletion and sepsis are a consideration. However, these patients are at risk of rapidly developing volume over load and edema. Careful monitoring is essential. In patients who develop symptomatic hypotension during aggressive diuresis, the diuretics should be held. Patients who are highly preload dependent (eg, severe aortic stenosis or severe concentric left ventricular hypertrophy and normal LVEF) are at a higher risk of hypotension with aggressive diuresis.

In patients with cardiogenic shock who do not have an adequate response to pharmacologic therapy, mechanical assist devices should be considered. These include intra-aortic balloon pump and ventricular assist devices. They can provide temporary hemodynamic support as a "bridge to decision" or bridge to longer-term intervention. The evidence behind using mechanical assist devices in these settings is limited and needs further study and validation.[1]

FLUID OVERLOAD

Symptoms of dyspnea in acute decompensated heart failure are attributed to elevated left-sided filling pressures. Most patients with decompensated heart failure are fluid overloaded owing to renal retention of sodium and water, whereas some patients with acute, especially precipitous, heart failure are normovolemic. Early diuresis and manipulation of preload are the most effective ways to bring symptomatic relief to those patients. Most patients with acute decompensated heart failure require intravenous loop diuretic therapy except "dry" patients and those with hypotension and shock. Patients with hypotension, severe acidosis, renal failure, and hyponatremia are less likely to respond to loop diuretics. The dosing of the intravenous loop diuretic (eg, furosemide) used in patients with acute decompensated heart failure should be based on the degree of fluid overload, renal function, and preadmission loop diuretic use (**Figure 10.3**). Interestingly, it has been shown that loop diuretics improve symptoms even before the diuretic effect by venodilation and a decrease in preload. Parameters that need to be monitored during diuretic therapy include volume status, intake and output, blood pressure, electrolytes, and renal function. Patients with decreasing renal function upon diuresis (a form of "cardiorenal syndrome") carry a worse prognosis. In patients who show suboptimal response to escalating doses of loop diuretics, the following options can be considered: addition of a thiazide diuretic, addition of mineralocorticoid receptor antagonist, inotropic therapy, and continuous infusion of a loop diuretic. In patients with renal dysfunction, metolazone added to loop diuretics might be used. Dopamine in low doses has been shown to improve renal perfusion, but the clinical implications of this finding were not supported in a large randomized clinical trial. Ultrafiltration is the last-resort therapy, especially in patients with severe renal dysfunction.

Preload reduction brings significant symptomatic relief in patients with acute decompensated heart failure by decreasing left-sided filling pressures. It can be achieved by using venodilators such as nitroglycerine, isosorbide dinitrate, and nitroprusside. Nitroglycerin, typically in the form of intravenous infusion, can be used as add-on therapy to diuretics if systolic blood pressure is >110 mm Hg. In patients with systolic blood pressure <90 mm Hg, vasodilators should be avoided, whereas in patients with systolic blood pressure of 90 to 110 mm Hg, they should be used with caution. Hypotension is the main side effect of nitroglycerine, especially in patients who are significantly preload dependent (eg, severe aortic stenosis, right ventricular infarction). Nitrates should be avoided in patients using phosphodiesterase inhibitors (eg, sildenafil). Headache is a common complaint, and tachyphylaxis develops with continuous use. Nitroprusside is a potent vasodilator that achieves significant afterload reduction along with preload reduction. This property is important in certain situations such as hypertensive emergencies and acute valvular pathology such as acute mitral regurgitation. Accumulation of cyanide is a potential side effect with continuous infusion. Nesiritide is an analog of brain natriuretic peptide. It produces vasodilation, reduces preload, and may bring symptomatic relief to patients with pulmonary congestion. However, a large randomized trial showed that nesiritide improves symptoms only marginally and does not improve the rates of death and rehospitalization.[9] Therefore, routine use of nesiritide is not recommended. Morphine reduces anxiety and sense of dyspnea and produces vasodilation in patients with pulmonary edema. However, retrospective studies raised some concerns regarding the use of morphine in these patients because of association with increased in-hospital mortality.[2] In patients with acute coronary syndrome and chest pain, morphine should not be withheld.

OTHER THERAPIES

Angiotensin-converting enzyme (ACE) inhibitors reduce morbidity and mortality in patients with chronic heart failure and decreased LVEF but their role in managing patients with acute decompensated heart failure is limited. They are generally avoided in these patients until they are stable due to the following concerns: ACE inhibitors can precipitate hypotension and worsening renal function in patients who are aggressively diuresed. Similarly, β-blockers are the mainstay of chronic heart failure treatment in patients with systolic left ventricular dysfunction, but they should be avoided in the settings of acute exacerbation. In patients who are already taking β-blockers, they can be cautiously resumed once

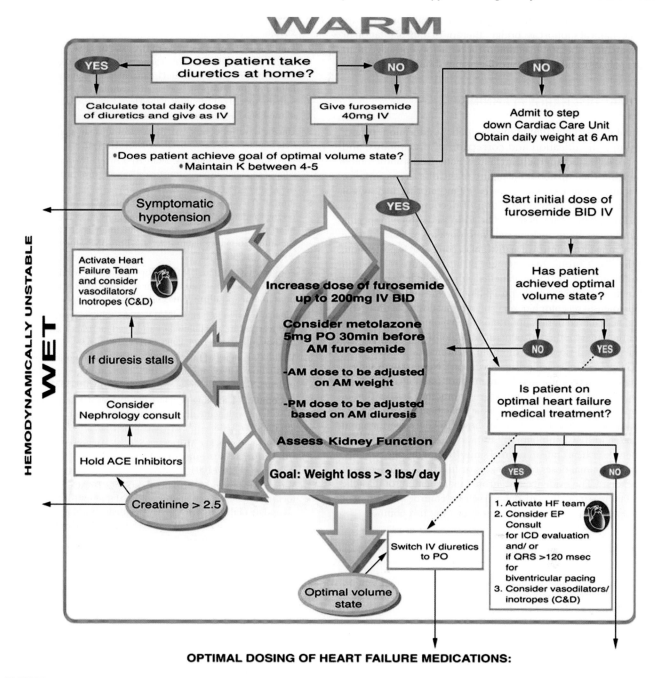

FIGURE 10.3 The "loop" concept of aggressive usage of loop diuretics to rapidly and safely diurese patients, shorten length of stay, and transition to oral therapy upon successful completion of diuresis. ACE, angiotensin converting enzyme; EP, electrophysiology; ICD, implantable cardioverter defibrillator.

the patients are stable. Thromboembolism prophylaxis should be ensured in all patients with acute decompensated heart failure.

PRECIPITANTS

Identifying the precipitating factors for acute decompensated heart failure should be the part of the initial thought process. The common precipitating factors are described above, and some of them should be actively sought and corrected such as myocardial ischemia, hypertensive crisis, arrhythmias, and acute valvular pathology (see specific chapters on how to address those issues). Medication and diet noncompliance is a common precipitant,

and it should be specifically inquired. Other precipitating factors such as infection, medications (eg, nonsteroidal antiinflammatory drugs), pulmonary disease, and so on could be more subtle and their identification requires a systematic approach to history taking, physical examination, and laboratory work-up.

END-STAGE HEART FAILURE

Patients with severe, "end-stage" heart failure that are resistant to optimal medical therapy often have symptoms at rest (NYHA functional class IV). They have frequent hospitalizations, long hospital stays, and poor quality of life. Options for those patients are limited to continuous inotrope infusion as palliative measure and mechanical support as "bridge" therapy to transplantation or as "destination" therapy. In addition, for refractory end-stage heart failure palliative and hospice care discussions should be initiated.[1,2]

OPTIMAL DISCHARGE PLANNING

Optimal discharge planning involves patient education, proper follow-up, identification and correction of precipitants, and evidence-based therapy for heart failure. Patient education should include information about the nature of the disease, importance of diet and medication compliance, self-monitoring (eg, weight and edema), and early recognition of decompensation symptoms. Precipitating factors should be addressed, which in specific circumstances might include ischemic work-up, valvular disease surgery, long-term control of arrhythmias, control of hypertension, and the like. Chronic management of heart failure is based on the estimation of the LVEF. Patients with systolic left ventricular dysfunction should be placed on a β-blocker and an ACE inhibitor (or angiotensin receptor blocker) and optimal dosing of the agents should be achieved by slow uptitration during outpatient follow-up. Other therapies for those patients include aldosterone antagonists, hydralazine and isosorbide dinitrate combination, and digoxin (see Chapter 19 for specific drug discussion). Newer agents such as an angiotensin receptor-neprilysin inhibitor (sacubitril-valsartan) and a selective sinus node inhibitor (ivabradine) have a role in the outpatient treatment of chronic systolic heart failure. Specifically, sacubitril-valsartan has been shown to be a superior agent compared with ACE inhibitor.[10,11] Ivabradine can be considered to further lower heart rate in normal sinus rhythm despite patients' being on optimal doses of β-blockers or in patients intolerant of β-blockers.[12] The evidence for chronic management of diastolic heart failure is more limited; optimal volume control and treatment of hypertension seem to be the best strategy at this point.

REFERENCES

1. Yancy CW, Jessup M, Bozkurt B, et al. 2013 ACCF/AHA guideline for the management of heart failure: a report of the American College of Cardiology Foundation/American Heart Association Task Force on Practice Guidelines. *J Am Coll Cardiol.* 2013;62(16):e147-e239.

2. Ponikowski P, Voors AA, Anker SD, et al. 2016 ESC Guidelines for the diagnosis and treatment of acute and chronic heart failure: the task force for the diagnosis and treatment of acute and chronic heart failure of the European Society of Cardiology (ESC). Developed with the special contribution of the Heart Failure Association (HFA) of the ESC. *Eur J Heart Fail.* 2016;18(8):891-975.

3. Herzog E, Varley C, Kukin M. Pathway for the management of acute heart failure. *Crit Pathw Cardiol.* 2005;4(1):37-42.

4. Forrester JS, Diamond GA, Swan HJ. Correlative classification of clinical and hemodynamic function after acute myocardial infarction. *Am J Cardiol.* 1977;39(2):137-145.

5. Januzzi JL, van Kimmenade R, Lainchbury J, et al. NT-proBNP testing for diagnosis and short-term prognosis in acute destabilized heart failure: an international pooled analysis of 1256 patients: the International Collaborative of NT-proBNP Study. *Eur Heart J.* 2006;27(3):330-337.

6. Fonarow GC, Peacock WF, Phillips CO, et al. Admission B-type natriuretic peptide levels and in-hospital mortality in acute decompensated heart failure. *J Am Coll Cardiol.* 2007;49(19):1943-1950.

7. Binanay C, Califf RM, Hasselblad V, et al. Evaluation study of congestive heart failure and pulmonary artery catheterization effectiveness: the ESCAPE trial. *JAMA.* 2005;294(13):1625-1633.

8. Vital FM, Ladeira MT, Atallah AN. Non-invasive positive pressure ventilation (CPAP or bilevel NPPV) for cardiogenic pulmonary oedema. *Cochrane Database Syst Rev.* 2013;(5):CD005351.

9. O'Connor CM, Starling RC, Hernandez AF, et al. Effect of nesiritide in patients with acute decompensated heart failure. *N Engl J Med.* 2011;365(1):32-43.

10. McMurray JJ, Packer M, Desai AS, et al. Angiotensin-neprilysin inhibition versus enalapril in heart failure. *N Engl J Med.* 2014;371(11):993-1004.

11. Yancy CW, Jessup M, Bozkurt B, et al. 2016 ACC/AHA/HFSA focused update on new pharmacological therapy for heart failure: an update of the 2013 ACCF/AHA guideline for the management of heart failure: a report of the American College of Cardiology/American Heart Association Task Force on Clinical Practice Guidelines and the Heart Failure Society of America. *J Am Coll Cardiol.* 2016;68(13):1476-1488.

12. Swedberg K, Komajda M, Bohm M, et al. Ivabradine and outcomes in chronic heart failure (SHIFT): a randomised placebo-controlled study. *Lancet.* 2010;376(9744):875-885.

Patient and Family Information for:
THE MANAGEMENT OF ACUTE HEART FAILURE

DEFINITION AND CAUSES

Heart failure is a common problem in the United States, especially in the elderly population. It is one of the most common reasons for hospital admission. Heart failure is a clinical syndrome and not a specific disease. It can have many causes. It results from decreased pumping function of the heart and its inability to propagate adequate amounts of blood to the tissues. Acute heart failure is a serious, life-threatening condition; it can be the presentation of newly diagnosed illness or an exacerbation of a preexisting disease. Shortness of breath is the most common symptom of acute heart failure. It results from fluid accumulation in the lungs. Other manifestations of heart failure include cough, swelling of the legs, fatigue, tiredness, and poor appetite. Some patients experience nighttime episodes of breathlessness and find it difficult to sleep flat in bed. Patients with preexisting chronic heart failure often experience slow and progressive shortness of breath on exertion, leg swelling, and weight gain, all symptoms of fluid accumulation in the body before they present to the hospital with breathlessness at rest. Acute heart failure is not synonymous to "heart attack," but it can sometimes be precipitated by heart attack. In that case, it is common for patients to have chest pain, chest discomfort, or pressure-like sensation in the chest. The severe form of acute heart failure is called "pulmonary edema"; it causes significant distress and breathing difficulty due to rapid build-up of the fluid in the lungs. Another extreme form of heart failure is called "cardiogenic shock"; it causes poor perfusion of the tissues due to significant impairment of heart function. The patients appear cold and clammy, their blood pressure is low, and their thinking can be impaired. Those patients are at a high risk of dying and often need drastic measures to correct the underlying problem and support the circulation.

Heart failure is not a single disease; it is a manifestation of a big variety of structural heart disorders. The most common disorder that results in heart failure is coronary artery disease. Blockage of the blood vessels that supply the heart muscle can result in a significant heart muscle damage, causing the heart to fail. High blood pressure, if unrecognized or untreated, causes pathologic changes in the heart muscle over months to years and can eventually result in heart failure. The heart valve narrowing or leakage is a relatively common cause of heart failure. Diseases of the heart muscle, itself termed "cardiomyopathy," manifest as heart failure. Some causes of cardiomyopathy are known (such as infection, alcohol, and illegal drugs) and some are genetically inherited. A well-described form of cardiomyopathy is associated with pregnancy. Sometimes, there is no obvious cause for the heart muscle weakness, and in medical literature, it is referred to as "idiopathic." Besides the structural heart disease that results in heart failure, it is important to realize that a variety of conditions can provoke an acute exacerbation of heart failure. Those conditions are called "precipitating factors." Precipitating factors superimposed on the underlying structural heart disease are responsible for acute onset of symptoms in otherwise stable patient. A "heart attack" or inadequate blood supply to the heart muscle called "ischemia" is a common precipitating factor. Poorly controlled blood pressure puts excessive strain on the heart and precipitates heart failure. Noncompliance with the diet and medications is among the most common precipitating factors for acute heart failure. Other conditions that can precipitate or worsen heart failure include infection, certain medications (including painkillers), low blood count, heart rhythm disturbances (called "arrhythmias"), kidney disease, etc.

DIAGNOSIS AND TREATMENT

The physician establishes the diagnosis of acute heart failure by taking history (asking questions about the patient's symptoms), performing physical examination, and ordering appropriate tests. Besides confirming the diagnosis, the physician needs to determine what the underlying structural heart disease is that causes heart failure and what the precipitating factor for the current acute exacerbation is. Blood tests are commonly sent, and ECG and chest X-ray are also typically performed. Ultrasound examination of the heart (also known as echocardiogram) helps to visualize cardiac chambers, and it is the most commonly used tool to evaluate the structure and function of the heart. Other tests are performed as deemed necessary by the physician. Cardiac catheterization is an invasive test that includes placing catheters into the heart chambers and major vessels to diagnose vessel blockage or get important pressure readings from various heart chambers. It is also used for interventions if vessel blockage seems to be causing patient's symptoms.

Treatment of heart failure has several important components. Patients are given oxygen by nasal prongs or a mask to ensure adequate oxygen delivery to the tissues. In patients with significant breathing difficulty, assisted ventilation via special mask is employed (commonly called "continuous positive airway pressure"). Occasionally, a breathing tube is placed in the airway and mechanical ventilation is initiated. In patients with low blood pressure and poor perfusion, medications are used to maintain blood pressure. In severe cases, medications that enhance heart muscle contractility are used; unfortunately, those medications are associated with significant adverse effects and therefore their use is limited to refractory cases. As explained above, fluid overload underlies many symptoms of heart failure; therefore, diuretic medications are commonly administered to increase water and sodium excretion from the body. Other medications that help to relieve the symptoms include vasodilators; these medications dilate the blood vessels in the body decreasing the workload on the heart. These are commonly administered as intravenous drips. Precipitating factors are also addressed. These could include controlling abnormal heart rhythm, lowering blood pressure, treating infection, etc.

FOLLOW-UP AND PREVENTION

Once the acute phase is over, the long-term management plan should be discussed in detail. Medications used to treat chronic heart failure are often different from those used to treat acute exacerbation. β-Blockers (such as metoprolol or carvedilol), ACE inhibitors (such as lisinopril and enalapril), sacubitril-valsartan, and spironolactone are commonly used in the treatment of chronic heart failure. They help to maintain heart function and prevent acute exacerbation. They have also been shown to decrease the risk of death in certain patients with heart failure. Proper education of the patient includes teaching them about the appropriate medication regimen, necessity of taking the medications daily, and compliance with low-salt diet. Sodium contained in salt retains fluid in the body and causes heart failure exacerbations. Besides, it commonly elevates blood pressure, putting excessive stain on the heart. Patients should not only follow appropriate diet but also be able to recognize early signs and symptoms of heart failure such as exertional shortness of breath, fatigue, inability to lay flat in bed, awakening from sleep short of breath, using several pillows to elevate the head and thereby making breathing at night easier, gradual weight gain, and ankle swelling. Weight gain is commonly the first manifestation of fluid build-up in the body; therefore, the patients should know their "dry weight" and try to follow their weight regularly. Proper follow-up after discharge is necessary to ensure stability of clinical symptoms and proper adjustment of medication doses. Some of the medications (such as β-blockers) need to be titrated up slowly during follow-up visits to avoid adverse effects. In case of coronary artery disease and valvular heart disease, certain interventions or surgery can fix the problem. Implantations of certain devices such as a pacemaker or defibrillator might be beneficial in certain groups of patients.

Yaron Hellman

11

Heart Failure with Reduced Ejection Fraction

INTRODUCTION

This chapter provides the basic definitions, pathophysiology, clinical presentation, and the basis of treatment in patients with heart failure (HF) with reduced ejection fraction (EF). From an epidemiologic standpoint, HF is a growing problem with a substantial impact affecting millions of patients worldwide. About 5.7 million adults in the United States have HF, and half of those affected will die within 5 years of diagnosis.[1] In fact, HF is the leading cause of hospitalization among patients over the age of 65 in the United States.[2] The economic burden of HF is reflected in costs estimated to be as much as $30.7 billion/year in the United States alone.[3] This total includes the cost of health care services, medications to treat HF, and missed days of work.

DEFINITION

HF has a broad definition with no single diagnostic test as a gold standard. Impaired contractility and reduced EF are not an adequate definition—at least half of the patients with HF have a preserved EF (impaired relaxation or "diastolic" HF). According to current clinical guidelines, the broadest definition of HF is "a complex clinical syndrome that results from any structural or functional impairment of ventricular filling or ejection of blood."[4]

Older definitions include the "classic" definition by Braunwald—"A pathophysiological state in which an abnormality of cardiac function is responsible for the failure of the heart to pump blood at a rate commensurate with the requirements of the metabolizing tissues."[5] Another classic definition emphasizing HF pathophysiology proposed by Poole-Wilson is "a clinical syndrome caused by an abnormality of the heart and recognized by a characteristic pattern of hemodynamic, renal, neural and hormonal responses."[6]

Currently, "heart failure" replaced the older term "congestive heart failure" because many patients present with symptoms of dyspnea and exercise intolerance rather than overt volume overload.[4]

SUBGROUPS

HF can be divided into several well-known subgroups. Left-sided HF refers to pulmonary congestion as opposed to right-sided HF

representing peripheral edema, pleural effusion, and ascites. Forward failure is used to describe low cardiac output and poor peripheral perfusion. In contrast, backward failure consists of peripheral edema, pulmonary edema, and splanchnic congestion (ascites, hepatomegaly, abdominal fullness).

CLASSIFICATION ACCORDING TO LEFT VENTRICULAR EJECTION FRACTION

EF is the percentage expressed by (left ventricular end-diastolic volume—end-systolic volume)/left ventricular end-diastolic volume. EF is considered as a load-independent factor that can identify patients with a primary defect in cardiac contractility—systolic function. Many HF trials selected patients according to reduced EF because it can be measured objectively by echocardiography, magnetic resonance imaging (MRI), or radionuclide imaging. However, as mentioned earlier, approximately half of the patients with HF have preserved EF—diastolic dysfunction. The etiology, comorbidities, demographics, and response to therapy differ between patients with reduced ejection fraction (HFrEF) and preserved EF (HFpEF). Therefore, patients with HF are generally divided into these two categories.[7] It is important to understand that diastolic dysfunction (impairment of myocardial relaxation) may coexist in the setting of systolic dysfunction. Conversely, patients with diastolic dysfunction may have impaired systolic function not identified by the EF. That is why the terms HFrEF and HFpEF are more accurate rather than systolic and diastolic HF. In addition, an intermediate group with a left ventricular ejection fraction (LVEF) of 40% to 50% has been added recently to reflect this mixture of systolic and diastolic dysfunction.[4,7]

ETIOLOGY

HF has a wide range of causes varying from common causes (coronary artery disease, hypertension) to rare infiltrative diseases (amyloidosis, Fabry disease). These etiologies are categorized phenotypically in **Figure 11.1**. The initial classification includes non-myocardial diseases—valvular disease, pericardial disease, and congenital heart disease. Pericardial disease mainly refers to constrictive pericarditis, which typically presents with right-sided

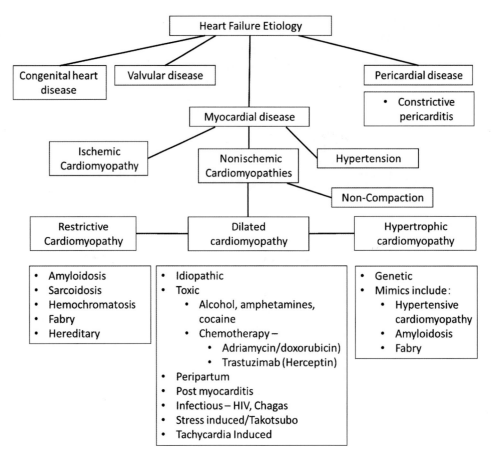

FIGURE 11.1 Heart failure etiologies.

HF, although many patients have dyspnea as well. Valvular heart disease often results in myocardial disease over time because of compensatory mechanisms such as hypertrophy (eg, aortic stenosis and left ventricular hypertrophy [LVH]) and dilation (aortic regurgitation and dilated left ventricle [LV]). Congenital heart disease represents a diverse category, often with myocardial changes, even after palliative or correctional surgery.

Primary myocardial disease can be roughly divided to ischemic cardiomyopathy and nonischemic cardiomyopathies. Although hypertension is not a primary myocardial disease, it causes LVH over time (depending on treatment) and results in diastolic dysfunction. When blood pressure elevation is at extreme levels, systolic dysfunction may also occur ("afterload mismatch")—reduced LVEF.

Coronary artery disease and myocardial infarction remain a leading cause of HFrEF even in the current era of timely reperfusion for ST-elevation myocardial infarction. Eventually, many patients post myocardial infarction will develop a global dilated cardiomyopathy after the initial insult (remodeling) or repeated insults—ischemic cardiomyopathy. Some of these patients may present with HF without preceding angina (usually diabetics with "silent" ischemia). Nonischemic cardiomyopathies include a variety of myocardial diseases. These can be divided into dilated, restrictive, hypertrophic, and non compaction cardiomyopathies.

Dilated cardiomyopathy can be subdivided into several groups—genetic/idiopathic, post myocarditis, toxic, and peripartum cardiomyopathy. Alcohol is a common cause of toxic cardiomyopathy, often partially reversible after cessation of alcohol intake. Chemotherapy-induced cardiomyopathy is increasing in prevalence, especially due to the relatively high success rate in the treatment of leukemia/lymphoma, and the use of doxorubicin and Herceptin in breast cancer. This set the ground for a new subspecialty in itself—cardio-oncology.

PATHOPHYSIOLOGY

Several key pathophysiologic concepts are important to understand when dealing with HF.[8] Cardiac output is determined by heart rate (HR) × stroke volume (SV). One important consequence of this equation is that tachycardia is a proper response to increase cardiac output. Therefore, beta-blockers and HR–lowering therapy in patients with a fixed SV may be detrimental (eg, acute systolic HF, amyloidosis, aortic stenosis). The hazardous effects of tachycardia in the long term are discussed later.

SV is determined by three factors: preload, cardiac contractility (inotropic state), and afterload.

Preload is defined as the ventricular end-diastolic volume. The left ventricular preload is determined by venous return, atrial contraction (20%), and right ventricular function. An important relationship is the force–volume curve, more commonly known as the Frank-Starling curve. A useful analogy is visualizing the basic myocardial unit, the actin–myosin complex, as a spring **(Figure 11.2)**. If the spring is stretched (ie, filling the LV with volume—preload), it will contract with increased force. When the preload is excessive, the spring will reach a certain limit and may

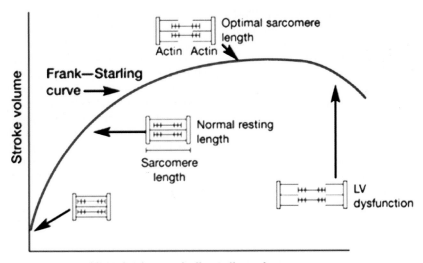

FIGURE 11.2 Relation between stroke volume and ventricular end-diastolic volume. LV, left ventricle.

even generate a reduced force of contraction. The final end of the Frank–Starling curve is also explained by the right ventricle–left ventricle (RV–LV) interaction and septal displacement.

Cardiac contractility is also known as the inotropic state. This is determined by the intrinsic ability of the myocardium to contract. Factors affecting the inotropic state are intracellular calcium, catecholamines, and pharmacologic agents at different levels (beta-adrenergic receptor, phosphodiesterase 3, NA/K exchanger, etc).

Afterload represents the resistance against which the heart ejects blood. This tension faced by the myocardium is determined by Laplace's law—$T = P*R/2D$, where P is the pressure faced by the LV, R is the radius of the ventricular chamber, and D is the wall thickness. Common situations of increased afterload are vasoconstriction, systemic hypertension, and aortic stenosis. Increased afterload results in reduced systolic function even in hearts with preserved cardiac contractility. This inverse relationship is markedly pronounced in patients with HFrEF **(Figure 11.3)**—patients with HFrEF are "afterload sensitive." This is why afterload reduction is such a crucial and important part of HF therapy.

REMODELING

Remodeling is a pathophysiologic concept describing the process in which an initial insult (eg, myocardial infarction, myocarditis) results in eccentric hypertrophy and LV enlargement. At first, LV enlargement increases SV and cardiac output allowing for initial compensation. However, the progressive ventricular enlargement (beyond the extent of the initial insult) results in thinning of the heart muscle and globally reduced contraction. This is analogous to a "bad remodeling" job done in the house. The official definition of remodeling is a "group of molecular, cellular and interstitial changes that clinically manifest as changes in size, shape and function of the heart resulting from cardiac injury," as published in an international consensus document.[9]

NEUROHORMONAL ACTIVATION AFTER MYOCARDIAL INSULT

The reduced SV in HFrEF along with elevated pressures lead to the activation of several neurohormonal pathways.

Activation of the sympathetic nervous system is an immediate consequence of any cardiac insult. Reduced cardiac output is sensed by baroreceptors, which in turn increase central nervous system sympathetic discharge and catecholamine production by the adrenal glands. Catecholamines act upon beta-receptors in the heart and alpha-receptors in the peripheral vasculature; resulting in tachycardia, increased venous return (preload), increased cardiac contractility (inotropic state), and peripheral vasoconstriction (which increases blood pressure and afterload). The sympathetic activation therefore increases cardiac output in the short term, allowing for compensation and meeting the body's metabolic demands. However, in the long term, catecholamines are detrimental with direct apoptotic effects on myocardial cells, pro-arrhythmia, and increase in afterload and cardiac work.

Another hormonal cascade activated post myocardial injury is the renin–angiotensin–aldosterone axis. Decreased cardiac output causes an increase in renin production, which in turn increases angiotensin production and vasoconstriction. In addition to

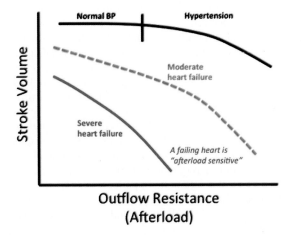

FIGURE 11.3 Relation between stroke volume and outflow resistance (afterload). BP, blood pressure.

vasoconstriction, angiotensin stimulates production of aldosterone. Aldosterone exerts its effect on the renal collecting ducts, promoting sodium reabsorption along with K and H secretion. Aldosterone also has a direct effect on myocardial cells, promoting apoptosis and fibrosis.

An inflammatory reaction occurs as well during HF, resulting in increased levels of cytokines such as tumor necrosis factor. In the long term, this is one of the causes of cardiac cachexia, similar to that in cancer patients.

In contrast to the deleterious "bad" neurohormones that cause salt and water retention and long-term damage to myocardial cells, there is a "positive" pathway providing natriuresis and vasodilation—the natriuretic peptides. These natriuretic peptides are secreted by the heart chambers and blood vessels. There are several natriuretic peptides; the most well known is the B-type natriuretic peptide (BNP) secreted mainly by the ventricles. Since natriuretic peptides are measurable, elevated BNP and N-terminal (NT)-pro-BNP levels provide a diagnosis of HF as well as an estimation of prognosis (extent of HF).

Myocardial energy metabolism is also modulated in HF—an "energy crisis."[10] Since free fatty acids require more O_2 and energy to derive adenosine triphosphate, glucose is a more efficient fuel for the failing heart. The implications of these energetic derangements are providing good nutritional support, in general, and appropriate glucose and insulin management during acute HF.

SYMPTOMS AND SIGNS OF HFrEF

Dyspnea is a cardinal manifestation of HF and may manifest in several forms. The basic underlying mechanism of dyspnea is increased hydrostatic pressure in the alveolar capillaries and transudation of fluids into the alveoli. Exertional dyspnea occurs because of the increased preload and cardiac demand. Dyspnea may also occur during the night, due to the supine position and increased preload. This is the mechanism of paroxysmal nocturnal dyspnea (PND) and orthopnea. PND is often described by patients as nightly rales or wheezing. Orthopnea is not as common as exertional dyspnea; but when it is described ("sleeping upright in a chair"), it is quite specific for HF rather than for other causes of dyspnea. A recently recognized symptom is bendopnea—dyspnea while bending over.[11] Bendopnea is quite common in HFrEF (especially in the patients with advanced HF), also due to increased preload. Many patients will complain of the inability to tie their shoe laces. Because the underlying cause of dyspnea in HF is increased hydrostatic pressure, it is not specific for HFrEF and is a common symptom of HFpEF as well. In addition, younger patients with a more compliant LV and atrium ("less stiff" compared to the aging fibrotic heart) may not necessarily complain of dyspnea. Dyspnea may also present as "cardiac asthma"—the alveolar fluid may cause bronchoconstriction and wheezing. This may sound exactly like asthma on clinical examination!

Patients with HFrEF may also manifest right-sided symptoms such as peripheral edema, abdominal fullness, or ascites. Often the liver/splanchnic congestion may cause right upper quadrant and epigastric pain, sometimes masquerading as cholecystitis (especially when the patient already has gallstones). Cachexia and unintended weight loss are late and ominous symptoms of advanced HF, usually marking the "point of no return" even with advanced therapies.

Important physical signs in patients with HFrEF include measurement of vital signs (HR, blood pressure), estimation of jugular venous pressure (JVP), lung auscultation (crackles and wheezing), heart auscultation (S3), and lower extremity edema. JVP is an essential component, with a particular emphasis on the abdominojugular test (abdominal compression resulting in jugular venous distension), which correlates well with wedge pressure (not only occult right atrial pressures as previously thought).[12] Weight is another physical sign that reflects changes in body volume/fluids in the short term. In the long term, weight loss and cachexia are signs of advanced HF. In fact, obesity seems to have a "protective" effect in HF—hence the term "obesity paradox."

DIAGNOSTIC TESTS

The single most important test in HF is the echocardiogram. First, the echocardiogram provides us with the major distinction between HFrEF and HFpEF. Second, the echocardiogram allows for evaluation beyond LV function—including valvular disease (eg, mitral regurgitation, aortic stenosis), hemodynamics (estimation of pulmonary artery pressure, cardiac output), presence of thrombus, and RV function.

Natriuretic peptide measurement in HF is the equivalent of the troponin measurement in myocardial infarction. As mentioned earlier, the natriuretic peptide system is activated as part of the neurohormonal response in HF. BNP is released from the ventricles in response to increased wall stress, and reflects the degree of HF. During the late 1990s and early 2000s, the natriuretic peptides transformed from a basic science neurohormonal marker to a clinically relevant biomarker allowing for rapid diagnosis of dyspnea in the emergency room.[13] BNP is measured directly or as NT-pro-BNP, depending on the commercial kit used by the hospital biochemistry laboratory. In addition to ruling in or ruling out HF in patients with dyspnea, natriuretic peptides are also a useful marker of prognosis. Lastly, BNP may be used to guide therapy, suggesting that several measurements of BNP during the HF hospitalization are warranted.

The electrocardiogram (ECG) is a basic cardiac test and contributes in the diagnosis and management of HF. Although most patients with HF will have a pathologic ECG, it does not always provide specific information. However, the ECG can help support possible etiologies—such as low voltage in amyloidosis, Q waves with or without ST elevation in myocardial infarction, and LVH in patients with hypertension, hypertrophic cardiomyopathy or aortic stenosis. Left bundle branch block (LBBB) is also important, because this is the main indication of biventricular pacing (cardiac resynchronization therapy). In addition, ECG findings are helpful in the diagnosis of hyperkalemia/hypokalemia, digoxin toxicity, and in the assessment of pacemaker function. Lastly, the ECG may demonstrate arrhythmias with important clinical implications. A common situation is the HF patient with atrial fibrillation, requiring the consideration of anticoagulation for the prevention of stroke and systemic thromboembolism.

The chest X-ray may demonstrate pulmonary congestion and an enlarged cardiac silhouette in patients with HF. In addition, the chest X-ray allows for further evaluation of other causes of dyspnea, such as lung disease, diaphragmatic paralysis, and pulmonary effusion.

MRI is a complex imaging modality that is currently used mainly for the diagnosis and risk stratification of infiltrative disorders (amyloidosis, hemochromatosis, and sarcoidosis), hypertrophic cardiomyopathy, myocarditis, and congenital heart disease. The MRI is useful in quantifying RV function (which is not always fully captured in the two-dimensional echo), presence of scar (late gadolinium enhancement), and LV chamber evaluation (non compaction, LVEF)

Cardiac catheterization is an essential part of evaluating HFrEF. Coronary artery disease is a common etiology of reduced LV systolic function. More importantly, revascularization (coronary artery bypass grafting, percutaneous coronary intervention) may significantly improve LV function and outcomes.[14] Therefore, coronary evaluation is mandated in most patients. In younger patients without significant coronary calcification, computed tomography (CT) angiography is a noninvasive alternative. Hemodynamic assessment via right heart catheterization is necessary in patients with borderline hemodynamics (precardiogenic shock, cardiogenic shock) and in candidates for ventricular assist device (VAD) or heart transplantation.

Cardiopulmonary exercise testing (CPET) offers a means of improved diagnosis (cardiogenic vs pulmonary vs other causes of dyspnea), as well as estimating prognosis. This test does not require the patient to reach a maximal HR because the anaerobic threshold is determined during the test itself. An important value to keep in mind is the VO_{2max} (peak oxygen consumption)—a value less than 14 mL/kg/min indicates a poor prognosis and a clear benefit from heart transplantation or left ventricular assist device (LVAD) rather than medical management.[15]

The 6-minute walk test is simpler and more readily available than the CPET. It provides useful prognostic information, although with limited accuracy and without the ability to differentiate between cardiac and noncardiac causes of exertional dyspnea and limitation.[16]

CLASSIFICATION OF HEART FAILURE

Patients with HF are typically categorized into two classification systems, in addition to the subgroups presented earlier.[4] The New York Heart Association (NYHA) functional classification allows semi-quantification of symptom severity. Class I patients have no symptoms, class II patients have symptoms during moderate to severe exertion, class III patients are symptomatic during mild to moderate exertion, and class IV patients are symptomatic at rest or with minimal exertion, including basic daily activities. The NYHA class serves as an important marker of prognosis and guides therapy accordingly.

A relatively recent classification scheme was introduced by the American College of Cardiology/American Heart Association (ACC/AHA), similar to the staging performed in oncology. Patients with stage A HF are only at risk for HF. These patients are asymptomatic; but if untreated, they might develop HF with time. Risk factors include hypertension, diabetes, and chemotherapy. Patients with stage B HF have already sustained a myocardial insult; however, they are still asymptomatic. Examples are patients post myocardial infarction, chemotherapy-induced cardiotoxicity with reduced LVEF. Stage C HF patients are the "typical" patients seen in clinical practice—symptomatic, requiring diuretics, angiotensin-converting enzyme inhibitors (ACEI), and beta-blockers. Stage D is an important distinction defining a subset of moribund patients who are repeatedly hospitalized and frequently inotrope dependent. These patients have a very limited prognosis, if not eligible for advanced HF therapy (LVAD, transplant). This recognition is also important to initiate proper palliative care.

HEART FAILURE TREATMENT

HF treatment requires several general measures, in addition to medical and device therapy. Sodium intake should be limited, because this is one of the major factors determining total body volume. However, recently the use of severe sodium restriction has been criticized and even linked to excess mortality. Practically, patients should be informed of the following—do not add salt, do not add salt substitutes (which contain potassium and pose a risk of hyperkalemia when treated with ACEI and aldosterone antagonists), beware of sodium-rich foods (anything preserved in a can or box, pickles, deli, soy sauce, etc). Water restriction was also a common practice; however, the ability to excrete water is relatively independent from the sodium balance and total body volume. Therefore, this is mainly relevant in patients with problems of water balance—hyponatremia. In a recent study of patients hospitalized with acute decompensated HF, the use of an aggressive sodium and water restriction approach had no effect on outcome, except for increased perceived thirst in the water-restricted group.[17]

Alcohol and smoking should be avoided. Alcohol is directly toxic to the myocardium, especially when myocardial injury is already established. In addition to vasodilation, which lowers blood pressure along with the patient's vasodilating medications, alcohol may contribute to the occurrence of both atrial and ventricular arrhythmia. Obviously, alcohol cessation is especially important in alcoholic cardiomyopathy.

Smoking should also be discouraged for several reasons. First, this may improve the patient's lung function and dyspnea. Second, smoking is a major risk factor for coronary artery disease and may provoke subsequent myocardial infarctions. Lastly, owing to increased cancer risk and as a marker of poor compliance with medical advice, smoking is considered in most transplant centers a contraindication for heart transplantation.

Dietary modifications are required when the patient is obese, although the obesity paradox should be kept in mind. Excessive weight loss also might be harmful.

Physical activity should be encouraged, within the limitations of the patient's ability to perform exercise. This is where the role of a formal cardiac rehabilitation program is extremely important.

The patients should also be informed of hazardous medications—nonsteroidal anti-inflammatory drugs (NSAIDs). These are one of the most common causes for HF decompensation. NSAIDs disrupt renal function and interfere with the whole renin–angiotensin–aldosterone axis.

Medical therapy and device therapy are discussed in the following chapters.

REFERENCES

1. Mozzafarian D, Benjamin EJ, Go AS, et al. On behalf of the American Heart Association Statistics Committee and Stroke Statistics Subcommittee. Heart disease and stroke statistics—2016 update: a report from the American Heart Association. *Circulation.* 2016;133:e38-360.

2. Desai AS, Stevenson LW. Rehospitalization for heart failure: predict or prevent? *Circulation.* 2012;126(4):501-506.

3. Heidenreich PA, Trogdon JG, Khavjou OA, et al. Forecasting the future of cardiovascular disease in the United States: a policy statement from the American Heart Association. *Circulation*. 2011;123(8):933-44.

4. Yancy CW, Jessup M, Bozkurt B, et al. 2013 ACCF/AHA guideline for the management of heart failure: a report of the American College of Cardiology Foundation/American Heart Association Task Force on practice guidelines. *Circulation*. 2013;128(16):e240-e327.

5. Braunwald E. Clinical manifestations of heart failure. In: Braunwald E, ed. *Heart Disease: A Textbook of Cardiovascular Medicine*. Philadelphia, PA: Saunders; 1988:471-484.

6. Purcell IF, Poole-Wilson PA. Heart failure: why and how to define it? *Eur J Heart Fail*. 1999;(1):7-10.

7. Ponikowski P, Voors AA, Anker SD, et al. 2016 ESC guidelines for the diagnosis and treatment of acute and chronic heart failure. *Eur Heart J*. 2016;37(27):2129-2200.

8. Heart Physiology: From Cell to Circulation. Lionel H. Opie. 4th edition; 2004.

9. Cohn JN, Ferrari R, Sharpe N. Cardiac remodeling-concepts and clinical implications: a consensus paper from an international forum on cardiac remodeling. Behalf of an International Forum on Cardiac Remodeling. *J Am CollCardiol*. 2000;35(3):569-582.

10. Ashrafian H, Frenneaux MP, Opie LH. Metabolic mechanisms in heart failure. *Circulation*. 2007;116(4):434-448.

11. Thibodeau JT, Turer AT, Gualano SK, et al. Characterization of a novel symptom of advanced heart failure: bendopnea. *JACC Heart Fail*. 2014;2(1):24-31.

12. Ewy GA. The abdominojugular test: technique and hemodynamic correlates. *Ann Intern Med*. 1988;109(6):456-460.

13. Maisel AS, Krishnaswamy P, Nowak RM, et al. Rapid measurement of B-type natriuretic peptide in the emergency diagnosis of heart failure. *N Engl J Med*. 2002;347(3):161-167.

14. Velazquez EJ, Lee KL, Jones RH, et al. Coronary-artery bypass surgery in patients with ischemic cardiomyopathy. *N Engl J Med*. 2016;374(16):1511-1520.

15. Mancini DM, Eisen H, Kussmaul W, et al. Value of peak exercise oxygen consumption for optimal timing of cardiac transplantation in ambulatory patients with heart failure. *Circulation*. 1991;83(3):778-786.

16. Forman DE, Fleg JL, Kitzman DW, et al. 6-Min walk test provides prognostic utility comparable to cardiopulmonary exercise testing in ambulatory outpatients with systolic heart failure. *J Am CollCardiol*. 2012;60(25):2653-2661.

17. Aliti GB, Rabelo ER, Clausell N, et al. Aggressive fluid and sodium restriction in acute decompensated heart failure: a randomized clinical trial. *JAMA Intern Med*. 2013;173(12):1058-1064.

Patient and Family Information for: HEART FAILURE WITH REDUCED EJECTION FRACTION

WHAT IS HEART FAILURE?

The heart is the organ responsible for pumping blood throughout the body, delivering oxygen and essential nutrients. This muscular pump is divided into the right and left sides. The right side of the heart receives blood without oxygen from the rest of the body and delivers the blood to the lungs. After the blood flows through the lungs and receives oxygen, it arrives at the left side of the heart. The left side of the heart is much more muscular, because it has to eject the blood (which now has oxygen) to the rest of the body—from head to toe, except for the lungs. The force of flow is powerful enough to generate a blood pressure, which is routinely measured.

HF is defined as a problem with the heart's ability to eject blood and/or fill with blood. Various diseases cause the heart to weaken as a muscular pump, thereby resulting in HF. The ability of the heart to contract and eject blood is measured by the term EF.

WHAT IS EJECTION FRACTION?

EF represents the percentage of blood flowing out of the heart during each contraction. The EF is never 100%, because the heart cannot contract, totally empty out all of its contents, and then refill. Actually, the heart is usually half filled even at the end of its contraction. Therefore, the normal EF is 55% to 60%. An EF below 50% is considered abnormal. When the EF is reduced below 30% to 35%, the heart's pumping action is considered severely reduced. HF can also occur with a "normal" EF—the heart can eject blood properly, but has trouble filling. A common cause of this situation is hypertension. After years of the heart trying to pump out blood against a high blood pressure, the heart muscle thickens (similar to the enlargement of muscles after lifting weights). The thickened heart muscle requires a much higher pressure to fill (think of trying to fill a balloon vs filling a tire). These high pressures cause the blood to go back to the lungs and fill with fluid, ending up with shortness of breath. The causes and treatment of HF differ according to EF—HFrEF and HFpEF. However, many of the symptoms and signs of HF are the same.

CAUSES OF HEART FAILURE

HF is the result of several diseases affecting the heart as a pump. Usually problems with the heart muscle cause HF. However, the heart as a pump also has valves and an encasement (pericardium). Therefore, diseases of the heart valves (aortic stenosis, aortic regurgitation, mitral stenosis, and mitral regurgitation) and pericardium (constrictive pericarditis) also result in HF.

Common diseases affecting the heart muscle include the following:

Coronary artery disease—Blockages in the heart's blood supply, previous "heart attacks."

Hypertension or high blood pressure—The EF is usually preserved in this situation.

Alcohol—The heart muscle can recover once alcohol intake is stopped.

Drugs—Cocaine, amphetamines; may result in irreversible damage.

Chemotherapy—There are several chemotherapies that are toxic to the heart muscle. Common examples include doxorubicin (Adriamycin) given for lymphoma and, sometimes, for breast cancer, and trastuzumab (Herceptin) given for breast cancer.

Familial/genetic heart disease—This may be a disease limited to the heart muscle, causing weakness and impaired contraction—dilated cardiomyopathy. Sometimes this is part of a general muscular disease (as in Duchenne muscular dystrophy).

Infection—Viruses can cause myocarditis, resulting in heart damage.

Congenital heart disease—These are complex diseases. HF is a problem even after palliative or corrective surgery.

Peripartum—This rare form of HF can present following pregnancy.

SYMPTOMS AND SIGNS OF HFrEF

Shortness of breath—dyspnea—is a common symptom of HF and may appear in several forms. Shortness of breath occurs because of the increased pressure in the heart muscle, causing a backward flow of blood toward the lungs. The lungs then fill with fluid, resulting in breathing difficulty. Shortness of breath is worsened during exercise—the heart cannot keep up with the increased need for blood flow, and more blood remains in the lungs.

Dyspnea may also occur when lying down—during the day, gravity helps pull blood away from the heart (standing and walking). When lying down, this effect is neutralized. This is known as orthopnea. Patients with severe HF will complain of sleeping upright in a chair during the night.

Bendopnea is a similar symptom—shortness of breath while bending over. Many patients with advanced HF will have trouble tying their shoe laces or picking up objects. This is also due to the blood flow to the heart being affected by gravity.

Shortness of breath during the night—PND. In this situation, the patient awakens at night with shortness of breath, sometimes even wheezing.

"Cardiac asthma"—sometimes the fluid in the lungs can cause wheezing, mimicking the sounds heard during an asthma attack. Many times, HF episodes (especially before diagnosis) can be mistaken for bronchitis, chronic obstructive pulmonary disease exacerbation, or an asthma attack.

Peripheral edema/swelling—fluid can accumulate in the rest of the body, not only in the lungs. This commonly occurs in the legs, due to gravity.

Abdominal pain—accumulation of fluid in the liver and gut area causes abdominal pain, abdominal swelling, and loss of appetite.

Weight gain—this can be due to fluid accumulation.

Weight loss can occur in patients with very advanced HF—because of increased energy requirements by the failing heart and changes in body metabolism.

DIAGNOSTIC TESTS

There is no single test for the diagnosis of HF. Several tests are required:

Echocardiogram—ultrasound of the heart. The single most important test in HF is the echocardiogram. First, the echocardiogram provides us with the EF—the major distinction between HFrEF and HFpEF. Again, this is important because the medical treatment for HFrEF is different from the treatment for HFpEF. Second, the echocardiogram allows for evaluation beyond the percentage of heart muscle contraction—including valves, the heart's encasement (pericardium), and other important measures of heart function (right-sided function, flow in the right and left sides, estimation of filling pressures, and muscle thickness).

BNP—This is a blood test. In response to increased pressures inside the heart, the heart secretes a hormone named BNP. This hormone is measurable and can help diagnose HF. In addition to diagnosis, BNP can also provide a rough measure of the extent of HF—in patients with congestion and fluid retention, the BNP levels are high. Once the HF is treated and congestion is relieved (compensated HF), BNP levels can return to lower values. Therefore, in addition to HF diagnosis and assessment of severity, BNP may help guide therapy.

The ECG is a basic cardiac test demonstrating the electrical activation of the heart. The ECG is helpful in HF, because it can hint at possible causes and also direct medical decisions. For example, the ECG can demonstrate previous heart attacks. The ECG may also demonstrate a conduction problem known as LBBB. When this occurs in the setting of HFrEF, a biventricular pacemaker, which can synchronize the heart's contraction between the right and left sides, should be considered. In patients who already have a pacemaker, the ECG can help determine pacemaker function. Lastly, the ECG may demonstrate heart rhythm disturbances, which are not always felt by the patient.

The chest X-ray is also a basic test—in HF it can demonstrate fluid in the lungs and an enlarged heart. More importantly, it can help the physician look for other causes of shortness of breath, such as pneumonia or lung disease.

MRI—In this test, use of a powerful magnet and the detection of energy waves released by provoked hydrogen atoms generate a high-resolution picture of the heart tissue. Advances in computer technology and quick processing of images allow evaluation of serial images and heart function. The advantage over echo/ultrasound technology is that MRI is not angle dependent. MRI can also characterize tissues and detect abnormalities not "seen" by echo. However, MRI is expensive, not always widely available, and requires time. In addition, the examination takes place within a tube, which might pose a problem in patients with claustrophobia. Lastly, metal objects are problematic because of the strong magnetic field. Therefore, only patients with MRI-safe pacemakers and without metal implants (orthopedic) are candidates for MRI.

Cardiac catheterization—this is usually an essential part of evaluating HFrEF. Coronary artery disease and heart attacks are a common cause of reduced heart function. More importantly, revascularization and opening of the blockages may improve heart function and outcomes. Therefore, coronary catheterization is mandated in most patients with reduced heart function. In younger patients, CT angiography is a noninvasive alternative. Direct measurement of pressures using a catheter inserted into the neck or groin veins is necessary in patients with advanced HF to determine medical therapy and plan for VAD or heart transplantation.

CPET is a test where the patient performs exercise (either on a bike or a treadmill) with a specialized mask measuring oxygen and carbon dioxide coming in and out of the lungs. This test does not require the patient to reach a maximal HR. The CPET offers a means of improved diagnosis whether the shortness of breath originates from HF, lung disease, muscle weakness, or a combination of problems. It is an objective test. One of the measurements is the peak oxygen consumption—a value less than 14 mL/kg/min indicates a clear benefit from heart transplantation or LVAD rather than medical management.

The 6-minute walk test is simpler and more readily available then the CPET. The patient is asked to walk for 6 minutes and the distance is measured. This test also provides useful information concerning the timing of heart transplantation or LVAD. However, it has limited accuracy and does not have the ability to differentiate between HF and other causes of shortness of breath.

CLASSIFICATION OF HEART FAILURE

Patients with HF are typically categorized into two classification systems.

The NYHA functional classification: NYHA class I patients have no symptoms, NYHA class II patients have symptoms during moderate to severe exercise, NYHA class III patients are symptomatic during mild to moderate activities, and class IV patients are symptomatic at rest or with minimal activities, including basic daily activities (bathing, toilet, etc).

A similar but different classification scheme was introduced by the ACC and AHA.

Patients with stage A HF are only at risk for HF. These patients are asymptomatic, but if untreated, they might develop HF with time. Risk factors include hypertension, diabetes, and chemotherapy. Patients with stage B HF have already sustained an injury to their heart muscle; however, they are still asymptomatic. Examples are patients after a heart attack, or patients after chemotherapy with a reduced EF. Stage C HF patients are the "typical" patients—symptomatic, requiring standard medical treatment with diuretics, ACE inhibitors, and beta-blockers. Stage D is an important distinction defining a subset of patients who are repeatedly hospitalized or cannot be discharged from the hospital. These patients are very sick—if they are not eligible for advanced HF therapy (LVAD, transplant), palliative care should be initiated. In addition to the importance of determining stage D, patients who feel well and are in stage A or B also deserve special attention—despite feeling well, they should receive medications to *prevent* future HF.

HEART FAILURE TREATMENT

HF treatment requires several general measures, in addition to medical and device therapy.

Salt—Sodium intake should be limited, because this is one of the major factors determining the amount of total body fluids. The basic rules: Do not add salt. Do not add salt substitutes (which contain potassium—this is usually a problem with the medications given in HF). Beware of sodium-rich foods (anything preserved in a can or box, pickles, deli, soy sauce, etc).

Water restriction was also a common practice; however, the ability to get rid of water is relatively independent from the ability to get rid of sodium. Therefore, this is mainly relevant in patients with problems in water balance—hyponatremia. In a recent study of patients hospitalized with acute HF, the use of an aggressive sodium and water restriction approach had no effect, except for increased perceived thirst in the water-restricted group.

Alcohol and smoking should be avoided. Alcohol is directly toxic to the heart, especially when injury to the heart muscle is already established. In addition, alcohol may lower blood pressure, which may be low anyway because of HF medications. Lastly, alcohol may contribute to the occurrence of electrical heart disturbances—arrhythmia. Obviously, alcohol cessation is especially important in HF resulting from alcoholism.

Smoking should also be discouraged for several reasons. First, this may improve the patient's lung function and decrease the sensation of shortness of breath. Second, smoking is a major risk factor for coronary artery disease and may provoke subsequent heart attacks. Lastly, owing to increased cancer risk and as a marker of poor compliance with medical advice, smoking is considered in most transplant centers a contraindication for heart transplantation.

Dietary modifications are required when the patient is obese. However, excessive weight loss also might be harmful.

Physical activity should be encouraged, within the limitations of the patient's ability to perform exercise. This is where the role of a formal cardiac rehabilitation program is extremely important.

Patients should also be informed of hazardous medications—NSAIDs. These medications (Advil, ibuprofen, naproxen) disrupt renal function and interfere with hormonal activation in HF. NSAIDs are a common cause of HF deterioration.

Medical therapy and device therapy are discussed elsewhere.

Manpreet Sabharwal
Eyal Herzog
Edgar Argulian

12

Heart Failure with Preserved Ejection Fraction

INTRODUCTION

Heart failure with preserved ejection fraction (HFpEF) is a clinical syndrome characterized by the impaired ability of the heart to meet the metabolic needs of the body, resulting in breathlessness, fatigue, and/or fluid retention. HFpEF is defined by the left ventricular ejection fraction (LVEF) $\geq 50\%$. Patients with LVEF <40% are defined as having heart failure with reduced ejection fraction (HFrEF). The subgroup of patients in the borderline range (LVEF 40% to 49%) is termed borderline, intermediate, or as having heart failure with mid-range LVEF with characteristics and treatment patterns that need further research.[1]

Historically, diastolic heart failure has been the term used synonymously with HFpEF; but, currently, with new insights into the pathophysiology of the disease, diastolic dysfunction is thought to be one of the several factors contributing to the development of HFpEF and it is not necessarily the only component of the syndrome.

EPIDEMIOLOGY

Heart failure is a major source of morbidity and mortality in the United States with the estimated prevalence of 5.7 million cases, and nearly half of these cases are patients with HFpEF.[2] It has been projected that the prevalence of heart failure will increase by 46% by 2030.[3] The prevalence increases dramatically with age, and it is more common in women than in men at any age. The mortality rates are grossly similar in patients with HFrEF and HFpEF, with recent data showing some improvement in survival for patients with HFrEF.[4] This has been attributed to the use of guideline-directed medical therapies. However, no such evidence-based treatment strategies exist for HFpEF. Therefore, the development of medical and device therapies for HFpEF is a major unmet medical need.

PATHOPHYSIOLOGY

The pathophysiology of HFpEF is complex and is the subject of active ongoing research. It is postulated that HFpEF is a heterogeneous syndrome to which various mechanisms contribute. These mechanisms can contribute to various degrees in each individual patient and can be divided into the following categories:

1. Cardiac abnormalities
   a. Diastolic dysfunction
   b. Systolic dysfunction
   c. Atrial fibrillation and atrial dysfunction
   d. Pulmonary hypertension and right ventricular dysfunction
   e. Chronotropic incompetence
2. Vascular abnormalities and impaired ventricular–vascular coupling
3. Extra cardiac abnormalities
4. Cardiovascular aging

CARDIAC ABNORMALITIES

Diastolic Dysfunction

In a normal person, diastole is the summation of an active process of relaxation related to calcium reuptake and myofilament dissociation and passive stretching resulting from mechanical properties of the sarcomere and extracellular matrix at the molecular level and the chamber and pericardium at the organ level. During the isovolumic relaxation phase of the cardiac cycle, the left ventricle relaxes and creates a sucking force that helps the ventricle fill up during diastole when the mitral valve opens. Many studies indicate that in HFpEF the rate of ventricular relaxation during isovolumic relaxation is decreased. Also, diastolic dysfunction is associated with reduced left ventricular compliance.[5] As a result, the left ventricle can only accommodate volumes similar to the normal heart at higher filling pressures. Also, due to impaired relaxation properties and chamber stiffening, patients with HFpEF poorly tolerate increased heart rates as seen with exercise and atrial fibrillation.

Systolic Dysfunction

The systolic function of the heart is commonly measured by LVEF, but LVEF does not reflect all aspects of the left ventricular systolic performance. The left ventricular systolic function is complex and can be fully evaluated using advanced echocardiographic techniques such as speckle tracking echocardiography. Several studies have demonstrated markedly impaired longitudinal systolic function in patients with HFpEF despite preserved LVEF.

Further studies will help subdivide the HFpEF syndrome based on the different aspects of the left ventricular systolic performance beyond the LVEF assessment.

Atrial Dysfunction

The left atrium contributes to about 20% of cardiac output in a normal individual, and this number has been shown to be up to 45% in patients with diastolic dysfunction because the left ventricular filling depends on the ability of the left atrium to push blood at higher pressures.[6] Left atrial dysfunction is common in patients with HFpEF as measured by advanced echocardiographic techniques and may contribute to transition from asymptomatic diastolic dysfunction to symptomatic heart failure.

Atrial fibrillation is common in patients with HFpEF. It is poorly tolerated in these patients and can precipitate acute decompensated heart failure.

Pulmonary Hypertension and Right Ventricular Dysfunction

Pulmonary hypertension is common in patients with HFpEF and is associated with worse prognosis. Elevated left atrial pressure leads to elevated pulmonary pressures and then chronic elevation in the left atrial pressure causes pulmonary arteriolar and venous remodeling, resulting in increased pulmonary vascular resistance. Right ventricular dysfunction can result from pulmonary hypertension and/or can be a part of the disease process independent of the elevated pulmonary pressures.

Chronotropic Incompetence

Studies have shown a blunted heart rate response to exercise and prolonged post-exercise heart rate recovery in patients with HFpEF.[7,8] These findings may contribute to the symptoms and they have also been linked to worse prognosis.[9]

VASCULAR ABNORMALITIES

Vascular remodeling is a part of aging, but it is greatly amplified by cardiovascular risk factors such as diabetes mellitus and hypertension. Vascular stiffening results in impaired ability to accommodate an increased systemic load during stress and exercise. Vascular remodeling is a part of the same systemic process that affects the diastolic properties of the left ventricle. As a result, the ability of the cardiovascular system to function efficiently under various loading conditions and maintain low filling pressures is compromised because of impaired ventricular–vascular coupling.

EXTRA CARDIAC FACTORS

A range of extra cardiac contributing factors have been implicated in the pathogenesis of HFpEF. These include anemia, pulmonary disease, renal disease, and obesity. Obesity and metabolic syndrome are especially important because of the high prevalence in the general population; also, weight loss may improve diastolic properties of the left ventricle.

CARDIOVASCULAR AGING

HFpEF is predominantly a disease of the elderly that emphasizes the importance of age-related cardiovascular changes in the disease pathogenesis. Aging leads to a wide range of changes within the cardiovascular system, including alteration in the left ventricular diastolic function and vascular stiffening. Aging does not invariably result in heart failure, but age-related changes are greatly amplified by cardiovascular risk factors and disease states (such as atherosclerosis) and contribute to the development of the HFpEF phenotype.

CLINICAL FEATURES

The clinical presentation of HFpEF can be variable: patients can present with mild symptoms of exercise intolerance and tiredness or be admitted with acute pulmonary edema if an immediate precipitating factor (such as atrial fibrillation or uncontrolled hypertension) is present. The range of symptoms is similar to HFrEF and includes dyspnea on exertion, orthopnea, paroxysmal nocturnal dyspnea, peripheral edema, and weight gain. As with HFrEF, it is important to characterize and quantify the functional status in a standardized way such as the New York Heart Association functional classification **(Table 12.1)**.

Physical examination can demonstrate signs of fluid overload such as elevated jugular venous pressure, lung rales, hepatomegaly and hepatojugular reflux, ascites, and peripheral edema. The lateral displacement of the apical impulse and the third heart sound usually point toward HFrEF.

Besides the symptoms and signs of heart failure, the history and physical examination should also be directed toward identifying the risk factors that can lead to the development of HFpEF such as hypertension, coronary artery disease, obesity, and diabetes mellitus. In cases of acute decompensated heart failure, the precipitating factors should be explored; these include medication noncompliance, poorly controlled hypertension, arrhythmia, and thyroid disease.

TABLE 12.1	New York Heart Association Functional Classification for Cardiac Diseases
I	Patients have cardiac disease without limitation of physical activity. Ordinary physical activity does not cause symptoms such as fatigue, palpitation, dyspnea, or chest pain
II	Patients have cardiac disease resulting in slight limitation of physical activity. Ordinary physical activity results in fatigue, palpitation, dyspnea, or chest pain
III	Patients have cardiac disease resulting in marked limitation of physical activity. Less than ordinary activity causes fatigue, palpitation, dyspnea, or chest pain
IV	Patients have cardiac disease resulting in symptoms at rest, and physical activity causes further discomfort

DIAGNOSIS

Diagnosis of HFpEF is not always straightforward. The following components should be considered in patients suspected to have HFpEF:[1,10]

1. Symptoms consistent with heart failure diagnosis
2. Presence of physical signs of heart failure, mostly evidence of fluid overload
3. Preserved LVEF (≥50%)
4. Elevated natriuretic peptide levels
5. Evidence of structural or functional alterations underlying heart failure as assessed by echocardiography

Natriuretic peptide levels are elevated in patients with HFpEF, but they are on average lower than the levels seen in patients with HFrEF. The structural alterations commonly observed in patients with HFpEF include left atrial enlargement and left ventricular hypertrophy; the functional alterations include decreased annular tissue velocities, elevated E/e' ratio, and pulmonary hypertension. Advanced echocardiographic assessment may demonstrate impaired longitudinal left ventricular systolic function. If the diagnosis remains uncertain after initial testing, invasive hemodynamic evaluation may be helpful. Elevated left ventricular filling pressures at rest support the diagnosis of HFpEF; however, many individuals demonstrate hemodynamic compromise only with stress. In these patients, hemodynamic measurements during exercise can be performed using either echocardiography (diastolic stress test) or uncommonly invasive hemodynamic testing.

A 12-lead electrocardiogram (ECG) should be performed initially on all patients presenting with heart failure. Initial laboratory evaluation of patients presenting with heart failure should include complete blood count, comprehensive metabolic panel, hemoglobin A1c, fasting lipid profile, urinalysis, ferritin and transferrin saturation, and thyroid-stimulating hormone. Serial monitoring, when indicated, should include serum electrolytes and renal function. Echocardiogram is the cornerstone of patient evaluation, as described earlier.

Further testing should be tailored to the clinical scenario and may identify specific causes, risk factors, or precipitating factors for HFpEF phenotype. These include coronary artery disease, systemic diseases (such as sarcoidosis), infiltrative disorders (such as amyloidosis), and so on. Also, further testing may be necessary to exclude other conditions presenting with a similar phenotype such as hypertrophic cardiomyopathy and constrictive pericarditis.

MANAGEMENT

There are no consistently proven treatment strategies that would reduce mortality in patients with HFpEF. The basics of management revolve around symptomatic treatment of volume overload with diuretics, control of hypertension, and treatment of risk factors such as atrial fibrillation, coronary artery disease, and diabetes mellitus.

DIURETICS

One of the main goals of HFpEF therapy is to achieve euvolemia by judicious use of diuretics. Diuretic treatment provides a symptomatic benefit similar to that in patients with HFrEF.

DRUGS AFFECTING RENIN-ANGIOTENSIN SYSTEM

Among the various drug therapies tested in HFpEF, several trials have targeted the renin–angiotensin system, but they have largely failed to show any significant mortality benefit. The trials specifically studied an angiotensin-converting enzyme inhibitor perindopril and angiotensin receptor antagonists candesartan and irbesartan. The summary of various trials is shown in **Table 12.2**.[11–13]

It is now clear that HFpEF is a heterogeneous disease with variable contribution by different pathophysiologic components; and the trials that studied renin–angiotensin system antagonists applied broad criteria for patient selection and did not target any specific pathophysiologic component. Currently, the use of these agents is necessary for hypertension control and diabetes management, but there is no convincing evidence to support their role as disease-modifying agents for HFpEF. Use of a neprilysin inhibitor in combination with an angiotensin receptor blocker is being studied now in the HFpEF phenotype.

TABLE 12.2	**Summary of Randomized Controlled Trials with Various Pharmacologic Agents in Patients with HFpEF**				
	PEP-CHF	**CHARM-PRESERVED**	**I-PRESERVE**	**TOPCAT**	**RELAX**
Patients, number	850	3023	4128	3445	216
Drug	Perindopril	Candesartan	Irbesartan	Spironolactone	Sildenafil
Mean follow up (years)	2.1	3	4.1	3.3	24 weeks
Primary end point	All-cause death/HF hospitalization	CV death/HF hospitalization	All-cause death/CV hospitalization	CV death/aborted cardiac arrest/HF hospitalization	Change in peak O_2 consumption, median
Hazard ratio	0.92 (0.70–1.21)	0.89 (0.77–1.03)	0.95 (0.86–1.05)	0.89 (0.77–1.04)	−0.2 (IQR, −1.7–1.11)
P value	0.54	0.12	0.35	0.14	0.9

CV, cardiovascular; HF, heart failure; HFpEF, heart failure with preserved ejection fraction.

ALDOSTERONE ANTAGONISTS

The mineralocorticoid receptor antagonist spironolactone has been studied in a large randomized controlled trial in HFpEF (TOPCAT). The study showed no significant reduction in the composite primary end point of cardiovascular death, hospitalization for heart failure, or aborted cardiac death as compared with placebo. From the components of the primary outcome, spironolactone did show benefit in reducing hospitalizations ($P = 0.04$). As the pathophysiologic components of HFpEF phenotype are further refined, it is possible that certain subgroups of patients with HFpEF may benefit from an aldosterone antagonist.

PHOSPHODIESTERASE 5 INHIBITORS

Early animal study data showed improvement in ventricular structure and function with the use of sildenafil in pressure overload hypertrophy. However, when sildenafil was tested in a clinical trial of 216 patients with HFpEF, no significant benefits regarding exercise capacity, clinical status, or quality of life were noted with the follow-up period of 24 weeks.[14]

β-BLOCKERS

There are limited data on the use of β-blockers in patients with HFpEF. The potential theoretical advantage of using β-blockers in HFpEF comes from the possibility of prolonging the diastolic period because of the negative chronotropic effect of β-blockers. However, there is significant prevalence of chronotropic incompetence in patients with HFpEF that offsets the potential benefit of β-blockers. Limited data comes from registries like the Organized Program to Initiate Life-saving Treatment in Hospitalized Patients with Heart Failure (OPTIMIZE-HF).[15] The study evaluated 7154 hospitalized patients and showed that β-blockers had no effect on 1-year mortality and hospitalization rates in patients with HFpEF but significantly improved both end points in the HFrEF group.

CONTROL OF HYPERTENSION AND OTHER CONTRIBUTING FACTORS

Hypertension is an important factor in the development of HFpEF and precedes the development of HFpEF in the majority of the cases. Early blood pressure treatment is the most important intervention that could possibly prevent the progression of hypertensive heart disease to symptomatic HFpEF. The choice of drugs should follow the common practices for hypertension control unless compelling indications are present for specific drug use (eg, rate control of atrial fibrillation with a β-blocker). Other contributing factors that should be addressed in the treatment strategy include anti-ischemic therapies in patients with coronary artery disease, proper diabetes control, and so on.

ROLE OF EXERCISE

Exercise training in HFpEF has shown benefit in improving exercise tolerance and managing obesity. The HF-ACTION trial focusing on patients with HFrEF showed that exercise had a modest reduction for both all-cause mortality and rehospitalization. In one meta-analysis, exercise training was associated with an improvement in cardiorespiratory fitness and quality of life.[16]

CONCLUSIONS

In the past decade there have been several advances in the management of HFrEF, but no breakthrough treatment discoveries have been made for HFpEF. The efforts to understand the pathophysiology of HFpEF have broadened our understanding of this phenotype from a disorder of diastolic function to a complex interplay of multiple abnormalities. Despite these advances, there is still a need to standardize the diagnostic criteria and better characterize the disease processes based on specific pathophysiologic features rather than LVEF alone. Future therapies targeting these pathophysiologic mechanisms may provide better clinical outcomes.

REFERENCES

1. Yancy CW, Jessup M, Bozkurt B, et al. 2013 ACCF/AHA guideline for the management of heart failure: a report of the American College of Cardiology Foundation/American Heart Association Task Force on Practice Guidelines. *J Am CollCardiol.* 2013;62(16):e147-e239. doi:10.1016/j.jacc.2013.05.019.

2. Mozzafarian D, Benjamin EJ, Go AS, et al. On behalf of the American Heart Association Statistics Committee and Stroke Statistics Subcommittee. Heart disease and stroke statistics—2016 update: a report from the American Heart Association. *Circulation.* 2016;133:e38-360.

3. Heidenreich PA, Albert NM, Allen LA. Forecasting the impact of heart failure in the United States: a policy statement from the American Heart Association. *Circ Heart Fail.* 2013;6(3):606-619.

4. Owan TE, Hodge DO, Herges RM, et al. Trends in prevalence and outcome of heart failure with preserved ejection fraction. *N Engl J Med.* 2006;355:251-259.

5. Braunwald E, Zipes DPLP. Heart Disease: *A Textbook of Cardiovascular Medicine.* 6th ed. Philadelphia, PA:Saunders; 2001.

6. Phan TT, Abozguia K, Shivu GN, etal. Increasedatrialcontributiontoleftventricular filling compensates for impaired early filling during exercise in heart failure with preserved ejection fraction. *J Card Fail.* 2009;15:890-897.

7. Borlaug BA, Melenovsky V, Russell SD, et al. Impaired chronotropic and vasodilator reserves limit exercise capacity in patients with heart failure and a preserved ejection fraction. *Circulation.* 2006;114;2138-2147.

8. Phan TT, Shivu GN, Abozguia K, et al. Impaired heart rate recovery and chronotropic incompetence in patients with heart failure with preserved ejection fraction. *Circ Heart Fail.* 2009;3:29-34.

9. Cole CR, Blackstone EH, Pashkow FJ, Snader CE, Lauer MS. Heart-rate recovery immediately after exercise as a predictor of mortality. *N Engl J Med.* 1999;341:1351-1357.

10. McMurray JJ, Adamopoulos S, Anker SD et al. *ESC Guidelines for the diagnosis and treatment of acute and chronic heart failure 2012: The Task Force for the Diagnosis and Treatment of Acute and Chronic Heart Failure 2012 of the European Society of Cardiology.* Developed in collaboration with the Heart Failure Association (HFA) of the ESC. Eur Heart J 2012;33:1787-847.

11. Yusuf S, Pfeffer MA, Swedberg K, et al. Effects of candesartan in patients with chronic heart failure and preserved left-ventricular ejection fraction: the CHARM-Preserved Trial. *Lancet.* 2003;362(9386):777-781. doi:10.1016/s0140-6736(03)14285.

12. Massie BM, Carson PE, McMurray JJ, et al. Irbesartan in patients with heart failure and preserved ejection fraction. *N Engl J Med.* 2008;359(23):2456-2467. doi:10.1056/NEJMoa0805450.

13. Pitt B, Pfeffer MA, Assmann SF, et al. Spironolactone for heart failure with preserved ejection fraction. *N Engl J Med.* 2014;370(15):1383-1392. doi:10.1056/NEJMoa1313731.

14. Redfield M, Chen HH, Borlaug BA, et al. RELAX trial. Effect of phosphodiesterase-5 inhibition on exercise capacity and clinical status in heart failure with preserved ejection fraction: a randomized clinical trial. *JAMA*. 2013;309:1268-1277.

15. Hernandez AF, Hammill BG, O'Connor CM, et al. Clinical effectiveness of beta blockers in heart failure: Findings from the OPTI-MIZE-HF (Organized Program to Initiate Lifesaving Treatment in Hospitalized Patients with Heart Failure) Registry. *J Am Coll Cardiol*. 2009;53(2):184-192. doi:10.1016/j.jacc.2008.09.031.

16. O'Connor CM, Whellan DJ, Lee KL, et al. Efficacy and safety of exercise training in patients with chronic heart failure: HF-ACTION randomized controlled trial. *JAMA*. 2009;301(14):1439-1450. doi:10.1001/jama.2009.454.

Patient and Family Information for: HEART FAILURE WITH PRESERVED EJECTION FRACTION

DESCRIPTION AND CAUSES

Heart failure with preserved ejection fraction, also known as HFpEF, is a disease of the heart caused by increased stiffness of the heart and blood vessels and inability of the heart to relax properly. As a result, the heart function does not meet the demands of the body even though the pumping function of the heart (measured as "ejection fraction") is preserved. Impaired heart function can cause fluid accumulation in the lungs and other organs of the body. Patients commonly feel shortness of breath and fatigue with exertion as initial symptoms. As the disease progresses, shortness of breath can develop at rest, commonly with inability to sleep lying flat. Patients can also notice swelling of the ankles and stomach discomfort due to fluid accumulation in the abdomen.

The exact cause of the disease is not quite clear, but several health problems are known to contribute to the development of HFpEF. Hypertension (high blood pressure) is considered the main one. High blood pressure over time causes abnormal thickening of the heart muscle and increased stiffness of blood vessels: these are the major contributors to HFpEF. Some patients have coexisting obesity and diabetes. Coronary artery disease (blockage of the arteries supplying blood to the heart) is seen in some patients and it can also precipitate HFpEF. Abnormal heart beats, most typically atrial fibrillation, commonly coexists with HFpEF and can contribute to inefficient pumping of the heart.

HFpEF is known as the disease of the elderly. The heart muscle and blood vessels become stiff as people age; therefore, aging increases the chances of developing HFpEF. Also, women are twice more likely to develop HFpEF as compared to men. The reason for this is not fully understood.

ASSESSMENT AND TESTING

The physician establishes the diagnosis of HFpEF by taking history (asking questions about the patient's symptoms), performing physical examination, and ordering appropriate tests. Besides confirming the diagnosis, the physician needs to determine the underlying structural heart disease that causes heart failure and its contributing factors so that it can be effectively treated. Blood tests are commonly done, and ECG and chest X-ray are also typically performed. Ultrasound examination of the heart (also known as echocardiogram) helps visualize cardiac chambers, and it is the most commonly used tool to evaluate the structure and function of the heart. Other tests are performed as deemed necessary by the physician. Cardiac catheterization is an invasive test that includes placing catheters into the heart chambers and major vessels to diagnose vessel blockage or get important pressure readings from various heart chambers. It is also used for interventions if vessel blockage seems to be causing the patient's symptoms.

TREATMENT

Treatment of HFpEF is challenging because there are no proven therapies that can change the natural cause of the disease. Therefore, therapies are focused on symptom relief and modification of risk factors for this condition. Diuretics (also known as water pills) are of great benefit because they remove excess fluid from the lungs and other organs of the body. They help decrease shortness of breath and leg swelling. Blood pressure medications are also important because hypertension has been identified as a major risk factor for developing HFpEF. The blood pressure control is individualized by the physician based on patient's age and coexisting medical conditions. The patient needs to follow closely with the physician because blood pressure control can be challenging and may involve multiple adjustments of medication types and dosages. Lifestyle modifications should be a routine part of patient management in HFpEF. Exercise training has shown to improve the exercise capacity and quality of life in patients with HFpEF. The physician may recommend a cardiac rehabilitation program with dynamic exercise training.

Salt restriction is recommended in patients who have symptoms of heart failure or have high blood pressure because excess salt can cause fluid buildup in the body.

The patient's weight should be monitored routinely because weight gain may be the early sign of excess fluid in the body. Patients should avoid smoking because it increases the chances of heart attack and can worsen heart failure. Alcohol is one of the important contributors to high blood pressure and its use should be restricted in any patient with heart disease.

Eyal Herzog
Indra Warren

Mechanical Complications of Myocardial Infarction

Mechanical complications of acute myocardial infarction (AMI) result in some of the deadliest cardiovascular outcomes. It is difficult to assess the true incidence of these complications because both clinical and autopsy series differ considerably. Nevertheless, they are thought to be responsible for about 15% of all AMI deaths.[1] It is important to realize that these catastrophic events can occur within minutes to hours of the inciting event, or even days to weeks later. Mechanical complications of AMIs can be divided into two major categories: acute phase complications and chronic phase complications. **Table 13.1** outlines these complications.

LEFT VENTRICULAR FREE WALL RUPTURE

Left ventricular free wall rupture (LVFWR) is almost an entirely fatal complication of myocardial infarction (MI). Despite great progress in the reduction of both mortality and morbidity from AMI, death related to LVFWR has been high.

Among patients who die after an AMI, many large studies have found a 14% to 26% incidence of cardiac rupture.[2] According to the National Registry of Myocardial Infarction, which reviewed data from 350,755 patients with AMI, the incidence of cardiac rupture was <1%.[3] Approximately 50% of the time, myocardial rupture occurs within the first 5 days of MI and within 2 weeks in over 90% of cases.[4,5] Regardless, acute or subacute myocardial rupture is a serious and predominantly fatal complication of AMI.[6]

Studies have also suggested a higher mortality from free wall rupture with thrombolytics because cardiac rupture was

responsible for 7.3% of all deaths and 12.1% with thrombolytic agents. Thrombolytic therapy does not necessarily increase the risk of rupture but it may accelerate occurrence, often within the first 24 hours of drug administration.[7] In contrast, the incidence of cardiac rupture may be lower in patients treated with percutaneous coronary intervention. This was suggested in an observational study of 1375 patients who received a thrombolytic agent or underwent primary angioplasty, the incidence of rupture was 3.3% and 1.8% respectively.[8] It is well known that myocardial rupture after MI is less common in patients with successful reperfusion.[9]

One study found that myocardial rupture was 9.2 times more likely to occur in patients who had no prior history of angina or MI, ST-segment elevation or Q-wave development on the initial electrocardiogram (ECG), and peak MB-creatine kinase above 150 IU/L.[4] Absence of collateral blood flow and greater size of infarct territory correlate with a higher risk of myocardial rupture. Other risk factors for rupture include anterior location of the infarction, age >70, and female sex.[8,10]

PATHOPHYSIOLOGY

Myocardial rupture more frequently involves the left ventricle than the right ventricle, and rarely involves the atria.[3] The infarct commonly affects the anterior and lateral walls of the left ventricle near the junction of the infarct and normal myocardium. Ventricular free wall rupture is defined as an acute, traumatic perforation of the ventricles, which may include pericardial rupture.[6] With unsuccessful or no reperfusion, coagulation necrosis develops within the first 3 to 5 days.[5] As the necrosis progresses, neutrophils infiltrate the myocardial space and release lytic enzymes that disintegrate the necrotic myocardium leading to perforation. The rupture thus is a result of transmural infarction and the actual perforation can range in size from millimeters to centimeters depending on infarct size.[5] Early phase rupture is defined as within 72 hours post MI and late rupture is greater than 4 days.

The hallmark of rapid deterioration is primarily due to the extravasation of blood into the pericardial space with resultant instantaneous, acute pericardial tamponade. Because these events occur so quickly, the condition of patients usually deteriorates before any therapeutic intervention. Less commonly, subacute rupture can provide a longer therapeutic window because the rupture may be

TABLE 13.1	Acute Phase Versus Chronic Phase Complications in Acute Myocardial Infarction	
ACUTE PHASE	**CHRONIC PHASE**
Left ventricular free wall rupture	True ventricular aneurysm
Ventricular septal rupture	Ventricular pseudoaneurysm
Right ventricular infarction	Left ventricular thrombus
Acute mitral regurgitation	

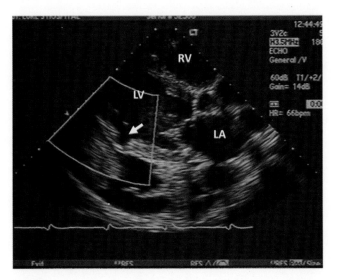

FIGURE 13.1 Parasternal long-axis view of a transthoracic echocardiogram demonstrating a posterior free wall rupture (*arrow*). LA, left atrium; LV, left ventricle; RV, right ventricle.

temporarily contained by pericardial adhesions or by thrombosis at the rupture site. It is in these patients that immediate, life-saving, cardiovascular surgery is possible **(Figure 13.1)**.[11]

CLINICAL PRESENTATION

The clinical course of myocardial rupture is variable and challenging to diagnose, because patients may rapidly decompensate. Their clinical course parallels that of any patient suffering from pericardial tamponade. Thus, the presentation of rupture can vary from sudden death in an undetected or silent MI to incomplete/subacute rupture in those with known MI.[12] **Figure 13.2** demonstrates a case of LVFWR causing pericardial tamponade with thrombus formation in the pericardial space.

Complete rupture of the left ventricular (LV) free wall usually leads to hemopericardium and death from cardiac tamponade. Patients may complain of transient chest pain or dyspnea. Acute

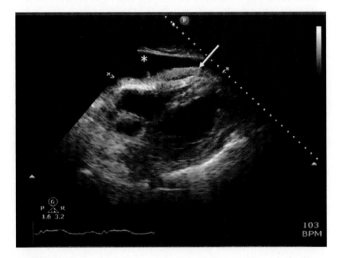

FIGURE 13.2 Subcostal view showing pericardial effusion (*asterisk*) with a thrombus in the pericardial space (*arrow*). This resulted from a ventricular free wall rupture after an acute myocardial infarction and the patient developed cardiac tamponade physiology.

tamponade can cause tachypnea, tachycardia, muffled heart sounds, elevated jugular venous pressure, and pulsus paradoxus. The presence of rupture is first suggested by the development of sudden profound right heart failure and shock, often progressing rapidly to pulseless electrical activity and death. Emergent transthoracic echocardiography (TTE) will confirm the diagnosis and emergent pericardiocentesis can transiently relieve the tamponade.[12]

Incomplete/subacute rupture of the LV free wall can occur when organized thrombus and the pericardium seal the ventricular perforation. Patients may present with persistent or recurrent chest pain (particularly pericardial pain), nausea, restlessness, agitation, abrupt hypotension, and/or electrocardiographic features of localized or regional pericarditis.[4,5] The diagnosis of incomplete/subacute rupture is again confirmed by TTE.[12]

There are three types of ventricular free wall rupture **(Figure 13.3)**. Type I is a slitlike or fissure full-thickness rupture, usually occurring within the first 24 hours with abrupt onset of symptoms. Type II is more subacute and occurs as a result of erosion of the myocardium at the infarct site. Type III has a later onset, occurring because of the expansion of the infarct zone with wall thinning and rupture through an aneurysmal segment.

TREATMENT

As mentioned, the mortality for acute and subacute free wall rupture is high because of rapid clinical deterioration. Survival depends primarily on the prompt recognition of myocardial rupture and provision of immediate therapy. Patients displaying suggestive symptoms, signs, and ECG changes require emergent bedside echocardiogram and echocardiographically guided pericardiocentesis if fluid is visualized. Immediate surgical intervention is indicated if the pericardiocentesis identifies the fluid as blood. Medical therapy aimed at hemodynamic stabilization

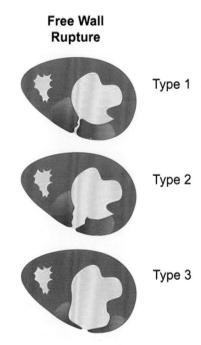

FIGURE 13.3 Classification of myocardial free wall rupture. (Adapted from Reynolds HR, Hochman JD. *Eur Heart J.* 2010;31:1433-1435, modified from Becker AE, van Mantgem JP. Cardiac tamponade. A study of 50 hearts. *Eur J Cardiol.* 1975;3:349-358.)

should also be instituted. In addition to pericardiocentesis, this includes fluids, inotropic support, vasopressors, and even intra-aortic balloon pump counterpulsation and percutaneous cardiopulmonary bypass when available and indicated.[4]

With rapid recognition and initiation of both medical and surgical therapy, the potential for survival, particularly with subacute rupture, can improve dramatically. In 1 study, 25 of 33 patients (76%) with subacute ventricular rupture survived the surgical procedure and 16 (48%) were long-term survivors.[13]

VENTRICULAR SEPTAL RUPTURE

Another deadly complication of AMI involves rupture of the interventricular septum. Rapid diagnosis, aggressive medical therapy, and prompt surgical intervention are essential to increase the chances of survival.

In the era before reperfusion therapy, rupture of the interventricular septum is thought to have occurred in 1% to 2% of patients with AMI and accounts for approximately 5% of deaths in this setting.[14] It typically occurs in the first week after infarction, with a mean time from symptom onset of 3 to 5 days.[15] The classic risk factors for septal rupture in the pre-reperfusion era include hypertension, advanced age, female sex, and the absence of a history of MI or angina.[16] Prognosis for ventricular septal rupture (VSR) in the prereperfusion era was very poor, with an in-hospital mortality of about 45% in those treated surgically and about 90% in those treated medically.[15] With the advent of thrombolysis and percutaneous intervention, incidence and outcomes have changed.

In the reperfusion era, studies show a much lower incidence and an accelerated time to diagnosis of interventricular septal rupture than had been previously reported. Early reperfusion therapy may prevent the extensive myocardial necrosis that is associated with ventricular rupture.[15] Patients generally have a mean time of 1 day from infarction to development of a VSR. Many have postulated that this acceleration of rupture may be due to thrombolysis causing hemorrhage during the "lytic state," so that if a VSR occurs, its time course may be accelerated.[15] In the reperfusion era, advanced age, anterior infarct location, female sex, and no previous history of smoking were found to be the most potent predictors of a VSR.[15]

PATHOPHYSIOLOGY

The pathophysiology of interventricular septal rupture is similar to that of free wall rupture. Without reperfusion, coagulation necrosis develops within the first 3 to 5 days. The septum becomes necrotic and is infiltrated by neutrophils, which release lytic enzymes, thereby disintegrating the necrotic myocardium.[16] A transmural septal infarction underlies the rupture of the interventricular septum, with the tear ranging in size from millimeters to centimeters.[14]

The ventricular septum is a very vascular structure. The rarity of septal rupture and the variable infarct location relate to the fact that the interventricular septum has a dual blood supply. The anterior two-thirds is supplied by the left anterior descending (LAD) coronary artery and its branches. The posterior one-third is supplied by branches of the posterior descending artery, which come from the right coronary or the left circumflex artery, depending on the dominance of the circulation.[17] Studies have been conflicting in terms of which artery is predominantly responsible for septal rupture, but anterior MIs are considered to be more frequent, followed by

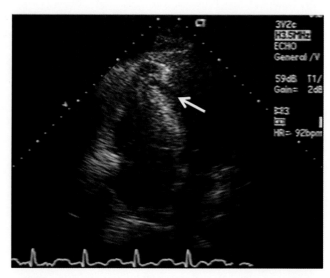

FIGURE 13.4 Apical four-chamber view of a transthoracic echocardiogram demonstrating a ventricular septal rupture in the distal portion of the interventricular septum (*arrow*).

inferior infarctions. Similar to free wall rupture, interventricular septal rupture occurs most frequently with a first MI when there is less likely to be collateral blood flow. In this setting, with an abrupt cessation of flow in the infarct-related artery, no collateral flow exists to support the infarcted zone, thereby making the septum prone to rupture **(Figure 13.4)**.

CLINICAL PRESENTATION

Symptoms of rupture include shortness of breath, chest pain, signs of low cardiac output, and shock.[16] In 1934, Sager proposed a set of clinical criteria for suspecting a ruptured septum. The sudden onset of a systolic murmur, often accompanied by a thrill, in a patient with rapid hemodynamic decompensation is highly suggestive of a ruptured interventricular septum.[18] The rupture produces a harsh, loud, holosystolic murmur along the left sternal border, radiating toward the base, apex, and right parasternal area with a palpable thrill present in half of the patients. Compared to acute mitral regurgitation (MR), initially there is often right ventricular (RV) failure and absence of severe pulmonary edema before LV failure ensues. As the disease progresses, complete biventricular failure invariably occurs.[16]

In the setting of cardiogenic shock, the thrill and murmur may be difficult to appreciate because turbulent flow across the defect is reduced. Pulmonary hypertension may cause the pulmonic component of the second heart sound to be accentuated. RV and LV S3 gallops are often heard. Tricuspid regurgitation may be present and biventricular failure generally occurs within hours to days.[16]

TREATMENT

In the correct clinical setting, immediate echocardiogram is crucial to confirm the diagnosis. After the diagnosis is made, medical therapy may consist of mechanical support with an intra-aortic balloon pump, afterload reduction, diuretics, and inotropic agents.[16] Prompt surgical intervention is essential because most patients have a rapid deterioration and die. It was previously believed that shortly after an AMI, the myocardium was too fragile for safe repair of the rupture. A waiting period of 3 to 6 weeks, to allow the margins of the infarcted muscle to develop a firm scar to facilitate surgical repair, was standard before surgical intervention.[19] Medical therapy carries close to 100% mortality. While surgical therapy is associated with poor results—only about 13% survival, it is still considered the primary therapy.[20] Surgical therapy consists of placing a myocardial patch across the ruptured septum with concomitant coronary artery bypass as needed. A recent review in the European Heart Journal shows reported 30-day mortality at various time points after AMI, and outlines an approach for the management of VSR shown in **Figures 13.5** and **13.6**.[21] **Figure 13.7** demonstrates a case of apical VSR in a patient with an acute LAD territory MI.

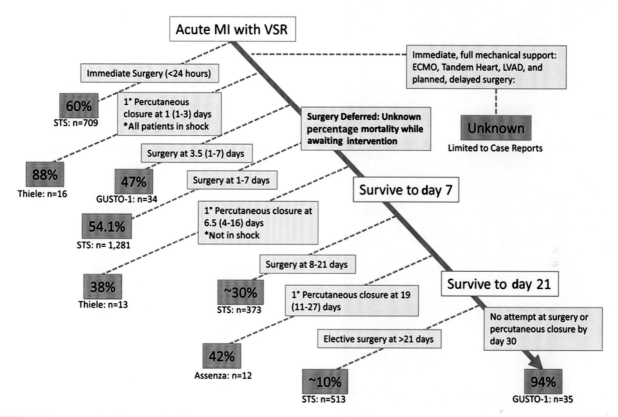

FIGURE 13.5 Reported 30-day mortality for VSR with immediate surgical management or at various time points of delayed intervention. ECMO, extracorporeal membrane oxygenation; LVAD, left ventricular assist device; MI, myocardial infarction; VSR, ventricular septal rupture. (Adapted from Jones BM, Kapadia SR, Smedira NG, et al. *Eur Heart J.* 2014;35:2060-2068.)

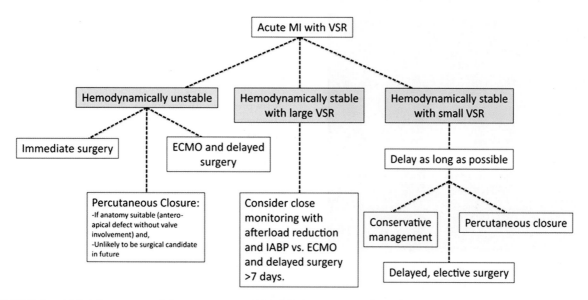

FIGURE 13.6 A multidisciplinary approach for managing acute VSR. ECMO, extracorporeal membrane oxygenation; IABP, intra-aortic balloon pump; MI, myocardial infarction; VSR, ventricular septal rupture. (Adapted from Jones BM, Kapadia SR, Smedira NG, et al. *Eur Heart J.* 2014;35:2060-2068.)

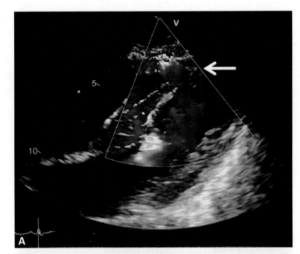

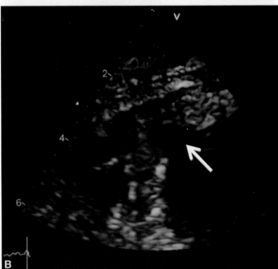

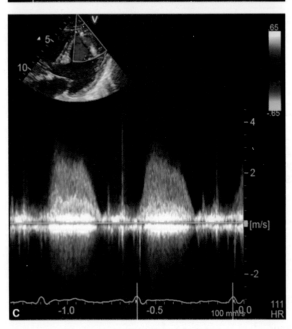

FIGURE 13.7 Subcostal view showing apical VSR with flow from left ventricle to right ventricle (A) color Doppler flow, (B) VSR defect seen with 2D imaging highlighted by an arrow, (C) continuous wave Doppler demonstrating gradient across VSR. 2D, two-dimensional; VSR, ventricular septal rupture.

RIGHT VENTRICULAR INFARCTION

Right ventricular infarction (RVI) was described over 60 years ago, but for decades it was not considered to be important because it showed no hemodynamic consequence in animal models.[22] Over time, it has become important to diagnose because it defines a specific clinical entity that is associated with considerable morbidity and mortality.[23] RVI complicates up to half of inferior wall LV infarctions.[22] Prompt recognition of this mechanical complication of AMI is crucial because its initial management differs from that of other types of infarction.

PATHOPHYSIOLOGY

The physiology of the right side of the heart varies considerably from that of the left. It is a low-pressure system that has one-sixth of the muscle mass of the left ventricle. Despite this, both ventricles have the same cardiac output.[22] This is due to the fact that the pulmonary vascular resistance is one-tenth that of the peripheral systemic resistance.[24] These factors are important in the hemodynamic consequences of RVI.

Coronary blood flow to the right ventricle is unique in that it occurs in both systole and diastole.[22] The right coronary artery (RCA) supplies the right ventricle through the acute marginal branches in the majority of patients, as well as the inferior wall and posterior interventricular septum through the posterior descending artery in right-dominant systems. Typically, RVI occurs when there is occlusion of the RCA proximal to the acute marginal branches. It can also occur with an occlusion of the left circumflex in those who have a left-dominant system. Although quite rare, occlusion of the LAD artery may result in infarction of the anterior right ventricle.[22]

The incidence of RVI in association with LV infarction ranges from 14% to 84% across different studies. Incidence of isolated RVI accounts for less than 3% of all cases of infarction.[22] When isolated to the right ventricle, the occlusion is usually in the acute marginal vessels or of a nondominant RCA.[24] Many RCA occlusions do not result in RV necrosis.[23] Less than half of inferior MIs involve the right ventricle. This may be due to lower RV myocardial oxygen demand as a result of its smaller muscle mass, or from its improved oxygen delivery from the biphasic nature of the coronary blood flow during both systole and diastole. A rich left-to-right collateral system is also thought to play a part.[22]

Acute underperfusion of the RV free wall and adjacent interventricular septum leads to a stunned and noncompliant right ventricle. Loss of RV contractility results in a serious deficit in LV preload with a resultant drop in cardiac output, thereby causing systemic hypotension.[25] Augmented atrial contractility is necessary to overcome the increased myocardial stiffness associated with RVI.[26] Factors that impair filling of the noncompliant right ventricle and cause decreased preload are likely to have profound adverse effects on hemodynamics in patients with large RVIs. These factors include volume depletion due to the use of diuretics and nitrates or any diminution in atrial function caused by concomitant atrial infarction or the loss of atrioventricular (AV) synchrony.[22]

To complicate matters, acute RV dilatation causes a leftward shift of the interventricular septum, increasing LV end-diastolic pressure with a resultant decrease in LV compliance and cardiac output. LV compliance is further aggravated by increased intrapericardial pressure as a result of RV dilatation **(Figure 13.8)**.

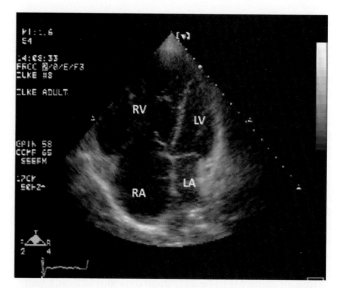

FIGURE 13.8 Apical four-chamber view of a transthoracic echocardiogram demonstrating a dilated and severely hypokinetic right ventricle with compression of the left ventricle. LA, left atrium; LV, left ventricle; RA, right atrium; RV, right ventricle.

As a consequence, the LV filling and systolic function may be below normal.[23] If significant LV dysfunction complicates RVI, the results can be disastrous.

CLINICAL PRESENTATION

Given that management of RVI is quite different from LV infarction, recognizing its clinical presentation is paramount. A patient presenting with an inferior MI and the triad of hypotension, clear lung fields, and elevated jugular venous pressure, is virtually pathognomonic for RVI.[22] This triad is very specific, but has a sensitivity of less than 25%.[27] Auscultation may reveal a right-sided S3 and S4.[28] Tricuspid regurgitation may also be noted if the right ventricle is sufficiently dilated.

Pulsus paradoxus (decreased systolic blood pressure with inspiration) and Kussmal sign (elevated jugular venous distension with inspiration) have also been reported in RVI.[28] Careful examination of neck veins in the setting of an inferior MI should alert the physician to the drastic consequences that use of nitrates, diuretics, and morphine can have. These agents should be avoided because they reduce preload and can promote or exacerbate hypotension.

The ECG is crucial for the diagnosis of RVI. The most frequent finding is any degree of ST elevation in leads II, III, and aVF with or without Q waves. Occlusion sufficiently proximal in the RCA to cause RV free wall injury also frequently compromises the blood supply to the sinoatrial node, atrium, and AV node, producing effects such as sinus bradycardia, atrial infarction, atrial fibrillation, and AV block.[25] Involvement of the RV free wall may be suspected with the presence of ST depression in precordial leads V2 and V3 when compared to V1. Confirmation of RV ischemia can be quickly obtained when right-sided leads V4R through V6R show ST-segment elevations greater than 1 mm **(Figure 13.9)**.[25] A 1-mm ST elevation in V4R is 70% sensitive and 100% specific for RVI.[22] ST-segment elevation in V4R has been shown to be a strong independent predictor of major complications and in-hospital mortality.[23] When the ECG shows signs of RVI, echocardiography can aid in the diagnosis.

TREATMENT

The treatment strategy of RVI includes early maintenance of RV preload, reduction of RV afterload, inotropic support of the dysfunctional right ventricle and early reperfusion.[22] When the right ventricle is ischemic, use of drugs such as nitrates and diuretics will reduce preload and may reduce cardiac output and cause severe hypotension. Volume loading alone with normal saline will often increase filling of the right ventricle and in turn increase filling of the underfilled left ventricle and increase cardiac output.[23]

Excessive fluid administration can further elevate right-sided filling pressures without improvement in cardiac output. In some cases, volume loading will cause further RV dilatation, which in turn further compromises LV output through pericardial restraining effects.[22] Inotropic support with dobutamine should be initiated if the cardiac output fails to improve with up to 1 L of fluid administration.[23]

Often, inferior MI can result in bradyarrhythmias and AV dyssynchrony. When stroke volume is impaired, cardiac output depends on heart rate; therefore, bradycardia can be deleterious. The development of a high-degree AV block has been reported in as many as 48% of patients with RVI.[29] AV

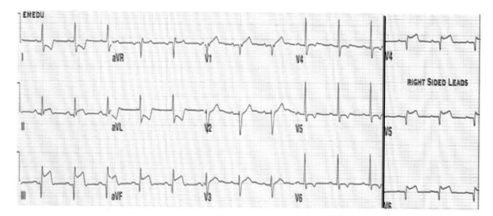

FIGURE 13.9 Electrocardiogram showing an inferior wall myocardial infarction with right-sided leads showing significant ST elevation in V4R through V6R.

dyssynchrony causes loss of right atrial contribution to preload and can lead to further hemodynamic compromise. Several investigators have shown that AV sequential pacing in patients with complete heart block leads to significant increase in cardiac output and reversal of shock when ventricular pacing alone has no benefit.[30] Prompt cardioversion for atrial fibrillation should be considered to restore AV synchrony at the earliest signs of hemodynamic compromise.[22]

Reperfusion should be considered in the initial management of RVI. Recent studies have shown that those patients with predominant RV failure who underwent revascularization with either percutaneous angioplasty or coronary artery bypass grafting (CABG) had much better outcomes. Mortality was 42% for those revascularized versus 65% for those not revascularized. These numbers were similar for those with predominant LV failure (40% and 73%). The conclusion was made that RV failure complicating AMI carries a very high mortality risk similar to that for LV failure. Revascularization helps improve these numbers and should be considered immediately.[31]

Long-term prognostic data for those suffering from RVI is conflicting. It is generally thought that when patients survive to discharge, prognosis is favorable but large-scale studies are needed to confirm this theory.[22]

ACUTE MITRAL REGURGITATION

Acute MR is another major fatal mechanical complication of AMI. As with the other complications of AMI, the rapid recognition, diagnosis, and treatment can result in significant improvement in survival. The three main causes of MR in the setting of an AMI include ischemic papillary muscle dysfunction, papillary muscle or chordal rupture, and LV dilatation.[32]

MR of mild-to-moderate severity occurs in 14% to 45% of patients following an AMI. Most MR is transient in nature but sudden papillary muscle rupture can be a life-threatening event. Fibrinolysis for reperfusion may decrease the incidence of rupture; however, when administered, rupture may occur earlier in the post-MI period than in the absence of reperfusion. In the prefibrinolytic era, papillary muscle rupture was reported to occur between days 2 and 7 post AMI. However, it is now thought that a median time to papillary muscle rupture is 13 hours.[33] Papillary muscle rupture is found in 7% of patients in cardiogenic shock and contributes to 5% of the mortality after acute MI.[34]

Studies have shown that the risk factors for acute MR with papillary muscle rupture include advanced age, female gender, and absence of previous angina, inferoposterior AMI, single-vessel disease, and no history of diabetes. When considering acute MR without papillary muscle rupture, the risk factors also include female gender and advanced age; however, these patients are likely to have had a prior MI, recurrent ischemia, and multivessel coronary artery disease.[35]

PATHOPHYSIOLOGY

The mitral valve is located retrosternally at the fourth costal space and consists of an anterior and posterior leaflet. Any portion of the mitral apparatus can become anatomically disrupted and result in a portion of the mitral valve becoming flail and dysfunctional. The degree of resultant regurgitation is directly related to the extent of anatomic disruption. Most of the time in the setting of acute MI, the rupture of an entire papillary muscle or muscle head typically results in acute severe MR.[36] In most patients, the anterolateral papillary muscle receives dual blood supply from the LAD and circumflex coronary arteries and is less likely to be involved by the ischemic process than is the posteromedial papillary muscle, which is supplied solely by the posterior descending artery. Because of its single-vessel blood supply the posteromedial papillary muscle is 6 to 12 times more vulnerable to vascular compromise and rupture than the anterolateral papillary muscle. Often, the infarct expansion is relatively small with poor collaterals, and up to 50% of patients have single-vessel disease, with many of them being a consequence of a first-time MI.[6,37] Several studies support that acute MR is not only a common complication post AMI, but also that the degree of MR is predictive of patient survival. Large studies calculate the mortality of patients with moderately severe to severe MR during an acute MI to be 24% at 30 days and 52% at 1 year.[38] Mild MR in the setting of AMI is however not associated with clinically adverse events because it is likely reversible and secondary to the acute ischemic insult.

Of note, select patients with moderate-to-severe MR, but without papillary muscle rupture, are hemodynamically stable. In this setting, patients respond well to medical therapy and revascularization with or without eventual surgical intervention (mitral valve repair or replacement or CABG).[39]

TREATMENT

As with all of the acute phase complications of AMI, the proper treatment of acute, severe MR is emergent surgical correction of the mitral valve and CABG when indicated. Prompt diagnosis with echocardiogram and aggressive medical therapy before surgery markedly improve patient outcomes. **Figure 13.10** demonstrates an apical four-chamber view of a transthoracic echocardiogram showing MR as a result of an inferior wall MI. When considering hemodynamic compromise secondary to significant, acute MR, aggressive medical resuscitation involves improving forward flow by afterload reduction and thus improving the regurgitant fraction. Afterload reduction is accomplished with the use of nitrates such as sodium nitroprusside, diuretics, and intra-aortic balloon pump counterpulsation.

The operative mortality for these patients is an estimated 20% to 25% and heavily dependent on the timing of diagnosis and treatment. Despite such a high mortality, survival in patients restricted to medical therapy alone is significantly lower. Thus, emergent surgical intervention remains the treatment of choice for papillary muscle rupture.[40] Of note, mitral valve repair rather than replacement should be attempted in centers experienced in performing this procedure[38,39]; and patients must meet the strict criteria for mitral valve repair, which includes the preserved integrity of the mitral apparatus (ie, intact papillary muscles and chordae). Interestingly, long-term results in 1 small study of 22 patients revealed a perioperative mortality of 27% and a 7-year survival for the survivors of surgery of 64% (the overall 7-year survival was 47%).[40] The only factor that improved both immediate and long-term survival was the concomitant performance of CABG. **Figure 13.11** shows a ruptured papillary muscle resulting in severe MR, requiring urgent surgical intervention.

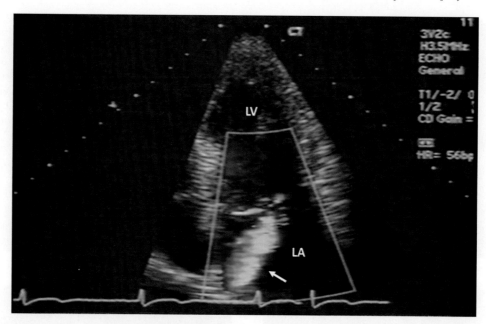

FIGURE 13.10 Apical four-chamber view of a transthoracic echocardiogram showing mitral regurgitation as a result of an inferior wall myocardial infarction (*arrow*). LA, left atrium; LV, left ventricle.

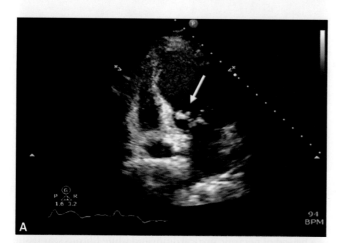

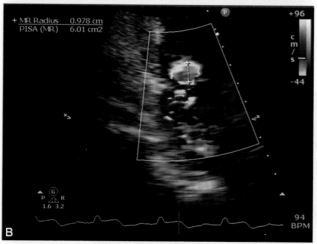

FIGURE 13.11 Papillary muscle rupture. A, Apical four-chamber view showing ruptured head of the papillary muscle (*arrow*). B, Apical three-chamber view with color Doppler demonstrating severe mitral regurgitation with large proximal isovelocity surface area (PISA) radius.

TRUE VENTRICULAR ANEURYSM

In contrast to the acute complications of MI, the chronic complications of AMI are not immediately life-threatening. They have very different presentations and require different treatments. True left ventricular aneurysm (LVA) is a common chronic complication of AMI that is important to diagnose.

LVA is a common mechanical complication following an AMI, often occurring between 10% and 15% of patients. Before the era of current management, which includes strategies such as thrombolytic therapy, percutaneous coronary intervention, and the administration of afterload reducing agents, the incidence of LVA approached 40%.[41,42] A recent analysis has shown that the incidence of LVA among 350 consecutive patients with ST-segment elevation MI, treated with thrombolytic therapy, was significantly lower in those with a patent infarct-related artery (7.2% vs 18.8%).[43] LVA of the apex and anterior wall are approximately four times more common than those of the inferior or inferoposterior walls.

Approximately 70% to 85% of LVAs are located in the anterior or apical walls, and in most cases are due to complete occlusion of the LAD coronary artery and the absence of collateralization. However, 10% to 15% of cases involve the inferior-basal walls because of RCA occlusion. A rare finding is a lateral LVA, which is the result of an occluded left circumflex coronary artery. Among patients with multivessel disease, LVA is uncommon if there is extensive collateralization or a nonoccluded LAD artery.

PATHOPHYSIOLOGY

LVA has been described as a well-delineated and distinct break, ("hinge point") in the LV geometry and contour present in both systole and diastole. The walls consist of thin, scarred, or fibrotic myocardium, completely devoid of muscle, the result of a healed transmural AMI. The pathognomonic features include a wide mouth that enables communication with the aneurysmal cavity. Often, this is evident at 4 to 6 weeks following an AMI.

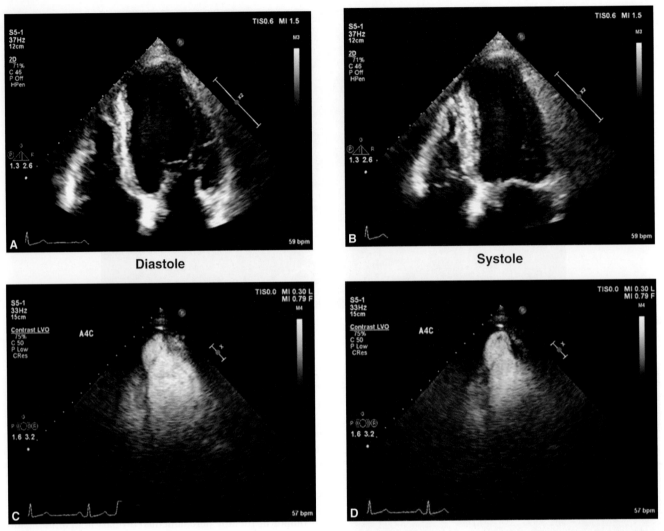

FIGURE 13.12 Apical four-chamber view in (A) diastole and (B) systole and (C and D) with echo contrast, respectively, showing a large apical acute myocardial infarction with a large apical aneurysm with no clot.

The involved wall segment is either akinetic or dyskinetic during systole, and collapses inward when the ventricle is fully vented during surgery (**Figures 13.12** and **13.13**).

Although the size of an aneurysm varies widely, most are within 1 to 8 cm in diameter. The wall of the aneurysm typically consists of a hybrid of necrotic myocardium and white fibrous scar tissue. This wall is extremely thin and delicate and may calcify over an extended period of time. Of note, it is imperative to distinguish between an LVA and a pseudoaneurysm, which is characterized by a narrow neck and a distinct "shelf-like" opening.

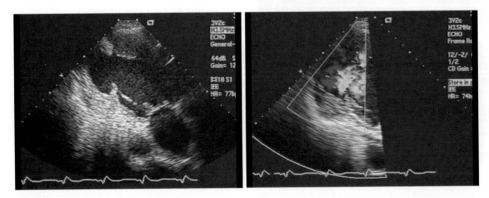

FIGURE 13.13 Apical three-chamber view **(left)** obtained from transthoracic echocardiogram revealing a large left ventricular aneurysm, enhanced with color flow Doppler **(right)** establishing an area of communication between the normal left ventricle and the aneurysmal portion.

The endocardial surface is smooth and nontrabeculated. The aneurysm is filled with organized thrombus in more than 50% of cases, which has the tendency to calcify over time.[44] Dense adhesions between the aneurysm and the overlying pericardium are common phenomena. On a molecular level, initially, the ventricular wall is characterized by myocardial muscle necrosis and a concomitant intense inflammatory reaction, which eventually is replaced with scar tissue formation, and a mature aneurysm consists mostly of hyalinized fibrous tissue. The "border zone," that is, the layer between the aneurysm and the healthy myocardium, is characterized by patchy fibrosis and abnormal alignment of the muscle fibers.

CLINICAL PRESENTATION

A prior history of AMI is almost universally present in patients with an LVA that is not associated with other etiologies such as hypertrophic cardiomyopathy or Chagas disease. The physical examination may reveal one or more of the following findings; however, it may prove to be somewhat difficult to diagnose an LVA by physical examination because the findings are nonspecific.

- Cardiac enlargement with a diffuse apical impulse located to the left of the midclavicular line.
- An area of dyskinesis can occasionally be appreciated with palpation of the left lateral chest wall, in the area of the apex and anterior wall of the left ventricle.
- A third and/or fourth heart sound (S3 or S4) is often heard, which represents the onset of blood flow into a dilated and stiffened LV chamber.
- A MR-like systolic murmur may be appreciated because of the distortion of LV geometry that results in the absence of leaflet apposition, papillary muscle dysfunction, and/or annular dilatation.

The presence of an LVA should be suspected when a patient with a large, predominantly, anterior AMI develops one of the aforementioned physical examination findings. The ECG usually reveals evidence of a large AMI and there may be persistent ST-segment elevation; however, this finding is usually the result of a large area of scar and does not necessarily imply an aneurysm **(Figure 13.14)**.

Although limited and rarely used today, chest radiography may aid in the diagnosis of an LVA; however, given the extreme limitations of chest radiography, the diagnosis is definitively made via two-dimensional echocardiography. A simple definition of an LVA on echocardiography imaging is the presence of a dyskinetic wall motion abnormality with the feature of diastolic deformity.[45,46] TTE is most often used and has globally emerged as the diagnostic tool of choice. Even before the diagnosis is made, there are a number of serious complications that can result from an LVA, such as heart failure, ventricular arrhythmias, and thrombus formation.

During ventricular systole, the paradoxical bulging of the aneurysmal segment results in "stealing" part of the LV stroke volume, resulting in decreasing cardiac output and predisposing to LV volume overload. LV dilatation and increase in wall stiffness can increase oxygen demand. In the setting of underlying coronary artery disease, the increase in oxygen demand may lead to myocardial ischemia with subsequent angina. The end result of long-standing volume overload and prolonged ischemia is a globally dilated, failing left ventricle. Heart failure symptoms are common.

The myocardial scarring present in LVA is a substrate for ventricular arrhythmias. Two mechanisms contribute to this possible deadly outcome. Firstly, myocardial ischemia and increased myocardial stretch can lead to enhanced cardiac automaticity. Secondly, the myocardium located at the border zone is made up of a mix of fibrotic tissue, inflammatory cells, and damaged muscle fibers, which is a suitable substrate for a reentrant tachycardia. Ventricular arrhythmias often result in sudden cardiac death.

As previously mentioned, a mural thrombus is identified in autopsy or surgery in >50% of patients with LVA. A possible

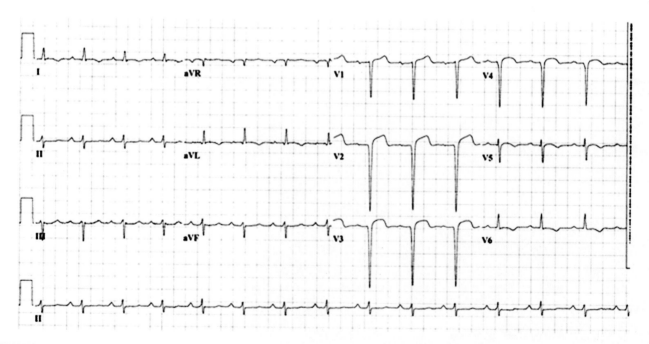

FIGURE 13.14 Electrocardiogram of a patient with a true left ventricular aneurysm displaying persistent ST elevation with Q waves in V1 through V4.

fatal consequence of thrombus formation is possible systemic embolization, which can result in stroke, ischemic colitis, ischemic limbs, and a variety of other disastrous complications.

It is important to note that true LVAs may enlarge over time. However, unlike false aneurysms, a true LVA rarely ruptures because of the dense fibrosis that comprises the walls.[47,48]

TREATMENT

Mild-to-moderate size asymptomatic aneurysms can be safely treated medically with an anticipated 5-year survival of up to 90%. Therapy includes reduction of afterload via angiotensin-converting enzyme inhibitors, nitrates, and anticoagulation (in the setting of significant LV dysfunction or evidence of thrombus formation). The optimal approach to the patient with a large, asymptomatic LVA remains a clinical dilemma. Concomitant repair of the aneurysm has been advocated when CABG or valve surgery is performed. In the absence of such indications for surgery, these patients should otherwise be treated with the same regimen as those with a small LVA; they should also be followed up closely for progressive LV dilation. Similar to other settings of chronic volume overload, a progressive increase in LV diameter and/or decrease in LV ejection fraction are a clear indication for surgery even before the presence of advanced heart failure or other symptoms.

As per the 2004 American College of Cardiology/American Heart Association (ACC/AHA) guidelines on ST-elevation MI, aneurysmectomy, accompanied by CABG, in patients with an LVA who have repetitive ventricular arrhythmias and/or heart failure unresponsive to medical and catheter-based therapy, is a Class IIa recommendation and is therefore reasonable.[49] Surgical repair should be considered for symptomatic patients with either akinetic or dyskinetic segments, because they represent variants in the spectrum of the same disease. Surgical repair of an LVA is very effective, and results in a significant improvement in patient survival, symptoms, and functional class compared to medical treatment.[50-52] Furthermore, a marked decrease in surgical mortality has been achieved in the past 25 years. Endocardial mapping with subsequent endocardial resection and possible cryoablation are performed in patients with malignant ventricular arrhythmias.

LEFT VENTRICULAR PSEUDOANEURYSM

A left ventricular pseudoaneurysm (LVPA) or false aneurysm is a less common form of a ventricular aneurysm present in <1% of patients post MI. It is briefly discussed here.

PATHOPHYSIOLOGY

An LVPA forms when cardiac rupture is more or less contained by adherent pericardium or scar tissue. Unlike a true aneurysm, an LVPA is devoid of endocardium or myocardium and because these aneurysms are prone to rupture, a quick and accurate diagnosis is of extreme importance. Unlike a true LVA whereby the walls consist of dense fibrous tissue with excellent tensile strength, the wall of an LVPA is comprised of thrombus and varying portions of the epicardium and parietal pericardium. It is the result of an AMI (typically an inferior or posterolateral wall AMI) with myocardial rupture and hemorrhage into the pericardial space, becoming progressively compressive. Cardiac tamponade occurs, thereby preventing further hemorrhage into the pericardium. Over time, thrombus organizes with overall poor structural integrity, and thus is prone to inevitable rupture, which is a fatal event.[53]

CLINICAL PRESENTATION

It has been suggested that the most frequent symptoms associated with LVPA include chest pain and dyspnea. However, often symptoms can be somewhat vague and nonspecific. The other symptomatology includes that of tamponade, heart failure, syncope, arrhythmia, or systemic embolism. Cardiac murmurs are present in about two-thirds of patients. The murmur is often indistinguishable from that of MR. Almost all patients have some degree of underlying ECG changes, which include ST-segment elevation and nonspecific T-wave changes. Evidence of a mass on chest X-ray is seen in more than one-half of patients; however, as previously mentioned, this is not specific or sensitive for the diagnosis of an LVPA.[54,55]

The most reliable method for diagnosis of an LVPA is via echocardiography. A TTE is a reasonable first step, but a definitive

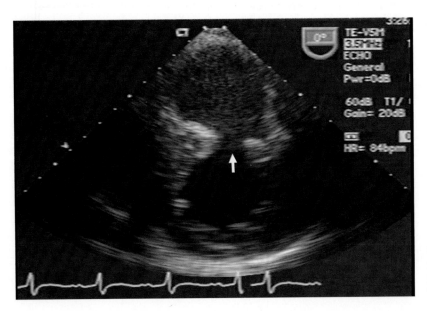

FIGURE 13.15 Short-axis view of the left ventricle (*lower cavity*) during transesophageal echocardiography. Large pseudoaneurysm (*higher cavity*). Notice the narrow "bottleneck" opening (*arrow*).

diagnosis is made in only a fraction of patients. Echocardiography can usually distinguish a pseudoaneurysm from a true aneurysm by the appearance of the connection between the aneurysm and ventricular cavity. LVPAs have a narrow neck, typically less than 40% of the maximal aneurysm diameter, which causes an abrupt interruption in the ventricular wall contour (**Figures 13.15** and **13.16**). In contrast, true aneurysms are nearly as wide at the neck as they are at the apex. **Figures 13.17** compares true aneurysms versus false/pseudoaneurysms.

TREATMENT

Untreated LVPAs have a 30% to 45% risk of rupture and, with medical therapy, a mortality of almost 50%. Thus, surgery is the preferred therapeutic option. With current techniques, the perioperative mortality is less than 10%, although the risk is greater among patients with severe MR requiring concomitant mitral valve replacement.

LEFT VENTRICULAR THROMBUS

A mural LV thrombus is a common sequela of an AMI and most commonly develops in the presence of a large infarction. Thrombi are prone to originate in regions of stasis; they are most commonly noted to occur in the apex but may also occur in lateral and inferior aneurysms. With extensive transmural infarction, mural thrombi may overlie the infarcted myocardium. Before current conventional medical therapy, the incidence ranged between 25% and 40%.[54] The initiation of heparin and perhaps thrombolysis can reduce the development of an LV thrombus by 50%. The major risk of a thrombus is subsequent distal embolization, which is highest during the first 2 weeks following an AMI with eventual reduction of risk by 6 to 8 weeks. This is attributed to a relative endothelialization of the thrombus with reduction in its embolic potential. Echocardiography has high sensitivity (95%) and high specificity (85%) for identification of an LV thrombus and has emerged as the diagnostic modality of choice. Characteristically, a thrombus has a nonhomogeneous echo density with a margin distinct from the underlying wall, which is akinetic to dyskinetic (**Figures 13.18** and **13.19**).[56] A thrombus is more likely to occur following an AMI in the LAD artery distribution (up to 33%) versus the right coronary or circumflex (<1%) coronary arteries.

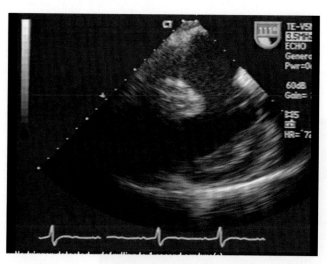

FIGURE 13.16 Short-axis view from transesophageal echocardiogram depicting a large pseudoaneurysm (*higher cavity*). Notice the narrow "shelf-like" opening into the aneurysmal cavity.

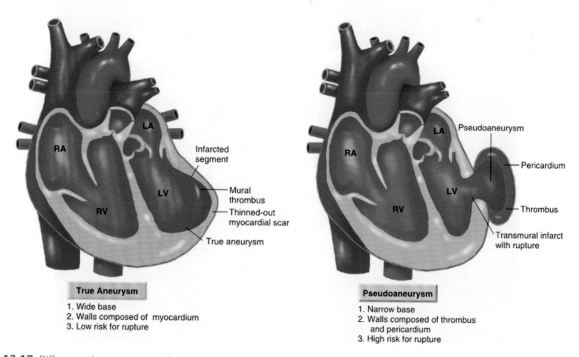

FIGURE 13.17 Differences between a pseudoaneurysm and a true aneurysm. LA, left atrium; LV, left ventricle; RA, right atrium; RV, right ventricle. (Adapted from Mann DL, Zipes DP, Libby P, Bonow RO: *Braunwald's Heart Disease: A Textbook of Cardiovascular Medicine.* Philadelphia, PA: Elsevier, 2015; and from Shah PK. Complications of acute myocardial infarction. In: Parley W, Chatterjee K, eds. *Cardiology.* Philadelphia, PA: JB Lippincott; 1987.)

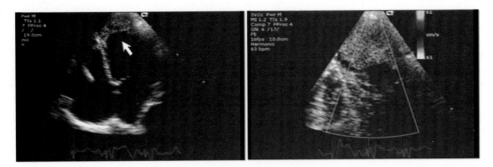

FIGURE 13.18 Apical four-chamber views of a transthoracic echocardiogram from a 74-year-old patient 3 months following AMI (*top*). Notice the large protruding apical thrombus (*arrow*). Color flow imaging (*bottom*) may be used to demonstrate abnormal flow patterns. AMI, acute myocardial infarction.

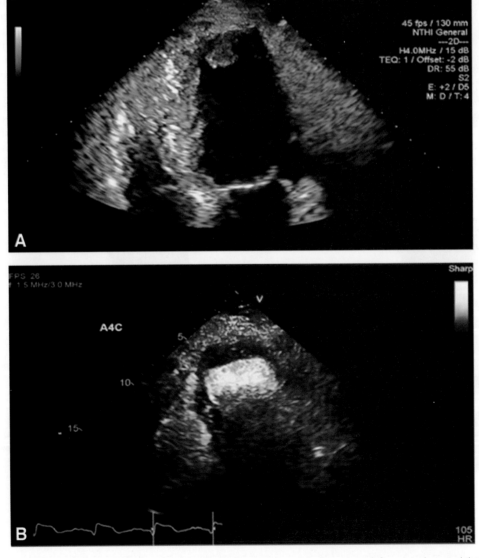

FIGURE 13.19 A, Apical four-chamber view of a transthoracic echocardiogram demonstrating a large left ventricular apical thrombus. B, Injection of an echo-contrast agent delineates the linear appearance of this large apical thrombus.

Current data on the correct treatment of LV thrombi is lacking. There are no large-scale trials that direct treatment; however, it is generally recommended that patients who have an apical clot will receive full anticoagulation with traditional anticoagulant therapy, that is, warfarin. They should be initiated with heparin and converted to full-dose warfarin for at least 3 months with a goal international normalized ratio between 2 and 3.[1]

CONCLUSION

As outlined, mechanical complications of an AMI are important to recognize, to diagnose, and, especially, to treat. Recognizing the most important signs and symptoms should prompt an immediate echocardiogram and, in most cases, this may lead to surgical intervention. Most therapies carry with them a poor prognosis, but surgery is clearly a better option with improved survival over medical therapy alone. Physicians in cardiac care units (CCUs) must grasp all of these concepts to provide proper medical care.

REFERENCES

1. Antman EM. ST elevation myocardial infarction. In: Libby P, Bonow R, Mann D, et al, eds. Braunwald's heart disease: a textbook of cardiovascular medicine. 8th ed. Philadelphia, PA: Elsevier Saunders; 2008l:1233-1299.

2. Pohjola-Sintonen S, Muller JE, Stone PH, et al. Ventricular septal and free wall rupture complicating acute myocardial infarction: Experience in the multicenter investigation of limitation of infarct size. *Am Heart J.* 1989;117:809.

3. Becker RC, Gore JM, Lambrew C, et al., for the National Registry of Myocardial Infarction Participants. A composite view of cardiac rupture in the United States National Registry of Myocardial Infarction. *J Am Coll Cardiol.* 1996;27:1321.

4. Purcaro A, Costantini C, Ciampani N, et al. Diagnostic criteria and management of subacute ventricular free wall rupture complicating acute myocardial infarction. *Am J Cardiol.* 1997;80:397.

5. Batts KP, Ackerman DM, Edwards WD. Postinfarction rupture of the left ventricular free wall: clinicopathologic correlates in 100 consecutive autopsy cases. *Hum Pathol.* 1990;21:530.

6. Reeder GS. Identification and treatment of complications of myocardial infarction. *Mayo Clin Proc.* 1995;70:880.

7. Becker RC, Charlesworth A. Wilcox RG, et al. Cardiac rupture associated with thrombolytic therapy: impact of time to treatment in the late assessment of thrombolytic efficacy (LATE) study. *J Am Coll Cardiol.* 1995;25:1063.

8. Moreno R, Lopez-Sendon J, Garcia E, et al. Primary angioplasty reduces the risk of left ventricular free wall rupture compared with thrombolysis in patients with acute myocardial infarction. *J Am Coll Cardiol.* 2002;39:598.

9. Cheriex EC, de Swart H, Dijkman LW, et al. Myocardial rupture after myocardial infarction is related to the perfusion status of the infarct-related coronary artery. *Am Heart J.* 1995;129:644.

10. Becker RC, Hochman JS, Cannon CP, et al., for the TIMI 9 Investigators. Fatal cardiac rupture among patients treated with thrombolytic agents and adjunctive thrombin antagonists. Observations from the Thrombolysis and Thrombin Inhibition in Myocardial Infarction 9 study. *J Am Coll Cardiol.* 1999;33:479.

11. Otto C. *The Practice of Clinical Echocardiography. Chapter 12: Echocardiography in the Coronary Care Unit.* Philadelphia, PA WB Saunders Co; 2002.

12. McMullan MH, Maples MD, Kilgore TL Jr, Hindman SH. Surgical experience with left ventricular free wall rupture. *Ann Thorac Surg.* 2001; 71:1894.

13. Lopez-Sendon J, Gonzalez A, Lopez de Sa E, et al. Diagnosis of subacute ventricular wall rupture after acute myocardial infarction: Sensitivity and specificity of clinical, hemodynamic and echocardiographic criteria. *J Am Coll Cardiol.* 1992;19:1145-1153.

14. Topaz O, Taylor AL. Interventricular septal rupture complicating acute myocardial infarction: from pathophysiologic features to the role of invasive and noninvasive diagnostic modalities in current management. *Am J Med.* 1992;93:683-688.

15. Crenshaw BS, Granger CB, Birnbaum Y, et al. Risk factors, angiographic patterns, and outcomes in patients with ventricular septal defect complicating acute myocardial infarction. *Circulation.* 2000;101:27-32.

16. Birnbaum Y, Fishbein MC, Blanche C, et al. Ventricular septal rupture after acute myocardial infarction. *N Engl J Med.* 2002;347(18):1426-1432.

17. Buda, AJ. The role of echocardiography in the evaluation of mechanical complications of acute myocardial infarction. *Circulation.* 1991;84(3, suppl I):109-121.

18. Sager RV. Coronary thrombosis; perforation of the infarcted interventricular septum. *Arch Intl Med.* 1934;53:140-148.

19. Giuliani ER, Danielson GK, Pluth JR, et al. Postinfarction ventricular septal rupture: Surgical considerations and results. *Circulation.* 1974;49:455-459.

20. Menon V, Webb JG, Hillis LD, et al. Outcome and profile of ventricular septal rupture with cardiogenic shock after myocardial infarction: a report from the SHOCK Trial Registry. *J Am Coll Cardiol.* 2000;36(suppl A):1110-1116.

21. Jones BM, Kapadia SR, Smedira NG, et al. Ventricular septal rupture complicating acute myocardial infarction: a contemporary review. *Eur Heart J.* 2014;35:2060-2068.

22. Kinch JW, Ryan TJ. Right ventricular infarction. *N Engl J Med.* 1994;330:1211-1219.

23. Haji SA, Movahed A. Right ventricular infarction—diagnosis and treatment. *Clin Cardiol.* 2000;23:473-482.

24. Lee FA. Hemodynamics of the right ventricle in normal and disease states. *Clin Cardiol.* 1992;10:59-67.

25. Horan LG, Flowers NC. Right ventricular infarction: specific requirements of management. *Am Fam Phys.* 1999;60(6):1727-1734.

26. Goldstein JA, Barzilai B, Rosamond TL, Eisenberg PR, Jaffe AS. Determinants of hemodynamic compromise with severe right ventricular infarction. *Circulation.* 1990;82:359-368.

27. Dell'Italia LJ, Starling MR, O'Rourke RA. Physical examination for exclusion of hemodynamically important right ventricular infarction. *Ann Intl Med.* 1983;99:608-611.

28. Cintron GB, Hernandez E, Linares E, et al. Bedside recognition, incidence and clinical course of right ventricular infarction. *Am J Cardiol.* 1981;47:224-227.

29. Braat SH, deZwann C, Brugada P, et al. Right ventricular involvement with acute inferior wall myocardial infarction identifies high risk of developing atrioventricular nodal conduction disturbances. *Am Heart J.* 1984;107:1183-1187.

30. Love JC, Haffajee CI, Gore JM, et al. Reversibility of hypotension and shock by atrial or atrioventricular sequential pacing in patients with right ventricular infarction. *am Heart J.* 1984;108:5-13.

31. Jacobs AK, Leopold JA, Bates E, et al. Cardiogenic shock caused by right ventricular infarction: a report from the SHOCK registry. *J Am Coll Cardiol.* 2003;41:1273-1279.

32. Tcheng JE, Jackman JD, Nelson CL, et al. Outcome of patients sustaining acute ischemic mitral regurgitation during myocardial infarction. *Ann Intern Med.* 1992;117:18.

33. Thompson CR, Buller CE, Sleeper LA, et al. Cardiogenic shock due to acute severe mitral regurgitation complicating acute myocardial infarction: a report from the SHOCK Trial Registry. SHould we use emergently revascularize Occluded Coronaries in cardiogenic shocK? *J Am Coll Cardiol.* 2000;36(3 suppl A):1104-1109.

34. Hochman JS, Buller CE, Sleeper LA, et al. Cardiogenic shock complicating acute myocardial infarction—etiologies, management and outcome: a report from the SHOCK Trial Registry. SHould we emergently revascularize Occluded Coronaries for cardiogenic shocK? *J Am Coll Cardiol.* 2000;36(3 suppl A):1063-1070.

35. Birnbaum Y, Chamoun AJ, Conti VR, et al. Mitral regurgitation following acute myocardial infarction. *Coron Artery Dis.* 2002;13(6): 337-344.

36. Feigenbaum H, Armstrong W, Ryan T. *6th edition Feigenbaum's Echocardiography. Chapter 15: Coronary Artery Disease.* Philadelphia, PA: Lippincott Williams and Wilkins; 2005.

37. Feigenbaum H, Armstrong W, Ryan T. *6th edition Feigenbaum's Echocardiography. Chapter 11: Mitral Valve Disease.* Philadelphia, PA: Lippincott Williams and Wilkins; 2005.

38. Lavie, CJ, Gersh, BJ. Mechanical and electrical complications of acute myocardial infarction. *Mayo Clin Proc.* 1990;65:709.

39. David, TE. Techniques and results of mitral valve repair for ischemic mitral regurgitation. *J Card Surg.* 1994;9:274.

40. Kishon, Y, Oh, JK, Schaff, HV, et al. Mitral valve operation in post-infarction rupture of a papillary muscle: immediate results and long-term follow-up of 22 patients. *Mayo Clin Proc.* 1992;67:1023.

41. Friedman BM, Dunn MI. Postinfarction ventricular aneurysms. *Clin Cardiol.* 1995;18(9):505-511.

42. Glower, DG, Lowe, EL. Left ventricular aneurysm. In: Edmunds LH, ed. *Cardiac Surgery in the Adult.* New York, NY: McGraw-Hill; 1997:677.

43. Tikiz, H, Balbay, Y, Atak, R, et al. The effect of thrombolytic therapy on left ventricular aneurysm formation in acute myocardial infarction: relationship to successful reperfusion and vessel patency. *Clin Cardiol.* 2001;24:656.

44. Feigenbaum H, Armstrong WF, Ryan T. *Feigenbaum's Echocardiography.* Philadelphia, PA: Lippincott, Williams and Wilkins; 2005:469-473.

45. Nicolosi, AC, Spotnitz, HM. Quantitative analysis of regional systolic function with left ventricular aneurysm. *Circulation.* 1988;78:856.

46. Matsumoto M, Watanabe F, Goto A, et al. Left ventricular aneurysm and the prediction of left ventricular enlargement studied by two-dimensional echocardiography: quantitative assessment of aneurysm size in relation to clinical course. *Circulation.* 1985;72:280.

47. Vlodaver, Z, Coe, JL, Edwards, JE. True and false left ventricular aneurysms: Propensity for the latter to rupture. *Circulation.* 1975;51:567.

48. Dubnow MH, Burchell HB, Titus JL. Postinfarction ventricular aneurysm. A clinicomorphologic and electrocardiographic study of 80 cases. *Am Heart J.* 1965;70:753.

49. Antman EM, Anbe DT, Armstrong PW, et al. ACC/AHA guidelines for the management of patients with ST-elevation myocardial infarction; A report of the American College of Cardiology/ American Heart Association Task Force on Practice Guidelines (Committee to Revise the 1999 Guidelines for the Management of patients with acute myocardial infarction). *J Am Coll Cardiol.* 2004;44(3):E1-E211.

50. Rao G, Zikria EA, Miller WH, et al. Experience with sixty consecutive ventricular aneurysm resections. *Circulation.* 1974;50:II149.

51. Antunes PE, Silva R, Ferrão de Oliveira J, et al. Left ventricular aneurysms: early and long-term results of two types of repair. *Eur J Cardiothorac Surg.* 2005;27(2):210-215.

52. Shapira, OM, Davidoff, R, Hilkert, RJ, et al. Repair of left ventricular aneurysm: long-term results of linear repair versus endoaneurysmorrhaphy. *Ann Thorac Surg.* 1997;63:701.

53. Frances C, Romero A, Grady D. Left ventricular pseudoaneurysm. *J Am Coll Cardiol.* 1998;32:557.

54. Dachman AH, Spindola-Franco H, Solomon N. Left ventricular pseudoaneurysm: Its recognition and significance. *JAMA.* 1981;246:1951.

55. Yeo, TC, Malouf, JF, Oh, JK, et al. Clinical profile and outcome in 52 patients with cardiac pseudoaneurysm. *Ann Intern Med.* 1998;128:299.

56. Mann, DL, Zipes, DP, Libby, P, et al. *Braunwald's Heart Disease A Textbook of Cardiovascular Medicine.* 10th ed. Philadelphia, PA: Elsevier Saunders; 2015.

Patient and Family Information for: MECHANICAL COMPLICATIONS OF MYOCARDIAL INFARCTION

For decades, heart disease has consistently been the leading killer in the world. When a family member or loved one has a heart attack, it can be a terrifying experience for everyone involved. Most of the time, everything goes smoothly, and that family member or loved one walks out of the hospital with a new outlook on life. However, there are occasions when a patient's condition can rapidly deteriorate and circumstances drastically change. These potential complications can happen at home, in transit to the hospital, in the emergency room, or even in the CCU. An understanding of the complications that go hand in hand with an acute heart attack is crucial for comprehending the nature of the disease.

The heart is the most important muscle in the human body. Like all muscles, it needs oxygen to live. However, unlike all muscles, it continuously beats around 100,000 times a day. A heart attack involves the blockage of blood flow to that muscle; this results in the cutting off its oxygen supply, for all intents and purposes, suffocating the muscle. Without oxygen, the heart muscle will die. The intense chest pain that a patient senses during an acute heart attack is due to this muscle death. Relieving that blockage will restore blood flow to the damaged muscle, replenish its oxygen supply, and hopefully allow it to live. The timely nature of this intervention is paramount to the heart's survival.

Prompt recognition and initiation of therapy for an acute heart attack is the most important factor in that patient's survival. The longer the heart muscle goes without oxygen, the faster it dies, and the worse the prognosis. The signs and symptoms of a heart attack include a left-sided or central chest pressure accompanied by any combination of shortness of breath, nausea, vomiting, sweating, and left arm or neck pain. The moment these symptoms commence, immediate medical attention should be sought.

Doctors have various methods to relieve the obstruction, including medications and direct intervention in the blocked vessel. Medical therapy involves the administration of an IV medication called a thrombolytic. This medicine will rapidly break up the blood clot in the coronary artery that has been blocked, thereby thwarting the heart attack. Interventional therapy involves the placement a tube or "catheter" into one of several arteries in the arms or the legs that lead to the heart. These catheters are then advanced to insert directly into the coronary arteries and through the use of a moving X-ray, the thrombosis can be directly visualized and extracted. Subsequently, a little piece of hollow metal, called a "stent," can be inserted in the artery and allow blood to freely flow to the dying heart muscle. The faster the therapy is delivered, the better. There are times when a substantial amount of irreversible damage has been done, causing the muscle to die and possibly tear, leading to life-threatening complications. There are other times when the muscle does not tear, but simply dies, and causes more chronic complications. In this chapter we discuss the disastrous complications of a heart attack.

When the heart muscle dies, it can eventually tear and cause sudden clinical deterioration and possibly death. If there is a delay in a patient's presentation to the emergency room, therapy cannot be initiated and the heart muscle will die. This delay can be from hours to days. If there is no delay, and therapy is administered immediately, there is always a possibility that the therapy may not be completely successful, the artery will remain blocked, and the heart muscle will die anyway. This is an unfortunate reality because not all treatments are successful. On these rare occasions, the area of the heart muscle between the dead and viable tissue will completely sever. This will result in free communication between two areas of the heart, causing brisk bleeding and inevitable death. There are three such scenarios that must be promptly recognized because surgical therapy usually provides the only means for survival. These three scenarios include ventricular free wall rupture, interventricular septal rupture, and papillary muscle rupture.

It is not as important to know the intricate details of these complications as it is important to understand their deadly potential. Any sudden deterioration in clinical condition should prompt suspicion of myocardial rupture. Development of increased chest pain or shortness of breath accompanied by a new murmur on physical examination, an accelerated heart rate, and a drop in blood pressure must be followed by an immediate echocardiogram, or ultrasound of the heart. This will provide visualization of the cardiac muscle and diagnosis of a myocardial tear. If the situation arises, IV medications can be administered to temporarily stabilize the patient, but emergent surgical intervention is paramount to provide any chance of survival.

Emergent surgery should be performed within hours of recognition of the rupture. IV medications will support the patient's blood pressure and heart rate until the operating room is ready for patient transfer. The surgical procedure will involve opening the chest wall, directly visualizing the heart, and repairing the torn tissue. Often, bypass of any blocked arteries will accompany repair of the damaged cardiac muscle. The procedure will take many hours to complete; and even if successful, the probability of eventual death is still very high. When the ruptured myocardium is repaired and the bypass complete, the patient still has a long and dangerous road ahead.

The postoperative period is every bit as important as the procedure itself. Making it out of the operating room does not mean that long-term survival is guaranteed. There are many factors such as age and comorbidities that complicate both the surgical procedure and the recovery period. The older a person is, the more unlikely it is for the person to survive such a difficult surgery and the more difficult it is to recover. Coexisting medical conditions such as asthma, emphysema, kidney disease, cancer, and diabetes, among others, all increase mortality. Friends and family must be realistic about the severity of the situation and expectations for survival. Most studies quote far less than 50% survival, with the actual numbers being less than 25%.

The left ventricle is the most important of the four heart chambers for survival. Most of what has been discussed involves damage to this all important chamber. The right ventricle is a less muscular part of the heart that can also be damaged during a heart attack. It is important to recognize RV injury, because its treatment is very different from that of garden variety LV injury. There are specific clinical signs and ECG findings that will lead to the diagnosis of an RVI. When present, a physician must be careful not to administer certain medications, such as nitroglycerin or diuretics, because they can lead to clinical deterioration. The astute medical professional can easily diagnose this situation and provide appropriate therapy. As with all heart attacks, restoring blood flow to the right ventricle will prevent poor clinical outcomes and improve survival. Surgical intervention is generally not necessary and if the patient survives to discharge, outlook is favorable.

Chronic complications of a heart attack are probably more common than the acute ones. Depending on the timing of the revascularization, a certain amount of heart muscle invariably dies. As described earlier, the longer the muscle goes without oxygen, the more of it dies. The most common phrase used is: "time is muscle." Patients who suffer large heart attacks and do not receive adequate therapy lose large amounts of muscle forever. The heart weakens, blood does not get pumped forward as it should, and over the following weeks an aneurysm can form. An aneurysm is described as a weakening of the muscle to the point that it forms a pocket within or outside the walls of the heart. To either side of the aneurysm is living tissue, and within the aneurysm is dead tissue. Aneurysms are divided into two categories that require different therapies: true aneurysms and pseudoaneurysms.

The more common and less dangerous of the two types of aneurysms are the true aneurysms. The entire aneurysm forms a pocket that is made of dead cardiac tissue. An indentation is created in the myocardium with a wide neck that contains the aneurysm. True aneurysms are entirely made of dead myocardial tissue. Because the muscle does not contract, there is invariably stasis of blood flow within the pocket, making it prone to forming blood clots. Often, a piece of the blood clot can break off and cause many complications including stroke. True aneurysms should be treated with the same aggressive medical therapy that all heart attack patients receive. This includes but is not limited to beta-blockers, angiotensin-converting enzyme inhibitors, and aspirin. If a blood clot is present, patients should be administered blood thinners to prevent against stroke. Rarely, surgical intervention is necessary to excise the aneurysm when there is evidence of deadly arrhythmias that are resistant to medical therapy.

Pseudoaneurysms are extremely rare and are very dangerous. A pseudoaneurysm represents a contained rupture of the cardiac tissue. As has been described previously, tearing of the heart muscle results in brisk bleeding and, often, death. Occasionally, this bleeding can be contained by the thin layer of tissue surrounding the heart called the pericardium. The pericardium is a rigid layer of tissue that encases the heart and at times will seal off a myocardial rupture, thereby preventing certain death. A pseudoaneurysm forms when the pericardium bubbles outward and contains a rupture during a heart attack.

Instead of the wide neck seen in true aneurysms, a pseudoaneurysm has a narrow neck that communicates with the left ventricle. There is no dead myocardium in the pseudoaneurysm because it is entirely made of pericardium. Invariably, the pocket of the pseudoaneurysm contains a blood clot, because there is complete stasis of blood flow. A pseudoaneurysm is prone to rupture because it consists of only the thin pericardium that has sealed off the prior rupture. When demonstrated by echocardiogram or computed tomography scan, surgical consultation is appropriate. Surgical excision of the pseudoaneurysm is the only treatment that can be offered to prevent rupture and certain death.

Both acute and chronic complications of a heart attack have become less common as medical therapy has advanced. The development of thrombolytics and interventional procedures have improved survival and drastically reduced the number of disastrous complications that can occur. In the unfortunate cases when they do occur, advancements in surgical technology and techniques have further improved the chances of survival. Even with all these advancements in therapy, however, prompt recognition and timely diagnosis can be the difference between life and death. Survival to hospital discharge is not certain when these complications occur and family members must realize that there is a long road ahead.

When a patient does survive a complication of an AMI, he or she must realize that great care must be taken to improve the likelihood of long-term survival. Outpatient follow-up with a cardiologist, surgeon, and medical doctor should be in place before discharge. The patient will invariably be on a new regimen of medications that can be extremely complicated. Survivors will often need a significant amount of rehabilitation before they can return to their pre–heart attack state. Social support and family encouragement both increase the likelihood of recovery. Patients should not leave the hospital without a strict understanding of what medications they are to take and who they are to follow up with. A structured regimen of medication compliance, physician follow-up, and cardiac rehabilitation can turn a life-threatening situation into a rewarding experience for patients, families, and all medical professionals involved.

Andrew Higgins
May Bakir
Venu Menon

14

Cardiogenic Shock Complicating Acute Myocardial Infarction

INTRODUCTION

Over the past several decades, both the incidence of acute myocardial infarction (AMI) and the mortality rate for AMI patients have shown a steady decline because of multiple factors, including effective risk factor modification as well as improved medical, surgical, and percutaneous therapies for coronary artery disease.[1–3] The incidence of cardiogenic shock complicating AMI, however, remains unaffected, and the mortality resulting from this condition remains high and is a leading cause of death among patients hospitalized for AMI.[4,5]

Myocardial infarction–related cardiogenic shock is a heterogeneous clinical entity in both etiology and presentation but is most commonly the result of acute left ventricular (LV) dysfunction caused by extensive cardiac muscle necrosis in the setting of an ST elevation myocardial infarction (STEMI). As the stroke volume acutely declines, the heart attempts to maintain cardiac output by increasing heart rate as a compensatory response. Once this compensatory mechanism becomes inadequate, tissue hypoperfusion ensues, leading to a systemic inflammatory response, multiorgan dysfunction, and eventually circulatory collapse. This may be further precipitated by a vasodilatory response of the peripheral circulatory system, resembling a systemic inflammatory state. Early signs of impending cardiovascular collapse may be evident on arrival at the hospital, but the majority of patients will present in a well-compensated state and progress to shock only after clinical presentation.[6]

In part because of the heterogeneity of its etiologies and manifestations, there is no universally accepted definition of cardiogenic shock. The SHOCK (SHould we emergently revascularize Occluded Coronaries for cardiogenic shocK) trial required patients to meet both clinical criteria of cardiogenic shock (sustained hypotension and end-organ hypoperfusion) and either hemodynamic confirmation with a pulmonary artery catheter or radiographic confirmation of pulmonary edema in the setting of anterior wall infarction (**Table 14.1**: SHOCK inclusion criteria for which patients should be revascularized early).[7] It is important to note that these are stringent criteria set for the purposes of a randomized control trial and that in clinical practice the myocardial dysfunction associated with ischemia exists along a spectrum: patients may meet only some of these criteria at the time of their initial evaluation.[8] In the setting of physical and biochemical findings of peripheral organ hypoperfusion despite adequate intravascular volume status, the clinician should suspect cardiogenic shock by the bedside. Recognition of early signs of falling cardiac output may facilitate earlier and more aggressive treatment of patients with a more grave prognosis (**Table 14.2**: Killip Classification, which outlines the early signs of decompensating cardiac function).[9]

TABLE 14.1	Shock Inclusion Criteria
INCLUSION CRITERIA	**PARAMETERS**
Ischemic criteria	ST-segment elevation, Q-wave infarction, new left bundle-branch block, or posterior infarction with anterior ST-segment depression
Clinical Criteria	Hypotension: SBP <90 mm Hg for at least 30 min or the need for supportive measures to maintain blood pressure End-organ hypoperfusion: cool extremities or urine output < 30 mL/h despite a heart rate of ≥ 60 beats/min
Hemodynamic criteria	Cardiac index ≤ 2.2 L/min/m^2, pulmonary capillary wedge pressure ≥ 15 mm Hg (not necessary if radiographic criteria are met)
Radiographic criteria	Pulmonary congestion on chest radiograph in setting of anterior wall myocardial infarction

SBP, systolic blood pressure.

TABLE 14.2	Killip Classification
KILLIP CLASS	**DESCRIPTION**
I	No evidence of heart failure
II	Mild heart failure: rales over one-third or less of posterior lung fields, systolic blood pressure of 90 mm Hg or higher
III	Pulmonary edema involving more than one-third of lung fields, systolic blood pressure of 90 mm Hg or higher
IV	Cardiogenic shock: extensive rales, systolic blood pressure less than 90 mm Hg

INCIDENCE

Cardiogenic shock remains an infrequent but life-threatening complication of AMI. Evidence of shock is either present on arrival or develops after admission in 4% to 10% of patients hospitalized for ST elevation AMI.[5,10] There is significant regional variation in temporal trends in incidence over time; it remains unclear to what extent this is driven by a changing burden of disease versus being reflective of changing definitions and evolving patterns of coding and classification.[11]

ETIOLOGY AND PATHOPHYSIOLOGY

Cardiac myocytes are among the most aerobically active cells in the body and are dependent on a blood supply commensurate with their relatively high oxygen demand.[12] When this relationship is disrupted through either acute plaque rupture (type 1 myocardial infarction) or through a mismatch in supply and demand (type 2), myocyte contractility is compromised, and the heart attempts to compensate through other mechanisms. When these mechanisms are inadequate, cardiac output begins to fall, and a downward spiral toward cardiogenic shock begins (**Figure 14.1**).[13]

Coronary perfusion occurs primarily during diastole and is dependent on the gradient between the proximal aortic pressure and the left ventricular end diastolic pressure (LVEDP). As cardiac output begins to fall, LVEDP begins to rise and diastolic pressures begin to decrease, further reducing the coronary perfusion gradient in the culprit vessel as well as the coronary circulation as a whole. This can result in remote ischemia in the noninfarct regions and further compromises cardiac output, creating a vicious spiral that culminates in frank circulatory collapse.

Beyond the immediate hemodynamic effects, a similarly injurious biochemical cascade begins. The fall in cardiac output leads to a reflexive activation of the sympathetic nervous system and an ensuant catecholamine surge; renal hypoperfusion also activates the renin–angiotensin–aldosterone axis. The resulting increase in heart rate and vasoconstriction lead to an increase in myocardial oxygen demand through increased wall stress, heart rate, and contractility.

In parallel to this, tissue destruction related to both local myocardial ischemia and systemic end-organ damage leads to acidemia and the release of inflammatory cytokines, including IL-6; these trigger an increase in nitric oxide synthase production in vascular smooth muscle cells. This vasodilator response may be

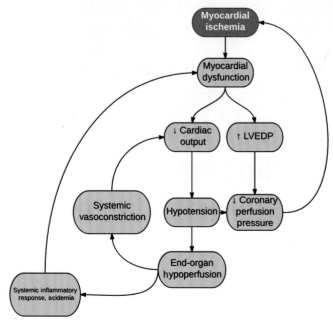

FIGURE 14.1 The hemodynamic and biochemical decompensation cascade of cardiogenic shock. LVEDP, left ventricular end diastolic pressure.

a dominant feature in a proportion of patients with cardiogenic shock. Both nitric oxide and acidemia itself may act as negative inotropes and exacerbate an acute decline in cardiac function.[14,15]

In addition to the direct myocardial dysfunction and sequelae described above, AMI may also result from several mechanical complications, including mitral regurgitation (caused by acute LV dilatation or papillary muscle ischemia/rupture), ventricular septal rupture, or ventricular free wall rupture. Although relatively uncommon, early comprehensive bedside echocardiography is critical to rule out these complications because they portend a worse prognosis and mandate consideration for surgical intervention.

It is important to maintain a wide differential in patients with hemodynamic instability to ensure that syndromes with similar presentations such as underresuscitated sepsis or hemorrhagic shock are not missed. Noncoronary cardiovascular emergencies such as acute thoracic aortic dissection, pulmonary embolism, myocarditis/pericarditis, tension pneumothorax, and tamponade should also be considered and ruled out with further testing if necessary.

MANAGEMENT

DIAGNOSIS

The cornerstone of management of cardiogenic shock is prompt recognition and accurate diagnosis of the dominant mechanism affecting circulatory instability. A quick but comprehensive history should be taken with a focus on determination of risk factors, comorbidities, medication use, and allergies (particularly to antiplatelet agents or to contrast medium). A focused physical exam should also be performed to screen for mechanical or valvular etiologies of shock (eg, a murmur suggestive of ventricular septal rupture or of acute mitral regurgitation) as well as to look for evidence of early cardiogenic shock (including but not limited to impaired mentation, cool extremities, pulmonary congestion, or an elevated jugular venous pressure).

STABILIZATION AND RESUSCITATION

In concurrence with planning for emergent revascularization, a physiologic baseline for the patient should be established and early resuscitative measures initiated. Initial measurements of relevant biomarkers such as cardiac enzymes (troponin T and CK-MB) and lactate should be made. Adequate intravascular volume status should be confirmed clinically if not invasively.

We perform routine invasive hemodynamic monitoring in this patient population. Placement of a pulmonary artery catheter receives a class I recommendation from the American College of Cardiology for patients with respiratory distress or clinical evidence of impaired perfusion in whom the adequacy or excess of intracardiac filling pressures cannot be determined from clinical assessment.[16,17] A right heart catheter enables continuous monitoring of vital hemodynamic parameters such as cardiac index, cardiac power, and mixed venous oxygen saturations, all of which are strong prognostic outcome variables. It also enables quantification of systemic vascular resistance (SVR), which helps gauge the response of the periphery to the acute myocardial insult. Similarly, invasive arterial blood pressure monitoring is useful to assess the real-time response to vasoactive therapies or when indirect blood pressure monitoring is unreliable.

If hypotension persists despite adequate filling pressures, pharmacologic or mechanical support should be initiated. If a vasopressor is required, norepinephrine should likely be used over dopamine. A recent randomized trial failed to show a significant difference between norepinephrine and dopamine across all subtypes of shock; however, a predefined subgroup analysis of patients with cardiogenic shock showed a significant increase in mortality with dopamine therapy.[18] Vasopressin may also be considered in cases with persistently low SVR.

MECHANICAL CIRCULATORY SUPPORT

Although vasopressor therapy may play a critical role in temporizing a patient with impending circulatory collapse, this must be weighed against the associated risks, including tachyarrhythmia, peripheral vasoconstriction leading to distal malperfusion, and an increase in myocardial oxygen demand triggering worsening myocardial ischemia. More definitive support can be offered by a mechanical assist device. Although mechanical support is not a new therapy and placement of an intra-aortic balloon pump (IABP) was an integral component of the early revascularization strategy of the SHOCK trial, other durable options have become available in recent years.

Mechanical circulatory support (MCS) devices fall into three primary categories: pulsatile flow devices (IABP), axial continuous-flow devices such as the Impella (with flow from left ventricle to aorta), and centrifugal continuous-flow devices such as the TandemHeart (with flow from left atrium to femoral artery) and venoarterial extracorporeal membrane oxygenation (VA-ECMO). In addition to different positions and modalities of support, each of these devices differs in the extent to which it is able to support the circulation of a patient with worsening left-sided cardiogenic shock (as seen in **Table 14.3**).[19]

The IABP is the most familiar, readily available, and easily insertable of the percutaneous MCS options. It is typically inserted transfemorally: arterial access is obtained via the femoral artery, followed by advancement of a guidewire into the aorta; the balloon pump is subsequently advanced over the wire and placed in the descending aorta distal to the takeoff of the left subclavian artery. Once connected, the balloon pump is controlled either through electrocardiogram (ECG) gating or through pressure transduction to inflate during diastole and actively deflate during systole. This leads to a decrease in afterload because of the active deflation during LV ejection, augmenting cardiac output and reducing myocardial oxygen demand. In addition, the inflation during diastole raises the coronary perfusion pressure. IABP utilization is contraindicated in patients with severe aortic regurgitation, severe peripheral arterial disease, or significant coagulopathy. The most commonly used balloon size shifts approximately 40 mL of blood per inflation and increases cardiac output by up to 1 L/min.[20]

The Impella family of devices is offered in three primary sizes, two of which may be inserted percutaneously (the Impella 2.5 and CP) and one that must be inserted via surgical cutdown (the Impella 5.0). As with the IABP, these are typically inserted transfemorally. Arterial access is obtained via the femoral artery,

TABLE 14.3	Mechanical Circulatory Support Devices			
	IABP	**IMPELLA**	**TANDEMHEART**	**VA-ECMO**
Output	0.3–1 L/min	1–5 L/min	2.5–5 L/min	3–7 L/min
Flow/mechanism	Aortic counterpulsation	LV to aorta continuous flow	LA to aorta continuous flow	Venous to arterial continuous flow (multiple configurations possible)
Preload	↓	↓↓	↓↓	↓
Afterload	↓	↓	↑	↑↑
Contraindications	Severe AI Severe PAD	Severe AI, critical AS, mechanical AVR Severe PAD Contraindication to anticoagulation LV thrombus	Severe AI Severe PAD Contraindication to anticoagulation VSD LA thrombus	Severe AI Severe PAD Contraindication to anticoagulation

AI, aortic insufficiency; AS, aortic stenosis; AVR, aortic valve replacement; IABP, intra-aortic balloon pump;; LA, left atrial; LV, left ventricular; PAD, peripheral arterial disease; VA-ECMO, venoarterial extracorporeal membrane oxygenation; VSD, ventricular septal defect..

followed by insertion of a guidewire. An introducer is advanced over the guidewire, and a diagnostic catheter is advanced into the left ventricle; a placement guidewire is then inserted into the apex of the ventricle, and the diagnostic catheter is removed. The Impella is then inserted over this guidewire and positioned so that it sits across the aortic valve with the inlet area 3 to 3.5 cm below the aortic annulus and the outlet in the ascending aorta. It is contraindicated in severe aortic stenosis or regurgitation; severe peripheral arterial disease; and in patients with mechanical aortic valves, LV thrombi, or contraindications to anticoagulation. The degree of support offered varies with device size: The Impella 2.5 offers up to 2.5 L/min of support, the CP offers up to 3.5 L/min, and the Impella 5.0 offers up to 5 L/min.[19] When long-term temporary support is anticipated, the Impella 5.0 is often placed via the axillary approach using a graft.

The TandemHeart device is also typically inserted transfemorally. Venous access is obtained via the femoral vein; a transseptal puncture technique is then used to enter the left atrium, and a guidewire is advanced into the left atrium. An inflow catheter is then inserted over this to access the left atrium, where it drains oxygenated blood back to the centrifugal pump of the TandemHeart. This oxygenated blood is then reintroduced into the circulation in the femoral artery. Contraindications include uncontrolled bleeding diatheses or contraindications to anticoagulation, severe aortic regurgitation, and left atrial thrombi. It offers up to 4.5 L/min of support.

VA-ECMO offers both the capability of biventricular support as well as treatment of concomitant respiratory and circulatory collapse. It is most often inserted in a femoral vein to femoral artery fashion but can be performed in a wide variety of configurations. Regardless of the site of insertion, deoxygenated blood is drained via a venous inflow catheter into a centrifugal pump, oxygenated, and reintroduced into the arterial circulation. Contraindications include severe aortic insufficiency, severe peripheral arterial disease, and contraindications to anticoagulation. It offers the most extensive hemodynamic support of current MCS devices, with up to 7 L/min of flow. When placed peripherally, it is important to place an antegrade cannula to perfuse the distal limb and avoid ischemic complications.

Most recently, percutaneous right ventricular assist devices have emerged as an option for patients with refractory cardiogenic shock in the context of isolated right ventricular failure. Early data suggest promising outcomes, but the technical difficulty of device insertion and relatively good prognosis for isolated right ventricular infarction may limit widespread use.[21]

Although options for MCS have proliferated in recent years and their use is rapidly becoming more widespread, the evidentiary base to support their more frequent use has lagged behind.[22] Trials comparing the newer MCS options versus IABP in cardiogenic shock complicating AMI have largely been underpowered, and although some have shown superiority in improvement of hemodynamic parameters, there is to date little evidence supporting a mortality benefit.[23,24] Given equivocal clinical benefits and significantly higher cost associated with percutaneous ventricular assist devices (VADs), IABP may remain the preferred first-line choice for cardiogenic shock, with escalation to more support only when necessary.[25]

REVASCULARIZATION

Early diagnostic angiography and subsequent percutaneous or surgical revascularization should be pursued in patients with cardiogenic shock complicating either STEMI or non–ST elevation acute coronary syndrome. This is a class I recommendation for both patient populations and is driven primarily by findings from the SHOCK trial.[7,26,27] The SHOCK trial randomized 302 patients with AMI complicated by cardiogenic shock to either medical therapy alone (with delayed revascularization if needed) or to emergent revascularization via either coronary artery bypass grafting (CABG) or percutaneous coronary intervention (PCI) within 6 hours of randomization. Compared with medical therapy alone, urgent revascularization was associated with a nonsignificant reduction in 30-day all-cause mortality (46.7% vs 56.0%, $P = 0.11$); a lasting survival benefit was conferred with revascularization and was found to be significant at 6 months postrandomization (50.3% vs 63.1%, $P = 0.027$).

The ideal mode and extent of revascularization is an area of ongoing debate. For patients with only one- or two-vessel disease (including isolated left main disease), PCI of the infarct-related artery can be performed at the time of initial angiography.[28] The role for revascularization of nonculprit lesions is less clear; although restoration of blood flow to a wider area of the myocardium has strong theoretical benefits, this must be balanced against the additional procedural risk and contrast exposure inherent to a more extensive coronary intervention. Current guidelines recommend consideration of nonculprit vessel revascularization in the setting of broadly defined hemodynamic instability; although this is supported by observational studies and registry analysis, there is a paucity of randomized data.[29,30] The ongoing CULPRIT-SHOCK trial will randomize patients with shock complicating AMI to either immediate multivessel PCI or to PCI of the culprit lesion only and should help to narrow this evidence gap.[31]

Emergent CABG offers definitive revascularization to patients with multivessel disease. In addition, prompt cardiopulmonary bypass may rescue a patient with impending circulatory collapse and halt the cycle of worsening end-organ perfusion described earlier. Within the SHOCK trial, CABG was recommended for patients with a left main stenosis of ≥ 50%, two or more total or subtotal occlusions, or stenoses of > 90% in two noninfarct major epicardial vessels. Based on these criteria, approximately 36% of patients in the emergent revascularization arm underwent CABG. Despite being a higher-risk population (higher incidence of diabetes, three-vessel disease, and left main disease), patients treated with CABG had similar rates of survival as those treated with PCI. In clinical practice, however, less than 5% of patients with cardiogenic shock currently receive early CABG.[11] Analysis of the National Cardiovascular Data Registry shows increasing rates of PCI in this setting, with only a small minority referred for CABG over a similar time frame.[32] Percutaneous intervention with its implicit commitment to dual antiplatelet therapy may preclude definitive surgical revascularization in these patients; it should thus be kept in mind that emergent CABG remains the treatment of choice and should be considered for patients with complex left main disease, severe three-vessel disease not amenable to PCI, or with concurrent mechanical complications of AMI.

PERSISTENT SHOCK

Cardiogenic shock may not resolve despite aggressive revascularization and appropriate initial support. Persistent shock despite revascularization should prompt a reevaluation of the patient's situation with a focused physical examination, consideration of

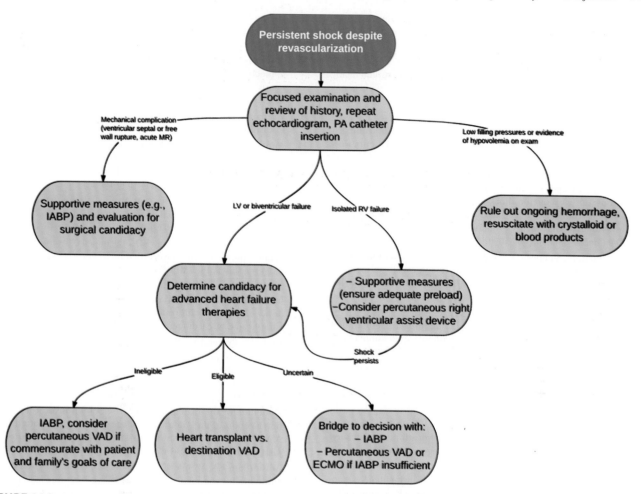

FIGURE 14.2 Management of persistent shock. ECMO, extracorporeal membrane oxygenation; IABP, intra-aortic balloon pump; LV, left ventricular; MR, mitral regurgitation; PA, pulmonary artery; RV, right ventricular; VAD, ventricular assist device.

pulmonary artery catheter insertion if not already performed, and repeat echocardiography (**Figure 14.2** outlines the management of persistent shock).

If persistent shock resulting from LV failure is confirmed, the patient's eligibility for advanced heart failure therapies (ie, transplantation or destination left ventricular assist device) should be assessed; if they are an appropriate candidate, an expedited evaluation should be initiated. If the patient is ineligible, a percutaneous VAD may still be an option, but this should be discussed in the context of the goals of care of the patient and family. If candidacy is unclear initially, consideration should be given to deploying a bridge-to-decision MCS. In patients with a dismal prognosis, especially those with poor prior functional status, significant comorbidities, especially established renal failure, palliative options should be considered.

DISCHARGE PLANNING

Survivors of cardiogenic shock after AMI will require aggressive medical management for secondary prevention. High-intensity statin therapy, smoking cessation, weight loss, and management of other risk factors should be emphasized before their discharge. All patients should be referred to cardiac rehabilitation at discharge.

LV ejection fraction should be assessed both before discharge and again 6 weeks after their acute event to determine eligibility for implantable cardiac defibrillator insertion.

SUMMARY

Despite advances in medical therapy and revascularization techniques for coronary artery disease, cardiogenic shock remains a major source of morbidity and mortality among patients hospitalized with AMI. The mainstay of treatment of cardiogenic shock is early recognition, followed by prompt treatment of the underlying cause (with surgical or percutaneous revascularization) while providing appropriate hemodynamic support.

REFERENCES

1. Ford ES, Ajani UA, Croft JB, et al. Explaining the decrease in U.S. deaths from coronary disease, 1980–2000. *N Engl J Med.* 2007;356:2388-2398.

2. Gerber Y, Weston SA, Jiang R, et al. The changing epidemiology of myocardial infarction in Olmsted County, Minnesota, 1995–2012. *Am J Med.* 2015;128:144-151.

3. Mozaffarian D, Benjamin EJ, Go AS, et al. Heart disease and stroke statistics-2016 update: a report from the American Heart Association. *Circulation.* 2016;133:e38-360.

4. Goldberg RJ, Spencer FA, Gore JM, et al. Thirty-year trends (1975 to 2005) in the magnitude of, management of, and hospital death rates associated with cardiogenic shock in patients with acute myocardial infarction: a population-based perspective. *Circulation.* 2009;119:1211-1219.

5. Redfors B, Angerås O, Råmunddal T, et al. 17-year trends in incidence and prognosis of cardiogenic shock in patients with acute myocardial infarction in western Sweden. *Int J Cardiol.* 2015;185:256-262.

6. Webb JG, Sleeper LA, Buller CE, et al. Implications of the timing of onset of cardiogenic shock after acute myocardial infarction: a report from the SHOCK Trial Registry. SHould we emergently revascularize Occluded Coronaries for cardiogenic shocK? *J Am Coll Cardiol.* 2000;36:1084-1090.

7. Hochman JS, Sleeper LA, Webb JG, et al. Early revascularization in acute myocardial infarction complicated by cardiogenic shock. SHOCK Investigators. Should We Emergently Revascularize Occluded Coronaries for Cardiogenic Shock. *N Engl J Med.* 1999;341:625-634.

8. Menon V, Slater JN, White HD, et al. Acute myocardial infarction complicated by systemic hypoperfusion without hypotension: report of the SHOCK trial registry. *Am J Med.* 2000;108:374-380.

9. Khot UN, Jia G, Moliterno DJ, et al. Prognostic importance of physical examination for heart failure in non-ST-elevation acute coronary syndromes: the enduring value of Killip classification. *JAMA.* 2003;290:2174-2181.

10. Goldberg RJ, Makam RCP, Yarzebski J, et al. Decade-long trends (2001–2011) in the incidence and hospital death rates associated with the in-hospital development of cardiogenic shock after acute myocardial infarction. *Circ Cardiovasc Qual Outcomes.* 2016;9:117-125.

11. Kolte D, Khera S, Aronow WS, et al. Trends in incidence, management, and outcomes of cardiogenic shock complicating ST-elevation myocardial infarction in the United States. *J Am Heart Assoc.* 2014;3:e000590.

12. Mann D, Zipes D, Libby P, et al. *Braunwald's Heart Disease: A Textbook of Cardiovascular Medicine.* 10th ed. Philadelphia, PA: Saunders/Elsevier; 2015.

13. Reyentovich A, Barghash MH, Hochman JS. Management of refractory cardiogenic shock. *Nat Rev Cardiol.* 2016;13:481-492.

14. Kimmoun A, Novy E, Auchet T, et al. Hemodynamic consequences of severe lactic acidosis in shock states: from bench to bedside. *Crit Care.* 2015;19:175.

15. Hare JM, Loh E, Creager MA, et al. Nitric oxide inhibits the positive inotropic response to β-adrenergic stimulation in humans with left ventricular dysfunction. *Circulation.* 1995;92:2198-2203.

16. Yancy CW, Jessup M, Bozkurt B, et al. 2013 ACCF/AHA guideline for the management of heart failure: Executive summary report of the American College of Cardiology Foundation/American Heart Association task force on practice guidelines. *J Am Coll Cardiol.* 2013;62:1495-1539.

17. Binanay C, Califf RM, Hasselblad V, et al. Evaluation study of congestive heart failure and pulmonary artery catheterization effectiveness: the ESCAPE trial. *JAMA.* 2005;294:1625-1633.

18. De Backer D, Biston P, Devriendt J, et al. Comparison of dopamine and norepinephrine in the treatment of shock. *N Engl J Med.* 2010;362:779-789.

19. Atkinson TM, Ohman EM, O'Neill WW, et al. A practical approach to mechanical circulatory support in patients undergoing percutaneous coronary intervention: an interventional perspective. *JACC Cardiovasc Interv.* 2016;9:871-883.

20. Werdan K, Gielen S, Ebelt H, et al. Mechanical circulatory support in cardiogenic shock. *Eur Heart J.* 2014;35:156.

21. Anderson MB, Goldstein J, Milano C, et al. Benefits of a novel percutaneous ventricular assist device for right heart failure: the prospective RECOVER RIGHT study of the Impella RP device. *J Heart Lung Transplant.* 2015;34:1549-1560.

22. Stretch R, Sauer CM, Yuh DD, et al. National trends in the utilization of short-term mechanical circulatory support: incidence, outcomes, and cost analysis. *J Am Coll Cardiol.* 2014;64:1407-1415.

23. Ouweneel DM, Eriksen E, Sjauw KD, et al. Impella CP versus intra-aortic balloon pump in acute myocardial infarction complicated by cardiogenic shock: the IMPRESS trial. *J Am Coll Cardiol.* 2016;23127.

24. Thiele H, Sick P, Boudriot E, et al. Randomized comparison of intra-aortic balloon support with a percutaneous left ventricular assist device in patients with revascularized acute myocardial infarction complicated by cardiogenic shock. *Eur Heart J.* 2005;26:1276-1283.

25. Shah AP, Retzer EM, Nathan S, et al. Clinical and economic effectiveness of percutaneous ventricular assist devices for high-risk patients undergoing percutaneous coronary intervention. *J Invasive Cardiol.* 2015;27:148-154.

26. O'Gara PT, Kushner FG, Ascheim DD, et al. 2013 ACCF/AHA guideline for the management of ST-elevation myocardial infarction a report of the American College of Cardiology Foundation/American Heart Association Task Force on Practice Guidelines. *J Am Coll Cardiol.* 2013;61:e78-e140.

27. Amsterdam EA, Wenger NK, Brindis RG, et al. 2014 AHA/ACC guideline for the management of patients with non–ST-elevation acute coronary syndromes a report of the American college of cardiology/American heart association task force on practice guidelines. *J Am Coll Cardiol.* 2014;64:e139-e228.

28. Stone GW, Sabik JF, Serruys PW, et al. Everolimus-eluting stents or bypass surgery for left main coronary artery disease. *N Engl J Med.* 2016; 375:2223-2235.

29. Park JS, Cha KS, Lee DS, et al. Culprit or multivessel revascularisation in ST-elevation myocardial infarction with cardiogenic shock. *Heart Br Card Soc.* 2015;101:1225-1232.

30. Yang JH, Hahn J-Y, Song PS, et al. Percutaneous coronary intervention for nonculprit vessels in cardiogenic shock complicating ST-segment elevation acute myocardial infarction. *Crit Care Med.* 2014;42:17-25.

31. Thiele H, Desch S, Piek JJ, et al. Multivessel versus culprit lesion only percutaneous revascularization plus potential staged revascularization in patients with acute myocardial infarction complicated by cardiogenic shock: design and rationale of CULPRIT-SHOCK trial. *Am Heart J.* 2016;172:160-169.

32. Frutkin AD, Lindsey JB, Mehta SK, et al. Drug-eluting stents and the use of percutaneous coronary intervention among patients with class I indications for coronary artery bypass surgery undergoing index revascularization: analysis from the NCDR (National Cardiovascular Data Registry). *JACC Cardiovasc Interv.* 2009;2:614-621.

Patient and Family Information for: CARDIOGENIC SHOCK COMPLICATING ACUTE MYOCARDIAL INFARCTION

DEFINITION

Every organ in the body requires a continuous supply of oxygen in order to function properly. Blood, pumped by the heart, is what carries oxygen to all the organs. If the pumping function of the heart becomes weak enough that it is unable to provide sufficient blood flow to the organs, the body begins to shut down, and this is known as *cardiogenic shock*. Many different conditions can cause cardiogenic shock, but the most common one is *myocardial infarction*, also known as a heart attack.

As with the rest of the organs in the body, the human heart also requires a constant supply of oxygen. The *coronary arteries* carry the oxygen-carrying blood to the heart tissue. If this blood flow is interrupted by a blockage in one or more of the coronary arteries, a heart attack results because oxygen cannot get to the portion of the heart that has the blockage. The heart tissue stops functioning properly when blood flow is disrupted, and it can die if it lacks blood flow for long enough. Large heart attacks can cause such significant damage to the heart that it is unable to pump strongly enough for the blood to reach all the organs in sufficient amounts. When this occurs, it is known as cardiogenic shock.

SIGNS AND SYMPTOMS OF CARDIOGENIC SHOCK

Patients with cardiogenic shock will often complain of shortness of breath. Other symptoms such as chest, neck/jaw, or arm pain are also common in patients with cardiogenic shock caused by a heart attack. As a result of the weak condition of the heart, patients with cardiogenic shock will often have low blood pressures and high heart rates. It is also common for patients to be confused, have cool skin, and make only minimal amounts of urine.

MANAGEMENT AND TREATMENT

Cardiogenic shock is a medical emergency, and patients with this condition need urgent care in a critical care unit. When physicians are concerned that cardiogenic shock is present, they will act quickly in an attempt to gather information to see the cause of the shock. Blood work will be obtained to determine the amount of red blood cells in the body, how well the kidneys are functioning, and an ECG, which is a tracing of the heart rhythm, will be done to see if a patient is having a heart attack. Patients will have intravenous (IV) lines placed in their blood vessels so that medicines that act quickly can be given. At times, it may even be necessary to place a large (IV) line, known as a central venous line, so that numerous medications can be given at the same time. Patients will also receive an echocardiogram, which is an ultrasound, to be able to see the pumping function of the heart and to be able to evaluate the heart structures.

Patients who have evidence of an ongoing heart attack need blood flow to the heart restored quickly in order to minimize the amount of heart damage. Some hospitals have the ability to perform cardiac angiography, which is a procedure that allows for identification of the blocked artery. If there is a blockage, using balloons and *stents*, which are devices that prop the blood vessel open, blood flow can be restored to the heart. Some patients have such severe blockages that they require emergency *coronary artery bypass surgery* to restore blood flow or fix defects in the heart caused by the heart attack. If the nearest hospital that performs catheterization is too far away or not available in a timely manner, some patients may be treated with medications designed to dissolve the blood clot in the coronary artery.

Patients who have blood flow restored through one of these methods (or in patients with cardiogenic shock resulting from a cause other than a myocardial infarction) may require a mechanical assist device that improves the heart's ability to pump blood to the remainder of the body. The oldest and most commonly used device is an *IABP*. The IABP sits in a large blood vessel near the heart and inflates and deflates in a way that maximizes blood flow to both the heart and the rest of the body. Other types of mechanical assist devices are the Impella, TandemHeart, and ECMO, which are catheter-based heart pumps. The Impella is placed inside the heart chamber and uses a motor to pump the blood from the heart to the arteries that will carry the blood to the rest of the body. TandemHeart is a continuous-flow assist device that sits outside the heart. The pump withdraws oxygenated blood from the left upper chamber of the heart (the left atrium) and propels it by a magnetically driven, six-bladed impeller through the outflow port, and returns it to the arteries. ECMO uses technology derived from heart and lung bypass that allows gas exchange outside the body as well as providing circulatory support. Patients with cardiogenic shock are also often treated with *mechanical ventilators* to assist with breathing, have *pulmonary artery catheters* placed to measure blood pressures, and are given medications that improve the function of the heart.

OUTCOMES/QUALITY OF LIFE

Cardiogenic shock is a serious problem that results in the death of one out of every two patients; however, survival in patients with heart attacks can be improved with the rapid restoration of blood flow to the heart. The amount of time, size, and area of the heart that is without blood flow are the most important factors in determining whether patients will survive heart attacks complicated by cardiogenic shock. Other factors that are critical in determining how well a patient will do is the heart function, age of the patient, kidney function, and other illnesses or comorbidities that the patient has to simultaneously battle.

Although patients with cardiogenic shock are at high risk of death, about half of all patients will survive. Patients who had a normally functioning heart before the event that led to the cardiac shock and who survive their hospitalization have good outcomes and can live for long periods of time. In fact, the vast majority of patients who survive cardiogenic shock and are discharged home will have minimal signs of heart failure one year after their hospitalization.

SUMMARY

Cardiogenic shock is a serious problem that can result in death. The most common cause of cardiogenic shock is a major heart attack. The treatment of patients with heart attacks begins with rapid restoration of blood flow to the heart by either opening up a blocked coronary artery or by bypassing the diseased arteries with surgery. After blood flow is restored, patients are treated supportively with MCS devices and medicines to improve the function of the heart. Despite the high risk of death, patients who were healthy before their illness and can survive the hospitalization have a good chance of resuming a normal life.

Richard Ro
Patricia Chavez
Bette Kim

15

Hypertrophic Cardiomyopathy

INTRODUCTION

Hypertrophic cardiomyopathy (HCM) is characterized by hypertrophy of the left ventricular (LV) myocardium without ventricular dilatation. It occurs without a secondary cause such as hypertension or systemic disease, and is marked by variable morphologic, clinical, and hemodynamic abnormalities. HCM is one of the great masqueraders of cardiology. It may be mistaken for coronary artery disease as it presents with typical angina chest pain owing to myocardial ischemia in the absence of epicardial coronary stenosis resulting from supply and demand mismatch. It is additionally misleading when HCM presents with ST depressions, T-wave inversions, or pathologic Q waves. It may masquerade as mitral or aortic valve disease with a systolic murmur and heart failure symptoms. It can also be mistaken as pulmonary disease with symptoms of dyspnea on exertion. Tragically, patients with HCM can be asymptomatic until their initial presentation is sudden death, which can occur at rest or on the athletic playing field. With this wide diversity of possible presentations, HCM patients are not infrequently encountered in the cardiac care unit (CCU), and therefore an understanding of the disease is vital in its diagnosis and therapy. The pathophysiology includes the understanding and interplay of the following factors: LV outflow obstruction, concurrent mitral regurgitation, myocardial ischemia, atrial fibrillation (if present), sudden death, diastolic dysfunction, and aspects of molecular biology and genetics. Diagnostic testing with transthoracic echocardiography (TTE), nuclear scintigraphy, exercise stress testing, cardiac catheterization, 24-hour electrocardiogram (ECG), and cardiac magnetic resonance imaging (cMRI) may be applied. Treatment may involve pharmacologic agents, the implanted defibrillator, surgical septal myectomy, transcoronary intervention in the form of alcohol septal ablation (ASA), or, in very rare cases, pacing.[1]

GENETICS

HCM is inherited as an autosomal dominant trait and occurs in 1:500, or about 0.2% of the general population. Emerging data from genetic population-based studies suggest an increased prevalence of HCM estimated to be 1:200 people or greater.[2] The risk of transmission is 50% from an affected parent, but the mutation may also occur sporadically. Missense (insertions or deletions occur less frequently) mutations of at least 11 genes that code for components of the myocardial sarcomere such as the thick myosin filament, intermediate filament, thin actin filament, Z-disc, or supporting proteins have been identified as a cause of HCM. The most common mutations (accounting for the majority of established mutations) found are in the β-myosin heavy chain and myosin-binding protein C. Despite the presence of a known gene mutation, there is a wide variation in phenotype, and some genes demonstrate higher penetrance compared to others.[3] In a cohort of referred, unrelated patients with HCM who underwent gene testing for the eight most common mutations, 38% of the patients were found to have sarcomeric mutations. The remainder were noted to be genotype negative. Younger age at diagnosis, marked wall thickness, and a family history of HCM increased the frequency that a patient will be found to be gene positive.[4] Once a patient is identified to have HCM, all first-degree family members should be referred for clinical or genetic screening. Genetic screening should be performed in an experienced laboratory, and preceded by genetic counseling so that an informed decision can be made by the patient and their family regarding the possible results and subsequent management. In addition, multiple concurrent mutations may portend increased severity of disease.[1] In patients who have a positive genotype with negative phenotype (absence of hypertrophy), first-degree family members where a known mutation was not identified in the index case, or if genetic screening was discussed and declined, regular clinical screening via physical examination, ECG, and transthoracic echocardiogram should be utilized. This should be performed every 12 to 18 months for children and adolescents, and transitioned to every 5 years in adulthood.

Echocardiographic appearance also appears to predict a high likelihood of sarcomeric mutation in HCM; a reversed septal curvature causing a crescent-shaped LV cavity predicts gene-positive patients as compared with those with localized subaortic bulge and preserved septal curvature.[5] Although most genetically determined HCM occur on eight genes, many hundreds of HCM-causing mutations are dispersed over many gene loci. These genes may cause different phenotypes and may have different prognoses. Even among families with the same mutation on a particular locus, individuals vary with respect to phenotype and prognosis. This has markedly delayed genotype–phenotype correlation. The pathophysiologic linkage between mutations and hypertrophy appears to be mediated by mutation-induced functional abnormalities, most often because of increased contractile function. Recent theories about cause of hypertrophy have focused on inefficient utilization of ATP.

PATHOPHYSIOLOGY

On light microscopy, myocyte hypertrophy is noted, particularly in the subendocardium, as well as extensive myocardial fiber disarray—the combination of the two represent the pathognomonic abnormality. In normal individuals, myocytes are arranged in a linear and parallel configuration. However, patients with HCM demonstrate myocytes that are oblique or perpendicular to each other **(Figure 15.1)**. Furthermore, the nucleus of the cardiac myocyte is affected. Rather than having a central nucleus, enlarged nuclei are noted with pleomorphism and hyperchromasia. The myocyte myofibrillary architecture, which can be observed with phosphotungstic acid hematoxylin stain, is also disordered. Myocyte fiber disarray can be noted in other diseases, but myocyte hypertrophy and the percentage of the involved myocardium is less than 10%.[6] The interstitial connective tissue is also overly prolific with extensive fibrosis and is thought to account for the reduced LV chamber compliance and diastolic dysfunction seen **(Figure 15.2)**. Fiber disarray and myocardial fibrosis are thought to predispose to electrical reentry and sudden cardiac death (SCD). The coronary vasculature is

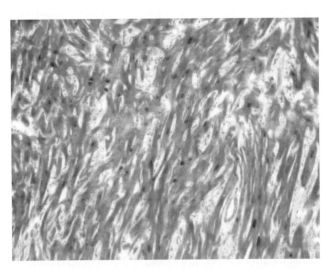

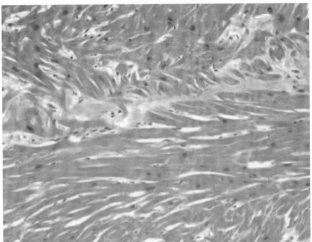

FIGURE 15.1 On light microscopy, myocyte hypertrophy is noted with extensive myocardial fiber disarray—the myocytes are oblique or perpendicular to each other, rather than being arranged in a linear and parallel configuration.

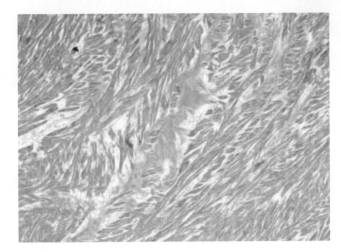

FIGURE 15.2 A modified Masson's trichrome stain of the myocardium is shown above and demonstrates extensive interstitial fibrosis with myocyte disarray.

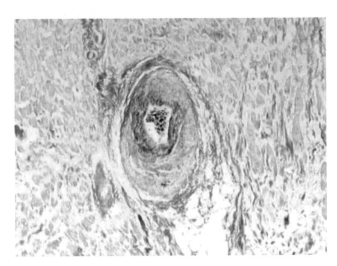

FIGURE 15.3 An intramural artery is shown above with intimal and medial smooth muscle hyperplasia and medial fibrosis, resulting in luminal narrowing. The capillaries are similarly affected. These narrowings are thought to contribute to ischemia.

not exempt from adverse changes—smaller intramural arteries show intimal and medial smooth muscle hyperplasia and medial fibrosis, resulting in luminal narrowing **(Figure 15.3)**. The capillaries are similarly affected. These narrowings are thought to contribute to ischemia, which is well documented in HCM. Epicardial arteries can also be involved, less likely with stenosis than with myocardial bridging, which is noted in 15% to 30% of patients with HCM.

DIAGNOSIS

The most common imaging modality used to establish a clinical diagnosis of HCM is TTE with an emerging role of cMRI. Additional testing in the initial evaluation of HCM should include an ECG, which is abnormal in up to 95% of patients.[7] A 24-hour ambulatory Holter monitor should be obtained to rule out episodes of nonsustained ventricular tachycardia, which generally adds prognostic information about risk of SCD. HCM is diagnosed when LV hypertrophy without dilatation occurs in the absence of a clinical condition that would cause the degree of hypertrophy noted.[1] Therefore, to make the diagnosis of HCM, it is important to evaluate for other cardiac or systemic conditions capable of producing the magnitude of hypertrophy evident (eg, aortic valve stenosis, systemic hypertension, athlete's heart). Athlete's heart occurs in elite, highly trained competitive athletes, where wall thickness is increased but is usually less than 15 mm.[8] Compared to patients with HCM, these patients have normal or enlarged cardiac chambers, normal diastolic function, and have regression of their LV hypertrophy with temporary cessation of training. The location of abnormal hypertrophy in patients with HCM is most often the anterior septum, although the posterior septum and anterior wall can be involved as well. Typical of the heterogeneity of HCM is that hypertrophy can occur in any segment, even among relatives known to have the same genotype. Truly atypical HCM variants include thickening isolated to the lateral or posterior wall. Wall thickness should be evaluated for all patients with TTE, but may be limited by the obtained ultrasound window. MRI, which has become an important diagnostic tool in HCM, is useful in this situation. In a subset of patients, the site and extent of cardiac hypertrophy and abnormalities of the mitral valve result in obstruction to LV outflow. LV outflow tract (LVOT) obstruction is an important determinant of symptoms and is associated with adverse outcomes. This is caused by systolic anterior motion (SAM) of the mitral valve and contact of the valve with the hypertrophied septum (mitral–septal contact), which is demonstrated through echocardiography (**Figure 15.4**).[9] The phenomenon of dynamic SAM is caused by a crucial anatomic overlap between the inflow and outflow portions of the left ventricle. **Figure 15.5** shows dynamic SAM as it progresses through the early moments of systole. The narrowing of the LVOT and the anteriorly positioned coaptation point of the mitral valve places the protruding leaflet into the edge of the flow stream, subjecting the undersurface of the leaflet to the pushing force of flow, as illustrated in **Figure 15.6**.

cMRI can provide additional clinically relevant information by quantifying LV mass, evaluating the right ventricle and mitral valve, identifying aberrant muscle bundles within the left ventricle (LV), and identifying myocardial fibrosis/scarring by late gadolinium enhancement (LGE). If myocardial mass has at least 15% with LGE, there is a 2-fold risk in SCD compared with those who are otherwise considered low risk. Finally, CMR can also play a role in distinguishing HCM from other cardiac pathology that may similarly demonstrate LV hypertrophy on echocardiography.[10]

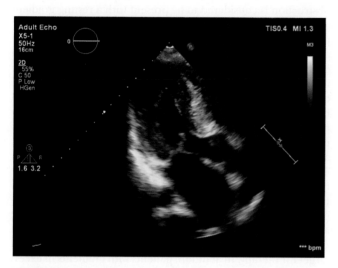

FIGURE 15.4 This apical three-chamber view on transthoracic echocardiography demonstrates systolic motion of the mitral valve with resulting mitral–septal contact. Note the hypertrophy of the left ventricular walls, particularly the anteroseptum.

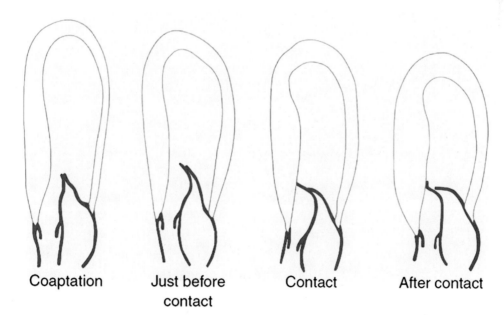

Coaptation   Just before contact   Contact   After contact

FIGURE 15.5 Systolic anterior motion of the mitral valve, schematically drawn from apical five-chamber view, as it proceeds in early systole. (Adapted from Sherrid MV, Chu CK, Delia E, et al. An echocardiographic study of the fluid mechanics of obstruction in hypertrophic cardiomyopathy. *J Am Coll Cardiol.* 1993;22:816-825.)

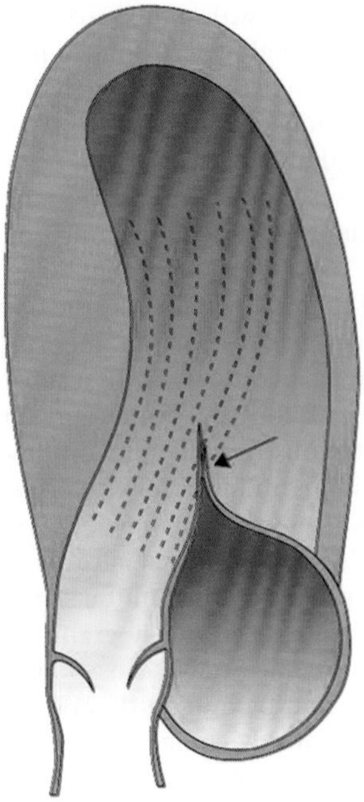

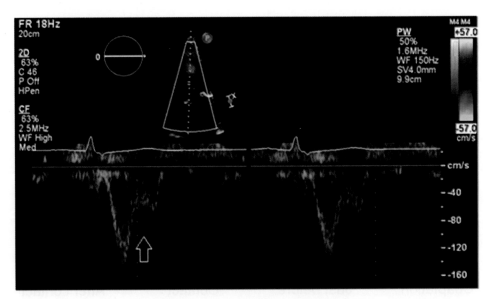

FIGURE 15.6 The pushing force of flow in the left ventricle is shown schematically above relative to the mitral valve in the apical five-chamber view. In obstructive hypertrophic cardiomyopathy, the mitral leaflet coaptation point is closer to the septum than normal. The protruding leaflets extend into the edge of the flow stream and are swept by the pushing force of flow toward the septum. Flow pushes the underside of the leaflets (*arrow*). Note that the midseptal bulge redirects flow so that it comes from a relatively lateral and posterior direction; on the five-chamber view, flow comes from the "1 o'clock" direction. This contributes to the high angle of attack relative to the protruding leaflets. (Adapted from Sherrid MV, Gunsburg DZ, Moldenhauer S, et al. Systolic anterior motion begins at low left ventricular outflow tract velocity in obstructive hypertrophic cardiomyopathy. *J Am Coll Cardiol*. 2000;36:1344-1354.)

LEFT VENTRICULAR OUTFLOW TRACT OBSTRUCTION

The degree of obstruction is quantified by measuring the pressure drop and the gradient across the LVOT. This is most commonly done noninvasively with continuous wave Doppler echocardiography. Pulsed wave Doppler correlation with the two-dimensional echocardiogram allows for determination of the site of obstruction, which must be ascertained in every patient, especially if intervention is contemplated. LV outflow obstruction causes a midsystolic drop in LV ejection velocities and flow when the gradient is >60 mm Hg. This echocardiographic pattern has been termed the "lobster claw" abnormality because of its characteristic appearance (**Figure 15.7**). Significant obstruction is considered to be present with a resting gradient greater than 30 mm Hg. Changing preload and afterload may provoke a gradient by increasing the overlap between the inflow and outflow portions of the LV, reflecting the dynamic nature of the obstruction. After completing initial echocardiographic imaging with no evidence of a resting gradient, patients with concern for HCM such as septal hypertrophy or SAM should be additionally imaged while asked to perform the Valsalva maneuver or standing to elicit a possible gradient. Two-thirds of patients with HCM have resting or provokable LVOT obstruction, and one-third are nonobstructive. Exercise, and on occasion exercise in the postprandial state, can also be used to uncover latent obstruction. However, exercise testing is not indicated in patients with gradients over 4 m/s at rest, New York Heart Association class III or IV symptoms, or prior history of ventricular arrhythmia.[11] These maneuvers are helpful in order to correlate patient symptoms with degree of obstruction and to provide a target for therapy. In addition, patients with gradients in excess of 50 mm Hg at rest or with provocation should be considered for invasive intervention if they remain symptomatic despite medical management.

FIGURE 15.7 Midsystolic drop in LV ejection velocity in obstructive hypertrophic cardiomyopathy. On a pulsed wave Doppler recording just apical of the entrance to the LVOT in a patient with severe dynamic obstruction caused by systolic anterior motion and mitral–septal contact. The arrow points to the LV midsystolic drop in LV ejection flow velocity. This drop in velocity has been called the "lobster claw abnormality" because of its characteristic appearance. The drop in velocity results from the sudden imposition of afterload because of the mitral–septal contact and the gradient. LV, left ventricular; LVOT, left ventricular outflow tract.

TREATMENT

There are five aspects of care that should be covered in the treatment of every HCM patient, some of which may not necessarily be applicable in the setting of the CCU: (1) Risk of sudden death should be discussed, and individual stratification of risk should be done. The average risk of dying suddenly is 1% per year for HCM patient populations, but the risk may be higher or lower depending on whether risk factors for sudden death are present. For patients deemed by their physicians to be at high risk, discussion of implantation of a defibrillator should be considered. (2) Treatment in hopes of alleviating symptoms should be initiated. (3) A discussion to avoid athletic competition and extremes of exertion should be conducted, as well as lifestyle modifications to avoid exacerbation of LVOT obstruction. (4) There should be an effort to detect and manage risk factors contributing to coronary artery disease such as hypercholesterolemia, diabetes mellitus, and cigarette smoking (HCM and coronary disease have an adverse synergistic effect on prognosis). (5) Clinical screening (physical exam, transthoracic echocardiogram and

ECG) or genetic testing of first-degree family members should be performed to assess who is at risk or has inherited the gene mutation. Although many aspects of this evaluation can wait until a patient is stabilized after the CCU stay, it must be remembered that HCM is a lifelong condition and that these issues need discussion, management, and follow-up.

PHARMACOLOGIC TREATMENT OF SYMPTOMS

Figure 15.8 outlines an algorithm for the management of symptomatic HCM in patients grouped into obstructive and nonobstructive HCM categories.

NONOBSTRUCTIVE HCM

In nonobstructive HCM, symptoms are caused by diastolic dysfunction with impaired relaxation early in diastole and decreased chamber compliance in late diastole. This is coupled with small LV volumes and hypertrophy.

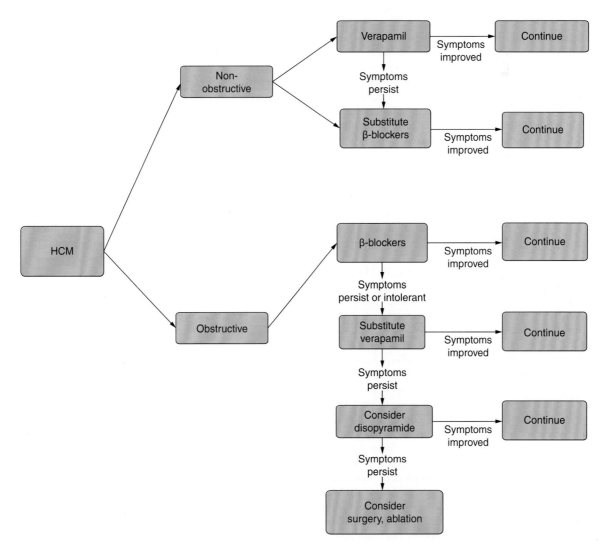

FIGURE 15.8 The management of patients with either obstructive or nonobstructive hypertrophic cardiomyopathy is detailed above. Pharmacologic therapy is driven by symptom response, and patients with obstruction who are refractory to medications are indicated for advanced intervention. HCM, hypertrophic cardiomyopathy.

Few agents are available, and they are not particularly effective in improving severe symptoms owing to diastolic dysfunction. No pharmacologic agent has been consistently shown to improve LV relaxation and chamber compliance in HCM.[12] Therefore, treatment options for symptomatic nonobstructive HCM are limited.[13] Two treatment goals are to improve LV diastolic function and to improve ischemia. Two classes of agents are currently used—β-blockade and calcium channel blockade. Neither class of agents has been shown to improve diastolic chamber compliance.[14] Verapamil's positive contribution in the pathophysiology of nonobstructive HCM appears to be relief of ischemia. Verapamil improves myocardial perfusion as assessed by stress radionuclide perfusion imaging and may thus improve symptoms.[15] Beta-blockade and, to a lesser degree, verapamil may cause chronotropic incompetence in HCM.[16] As diastolic dysfunction may limit the exercise-induced increase in stroke volume, patients with HCM often rely on increased heart rate to increase cardiac output. In such patients, pharmacologic limitation of increase in heart rate may impair exercise capacity. Whereas disopyramide has been shown to improve diastolic function in obstructed patients, by decreasing gradient and systolic load, it has not been shown to improve diastolic function in nonobstructed patients and should be avoided in this group, pending further investigation.[17,18] For the patient with fluid retention, with edema or rales, diuretics may be helpful by relieving dyspnea and uncommon edema. Overdiuresis should be avoided because patients with HCM are often preload dependent for adequate cardiac output. If patients initially present with significant edema, another diagnosis should be sought as this is very unusual. Amyloid may be suspected in this clinical situation, especially if the ECG QRS voltage is low. The use of angiotensin receptor blocker losartan did not demonstrate improvement in exercise capacity or cardiac function. Clinical trials are ongoing because there is currently no good pharmacologic treatment for advanced symptoms in nonobstructive HCM.[19] Fortunately, patients with nonobstructive HCM appear to have a more benign clinical course compared with obstructed patients.[20]

OBSTRUCTIVE HCM

Pharmacologic therapy of symptoms in obstructive HCM (OHCM) is successful in two-thirds of patients. β-blockers are initially used because of their negative inotropic effect. This improves dynamic LV outflow obstruction by decreasing ejection acceleration, which in turn lowers flow velocities early in systole and decreases early drag forces on the mitral valve. SAM and mitral–septal contact are delayed, thereby reducing the LVOT gradient. In addition, decreased myocardial tissue oxygen consumption alleviates possible myocardial ischemia, and negative chronotropy increases diastolic filling time.[13] β-blockers also decrease the sympathetically mediated rise in gradient and tachycardia. The doses should be titrated to cessation of symptoms, a heart rate ranging from 60 to 65 beats/min, or recommended maximum doses. However, β-blockade is not expected to reduce resting gradient, and less than half of patients have sustained improvement in symptoms.[21] β-blockers are effective in reducing exercise-induced LVOT obstruction.[22] For patients who are intolerant of β-blockers or remain symptomatic verapamil therapy can be attempted in doses as high as 480 mg/day. Verapamil, a potent calcium channel blocker (CCB), also has negative inotropic properties but is also a vasodilator. It has been shown to decrease gradient and improve symptoms. Some studies have demonstrated an improvement in

exercise tolerance as well. However, it is not used in patients with severe obstruction and severe symptoms because, on occasion, its vasodilating effects outweigh its negatively inotropic effects: the LVOT gradient may rise, and pulmonary edema and death have been reported. In addition, heart block and bradycardia may complicate its use. If there is no improvement with verapamil, disopyramide can be added to beta-blockade or verapamil.[23,24] Disopyramide is a type I antiarrhythmic drug with potent negatively inotropic properties; in normal individuals, it can decrease echocardiographic fractional shortening by 28%. It is a sodium channel blocker and may have calcium channel blocking properties as well; however, it is not a vasodilator. Disopyramide is generally given to patients who are refractory to β-blockade or verapamil and would otherwise require intervention with surgical septal myectomy or ASA. In a multicenter study, two-thirds of patients with OHCM treated with disopyramide combined with a β-blocker could be managed medically with amelioration of symptoms and 50% reduction in LVOT gradient when followed for 3 years. The remaining one-third of patients could not be managed successfully with disopyramide and required invasive therapy secondary to inadequate symptom and gradient control or vagolytic side effects. There was a trend toward lower cardiac mortality and sudden death in the disopyramide group, without an increased risk of arrhythmia. The starting dose of disopyramide is 250 mg twice a day using the controlled-release preparation, and can be increased to 300 mg twice daily.[25] Disopyramide is generally given with a β-blocker or verapamil to limit exercise-induced adrenergic response and to slow ventricular response, should atrial fibrillation occur. Mild vagolytic side effects, dry mouth, blurred vision, and constipation are common but generally subside. If they prove troubling, the dosage may be reduced, or controlled-release pyridostigmine may be added, 180 mg/day. A more serious vagolytic side effect is urinary retention. Vagolytic side effects cause discontinuation of disopyramide in 7% of patients. Because of its impaired elimination in renal failure, disopyramide should be administered in reduced dosage or with serum monitoring. ECG surveillance of the QTc interval should be performed, and QTc prolonging medications should be carefully considered prior to initiation in patients who are on disopyramide.

DRUGS TO AVOID (OR DISCONTINUE) IN OBSTRUCTIVE HYPERTROPHIC CARDIOMYOPATHY

All vasodilators should be avoided in OHCM, a drug class that is commonly used in the CCU. Vasodilators will worsen LVOT obstruction. These include all nitrate preparations (sublingual, topical, and IV), dihydropyridine CCBs (amlodipine and nifedipine), angiotensin-converting enzyme inhibitors, angiotensin receptor blockers, and alpha-adrenergic blockers that are used for prostatism. Furthermore, drugs that increase contractility will worsen obstruction and should also be avoided in OHCM such as dopamine, dobutamine, milrinone, and digoxin.

SURGICAL SEPTAL MYECTOMY

Myectomy is the treatment of choice for patients who fail medical therapy.[24,25] Candidates for myectomy have persistent disabling symptoms and gradients of >50 mm Hg at rest or after physiologic provocation. Myectomy has been successfully performed for 30 years, and in experienced centers it can be performed with low surgical mortality of 1%. It is uniformly successful in reducing both gradient and symptoms.

Interventions are not always successful, and the reason for heterogeneity in response is not clear. Understanding the central role of flow drag in the pathogenesis of SAM may prevent treatment failures. Inadequate myectomy resection focused on just the subvalvular septum, targeted to widen the outflow tract and to reduce Venturi forces, may result in persistent SAM and obstruction. A limited myectomy misses the impact of the mid-ventricular septal bulge that redirects LV flow so that it comes from a relatively posterolateral direction. This sort of resection results in persistent SAM and either outflow obstruction or mitral regurgitation because flow must still course around the remaining septal hypertrophy, and it still catches the mitral valve and pushes it into the septum, causing mitral regurgitation. To alleviate this sort of residual SAM, investigators from Germany have popularized the extended myectomy. More extensive resection redirects flow away from the mitral valve, precluding drag-induced SAM. A large decrease in the angle of attack of flow relative to the mitral valve has been shown after successful myectomy; flow is made more parallel to the mitral valve. The myectomy resection must be extended far enough down toward the apex to allow flow to track anteriorly along the surgically reduced septum away from the mitral valve. Surgical septal myectomy also addresses abnormalities in the attachments of the papillary muscles, which are common in HCM and which can often contribute to LVOT obstruction.[25] In addition, HCM patients typically have intrinsic mitral valve pathology such as mitral valve prolapse, increased leaflet length, and abnormal chordal attachments that contribute to obstruction. Surgical myectomy has the advantage of addressing mitral valve abnormalities with a repair.[26,27] Targeting the basal septum alone is unlikely to completely relieve SAM, obstruction, and mitral regurgitation. When surgery is selected, myectomy is preferred over mitral replacement for relief of LVOT obstruction in HCM patients refractory to pharmacotherapy.

ALCOHOL SEPTAL ABLATION

Percutaneous Alcohol Septal Ablation (ASA) can be considered an alternative to surgical septal myectomy for patients at high operative risk and advanced age. It can be done only if there is suitable anatomy. This procedure offers the attractive promise of septal reduction without cardiopulmonary bypass and its complications. After placement of a temporary right ventricular pacing lead, a small diameter balloon catheter is placed in a selected left anterior descending (LAD) septal branch, and after inflating the balloon, angiographic contrast is injected to ensure that contrast does not reflux back into the LAD. Diluted echo contrast is then injected during transthoracic or transesophageal echocardiographic imaging. In 8% of such injections, contrast is seen to flow to structures where alcohol injection would be disastrous: posterior LV wall, RV free wall, mitral papillary muscles, or the entire septum. With this information, the operator searches for a septal branch that can be demonstrated to supply just the upper septum, preferably including and extending past the point of mitral–septal contact. A dose of 1 to 3 mL of absolute alcohol is instilled into the septal branch. Optimally, a

controlled myocardial infarction occurs. This is accompanied by typical chest pain, enzyme elevation, and risk for potentially lethal ventricular arrhythmia. The acute gradient reduction of ASA is caused by reduced ejection acceleration from the infarct and decreased hemodynamic force on the mitral valve decreasing SAM identically as in negatively inotropic medications. Late improvement stems from septal thinning owing to septal scar. ASA is associated with a risk of pacemaker dependency in 10% to 15% of cases, and an increase in ventricular arrhythmias has been reported. In addition, ASA does not offer as complete relief of obstruction compared with surgical myectomy.[28,29]

DUAL-CHAMBER PACING

Dual-chamber pacing with complete ventricular preexcitation through a short atrioventricular (AV) delay to reduce outflow tract gradient is not considered primary therapy for obstruction.[30] Select older patients who are ≥65 years old may benefit with modest improvement on LVOT gradient and functional improvement.[30] Therapeutic effect is often incomplete; SAM persists with mean gradients of 30 to 55 mm Hg after 3 months of pacing. The mechanism by which pacing benefits SAM is unclear at this time. It may be because of the dyssynchrony caused by the right ventricular pacing, or because of the short AV delay. It is usually considered for patients who already have a dual-chamber pacemaker present with comorbid medical conditions or old age given in conjunction with disopyramide and a β-blocker.

IMPLANTABLE CARDIOVERTER DEFIBRILLATOR

Although not a decision made solely in the CCU, the Implantable defibrillator has a role in the spectrum of care for HCM patients. Situations may arise in CCU patients that may prompt the recommendation of implantable cardioverter defibrillator (ICD) insertion. These include presentation with syncope or ventricular tachycardia—nonsustained or persistent. Other risk factors that are associated with higher risk for SCD and may prompt ICD include massive segmental wall thickening ≥30 mm, family history of SCD from HCM in a young family member, and apical akinetic aneurysm owing to mid-LV obstruction.

MANAGEMENT OF ACUTE DECOMPENSATION OF PATIENTS WITH HCM

The initial step in the management of acute decompensated HCM patients with obstruction should be discontinuation of any possible offending agents such as vasodilators. The clinician should also keep in mind that positive inotropes in this setting of hemodynamic instability secondary to obstruction may be deleterious and should also be avoided. When hemodynamics stability is preserved, β-blockers constitute the first line of treatment. If hemodynamic stability is compromised (systolic blood pressure <90 mmHg), increasing afterload and preload is in order. **Figure 15.9** shows the progression of management in these patients. In the event atrial fibrillation ensues, rate and rhythm control are imperative.

The most common cause of acute decompensation in HCM patients is the acute onset of atrial fibrillation. The loss of the atrial kick and rapid heart rate on top of diastolic dysfunction can provoke

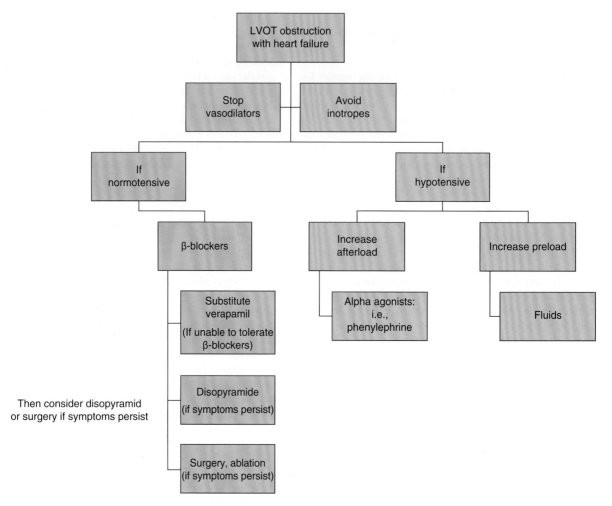

FIGURE 15.9 The management of patients being admitted into the cardiac care unit with heart failure symptoms secondary to left ventricular outflow tract obstruction is demonstrated above. Cessation of offending agents is the first step, and patients with hypotension should be treated with intravenous fluids and phenylephrine, if needed. Positive inotropes should be avoided because they can worsen obstruction. LVOT, left ventricular outflow tract.

heart failure symptoms. The first consideration should be whether the patient needs acute direct current cardioversion for severe heart failure or hemodynamic instability. For most other patients, slowing the ventricular rate with beta-blockade or nondihydropyridine CCBs is generally the best first treatment option. Verapamil may be used in nonobstructed patients but not in patients with resting obstruction because it has vasodilatory properties with a risk of pulmonary edema in severely obstructed patients. Amiodarone may be used to slow ventricular rate, but in non-anticoagulated patients it should be used only in those who have recent (<48 hours) atrial fibrillation because the drug has the potential to restore sinus rhythm. Anticoagulation with parenteral heparin or low-molecular-weight heparin is indicated, because systemic embolism is very common in HCM patients. There should be a low threshold to refer patients for transesophageal echocardiogram (TEE) to exclude the presence of left atrial appendage thrombus before cardioversion. If there is no left atrial appendage thrombus noted, cardioversion may be performed either electrically or pharmacologically with a plan to continue warfarin or newer oral anticoagulants as an outpatient. The use of a newer oral anticoagulant agent should be considered, and although there are no data specifically looking at their use in this patient population, they are used in clinical practice with HCM patients who have atrial fibrillation. Frequent episodes of

atrial fibrillation may warrant referral for catheter-based ablation, which may be an option for these patients. All patients with HCM and atrial fibrillation should continue long-term anticoagulation to reduce the risk of stroke and embolic events. In HCM patients who develop atrial fibrillation, the risk of embolic events is high (ie, incidence is 2.5%/year). Long-term anticoagulation regardless of CHADS–VASC score is indicated in these patients to reduce stroke and peripheral embolic events.[31]

ACUTE LVOT OBSTRUCTION AND TAKOTSUBO CARDIOMYOPATHY

Patients with HCM and latent obstruction may rarely present with acute, severe LV dysfunction consistent with apical ballooning, pulmonary congestion, and cardiogenic shock similar to Takotsubo cardiomyopathy. Besides apical ballooning and hypercontractile basal LV function, these patients are also noted to have SAM of the mitral valve and mitral–septal contact. Around 10% to 25% of Takotsubo cardiomyopathy cases have been documented showing SAM, with the etiology of this being unclear. It has been theorized that the hypercontractility of the basal myocardium narrows the LVOT, causes flow to course around the basilar septum posterior and laterally, and positions the mitral valve leaflets to be swept into the outflow tract by a Venturi or flow-drag mechanism.[32] Another proposed mechanism is that patients initially presenting with this variant of Takotsubo cardiomyopathy have underlying, undiagnosed HCM with latent obstruction. Severe increased afterload mismatch from SAM can cause subendocardial ischemia with resulting LV dysfunction.[33] The complete reversal of these findings after relief of LVOT obstruction indicates that they were caused by the dynamic obstruction caused by SAM of the mitral valve and mitral–septal contact. These patients should be admitted to the CCU after cardiac catheterization to exclude severe coronary artery disease with a left ventriculogram (if able to be clinically tolerated). Intravenous fluids, beta-blockade, and phenylephrine should be administered so as not to exacerbate LVOT obstruction and for hemodynamic support.

ACKNOWLEDGMENT: We acknowledge the guidance and mentorship of Dr. Mark Sherrid without whose support this chapter would not be possible.

REFERENCES

1. Gersh BJ, Maron BJ, Bonow RO, et al. 2011 ACCF/AHA guideline for the diagnosis and treatment of hypertrophic cardiomyopathy: Areport of the American College of Cardiology Foundation/American Heart Association task force on practice guidelines. *Circulation.* 2011;24:e785-e831.

2. Semsarian C, Ingles J, Maron MS, et al. New perspectives on the prevalence of hypertrophic cardiomyopathy. *J Am Coll Cardiol.* 2015;65:1249-1254.

3. Kacem S, Cheniti G. Genetic testing in management of hypertrophic cardiomyopathy—fifth in series (2015, July 21). Retrieved from https://www.escardio.org/Guidelines-&-Education/Journals-and-publications/ESC-journals-family/E-journal-of-Cardiology-Practice/Volume-13/genetic-testing-in-management-of-hypertrophic-cardiomyopathy-fifth-in-series.

4. Van Driest SL, Ommen SR, Tajik AJ, et al. Yield of genetic testing in hypertrophic cardiomyopathy. *Mayo Clin Proc.* 2005;80:739-744.

5. Binder J, Ommen SR, Gersh BJ, et al. Echocardiography-guided genetic testing in hypertrophic cardiomyopathy: septal morphological features predict the presence of myofilament mutations. *Mayo Clin Proc.* 2006;4:459-467.

6. Hughes SE. The pathology of hypertrophic cardiomyopathy. *Histopathology.* 2004;44:412-427.

7. McLeod CJ, Ackerman MJ, Nishimura RA, et al. Outcomes of patients with hypertrophic cardiomyopathy and a normal electrocardiogram. *J Am Coll Cardiol.* 2009;54:229-33.

8. Pelliccia A, Maron BJ, Spataro A, et al. The upper limit of physiologic cardiac hypertrophy in highly trained elite athletes. *N Engl J Med.* 1991;324:295-301.

9. Sherrid MV, Gunsburg DZ, Moldenhauer S, et al. Systolic anterior motion begins at low left ventricular outflow tract velocity in obstructive hypertrophic cardiomyopathy. *J Am Coll Cardiol.* 2000;36:1344-1354.

10. Maron BJ, Maron MS. The remarkable 50 years of imaging in HCM and how it has changed diagnosis and management from m-mode echocardiography to CMR. *J Am Coll Cardiol Img.* 2016;9(7):858-872.

11. Drinko JK, Nash PJ, Lever HM, et al. Safety of stress testing in patients with hypertrophic cardiomyopathy. *Am J Cardiol.* 2004;93:1443-1444.

12. Kass DA, Wolff MR, Ting CT, et al. Diastolic compliance of hypertrophied ventricle is not acutely altered by pharmacologic agents influencing active processes. *Ann Intern Med.* 1993;119:466-473.

13. Sherrid M, Barac I. Pharmacologic treatment of symptomatic hypertrophic cardiomyopathy. In: Maron B, ed. *Diagnosis and Management of Hypertrophic Cardiomyopathy.* London, UK: Blackwell-Futura; 2004:200-219.

14. Nishimura RA, Holmes DR, Tajik AJ. Failure of calcium channel blockers to improve ventricular relaxation in humans. *J Am Coll Cardiol.* 1993;21:182-188.

15. Udelson JE, Bonow RO, O'Gara PT, et al. Verapamil prevents silent myocardial perfusion abnormalities during exercise in asymptomatic patients with hypertrophic cardiomyopathy. *Circulation.* 1989;79:1052-1060.

16. Gilligan DM, Chan WL, Joshi J, et al. A double-blind, placebo-controlled crossover trial of nadolol and verapamil in mild and moderately symptomatic hypertrophic cardiomyopathy. *J Am Coll Cardiol.* 1993;21:1672-1679.

17. Matsubara H, Nakatani S, Nagata S, et al. Salutary effect of disopyramide on left ventricular diastolic function in hypertrophic obstructive cardiomyopathy. *J Am Coll Cardiol.* 1995;26:768-775.

18. Pollick C, Kimball B, Henderson M, et al. Disopyramide in hypertrophic cardiomyopathy. I. Hemodynamic assessment after intravenous administration. *Am J Cardiol.* 1988;62: 1248-1251.

19. Axelsson A, Iversen K, Vejlstrup N, et al. Functional effects of losartan in hypertrophic cardiomyopathy—a randomized clinical trial. *Heart.* 2016;102:285-291.

20. Maron MS, Rowin EJ, Olivotto I, et al. Contemporary natural history and management of nonobstructive hypertrophic cardiomyopathy. *J Am Coll Cardiol.* 2016;67(12):1399-1409.

21. Harrison DC, Braunwald E, Glick G, et al. Effects of beta adrenergic blockade on the circulation, with particular reference to observations in patients with hypertrophic subaortic stenosis. *Circulation.* 1964;29:84-98.

22. Nistri S, Olivotto I, Maron MS, et al. β Blockers for prevention of exercise-induced left ventricular outflow tract obstruction in patients with hypertrophic cardiomyopathy. *Am J Cardiol.* 2012;110;715-719.

23. Sherrid MV, Barac I, McKenna WJ, et al. Multicenter study of the efficacy and safety of disopyramide in obstructive hypertrophic cardiomyopathy. *J Am Coll Cardiol.* 2005;45:1251-1258.

24. Sherrid M, Delia E, Dwyer E. Oral disopyramide therapy for obstructive hypertrophic cardiomyopathy. *Am J Cardiol.* 1988;62:1085-1088.

25. Maron BJ, Nishimura RA, Danileson GK. Pitfalls in clinical recognition and a novel operative approach for hypertrophic cardiomyopathy with severe outflow obstruction due to anomalous papillary muscle. *Circulation.* 1998;98:2505-2508.

26. Kaple RK, Murphy RT, DiPaola LM, et al. Mitral valve abnormalities in hypertrophic cardiomyopathy: echocardiographic features and surgical outcomes. *Ann Thorac Surg.* 2008;85:1527-1536.

27. Sherrid MV, Balaram S, Kim B, et al. The mitral valve in obstructive hypertrophic cardiomyopathy. *J Am Coll Cardiol.* 2016;67:1848-1858.

28. Maron BJ, Nishimura RA. Sursgical septal myectomy versus alcohol septal ablation. *Circulation.* 2014;130:1617-1624.

29. Qin JX, Shiota T, Lever HM, et al. Outcome of patients with hypertrophic obstructive cardiomyopathy after percutaneous transluminal septal myocardial ablation and septal myectomy surgery. *J Am Coll Cardiol.* 2001;38:1994-2000.

30. Maron BJ, Nishimura RA, McKenna WJ, et al. Assessment of permanent dual-chamber pacing as a treatment for drug-refractory symptomatic patients with obstructive hypertrophic cardiomyopathy. *Circulation.*1999;22:2927-2933.

31. Maron BJ, Olivotto I, Bellone P, et al. Clinical profile of stroke in 900 patients with hypertrophic cardiomyopathy. *J Am Coll Cardiol.* 2002;39:301-307.

32. Mahmoud RE, Mansencal N, Pilliere R, et al. Prevalence and characteristics of left ventricular outflow tract obstruction in Tako-Tsubo syndrome. *Am Heart J.* 2008;156:543-548.

33. Sherrid MV, Balaram SK. Reversal of acute systolic dysfunction and cardiogenic shock in hypertrophic cardiomyopathy by surgical relief of obstruction. *Echocardiography.* 2011;28:E174-E179.

Patient and Family Information for:
HYPERTROPHIC CARDIOMYOPATHY

HCM is characterized by thickening of the left ventricle that occurs without clinical cause such as high blood pressure or aortic valve disease. It is marked by varying symptoms and abnormalities. HCM is the great masquerader of cardiology. It often masquerades as coronary artery disease because it presents with chest pain, but without significant coronary narrowings. It is particularly confusing when HCM may present with ECG abnormalities mimicking those found in coronary disease. HCM is characterized by thickening of the heart muscle, most commonly at the septum between the ventricles. This leads to stiffening of the walls of the heart and abnormal mitral valve function that may obstruct normal blood flow out of the heart. Many people with HCM have no symptoms or only minor symptoms and live a normal life. Other people develop symptoms that progress and worsen as heart function worsens. Symptoms of HCM can occur at any age and may include chest pain or pressure that can occur with exercise or physical activity or at rest as well. Shortness of breath especially with exertion and fatigue (feeling overly tired) are often experienced. Initial presenting symptom could be a fainting episode (syncope) caused by irregular heart rhythms or abnormal responses of the blood vessels. Some patients may experience palpitations (fluttering in the chest) because of abnormal heart rhythms (arrhythmias), such as atrial fibrillation or ventricular tachycardia. Sudden death may occur as the presenting symptom in a small number of patients with HCM. HCM can run in families as a dominant genetic trait, owing to a gene that is inherited in half of the first degree relatives. In other instances, the cause is unknown. HCM is diagnosed on the basis of medical history (symptoms and family history), a physical exam, and echocardiogram results. Additional tests may include blood tests, ECG, chest X-ray, exercise stress test, cardiac catheterization, CT scan, and MRI. In a subset of patients, the site and extent of cardiac thickening and abnormalities of the mitral valve result in obstruction to LV outflow. LVOT obstruction is an important determinant of symptoms and is associated with adverse outcome. Obstruction is an important therapeutic target in HCM because relief of obstruction often leads to improved symptoms. The most common location of obstruction is in the LVOT, caused by SAM of the mitral valve and mitral–septal contact. The phenomenon of dynamic SAM is caused by a crucial anatomic overlap between the inflow and outflow portions of the left ventricle. There are five aspects of care that should be covered in the treatment of every HCM patient: (1) Risk of sudden death should be discussed, and individual stratification of risk should be done. The average risk of dying suddenly is 1%/year for HCM patient populations, but the risk may be higher or lower depending on other risk factors for sudden death that may be present. For patients deemed by their physicians to be at high risk, discussion of implantation of a defibrillator should be considered. (2) Treatment in hopes of alleviating symptoms should be initiated. (3) A discussion to avoid athletic competition and extremes of exertion should

be conducted, as well as lifestyle modifications to avoid exacerbation of LVOT obstruction. (4) There should be an effort to detect and manage risk factors of coronary artery disease such as hypercholesterolemia, diabetes mellitus, and cigarette smoking (HCM and coronary disease have an adverse synergistic effect on prognosis). (5) Clinical screening (physical exam, transthoracic echocardiogram, and ECG) or genetic testing of first degree family members should be performed to assess who is at risk or has inherited the gene mutation. Although many aspects of this evaluation can wait until a patient is stabilized after the CCU stay, it must be remembered that HCM is a lifelong condition and that these issues need discussion and management when the dust clears. Lifestyle changes may alter the course of HCM. Simple things like drinking adequate amounts of fluids, and avoiding competitive sports are important. Regular visits with a cardiologist are highly important. Patients with HCM should seek at least one consultation with a cardiologist at a specialized HCM treatment center—such doctors treat many HCM patients, whereas the usual cardiologist will see few in his/her career. Patients with HCM may find themselves in a CCU setting because of acute onset of symptoms of chest pain, shortness of breath or syncope, or the new onset of atrial fibrillation, a rapid irregular heart rhythm. Pharmacologic therapy is the first line of treatment for symptoms of HCM. Drugs are used to treat symptoms and prevent further complications of HCM. Medications are used to reduce the degree of obstruction in the heart so that it can pump more efficiently. β-blockers, disopyramide, and CCB are medications that may be prescribed for obstruction. If there is an arrhythmia, medications to control heart rate or decrease the occurrence of arrhythmias may be prescribed. Certain medications may need to be avoided; these include nitrates (because they lower blood pressure and worsen obstruction in the heart) or digoxin, dopamine, and dobutamine (because they increase the force of the heart's contraction and worsen obstruction).

If fluid collection in the lungs occurs, treatment is aimed at controlling it through diuretics. Surgical procedures are used to treat HCM when pharmacologic therapy fails to improve symptoms and obstruction. The "gold standard" is surgical septal myectomy. During this open heart surgical procedure, the surgeon removes a small amount of the thickened septal wall of the heart to widen the outflow tract (the path the blood takes) from the left ventricle to the aorta. This highly effective operation is done at specialized centers with a surgical mortality of <1%. Another important complication is the need for permanent pacing because of interruption of the normal electrical pathway of the heart. Alcohol Septal Ablation is another approach that involves cardiac catheterization to locate the small coronary artery that supplies blood flow to the septum. Small amounts of pure alcohol are injected through the catheter, which kills the cells on contact, causing a small "controlled" heart attack. This therapy decreases the contractile force of the heart and decreases obstruction in that way acutely. Later, the septum shrinks back to a more normal size over the following months, widening the passage for blood flow. Most HCM centers reserve ASA for patients who have substantial complicating medical illnesses or old age and frailty because the procedural risks are comparable to surgical myectomy, but the results are overall not as satisfactory.

IMPLANTABLE CARDIOVERTER DEFIBRILLATORS

ICD are suggested for people at risk for life-threatening arrhythmias or SCD. The ICD constantly monitors the heart rhythm. When it detects a very fast, abnormal heart rhythm, it delivers small electric currents or shocks to the heart muscle to cause the heart to beat in a normal rhythm again. A small number of people with HCM have an increased risk of SCD. People at risk include the following: (1) Patients with massive thickening of the left ventricle wall (exceeding 3 cm). (2) Those who have family members who have had SCD at a young age, thought to be because of HCM. (3) Young patients with HCM with fainting without cause. Generally, this is considered most important when blackout has happened within the last 6 months. (4) Adults who have a history of arrhythmia with a fast heart rate originating from the ventricles, called ventricular tachycardia. (5) Those with severe symptoms and poor contractile heart function. If risk factors are present, the strategy of the ICD is discussed with the patient, and the decision to implant depends on physician judgment and patient choice.

MANAGEMENT OF ACUTE DECOMPENSATION IN PATIENTS WITH HCM

The initial step in treating patients with acute decompensated HCM with obstruction involves discontinuing any medications that could dilate the peripheral vessels and cause the blood pressure to drop. The most common cause of acute decompensation in HCM patients is an arrhythmia called atrial fibrillation. This arrhythmia may speed up the heart rate. Usually, slowing it with medications is sufficient. However atrial fibrillation may cause the heart to fail, which translates into a dramatic drop in blood pressure. In this case, the arrhythmia might need to be stopped by performing a cardioversion. Anticoagulation with blood thinners such as heparin or low-molecular-weight heparin is indicated because emboli are very common in HCM patients. There should be a low threshold to refer patients for TEE to exclude the presence of thrombus prior to cardioversion. If there is no left atrial appendage thrombus noted, cardioversion may be performed either electrically or with medications with a plan to continue oral blood thinners, such as warfarin or other newer oral anticoagulants. Frequent episodes of atrial fibrillation may warrant referral for definitive treatment of the arrhythmia with procedures such as catheter-based ablations. In HCM patients who develop atrial fibrillation, the risk of embolic events is high (ie, incidence is 2.5%/year). All patients with HCM and atrial fibrillation should continue lifelong anticoagulation to reduce the risk of stroke and embolic events.

Nina Kukar
Gina LaRocca
Ziad Sergie
Javier Sanz

16

Cardiac Magnetic Resonance Imaging in the Cardiac Care Unit

INTRODUCTION

The diagnosis and management of patients in the cardiac care unit (CCU) often requires the inclusion of data obtained by cardiac imaging. Although echocardiography and catheter-based coronary angiography are more commonly used, noninvasive cross-sectional imaging modalities such as cardiac computed tomography (CT) and cardiac magnetic resonance (CMR) are frequently necessary for clinical care as well. Without the use of ionizing radiation, CMR generates a signal (image) by altering the magnetic properties of hydrogen protons in the body through the application of radiofrequency pulses and magnetic gradients within a static magnetic field. The images generated can be very helpful in defining anatomy, function, and tissue characteristics of cardiac structures and the great vessels. In this chapter, we focus on CMR techniques and evaluations that would be relevant to the house staff who are on CCU rotation.

CARDIAC MAGNETIC RESONANCE SEQUENCES IN BRIEF

Different combinations of radiofrequency pulses and magnetic gradients, generically termed sequences, enable acquisition of different types of images. Basic CMR sequences **(Figure 16.1)** include cine imaging, first-pass perfusion, phase-contrast, T1-, T2- and T2*-weighted imaging, early and late gadolinium enhancement (LGE) and magnetic resonance angiography (MRA).[1]

- **Cine** imaging provides anatomic and functional details on chamber volumes and wall motion.
- **First-pass perfusion imaging** demonstrates perfusion defects, including microvascular obstruction (MVO).
- **Phase-contrast** imaging provides accurate data on the flow through the valves, including peak velocities, regurgitant volumes, and the ratio of pulmonary to systemic blood flows (Qp/Qs) as in the case of shunts.
- **T1- and T2-weighted** sequences assist with characterization of myocardial tissue, including myocardial edema, blood, thrombus, and fat. **T1- and T2-mapping** sequences provide more accurate and objective measures of tissue characterization compared to more subjective visual assessments. Although currently restricted largely to investigational use in the United States,

these sequences are increasingly demonstrating abnormal myocardial parameters in various pathologies including, but not limited to, amyloidosis, cardiomyopathies, myocarditis, and autoimmune diseases.
- **T2*-weighted** sequences demonstrate the presence of myocardial iron and can assist with identification of myocardial hemorrhage.
- **Early gadolinium enhancement** shows areas of no reflow and the presence of MVO, as well as increased myocardial signal intensity in myocarditis due to increased capillary leakage.
- **LGE** demonstrates areas of infiltration, necrosis, or fibrosis in characteristic patterns that can help diagnose the etiology of cardiac pathology.

MAGNETIC RESONANCE IMAGING SAFETY— PRACTICAL ASPECTS

CMR is a safe and valuable modality for the practicing cardiologist, but there are several important safety parameters to consider. To maximize image quality and minimize adverse events (which are rare), careful patient selection is crucial. The CCU patient will usually require an accompanying nurse and/or a physician for close monitoring and/or to administer medications as needed. The patient should be able to lie down flat for the duration of the examination up to 30 to 60 minutes, and he/she should ideally be able to follow breathing instructions. Typically, the patient is instructed to hold his/her breath for 10 to 15 seconds. Lack of cooperation can significantly impact image quality and even render the examination nondiagnostic. This may occur in patients who are in decompensated heart failure (HF) or who have underlying lung disease, altered mental status, or significant language barriers. The latter can be overcome by having a translator communicate with the patient from the control room. When patients are unable to the hold their breath, free-breathing alternatives such as real-time cine imaging often provide diagnostic image quality at the possible expense of a longer examination time.

A small proportion of patients (estimated around 2% to 4%) have significant claustrophobia. Of those, about half can be scanned by maximizing patient comfort with the use of blindfolds, appropriate lighting, and temperature control, or by having a family member available and maintaining verbal contact. Severe claustrophobia can be mitigated with a short-acting anxiolytic to

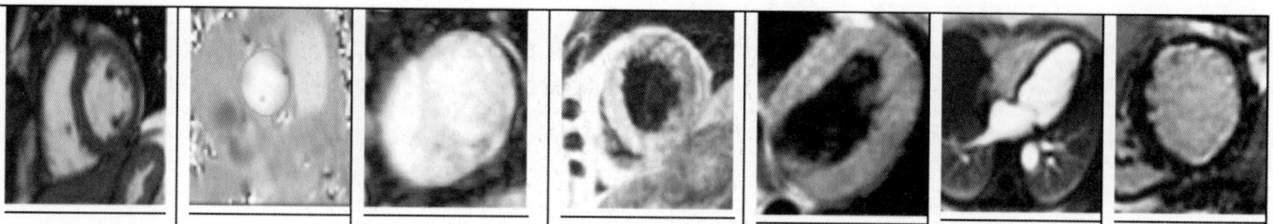

Cine	Phase Contrast	T2 *	T2 weighted	T1 weighted	First pass perfusion	LGE
Ventricular volumes, mass, ejection fraction, and wall motion assessment	Valvular stenosis and regurgitation, Qp/Qs	Iron deposition, intramyocardial hemorrhage	Presence of edema	Identification of fat, differentiation of chylous fluid and hemorrhage from simple fluid	Assessment of blood flow, microvascular obstruction	Assess for fibrosis/inf arction

FIGURE 16.1 Common cardiac magnetic resonance sequences. LGE, late gadolinium enhancement.

be taken before the study (such as a low-dose benzodiazepine), avoiding oversedation that will impact cooperation with breathing instructions. Cardiac rhythm abnormalities are also important to consider. Tachyarrhythmias, including rapid atrial fibrillation/flutter and sinus tachycardia, can lead to blurry images, particularly on specific sequences. It may be helpful to control the heart rate with oral and/or intravenous (IV) beta-blocker before the examination, if medically appropriate. Frequent premature beats or bigeminy can have an impact on image quality. In these cases, real-time cine imaging can also be helpful in improving image quality. While arrhythmias can reduce the accuracy of volumetric measurements, a diagnostic CMR study can be obtained in most cases.

The risks of CMR are primarily related to the generated static magnetic field, at a magnitude of 1.5 or 3.0 Tesla, representing 30,000 to 60,000 times the Earth's magnetic field strength. This can lead to ferromagnetic interactions causing motion or dislodgement of a ferromagnetic device or implant within the magnetic bore. Radiofrequency pulses can also result in local heating by concentrating energy around implanted wires or leads. Because of these risks, there are several devices that are categorized as unsafe because of their known hazard in all CMR environments. These are considered contraindicated and they include pacemakers (permanent or temporary), implantable cardioverter defibrillators (ICDs), and Swanz-Ganz catheters. A number of the newer pacemaker/ICDs are deemed magnetic resonance safe and are characterized as "MRI conditional" (magnetic resonance imaging conditional—meaning they can be scanned

safely under specific conditions). Even though these devices are relatively safer, they can still produce significant artifacts that may render a cardiac scan nondiagnostic. Patients with these devices should be evaluated on a case-by-case basis and imaged at experienced CMR centers. Some of the transdermal medications (such as nitroglycerine patches) contain ferromagnetic components and should be removed before the CMR study. **Table 16.1** provides a comprehensive list of MRI-unsafe and MRI-safe or MRI-conditional devices.

One of the most significant (and avoidable) complications of contrast-enhanced CMR is nephrogenic systemic fibrosis (NSF). This occurs in patients with advanced renal insufficiency receiving gadolinium-contrast agents. Gadolinium is a lanthanide metal containing paramagnetic Gd^{3+} ions that enhances image contrast when administered intravenously. It is renally excreted with an elimination half-life of 60 to 90 minutes (18 to 34 hours in patients with renal insufficiency). NSF may occur in patients with advanced (stage 4 to 5) chronic kidney disease or acute kidney injury (AKI), particularly AKI of any severity in the setting of hepatorenal syndrome or in the liver peri-transplant period. It is characterized by fibrosis of skin, joints, eyes, and internal organs; approximately 5% of patients will have a debilitating course and, rarely, die.[2] Recommendations for NSF prevention are summarized in **Table 16.2**.

To enhance patient safety and selection for CMR, dedicated questionnaires that address all the important safety precautions have been developed. It is important to have a trained professional

TABLE 16.1	MRI Safety of Devices and Implants
MRI UNSAFE	**MRI SAFE AND/OR CONDITIONAL (≤3.0 TESLA)**
Permanent pacemakers[a]	Prosthetic heart valves
Implantable cardioverter defibrillators[a]	Intracoronary stents
Temporary transvenous pacemakers	Prosthetic joints
Insulin pumps	Dentures
Some medication patches	Implantable rhythm monitors[c]
Swan-Ganz catheters	Retained epicardial leads
Metal foreign bodies in the eyes	Occluder devices[d]
Brain aneurysm clips[b]	Peripheral stents[d]
Cochlear implants	Aortic aneurysm stents[d]
	Inferior vena cava filters[d]

[a]MRI-compatible pacemakers and implantable cardioverter defibrillators are now approved by the Food and Drug Administration and can be scanned under certain conditions at experienced cardiac magnetic resonance centers.
[b]More contemporary aneurysm clips are nonferromagnetic; however, confirmation with the implanting physician and manufacturer is absolutely required.
[c]Rhythm monitors can be conditional or unsafe, check with the manufacturer.
[d]If weakly ferromagnetic, it is recommended to wait 6 weeks post implantation.
MRI, magnetic resonance imaging.

TABLE 16.2	MRI in Specific Patient Populations
Chronic kidney disease, renal insufficiency	eGFR <30 mL/min/1.73 m²: use lowest possible dose (≤0.1 mmol/kg), avoid high-risk[a] contrast agents
	ESRD: avoid contrast agents; if absolutely necessary, use lowest dose, avoid high-risk agents, consider hemodialysis 2 h afterward, and the following day
	AKI: avoid contrast agents (regardless of eGFR); if absolutely necessary, use lowest dose, avoid high-risk agents
Pregnancy	Gadolinium contrast agents should be avoided
	No evidence of teratogenic effects of noncontrast MRI studies

[a]High-risk contrast agents have a linear chemical structure, as compared with the safer macrocyclical contrast agents.
AKI, acute kidney injury; eGFR, estimated glomerular filtration rate; ESRD, end-stage renal disease; MRI, magnetic resonance imaging.

carefully administer these questionnaires and instruct the patient to provide accurate answers to all questions. It is also important to consider specific patient populations such as pregnant patients or patients with renal insufficiency (**Table 16.2**).

CARDIAC MAGNETIC RESONANCE IN ACUTE CHEST PAIN

The differential diagnosis for acute chest pain (often with troponin elevation) is extensive and can be broadly divided into cardiac and noncardiac etiologies. In this chapter, we focus on the coronary causes of chest pain with troponin elevation in the acute and subacute phases as well as explore common noncoronary causes of chest pain and troponin elevation that are often seen in the CCU. **Table 16.3** briefly outlines some of the more common causes of chest pain, highlighting the disorders where CMR plays a significant role. It is important to realize that

troponin elevation is sensitive but not specific for the detection of cardiac damage. It does not completely differentiate coronary from noncoronary causes of chest pain. Virtually any strain on the heart, whether from coronary occlusion, pulmonary embolism, or pneumonia, for example, can cause a troponin elevation. The decreased clearance of troponin in renal insufficiency can also lead to troponin elevation in nearly any setting.

ACUTE CORONARY SYNDROME

One of the most common presentations seen in the CCU is the acute coronary syndrome (ACS). Thankfully, the mortality and morbidity rates have consistently declined for acute myocardial infarction (MI), in large part because of better diagnostics and treatment, such as statin therapy and early invasive angiography. Although the incidence of ST-segment elevation myocardial infarction (STEMI) has decreased, as the population ages, the consequences of ACS will continue to grow.

TABLE 16.3	Differential Diagnosis of Chest Pain			
CARDIAC	**VASCULAR**	**GI**	**PULMONARY**	**OTHER**
Acute coronary syndrome*	Aortic dissection*	Esophageal spasm	Pulmonary embolus	Rib fracture
Myocarditis*	Intramural hematoma*	Esophagitis	Pneumothorax	Costochondritis
Pericarditis*	Aortic ulcer*	Peptic ulcer disease	Pneumonia	Herpes zoster
Cardiac trauma*	Aortic aneurysm	Pancreatitis	Pleuritis	
Takotsubo cardiomyopathy*		Cholecystitis		
		Boerhaave syndrome		

* Conditions in which CMR is potentially useful for diagnosis

Cardiac Magnetic Resonance in Acute Coronary Syndrome

For the patient with acute STEMI or non-STEMI (NSTEMI)/unstable angina with high-risk features, an early invasive approach is favored. The initial use of CMR in these patients is limited because any delay in revascularization can lead to worse outcomes. CMR after revascularization, however, can provide important prognostic information after an ACS. For stable patients without a diagnosed ACS, an imaging modality initially can be very beneficial in determining the etiology of symptoms. CMR may prevent unnecessary invasive angiography as well as identify patients who would receive greater benefit from an early invasive strategy. Kwong et al[3] studied 161 patients with chest pain and a nondiagnostic electrocardiogram (ECG) who had a CMR combining different sequences within 12 hours of presentation. The sensitivity and specificity for acute MI or unstable angina was 84% and 85%, respectively. CMR was far more sensitive than strict ECG criteria for ischemia, peak troponin-I, and thrombolysis in myocardial infarction (TIMI) risk score, and was more specific than an abnormal ECG.[3] Plein et al[4] showed that CMR, also by combining different sequences, can identify high-risk patients with significant coronary stenosis in patients with chest pain in the absence of STEMI. In a study with 72 patients with NSTEMI/unstable angina, a comprehensive CMR protocol predicted the presence of coronary stenosis with greater accuracy than did the TIMI risk score.[4]

Outside of the acute phase of presentation, CMR also adds significant information in determining the extent of MI, ventricular remodeling, the presence of MVO, and the degree of viability. These parameters provide useful information that can assist with prognosis and treatment.

Functional Assessment

Using CMR to detect the presence and extent of wall motion abnormalities can be a helpful tool to determine patients most at risk, who would then benefit from more aggressive medical therapy and an early invasive strategy.

Subtle wall motion abnormalities that may be missed on echocardiography can often easily be seen on cine imaging in CMR because of its superior image quality. Wall motion abnormalities that correlate with a coronary distribution can further provide support for ACS in patients without STEMI.

In stable, low-risk patients who present with acute chest pain, CMR can be highly predictive of ACS in the near future. In one study, the presence of wall motion abnormalities on CMR, regardless of perfusion abnormalities and infarction, had greater sensitivity and specificity than did troponin elevation in predicting ACS or a positive stress test within 8 weeks.[3]

Common sequelae of ACS include left ventricular (LV) dilation **(Figure 16.2)**, wall motion abnormalities, and the formation of aneurysms. Cine imaging provides quantitative assessment of LV volumes, wall motion abnormalities, and LV and right ventricular (RV) function with greater accuracy and reproducibility than two-dimensional echocardiography. The degree of LV dilatation and reduction in left ventricular ejection fraction (LVEF), in addition to scar burden and MVO, significantly predicts patients at risk for future cardiovascular events.[5]

Ischemia

The detection of ischemia on first-pass perfusion imaging can also reliably detect coronary disease even before wall motion abnormalities may be seen. Using a bolus of contrast with fast

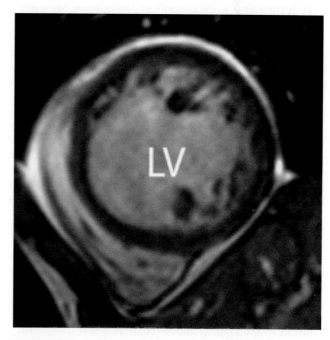

FIGURE 16.2 Short-axis view demonstrating a dilated left ventricle with a measured diastolic volume of 351 cc. LV, left ventricle.

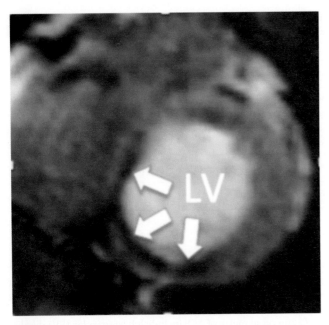

FIGURE 16.3 Short-axis view showing perfusion defects in the inferoseptal and inferior walls on first-pass perfusion imaging (white arrows). LV, left ventricle.

CMR sequences **(Figure 16.3)**, perfusion defects can become readily apparent. Normal myocardium will enhance, whereas relatively underperfused areas will appear dark for a certain amount of time.

Myocardial Edema

Myocardial edema can be seen in many forms of myocardial injury and is not specific to acute MI. It can, however, be helpful in determining the acuity of an MI as well as the extent of injury. T2 relaxation time is a useful MRI parameter and is directly correlated to the percentage of free water. Myocardial edema in the setting of acute/subacute injury, myocyte swelling, and increased cell permeability in necrotic and ischemic areas accounts for the increase in free water and signal seen on T2-weighted imaging **(Figure 16.4)**. Of note, edema after an ACS occurs in areas of both irreversibly and reversibly injured tissue and can overestimate the degree of myocardial necrosis. Myocardial edema may persist for weeks after infarction even after troponin levels have decreased to normal levels. A chronic infarct, on the other hand, will not have features of myocardial edema because water is resorbed and a fibrotic scar is formed, thus allowing CMR to distinguish between acute and chronic infarction. Cury et al[6] studied 64 patients presenting with chest pain, a normal ECG, and negative cardiac enzymes. Adding a T2-weighted sequence to cine imaging and LGE improved the specificity, positive predictive value, and accuracy in detecting ACS before a rise in serum biomarkers.[6]

In addition, combining T2-weighted imaging with LGE, a myocardial salvage index (MSI) can be calculated as the difference between the T2-intense region (area at risk) and final infarct (LGE), and used to predict outcomes after STEMI. Eitel et al[7] studied 208 patients with STEMI who had angioplasty within 12 hours of symptom onset and demonstrated that CMR-derived MSI can predict long-term clinical outcomes, including major adverse cardiovascular events (MACE) and mortality.

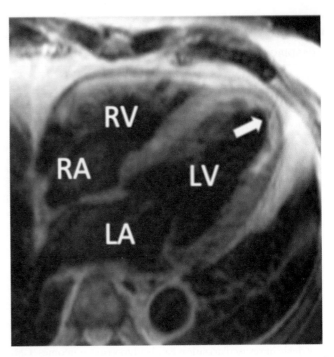

FIGURE 16.4 T2-weighted imaging demonstrating the presence of myocardial edema in the apical, apical lateral, and apical septal walls (*white arrow*) after acute myocardial infarction. LA, left atrium; LV, left ventricle; RA, right atrium; RV, right ventricle.

Myocardial Infarction (Late Gadolinium Enhancement)

Gadolinium-contrast agents accumulate in extracellular space and do not enter healthy cells. In the acute MI phase, degradation of myocardial cell membranes allows contrast to enter the damaged cells if given enough time, appearing bright on LGE imaging. In the chronic setting, the contrast accumulates temporarily in the enlarged interstitial space occupied by fibrotic tissue **(Figure 16.5)**. Assessment of scar and viability is discussed subsequently.

Multiple studies have demonstrated the close correlation between LGE and histopathologic specimens of necrotic tissue. LGE is capable of detecting infarctions as small as 1 g due to the outstanding spatial resolution of CMR. Other imaging modalities are limited in their ability to differentiate small infarctions because of lower spatial resolution. The right ventricle, in particular, is poorly imaged by echocardiography, and acute RV infarction is more often demonstrated by LGE on CMR **(Figure 16.6)** than with the combination of ECG and echocardiography.

Microvascular Obstruction and Intramyocardial Hemorrhage

Despite successful revascularization of their coronary arteries, subsets of patients have MVO. First-pass perfusion, early gadolinium enhancement, and/or LGE imaging can delineate these areas as a region without enhancement within the infarct core **(Figure 16.7)**, as a consequence of the lack of blood flow depositing contrast in these areas.

The presence of MVO has been demonstrated as an independent predictor of adverse LV remodeling and MACE. Hombach et al[5] studied 89 patients within 10 days of acute MI and concluded that, in addition to LV end-diastolic volume and LVEF, persistent MVO was a significant predictor of MACE.[5]

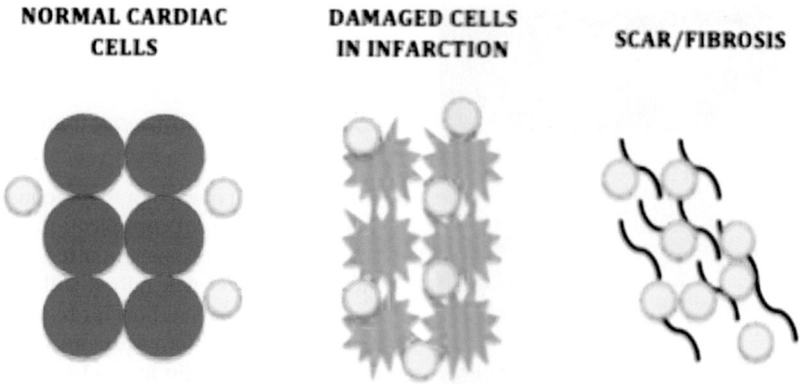

NORMAL CARDIAC CELLS **DAMAGED CELLS IN INFARCTION** **SCAR/FIBROSIS**

FIGURE 16.5 Deposition of gadolinium-contrast agents. Red—healthy cells; blue—acutely damaged cells; black—scar/fibrosis; yellow—gadolinium contrast.

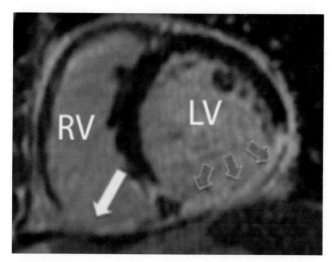

FIGURE 16.6 Short-axis view in delayed enhancement images demonstrating near transmural infarction of the inferior and inferolateral walls of the left ventricle (LV; *red arrows*) and near-transmural infarction of the inferior wall of the right ventricle (RV; *yellow arrow*). LV, left ventricle; RV, right ventricle.

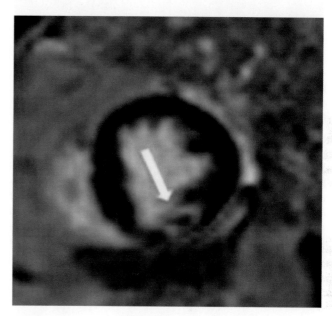

FIGURE 16.7 Short-axis view demonstrating a central hypointense core within an area of enhancement (*arrow*), signifying the presence of microvascular obstruction.

Viability

LGE is a useful tool to evaluate viability after ACS as well as provide prognostic information. The extent of the fibrosis is assessed by measuring the number of segments affected using a 17-segment model, as well as the percentage of thickness involved in each segment. Segments with a small amount of fibrosis are often viable and can recover spontaneously if stunned and with revascularization in hibernating myocardium. Conversely, segments that have near transmural or transmural fibrosis are unlikely to recover. This can be a very helpful tool in determining which patients will benefit from revascularization.[8] Subendocardial enhancement that can progress to full transmural enhancement is characteristic of ischemic coronary disease. This is easily differentiated from nonischemic patterns of scar (**Figure 16.8**) that are described in more detail in section "Cardiac Magnetic Resonance in Heart Failure."

Cardiac segments with LGE evident in less than 25% to 50% thickness (**Figure 16.9**) are likely to regain function after revascularization, whereas segments with ≥75% enhancement (**Figure 16.10**) are most likely scarred and unlikely to benefit

from further intervention. In addition, the amount of transmural infarction on LGE also predicts adverse LV remodeling.

The peri-infarct region (also known as "gray zone" or "border zone") on LGE imaging, is defined as an area with signal intensity above that of normal myocardium but less than dense scar.

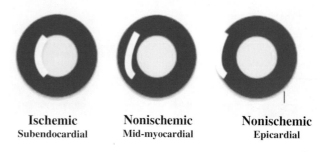

Ischemic
Subendocardial

Nonischemic
Mid-myocardial

Nonischemic
Epicardial

FIGURE 16.8 Fibrosis patterns in ischemic cardiomyopathies compared to nonischemic cardiomyopathies. Green—left ventricular (LV) cavity; blue—myocardium; white—fibrosis.

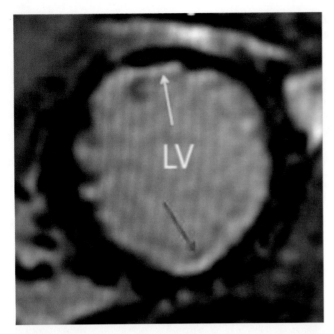

FIGURE 16.9 Short-axis view showing subendocardial infarctions of the anterior wall (*yellow arrow*) and inferior wall (*red arrow*) with a large area of preserved myocardium. LV, left ventricle.

It has been recognized as a marker of arrhythmia risk. Whether the peri-infarct zone, overall scar amount, or LVEF alone are better predictors of spontaneous ventricular arrhythmias remains a question. Gouda et al[9] studied 48 patients post MI, half of whom had sustained monomorphic ventricular tachycardia (VT), and evaluated total scar, scar core, mean infarct transmurality, peri-infarct zone, and number of segments with LGE. In multivariable analysis, total infarct size as percentage of LV mass was the only significant independent predictor of spontaneous and inducible VT.[9]

Post–Myocardial Infarction and Procedural Complications

With the advent of early percutaneous coronary intervention, the incidence of post-MI complications has dramatically decreased. When patients present late after onset of coronary occlusion, there is a greater risk (albeit still small) of dangerous post-MI complications. It is important to be aware of these phenomena because they are often acute and any delay in diagnosis can be fatal. Given the rapidity in onset and clinical deterioration, portable echocardiography is typically the most useful tool. However, if the patient is stable enough, post-MI complications can be more accurately assessed utilizing CMR.

Left Ventricular Thrombus

One of the most common complications of MI is the development of LV thrombus. Thrombus is most common in large anterior infarcts but can develop even in small isolated apical infarctions, as well as in other locations, particularly the septal and inferolateral walls.

Diagnosis by echocardiography, even with contrast administration, is far less sensitive than detection by CMR. Using simple CMR techniques, an LV thrombus can rapidly be distinguished from normal adjacent myocardium. Although contrast echocardiography significantly increased detection of thrombi compared to noncontrast echocardiography, LGE more accurately detected smaller and/or mural thrombi (**Figure 16.11**).[10] Differentiation between thrombi and other cardiac masses is discussed in section "Miscellaneous."

Left Ventricular Aneurysm

Another common complication of acute MI is the development of an LV aneurysm. Typically, an infarcted, thin-walled left ventricle that has remodeled extensively causes the formation of aneurysms. Persistent ST-segment elevations on an ECG in the absence of chest pain or acute MI can indicate the presence of an LV aneurysm. Cine imaging and/or LGE sequences (**Figure 16.12**) can demonstrate the extent of aneurysm formation and clearly delineate the wide orifice that is characteristic of them.

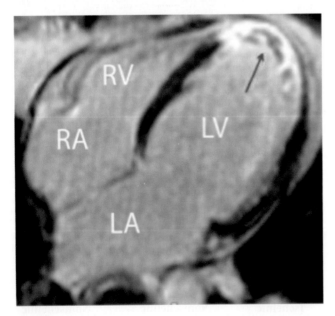

FIGURE 16.10 Four-chamber view demonstrating a large area of transmural infarction involving the LV apex, apical septal, and apical lateral walls (*arrow*). Note the central hypointensity within the area of enhancement, indicating the presence of microvascular obstruction. LA, left atrium; LV, left ventricle; RA, right atrium; RV, right ventricle.

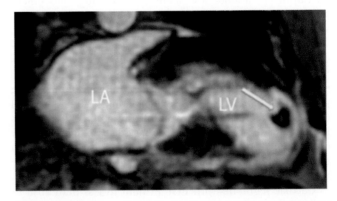

FIGURE 16.11 Two-chamber view demonstrating hypointense LV thrombus (*yellow arrow*) on late gadolinium enhancement imaging. LA, left atrium; LV, left ventricle.

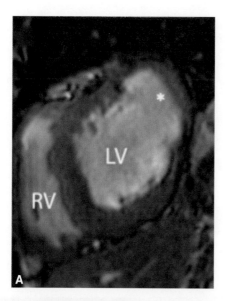

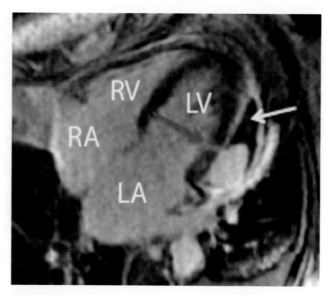

FIGURE 16.13 Free wall rupture contained only by thrombus (*yellow arrow*) and pericardium. Note the narrow neck at the point of rupture (*red arrow*). (Image courtesy of Jiwon Kim, MD, Weill Cornell Medical Center, New York, NY.) LA, left atrium; LV, left ventricle; RA, right atrium; RV, right ventricle.

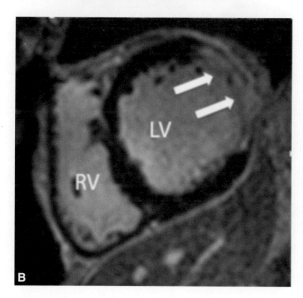

FIGURE 16.12 A, Short-axis view in cine images demonstrating a large aneurysm of the anterolateral wall. B, Short-axis late enhancement view demonstrating near-transmural infarction of the aneurysmal myocardial territory. LV, left ventricle; RV, right ventricle.

Left Ventricular Pseudoaneurysm/Free Wall Rupture

Less common, but more urgent, is the diagnosis of pseudoaneurysm/contained wall rupture. A true aneurysm contains all three layers of myocardial tissue (subendocardial, endocardial, and epicardial), whereas a pseudoaneurysm wall is constituted only by pericardium and fibrotic/inflammatory tissue (in essence, a contained free wall rupture) and is at high risk of losing that containment. A pseudoaneurysm typically has a narrow neck.

Uncontained free wall rupture is another rare post-MI complication that can be rapidly fatal. When suspected, immediate diagnosis with portable echocardiography and surgical intervention is often the only chance of survival. Patients are rarely, if ever, stable enough to have a CMR. In the rare case that a patient has a contained free wall rupture, CMR can provide detailed anatomic assessment of the rupture, including site,

orifice, material containing the rupture, and other important parameters **(Figure 16.13)**.

Ventricular Septal Defect

Ventricular septal defect (VSD) is another rare but potentially fatal complication that typically occurs within 1 week of acute MI. Patients typically present with a new holosystolic murmur, biventricular failure, and cardiogenic shock. Rapid diagnosis and surgical intervention are key to ensuring a patient's survival. Echocardiography is the diagnostic imaging modality of choice when VSD is suspected because of its portability and rapid image acquisition. Very rarely will a patient be stable enough to acquire a CMR to assist with diagnosis. If the patient is stable and there are poor acoustic windows on echocardiography, CMR can provide excellent anatomic detail of the VSD and calculate the Qp/Qs for shunt quantification.

CARDIAC MAGNETIC RESONANCE IN NONCORONARY CAUSES OF ACUTE CHEST PAIN (WITH OR WITHOUT TROPONIN ELEVATION)

The most common cardiac causes of chest pain and troponin elevation in patients with nonobstructive coronary artery disease are myocarditis, myopericarditis, Takotsubo cardiomyopathy, and acute aortic syndromes.

Myocarditis

Myocarditis (both acute and chronic) remains a diagnostic challenge in clinical cardiology. Myocarditis should be considered in any patient with chest pain, elevated cardiac biomarkers, and normal coronary arteries. In addition, cardiomyopathy may result from chronic inflammatory disease in patients with inadequate immune response. Endomyocardial biopsy (EMB) with immunohistology is the "gold standard" for the diagnosis of myocarditis, but it is an invasive procedure with risks of complications.

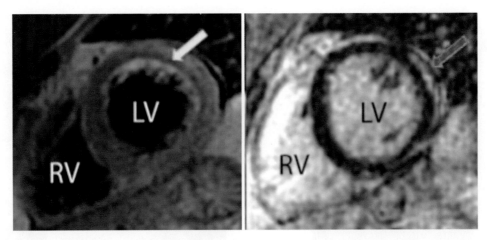

FIGURE 16.14 Myocardial edema on T2-weighted imaging (*yellow arrow*) and subepicardial late gadolinium enhancement (*red arrow*) in a patient with myocarditis. LV, left ventricle; RV, right ventricle.

CMR has been increasingly used as an aid in the diagnosis of myocardial inflammation in patients with suspected myocarditis. The International Consensus Group on CMR Diagnosis of Myocarditis was founded to establish recommendations on CMR techniques for myocarditis.[11] Infections are one of the most common etiologies of myocarditis, predominantly viral infections or post-viral immune-mediated reactions. Myocardial inflammation may also be triggered by reversible or irreversible toxic, ischemic, or mechanical injury, drug-related inflammation, transplant rejection, or some other immune response.[11] No single clinical or imaging finding confirms the diagnosis of myocarditis. The diagnostic approach should be an integrated synopsis of history, physical examination, noninvasive and invasive testing (LV function and volume as well as CMR tissue characterization) to guide medical therapy.

CMR has the ability to characterize inflammatory tissue changes. One approach is the Lake Louise Criteria (LLC): edema with T2-weighted imaging, hyperemia, or capillary leak with early gadolinium enhancement, and irreversible cell injury with LGE (besides other nonspecific findings such as LV dysfunction and pericardial effusion).[11] These CMR imaging techniques are used to determine the presence of edema, hyperemia, and myocardial necrosis/fibrosis, which are part of the pathological process seen in myocarditis **(Figure 16.14)**. Several patterns of LGE may be seen in myocarditis, which usually follows a nonischemic pattern. Focal signal intensity may be seen in a subepicardial or intramyocardial pattern and can involve part or the entire extent of the myocardial wall **(Figures 16.15** and **16.16)**.

More recently, T1 and T2 mapping with quantification of extracellular volume have provided additional information in the CMR diagnosis of myocarditis. Myocardial T1- and T2- relaxation times are significant parameters of active inflammation and edema in patients with acute myocarditis, as well as during the convalescent stage of the disease. In a recent publication, the MyoRacer Trial, Lurz et al[12] compared the diagnostic performance of CMR using T1 and T2 mapping versus the reference standard, EMB. They noted that in patients with acute myocarditis symptoms, T1- and T2-mapping techniques were even superior to the LLC (which have a sensitivity of 82% and a specificity of 98% for acute myocarditis). Therefore, T1 and T2 mapping may add useful information over T1- and T2-weighted imaging in the diagnosis of myocarditis.[12]

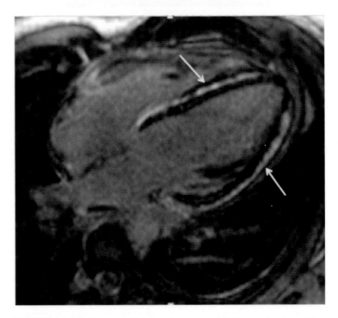

FIGURE 16.15 Late gadolinium enhancement (LGE) imaging in a patient with acute myocarditis. Note the diffuse subepicardial and intramyocardial enhancement, indicated by yellow arrows. (Image courtesy of Adam Jacobi, MD, Mount Sinai Hospital, New York, NY.)

In summary, in patients suspected of having acute myocarditis, a comprehensive quantitative CMR is a useful tool that can reliably detect inflammatory alterations in the myocardium and should be implemented early if myocarditis is suspected.

Acute Pericarditis

Inflammation of the pericardium often presents as acute chest pain, with possible troponin elevation if there is concomitant myocardial involvement. The causes of acute pericarditis are vast and include infectious (viral, bacterial, fungal, and mycobacterial), rheumatologic (eg, scleroderma, lupus, and rheumatoid arthritis), sequelae of radiation therapy, post-MI (ie, Dressler syndrome), trauma, and uremia.

Although systematic evaluation of the role of CMR in acute pericarditis is lacking, T2-weighted and LGE imaging can

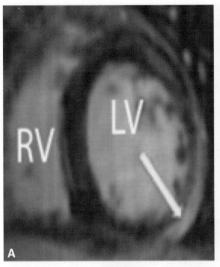 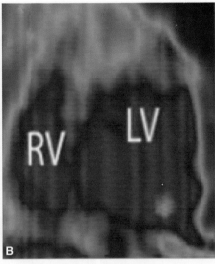 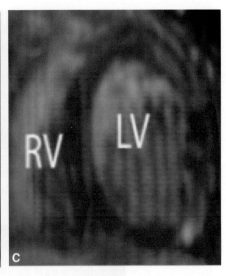

FIGURE 16.16 Panel (A) demonstrates a short-axis view of the LV with subepicardial (nonischemic) pattern of late gadolinium enhancement in the inferolateral wall in a patient with suspected myocarditis. Panel (B) demonstrates positron emission tomography (PET) imaging of the same patient. Panel (C) demonstrates fused PET magnetic resonance imaging (MRI): noteice the inflammatory activity in the area of LGE, consistent with active myocarditis. LV, left ventricle; RV, right ventricle. (Figure courtesy of Zahi Fayad, PhD, Maria Giovanna Trivieri, MD, and Phil Robson, PhD, Icahn School of Medicine, Mount Sinai Medical Center, New York, NY.)

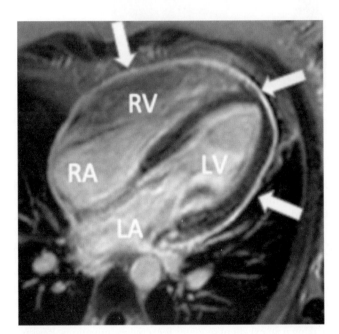

FIGURE 16.17 Diffuse delayed enhancement of the pericardium (*arrows*) in a patient with acute pericarditis. LA, left atrium; LV, left ventricle; RA, right atrium; RV, right ventricle.

respectively demonstrate edema and enhancement of the pericardium **(Figure 16.17)** when there is ongoing inflammation.[13]

Takotsubo Cardiomyopathy

Takotsubo cardiomyopathy, also known as "apical ballooning syndrome" or "stress-induced cardiomyopathy," is a unique syndrome that often presents similarly to an ACS or myocarditis **(Table 16.4)**. Among the hallmarks of the syndrome are wall motion abnormalities that do not correlate with a single coronary arterial territory. Takotsubo cardiomyopathy is classically described as a consequence of severe emotional stress, but virtually any stress, emotional or physical, can lead to this clinical entity. In some cases, no inciting event can be identified.

As of yet, the pathophysiology of Takotsubo cardiomyopathy is not well understood; theories range from multivessel spasm to catecholamine toxicity. Patients with Takotsubo cardiomyopathy often present with chest pain, ST-segment changes such as ST elevation or diffuse ST depression and prolongation of the QT interval. The classic wall motion abnormalities described are LV basal segment hyperkinesis with severe hypokinesis of the apical segments, and hence the term "apical ballooning." Multiple variants of Takotsubo have been described including reverse Takotsubo with hyperkinesis of the apex and severe hypokinesis of the mid segments and a midwall variant where only the mid segments are hypokinetic.

Takotsubo cardiomyopathy remains a diagnosis of exclusion. The diagnosis is only in the absence of coronary artery disease on invasive or noninvasive angiography that matches with wall motion abnormalities. CMR is emerging as a useful tool to readily distinguish between other causes of ACS and Takotsubo cardiomyopathy.

Cine imaging on CMR can accurately depict wall motion abnormalities that do not correlate with a coronary territory **(Figure 16.18)**. Myocardial edema on T2-weighted imaging, as described earlier, is often prominent in areas of wall motion abnormality. Edema and wall motion abnormalities can also be seen in the right ventricle.

The lack of significant LGE in the areas of wall motion abnormality confirms the absence of MI. The degree of enhancement is almost never to the extent of a true MI and is sometimes termed "low-intensity LGE" **(Figure 16.19)**.[14]

This constellation of findings (wall motion abnormalities beyond a coronary distribution, myocardial edema, and the lack of intense LGE) can assist in the diagnosis of Takotsubo cardiomyopathy. Patients often have a good prognosis, with the majority recovering LV function at 3 months.

TABLE 16.4	Comparison of MRI Findings in Takatsubo Cardiomyopathy, Myocardial Infarction, and Myocarditis		
	TAKOTSUBO	**MYOCARDIAL INFARCTION**	**MYOCARDITIS**
WMA in a coronary distribution	No	Yes	No
Edema	Yes (typically in areas of WMA)	Yes (typically in areas of WMA)	Yes (subepicardial/ midmyocardial or transmural)
Late gadolinium enhancement	No or low intensity	Yes (subendocardial to transmural)	Yes (subepicardial/ midmyocardial or "patchy")
Resolution or follow up to 3 months	Majority = Yes	No	Majority = Yes

WMA, wall motion abnormality.

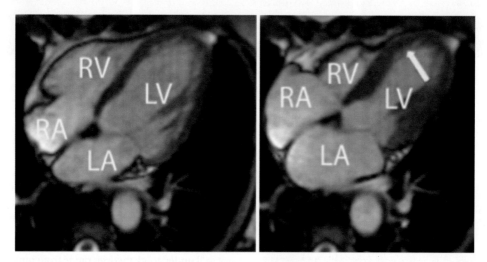

FIGURE 16.18 Four-chamber cine view (**left:** diastole; **right:** systole) demonstrating wall motion abnormalities in a patient with Takotsubo cardiomyopathy. Note the lack of movement of the mid-distal segments (*arrow*) compared to the basal segments. LA, left atrium; LV, left ventricle; RA, right atrium; RV, right ventricle.

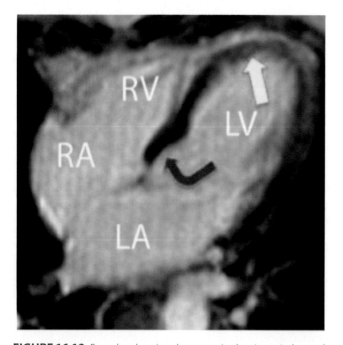

FIGURE 16.19 Four-chamber view demonstrating low-intensity late gadolinium enhancement (LGE) (*yellow arrow*) compared to normal myocardium (*blue arrow*) in the same patient as in the previous figure with Takotsubo cardiomyopathy. LA, left atrium; LV, left ventricle; RA, right atrium; RV, right ventricle.

Acute Aortic Syndromes

MRI can play an important role in determining the location and extent of involvement in patients with aortic dissection. When utilized, MRI provides a complete anatomic assessment of the intimal flap (**Figure 16.20**), aortic valve morphology and severity of insufficiency, the presence of hemopericardium indicating impending aortic wall rupture, branch involvement of the great vessels, and the presence of an MI due to dissection into a coronary artery (usually the right coronary). MRI is also one of the most valuable imaging techniques for imaging aortic dissections after surgical intervention. Images are highly reproducible, making it an excellent modality for serial examinations. Residual dissection, thrombosis of the false lumen, suture dehiscence, and anastomotic leaks can be easily identified and help guide further management.[15]

CARDIAC MAGNETIC RESONANCE IN VENTRICULAR ARRHYTHMIAS

Sudden cardiac death (SCD) has been the leading cause of death in North America. It has been well documented that severely depressed LVEF (<35%) has been associated with SCD. Ventricular fibrosis or myocardial "scar" is the nidus or "anatomic substrate" for ventricular arrhythmias in patients with ischemic cardiomyopathy

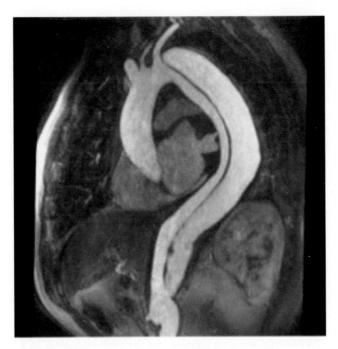

FIGURE 16.20 Contrast-enhanced aortic magnetic resonance angiography (MRA) demonstrating a type-B dissection flap extending from the origin of the left subclavian artery to the abdominal aorta.

(ICM) and nonischemic cardiomyopathy (NICM). In multiple randomized, controlled trials, with inclusion based on LVEF, the use of an ICD has reduced mortality. These studies are the basis of our current guidelines in primary prevention. However, only a fraction of patients (approximately 30%) receiving an ICD for primary prevention of SCD get appropriate therapy. The use of LVEF solely as the marker for ICD implantation is not ideal. SCD can occur also in patients with normal and mildly depressed LVEF. Therefore, a more in-depth need for risk stratification for primary prevention in patients with ICM and NICM (ie, myocarditis, sarcoidosis, and arrhythmogenic right ventricular cardiomyopathy [ARVC]) is necessary. CMR with LGE can be used to detect myocardial scar size and heterogeneity. Because myocardial scar is an important substrate for developing VT, CMR may be useful in predicting future ventricular arrhythmias.[16] CMR with contrast can be used to assess myocardial scar characteristics including scar transmurality, the border zone, and variations in the density of scar tissue and heterogeneity versus homogeneous scar appearance.

Disertori et al[16] performed a meta-analysis to evaluate the predictive value of LGE in CMR for ventricular tachyarrhythmia in ventricular dysfunction. Nineteen studies enrolling 2850 patients with ICM and NICM were included in the meta-analysis. The study demonstrated that LGE is a powerful predictor of ventricular tachyarrhythmic events in patients with ventricular dysfunction of ischemic and nonischemic etiology. The prognostic power of LGE for ventricular arrhythmias is particularly strong in patients with severely depressed LVEF (≤30%).

Regions of viable tissue within the gray zone detected by three-dimensional LGE-CMR correspond to conduction channels on endocardial voltage mapping and, therefore, may play a role in arrhythmia management and therapy.[16] As discussed also in section "Cardiac Magnetic Resonance in Heart Failure," the presence or absence of fibrosis or, particularly, mid-wall

fibrosis in NICM are indicators of high versus low risk of arrhythmic events.

HYPERTROPHIC CARDIOMYOPATHY

Hypertrophic cardiomyopathy (HCM) remains the most common cause of SCD in young adults. Contrast-enhanced CMR with LGE has emerged as an in vivo marker of myocardial fibrosis and perhaps a marker for ventricular arrhythmias and SCD **(Figure 16.21)**.[17]

In a recent publication by Chan et al,[17] the correlation between LGE and cardiovascular events were assessed in over 1200 patients with HCM. SCD events occurred in 37 patients (3%). The extent of LGE was associated with an increased risk of SCD events. LGE ≥15% of LV mass demonstrated a 2-fold increase in SCD event risk in those patients otherwise considered to be at lower risk. Performance of the SCD event risk model was enhanced by LGE (net reclassification index, 12.9%; 95% confidence interval, 0.3 to 38.3).[17] Absence of LGE was associated with lower risk for SCD events in these patients.

CARDIAC SARCOIDOSIS

Inflammatory cardiomyopathies can be associated with ventricular arrhythmias at any time throughout their clinical course. Myocarditis is discussed in section "Cardiac Magnetic Resonance "Acute Chest Pain." Another potential cause of inflammatory cardiomyopathy is sarcoidosis, a systemic non-necrotizing granulomatous disease. This CD4+–mediated disease has multiorgan system involvement. The lungs are affected in more than 90% of patients, and the disease can also involve the heart, liver, spleen, skin, eyes, parotid gland, or other organs and tissues. An estimated 20% to 25% of patients with pulmonary or systemic sarcoidosis have asymptomatic cardiac involvement.[18] This finding was initially established on the basis of autopsy studies, which estimated the prevalence of cardiac involvement to be at least 25% among patients with sarcoidosis. These autopsy findings are consistent with recent data using LGE-CMR technology.

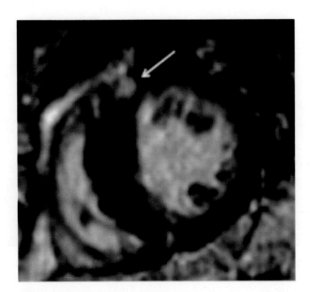

FIGURE 16.21 Short-axis view demonstrating mid-wall septal fibrosis at the right ventricular insertion point (*yellow arrow*), a characteristic pattern seen in hypertrophic cardiomyopathy.

Cardiac involvement can include atrioventricular conduction disorders, atrial and life-threatening ventricular arrhythmias, and biventricular HF. Approximately 60% to 70% of patients with sarcoid-related deaths have evidence of intramyocardial infiltration. Although rare, isolated cardiac sarcoidosis does exist. Between 16% and 35% of patients presenting with complete atrioventricular block (age <60 years) or VT of unknown etiology have previously undiagnosed cardiac sarcoidosis as the underlying etiology.[18] EMB is considered to be the gold standard when positive. EMB is highly specific, but it is an invasive procedure. As cardiac involvement is not homogeneous and lesions are usually in a patchy distribution, EMB has poor sensitivity with a diagnostic yield as low as 19%. Thus, CMR is becoming the imaging modality of choice for the diagnosis of cardiac sarcoidosis and to guide the EMB to active intracavitary inflammatory lesions to increase the yield of biopsy.

There is no specific pattern of LGE on CMR that is diagnostic for cardiac sarcoidosis, although usually it is patchy and multifocal, with sparing of the endocardial border. CMR is increasingly utilized for assessment of clinically silent cardiac sarcoidosis, in view of its ability to identify small regions of myocardial damage, even in subjects with preserved LV systolic function.[18] In a recent meta-analysis including 760 patients, Coleman et al[19] noted that the presence of LGE on CMR imaging is associated with increased odds of both all-cause mortality and arrhythmogenic events compared to those without myocardial involvement on LGE.

Positron emission tomography (PET)/CMR, which enables concurrent imaging of the two stages of the disease (inflammation and fibrosis/scar), has been also used recently in the diagnosis and management of cardiac sarcoidosis **(Figure 16.22)**.

The clinical situations where immunosuppression should be considered in patients with known cardiac sarcoidosis and myocardial inflammation include Mobitz II or third-degree heart block, frequent ventricular ectopy or nonsustained ventricular arrhythmias, sustained ventricular arrhythmias, and LV dysfunction.[18]

An electrophysiological study for SCD risk stratification may be considered in patients with LVEF >35% despite optimal

medical therapy. ICD implantation should be considered when LVEF is <35% despite optimal medical therapy.[18] Patients with cardiac sarcoidosis have a worse prognosis than patients without cardiac involvement. Cardiac death is due to progressive HF or SCD. In patients with clinically manifest disease, the extent of LV dysfunction is the most important predictor of survival.

ARRYTHMOGENIC RIGHT VENTRICULAR CARDIOMYOPATHY

Also known as arrythmogenic right ventricular dysplasia, ARVC is an inherited cardiomyopathy characterized by fibrofatty infiltration predominantly involving the right ventricle but that can also affect the left ventricle. Both can predispose patients to life-threatening ventricular arrhythmias. ARVC has a prevalence of 1 in 2000 to 5000 people, but can be as high as 1 in 1000 in certain regions because of underdiagnosis. Genetic testing for ARVC has developed over the past decade with associated mutations in desmosomal genes and non-desmosomal genes. Inheritance varies depending on the genes involved but most commonly is autosomal dominant with incomplete penetrance and variable expressivity.[20] Over the past decade, CMR has emerged as the gold standard imaging modality for in-depth evaluation of RV morphology, function, and tissue characterization.[20]

The diagnosis of ARVC is challenging and is based on the International Task Force criteria.[21] The Task Force set out to establish the major and minor CMR criteria for ARVC. Liu et al[21] evaluated the revised 2010 criteria in 968 consecutive patients referred for CMR with clinical suspicion for ARVC. The revised criteria in 2010 resulted in a reduction of total patients meeting any diagnostic CMR criteria for ARVC from 22.7% to 2.6% compared to the 1994 Task Force criteria.[21] This reinforced that perhaps ARVC was originally overdiagnosed before the 2010 revision. The new CMR major criteria include regional RV akinesia or dyskinesia plus RV enlargement (RV end-diastolic volume ≥110 ml/m² in males and ≥ 100 ml/m² in females) or RV ejection fraction ≤ 40%

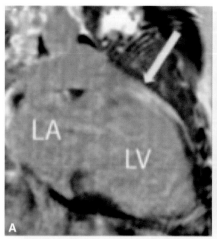 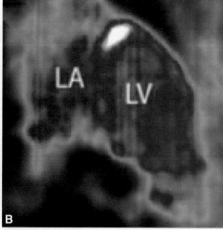 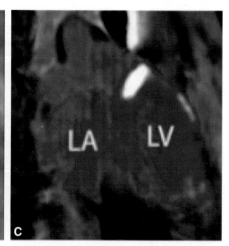

FIGURE 16.22 A, Two-chamber cardiac magnetic resonance (CMR) view of the LV with subepicardial (nonischemic) pattern of late gadolinium enhancement (LGE) in the basal to mid-anterior wall in a patient with known pulmonary sarcoidosis. B, Positron emission tomography (PET) imaging of the same patient. C, PET-CMR imaging: notice the inflammatory activity in the area of LGE consistent with active cardiac sarcoidosis. LA, left atrium; LV, left ventricle. (Image courtesy of Zahi Fayad, PhD, Maria Giovanna Trivieri, MD, and Phil Robson, PhD, Icahn School of Medicine, Mount Sinai Medical Center, New York, NY.)

TABLE 16.5	Revised Imaging Task Force Criteria for the Diagnosis of ARVC[22]

2010 TASK FORCE CRITERIA

MAJOR CRITERIA

Two-dimensional echocardiographic criteria

Regional RV akinesia, dyskinesia, or aneurysm
Plus one of the following (end-diastole):
- PLAX RVOT $\geq$32 mm (corrected for body size [PLAX/BSA] $\geq$19 mm/m^2)
- PSAX RVOT $\geq$36 mm (corrected for body size [PSAX/BSA] $\geq$21 mm/m^2) or fractional area change $\leq$33%

MRI imaging criteria

Regional RV akinesia, dyskinesia, or dyssynchrony
Plus one of the following:
- ratio of RV end-diastolic volume to BSA $\geq$110 mL/m^2 (male) or $\geq$100 mL/m^2 (female)
- or RV ejection fraction $\leq$40%

RV angiographic criteria

Regional RV akinesia, dyskinesia, or aneurysm

MINOR CRITERIA

Two-dimensional echocardiography criteria

Regional RV akinesia, dyskinesia, or aneurysm
Plus one of the following (end-diastolic):
- PLAX RVOT $\geq$29 to <32 mm (corrected for body size [PLAX/BSA] $\geq$16 to <19 mm/m^2)
- PSAX RVOT $\geq$32 to <36 mm (corrected for body size [PSAX/BSA] $\geq$18 to <21 mm/m^2) or fractional area change >33% to $\leq$40%

MRI criteria

Regional RV akinesia, dyskinesia, or dyssynchrony
Plus one of the following:
- ratio of RV end-diastolic volume to BSA $\geq$100 to <110 mL/m^2 (male) or $\geq$90 to <100 mL/m^2 (female)
- or RV ejection fraction >40% to $\leq$45%

ARVD, arrythmogenic right ventricular dysplasia; MRI, magnetic resonance imaging; RV, right ventricular.

(Table 16.5). Microaneurysms can also be present in the RV wall and are best seen on CMR cine imaging **(Figure 16.23C)**.

Infiltration of fat in the right ventricle can be seen on T1-weighted CMR imaging, which is demonstrated as regions of increased signal intensity in the myocardium **(Figure 16.23A)**. Fat–water separation imaging can further aid in the diagnosis of the fibrofatty infiltration. In addition, LGE of the RV myocardium can sometimes be seen **(Figure 16.23B)**. New CMR sequences including high-resolution T1 mapping are evolving tools that may detect early and subtle changes in the right ventricle. In addition, quantification of RV regional wall motion abnormalities and evaluation of inter- and intraventricular dyssynchrony can provide novel tools for early detection of ARVC. Genetic testing using comprehensive cardiomyopathy panels and whole exome sequencing are also likely to significantly impact the diagnosis of ARVC and prevention of SCD. The diagnosis of ARVC with CMR is difficult and requires experienced imaging specialists for accurate diagnosis of the disease.

CARDIAC MAGNETIC RESONANCE IN HEART FAILURE

The presence of HF is a common indication of admission in the CCU. As discussed previously, CMR is most commonly reserved for the stable patient who is able to tolerate a decubitus position. The main roles of CMR include providing accurate quantification of biventricular size and function, and characterization of the myocardium for the presence of scar, necrosis, infiltration, or edema. Although reduced LVEF as measured with a variety of imaging modalities is a well-known marker of risk in HF, during the past few years, the presence of myocardial scar as demonstrated by LGE has emerged as an important powerful prognosticator independent of LVEF. In a series of 857 consecutive patients with HF, survival free from death or heart transplantation was similar in patients with severe LV dysfunction but no scar compared with those with preserved LVEF but evidence of LGE.[23] These findings, subsequently confirmed in other studies, suggest that myocardial scarring may be as powerful a prognosticator as measures of LV dysfunction.

For the purpose of the discussion, this section is divided into predominantly left-sided or right-sided HF, although there is certainly overlap between the two syndromes and their underlying etiologies. Additional information that can be obtained from CMR includes pericardial involvement, valvular disease severity, or quantification of systemic to pulmonary shunts. It must be emphasized that data on CMR diagnostic and prognostic ability in HF has been obtained largely from stable cohorts and not from patients admitted to the CCU.

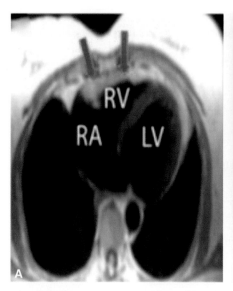
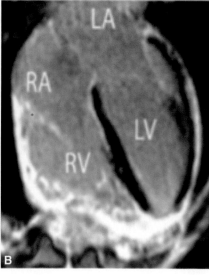
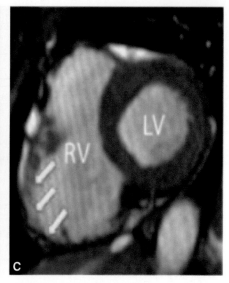

FIGURE 16.23 Axial black-blood imaging demonstrating fatty infiltration of the right ventricle (*red arrows*, A). Four-chamber view showing extensive late gadolinium enhancement (LGE) of the right ventricular free wall and apex (B). Short-axis cine view of the left and right ventricles with a large focal aneurysm of the right ventricular free wall (*yellow arrows*, C). LA, left atrium; LV, left ventricle; RA, right atrium; RV, right ventricle.

LEFT-SIDED HEART FAILURE

Dilated Cardiomyopathy

One of the most common causes of left-sided HF is dilated cardiomyopathy (DCM). DCM of specific etiologies, such as ischemia or sarcoid, have been discussed in section "Cardiac Magnetic Resonance in Ventricular Arrhythmias," so here we address mainly DCM of unknown cause. In idiopathic DCM, two patterns of LGE are commonly observed: absent (approximately 65% to 70%) or nonischemic (approximately 20% to 25%). As described in sections "Cardiac Magnetic Resonance in Acute Chest Pain" and "Cardiac Magnetic Resonance in Ventricular Arrhythmias," nonischemic LGE refers to areas of scar with a predominantly intramyocardial or subepicardial location, or transmural or subendocardial areas that do not conform to a coronary territory. Occasionally (around 10% of cases), "ischemic" LGE can be seen in patients with DCM and normal or nonobstructive coronary artery disease, raising the possibility of an ischemic etiology despite the absence of significant coronary stenoses (ie, embolization, vasospasm, thrombus autolysis, etc). A pattern of nonischemic, linear intramyocardial LGE in the interventricular septum can be often seen in idiopathic DCM and has received particular attention **(Figure 16.24)**.

In a meta-analysis of nine studies including ≈1500 patients,[24] this pattern was associated with increased midterm risk of mortality (odds ratio = 3.27), malignant ventricular arrhythmias (odds ratio = 5.32), or HF hospitalization (odds ratio = 2.91; $P<0.001$ for all), independent of other conventional risk markers including LVEF. RV ejection fraction is also of prognostic value in these patients.

HEART FAILURE WITH PRESERVED EJECTION FRACTION

Many cases of HF do not have reduced LVEF, a situation commonly referred to as heart failure with preserved ejection fraction (HF-pEF). HFpEF is a multifactorial syndrome in which diastolic LV

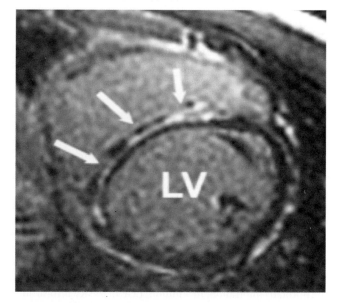

FIGURE 16.24 Short-axis image demonstrating linear intramyocardial late gadolinium enhancement (*arrows*) in a patient with idiopathic dilated cardiomyopathy. LV, left ventricle.

dysfunction is believed to represent a common pathophysiologic pathway. The role of CMR in HFpEF is not well defined because diastolic function is often better evaluated with echocardiography, although preliminary data suggest an association between localized scar (using LGE) or diffuse myocardial fibrosis (using novel T1-mapping sequences) with abnormalities in LV stiffness and impaired outcomes.[25]

RIGHT-SIDED HEART FAILURE

Restrictive Cardiomyopathy

CMR plays an increasingly important role in the evaluation of restrictive cardiomyopathy, one form of HFpEF associated

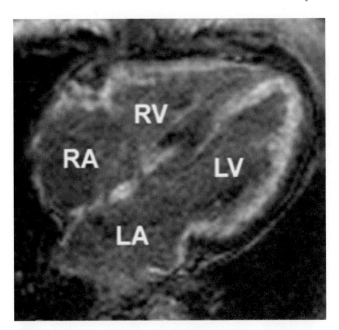

FIGURE 16.25 Four-chamber view demonstrating diffuse, predominantly subendocardial late gadolinium enhancement (LGE) in the LV of a patient with cardiac amyloidosis. LGE also noted in the RV and both atria. LA, left atrium; LV, left ventricle; RA, right atrium; RV, right ventricle.

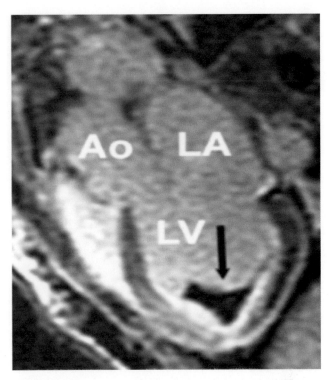

FIGURE 16.26 Three-chamber view in a patient with endomyocardial fibrosis demonstrating apical late gadolinium enhancement with superimposed thrombus (*arrow*). Ao, aorta; LA, left atrium; LV, left ventricle.

with congestive symptoms, related to infiltrative heart disease. In developed countries, the most common cause of restrictive cardiomyopathy is cardiac amyloidosis. The typical features of amyloidosis include increased ventricular wall thickness in the absence of electrocardiographic hypertrophy, relatively preserved LVEF, biatrial enlargement, thickening of the mitral and tricuspid leaflets as well as of the interatrial septum, and pericardial and pleural effusions. These features are specific but have low sensitivity. Cardiac amyloid is associated with a typical pattern of diffuse LGE, more prominent toward the base of the heart, with a predominantly intramyocardial and subendocardial distribution (**Figure 16.25**).

In addition, abnormal contrast kinetics between the blood and the myocardium can be observed and quantified. This pattern is highly specific to cardiac amyloidosis and, importantly, has been associated with increased mortality (hazard ratio = 5.2; $P<0.001$) after adjusting for LV systolic and diastolic function, LV mass index, and N-terminal pro-brain natriuretic peptide.[26] Some distinguishing CMR features may help in the differential diagnosis between light-chain and transthyretin amyloid, which has both prognostic and therapeutic implications. Other less common etiologies of restrictive heart disease such as iron deposition or endomyocardial fibrosis (**Figure 16.26**) can also be accurately identified with CMR.

Constrictive Pericarditis

Constrictive pericarditis can be idiopathic as well as the end result of virtually any progressive inflammatory pericarditis process. The diagnostic standard of pericardial constriction is equalization of end-diastolic pressures in all cardiac chambers due to the pressure exerted by the thickened, and/or inflamed pericardium as well as increased ventricular interdependence. It is important to distinguish this entity from restrictive cardiomyopathies, which can present similarly, because patients with constrictive pericarditis, unlike those with restrictive cardiomyopathy, may benefit from

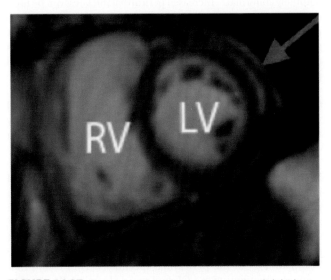

FIGURE 16.27 Short-axis view with prominent pericardial thickening (*arrow*) in a patient with constrictive pericarditis. LV, left ventricle; RV, right ventricle.

pericardiectomy or anti-inflammatory therapy. CMR can assess the thickness of the pericardium; the presence of pericardial edema, effusion and inflammation; as well as demonstrate exaggerated ventricular interdependence. Other sequelae of constriction that support the diagnosis may also be seen, such as a dilated inferior vena cava and pleural effusions.

CMR is well suited for direct quantification of pericardial thickness (**Figure 16.27**). Normal pericardial thickness in CMR

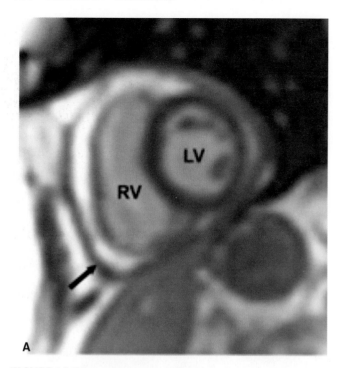
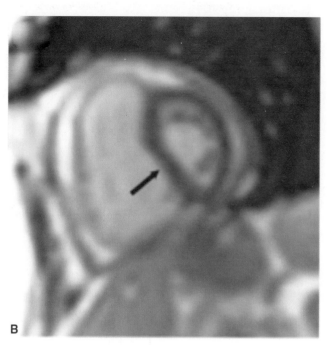

FIGURE 16.28 Expiratory (A) and inspiratory (B) short-axis views in a patient with pericardial constriction, demonstrating prominent flattening of the interventricular septum (*arrow* in B) with inspiration. Note also the thickened pericardium (*arrow* in A). LV, left ventricle; RV, right ventricle.

(due to limitations in spatial resolution) is 1 to 2 mm. A thickness of 3 mm is considered borderline, whereas ≥4 mm is considered definitely abnormal.[13] Increased pericardial thickness can be focal or diffuse. The most common pattern of thickening includes prominence over the right heart as well as the atrioventricular groove. It is important to realize that constriction can occur with normal pericardial thickness in the presence of focally inflamed pericardium that significantly impairs filling. Similarly, the presence of pericardial thickening is not synonymous with constriction. Constrictive physiology can be assessed with CMR as increased ventricular interdependence with respiration, manifested by marked inspiratory flattening of the interventricular septum during free-breathing cine imaging (**Figure 16.28**).[13]

As in the case of acute pericarditis (see section "Cardiac Magnetic Resonance in Acute Chest Pain"), increased T2 signal intensity (compatible with edema) and post-contrast LGE in the pericardium (**Figure 16.29**) are indicative of active inflammation and can be seen in constrictive effusive pericarditis. Zurick et al[27] studied 25 patients with constrictive pericarditis who underwent pericardiectomy, imaging them with CMR and examining the histopathology of the pericardial specimens. They found that a subset of patients with LGE had more chronic inflammation and fibroblastic proliferation. These patients often had increased pericardial thickness compared to patients with a fibrotic, less inflamed pericardium. These findings may help guide treatment and identify patients who may benefit from anti-inflammatory therapies in lieu of immediate surgical treatment.[27]

CMR can help not only diagnose constriction but also provide important prognostic information. Aquaro et al[28] studied 70 patients with clinical suspicion of constrictive hemodynamics on echocardiography and/or catheterization. Constrictive pericarditis was present in 53 patients, whereas 12 had active inflammation, suggestive of a transient constrictive process. LGE was correlated with adverse events.[28]

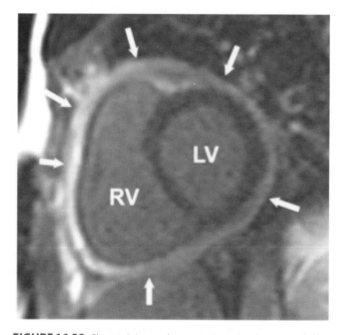

FIGURE 16.29 Short-axis image demonstrating extensive pericardial late gadolinium enhancement (*arrows*) in a patient with constrictive pericarditis. LV, left ventricle; RV, right ventricle.

Right Ventricular Dilatation

Dilatation involving only or predominantly the RV can be seen in ARVC (see section "Cardiac Magnetic Resonance in Ventricular Arrhythmias"), and in RV pressure or volume overload. In RV pressure overload (pulmonary hypertension, stenosis, and embolism), RV dilatation, hypertrophy (if chronic), predominantly systolic septal flattening and, eventually, reduced RV ejection

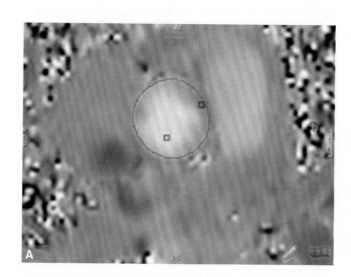

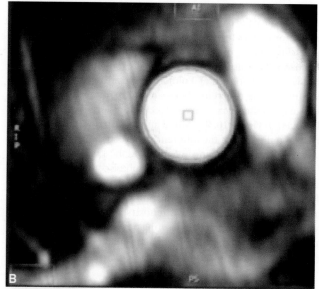

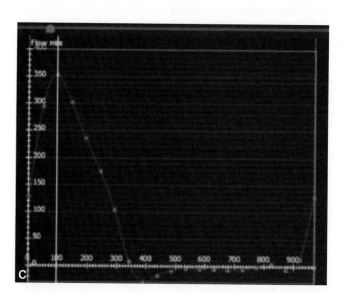

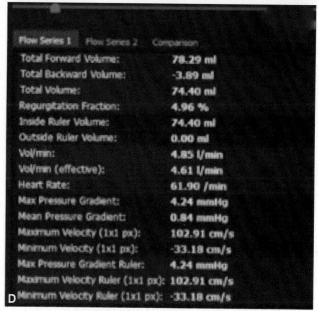

FIGURE 16.30 Phase-contrast imaging demonstrating a cross-section of the ascending aorta (*green contours*) in both the (A) velocity map and (B) anatomic reconstruction. C, Integration of the velocities within the aortic area enables determination of flow throughout the cardiac cycle and (D) quantification of parameters such as output, stroke volume, or degree of regurgitation. For example, the regurgitant fraction in this case is 5%.

fraction can all be identified with CMR and have been linked to impaired outcome.[29] Although identification of pulmonary embolism with MRA is feasible, CT is usually preferred for this application because of increased accuracy and speed of acquisition. RV volume overload is characterized by RV dilatation and dysfunction without hypertrophy and predominantly diastolic flattening of the interventricular septum. A common cause of RV volume overload is right-sided valvular regurgitation, such as can be seen in carcinoid heart disease. Both pulmonary and tricuspid insufficiency can be accurately quantified with CMR. If no valvular regurgitation is present, a systemic-to-pulmonary shunt should be suspected. CMR is well suited to depict shunts that may not be readily identified with echocardiography such as some ventricular and atrial septal defects, anomalous pulmonary vein drainage, or patent ductus arteriosus. CMR is the most accurate

noninvasive modality for the quantification of shunt severity, which is accomplished by measuring systemic (aortic) and pulmonary output using phase-contrast imaging as described here.

FLOW IMAGING—VALVULAR HEART DISEASE

Phase-contrast (or flow) imaging is a technique that can quantify blood velocity and flow within a vessel and that, when applied to the pulmonary artery or the aorta, can respectively provide right- and left-sided stroke volume/output **(Figure 16.30)**.

As indicated, the difference between the two is used in congenital abnormalities to calculate the Qp/Qs. In addition, phase-contrast imaging in the same locations can be employed to assess valvular heart disease. Evaluation of valvular abnormalities is rarely the primary indication for CMR, so a detailed description of available techniques is beyond the scope of this chapter. Nonetheless, valvular assessment is appropriate if the patient is undergoing CMR for other reasons, or in situations where test results are discordant or echocardiography may be limited (eg, quantification of pulmonary regurgitation, differentiation of bicuspid from trileaflet valves, identification of sub- or supravalvular stenoses, etc). Pulmonary and aortic regurgitation are measured as the difference between anterograde and retrograde flows in the pulmonary artery and ascending aorta, respectively (as illustrated in **Figure 16.30**). Mitral and tricuspid regurgitation are graded on the basis of the difference between the LV or RV stroke volume calculated with cine imaging, and the stroke volume in the aorta or pulmonary artery measured by phase contrast. Preliminary data indicate meaningful prognostic value of CMR-based indices of aortic and mitral regurgitation, although further confirmatory studies are needed. Finally, valve stenosis severity can be quantified by direct valve planimetry or measuring peak transvalvular gradients in a manner comparable to Doppler ultrasound (although gradients tend to be underestimated with CMR).

MISCELLANEOUS

CARDIAC CAUSES OF HYPOTENSION—BEYOND HEART FAILURE

In the reasonably stable patient with unexplained hypotension, and in the appropriate clinical scenario, CMR may be helpful to investigate potential underlying etiologies. A possible cause of unexplained hypotension in the CCU patient includes pericardial effusion and tamponade. Although this is more readily and efficiently evaluated with ultrasound, localized effusions or pericardial hematomas such as those seen after cardiac surgery may be difficult to identify on echocardiography. In addition, if CMR is performed in a patient with pericardial effusion, fluid signal characteristics can provide gross characterization on whether fluid is simple (ie, transudate) or complex (hemorrhagic, purulent, etc).[13]

Dynamic LV outflow tract obstruction can also cause hypotension, particularly in the postoperative settings after mitral valve replacement, or in patients with HCM, hypovolemia, and/or increased inotropic state. This complication is again usually identified with echocardiography, but CMR can be considered as an alternative if the ultrasound is not diagnostic.

ADULT CONGENITAL HEART DISEASE

Although a relatively uncommon indication for admission in the CCU, the increasing population of adults with surgically corrected complex congenital heart disease is likely to result in an increasing number of patients presenting with decompensated HF, arrhythmias, or thromboembolic disease.

As mentioned in section "Cardiac Magnetic Resonance in Heart Failure," CMR can be used to quantify the severity of systemic-to-pulmonary shunting, including Eisenmenger physiology, in simple and complex disorders. Additional important roles of CMR in these patients include the quantification of the volumes and function of the RV or the systemic ventricle, the evaluation of patency of surgical baffles and conduits, and the assessment of extracardiac structures such as the pulmonary arteries that can be difficult to study with echocardiography.

Regarding some specific malformations, Ebstein anomaly can present with right-sided HF, and the abnormal insertion of the tricuspid leaflets into the RV can be characterized with echocardiography and/or CMR. Patients with a repaired tetralogy of Fallot often develop RV dilatation and systolic dysfunction secondary to significant pulmonary insufficiency. CMR can provide absolute quantification of regurgitation severity, and guide the optimal timing of surgical or percutaneous pulmonary valve implantation before irreversible RV deterioration occurs. In addition, the presence of an RV scar has been linked to an increased risk of HF and ventricular arrhythmias. Patients with corrected transposition may develop dilatation and dysfunction of the systemic right ventricle in cases of atrial baffles, or narrowing of the pulmonary and reimplanted coronary arteries after arterial switch operations. Finally, in patients with a single-ventricle physiology, CMR can be used to determine ventricular performance (including dilatation, dysfunction, and LGE), patency of the Fontan circulation, and presence of cardiac or venous thrombi that is a common complication of associated chronic venous stasis.

CARDIAC MASSES

CMR can be very useful in the diagnostic evaluation of a cardiac mass, and in the differentiation between benign and malignant tumors. The most common primary cardiac tumors are benign, and they include myxomas, lipomas, and papillary fibroelastomas. Myxomas are mobile, pedunculated masses commonly in the atria and frequently attached to the interatrial septum **(Figure 16.31)**.

Fibroelastomas are valvular tumors that are small (<1 cm) and commonly involve the aortic side of the aortic valve. Cardiac lipomas are usually in the epicardial space, slow growing, and should be distinguished from the more prevalent lipomatous hypertrophy of the interatrial septum. The most common primary malignant cardiac mass is angiosarcoma, which classically involves the right atrium with extension into adjacent structures (pericardium, with associated pericardial effusion). Secondary tumors are much more common than primary cardiac tumors, and they involve the heart or pericardium either via direct invasion (lung and renal cell carcinoma) or by hematogenous spread (breast cancer, melanoma).

CMR offers several advantages in the imaging of cardiac masses over echocardiography. The combination of high resolution with a wide field of view can help define anatomy of the mass, attachment site, and adjacent structures. For example, the presence of a large pericardial effusion, lymphadenopathy, or involvement of more than one cardiac chamber or other mediastinal structures is consistent with a malignant process. The high temporal resolution of CMR (albeit less than that of echocardiography) can help assess mobility of the mass. Most importantly, CMR can delineate tissue characterization with the use of T1-weighted, T2-weighted, and fat-saturation sequences. With IV contrast administration and evaluation of first-pass perfusion, CMR can demonstrate vascularity of a mass, and LGE allows further tissue characterization **(Figure 16.32)**. The post-contrast inversion time (TI) scout images are also helpful, and a combination of these findings can narrow the differential diagnosis (see subsequent text).

In the CCU setting, one of the most relevant applications of CMR for cardiac masses is the differentiation between tumor and thrombus. This is important in patients who present with ischemic cardioembolic stroke with underlying atrial fibrillation, prior MI (see section "Cardiac Magnetic Resonance in Acute Chest Pain"), LV aneurysm, rheumatic heart disease, or DCM. In such patients, several findings can identify thrombus with reasonable accuracy, as demonstrated in a recent retrospective CMR analysis

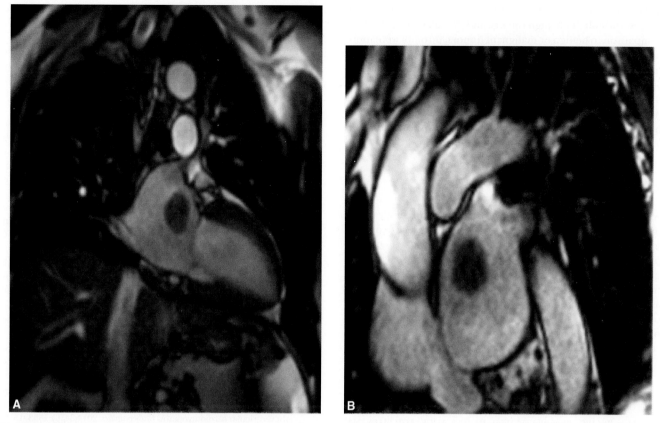

FIGURE 16.31 Two-chamber view demonstrating a left atrial myxoma (A). Short-axis stack at the level of the atria showing the large mass in the left atrium (B). Pathology confirmed the diagnosis of myxoma.

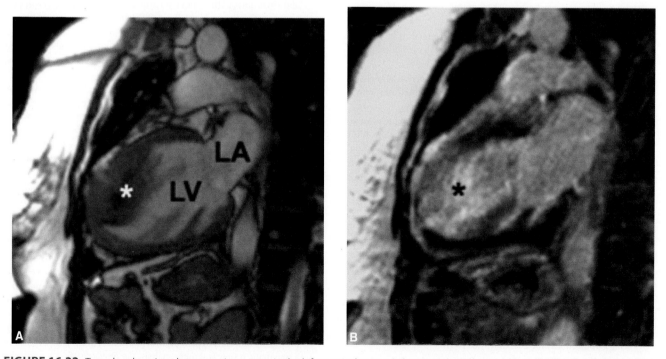

FIGURE 16.32 Two-chamber view demonstrating a mass in the left ventricular apex (*white asterisk*, A). Two-chamber view illustrating that the mass is a vascular structure on long TI imaging (B). Contrast this with the avascular thrombus in Figure 16.11. Pathology was consistent with a hamartoma. LA, left atrium; LV, left ventricle.

of 116 patients with a definite cardiac mass.[30] In this study there were 84 thrombi, 17 benign tumors, and 25 malignant tumors. In comparison to benign or malignant tumors, thrombi were more often smaller, more homogeneous and less mobile. On the other hand, tumors were more often hyperintense on T2-weighted imaging, first-pass perfusion, and LGE imaging when compared to thrombi. A key distinguishing characteristic with 95% accuracy was demonstrated on the TI scout images, where thrombi appeared hyperintense or isointense with short TI, and hypointense with long TI, whereas tumors demonstrated the opposite behavior.[30]

CONCLUSION

As demonstrated in this chapter, CMR is an increasingly useful imaging modality that can help diagnose and direct treatment in patients in the CCU. CMR can assist in the diagnosis of ACS, provide excellent tissue characterization, lend insights into HF etiology, precisely quantify LV and RV volumes and ejection fractions, demonstrate intracardiac shunts with precision, and assist with the identification of extracardiac structures, among other capabilities. Although not available at all cardiac centers because of its expense, it is a valuable tool when performed and read by experienced physicians.

REFERENCES

1. Hundley WG, Bluemke DA, Finn JP, et al. ACCF/ACR/AHA/NASCI/SCMR 2010 expert consensus document on cardiovascular magnetic resonance: a report of the American College of Cardiology Foundation Task Force on Expert Consensus Documents. *J Am Coll Cardiol.* 2010;55(23):2614–2662.

2. Reiter T, Ritter O, Prince MR, et al. Minimizing risk of nephrogenic systemic fibrosis in cardiovascular magnetic resonance. *J Cardiovasc Magn Reson.* 2012;14:31.

3. Kwong RY, Schussheim AE, Rekhraj S, et al. Detecting acute coronary syndrome in the emergency department with cardiac magnetic resonance imaging. *Circulation.* 2003;107(4):531–537.

4. Plein S, Greenwood JP, Ridgway JP, et al. Assessment of non-ST-segment elevation acute coronary syndromes with cardiac magnetic resonance imaging. *J Am Coll Cardiol.* 2004;44(11):2173–2181.

5. wwHombach V, Grebe O, Merkle N, et al. Sequelae of acute myocardial infarction regarding cardiac structure and function and their prognostic significance as assessed by magnetic resonance imaging. *Eur Heart J.* 2005;26(6):549–557.

6. Cury RC, Shash K, Nagurney JT, et al. Cardiac magnetic resonance with T2-weighted imaging improves detection of patients with acute coronary syndrome in the emergency department. *Circulation.* 2008;118(8):837–844.

7. Eitel I, Desch S, de Waha S, et al. Long-term prognostic value of myocardial salvage assessed by cardiovascular magnetic resonance in acute reperfused myocardial infarction. *Heart.* 2011;97(24):2038–2045.

8. Kim RJ, Wu E, Rafael A, et al. The use of contrast-enhanced magnetic resonance imaging to identify reversible myocardial dysfunction. *N Engl J Med.* 2000;343(20):1445–1453.

9. Gouda S, Abdelwahab A, Salem M, et al. Scar characteristics for prediction of ventricular arrhythmia in ischemic cardiomyopathy. *Pacing Clin Electrophysiol.* 2015;38(3):311–318.

10. Weinsaft JW, Kim RJ, Ross M, et al. Contrast-enhanced anatomic imaging as compared to contrast-enhanced tissue characterization for detection of left ventricular thrombus. *JACC Cardiovasc Imaging.* 2009;2(8):969–979.

11. Friedrich MG, Sechtem U, Schulz-Menger J, et al. Cardiovascular magnetic resonance in myocarditis: a JACC White Paper. *J Am Coll Cardiol.* 2009;53(17):1475–1487.

12. Lurz P, Luecke C, Eitel I, et al. Comprehensive cardiac magnetic resonance imaging in patients with suspected myocarditis: the MyoRacer-Trial. *J Am Coll Cardiol.* 2016;67(15):1800–1811.

13. Bogaert J, Francone M. Pericardial disease: value of CT and MR imaging. *Radiology.* 2013;267(2):340–356.

14. Eitel I, von Knobelsdorff-Brenkenhoff F, Bernhardt P, et al. Clinical characteristics and cardiovascular magnetic resonance findings in stress (takotsubo) cardiomyopathy. *JAMA.* 2011;306(3):277–286.

15. Baliga RR, Nienaber CA, Bossone E, et al. The role of imaging in aortic dissection and related syndromes. *JACC Cardiovasc Imaging.* 2014;7(4):406–424.

16. Disertori M, Rigoni M, Pace N, et al. Myocardial fibrosis assessment by LGE Is a powerful predictor of ventricular tachyarrhythmias in ischemic and nonischemic LV dysfunction: a meta-analysis. *JACC Cardiovasc Imaging.* 2016;9(9):1046–1055.

17. Chan RH, Maron BJ, Olivotto I, et al. Prognostic value of quantitative contrast-enhanced cardiovascular magnetic resonance for the evaluation of sudden death risk in patients with hypertrophic cardiomyopathy. *Circulation.* 2014;130(6):484–495.

18. Birnie DH, Nery PB, Ha AC, et al. Cardiac sarcoidosis. *J Am Coll Cardiol.* 2016;68(4):411–421.

19. Coleman GC, Shaw PW, Balfour PC, et al. Prognostic Value of Myocardial Scarring on CMR in Patients With Cardiac Sarcoidosis. *JACC Cardiovasc Imaging.* 2017;10(4):411–420.

20. Rastegar N, Burt JR, Corona-Villalobos CP, et al. Cardiac MR findings and potential diagnostic pitfalls in patients evaluated for arrhythmogenic right ventricular cardiomyopathy. *Radiographics.* 2014;34(6):1553–1570.

21. Liu T, Pursnani A, Sharma UC, et al. Effect of the 2010 task force criteria on reclassification of cardiovascular magnetic resonance criteria for arrhythmogenic right ventricular cardiomyopathy. *J Cardiovasc Magn Reson.* 2014;16:47.

22. te Riele AS, Tandri H, Bluemke DA. Arrhythmogenic right ventricular cardiomyopathy (ARVC): cardiovascular magnetic resonance update. *J Cardiovasc Magn Reson.* 2014;16:50.

23. Cheong BYC, Muthupillai R, Wilson JM, et al. Prognostic significance of delayed-enhancement magnetic resonance imaging: survival of 857 patients with and without left ventricular dysfunction. *Circulation.* 2009;120(21):2069–2076.

24. Kuruvilla S, Adenaw N, Katwal AB, et al. Late gadolinium enhancement on cardiac magnetic resonance predicts adverse cardiovascular outcomes in nonischemic cardiomyopathy: a systematic review and meta-analysis. *Circ Cardiovasc Imaging.* 2014;7(2):250–258.

25. Rommel KP, von Roeder M, Latuscynski K, et al. Extracellular volume fraction for characterization of patients with heart failure and preserved ejection fraction. *J Am Coll Cardiol.* 2016;67(15):1815–1825.

26. Fontana M, Pica S, Reant P, et al. Prognostic value of late gadolinium enhancement cardiovascular magnetic resonance in cardiac amyloidosis. *Circulation.* 2015;132(16):1570–1579.

27. Zurick AO, Bolen MA, Kwon DH, et al. Pericardial delayed hyperenhancement with CMR imaging in patients with constrictive pericarditis undergoing surgical pericardiectomy: a case series with histopathological correlation. *JACC Cardiovasc Imaging.* 2011;4(11):1180–1191.

28. Aquaro GD, Barison A, Cagnolo A, et al. Role of tissue characterization by Cardiac Magnetic Resonance in the diagnosis of constrictive pericarditis. *Int J Cardiovasc Imaging.* 2015;31(5):1021–1031.

29. Baggen VJ, Leiner T, Post MC, et al. Cardiac magnetic resonance findings predicting mortality in patients with pulmonary arterial hypertension: a systematic review and meta-analysis. *Eur Radiol.* 2016.

30. Pazos-López P, Pozo E, Siqueira ME, et al. Value of CMR for the differential diagnosis of cardiac masses. *JACC Cardiovasc Imaging.* 2014;7(9):896–905.

Patient and Family Information for: CARDIAC MAGNETIC RESONANCE IMAGING

MRI stands for magnetic resonance imaging. Cardiac MRI is a safe and painless imaging modality that uses a strong magnet to create pictures of the inner structures of the heart and help the referring physician determine many aspects of heart health. Unlike other types of imaging, MRI does not use harmful ionizing radiations such as X-rays or gamma rays. It can accurately determine the function of both sides of the heart, identify problems with valves, assess the presence of scar tissue in the heart, and provide information on many more structural and functional aspects of the heart.

PREPARATION FOR THE PROCEDURE

Some imaging facilities request that patients do not eat or drink anything before the procedure. It is important to check with the imaging facility to determine what their pre-MRI dietary guidelines are.

The magnetic field of an MRI machine extends beyond its physical boundaries and usually includes the room where the machine is placed. Any metallic object placed inside or close to the magnetic field can interfere with its function. As a result, jewelry and metal accessories, cell phones, electronic devices, and wallets containing credit or debit cards should be removed before the examination and preferably left at home.

A few types of metal implants are not safe for cardiac MRIs. Certain types of metal coils in brain aneurysms, cochlear implants (hearing aid implants placed inside the inner ear), "Triggerfish" contact lenses, insulin pumps, defibrillators, and pacemakers are not MRI compatible. Virtually any metal-containing material can interfere with an MRI. These include, but are not limited to, bullets or shrapnels left in place and metallic rods, plates, or screws used in fixing fractured bones. All implantable and external devices should be reported to the physician before undergoing a cardiac MRI.

The examination requires that patients are able to lie flat for 30 to 60 minutes and hold their breath for 10 to 15 seconds multiple times over the course of the examination. If a patient has any difficulty lying flat or is unable to hold his/her breath, the referring physician should be informed.

Some patients will need injectable contrast with the examination depending on the clinical indication. The contrast used in cardiac MRI examinations is a gadolinium-based agent, which is distinctly different from the contrast used in CT scans. It should not be used if the patient's kidney function is very low. Gadolinium-based contrast agents have a much lower incidence of allergic reactions compared to iodinated contrast agents used in CT scans. If the patient has had an allergy to the iodinated contrast used in CT scans and has any other allergies, the physician should be informed to determine the best course of action.

If the patients have claustrophobia, which is a fear of being in enclosed spaces, they should alert their physician because some MRIs can appear to the patients as small and enclosed. In some cases, the physician may prescribe a medication to help with the claustrophobia.

Patients who are pregnant or think that they may be pregnant should alert their physician before having an MRI. There have been limited studies to determine the safety of an MRI in pregnant patients. The decision to do the examination is made individually in each case after careful consultation between the physician conducting the MRI and the referring physician.

THE DAY OF THE EXAMINATION

MRI units vary in size but are often quite large, with a cylinder-shaped tube where the patient will lie down. Some MRI units are open on the sides, "open MRI," whereas others are closed. Closed MRIs can make some patients claustrophobic. Many imaging facilities have headphones and some have videos that the patient can watch during the examination to ease the claustrophobia. The patients are given a handheld device that they can squeeze if they feel uncomfortable at any point during the examination. This device alerts the technician to stop the examination and come into the room to check on the patient. The MRI technician will be able to speak with, and hear, the patient from the control room. While the patient will be alone in the MRI room, the control room is immediately adjacent to the MRI room with large windows so that the technician can see the patient at all times.

The patients will have stickers attached to their chest that will connect to a monitor to observe the heart rate and correlate the imaging with the cardiac cycle to obtain the best possible images. The examination has many sequences that require the patient to hold his/her breath for 7 to 8 seconds at a time. The breath-holding instructions will be clearly given by the technician. If the patient becomes tired with the breath holding, some sequences can be obtained with normal breathing, but this may affect the quality of the images.

Some patients will have an IV line placed if they need contrast. A series of images are often taken before the contrast is given, with another series of images taken afterward. The gadolinium-based contrast is usually well tolerated, but may make some patients feel warm, nauseous, and/or leave them with a metallic taste in their mouth. If the patient experiences any itching, hives, difficulty breathing, he/she should immediately press the handheld button and alert the technician.

The entire examination typically lasts between 30 and 60 minutes depending on the sequences that need to be obtained and whether contrast is being used.

AFTER THE EXAMINATION

After the examination, the patients can go about their normal day as long as they did not get any sedating medications. If they were given medication to ease anxiety, they should be accompanied by another person who would be able to safely take the patient home and monitor them for a few hours. The radiologist or cardiologist interpreting the examination will analyze the images and send a report to the referring physician. The referring physician will share the results with the patient. The time of reporting varies according to the policies at each imaging facility.

Noah Moss
Sean P. Pinney

17

Mechanical Circulatory Support in the Cardiac Care Unit

Cardiogenic shock refers to the disorder where cardiac dysfunction results in inadequate end-organ perfusion. The classic condition involves systemic hypotension and symptoms or signs of organ hypoperfusion despite adequate intravascular volume. Initial management is focused on treatment of reversible causes such as revascularization when appropriate in acute coronary syndromes. Following this or simultaneously, inotropic and vasopressor agents are administered to improve hemodynamics. Despite these measures, adequate perfusion to prevent end-organ dysfunction is often not restored or able to be maintained. As a result, morbidity and mortality from this disorder remain high, with a 30-day mortality, across many studies, exceeding 40%.[1] This has led to the development of mechanical circulatory support (MCS) devices that have been proven to reverse the poor hemodynamic profile of cardiogenic shock. It is important to note that although use of MCS clearly improves hemodynamics, data demonstrating a mortality benefit are lacking.

The decision to initiate MCS must not be taken lightly. Its use demands substantial resource allocation and carries tremendous cost. In addition, there is a high rate of serious complications when MCS is employed. Appropriate patient selection is of utmost importance. It is imperative that patients for whom temporary MCS is considered are thought to have a long-term option for survival, because temporary MCS is merely a bridging therapy. Therefore, the medical providers must have a high index of suspicion that survival with the capacity for meaningful recovery of end-organ function and quality of life is possible. This may be accomplished by eventual improvement of native cardiac function, by placement of long-term MCS or through cardiac transplantation.

The MCS devices currently available differ in several ways, including the level of support provided, hemodynamic effects, site of vascular access, vessel size required for delivery, and associated complications (**Table 17.1**). In this chapter, we will discuss the most commonly used devices and highlight their important distinctive features.

INTRA-AORTIC BALLOON PUMP

The intra-aortic balloon pump (IABP) was the first mechanical device developed, and its use has become widespread since its inception in the 1960s. It is placed in the descending thoracic aorta and acts by balloon inflation during diastole and active deflation in systole (see **Figure 17.1**). This results in a higher perfusion pressure in the coronary arteries during diastole and a reduction in left ventricular afterload during systole. The hemodynamic effects are variable and depend on the position in the aorta, heart rate, rhythm, aortic compliance, and systemic resistance. Overall, the potential hemodynamic effects include an increase in cardiac output (CO) of approximately 500 cc minute, an increase in mean arterial blood pressure (MAP), and a reduction in left ventricular end-diastolic pressure (LVEDP) with a resulting decrease in left ventricle (LV) wall stress and myocardial oxygen demand. Given the mechanism of action already described, the use of IABP has generally been studied in patients with cardiogenic shock resulting from myocardial infarction. The largest randomized trial evaluating the use of IABP in this group of patients was the IABP-SHOCK II Trial.[1] Six hundred patients with cardiogenic shock complicating acute myocardial infarction expected to undergo early revascularization were randomly assigned to IABP or usual care. No difference in the primary end point of 30-day all-cause mortality was found. Several smaller studies and meta-analyses have failed to show convincing evidence of a mortality benefit with the use of IABP in this setting. Of note, some benefit has been demonstrated with the use of an IABP in patients with myocardial infarction complicated by shock treated with thrombolytic therapy.[2,3]

CLINICAL USE

The IABP is typically placed in the femoral artery, although placement in the left axillary/subclavian artery has been used when long-term support is planned. Its tip is advanced to the descending thoracic aorta up to the level of the carina and at least 2 cm below the aortic knob. An IABP should not be placed in patients with more than mild aortic regurgitation, because the degree of regurgitation will be increased by counterpulsation from the device. Aortic pathology such as dissection or a significant aneurysm would preclude the insertion of an IABP because of the risk of furthering aortic disease. In addition, severe peripheral vascular disease (or small vasculature) will limit its use in view of the development of ipsilateral limb ischemia.

A chest X-ray should be performed daily to confirm proper position. Distal pulses must be regularly checked following placement to screen for limb ischemia. The pressure waveform should be reviewed to ensure proper device function and timing (see **Figure 17.2**).

TABLE 17.1	Characteristics of Mechanical Circulatory Support Devices			
DEVICE	**MECHANISM**	**HEMODYNAMIC SUPPORT (L/min)**	**DEVICE SIZE (Fr)**	**INSERTION**
IABP	Pneumatic	0–1	8	Percutaneous: femoral or axillary artery
TandemHeart	Centrifugal	4	Inflow 21 Outflow 12–17	Percutaneous: inflow femoral vein (to left atrium via transseptal puncture), outflow femoral artery
Impella 2.5	Axial	2.5	13	Percutaneous: femoral artery
Impella CP	Axial	4	14	Percutaneous: femoral artery
Impella 5.0	Axial	5	23	Surgical cutdown: femoral or axillary artery
Impella RP	Axial	4	22	Percutaneous: femoral vein
VA-ECMO	Centrifugal	>4.5	Inflow 18–21 Outflow 15–22	Percutaneous ± cutdown: inflow femoral vein, outflow femoral artery
Durable LVAD	Axial or Centrifugal	>7	NA	Surgical: inflow from LV, outflow ascending aorta

Fr, French; IABP, intra-aortic balloon pump; LV, left ventricular; LVAD, left ventricular assist device; L/min, liters per minute; VA-ECMO, venoarterial-extracorporeal membrane oxygenation.

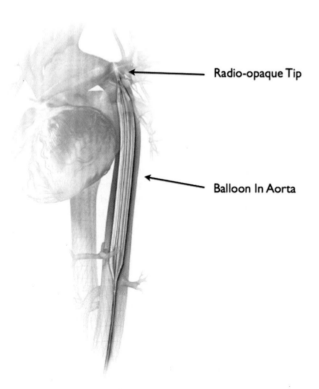

FIGURE 17.1 Intra-aortic balloon pump. It is shown placed in the descending thoracic aorta below the aortic knob. The radio-opaque tip is used to assess placement by X-ray.

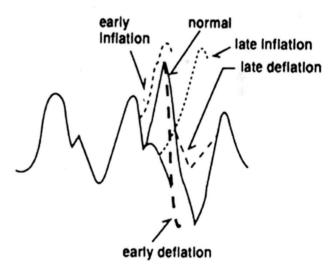

FIGURE 17.2 IABP tracing displaying normal and improper timings of balloon inflation. In a normal waveform, balloon inflation occurs at or slightly above the dicrotic notch, which represents the onset of diastole after aortic valve closure. Deflation occurs during isovolumetric contraction, just before the aortic valve opens. Early inflation, balloon inflation before aortic valve closure, can result in premature aortic valve closure and a reduced cardiac output. Late inflation, where the inflation point follows the dicrotic notch, leads to a reduction in coronary perfusion pressure. Early deflation will prevent the intended decrease in assisted systolic pressure and the resulting afterload reduction from occurring. Late deflation, occurring following aortic valve opening, will increase afterload and myocardial oxygen demand. IABP, intra-aortic balloon pump.

The use of anticoagulation with IABP support can be weighed in the context of patient-specific factors or based on institutional guidelines. Studies evaluating the routine use of anticoagulation have not demonstrated a reduced risk of thrombus formation, thromboembolism, or limb ischemia. Only an increased risk of bleeding has been found.[4]

COMPLICATIONS

The most common complications of IABP use are vascular in nature. These include limb ischemia and hemorrhage from the access site. A rare but serious complication resulting from the IABP is compromised perfusion in the aorta, leading to visceral (including renal) and spinal cord ischemia. These can be mitigated by proper placement, as discussed above.

INDICATIONS

The 2013 ACC/AHA guidelines for the management of ST-elevation myocardial infarction (STEMI) state, as a class IIa (level of evidence B) recommendation, that "the use of an IABP can be useful for patients with cardiogenic shock after STEMI who do not quickly stabilize with pharmacological therapy."[5] In addition, they highlight its use as a temporizing measure in mechanical complications of shock such as papillary muscle rupture with resulting mitral regurgitation and ventricular septal rupture.

TANDEMHEART

The TandemHeart (Cardiac Assist, Inc, Pittsburgh, PA) percutaneous assist device is a left atrial to femoral artery bypass continuous flow centrifugal pump system designed to provide complete hemodynamic support. It has been studied in a randomized fashion for patients presenting with cardiogenic shock caused by ischemic[6] and nonischemic disease.[7] When compared to the IABP it has demonstrated superior hemodynamic effects and, among other parameters, results in larger increases in CO and MAP and a greater reduction in pulmonary capillary wedge pressure (PCWP). It was also evaluated in patients with severe refractory cardiogenic shock, a scenario in which its use would likely be of the greatest benefit, and it was shown to dramatically improve hemodynamic and clinical parameters.[8] No mortality benefit has been demonstrated, but the trials were not adequately powered to evaluate this outcome.

CLINICAL USE

An atrial drainage cannula (21F) is placed in the left atrium by means of a transeptal puncture, and oxygenated blood is drawn from there and returned via a centrifugal pump to an arterial cannula (most often 17 French) in the femoral artery (see **Figure 17.3**). Aortoiliac and femoral angiography is recommended before insertion to assess vessel size, as a 12F bilateral femoral artery access system is available to accommodate smaller vasculature. It is powered by an electromagnetic motor that drives a plastic impeller at a speed of 3000 to 7500 rpm and is capable of delivering flows up to 4.0 L/min. During use, anticoagulation is administered continuously to achieve a target partial thromboplastin time of 65–80 seconds or an activated clotting time (ACT) between 180 and 220 seconds.

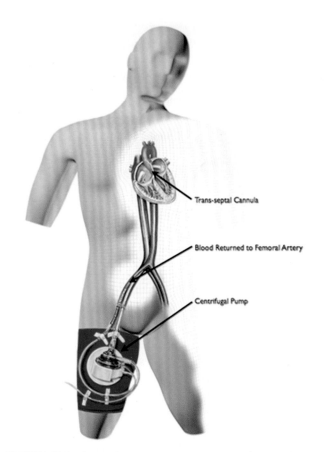

Trans-septal Cannula

Blood Returned to Femoral Artery

Centrifugal Pump

FIGURE 17.3 The TandemHeart percutaneous assist device. A drainage cannula is placed in the left atrium by means of a transseptal puncture, and oxygenated blood is drawn from there and returned via the centrifugal pump to a cannula in the femoral artery.

Despite the impressive hemodynamic benefits observed with the use of TandemHeart, its implementation is ultimately limited by the complexities of device insertion, which can be particularly challenging in emergency situations.

COMPLICATIONS

The most common complications of TandemHeart use are device-related limb ischemia and bleeding. These occur as a result of vascular access site trauma and the development of a coagulopathy. In trials, a high rate of blood transfusions was noted.

INDICATIONS

The 2013 ACC/AHA STEMI guidelines state, as a class IIa (level of evidence C) recommendation, that "LV assist devices for circulatory support may be considered in patients with refractory cardiogenic shock."[5]

The 2013 International Society for Heart and Lung Transplantation (ISHLT) guidelines for MCS state, as a class I (level of evidence C) recommendation, that the use of temporary mechanical support should be strongly considered in patients with multiorgan failure, sepsis, or on mechanical ventilation to allow successful optimization of clinical status and neurologic assessment before placement of a long-term MCSD.[9]

A 2015 clinical expert statement, endorsed by multiple organizations, concludes that patients with acute decompensated heart failure may benefit from early use of percutaneous MCS when they continue to deteriorate despite initial interventions.[10]

IMPELLA

The Impella (Abiomed, Inc, Danvers, MA) families of devices are axial flow pumps that work on the principle of the Archimedes screw. These devices deliver blood from the inlet area, which sits in the LV, through the impeller to the outlet opening in the ascending aorta (**Figure 17.4**). The left-sided Impella device comes in three different sizes that differ on the basis of the degree of support it can deliver. The Impella 2.5 can provide up to 2.5 L/min, the Impella CP can deliver up to 4 L/min, and the Impella 5.0 up to 5 L/min. The family of devices has been shown to improve the hemodynamics of cardiogenic shock by unloading the LV, which results in an increased MAP, reduced myocardial oxygen demand, and a reduced PCWP. The Impella 2.5 is the only device of the group to be studied in a randomized fashion and has been shown to provide greater hemodynamic support compared to the IABP in patients with cardiogenic shock complicating AMI.[11] The Impella 5.0 was evaluated for use in postcardiotomy cardiogenic shock and was found to yield favorable outcomes.[12]

CLINICAL USE

The Impella is inserted via arterial access and is advanced retrograde across the aortic valve until the catheter with a pigtail tip, which helps avoid myocardial injury and ensures a stable position, sits in the LV. The Impella 2.5 and Impella CP can be

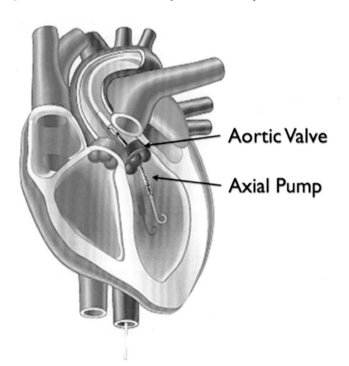

FIGURE 17.4 The Impella axial flow pump. The Impella is advanced retrograde across the aortic valve until the catheter with a pigtail tip sits in the LV. Blood is delivered from the inlet area through the impeller to the outlet area in the ascending aorta. LV, left ventricle.

inserted through a 14Fr introducer sheath using a percutaneous approach via the femoral artery. The Impella 5.0 uses a larger introducer sheath (23Fr) that requires a surgical cutdown for insertion and is often placed in the axillary artery. The Impella devices are typically placed under fluoroscopic guidance in the catheterization laboratory. To optimize device flow and avoid complications, proper positioning of the Impella tip in the LV is of utmost importance. Echocardiography can be used at the patient's bedside to confirm proper positioning of the device in the LV cavity. The degree of support is managed by graduation of pump speed.

The Impella requires sufficient LV preload for proper function, and its use is therefore contraindicated with significant right heart failure. Given the need for the system to cross the aortic valve, a mechanical prosthesis or severe AS precludes its use. It should be avoided when more than mild aortic insufficiency is present because a significant amount of blood that is pumped in the ascending aorta can flow back into the LV and reduce systemic perfusion. As with other devices that require arterial access, severe peripheral vascular disease limits its use. In addition, use of the Impella is contraindicated in the presence of an LV thrombus or a ventricular septal defect.

COMPLICATIONS

Major bleeding at the vascular access site is the most common complication of Impella use. Hemolysis is frequently seen owing to the high rotational speed of the impeller. If the catheter is advanced too far into the LV apex, there is a risk of ventricular arrhythmias and perforation, which may result in pericardial tamponade.[13] Limb ischemia remains a concern given the large arterial sheath required for placement.

INDICATIONS

In general, the recommendations from major society guidelines discuss all temporary mechanical support devices under the same heading. Therefore, the recommendations for Impella use in cardiogenic shock are identical to those listed for the TandemHeart.

The Impella 2.5 has received a separate indication from the FDA for use during high-risk percutaneous coronary interventions (PCI) performed in elective or urgent hemodynamically stable patients with severe coronary artery disease and depressed left ventricular ejection fraction, when a heart team, including a cardiac surgeon, has determined high-risk PCI is the appropriate therapeutic option.

RIGHT VENTRICULAR SUPPORT

Right ventricular failure (RVF) can occur in multiple settings. It can be particularly devastating during the use of left-sided MCS devices because they rely on sufficient LV preload for proper function. The right ventricle (RV) can be placed under exceptional stress during MCS use for several reasons, including the rise in RV preload with normalization of CO, the alteration of normal RV geometry caused by septal shift resulting from LV unloading and an increase in pulmonary vascular resistance, which can typically be seen with critically ill patients and in the postoperative period. The RV often recovers over a short period of time, and patients can typically be stabilized with volume optimization along with the use of inotropes and pulmonary vasodilators. Right-sided MCS devices have been developed for use in RVF refractory to medical therapy. The Impella RP system works on the same principles previously described for the Impella family of pumps and can provide flow greater than 4 L/min at an impeller speed of 33,000 rpm. The device delivers blood from the inlet area, which sits in the inferior vena cava, through the cannula to the outlet opening in the pulmonary artery (PA). Its use was evaluated in a prospective trial comprising patients with RVF complicating left ventricular assist device (LVAD) implant and myocardial infarction or postcardiotomy.[14] Following initiation of support, there was a significant increase in cardiac index (CI) and a reduction in central venous pressure (CVP).

The TandemHeart system, described earlier, has been successfully converted to a right-sided support device. The inflow cannula draws blood from the right atrium (RA), and it is returned to the PA. Analysis of a registry of patients who received the device for management of RV failure found that its use led to an improvement in MAP, CVP, PA systolic pressure, and CI.[15]

CLINICAL USE

The Impella RP is inserted into the femoral vein via a 23Fr sheath and advance to the right heart with its tip passing through the RA, tricuspid valve, and pulmonic valve. During pump operation, an ACT of 160 to 180 is recommended. Its use is contraindicated with right-sided mechanical valves, severe valvular stenosis or regurgitation of the tricuspid or pulmonary valve, and mural thrombus in the RA or vena cava.

The TandemHeart system can be placed percutaneously or surgically. Percutaneous implantation requires two areas of venous cannulation, and this can be accomplished via bifemoral or right internal jugular approaches using 21Fr cannulas. Surgical implantation is performed by direct cannulation of the RA and PA or by peripheral cannulation of the femoral vein and direct cannulation of the PA.

COMPLICATIONS

The most frequent complication with both devices is major bleeding. As described with the Impella systems above, hemolysis is seen with Impella RP use.

INDICATIONS

There are no societal recommendations for use of temporary right-sided mechanical support devices. The Impella RP is FDA approved for use in patients who develop acute right heart failure or decompensation following LVAD implantation, myocardial infarction, heart transplantation, or open-heart surgery.

EXTRACORPOREAL MEMBRANE OXYGENATION

Extracorporeal membrane oxygenation (ECMO) differs from the temporary devices already discussed in that it is able to provide full support in cases of severe biventricular failure. There are two forms of extracorporeal support, veno-venous (VV) and venoarterial (VA). The VV system provides only oxygenation. However, VA ECMO can provide complete cardiopulmonary

support. The system consists of a continuous flow centrifugal pump and a membrane oxygenator (**Figure 17.5**). Blood is aspirated from the RA into the venous inflow cannula and, via the pump, is circulated through the membrane oxygenator. Oxygenated blood is then directed into the arterial circulation via the outflow cannula. ECMO can provide substantial hemodynamic support, with flows up to 6 L per minute, and increased LV afterload, which can have negative consequences discussed later. ECMO has been applied clinically in many forms of circulatory failure, including cardiogenic shock from various etiologies and cardiac arrest, but no randomized controlled trials have been performed to study its use. For the most part, the data supporting its implementation come from prospective and retrospective single center experiences or pooled analysis of this data. In these, it has been suggested that ECMO use improves 30-day survival and neurologic outcomes in the cardiac arrest population but resulted in similar outcomes when compared to other forms of mechanical support, aside from IABP, in the cardiogenic shock patients.[16] When considering these data, one must recognize the nonrandomized nature of these studies and the potential large influence that confounders have on these results.

CLINICAL USE

The appeal of the ECMO system is the ability to provide complete cardiopulmonary support with rapid insertion peripherally at the bedside. A venous inflow cannula (ranging from 15 to 29 Fr) is inserted into the femoral vein and advanced to the RA; this is usually performed under transesophageal echocardiography guidance. The arterial outflow cannula (ranging from 15 to 23Fr) is typically placed in the femoral artery, but other arterial sites of cannulation have been used. Adjusting the rotational speed of the device controls flow, and it should be placed at the lowest speed necessary to provide adequate perfusion. As flow is increased, the afterload rises as well. This results in a reduction in the heart's ability to unload and increases myocardial oxygen demand. In turn, there is an increase in the LVEDP/PCWP that can lead to the development of pulmonary congestion. In addition, it is thought that the unfavorable LV loading conditions created by ECMO use may adversely affect myocardial recovery. Several strategies can be employed to decompress or "vent" the LV when deemed necessary. These include inotropic support, IABP placement, Impella use, atrial septostomy, or direct LA or LV cannulation. When femoral cannulation is employed, arterial blood gases and pulse oximetry should be checked in the right arm, the farthest area from the cannulation site, to confirm uniform oxygenation throughout the arterial system. This is necessary because the ECMO device will preferentially perfuse the lower extremities with its fully saturated blood, whereas blood ejected from the heart will selectively perfuse the brain, coronaries, and upper extremities. This phenomenon can be exacerbated by improvement in native CO and IABP use.

Anticoagulation is necessary to prevent thrombus formation in the system, particularly in the membrane oxygenator, and ACTs are typically maintained between 180 and 250 seconds.

One disadvantage to ECMO use is that a cardiac perfusionist, whose availability is limited at many centers, is required for management of the system. The perfusionist plays an integral role in the ECMO circuit setup, priming, and optimization of settings during use.

VA-ECMO

VV-ECMO

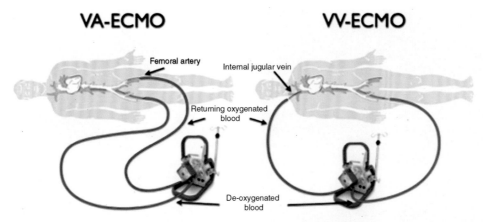

FIGURE 17.5 Diagrammatic representation of peripheral veno-venous (VV-ECMO) and peripheral veno-arterial (VA-ECMO) extracorporeal membrane oxygenation. With VA-ECMO, venous blood is circulated through the membrane oxygenator, and oxygenated blood is directed into the arterial circulation. With VV-ECMO, venous blood flows through the membrane oxygenator, and oxygenated blood is returned to the venous circulation. (From Cove ME, MacLaren G. Clinical review: MCS for cardiogenic shock complicating acute myocardial infarction. *Crit Care.* 2010;14:235.)

COMPLICATIONS

The most frequent complication during ECMO use is hemorrhage that can occur at the sites of cannulation or other. Neurologic complications such as seizures, cerebral infarction, and hemorrhage have been reported. Cardiac thrombus formation, especially when CO remains low, is seen. Renal failure has been observed with a notable oliguric phase following implant. As with the other devices placed peripherally, limb ischemia is of concern, and in order to decrease the occurrence an additional cannula can be placed to perfuse the distal extremity. Given the multiple entry sites and large-size catheters, close monitoring for infectious complications is required.

INDICATIONS

ECMO carries a society recommendation similar to the other forms of percutaneous MCS, but strong consideration should be given to ECMO use when there is significant impairment in respiratory gas exchange.[10]

DURABLE MCS

Implantable MCS devices have become integral to the management of patients with end-stage heart failure. They have been shown to improve both survival and quality of life when compared to traditional care in this group of patients.[17] The newer-generation continuous flow pumps have proven to be more durable and carry a superior adverse event profile than the original pulsatile devices.[18] The two main indications for implantation are bridge to transplantation (BTT) and destination therapy (DT). The hope that these devices would routinely offer a path to recovery has been unrealized because this occurs in few cases.[19] BTT refers to implanting an LVAD to maintain hemodynamic support in those patients who are listed for cardiac transplantation. Given the prolonged wait times for donor organs, bridging is necessary, because many patients would not survive to the time of transplantation. Devices are placed as DT with the intent of providing prolonged support in patients who are ineligible for cardiac transplantation.

Implantation of durable mechanical support devices in patients with cardiogenic shock and multiorgan failure has traditionally been avoided in view of the concern that these critically ill patients would not tolerate the rigors of surgery and extended cardiopulmonary bypass. Registry data have indeed shown that early and midterm survival for patients implanted at INTERMACS profile 1, defined as critical cardiogenic shock, is significantly worse than for less sick patients, but despite the advanced disease state, 1-year survival is reported to be 76%.[20] Some centers have adopted strategies of inserting implantable LVADs as the primary therapy for refractory cardiogenic shock rather than attempts at hemodynamic stabilization with short-term mechanical devices.[21] This approach restores consistent CO to a greater degree and avoids the exposure to the multiple complications associated with the short-term devices.

CLINICAL USE

The two most commonly used commercially available LVADs are the Heartmate II (St. Jude Medical, St. Paul, MN) and the HVAD (Medtronic Inc., Minneapolis, MN). Both pumps consist of a blood inlet, termed the inflow cannula, traditionally placed in the left ventricular apex, and an outlet, termed the outflow cannula, typically placed in the ascending aorta, separated by a single rotating element that imparts energy on the blood to increase flow and pressure. There is a percutaneous driveline connected to the LVAD pump that is tunneled outside the body and linked to a controller that is powered by connecting battery packs (**Figure 17.6**). The primary differences between the two devices lie in the mechanics of the rotating element and implant location. The Heartmate II is an axial flow pump whose impeller with its housing is positioned below the left rectus abdominis muscle or in the peritoneal cavity. The HeartWare HVAD is a centrifugal flow device with the impeller and its housing in the pericardial space (**Figure 17.7**). Of note, the Heartmate 3 (St. Jude Medical, Inc., St. Paul, MN), a centrifugal flow intrapericardial pump, is currently being studied in a clinical trial. Because of the continuous LV unloading and flow generated by these devices, patients most often lack a palpable pulse. Measurement of systemic pressure requires the use of a doppler device and manual blood pressure cuff, and in critically ill patients, the use of an

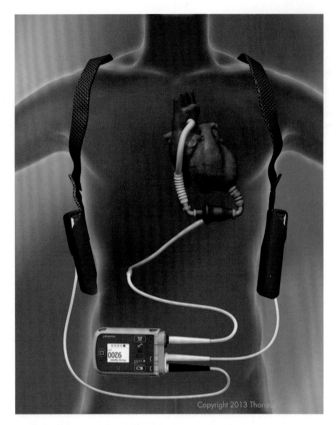

FIGURE 17.6 Components of a ventricular assist device system. Pictured here is the Thoratec Heartmate II Left Ventricular Assist Device (HM-II LVAD). A, Pump, B, batteries, C, system controller, D, driveline, E, position of inflow cannula, F, position of outflow cannula. (Permission requested from Thoratec Corporation of SJM.)

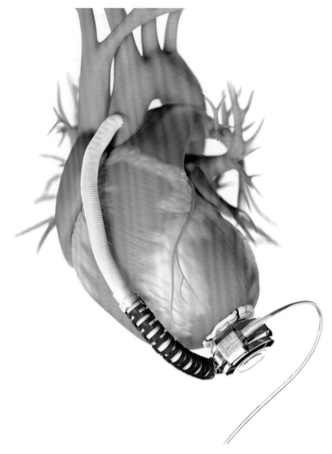

FIGURE 17.7 Position of an intrapericardial ventricular assist device. Pictured here is the HeartWare HVAD system. A, Pump, B, driveline, C, position of outflow cannula. (Permission requested from HeartWare.)

arterial line is prudent. Patients are chronically maintained on warfarin with a goal international normalized ratio in the range of 2 to 3 and antiplatelet therapy to prevent device thrombosis.

COMPLICATIONS

Several serious complications, including stroke, bleeding, and pump thrombosis, have been noted to occur both in the initial trials and in registry data.[20] Readmissions are common, and some adverse events require management in the CCU.

Bleeding requiring transfusion of packed red blood cells, most often from a gastrointestinal source, occurs at high rates. Formation of arteriovenous malformations and acquired von Willenbrand syndrome are thought to be responsible for these events. These typically resolve with brief periods off anticoagulation or with endoscopic treatment but can continue to occur at high rates in certain individuals.

Pump thrombosis can present with a wide range of clinical manifestations, depending on the extent of the clot. In its most benign form, only elevated markers of hemolysis with little change in device function or patient symptoms are found. On the other end of the spectrum, severe hemolysis with pump failure and resulting heart failure can occur. Features suggestive of thrombosis include signs of hemolysis such as red or reddish-brown urine, elevated serum lactate dehydrogenase, decreased serum haptoglobin, and increased plasma-free hemoglobin. The change in pump performance most suggestive of thrombosis is the development

of a marked or gradual increase in pump power. Given the decline in output through the pump, increased pump speed may be required to maintain adequate flow. Pump thrombosis can initially be managed with intensification of anticoagulation, but pump exchange may be indicated depending on the severity and clinical scenario.

Right heart failure can be an early or late complication of LVAD support. For proper LVAD function, the RV must supply adequate preload across the pulmonary circuit. RV failure can manifest as low flow through the device, volume overload and end-organ dysfunction. It is thought that LVAD support can further weaken an already compromised RV by increasing systemic venous return and inducing geometric changes that can increase tricuspid regurgitation or reduce the septal contribution to RV stroke volume. In the perioperative period post-LVAD implant, management of right heart failure will include high doses of intotropic support or, in refractory cases, implantation of a temporary right ventricular assist device.

Ventricular arrhythmias, typically sustained ventricular tachycardia (VT), have been observed to occur at high rates post-LVAD implant, even in patients who had not experienced these previously.[22] These can occur in the immediate postoperative period, when electrolyte imbalances and the use of arrythmogenic inotropes contribute to their cause, or later in the course. An echocardiogram should be performed to evaluate whether endocardial irritation in the setting of excessive ventricular unloading resulting in direct contact of the LVAD outflow cannula and endocardium, termed a "suction event," is the culprit. Initially, sustained VT is typically well tolerated, as the device will continue to provide support. When the event is protracted, right heart failure can develop, and the accompanying clinical manifestations previously discussed can follow. The management of VT in an LVAD patient is similar to that employed in the typical patient. First, reversal of inciting factors and correction of electrolyte imbalances should be tried. This may include cessation of proarrythmic medications or a speed reduction to prevent approximation of the outflow cannula and endocardium. Following this, treatment with antiarrhythmics, antitachycardia pacing or defibrillation should be implemented. Only rarely, in cases repeatedly refractory to the above treatments, is ablation considered.

INDICATIONS

The 2013 ISHLT guidelines[9] for MCS state, as a class IIa (level of evidence C) recommendation, that long-term MCS for patients who are in acute cardiogenic shock should be reserved for the following:

1. Patients whose ventricular function is deemed unrecoverable or unlikely to recover without long-term device support.
2. Patients who are deemed too ill to maintain normal hemodynamics and vital organ function with temporary MCS devices (MCSDs), or who cannot be weaned from temporary MCSDs or inotropic support.
3. Patients with the capacity for meaningful recovery of end-organ function and quality of life.
4. Patients without irreversible end-organ damage.

The Centers for Medicare and Medicaid Services (CMS) has laid down the following criteria for LVAD implantation as DT:

1. New York Heart Association class IV patients with end-stage heart failure that are not candidates for transplantation.
2. Patients who have failed to respond to optimal medical management for at least 45 of the last 60 days or have been balloon pump dependent for 7 days or IV inotrope dependent for 14 days.
3. Patients who have a left ventricular ejection fraction < 25% and have demonstrated functional limitation with a peak oxygen consumption of ≤14 mL/kg/min unless balloon pump or inotrope dependent or physically unable to perform the test.

CONCLUSION

Cardiogenic shock remains a devastating condition with high rates of morbidity and mortality. Over the past several decades, we have seen the development of MCS devices that are able to offer excellent hemodynamic support. The choice of device can be tailored to patient characteristics, degree of desired support, and institutional resources. **Figure 17.8** outlines an algorithm for deciding on the proper implementation of these therapies. Their use has become widespread, and the costs associated with them continue to rise. This is all occurring without concrete evidence of improvement in mortality with the use of these devices. Whether the benefit of reversing the hemodynamics of cardiogenic shock has not translated into improved long-term outcomes because of the high rate of complications associated with these devices or as a result of delayed initiation, to a time when multiorgan

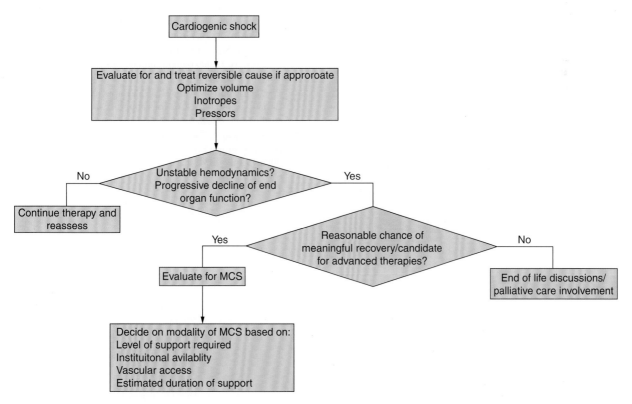

FIGURE 17.8 An algorithm for deciding on the use of mechanical circulatory support.

dysfunction has already developed, needs further evaluation in well-designed clinical trials. In addition, before instituting support it must be confirmed that there is a reasonable chance that a pathway to a meaningful recovery will be established.

REFERENCES

1. Thiele H, Zeymer U, Neumann FJ, et al. Intraaortic balloon support for myocardial infarction with cardiogenic shock. *N Engl J Med.* 2012;367:1287-1296.

2. Barron HV, Every NR, Parsons LS, et al. The use of intra-aortic balloon counterpulsation in patients with cardiogenic shock complicating acute myocardial infarction: data from the National Registry of Myocardial Infarction 2. *Am Heart J.* 2001;141:933-939.

3. Sjauw KD, Engstrom AE, Vis MM, et al. A systematic review and meta-analysis of intra-aortic balloon pump therapy in ST-elevation myocardial infarction: should we change the guidelines? *Eur Heart J.* 2009;30:459-468.

4. Jiang CY, Zhao LL, Wang JA, Mohammod B. Anticoagulation therapy in intra-aortic balloon counterpulsation: does IABP really need anti-coagulation? *J Zhejiang Univ Sci.* 2003;4:607-611.

5. American College of Emergency P, Society for Cardiovascular A, Interventions, et al. 2013 ACCF/AHA guideline for the management of ST-elevation myocardial infarction: a report of the American College of Cardiology Foundation/American Heart Association Task Force on Practice Guidelines. *J Am Coll Cardiol.* 2013;61:e78-140.

6. Thiele H, Sick P, Boudriot E, et al. Randomized comparison of intra-aortic balloon support with a percutaneous left ventricular assist device in patients with revascularized acute myocardial infarction complicated by cardiogenic shock. *Eur Heart J.* 2005;26:1276-1283.

7. Burkhoff D, Cohen H, Brunckhorst C, et al. A randomized multicenter clinical study to evaluate the safety and efficacy of the TandemHeart percutaneous ventricular assist device versus conventional therapy with intraaortic balloon pumping for treatment of cardiogenic shock. *Am Heart J.* 2006;152:469 e1-e8.

8. Kar B, Gregoric ID, Basra SS, et al. The percutaneous ventricular assist device in severe refractory cardiogenic shock. *J Am Coll Cardiol.* 2011;57:688-696.

9. Feldman D, Pamboukian SV, Teuteberg JJ, et al. The 2013 International Society for Heart and Lung Transplantation Guidelines for mechanical circulatory support: Executive summary. *J Heart Lung Transpl.* 2013;32:157-187.

10. Rihal CS, Naidu SS, Givertz MM, et al. 2015 SCAI/ACC/HFSA/STS clinical expert consensus statement on the use of percutaneous mechanical circulatory support devices in cardiovascular care: endorsed by the American Heart Assocation, the Cardiological Society of India, and Sociedad Latino Americana de Cardiologia Intervencion; Affirmation of Value by the Canadian Association of Interventional Cardiology-Association Canadienne de Cardiologie d'intervention. *J Am Coll Cardiol.* 2015;65:e7-e26.

11. Seyfarth M, Sibbing D, Bauer I, et al. A randomized clinical trial to evaluate the safety and efficacy of a percutaneous left ventricular assist device versus intra-aortic balloon pumping for treatment of cardiogenic shock caused by myocardial infarction. *J Am Coll Cardiol.* 2008;52:1584-1588.

12. Griffith BP, Anderson MB, Samuels LE, et al. The RECOVER I: a multicenter prospective study of Impella 5.0/LD for postcardiotomy circulatory support. *J Thorac Cardiovasc Surg.* 2013;145:548-554.

13. Lauten A, Engstrom AE, Jung C, et al. Percutaneous left-ventricular support with the Impella-2.5-assist device in acute cardiogenic shock: Results of the Impella-EUROSHOCK-registry. *Circ Heart Fail.* 2013;6:23-30.

14. Anderson MB, Goldstein J, Milano C, et al. Benefits of a novel percutaneous ventricular assist device for right heart failure: the prospective RECOVER RIGHT study of the Impella RP device. *J Heart Lung Transplant.* 2015;34:1549-1560.

15. Kapur NK, Paruchuri V, Jagannathan A, et al. Mechanical circulatory support for right ventricular failure. *JACC Heart Fail.* 2013;1:127-134.

16. Ouweneel DM, Schotborgh JV, Limpens J, et al. Extracorporeal life support during cardiac arrest and cardiogenic shock: a systematic review and meta-analysis. *Intensive Care Med.* 2016;42(12):1922-1934.

17. Rose EA, Gelijns AC, Moskowitz AJ, et al. Long-term use of a left ventricular assist device for end-stage heart failure. *N Engl J Med.* 2001;345:1435-1443.

18. Slaughter MS, Rogers JG, Milano CA, et al. Advanced heart failure treated with continuous-flow left ventricular assist device. *N Engl J Med.* 2009;361:2241-2251.

19. Maybaum S, Mancini D, Xydas S, et al. Cardiac improvement during mechanical circulatory support: a prospective multicenter study of the LVAD Working Group. *Circulation.* 2007;115:2497-2505.

20. Kirklin JK, Naftel DC, Pagani FD, et al. Seventh INTERMACS annual report: 15,000 patients and counting. *J Heart Lung Transplant.* 2015;34:1495-504.

21. Pawale A, Pinney S, Ashley K, et al. Implantable left ventricular assist devices as initial therapy for refractory postmyocardial infarction cardiogenic shock. *Eur J Cardiothorac Surg.* 2013;44:213-216.

22. Ziv O, Dizon J, Thosani A, et al. Effects of left ventricular assist device therapy on ventricular arrhythmias. *J Am Coll Cardiol.* 2005;45:1428-1434.

Patient and Family Information for: MECHANICAL CIRCULATORY SUPPORT

The heart is responsible for providing the force to deliver oxygenated blood to the body's organs and tissues. The heart has a right and left side that serve different functions but work in tandem to maintain the circulation of blood. The right side of the heart sends blood through the lungs, where it picks up oxygen. The oxygenated blood then passes to the left side, where it is pumped to the rest of the body. When the heart suffers a serious injury, an insufficient amount of blood is delivered to the organs to meet their demands, and organ dysfunction follows. This clinical situation is termed cardiogenic shock. The heart can be weakened to this extent either by a new cardiac event, such as a heart attack, by progression of existing heart disease, or by an insult to an already impaired heart. Signs of cardiogenic shock include fatigue, altered mental state, cool extremities, low blood pressure, kidney failure, and liver failure. Initial management is focused on treatment of reversible causes, such as opening up blocked arteries, and attempting to augment heart function with intravenous medications. At times, these maneuvers are not sufficient to restore adequate circulation. It is in these situations that the use of mechanical circulatory support (MCS) is considered. MCS refers to a variety of devices that aim to improve or replace the heart's pumping function. They are placed in order to allow the heart to recover adequate function or until a more definitive treatment is implemented. These devices differ in several ways, including the way they function, the level of support provided, the manner in which they are placed, and the associated complications.

The *IABP* is typically used and is the best studied device in patients with cardiogenic shock resulting from a heart attack. The device imparts its impact by timed inflation and deflation of a balloon that sits at its tip. It supports the failing heart by decreasing the pressure that the heart has to pump against and increasing blood flow to the coronary arteries. It is usually placed in the arteries of the lower extremities and advanced up the aorta to its proper position. The most common complications of IABP use are related to the artery in which it is placed. Complications include disruption of blood flow to the lower extremities and bleeding from the site of access.

The *TandemHeart* assist device is a continuous flow pump designed to provide a high level of support. A catheter is placed in the veins of the lower extremities and advanced to the heart, where its tip crosses from the right to the left side. Blood is drained from the left side of the heart and directed, using the force of the pump, to a catheter in the arteries of the lower extremities where it enters circulation. The most common complications of TandemHeart use are related to the blood vessels in which the catheters are placed. Complications include disruption of blood flow to the lower extremities and bleeding from the site of access. It is not uncommon to require a blood transfusion as a result of significant bleeding.

The *Impella* system is available in three distinct sizes that differ in the amount of support they can provide. They all function on the same principle. The system is inserted into the peripheral arteries, and its tip is advanced into the LV of the heart. Using the force of the pump, blood is pulled through the opening at the tip seated in the LV and pushed to the aorta. Complications include disruption of blood flow to the lower extremities and bleeding from the site of access. In addition, it is common to induce breakdown of blood cells given the force placed on them when passing through the pump.

ECMO is the only device system able to provide full cardiac support and oxygenate blood. A catheter is placed in the veins of the lower extremities and advanced to the right side of the heart. Blood is drained from the right side and directed, using the force of the pump, to a device that provides oxygen to the blood. The oxygenated blood is then passed to a catheter in the arteries, typically in the lower extremities, where it enters circulation. Complications include disruption of blood flow to the lower extremities and bleeding from the site of access. As a result of the disruption to normal blood flow, clot formation in the heart can occur. In addition, neurologic events such as seizures and strokes have been documented during use.

Placement of a long-term support device, called a *LVAD*, can be considered in cases where there is little hope of restoring adequate heart function in a relatively short period of time. These pumps restore blood circulation in a reliable manner and are quite durable. They must be implanted surgically in the operating room with use of the heart–lung machine. Blood enters the system through a tube in the LV and flows through the pump. From the pump, it is passed through tubing and exits the system in the aorta, where it circulates to the rest of the body. LVADs can remain in place for months to years. They remain in use until the heart recovers its native function or until a heart transplant is available or permanently remain for those patients not eligible for heart transplantation. They have been proven to both improve survival and quality of life in patients with advanced heart failure. The impressive benefits of the device do not come without cost. There are several complications associated with LVAD support. These include bleeding, infection, stroke, device malfunction requiring exchange and ventricular arrhythmias.

The condition of cardiogenic shock, resulting from severely impaired cardiac function, carries a high risk of morbidity and mortality. This has led to the development of novel devices with the hope of improving outcomes. These mechanical devices have repeatedly been proven to enhance blood circulation dramatically, but studies have yet to demonstrate an overall improvement in survival. It is important to understand that it is not appropriate to employ MCS in all cases. Use of these devices comes with a high rate of complications, many of them serious, which can place further stress on an already critically ill patient. In addition, the health care costs associated with their use are significant. The physicians must have a high index of suspicion that the patient can recover from their critically ill state and enjoy a meaningful quality of life in the future. To reach this end, these devices can serve as a bridge to recovery of native heart function, to placement of a long-term mechanical device, or to cardiac transplantation.

Eric Adler
Johanna Contreras
Sean P. Pinney

18

Selection and Care of the Heart Transplant Patient

INTRODUCTION

Despite making great advances in the medical treatment of heart failure over the last several decades, heart transplantation remains the definitive therapy for end-stage heart failure by extending survival and improving quality of life.[1,2] Although the number of heart transplantations performed annually in the United States has remained static over the last decade, both short- and long-term survival rates have increased significantly.[3]

This chapter will discuss patient selection for transplantation as well as postoperative and follow-up care. It will focus on the first 6 months after transplantation, making references to later time points.

PATIENT SELECTION

Heart transplantation is indicated for the treatment of Stage D heart failure according to the American Heart Association/American College of Cardiology comprehensive heart failure guidelines. Transplantation may also be considered for the treatment of refractory arrhythmias; hypertrophic cardiomyopathy; severe angina, valvular heart disease, or congenital heart disease not amendable to surgical repair; and, less frequently, selected cardiac neoplasms. A second transplant may be considered for patients with a history of heart transplant who develop allograft failure from vasculopathy, rejection, or other causes.

The specific criteria employed by transplant centers to decide patient eligibility may vary somewhat. The International Society for Heart and Lung Transplantation (ISHLT) has published consensus guidelines regarding patient selection.[4] Among the many criteria used, perhaps none is as variable as age. The ISHLT recommends that patients should be less than or equal to 70 years of age. Some centers draw the line at 65 years, whereas others have no absolute age criteria. Notably, in 2006, of the 2192 transplants performed in the United States, 243 (11%) occurred in patients over 65. Given that the majority of heart failure cases occur in patients older than 65, there is an implicit need for either transplantation or other destination therapies for patients in their seventh and eighth decades of life.

All patients should be without neoplasm. Select patients with recently treated localized cancers with a low chance of recurrence may be eligible if they are free of metastatic disease. Cancer screening includes colonoscopy in all patients over 50 years, a prostate-specific antigen in men, and mammography and a PAP smear in women. Cardiac transplantation has been successfully performed to treat cardiac neoplasms such as large atrial myxomas, and cardiac sarcomas without evidence of metastatic disease. Primary amyloidosis is an emerging indication for transplantation. Transplantation using extended-donor criteria followed by chemotherapy alone or in conjunction with bone marrow transplantation has been shown to extend survival in these patients.[5]

Although once excluded from consideration, diabetic patients can now be listed for transplant provided they have little or no evidence of end organ disease such as retinopathy, nephropathy or peripheral vascular disease. Patients with other debilitating chronic illnesses that may impact survival and those who lack the ability to provide self-care are generally excluded. Examples include dementia or hemiplegia after stroke. Patients with severe peripheral or cerebral vascular disease are excluded, as are those patients with significant restrictive or obstructive pulmonary disease (FEV_1 <1 L).

Evaluation of liver and kidney function should be done at baseline and repeated at regular intervals. Patients with chronic kidney disease with a creatinine clearance of less than 34 mL/min face a high risk for developing chronic renal failure and should be considered for combined heart–kidney transplantation. Patients with significant liver dysfunction are at risk for perioperative bleeding, vasoplegia, and organ failure. A transjugular liver biopsy may be required in those patients with significant liver dysfunction in order to exclude cirrhosis. This also permits measurement of hepatocaval and hepatic vein pressures to clarify the etiology and severity of the disease. Patients with significant irreversible disease, defined by bilirubin >2.5 or alanine transaminase/aspartate transaminase >3x normal, may be declined listing or, at select centers, considered for heart–liver transplant. Patients with reversible hepatic dysfunction with "nutmeg liver" from outflow obstruction may still be considered eligible for transplant because central venous pressure should fall with transplantation of a new cardiac allograft.

Screening for chronic viral infection should be performed before listing. Testing for herpes simplex virus (HSV), Epstein Barr virus (EBV), cytomegalovirus (CMV), hepatitis A, B, and C as well as HIV is recommended. Prophylaxis against reactivation of CMV and HSV is determined on the basis of the results of serologic testing. Controversy remains as to whether patients infected with hepatitis B and C should be transplanted in view of the risk of increased viral replication in the setting of immunosuppression. Infected patients with HIV have recently been considered eligible at some centers using extended-donor criteria. Eligible patients must have an undetectable viral load and a reconstituted immune system with normal CD4 count.[6,7] Titers for *Trypanosoma cruzi* (Chagas) should be tested in all patients with nonischemic cardiomyopathy who are native or resided in South or Central America. Screening for strongyloides is recommended for those patients who lived or visited an endemic area such as Puerto Rico or the Dominican Republic.

Selection of heart transplant recipients should be reserved for those patients with a significant cardiovascular limitation resulting in reduced 1-year survival. Identifying such patients can be challenging, particularly in ambulatory patients. Cardiopulmonary exercise testing to measure peak oxygen consumption (VO_2 max) is a proven risk stratifying method and should be performed in all ambulatory patients.[8] A peak oxygen consumption of less than 12 mL/min/kg, or less than 14 mL/kg/min if intolerant of a beta-blocker, is considered the threshold for listing because it is predictive of reduced 1-year survival. Other noninvasive predictive models include the heart failure survival score, which incorporates peak oxygen consumption, or the Seattle Heart Failure model.[9,10]

Patients with pulmonary hypertension are at increased risk for right heart failure following transplant because the unconditioned donor right ventricle (RV) may struggle and fail in the face of increased afterload. Generally speaking, a pulmonary vascular resistance (PVR) of greater than 6 Wood Units or greater than 3 Wood Units following vasodilator testing with nitroprusside is considered a contraindication to transplantation. Long-term treatment with an inodilator, such as milrinone, or a ventricular assist device may help reduce PVR to safely allow transplantation. When PVR remains fixed, heart–lung transplantation may be considered. A summary of our transplant listing algorithm can be found in **Figure 18.1.**

The presence of alloantibodies increases the risk of experiencing either acute or chronic rejection. All potential recipients are screened against a panel of reactive antibodies (PRA). It is our practice to perform a donor-specific prospective crossmatch for all recipients with a PRA greater than 10% to reduce the chance of developing acute or hyperacute rejection. This step reduces the risk of allograft loss, but, because of the mechanics of performing the test, effectively reduces the donor pool. Further steps to minimize the risk of humoral sensitization include limiting blood product transfusion while awaiting transplantation. Patients who are more likely to have elevated levels of alloantibodies include postpartum women and prior recipients of organ transplants. A program of desensitization can be performed in patients whose PRA remains elevated. Both plasmapheresis and infusions of immunomodulatory drugs, such as intravenous gamma globulin (IVIG) and rituximab, have been employed with varying degrees of success.[11]

Obese patients experience a greater number of complications following cardiac surgery, including prolonged ventilatory times, renal failure, and wound infection.[12] The presence of obesity in heart transplant recipients is associated with poorer survival compared with nonobese patients. A body mass index (BMI) greater than 35 is considered a relative contraindication to transplantation at our center, and all patients are encouraged to reduce their BMI to less than 30 to improve their odds of long-term survival.

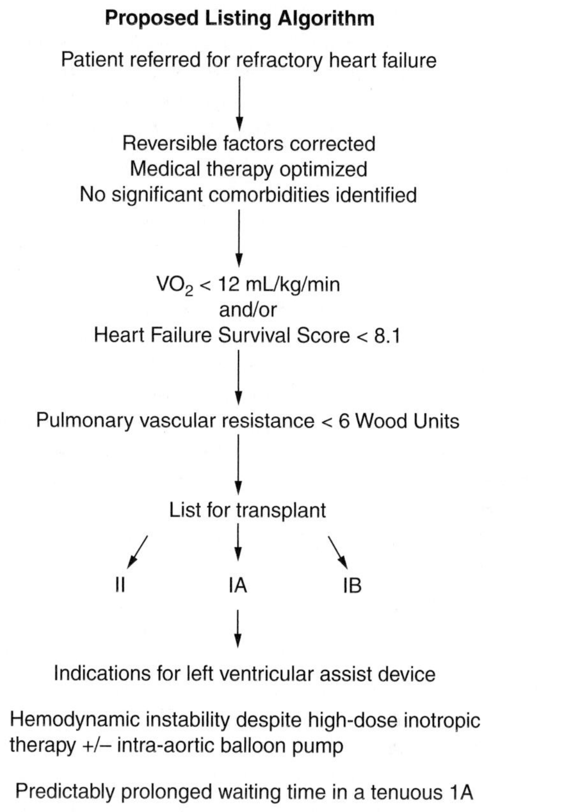

Proposed Listing Algorithm

FIGURE 18.1 The approach to evaluating patients for heart transplantation begins with referral to an advanced heart failure program. Reversible factors are corrected and medications are optimized. Persistently symptomatic patients will be risk stratified with a cardiopulmonary stress test and multivariable risk scores. Those with predicted high 1-year mortality will be formally evaluated, a process that includes right heart catheterization to screen for fixed pulmonary hypertension. Acceptable candidates will be listed for transplant and further stratified as 1A if they require intensive care hospitalization, 1B if they require continuous inotrope infusion, or II if they are otherwise stable.

Other contraindications to heart transplantation include any psychological or social barrier that would preclude one's ability to reliably comply with medical therapy and follow-up examinations. Active drug, alcohol, or tobacco use excludes consideration for transplantation. Nicotine blood levels, as well as blood alcohol levels and urine toxicology screens, can be used to test for compliance. Decisions about the severity of a patient's substance dependency are generally made as part of a general evaluation of all patients by a psychiatrist. Social support is critical for the patient posttransplantation given the physical and psychosocial stressors encountered.

It is recommended that patients on the waiting list be formally reevaluated every 6 months to ensure that they still fulfill the necessary listing criteria. Occasionally, a patient's clinical condition will improve as a result of medical or device therapy. Those patients with significant improvement in cardiac function and symptoms should be considered for removal from the waiting list.

DONOR SELECTION

Following the establishment of brain death, organs are offered for transplantation by local organ donor networks following the rules established by the United Network for Organ Sharing. Because the specific criteria used to accept donor organs remain variable between transplant centers, a recent consensus statement provided recommendations to improve the evaluation and successful utilization of potential cardiac donors.[13] In general, donors should be younger than 50 years old, but older donors may be considered for extended criteria recipients. Donors with significant chest wall trauma are excluded from transplantation, although short periods of cardiopulmonary resuscitation or isolated rib fractures are acceptable. To ensure that the heart is of a sufficient size to match the recipient's needs, a donor's weight should not be less than 80% of that of the recipient, and the donor should be no more than 6 inches smaller than the recipient. Some believe that a male donor whose height exceeds 66 inches is sufficient for all recipients regardless of their height. Donors should be free of malignancy and should have negative blood and sputum cultures to reduce the risk of bacterial transmission. Donors with HIV or active hepatitis B infection are excluded from consideration. Although in the past donors with serologic evidence of hepatitis C infection have been used in some centers, a recent study called this practice into question. Gasink et al investigated the impact of transplanted hearts from hepatitis C seropositive patients into seronegative recipients.[14] One-, five- and ten-year mortality rates were significantly higher in those patients who received organs from seropositive donors. Donors who are seronegative for hepatitis B surface antigen but seropositive for the core antibody may be acceptable donors. When these hearts are used, recipients should receive prophylactic treatment with lamivudine and hepatitis B immune globulin to further reduce the risk of viral transmission. All patients should be offered hepatitis B vaccination while awaiting transplantation.[15] Patients infected with HIV or HTLV (Human T-lymphotropic Virus) are not acceptable donors.

To assess the heart's suitability for donation, one typically performs an electrocardiogram (ECG), echocardiogram, and, on occasion, coronary angiography. Cardiac enzymes may be minimally elevated in the setting of brain death because of the occurrence of myocardial contraction band necrosis. Markedly elevated levels of the MB fraction of creatine phosphokinase or troponin-I are more consistent with myocardial injury or infarction.

Echocardiography is particularly useful for evaluating cardiac structure and function. Left ventricular hypertrophy with a septal or posterior wall thickness greater than 13 mm is frequently a contraindication to donation because of the difficulty in preserving such a thickened myocardium. A significantly reduced ejection fraction or regional wall motion abnormalities suggestive of infarction will similarly exclude donation, as will severe regurgitant or stenotic valvular lesions.

Coronary angiography is recommended for male donors over 45 and females over 55 as well as younger patients with significant atherosclerotic risk factors. The use of computed tomography (CT) angiography in lieu of percutaneous angiography may be considered in those centers unable to provide coronary angiography. The presence of coronary disease can also be assessed by palpation of the coronary arteries at the time of harvesting. Inspection should include evaluation of significant valvular disease and the presence of congenital lesions or a large patent foramen ovale (PFO). Such PFOs are generally sutured closed at the time of transplantation to prevent paradoxical embolization. A summary of absolute and relative contraindications to donation can be found in **Table 18.1**.

TABLE 18.1	**Absolute and Relative Contraindications to Donor Heart Selection**

ABSOLUTE CONTRAINDICATIONS
Organ transport time > 4 h
Confirmed myocardial infarction with systolic dysfunction
LVEF < 30%
Severe valvular disease not amenable to repair
Active infection with transmissible pathogens including, but not limited to, HIV hepatitis B (HBSAg +) or C virus, or highly resistant bacteria
Bacterial endocarditis
A history of major extracranial or metastatic malignancy
Age > 65 years
Significant penetrating cardiac trauma

RELATIVE CONTRAINDICATIONS
Donor–recipient height mismatch > 6 inches
Age 50–65 years
Male donors > 45 years and female donors > 50 years with cardiovascular risk factors and an inability to perform coronary angiography
Previous high-risk behavior including intravenous drug use or risky sexual activity
Donor instability manifested by hypoxia, severe acidosis with pH < 7.2, hypotension requiring high-dose vasoconstrictors
Organ transport time 3–4 hours

LVEF, left ventricular ejection fraction.

PATIENT MANAGEMENT

The patient with a newly transplanted heart faces a number of physiologic challenges. Without having time to recover from cold ischemia and facing reperfusion injury, the denervated heart is expected to function fully and provide an adequate cardiac output as soon as possible after being weaned from cardiopulmonary bypass. The loss of sympathetic innervation makes the allograft dependent on circulating catecholamines in order to sustain cardiac output. Infusions of positive inotropic medicines, such as dobutamine or milrinone, are always given in sufficient quantity to assist the heart in providing an adequate cardiac output. This obligatorily requires continuous patient monitoring with arterial lines and a pulmonary artery catheter in an intensive care unit. Vasoconstrictors such as arginine vasopressin (AVP) and norepinephrine may be temporarily employed to counter the vasoplegia that often occurs after cardiopulmonary bypass in advanced heart failure patients. Because of their deleterious effects on the microcirculation, vasoconstrictors should be weaned and discontinued at the earliest possible time. Weaning of positive inotropic medicines generally begins 48 hours after transplantation after allowing the sinus node to recover from cold ischemia, and for the RV to accommodate itself to the increased afterload in those patients with preexisting pulmonary hypertension. Transfer out of the intensive care unit to a floor with continuous telemetry monitoring commonly occurs before weaning is completed.

Vasodilatory hypotension is commonly encountered postoperatively. The mechanism for this may be related to the pretransplant use of vasodilatory drugs, such as angiotensin converting enzyme inhibitors, and inodilators such as milrinone. Other suspected factors include a systemic inflammatory response to prolonged cardiopulmonary bypass and a reported depletion of AVP that occurs as consequence of long-standing advanced heart failure. Although vasoconstrictors such as norepinephrine have generally been used to treat vasodilatory hypotension, synthetic AVP may be more effective in this patient population because it does not constrict pulmonary arteries or compromise renal function.

Renal dysfunction is a common posttransplant occurrence and contributes to both a prolonged hospital stay and increased risk of mortality. Postoperative renal failure is usually a consequence of ischemic injury that results from diminished renal perfusion during cardiopulmonary bypass, perioperative hypotension, and perhaps from embolization from an atherosclerotic aorta. Its presence not only contributes to the volume-overloaded state, but may also delay the initiation of immunosuppressive therapy, particularly the use of calcineurin inhibitors. Temporarily withholding the calcineurin inhibitor may allow time for renal function to improve.[16] When patients with reduced urine output are unable to match their obligatory inputs, such as blood products and intravenous medications, diuretics may be used. Frequently, oliguric renal failure will require mechanical renal replacement therapy. When clearance is not required, aquapheresis (Aquadex FlexFlow System, Sunshine Heart Inc., Eden Prairie, MN) may be employed. Slow, low efficiency dialysis or continuous veno-venous hemofiltration (CVVH) allows for removal of large volumes of fluid, provides clearance, and may facilitate renal recovery. Rarely, patients will develop fulminant renal failure postoperatively. These patients are typically patients with preexisting chronic kidney disease. Such patients may be managed with dialysis, but in consideration of poor long-term outcomes, renal transplantation is preferred.[17,18]

Right heart failure is common in the posttransplant patient. Reasons for its occurrence include ischemia–reperfusion injury, preexisting pulmonary hypertension, and volume overload from infusion of intravenous fluids. Multiple blood product infusions, including packed red blood cells and fresh frozen plasma, may further volume load an already distended RV. In the face of this additional preload, ventricular function may deteriorate. A rising central venous pressure (CVP) in the setting of systemic hypotension will compromise myocardial perfusion and lead to ventricular ischemia with contractile dysfunction. Release of cytokines such as thromboxane from transfused platelets may further increase pulmonary arteriolar pressure and place additional afterload on a straining RV. Furthermore, transplantation of a smaller donor heart into a larger recipient predisposes to RV dysfunction more than to left ventricle (LV) dysfunction. RV failure should be suspected when CVP rises and cardiac output falls. Transthoracic echocardiography may not offer adequate RV visualization in postoperative patients because of an inability to obtain sufficient echocardiographic windows or position the patient properly; thus, transesophageal echocardiography is preferred in endotracheally intubated patients.

Treatment is directed at improving the loading conditions for the RV while providing adequate inotropic support to maintain circulation. Aggressive diuresis to achieve a CVP of 12 to 15 mm Hg will lower RV preload and may help to reduce tricuspid regurgitation. When patients are diuretic resistant or in overt renal failure, or simply need large volumes of fluid removed quickly, aquapheresis or CVVH is indicated. Inhaled nitric oxide will reduce RV afterload by dilating pulmonary arteries. Nitric oxide also improves oxygenation and V/Q matching. When patients require positive inotropic support for a prolonged period

of time, milrinone is preferred over dobutamine, because of its superior ability to dilate the pulmonary vasculature. Mechanical support, using a right ventricular assist device, may be necessary for some patients as a means of providing longer-term support. The ventricular assist device can be slowly weaned over a period of days or weeks as right heart function improves.

Bradyarrhythmias are frequently encountered, but their incidence has decreased with the use of bicaval anastamoses, which tend to spare the sinus node. Given that resting heart rate of a denervated heart is between 90 and 120 beats per minute (bpm), rates lower than this may be a result of sinus node dysfunction, ischemia, or preoperative use of amiodarone. Both isoproterenol and aminophylline were widely used in the past to elevate resting heart rate, but nowadays electronic pacing through temporary wires is preferred. Temporary pacing wires should remain in place long enough to ensure that sinus node function has adequately recovered. Temporary pacing can be considered for patients whose heart rates are below 90 bpm, especially if the patient has evidence of low cardiac output. Permanent pacemakers are reserved for patients with persistent sinus or atrioventricular nodal dysfunction.

Although infrequently encountered, tachyarrhythmias are usually a sign of an injured allograft. Atrial fibrillation is commonly seen in cardiac surgery, but less so following heart transplantation. This is believed to be a result of the left atrial anastamosis, which effectively isolates the pulmonary veins and prevents atrial fibrillation. When present, atrial arrhythmias are a sign of either ischemic injury or early rejection. Ventricular arrhythmias are also rare, but are generally not a sign of rejection but of myocardial ischemia or infarction. Congenital arrhythmias in the donor heart, such as Wolf Parkinson White syndrome, are occasionally seen and can be treated with catheter ablation.

ACUTE ALLOGRAFT DYSFUNCTION

Acute allograft dysfunction remains one of the most common causes of early posttransplant death. It occurs in up to 5% of transplants and has multiple etiologies. These include ischemia–reperfusion injury, poor preservation, and unrecognized or underappreciated predonation dysfunction. Both prolonged ischemia and the use of high-dose catecholamine infusions predispose to allograft dysfunction, perhaps by depleting myocardial energy stores. Hyperacute rejection, which occurs because of the presence of preformed antibodies to human leukocyte antigens, is now rarely seen because of the routine use of PRA screening. The struggling allograft can usually be adequately supported with infusions of epinephrine, dobutamine, or milrinone. More severe degrees of dysfunction require mechanical support with the use of intra-aortic balloon counterpulsation, or the placement of ventricular assist devices to rest the allograft and provide adequate organ perfusion. Patients who can be weaned successfully from the device have a survival rate similar to that of the general transplant population. Although urgent repeat transplantation is an option for these patients, the presence of multiorgan dysfunction often limits their candidacy. Causes of death in the posttransplant period are listed in **Table 18.2**.

IMMUNOSUPPRESSION

Prior to the routine use of cyclosporine (CyA) in the early 1980s, heart transplantation survival was so poor that many physicians called for a moratorium on the procedure. Although advances

TABLE 18.2	Causes of Death in the Posttransplant Period
Cardiac allograft vasculopathy	54 (1.7%)
Acute rejection	208 (6.5%)
Lymphoma	2 (0.1%)
Malignancy, other	2 (0.1%)
CMV	4 (0.1%)
Infection, non-CMV	414 (12.9%)
Primary graft failure	831 (26.0%)
Graft failure	445 (13.9%)
Technical	237 (7.4%)
Other	213 (6.7%)
Multiple organ failure	431 (13.5%)
Renal failure	18 (0.6%)
Pulmonary	134 (4.2%)
Cerebrovascular	205 (6.4%)

CMV, cytomegalovirus.

From Taylor DO, Edwards LB, Boucek MM, et al. Registry of the International Society for Heart and Lung Transplantation: twenty-third official adult heart transplantation report—2006. *J Heart Lung Transplant.* 2006;25:869–879.

in immunosuppression have improved outcomes dramatically, allograft rejection still accounts for 6.5% of early deaths following transplantation. Typical maintenance immunosuppression in the current era consists of a calcineurin inhibitor in combination with an antimetabolite and corticosteroids.

The use of induction immunosuppression, although once routine, has lately been called into question. It was thought that by passivating the immune system through the use of either monoclonal or polyclonal antibodies, induction therapy allowed time for the allograft to recover function without facing the threat of rejection. This period of induction also allowed for postoperative recovery of renal function prior to the initiation of a calcineurin inhibitor with its attendant risk of nephrotoxicity. In retrospect, this approach was limited by the fact that induction therapy induced T-cell anergy, but not clonal depletion. In effect, moderate-to-severe rejection was not prevented, but only delayed by 6 to 12 months. Nonetheless, upward of half of all transplant centers continue to use induction immunosuppression, although use of OKT3 and polyclonal antibodies, such as thymoglobulin, has declined, whereas use of selective interleukin-2 (IL-2) receptor antibodies has increased. The IL-2 receptor blocker basiliximab has been shown to reduce both the severity and the frequency of cardiac rejection as well as increase the time to a first rejection episode. Its use is not associated with the cytokine release syndrome or the significant side effects associated with OKT3.[19]

Cell cycle antagonists, either aziothioprine or mycophenelate mofetil (MMF), are started intraoperatively or on postoperative day one. Both drugs work by inhibiting the de novo pathway of purine synthesis, a step crucial to cellular proliferation. Because leukocytes and lymphocytes lack the salvage pathway, these drugs particularly inhibit their proliferation. Azathioprine produces a

greater degree of bone marrow suppression than does MMF. It is given as a single dose of 1.5 to 5 mg/kg adjusted for white blood cell and liver function. Azathioprine is metabolized by thiopurine methyltransferase (TPMT) in vivo. Small proportions of patients have very low levels of TPMT (roughly 0.3% of the general population) and are at greater risk of experiencing myelosuppresion.

Following the results of a large multicenter randomized clinical trial showing its benefits over azathioprine, MMF has become the preferred antiproliferative agent at most transplant centers.[20] Patients receiving MMF experienced fewer episodes of hemodynamically significant rejection and enjoyed a higher survival rate at the first year of follow-up, as well as a trend toward a lesser incidence of severe rejection. Opportunistic infections were seen more commonly in patients receiving MMF, but most of these resulted from either HSV or herpes zoster and were not life threatening. MMF is given as a fixed dose of 1500 mg twice daily for patients with preserved renal function. Lower doses of 500 to 1000 mg bid are used for patients with estimated creatinine clearance of less than 50 mL/kg/min. The dose of MMF may need to be reduced in the setting of gastrointestinal upset or leucopenia. Blood levels of mycophenolate and its metabolite can be measured, but are not available at all centers.

Inhibition of the calcineurin pathway is the cornerstone of solid organ transplantation. The introduction of the first calcineurin inhibitor, CyA, in 1983 revolutionized solid organ transplantation, essentially doubling the 1 and 5-year survival rates. They work by inhibiting calcineurin, a calcium calmodulin–dependent phosphatase that activates transcription factors responsible for transcription of IL-2. Calcineurin inhibition prevents both IL-2 transcription and T-lymphocyte activation.

CyA is a cyclic decapeptide that is derived from the fungus *Trichoderma polysporin.* Its major immunosuppressive effect is to inhibit the production of IL-2 and other cytokines by activated lymphocytes. CyA binds to cyclophilin in the cytoplasm of T-lymphocytes, and this complex then binds to and inhibits calcineurin, ultimately preventing transcription of IL-2. CyA affects T-helper and cytotoxic T-cells but has little or no effect on suppressor T-cells. The drug is metabolized by cytochrome P450 3A4, located in the liver and along the gastrointestinal tract. Approximately 5% to 10% of the parent compound is excreted unchanged in the urine. CyA has a half-life of 19 hours. Different formulations of CyA are supplied for both intravenous and oral administration. When given intravenously, CyA is mixed in a 1:1 concentration in either normal saline or 5% dextrose and infused continuously. CyA (Sandimmune, Novartis, East Hanover, NJ) for oral use is provided in liquid (100 mg/mL) and capsule form and is administered 2 or 3 times daily. Neoral (Novartis, East Hanover, NJ) is a microemulsion formulation of CyA that has improved absorption and bioavailability and is given in two daily doses. CyA can be given as a continuous infusion immediately after transplant or delayed for 24 to 48 hours until it can be given enterally. A typical continuous infusion begins at 0.5 to 1.0 mg/h and is adjusted accordingly. When converting to oral CyA, approximately 3 times the total daily intravenous dose is given. In the early posttransplant period, CyA is administered to achieve a trough whole blood level of 300 to 350 ng/mL. Target levels decrease with time as rejection risk begins to wane. Typical target levels are 250 to 350 in the first 6 months, 150 to 250 in months 6 to 12, and 100 to 150 long-term. Side effects include nephrotoxicity, hypertension, hypertrichosis, gingival hyperplasia, tremor, and seizures. Serum levels of CyA are affected by many medications. Those that elevate levels are drugs that inhibit its metabolism through the cytochrome P450 system, such as erythromycin, fluconazole, and amiodarone and the antihypertensive diltiazem.

Tacrolimus (Prograf, also known as FK-506) is a macrolide antibiotic derived from the bacteria Streptomyces tsukubaensis. It has now become the preferred drug at many transplant centers. The major advantage of tacrolimus over CyA is the lesser degree of hypertension and hyperlipidemia. Some prescribers prefer its use in women for cosmetic reasons, because it produces less hirsutism and gingival hyperplasia than CyA. After binding with FKBP-12 (also referred to as the FK506 binding protein), tacrolimus inhibits calcineurin. Although its mechanism of activation is similar to that of CyA, it is much more potent but appears to produce less nephrotoxicity. Other side effects include seizures, insomnia, tremor, and hypertension. Tacrolimus is also associated with an increased risk of hyperglycemia, although whether the long-term incidence of diabetes is increased remains controversial. Tacrolimus can be administered either orally or intravenously. When given intravenously, an initial dose of 0.01 to 0.05 mg/kg/d is infused continuously and adjusted to achieve a level of around 12 to 15 ng/mL. When given enterally, a 1 mg dose test of tacrolimus is given to all patients because clearance of the drug may vary significantly between patients. Typical trough target levels are 10 to 15 ng/mL in the first 2 months, 8 to 12 ng/mL for the next 3 to 6 months, and 5 to 10 ng/mL thereafter.

Rapamycin (Rapamune) and everolimus (Zortress, Certican) are reserved for patients with transplant vasculopathy. When initiating these proliferation signal inhibitors, one should discontinue antiproliferative drugs such as MMF or azathioprine. Doses of tacrolimus should be reduced to achieve trough levels of approximately 4 to 6 ng/mL. An initial rapamycin dose of 6 mg is given 6 hours after tacrolimus and is followed by a daily dose of 2 mg. This daily dose should be adjusted to achieve rapamycin levels of approximately 10 ng/mL in the first year of transplant and between 5 and 10 ng/mL thereafter.

Corticosteroids are the third class of medications used for maintenance immunosuppression. Intravenous methylprednisolone is given preoperatively and switched to prednisone once the patient can tolerate oral agents. Prednisone dosing is tapered down during the first several months of transplant. Corticosteroids have numerous troublesome side effects: they worsen glycemic control, increase serum lipids, and stimulate appetite, leading to obesity. They have profound effects on bone absorption, producing osteoporosis and a susceptibility to fracture. Avascular necrosis of the hips and shoulders from steroid use necessitates joint replacement surgery in some patients. Other debilitating side effects include cataract formation, colonic perforation, and, especially with higher doses, mood disorders such as psychosis. Motivated to limit these toxicities, many centers attempt to wean patients entirely off corticosteroids after 6 to 12 months.[21] The optimal timing of complete steroid withdrawal has yet to be determined, and the majority of patients remain on steroids indefinitely.

REJECTION SURVEILLANCE

Endomyocardial biopsy remains the gold standard for the diagnosis rejection. Biopsies are taken from the RV via the transvenous approach (**Figure 18.2**). At the time of each biopsy, four to five samples are taken and graded using the 2004 revised ISHLT system. Both the revised and standard system, published in 1990, are summarized in **Table 18.3**. Biopsies are performed at

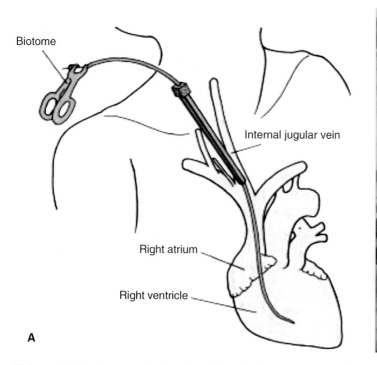

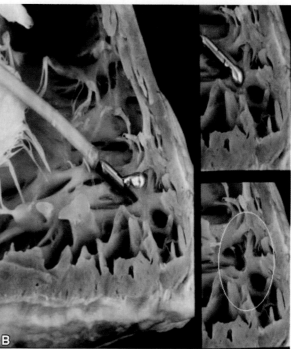

FIGURE 18.2 Endomyocardial biopsy is performed under fluoroscopic guidance. A bioptome is advanced through the jugular vein and directed across the tricuspid valve into the right ventricle and positioned against the interventricular septum (A). After the bioptome is closed and withdrawn, a small defect remains within the myocardium (B). During a typical biopsy session, four to six pieces of myocardium will be sampled and sent to pathology for review.

TABLE 18.3	Standardized ISHLT Cardiac Biopsy Grading Scales (2005 Revised Version in Comparison with 1990 Version)		
1990 SCALE		**2005 SCALE**	
Grade	*Description*	*Grade*	*Description*
0	No rejection	0	No rejection
1A	Focal perivascular or interstitial infiltrate without	1R	Interstitial and/or perivascular infiltrate with up to 1
1B	necrosis	2R	focus of myocyte damage
2	Diffuse but sparse infiltrate without necrosis	3R	Two or more foci of infiltrate with associated myocyte
3A	One focus only with aggressive infiltration and/or		damage
3B	focal myocyte damage		Diffuse infiltrate with multifocal myocyte damage,
4	Multifocal aggressive infiltrates and/or myocyte		edema, hemorrhage, vasculitis
	damage		
	Diffuse inflammatory process with necrosis		
	Diffuse aggressive polymorphous infiltrate, with		
	or without edema, hemorrhage or vasculitis; with		
	necrosis		

ISHLT, The International Society for Heart and Lung Transplantation.

a frequency that matches the time-dependent risk of rejection. A typical schedule would require biopsies on a weekly basis for the first month, then on a biweekly basis for the second and third months, and on a monthly basis for the fourth through sixth months, with the frequency diminishing thereafter. Routine performance of endomyocardial biopsy after the fifth transplant year is no longer required. Biopsies should be performed anytime rejection is suspected.

Symptoms of rejection are often absent, but can be insidious when present. They may include malaise or generalized fatigue, symptoms of heart failure (shortness of breath, peripheral edema), and palpitations. Arrhythmias, such as atrial fibrillation, may be present. Biopsy should be promptly arranged for in any patient in whom rejection is suspected. Assessment of ventricular dysfunction should be performed using either echocardiography or magnetic resonance imaging. Depending on the degree of suspicion for rejection, empiric therapy may need to be given while awaiting endomyocardial biopsy results. A typical biopsy schedule is shown in **Table 18.4**.

Recent work suggests that detection of cellular rejection may be possible using less invasive methods. The Cargo Study evaluated the gene expression profile of peripheral blood mononuclear cells obtained from patients a minimum of one year after transplantation. Using this profile, a scoring system was created that could exclude the presence of ≥ ISHLT 2R (previously 3A) rejection with a negative predictive value of 99.6%. The system is currently approved for clinical use, and studies are ongoing to predict whether the test is useful in patients during the first year posttransplant.[22]

TABLE 18.4	Typical Endomyocardial Biopsy Schedule for Rejection Surveillance
TIME POSTTRANSPLANT	**FREQUENCY**
1 month	Weekly
2 months	Biweekly
3–6 months	Monthly
7–12 months	Every 2 months
12–18 months	Every 3 months
>18 months	Every 6–12 months

TREATMENT OF CELLULAR REJECTION

Strategies for the treatment of rejection differ significantly from center to center. Factors influencing one's decision to treat include grade of rejection, impact on cardiac function (as determined by echocardiogram and/or right heart catheterization), and time from transplantation. At our center, patients are treated as follows: Grade 0 and Grade 1R (previous grades 1A, 1B, and 2) biopsies do not require treatment in the absence of symptoms or abnormal hemodynamics. Care is taken to ensure that doses and levels of immunosuppressive medications are at their therapeutic targets. Patients with symptomatic rejection are treated with corticosteroids. Grade 2R (previous grade 3A) rejection may be treated with a short pulse of oral steroids, for example, prednisone 50 mg bid, if occurring more than 3 months posttransplant. Patients with grade 2R rejection that are symptomatic or have hemodynamic consequences of rejection, as well as those patients less than 3 months posttransplant, are treated with intravenous methylprednisolone (1000 mg/d for 3 days) followed by a prednisone taper. Repeat biopsy is typically performed in 2 weeks. Hemodynamically severe rejection occurs in fewer than 5% of patients, but requires inpatient admission and treatment with cytolytic therapy consisting of thymoglobulin. Inpatient admission and hemodynamic monitoring are essential because patients are at risk of rapidly progressing cardiac failure and circulatory collapse.

HUMORAL REJECTION

Humoral rejection is a B-cell mediated process in which alloantibodies attach to major histocompatibility complex class I or II antigens usually in a perivascular pattern. It can present in a variety of ways, from an insidious process to fulminant hyperacute rejection. Its diagnosis is confirmed with either immunofluorescence or immunoperoxidase staining for the complement degradation products C4D or C3D. When the latter is used, a positive stain must be present in the setting of symptoms or other signs of rejection such as abnormal hemodynamics or left ventricular dysfunction to complete the diagnosis. Risk factors for its development include having an elevated pretransplant PRA, the development of specific antidonor antibodies, or the preoperative use of a left ventricular assist device. Treatment of humoral rejection is targeted at three distinct processes: clearance or neutralization of circulating antibodies, eradication of plasma cells, and prevention of sensitized B-cells transforming into plasma cells. Plasmapheresis with plasma exchange can quickly remove circulating alloantibodies and allow graft function to recover.[23] Up to 40% of circulating immunoglobulin G may not be cleared by plasmapheresis, but may be neutralized by administering IVIG. We typically prefer a sucrose-free preparation in order to avoid nephrotoxicity. Intravenous cyclophosphamide (0.5 to 1.0 g/m^2) may be given following plasmapheresis to eliminate alloantibody-producing plasma cells. More recently, the anti-CD20 monoclonal antibody rituximab (Genentech, San Francisco, CA), a chimeric humanized antibody directed against the pan–B-cell surface molecule CD20, has been used as the third component of therapy. It targets sensitized B-cells and interferes with their ability to transform into antibody-producing plasma cells. Ultimately, rituximab may provide long-term benefit by eliminating "memory" B cells and preventing the adverse late sequelae of humoral rejection.

CARDIAC ALLOGRAFT VASCULOPATHY

Cardiac allograft vasculopathy (CAV) is a diffuse arteriosclerosis that remains one of the most common long-term complications of cardiac transplantation. CAV resembles the arteriopathy of restenosis following balloon angioplasty **(Figure 18.3)**. Both processes represent an abnormal response to vessel injury. In the case of CAV, both immunologic and nonimmunologic arterial injury contributes to its development. The arteriopathy comprises both intimal proliferation and negative remodeling of the external elastic lamina. Because it produces concentric rather than eccentric luminal stenoses, the presence of CAV is often underestimated, but its prevalence may be as high as 55% by the third posttransplant year.[24] The presence of CAV limits the long-term success of cardiac transplantation. In a multi-center study of 2609 heart transplantation recipients, 42% had angiographic evidence of graft vasculopathy by 5 years following transplantation.[25] Up to 7% of transplant recipients will die or require repeat transplantation because of CAV.

The development of CAV is an insidious process. Because the transplanted heart is denervated, patients will rarely, if ever, present with angina. Instead, they may experience atypical exertional symptoms, such as malaise or generalized discomfort, or, when allograft dysfunction is pronounced, symptoms of heart failure. Frequently, CAV remains asymptomatic, and therefore yearly screening is encouraged. Coronary angiography is the accepted method of assessing CAV. For those patients whose baseline angiogram is free of disease, angiography can be performed on an alternate year basis. In the intervening years, noninvasive imaging with either positron emission tomography or dobutamine echocardiography is acceptable. For those patients in whom CAV is detected, yearly angiography should be performed to track its progression. More recently, CT angiography has been employed for routine detection of CAV, avoiding the need for invasive angiography.[26]

Effective prevention of CAV includes the use of aspirin and HMG-CoA reductase inhibitors (statins). Pravachol is preferred because it is not metabolized by CYP 3A4, but other statins are equally effective in preventing CAV. Unfortunately, treatment

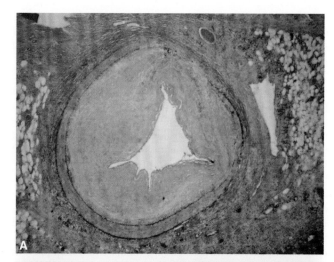

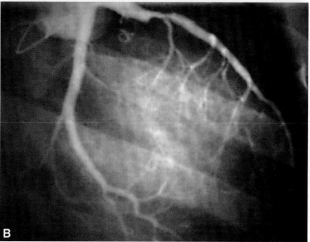

FIGURE 18.3 Cardiac allograft vasculopathy (CAV) is a proliferative disorder that typically arises in the branches and distal vessels in response to both immunologic and nonimmunologic forms of injury. A cross section of an artery affected by CAV shows near obliteration of the lumen (A). Coronary angiography remains the most common modality to diagnose CAV. Typical pruning of the branch and distal vessels (B).

options remain limited. Target of rapamycin inhibitors, such as sirolimus and evorolimus, have been shown to slow, and in some cases prevent, the progression of vasculopathy.[27] Revascularization with either coronary stenting or bypass surgery is frequently not an option because secondary and tertiary branches of the coronary arteries are often involved, reducing "downstream" blood flow. Intracoronary stenting may be an option for treating focal symptomatic lesions. Rates of restenosis are higher for CAV than for typical atherosclerotic lesions. The use of drug-eluting stents produces lower restenosis rates as compared to bare metal stents, but both have rates that are higher than those seen in nontransplant patients. For severe disease, retransplantation remains the only definitive treatment option.

ANTIMICROBIAL PROPHYLAXIS AND TREATMENT

Transplanted patients are at risk for infection from both common and opportunistic pathogens. Typical signs of infection may be less prominent in the setting of immune suppression, and fever may be suppressed by the use of corticosteroids. The prevalence of infection in the early transplant period is 47% for bacterial infections, followed by viral (42%), fungal (8%), and protozoal (4%) infections.[28]

The risk of bacterial infection is particularly high during the immediate postoperative period and slowly abates over a 6-month period. Antibiotic prophylaxis to prevent surgical wound infection using an agent against gram-positive cocci (ie, cefazolin or vancomycin) is routinely used in all patients. Contact isolation with the use of gowns and gloves is recommended to prevent nosocomial infection. Respiratory isolation is not required for patients, but hand washing before and after patient contact is encouraged, as is the early removal of support lines and tubes. Visitors are certainly allowed, but they should also perform hand washing. Patients should not be exposed to fresh cut flowers and should handle fruit and vegetables only after they have been thoroughly cleaned or peeled. The use of a surgical mask may help prevent airborne transmission when venturing out of the hospital room.

The risk of fungal infection is greatest during the period of maximal immune suppression and tails off by the sixth postoperative month. The most commonly encountered infection is candidiasis, particularly oral thrush. It is easily prevented with nystatin swish and swallow or mycelex troches. Deep tissue infections require more aggressive treatment with systemic antimicrobial drugs such as fluconazole. Pneumocystis carinii is an opportunistic fungal pathogen that classically presents as an interstitial pneumonia producing cough and hypoxemia, particularly with exertion. Prophylaxis with trimethaprim/sulfamethoxazole is given throughout the first year to prevent fulminant infection. Dapsone or atovaqoune can be used as a substitute in the sulfa allergic patient. Other fungal pathogens like aspergillus or cryptococcus can produce life-threatening infections. Therapy for these more severe infections requires aggressive care with intravenous azole therapy or amphotericin.

The risk of protozoal infection peaks at month 3 and dissipates over the first year. All transplant donors and recipients should be tested for exposure to toxoplasmosis gondii. Seronegative recipients from a positive donor should receive pyrimethamine prophylaxis or high-dose trimethoprim/sulfamethoxazole for 6 weeks. Folinic acid is given concomitantly to prevent pyrimethamine hepatotoxicity. As more patients from endemic areas receive transplants, it is incumbent on the transplant team to consider reactivation of a broad spectrum of pathogens. These include strongyloides hyperinfection in those patients who lived for a time in Puerto Rico or the Dominican Republic. Reactivation of *Trypanosoma cruzi* may be encountered in patients from South or Central America where Chagas cardiomyopathy is the leading cause of heart failure. Screening for both these pathogens should take place before listing for transplant.

Risk of viral infection, particularly from HSV, CMV, and varicella zoster virus, increases over the first 6 weeks after transplant, but falls by the sixth month coincident with the reduced dose of immunosuppressive therapy. Chronic infection may persist, particularly from viruses such as CMV, HBV, and EBV, and the latter may contribute to the risk of malignancy, particularly posttransplant lymphoproliferative disorder.[4]

Infection with CMV is of particular concern because it can occur from either latent viral reactivation or direct donor transmission. Seronegative patients who receive a heart from a seropositive donor have a 50% risk of developing infection. Symptoms of CMV can vary considerably, including flulike symptoms or a gastrointestinal syndrome with profuse watery diarrhea and elevation of liver transaminases. Leucopenia may be present as a consequence of bone marrow suppression. Other manifestations of CMV include pneumonitis, pancreatitis, retinitis, and encephalitis. Polymerase chain reaction is the most sensitive diagnostic test for the detection of viremeia, but the diagnosis can also be made from identification of virus from tissue biopsy (usually stomach or colon) or from the serum buffy coat.

ADJUVANT THERAPY FOR THE TRANSPLANT PATIENT

Routine treatment of the posttransplant patient with HMG-CoA reductase inhibitors (statins) decreases the incidence of CAV and increases long-term survival. In a landmark 1995 trial, cardiac transplant patients randomized to pravastatin had less rejection and CAV, and improved survival compared to controls.[29] These results were recently reconfirmed in a "real world" analysis of over 1000 transplant patients.[30] It is unclear whether the results are secondary to the anti-inflammatory effects of statins or to their lipid-lowering properties. Aspirin is routinely given to all heart transplant patients. Although data supporting antiplatelet therapy are not as robust as those for the statins, transplant patients are thought to be more likely to have activated platelets. Aspirin prophylaxis may consequently decrease the risk of myocardial infarction.[31,32]

Concomitant use of corticosteroids and calcineurin inhibitors places the transplant patient at increased risk for developing osteoporosis. To lower this risk, patients receiving chronic corticosteroid therapy should take a calcium and vitamin D supplement. Patients with dexa scan evidence of either osteopenia or osteoporosis, and any patient considered at increased risk for fracture, are encouraged to take one of the bisphosphanates, such as alendronate or risedronate. Calcitonin may be considered an alternative to the bisphosphonates.[33]

HOSPITAL DISCHARGE

Discharge planning should begin shortly after the patient leaves the intensive care unit. Physical therapy should be initiated as soon as the patient is medically clear to participate. Nutritionists should be consulted to provide education to patients about heart-healthy diets as well as drug–food interactions. Medical regimens are reviewed with the patient and family members. Before being cleared for discharge, patients must be hemodynamically stable without any need for vasoactive medicines, must have an endomyocardial biopsy free of rejection, and must have a therapeutic tacrolimus or CyA drug level. It is our general practice to ensure that patients can successfully recite the names of their immunosuppressive drugs before allowing home discharge. Follow-up appointments in the transplant clinic are generally performed within 1 week of discharge. Patients are instructed to stay near the transplant center for several months should the need for urgent hospitalization arise.

The goal of cardiac transplantation is to both extend life and restore productivity. Unfortunately, less than 30% of transplant recipients return to full-time employment. Although this is partially attributable to the advancing age of the transplant population, other obstacles exist. Patients may be severely deconditioned from their previous heart failure condition, and may require intensive physical therapy to regain full function. Chronic corticosteroid therapy, which produces proximal muscle weakness and central obesity, may contribute to this deconditioning. It is possible that a strategy that employs earlier implantation of bridging left ventricular assist devices will allow sufficient reconditioning prior to transplant to allow for quicker postoperative recovery. The denervated heart also limits full cardiovascular performance, because it produces a slightly diminished maximal cardiac output. This is particularly evident in size-mismatched recipients. Despite these limitations, the majority of heart transplant recipients enjoy a physically active lifestyle and an improvement in quality of life, especially when compared to their pretransplant state.

REFERENCES

1. Jalowiec A, Grady KL, White-Williams C. Functional status one year after heart transplant. *J Cardiopulm Rehabil.* 2007;27:24-32; discussion 33-34.

2. Triffaux JM, Wauthy J, Bertrand J, et al. Psychological evolution and assessment in patients undergoing orthotopic heart transplantation. *Eur Psychiatry.* 2001;16:180-185.

3. McGiffin DC, Kirklin JK, Naftel DC, et al. Competing outcomes after heart transplantation: a comparison of eras and outcomes. *J Heart Lung Transplant.* 1997;16:190-198.

4. Mehra MR, Canter CE, Hannan MM, et al. The 2016 International Society for Heart Lung Transplantation listing criteria for heart transplantation: a 10-year update. *J Heart Lung Transplant.* 2016;35: 1-23.

5. Maurer MS, Raina A, Hesdorffer C, et al. Cardiac transplantation using extended-donor criteria organs for systemic amyloidosis complicated by heart failure. *Transplantation.* 2007;83:539-545.

6. Uriel N, Jorde UP, Cotarlan V, et al. Heart transplantation in human immunodeficiency virus-positive patients. *J Heart Lung Transplant.* 2009;28:667-669.

7. Aberegg SK. Cardiac transplantation in an HIV-1-infected patient. *N Engl J Med.* 2003;349:1388-1389.

8. Mancini DM. Cardiopulmonary exercise testing for heart transplant candidate selection. *Cardiologia.* 1997;42:579-584.

9. Aaronson KD, Schwartz JS, Chen TM, et al. Development and prospective validation of a clinical index to predict survival in ambulatory patients referred for cardiac transplant evaluation. *Circulation.* 1997;95:2660-2667.

10. Levy WC, Mozaffarian D, Linker DT, et al. The Seattle Heart Failure Model: prediction of survival in heart failure. *Circulation.* 2006;113:1424-1433.

11. Kobashigawa J, Mehra M, West L, et al. Report from a consensus conference on the sensitized patient awaiting heart transplantation. *J Heart Lung Transplant.* 2009;28:213-225.

12. Yap CH, Zimmet A, Mohajeri M, et al. Effect of obesity on early morbidity and mortality following cardiac surgery. *Heart Lung Circ.* 2007;16:31-36.

13. Zaroff JG, Rosengard BR, Armstrong WF, et al. Maximizing use of organs recovered from the cadaver donor: Cardiac recommendations. *J Heart Lung Transplant.* 2002;21:1153-1160.

14. Gasink LB, Blumberg EA, Localio AR, et al. Hepatitis C virus seropositivity in organ donors and survival in heart transplant recipients. *JAMA.* 2006;296:1843-1850.

15. Foster WQ, Murphy A, Vega DJ, et al. Hepatitis B vaccination in heart transplant candidates. *J Heart Lung Transplant.* 2006;25:106-109.

16. Groetzner J, Kaczmarek I, Landwehr P, et al. Renal recovery after conversion to a calcineurin inhibitor-free immunosuppression in late cardiac transplant recipients. *Eur J Cardiothorac Surg.* 2004;25:333-341.

17. Ojo AO, Held PJ, Port FK, et al. Chronic renal failure after transplantation of a nonrenal organ. *N Engl J Med.* 2003;349:931-940.

18. Nardo B, Beltempo P, Montalti R, et al. Kidney transplantation combined with other organs: experience of Bologna s. Orsola hospital. *Transplant Proc.* 2005;37:2469-2471.

19. Carrier M, Leblanc MH, Perrault LP, et al. Basiliximab and rabbit anti-thymocyte globulin for prophylaxis of acute rejection after heart transplantation: a non-inferiority study. *J Heart Lung Transplant.* 2007;26:258-263.

20. Kobashigawa J, Miller L, Renlund D, et al. A randomized active-controlled trial of mycophenolate mofetil in heart transplant recipients. Mycophenolate Mofetil Investigators. *Transplantation.* 1998;66:507-515.

21. Lubitz SA, Baran DA, Alwarshetty MM, et al. Improved survival with statins, angiotensin receptor blockers, and steroid weaning after heart transplantation. *Transplant Proc.* 2006;38:1501-1506.

22. Pham MX, Teuteberg JJ, Kfoury AG, et al. Gene expression profiling for rejection surveillance after cardiac transplantation. *N Engl J Med.* 2010;362:1890-1900.

23. Olivari MT, May CB, Johnson NA, et al. Treatment of acute vascular rejection with immunoadsorption. *Circulation.* 1994;90:II70-II73.

24. Pinney SP, Mancini D. Cardiac allograft vasculopathy: advances in understanding its pathophysiology, prevention, and treatment. *Curr Opin Cardiol.* 2004;19:170-176.

25. Costanzo MR, Naftel DC, Pritzker MR, et al. Heart transplant coronary artery disease detected by coronary angiography: a multiinstitutional study of preoperative donor and recipient risk factors. Cardiac Transplant Research Database. *J Heart Lung Transplant.* 1998;17:744-753.

26. Knollmann FD, Bocksch W, Spiegelsberger S, et al. Electron-beam computed tomography in the assessment of coronary artery disease after heart transplantation. *Circulation.* 2000;101:2078-2082.

27. Eisen HJ, Tuzcu EM, Dorent R, et al. Everolimus for the prevention of allograft rejection and vasculopathy in cardiac-transplant recipients. *N Engl J Med.* 2003;349:847-858.

28. Smart FW, Naftel DC, Costanzo MR, et al. Risk factors for early, cumulative, and fatal infections after heart transplantation: a multi-institutional study. *J Heart Lung Transplant.* 1996;15:329-341.

29. Kobashigawa JA, Katznelson S, Laks H, et al. Effect of pravastatin on outcomes after cardiac transplantation. *N Engl J Med.* 1995;333:621-627.

30. Wu AH, Ballantyne CM, Short BC, et al. Statin use and risks of death or fatal rejection in the Heart Transplant Lipid Registry. *Am J Cardiol.* 2005;95:367-372.

31. de Lorgeril M, Dureau G, Boissonnat P, et al. Increased platelet aggregation after heart transplantation: influence of aspirin. *J Heart Lung Transplant.* 1991;10:600-603.

32. de Lorgeril M, Boissonnat P, Dureau G, et al. Low-dose aspirin and accelerated coronary disease in heart transplant recipients. *J Heart Transplant.* 1990;9:449-450.

33. Braith RW, Magyari PM, Fulton MN, et al. Comparison of calcitonin versus calcitonin + resistance exercise as prophylaxis for osteoporosis in heart transplant recipients. *Transplantation.* 2006;81:1191-1195.

Patient and Family Information for: SELECTION AND CARE OF THE HEART TRANSPLANT PATIENT

Patients with advanced heart failure (also referred to as Stage D or end-stage heart failure) experience symptoms of fatigue and shortness of breath in spite of optimal medical therapy. Once heart failure has progressed to this point, few treatment options remain. Heart transplantation has been performed since the 1960s. Over the years, refinements in both surgical technique and medical management have significantly improved patient survival and quality of life. In the early days of transplantation, most patients lived only a few months, whereas now heart transplant patients can expect to live many years with a good quality of life. About 90% of heart transplant recipients survive the first year. More than half of all recipients live for more than 10 years, and some live for more than 20 years with the same transplanted heart. The major downside to heart transplantation is that there simply are not enough donor hearts to go around. Currently in the United States, there are close to 200,000 patients living with advanced heart failure, but only 2000 heart transplants will be performed annually. This means that there is a constant need to increase awareness of organ donation to increase the pool of available organs.

Patients who are referred to an advanced heart failure program for consideration of heart transplantation must first undergo a standard evaluation. This evaluation is designed to answer two questions: first, is the patient sick enough to require transplant, and, second, are there any reasons why this patient should not receive a heart transplant. The typical evaluation includes consultations with a cardiologist, surgeon, and transplant coordinator. Additional visits with social work and psychiatry are necessary to screen for potential psychological, financial, or social barriers to living with a transplant. Typical tests include a CT scan, ultrasound, and age-appropriate cancer screening. One invasive test, a right heart catheterization, will measure the pressures inside the heart and lungs to ensure that it is safe to perform the operation.

The decision to place a patient on the heart transplant waiting list is made by a committee of transplant professionals, the same individuals who met the patient during the evaluation process. Waiting times vary from state to state and are determined by a patient's body size, blood type, and heart failure severity. Those patients who require admission to an intensive care unit or who have a failing ventricular assist device are moved to the top of the list because they face the highest risk of dying in the near future.

The transplant operation takes about 6 to 8 hours to perform. Most patients will remain in the intensive care unit for at least 4 or 5 days and in the hospital for about 10 to 14 days. During this time, the transplanted heart will be supported by a number of intravenous medications and occasionally a temporary pacemaker to ensure that it beats fast enough. This is also the time when patients start to receive medications that suppress the immune system and prevent the heart from being rejected by the body. Even though it sounds severe, heart transplant rejection is rarely severe and can almost always be treated simply by increasing the dose of immune suppressive medications.

Before leaving the hospital, all patients must have a heart biopsy to check for rejection. This procedure takes less than half an hour to perform. A physician will place a tube in the jugular vein and pass a bioptome (a small scissor-like instrument) through it to sample a few pieces of heart tissue. These samples will be looked at by a pathologist to make sure there is no sign of rejection. This procedure is repeated throughout the first year at regular intervals to make sure the heart is not being rejected and to safely allow reductions in immune suppressive medications.

Most patients feel very well living with a transplant. Although some have run marathons and climbed mountains, most heart transplant recipients simply live life without experiencing fatigue and shortness of breath as they did when they had heart failure. To make sure that the transplanted heart continues to function well, patients will have to return for check-ups several times each year. Everyone will have an echocardiogram performed annually to make sure that the heart is still beating well. Patients will also have an annual angiogram to make sure that the transplanted arteries remain free of blockages that could weaken the heart over time. All patients who take immune suppressive medications are more vulnerable to infections. In addition to taking antibiotics to prevent infection, transplant recipients should use common sense and avoid close contact with family or friends who are sick.

There are a number of long-term complications that can limit the success of heart transplantation. Some of the immune suppressive medicines can weaken the kidneys. About 5% of heart transplant recipients will have advanced kidney disease requiring dialysis or a kidney transplant. Although the immune suppressive drugs do not cause cancer, they do place transplant patients at higher risk for developing cancers. These include a rare form of lymphoma, which affects the immune system. Skin cancer is the most common form of cancer and should be prevented by wearing a hat, long-sleeved shirts, and sunscreen when outdoors.

Yaron Hellman
Ashish Correa
Eyal Herzog

Medications Used in the Management of Heart Failure

The past 30 years have provided remarkable advances in the pharmacotherapeutic management of patients with acute and chronic heart failure (HF). Major improvements in both survival and symptom management now provide practitioners with the ability to provide therapy that is well tolerated, decreases recurrent hospitalizations, and improves quality of life. As the incidence of HF continues to increase with the advancing age of the population, and there is improved post-infarction survival, maximizing the use of currently available agents, development of new class of drugs, and the continued development of implantable devices for treatment of mechanical and electrical complications of HF should further our ability to improve patient care.

In this chapter, we explore the various agents currently available for the management of HF.

INOTROPES

Intravenous inotropes dobutamine and milrinone are useful in patients with severe systolic dysfunction with relative hypotension and evidence of inadequate end-organ perfusion, who are not responsive to, or are intolerant of, vasodilators and diuretics. Inotropic agents relieve acute HF symptoms and may preserve end-organ function, but have not been demonstrated to improve survival. On the contrary, several studies have demonstrated increased adverse outcomes, including increased mortality with chronic intravenous inotropic therapy.

DOBUTAMINE

Dobutamine, a synthetic catecholamine, is primarily a β adrenergic stimulant with minimal α_1 cardiac sympathetic activity. Its β_1 sympathetic activity accounts for its inotropic activity through β-receptor–mediated activation of intracellular cyclic-adenosine monophosphate (c-AMP). The resulting sarcoplasmic reticulum calcium release mediates myocardial contractility. Similar β_1 activity at the sinoatrial (SA) node accounts for its modest chronotropic activity. Patients taking β-blockers on admission may have an attenuated initial response to dobutamine, until the β-blocker has been metabolized or renally eliminated.[1] However, cardiac output response to increasing doses of dobutamine has been observed in patients on chronic carvedilol.[2] The dose-dependent β_2 effect produces mild peripheral arteriolar dilation. As with most intravenous sympathetic stimulants, dobutamine has a rapid onset of action (1 to 2 minutes) and has a peak effect within 10 minutes. The drug is rapidly methylated providing for a short duration of action ($t_{1/2}$—2 minutes), ideal for a drug requiring titration based on hemodynamic effects.

The hemodynamic effects of dobutamine in patients with HF include increased cardiac output, arteriolar dilation, reduction of pulmonary artery occlusion pressure (PAOP or wedge pressure), and small but variable change in blood pressure (**Table 19.1**). In responsive patients, the hemodynamic benefits of the drug increase end-organ perfusion, manifest by improving renal function and urine output, decreased pulmonary vascular congestion, and improved skin perfusion and mentation.

The adverse effects that should be monitored in patients with HF include dose-related tachycardia – most concerning in ischemic cardiomyopathy – as well as atrial arrhythmias (like atrial fibrillation) and ventricular arrhythmias (like ventricular tachycardia).

Dobutamine dosing begins at 2.5 to 5 µg/kg/min and is progressively increased on the basis of clinical and hemodynamic response. Because it is not a vasoconstrictor (pressor), dobutamine does not need to be administered through a central line. Dosing may be increased to 15 µg/kg/min, although maximum hemodynamic benefit may be achieved at lower doses, and ventricular ectopy risk increases as the dose is increased. Once hemodynamic stability has been accomplished, dobutamine infusions should be gradually tapered off. Although intermittent ambulatory dobutamine infusions have been used for quality-of-life enhancement in patients who are not candidates for transplantation or pump implantation, or as a pharmacologic bridge to cardiac transplantation, the practice has generally been replaced by implantation of ventricular assist devices.[3] In addition, randomized trials have demonstrated increased mortality with the use of ambulatory dobutamine infusions.[4]

MILRINONE

Milrinone is a selective inhibitor of phosphodiesterase III, an enzyme responsible for the intracellular breakdown of c-AMP. c-AMP accumulation increases intracellular calcium and thereby facilitates myocardial contractility. Although milrinone's hemodynamic effects are similar to those of dobutamine, milrinone

TABLE 19.1	Hemodynamic Effects of Intravenous Agents Used in the Treatment of Acute Decompensated Heart Failure					
DRUG	DOSE	HR	MAP	PAOP	CO	SVR
Dobutamine	2.5–15 µg/kg/min	0/+	0	−	+	−
Milrinone	0.375–0.75 µg/kg/min	0/+	0/−	−	+	−
Dopamine	0.5–3 µg/kg/min	0	0	0	0/+	−
Dopamine	3–10 µg/kg/min	+	+	0	+	0
Dopamine	>10 µg/kg/min	+	+	+	+	+
Nesiritide	Bolus: 2 µg/kg Infusion: 0.01 µg/kg/min	0	0/−	−	+	−
Nitroglycerin	5–200 µg/min	0/+	0/−	−	0/+	0/−
Nitroprusside	0.25–3.0 µg/kg/min	0/+	0/−	−	+	−

CO, cardiac output; HR, heart rate; MAP, mean arterial pressure; PAOP, pulmonary artery occlusive pressure; SVR, systemic vascular resistance.
Adapted from DiPiro JT, Talbert RL, Yee GC, et al. *Pharmacotherapy: A Pathophysiologic Approach.* 7th ed. New York, NY: McGraw Hill; 1999.

produces more arterial and venous dilation, earning it the label "inodilator" (**Table 19.1**). Theoretical advantages of milrinone as compared to dobutamine include greater afterload reduction, augmenting the cardiac output produced by its inotropic effect, and its post-receptor mechanism of action, a potential benefit in patients receiving β-blockers for chronic HF. Hemodynamic improvement is usually observed within 15 minutes of initiation of therapy. The drug is renally eliminated with an elimination half-life of approximately 3 hours in patients with HF, and the maintenance infusion should be adjusted on the basis of creatinine clearance.

Although the package insert recommends a 50 µg/kg loading dose, many practitioners refrain from administering the loading dose to reduce the risk of hypotension. Typical maintenance doses of milrinone range from 0.375 to 0.75 µg/kg/min (**Table 19.2**). At maintenance doses above 0.5 µg/kg/min, once hemodynamic and clinical stability has been achieved, the infusion should be gradually tapered off. However, because the drug has a longer elimination half-life than does dobutamine, lower milrinone maintenance doses may be reduced more rapidly than dobutamine doses, provided hemodynamic stability has been achieved. In addition to hypotension, the most common side effects are

TABLE 19.2	Renal Dosing of Milrinone
CREATININE CLEARANCE (mL/min/1.73 m²)	MILRINONE INFUSION RATE (µg/kg/min)
5	0.20
10	0.23
20	0.28
30	0.33
40	0.38
50	0.43

tachyarrhythmias. Milrinone may produce less tachycardia than does dobutamine, but it also has the potential to produce both atrial and ventricular arrhythmias.

Despite the potential adverse long-term impact on morbidity and mortality related to intravenous inotropic therapy, patients with acute decompensated HF benefit from the short-term hemodynamic improvement associated with the administration of these agents, pending the resolution of the underlying events that precipitated their hemodynamic deterioration.

DOPAMINE

Dopamine possesses dose-dependent hemodynamic effects, stimulating D_1 dopamine receptors, α_1-, β_1-, and β_2-receptors. Other than the diuretic effect of low-dose (renal dose) dopamine to enhance volume loss in patients with diuretic-resistant HF, dopamine use is typically reserved for use in patients with marked hypotension including those with cardiogenic shock. Inotropic doses in the 2 to 5 µg/kg/min range promote increase in cardiac output; however, intermediate- and high-dose dopamine increase systemic vascular resistance, increasing afterload and PAOP, and impeding cardiac output (**Table 19.1**). In the setting of cardiogenic shock, dopamine may be required to maintain mean arterial pressure and coronary perfusion pressure until the underlying etiology can be treated or resolved.

DIGOXIN

Digoxin is a moderately potent inotrope with additional neurohormonal modulating effects producing increased parasympathetic nervous system activity and decreased central sympathetic nervous system drive. Its inotropic effect is related to inhibition of sarcolemmal sodium-potassium-ATP-ase, resulting in increased myocardial cell calcium, the final common pathway for all currently available inotropic agents. The benefit of digoxin in HF was debated for most of its first 200-year history. The drug has little use in the treatment of acute HF in patients with sinus rhythm. Perhaps the least controversial use of the drug in patients with

HF is to assist (in combination with β-blockers or amiodarone) in the management of rate control in patients with atrial fibrillation. The Digoxin Investigation Group (DIG) clarified the role of digoxin in the management of patients with HF with normal sinus rhythm.[5] This study demonstrated that digoxin, in addition to background angiotensin-converting enzyme inhibitor (ACEI) and diuretic therapy, improved exercise tolerance, and reduced HF-related hospitalizations, but did not improve survival. Therefore, digoxin therapy for HF may be considered in patients with atrial fibrillation or in patients in sinus rhythm on target doses (if tolerated) of angiotensin-converting enzyme inhibitor/angiotensin receptor blocker (ACEI/ARB) and β-blockers who exhibit continued exercise intolerance or recurrent HF-related hospitalizations.

Digoxin is primarily renally eliminated with a serum elimination half-life of 1.6 days in patients with normal renal function. Recent trials have demonstrated that the efficacy of digoxin in HF can be achieved with doses that produce serum concentrations of 0.5 to 1.0 ng/mL, lower than those previously defined as "therapeutic."[6] Higher serum concentrations provide no added benefit and increase the risk of digoxin toxicity.

Digoxin Toxicity

Digitalis intoxication is a clinical diagnosis based on the presence of signs and/or symptoms including anorexia, nausea, and vomiting, and atrial or ventricular arrhythmias. Given the establishment of lower effective serum concentration, the incidence of digoxin toxicity has likely diminished. It is important to understand that the diagnosis of digoxin toxicity is never based solely on the digoxin concentration. Elevated serum digoxin concentrations are only one etiology of drug toxicity, usually related to maintenance doses inappropriate for the level of renal function. Most patients with normal renal function require 0.125 mg digoxin daily. Patients with renal insufficiency typically require 0.125 mg every other day or less. Many other factors that do not produce elevated serum digoxin concentrations are capable of causing digoxin toxicity

including diuretic-induced hypokalemia or hypomagnesemia, hypoxemia, acidosis, hyperthyroidism, and others. Concurrent amiodarone therapy may double the serum digoxin concentration, and typical digoxin dosing in these patients should be reduced by 50% of the usual dose, considering renal function.

DIURETICS

Classical descriptions of acute decompensated HF characterize patients as volume overloaded, but well perfused ("wet and warm") or hypoperfused and not volume overloaded ("cool and dry"). However, the majority of hospitalized patients will require acute diuretic therapy to relieve signs and symptoms associated with their acute presentation. Much of the efficacy data associated with diuretic therapy for acute HF has been derived from experience before the era of randomized controlled trials. Despite their effectiveness for symptom relief, diuretics have not been demonstrated to improve survival in HF. Because of their potency, and rapid onset of action, loop diuretics (furosemide, torsemide, and bumetanide) are considered the mainstay of treatment (**Table 19.3**). These agents inhibit sodium and chloride reabsorption in the ascending limb of the loop of Henle. Their effect of reducing venous tone and therefore pulmonary capillary wedge pressure often begins to improve pulmonary symptoms before a significant increase in urinary output. It is important to recognize that patients with chronic HF may have increased pulmonary capillary pressures and progressive dyspnea in the absence of significant pulmonary crackles on physical examination. Conversely, patients with new-onset HF are more likely to demonstrate pulmonary vascular congestion (crackles) on examination.

Dosing of loop diuretics is empiric. In general, a 40-mg oral dose is equivalent to a 20-mg intravenous dose. In volume-overloaded patients with normal renal function, an initial intravenous dose should be 1 to 2 times the chronic oral dose. Response to an individual intravenous dose can be assessed in several hours. Patient

TABLE 19.3	Diuretics Used in the Treatment of Heart Failure		
DRUG	INITIAL DAILY DOSE(S)	MAXIMUM TOTAL DAILY DOSE	DURATION OF ACTION
Loop diuretics			
Bumetanide	0.5–1.0 mg once or twice	10 mg	4–6 h
Furosemide	20–40 mg once or twice	600 mg	6–8 h
Torsemide	10–20 mg once	200 mg	12–16 h
Potassium sparing diuretics			
Eplerenone	25 mg once	50 mg once	24 h
Spironolactone	12.5–25 mg once	50 mg	2–3 d
Triamterene	50–75 mg	200 mg	7–9 h
Sequential nephron blockade			
Metolazone	2.5–10 mg once plus loop diuretic		
Chlorothiazide (IV)	500–1000 mg once plus loop diuretic		

response is based on relief of pulmonary vascular congestion, daily weight, hepatic congestion, and peripheral edema. Because loop diuretics require a threshold serum concentration to affect their natriuretic response, patients with chronic HF, and those with moderate-to-severe renal insufficiency will usually require higher initial doses than patients with normal renal function or new-onset HF (diuretic-naive patients). Alternative furosemide dosing strategies comparing bolus dosing to continuous infusions have been evaluated in a number of small uncontrolled trials. Earlier studies, in addition to a review of eight randomized trials, suggest that continuous intravenous infusions of furosemide ranging from 10 to 40 mg/h, depending on renal function, produce a greater diuretic effect than similar total doses administered by intermittent bolus dosing, with fewer adverse effects.[7] The DOSE (Diuretic Optimization Strategies Evaluation) trial, a randomized, open-label comparison between twice-daily bolus furosemide versus continuous infusion demonstrated no differences in outcomes in hospitalized, volume-overloaded patients with HF.[8] There was a trend toward less hypokalemia and hypotension in the continuous infusion group. Although no definitive data currently resolve the dosing route of administration controversy, it does not appear that continuous infusion offers a significant advantage over traditional bolus dosing of furosemide.

Monitoring of adverse effects of diuresis such as abnormal electrolytes, orthostatic hypotension, prerenal azotemia or increasing serum creatinine, is essential. Less commonly, patients with a history of chronic gout may experience an acute gout exacerbation. Excessive diuresis can enhance undesired neurohormonal activation, increasing the risk of excessive hypotensive effects from ACEI and β-blockers.

Diuretic resistance is not uncommon in patients with an acute exacerbation of chronic HF. A number of factors predispose to lack of diuretic response including worsening renal function, agents such as nonsteroidal anti-inflammatory drugs (NSAIDs) that antagonize the effects of diuretics, or renal hypoperfusion secondary to HF or overly aggressive diuresis or vasodilators. A number of strategies to produce effective diuresis in nonresponsive patients have been employed. First, if appropriate diuretic response is not achieved within 4 hours, the intravenous dose can be successively doubled until an intravenous dose of 120 mg is reached. Higher single doses are unlikely to enhance diuresis and are more likely to risk ototoxicity. Despite the lack of controlled data, anecdotal reports of successful diuresis with continuous furosemide infusions in diuretic-resistant patients may promote successful diuresis. Oral metolazone, unlike other oral thiazide diuretics, can be effective in patients with renal insufficiency. An oral dose of 5 to 10 mg should be administered before intravenous furosemide—30 to 60 minutes is the accepted time frame, although pharmokinetically the distal tubule blockade requires at least several hours. Other distal convoluted tubule diuretics include oral hydrochlorothiazide, chlorthalidone, or intravenous chlorothiazide. However, metolazone, perhaps related to its efficacy in patients with renal insufficiency and its longer elimination half-life, seems to be preferred by most clinicians.

Diuretics that act more distally, such as spironolactone or amiloride, are less likely to overcome diuretic resistance, but may have a role in limiting hypokalemia and hypomagnesemia provoked by loop diuretics. These acute electrolyte disturbances in patients with HF increase the risk of hemodynamically compromising, or potentially life-threatening arrhythmias. Intravenous low-dose dopamine stimulates renal dopamine receptors and has been demonstrated to increase urine output; however, no controlled studies in patients with diuretic-resistant HF have been undertaken. Interpatient variability in response to the β1 adrenergic inotropic effects of dopamine may play a role in its ability to increase urinary output in HF. The UNLOAD (*UN*load the *L*eft ventricle in patients with *AD*vanced heart failure) trial demonstrated that ultrafiltration produced greater weight and fluid loss, as well as fewer HF-related hospitalizations than intravenous diuretics in patients hospitalized for HF.[9] The CARRESS-HF (*CA*rdiorenal *RES*cue *S*tudy in Acute Decompensated *H*eart *F*ailure) trial was undertaken to demonstrate the efficacy of ultrafiltration in patients with HF having persistent congestion and worsening renal function. Unfortunately, the ultrafiltration had no benefit over stepped pharmacological therapy (diuretics).[10] In fact, ultrafiltration was associated with more adverse events—worsening renal failure, bleeding, and catheter-related events. Therefore, ultrafiltration is reserved for patients with refractory congestion who have failed to respond to diuretic-based strategies.[11]

ALDOSTERONE ANTAGONISTS

The adverse effects of aldosterone in HF are related to its sodium- and water-retaining potential initiated by activation of the rennin–angiotensin–aldosterone system (RAAS), and from decreased hepatic aldosterone clearance. As important is the impact of aldosterone on myocardial and vascular remodeling that produces increased collagen deposition and fibrosis. These effects produce ventricular systolic and diastolic dysfunction and contribute to the progressive nature of chronic HF. Although both ACEIs and ARBs lower aldosterone production in the short term, long-term suppression may not be maintained. Aldosterone antagonists spironolactone and eplerenone have both been demonstrated to improve symptoms, reduce HF-related hospitalizations, and improve survival in selected patients. The *R*andomized *AL*dactone *E*valuation *S*tudy (RALES) trial evaluated the effect of spironolactone (maximum dose 25 mg daily) in patients with New York Heart Association (NYHA) class IV symptoms, or class III symptoms in recently hospitalized patients.[12] The EPHESUS (*E*plerenone *P*ost-Acute Myocardial Infarction *H*eart *F*ailure *E*fficacy and *SU*rvival *S*tudy) trial studied eplerenone (maximum dose 50 mg daily) in patients with HF or diabetes and left ventricular ejection fraction (LVEF) <40% within 14 days of myocardial infarction (MI). Both drugs demonstrated an improvement in survival and reduction in HF-related hospitalization.[13] The EMPHASIS (*E*plerenone in *M*ild *P*atients *H*ospitalization *A*nd *S*urv*I*val *S*tudy) trial expanded the use of aldosterone antagonists by evaluating the effect of eplerenone in patients with NYHA II symptoms and LVEF ≤35%, again resulting in reduction of mortality and hospitalizations.[14]

The benefits associated with the use of aldosterone antagonists must be carefully weighed against the potential for life-threatening hyperkalemia. Given that ACEI therapy has become a mainstay in the treatment of HF, and because some degree of renal insufficiency is common as the severity of HF increases, it is imperative that patients be chosen carefully, and that appropriate monitoring of serum potassium concentrations takes place. The major trials excluded patients with serum creatinine >2.5 mg/dL; however, serum creatinine is a poor predictor of creatinine clearance, especially in elderly patients. Aldosterone antagonists should not be administered to patients with creatinine clearances below 30 mL/min, and the dose should be reduced at creatinine clearances less than 50 mL/min. More frequent use of aldosterone antagonists in the general HF population, as opposed to patients enrolled in clinical trials, subsequent to the publication of the two major trials, has resulted in an incidence of hyperkalemia up to 24%.[15] Serum potassium concentrations should be monitored within 3 days of drug initiation and again at 1 week. Serum potassium concentrations greater than 5.5 mEq/L should promote discontinuation of the drug. The lack of routine monitoring has been well documented in the ambulatory care setting.[16]

Spironolactone may cause painful gynecomastia in approximately 10% of patients, according to the RALES study, and probably increased rates in higher doses. This is attributed to the anti-androgenic and indirect estrogenic effect of spironolactone. Eplerenone is much more selective than spironolactone in aldosterone receptor blockade and does not exert anti-androgenic and estrogenic effects. However, it is less potent than its corresponding dose of spironolactone. Eplerenone is also more expensive than spironolactone, and is therefore usually administered when patients complain of spironolactone-related side effects.

VASODILATORS

Nitroglycerin, nitroprusside, and nesiritide are all effective in improving hemodynamic and symptoms of pulmonary vascular congestions in patients who are not hypotensive. These agents are indicated in patients with ongoing pulmonary vascular congestion not responsive to diuretic therapy and standard oral therapy. Additional indications for intravenous vasodilator therapy include patients with HF and ongoing ischemia, hypertension, or significant mitral regurgitation.

NITROGLYCERIN

Nitroglycerin is primarily a venodilator with dose-dependent arteriolar dilating properties. At higher doses, nitroglycerin is a potent coronary vasodilator, making it an ideal agent for patients with ischemic cardiomyopathy. Nitrate-induced preload reduction results in reduced PAOP, myocardial oxygen demand, and improvement in dyspnea. Because of its short onset and duration of action, the infusion rate can be quickly adjusted, allowing easy titration toward maximal beneficial hemodynamic effects, and rapid correction of adverse effects. The risk of hypotension with nitroglycerin as with the other intravenous vasodilators is critically dependent on intravascular volume. Hemodynamic monitoring may be useful to assess the beneficial effects, and limit the risk of hemodynamic adverse effects with both nitroglycerin and nitroprusside, as well as with intravenous inotropes. Tolerance to the hemodynamic effects of nitroglycerin can be seen in 12 to 72 hours in patients on continuous nitroglycerin infusions.[17]

NITROPRUSSIDE

Nitroprusside is a more balanced arteriolar and venous dilator than nitroglycerin. As a more potent arteriolar dilator, it has greater effect in increasing cardiac output in patients with elevated systemic vascular resistance, while retaining the preload lowering benefit of reducing PAOP and pulmonary congestion. Although nitroprusside has been associated with coronary steal in patients with obstructive coronary disease, in patients with HF

the reduction in both preload and afterload generally decreases myocardial oxygen demand.[18] Obviously a significant reduction in aortic diastolic pressure has the potential to decrease coronary perfusion pressure and increase ischemia. As with nitroglycerin, nitroprusside is short acting, providing for easy titration. The most common side effect is hypotension. Two biochemical toxicities have potentially led to the underutilization of nitroprusside in acute decompensated HF—cyanide and thiocyanate toxicity. Malnourished patients or patients with liver disease are more prone to cyanide intoxication because of their inability to combine cyanide produced in the serum from nitroprusside with the hepatically produced sulfhydryl group to form thiocyanate. The accumulated cyanide produces elevated lactate levels and metabolic acidosis. Patients with decrease renal function are unable to eliminate the thiocyanate metabolite and develop neurotoxicity including headache, altered mental status, and seizures. Because thiocyanate has an elimination half-life of 4 days in patients with normal renal function, infusions of less than 3 µg/kg/min administered for less than 3 days in patients with a serum creatinine less than 3.0 mg/dL are unlikely to result in toxicity. Serum thiocyanate concentrations can be measured in the hospital laboratory.

NESIRITIDE

Nesiritide is an intravenous form of recombinant human brain natriuretic peptide (BNP). It produces a dose-dependent reduction in venous and arterial pressures, natriuresis, and diuresis. Its most consistent effect is decreased dyspnea and POAP, much like nitroglycerin. Questions remain as to the impact of nesiritide on hospitalization rates and mortality, especially in the face of its relatively high cost compared to nitroglycerin. In addition, in a review of a series of publications, nesiritide significantly increased the risk of worsening renal function.[19] The ASCEND-HF (Acute Study of Clinical Effectiveness of Nesiritide in Decompensated Heart Failure) trial enrolled 7141 patients hospitalized with acute HF randomly assigned to nesiritide or placebo. Nesiritide did not impact mortality or rehospitalization, and was not associated with worsening renal function, but it was associated with an increase in rates of hypotension.[20]

ANGIOTENSIN-CONVERTING ENZYME INHIBITORS/ ANGIOTENSIN RECEPTOR BLOCKING AGENTS

ACEIs have been demonstrated to improve survival in NYHA Class II to IV patients with systolic dysfunction, and improve symptoms in many patients (**Table 19.4**). Their pharmacologic effects, inhibiting the conversion of angiotensin I to angiotensin II, result in a decreased production of angiotensin II and aldosterone. Limiting aldosterone production decreases the progression of left ventricular dysfunction and reduces ventricular remodeling, myocardial fibrosis, cardiac hypertrophy, and dilatation. The chronic hemodynamic effects of ACEIs to reduce afterload (angiotensin is a potent vasoconstrictor), and, to a lesser extent, preload, improves exercise tolerance and quality of life. In addition to improving survival, ACEIs decrease the rate of HF-related hospitalizations, and limit the need for increasing diuretic doses. For post-MI patients, ACEIs reduce the risk of developing HF, recurrent MI, and HF-related hospitalizations. Angiotensin-converting enzyme is also responsible for the degradation of bradykinin. The cough and rare cases of angioedema observed in patients treated with ACEI are attributed to this elevation of bradykinin. Therefore, substitution of an ACEI with a direct ARB can bypass this effect without raising bradykinin levels. Owing to the significant cumulative data demonstrating the benefit for ACEI in the treatment of chronic HF, these drugs, as opposed to ARBs, are recommended as first-line therapy for chronic HF. ARBs, which probably possess similar symptom and survival benefit, should be reserved for the 10% to 15% of patients who develop ACEI-induced cough.

ACEI therapy for ischemic or nonischemic cardiomyopathy should be initiated at low doses, but may be titrated to maximum doses within a few days to weeks, provided blood pressure and renal function remain stable. It is important to note that patients with more severe HF may have relatively low blood pressures (systolic pressures in the 100 mm Hg range), and as long as symptomatic hypotension is not present, ACEI therapy should be maintained. Dose reduction or transient withholding of ACEI administration should not be based only on the systolic blood pressure reading, but on the presence of symptomatic hypotension. In addition, new-onset hypotension or an increase in serum creatinine, in the setting of ACEI therapy, warrants an evaluation for cause, especially overly aggressive diuretic therapy, or hyponatremia in the setting of NYHA Class IV HF. Although survival enhancement can be achieved with low doses of ACEIs (lisinopril 5 mg or its equivalent), maximum symptom improvement and limitation of HF-related hospitalizations are best achieved with higher doses (20 to 40 mg lisinopril).

For patients with acute decompensations of chronic HF, ACEIs or ARBs have minimal acute hemodynamic benefit, but should remain part of the therapeutic regimen as long as they are hemodynamically tolerated.

The two most likely adverse effects associated with ACEI/ARB administration in hospitalized patients are hypotension and worsening renal function. The risks of both of these outcomes are enhanced by overly aggressive diuresis. Small (10%) increases in serum creatinine are commonly associated with initiating ACEI/ARB therapy in patients with HF, and should not provoke dosage reduction or drug withdrawal. Progressive increases in serum creatinine, however, are a typical manifestation of decreased renal blood flow, commonly the result of aggressive diuretic therapy, or worsening HF. Reducing the rate of diuresis, rather than holding the dose of ACEI/ARB, will usually allow renal function and/or blood pressure to return to its baseline level. It is not usually necessary to temporarily withhold administration of the ACEI/ARB, unless the rise in serum creatinine continues. Drug-induced hypotension, even in the face of total body volume overload, will usually require holding the diuretic until intravascular volume equilibrates.

A second common cause of worsening renal function associated with the administration of ACEIs/ARBs is the concomitant use of other nephrotoxic agents, most notably, intravenous contrast administered for coronary artery imaging. Because of the risk of nephrotoxicity associated with iodinated contrast, especially in the diabetic patient, withholding ACEIs/ARBs for patients with suspected dye-induced nephrotoxicity is appropriate until renal function returns to baseline. Although volume repletion is an effective method of reducing the risk of dye-induced nephrotoxicity, this may be more difficult in patients with HF than in patients with coronary artery disease without HF.[21] The presence of preexisting renal disease in patients with HF should not be considered a contraindication to ACEI/ARB therapy in chronic

HF. Several trials in various patient populations including post-MI patients with decreased left ventricular function have demonstrated that ACEIs are more effective in the subset of patients with mild-to-moderate renal insufficiency than in patients with normal renal function.[22] Judicious routine monitoring of renal function is required in patients hospitalized for HF, irrespective of the addition of ACEIs/ARBs. Prevention of hyperkalemia is especially important in patients with HF with chronic kidney disease receiving ACEI/ARB therapy.

ANGIOTENSIN RECEPTOR–NEPRILYSIN INHIBITORS

A new class of drugs was recently developed, combining inhibition of the RAAS via an ARB with a molecule that inhibits the endogenous peptidase neprilysin—an enzyme responsible for the degradation of natriuretic peptides, bradykinin and adrenomedullin (counterregulatory substances released in HF, among other conditions). By inhibiting neprilysin, these counterregulatory substances are upregulated allowing for natriuresis, diuresis, vasodilation, and anti-fibrotic/antiremodeling effects. As with ACEIs, angiotensin receptor–neprilysin inhibitors reduce the degradation of bradykinin (**Table 19.4**). This is why the neprilysin inhibitor molecule was combined with an ARB and not an ACEI. This decision stemmed from the results of a study combining neprilysin inhibition and ACE inhibition in one molecule—omapatrilat, a "super ACE inhibitor." Trials with this molecule had a disturbing rate of angioedema, probably due to the double inhibition of bradykinin degradation causing marked bradykinin elevation.[23] Therefore, a molecule combining valsartan (ARB) and sacubitril (neprilysin inhibitor) was constructed and initially termed LCZ696. After preclinical testing, a large-scale trial (PARADIGM-HF, *P*rospective Comparison of *AR*NI with *ACE*I to *D*etermine *I*mpact on *G*lobal *M*ortality and *M*orbidity in *H*eart *F*ailure, trial) enrolling patients with HF having reduced LVEF (<40% and then 35% during the trial) and NYHA Class II to IV symptoms was initiated. This trial compared enalapril 10 mg bid versus LCZ696 (Sacubitril/Valsartan) in a randomized double-blind design after two single-blind run-in periods (where patients were tested with enalapril and then with LCZ696 individually).[24] The PARADIGM-HF trial demonstrated superiority of LCZ696, later named Entresto, over enalapril. This was reflected in reduced cardiovascular mortality, as well as in hospitalizations. The main side effects are similar to ACEI/ARB—hypotension and angioedema. Following this trial, HF guidelines began to endorse Entresto instead of ACEI/ARB if a patient is still symptomatic despite optimal medical therapy.[25]

β-BLOCKERS

β-Blockers were originally considered contraindicated in patients with HF because of their negative inotropic effects (**Table 19.4**). Once the paradigm for the pathogenesis of HF shifted away from primary myocardial dysfunction to a syndrome resulting from the action of "compensatory" mechanisms related to the sympathetic nervous system and the renin–angiotensin–aldosterone axis, it became clear that agents that antagonize these mechanisms might be beneficial. Several large randomized trials in the 1990s demonstrated that β-blockers improve survival in patients with NYHA Class II to IV HF.[26–28] In addition, they decrease the risk

TABLE 19.4	Oral Agents FDA Approved for Treatment of Chronic Heart Failure		
DRUG	**INITIAL DOSE**	**TARGET DOSE**	**ELIMINATION**
ACE inhibitors			
Captopril	6.25 mg tid	50 mg tid	Renal
Enalapril	2.5–5 mg bid	10 mg bid	Renal
Lisinopril	2.5–5 mg daily	20–40 mg daily	Renal
Quinapril	10 mg bid	20–40 mg bid	Renal
ARB			
Candesartan	4 mg daily	32 mg daily	Renal
Valsartan	40 mg bid	160 mg bid	Liver/some renal
ARNI			
Sacubitril-Valsartan	24–26 mg to 49–51 mg bid	97–103 mg bid	Sacubitril: renal/liver Valsartan: liver/some renal
β-Blockers			
Carvedilol	3.125 mg bid	<85 kg: 25 mg bid >85 kg: 50 mg bid	Liver
Carvedilol extended release	10 mg daily	80 mg daily	Liver
Metoprolol extended release	12.5 mg daily	200 mg daily	Liver
Ivabradine	2.5–5 mg bid	7.5mg bid	Liver/renal
Hydralazine-isosorbide dinitrate (Bidil)	Hydralazine 37.5 mg Isosorbide 20 mg tid	Hydralazine 75 mg Isosorbide 40 mg tid	Liver

ACE, angiotensin-converting enzyme; ARB, angiotensin receptor blocker; ARNI, angiotensin receptor–neprilysin inhibitor; FDA, U.S. Food and Drug Administration.

of overt HF in patients with asymptomatic left ventricular dysfunction. The progression and degree of chronic HF severity are associated with the serum concentration of norepinephrine. Patients with the highest norepinephrine concentrations have the poorest prognosis. Hemodynamically, norepinephrine-induced tachycardia and inotropic effects increase myocardial oxygen demand. In addition, the peripheral vasoconstriction increases left ventricular afterload, further increasing oxygen demand and decreasing cardiac output. Chronically, sympathetic stimulation produces myocardial cell loss through apoptosis and cell necrosis, as well as downregulation of myocardial β_1 receptors and loss of sensitivity to sympathetic stimulants. As had been previously discovered with the use of ACEIs to interfere with the adverse effects of the RAAS on progressive ventricular dysfunction, survival, and symptoms, blocking the detrimental effects of catecholamines on the failing ventricle with β-blockers resulted in improved left ventricular function, attenuating ventricular remodeling, decreasing the risk of life-threatening arrhythmias, and decreasing myocardial oxygen demand.

A number of issues are relevant to the use of β-blockers in the patient hospitalized for HF. These include timing of drug therapy initiation, methods for increasing doses toward chronic target dosing, strategies for dosing in patients on chronic β-blockers who are admitted for acute HF decompensation, and choosing between various β-blockers approved for use in chronic HF.

β-Blocker therapy should be initiated in patients with new-onset HF only after volume status has been optimized. Patients who remain volume overloaded are more likely to develop increasing HF symptoms, whereas patients who are intravascularly volume depleted are more like to become hypotensive. Several studies have addressed the order in which ACEI/ARB or β-blockers should be administered, because initiation of both agents is recommended within 24 hours of the onset of MI.[29] These studies, however, have been performed in patients with mild-to-moderate chronic HF, not patients hospitalized with new-onset or acutely decompensated HF. Although both β-blockers and ACEIs are effective for myocardial remodeling post MI, current guidelines recommend initiation of ACEI within 24 hours of the MI, and delaying the introduction of β-blockade until the signs and symptoms of HF have been resolved. It is not necessary to achieve the "target dose" of ACEI/ARB before initiating starting doses of the β-blocker.

Unlike the initial dosing strategy with ACEIs/ARBs, β-blockers should be titrated toward their target doses more gradually, with a minimum of 2-week intervals between dosage increases. It is well documented that many patients with chronic HF do not receive doses consistent with target doses determined by large controlled trials. As with ACEIs/ARBs, small doses of β-blockers do positively impact survival; however, greater reduction in HF hospitalizations and improvement in LVEF are achieved with dosing strategies intended to achieve target doses. It is common for ambulatory care providers to maintain patients on the low-dose β-blockers that were initiated during an acute hospitalization, presumptively based on concerns for worsening HF as the dose is increased, or assuming that the patient has achieved the ultimate level of symptom control. Clearly, monitoring for adverse effects such as worsening HF, symptomatic bradycardia, or hypotension are a requisite part of chronic monitoring during titration toward target doses of β-blocker therapy. Especially for patients with new-onset HF, however, maintaining a starting dose, without an attempt to titrate to target doses, diminishes the potential benefit that the combination of ACEI/ARB and β-blockers can achieve for prevention of disease progression.

Recent data have addressed the question of withdrawing β-blockers in patients on chronic therapy who present with an acute decompensation of HF. Until recently, the approaches have generally been either to temporarily discontinue the β-blocker or to decrease the chronic dose to some degree. The appropriate strategy clearly depends on the level of severity of the acute decompensation. Patients who present with severe hemodynamic decompensation (hypotensive, or approaching cardiogenic shock), or those with severe pulmonary vascular congestion are obvious candidates for transient withdrawal of β-blockers. Data prospectively analyzed from the OPTIMIZE-HF (Organized *P*rogram to Initiate Lifesaving Treatment in Hospitalized Patients with Heart Failure) demonstrated that patients who were withdrawn from β-blocker therapy had a higher risk for mortality, compared with those continued on β-blockers.[30] Patients who were eligible for β-blocker therapy, but did not receive them, had similar risk for mortality as those who had therapy withdrawn. During the 60- to 90-day follow-up period, 94% of patients remained on β-blockers after discharge. Only 57% of patients who had their β-blocker withdrawn received β-blocker treatment during the 60- to 90-day follow-up period. Of the patients maintained on therapy during hospitalization, only 12% had their maintenance dose reduced during follow-up. The remaining 88% were maintained on their preadmission dose, or had their dose increased (12%). It appears therefore from limited registry data that patients with chronic HF admitted to the hospital on β-blocker therapy should not have this therapy withdrawn unless they are hemodynamically compromised. An additional risk associated with β-blocker withdrawal is failure to reinstate the drug after hospital discharge.

Two β-blockers are currently approved in the United States for the treatment of HF—metoprolol controlled release/extended release (CR/XL) and carvedilol. Bisoprolol has also been demonstrated to reduce the incidence of sudden death and of HF-related death, but is not approved by the U.S. Food and Drug Administration for this indication in the United States. Metoprolol is a cardioselective β-blocker, whereas carvedilol is a nonselective β-blocker with α-adrenergic blocking activity. Both agents have demonstrated similar reductions in morbidity and mortality in large randomized controlled studies of patients with HF. Subtle pharmacodynamic features may influence the decision to use one drug or the other. The cardioselectivity of metoprolol may be beneficial in patients with reversible airway disease such as asthma; however, cardioselectivity diminishes with increasing dosage. The recommended target dose of metoprolol of 200 mg daily likely provides little cardioselectivity. The α-blocking property of carvedilol has a theoretical advantage in patients with a history of cocaine abuse in whom pure β-blocker pharmacology leaves unopposed coronary artery α-receptors susceptible to the vasospastic potential of cocaine. Both metoprolol XL and

carvedilol are available as once-daily dosing formulations to enhance patient compliance.

The most common adverse effects of β-blockers in patients with HF include worsening of HF symptoms, especially in volume-overloaded patients or in those whose dose titration has occurred too rapidly, symptomatic bradycardia, or hypotension.

IVABRADINE

Ivabradine is a drug that inhibits the If Current (If—"I funny"—because this sodium channel current is triggered by hyperpolarization, as opposed to other sodium channels) in the SA node. If is the "pacemaker current" responsible for spontaneous depolarization of the SA nodal tissue. The rationale behind the development of this agent was to produce further lowering of the heart rate, in addition to β-blockers. Ivabradine does not have negative inotropic effects, so patients with β-blocker intolerance can receive a lower dose of β-blocker with ivabradine or ivabradine alone as a heart-rate–lowering agent. The SHIFT (*S*ystolic *H*eart *F*ailure Treatment with the *I*f Inhibitor Ivabradine *T*rial) enrolled patients with HF having LVEF ≤35%, with NYHA class II to IV symptoms, and on optimal medical therapy with a heart rate >70. In this trial, ivabradine reduced the combined end point of hospitalizations and cardiovascular mortality.[31] Therefore, ivabradine (marketed as Corlanor) can be added on to optimal β-blocker therapy, along with ACEI/ARB and spironolactone in patients with LVEF ≤35% and are still symptomatic. Side effects include bradycardia and luminous phenomena—phosphenes, brightness in the visual fields. The visual changes are presumed to be the result of ivabradine inhibiting similar retinal channels.

HYDRALAZINE-ISOSORBIDE DINITRATE

The combination of the direct arteriolar dilator, hydralazine, and isosorbidedinitrate (ISDN), a long-acting nitrate venodilator was the first vasodilator regimen to demonstrate improved survival in chronic HF (V-HeFT, Vasodilator Heart Failure Trial).[32] Within a few years, ACEIs had been shown to enhance survival to a greater degree than did the original vasodilator combination, and had become the standard of care for chronic HF. A post hoc analysis of the original hydralazine-nitrate trial suggested that the combination was particularly effective in African-Americans. The A-HeFT (African-American Heart Failure Trial) compared a fixed combination of hydralazine and ISDN (maximum dose hydralazine 75 mg plus ISDN 40 mg 3 times a day) versus placebo in self-identified African-American patients on background ACEI, β-blocker, and a diuretic with or without digoxin and spironolactone.[33] The hydralazine-ISDN group had a significant reduction in mortality, in HF-related hospitalizations, and in an improvement in quality of life.

Oral vasodilator therapy with ACEIs and the combination of hydralazine have primarily been studied in patients with chronic HF. However, in patients hospitalized with acute HF for whom ACEIs may be transiently withheld because of acute elevations of serum creatinine, hydralazine-isosorbide has been substituted for its beneficial hemodynamic effect.[34] Once stable renal function has been reestablished, ACEIs are the preferred choice for chronic management. In addition to its use in African-American patients, chronic hydralazine-isosorbide therapy may be appropriate for patients who do not tolerate either ACEIs or ARBs because of renal insufficiency or hyperkalemia.

The frequency of side effects such as headache and gastrointestinal complaints from the hydralazine-isosorbide combination in large trials is significant, and in both vasodilator HF trials many patients did not tolerate target doses of these drugs. In addition, the necessity of 3 times daily dosing increases the risk of noncompliance.

REFERENCES

1. Dec GW. Management of acute decompensated heart failure. *Curr Probl Cardiol.* 2007;32:321-366.

2. Tsvetkova TFD, Abraham WT, Kelly P, et al. Comparative hemodynamic effects of milrinone and dobutamine in heart failure patients treated chronically with carvedilol. *J Card Fail.* 1998;4(suppl 1):36, Abstract.

3. Applefeld MM, Newman KA, Grove WR, et al. Intermittent continuous outpatient dobutamine infusion in the management of congestive heart failure. *Am J Cardiol.* 1983;51:455-458.

4. Silver AM, Horton DP, Ghali JK, et al. Effect of nesiritide versus dobutamine on short-term outcomes in the treatment of patients with acutely decompensated heart failure. *J Am Coll Cardiol.* 2002;39:798-803.

5. The Digitalis Investigation Group. The effect of digoxin on mortality and morbidity in patients with heart failure. *N Engl J Med.* 1997;336:525-533.

6. Adams KF, Gheorghiade M, Uretsky BF, et al. Clinical benefits of low serum digoxin concentrations in heart failure. *J Am Coll Cardiol.* 2002;39:946-953.

7. Salvador DR, Rey NR, Ramos GC, et al. Continuous infusion versus bolus injection of loop diuretics in congestive heart failure. *Cochrane Database Syst Rev.* 2005;CD003178.

8. Allen LA, Turer AT, DeWald T, et al. Continuous versus bolus dosing of furosemide for patients hospitalized for heart failure. *Am J Cardiol.* 2010;105:1794-1797.

9. Costanzo MR, Guglin ME, Saltzberg MT, et al. Ultrafiltration versus intravenous diuretics for patients hospitalized for acute decompensated heart failure. *J Am Coll Cardiol.* 2007;49:675-683.

10. Bart BA, Goldsmith SR, Lee KL, et al. Ultrafiltration in decompensated heart failure with cardiorenal syndrome. *N Engl J Med.* 2012;367(24):2296-2304.

11. Ponikowski P, Voors AA, Anker SD, et al. 2016 ESC guidelines for the diagnosis and treatment of acute and chronic heart failure: the Task Force for the diagnosis and treatment of acute and chronic heart failure of the European Society of Cardiology (ESC). Developed with the special contribution of the Heart Failure Association (HFA) of the ESC. *Eur Heart J.* 2016;37(27):2129-2200.

12. Pitt B, Zannad DF, Remme WJ, et al. The effect of spironolactone on morbidity and mortality in patients with severe heart failure. *N Engl J Med.* 1999;341:709-717.

13. Pitt B, Remme WJ, Zannad DF, et al. Eplerenone, a selective aldosterone blocker in patients with left ventricular dysfunction after myocardial infarction. *N Engl J Med.* 2003;348:1309-1321.

14. Zannad F, McMurray JJ, Krum H, et al; EMPHASIS-HF Study Group. Eplerenone in patients with systolic heart failure and mild symptoms. *N Engl J Med.* 2011;364(1):11-21.

15. Juurlink DM, Mamdani M, Kopp A, et al. Drug-drug interactions among elderly patients hospitalized for drug toxicity. *JAMA.* 2003;289:1652-1658.

16. Shah KB, Rao K, Sawyer R, Gottlieb SS. The adequacy of laboratory monitoring in patients treated with spironolactone for congestive heart failure. *J Am Coll Cardiol.* 2005;46:845-849.

17. Elkayam U, Kulick D, McIntosh N, et al. Incidence of early tolerance to hemodynamic effects of continuous infusion of nitroglycerin in patients with coronary artery disease and heart failure. *Circulation.* 1987;76:577-584.

18. Robertson RM, Robertson D. Drugs used for the treatment of ischemia. In: Limbird LE, Hardman JG, eds. *Goodman and Gillman's The Pharmacological Basis of Therapeutics.* 10th ed. New York, NY: McGraw Hill; 2001:840-871.

19. Sackner-Bernstein JD, Skopicki HA, Aaronson KD. Risk of worsening renal function with nesiritide in patients with acutely decompensated heart failure. *Circulation.* 2005;111:1487-1491.

20. O'Connor CM, Starling RC, Hernandez AF, et al. Effect of nesiritide in patients with acute decompensated heart failure. *N Engl J Med.* 2011;365(1):32-43.

21. Maeder M, Klein M, Fehr T, et al. Contrast nephropathy: review focusing on prevention. *J Am Coll Cardiol.* 2004;44:1763-1771.

22. Solomon SD, Rice MM, Jablonski KA, et al. Renal function and effectiveness of angiotensin-converting enzyme inhibitor treatment in patients with chronic stable coronary disease in the Prevention of Events with ACE inhibition (PEACE) trial. *Circulation.* 2006;114:26-31.

23. Packer M, Califf RM, Konstam MA, et al. Comparison of omapatrilat and enalapril in patients with chronic heart failure: the Omapatrilat Versus Enalapril Randomized Trial of Utility in Reducing Events (OVERTURE). *Circulation.* 2002;106(8):920-926.

24. McMurray JJ, Packer M, Desai AS, et al; PARADIGM-HF Investigators and Committees. Angiotensin-neprilysin inhibition versus enalapril in heart failure. *N Engl J Med.* 2014;371(11):993-1004.

25. Yancy CW, Jessup M, Bozkurt B, et al. 2016 ACC/AHA/HFSA focused update on new pharmacological therapy for heart failure: an update of the 2013 ACCF/AHA guideline for the management of heart failure: a report of the American College of Cardiology/American Heart Association Task Force on Clinical Practice Guidelines and the Heart Failure Society of America. *J Am Coll Cardiol.* 2016;68(13):1476-1488.

26. Packer M, Bristow MR, Cohn JN, et al. The effect of carvedilol on morbidity and mortality in patients with chronic heart failure. U.S. Carvedilol Heart Failure Study Group. *N Engl J Med.* 1996;334:1349-1355.

27. Effect of metoprolol CR/XL in chronic heart failure: metoprolol CR/XL Randomized Intervention Trial in Congestive Heart Failure (MERIT- HF). *Lancet.* 1999;353:2001-2007.

28. The Cardiac Insufficiency Bisoprolol Study II (CIBIS-II): a randomized trial. *Lancet.* 1999;353:9-13.

29. Willenheimer R, van Veldhuisen DJ, Silke B, et al. Effect on survival with hospitalization of initiating treatment for chronic heart failure with bisoprolol followed by enalapril, as compared with the opposite sequence: results of the randomized Cardiac Insufficiency Bisoprolol Study (CIBIS) III. *Circulation.* 2005;112:2426-2435.

30. Fonarow GC, Abrahan WT, Albert NM, et al. Influence of beta blocker continuation or withdrawal on outcomes in patients hospitalized with heart failure. Findings from the OPTIMIZE-HF Program. *J Am Coll Cardiol.* 2008;52:190-199.

31. Swedberg K, Komajda M, Böhm M, et al; SHIFT Investigators. Ivabradine and outcomes in chronic heart failure (SHIFT): a randomised placebo-controlled study. *Lancet.* 2010;376(9744):875-885.

32. Cohn JN, Archibald DG, Zeische S, et al. Effect of vasodilator therapy on mortality in chronic congestive heart failure. Results of a Veterans Administration Cooperative Study. *N Engl J Med.* 1986;314:1547-1552.

33. Taylor AL, Ziesche S, Yancy C, et al. Combination of isosorbidedinitrate and hydralazine in blacks with heart failure. *N Engl J Med.* 2004;351:2049-2057.

34. Verma SP, Silke B, Reynolds GW, et al. Vasodilator therapy for acute heart failure: haemodynamic comparison of hydralazine/isosorbide, alpha-adrenergic blockade, and angiotensin-converting enzyme inhibition. *J Cardiovasc Pharmacol.* 1992;20:274-281.

Patient and Family Information for: MEDICATIONS USED IN THE MANAGEMENT OF HEART FAILURE

DRUGS FOR PATIENTS HOSPITALIZED WITH HEART FAILURE

Patients with HF symptoms often need hospitalization when their symptoms become severe. Several drugs are useful to relieve the symptoms of HF and to return them to the quality of life they experienced before the need for hospitalization. For most patients, relieving symptoms related to shortness of breath and swelling of their extremities are important goals. For patients who are more severely ill, improving their heart function will provide better blood flow to their organs and muscles. There are three drug categories that are frequently used for patients hospitalized for HF: drugs that relieve swelling and shortness of breath—diuretics such as furosemide (Lasix), drugs that improve heart pumping function (dobutamine or milrinone), and drugs that relax blood vessels and make it easier for the heart to pump blood into the blood vessels (nitroglycerin or nitroprusside).

Diuretic drugs decrease the amount of volume that is in the bloodstream by increasing the amount of salt and water that is removed by the kidneys. Patients with HF are often short of breath because the amount of fluid in the lungs makes it difficult for them to breathe. In addition, many patients have fluid accumulation in their ankles, legs, and even in their abdomen. The primary goal in patients hospitalized for HF is to eliminate fluid from the lungs, followed by a reduction of fluid in other parts of the body. It is important for these patients to know their "dry weight," the target weight they should maintain as outpatients. Appropriate use of diuretic drugs in the hospital should bring patients close to their dry weight. It is equally important for patients with HF to weigh themselves daily at home, because this is a practical method to determine fluid accumulation. Weight gain of more than 2 to 3 pounds within a few days is an indication that their HF may not be well controlled. Dietary salt intake has the greatest potential to promote fluid accumulation. Patients should be aware of the salt (sodium) content of the foods they eat, especially prepared foods such as canned vegetables and soups, prepared meats, and snack foods such as pretzels, potato chips, and similar items. They should also avoid adding salt to their meals at the table. Excessive salt intake can easily overcome the effects of diuretic drugs, and result in fluid accumulation. Some physicians have successfully educated patient to increase the dose of their diuretic drugs (furosemide or Lasix) when their weight increases by several pounds. If weight gain continues, or patients become increasingly short of breath with exertion, or when lying down at night, they should contact their physician. The side effects of diuretics that are closely monitored are decreases in blood pressure, kidney function, and other body salts such as potassium and magnesium. A careful balance is maintained between too much volume in the circulation, producing symptoms of shortness of breath and swelling, and too little volume, resulting in diminished kidney function or low blood pressure.

In addition to diuretics such as furosemide, which are used in the hospital, and chronically to manage fluid balance, two other diuretic drugs may be used in selected patients with HF with moderate-to-severe forms of HF. Spironolactone (Aldactone) and eplerenone (Inspra) are diuretic drugs that work by a mechanism different from that of furosemide, and, unlike other diuretic agents, have been shown to improve survival in selected patients with HF. Although they add to the ability of diuretic drugs to maintain appropriate fluid balance, their major impact is to add to the survival benefit of drugs like ACEIs and β-blockers (see subsequent text). The most important side effect of these added diuretics is their ability to increase the level of potassium in the blood. Because ACE inhibitors or ARBs also have the ability to cause the kidneys to hold on to potassium, serum potassium level should be closely monitored, especially in patients whose kidney function is impaired.

Intravenous drugs that increase the force of contraction in patients with HF are sometimes required in hospitalized patients when more conservative therapy has failed to improve symptoms and blood flow. Dobutamine and milrinone are both drugs that increase the force with which the heart contracts, and therefore increase the amount of blood to the kidneys, muscles, and other vital organs. These drugs are intended for short-term use—several days—and are effective in improving blood flow, stabilizing blood pressure, and improving symptoms. Because these drugs have a short duration of action, doses can be easily adjusted to the heart pressures that are being closely monitored in severely ill patients. Most patients with HF have poorly contracting ventricles (lower heart chambers). Although it seems logical that drugs which improve the force of contraction of the heart should improve survival, the effect of these drugs is to improve symptoms and restore normal pressures in the circulation, rather than to benefit survival. The major side effect of dobutamine and milrinone include increased heart rate and heart rhythm disturbances. These potential side effects are closely monitored in patients in intensive care units. In rare cases, dobutamine may be used as an intermittent outpatient infusion to relieve symptoms in patients with severe HF who are not candidates for heart transplants or implantable heart pumps.

The only oral drug used in HF to increase the force of contraction is digoxin. The drug, used for more than 200 years in the treatment of HF, is much less powerful than agents such as dobutamine or milrinone. There are two circumstances in which digoxin may be used in HF. In hospitalized patients whose HF is complicated by the cardiac rhythm disturbance, atrial fibrillation, a rhythm disturbance of the upper chambers of the heart, digoxin may be used with other drugs to reduce pulse rate. In patients with chronic HF, digoxin may be added to other chronic HF medications to improve symptoms of exercise intolerance and to decrease the rate of hospitalizations for HF symptoms. Digoxin must be administered at lower dose or less frequently (every other day) to patients whose HF is complicated by reduced kidney function. Loss of appetite, nausea, and changes in heart rhythm are side effects that should be monitored in patients receiving digoxin therapy.

Nitroglycerin and nitroprusside are intravenous drugs that dilate arteries and/or veins and may also be used in patients with severe HF. By relaxing arteries, more blood can be ejected from the heart, increasing blood flow to vital organs. Because these drugs have the potential to lower blood pressure in patients whose heart function is already compromised, they must be administered under close supervision, making sure that blood flow is improved while blood pressure is maintained. Fortunately, both nitroprusside and nitroglycerin are very short-acting drugs, whose doses can be quickly altered if necessary. Because nitroprusside has some side effects that occur more commonly in patients whose kidneys are not functioning normally, some physicians prefer nitroglycerin in such patients. Because nitroprusside is better able to dilate arteries than nitroglycerin, it may be preferred in patients with normal kidney function. Nitroglycerin dilates veins, to a greater extent than arteries, and is especially useful in patients with significant shortness of breath due to fluid accumulation in the lungs, and in patients with coronary artery disease, who may be experiencing chest pain associated with their HF symptoms.

DRUGS FOR CHRONIC HEART FAILURE

Most drugs used for the treatment of chronic HF will be continued when patients are hospitalized. At times during a patient's hospitalization, especially if the blood pressure decreases, or the kidney function worsens, these drugs may be withheld for short periods of time. However, once the patient's symptoms and vital organ function (especially kidneys) have improved, these agents will be restarted before discharge from the hospital.

ACEIs (lisinopril and others) are drugs that relax (dilate) blood vessels, making it easier for the heart to eject blood into the circulation. They thereby decrease the amount of work that the heart has to perform to provide adequate blood flow to vital organs and muscles. Most importantly, these drugs reduce the rate of deterioration of heart function responsible for the progression of HF, and prolong survival. Patients with HF and their caretakers should understand that although most patients experience some symptom improvement, continued compliance with the medication is critical, even in those whose symptoms do not improve, or improve only slightly, because the drugs prolong life. About 10% of patients experience a dry cough with ACEI therapy. The cough may occur at any time during therapy, and the patient's caretaker may notice the symptoms before the patient. Should the cough become bothersome, replacing the ACEI with an ARB will provide the same benefit without the associated cough. Many HF experts, however, prefer ACEIs as first-line therapy for HF. Rarely, patients may experience swelling of the lips, tongue, or throat from ACEIs. This reaction is a medical emergency and the patient should be taken to an emergency department for treatment to make sure that the airway is not blocked.

ARBs provide similar benefit for patients with HF, but are generally reserved for patients who do not tolerate ACEIs. The incidence of swelling of the lips and throat is lower than with ACEIs, but there are rare cases of such swelling in patients receiving ARBs who had previous reactions with ACEIs. Patients receiving ACEIs of ARBs will require monitoring of blood pressure, kidney function, and potassium levels in the blood.

Similar to ACEIs, β-blocker drugs are an important part of the treatment of chronic HF. β-Blockers work in HF by preventing chemicals produced by the nervous system from interacting with heart muscle. This interaction is partially responsible for the chronic decrease in pump function with progression of symptoms experienced by patients with HF. β-Blockers, like ACE inhibitors and ARBs, may also be used to treat high blood pressure, but their use in HF is not primarily directed at blood pressure. Like ACEIs, β-blockers prevent the progression of pump function loss, improve survival, and, for most patients, improve exercise tolerance and other symptoms of HF. Also similar to ACEI therapy, lack of symptom improvement should not cause patients to stop taking the drug, because it also prolongs life. For patients with new-onset HF, β-blockers will be started at a low dose, whether the patient is in the hospital or is treated as an outpatient. However, β-blocker therapy will not be started until the patient's HF symptoms, especially fluid overload, have been treated, and the patient is considered stable. The dose of β-blocker will be gradually increased toward a maximum target dose no more frequently than every 2 weeks, provided no adverse effects are noticed. The most important β-blocker side effects are excessive slowing of heart rate or reduction of blood pressure, producing symptoms of dizziness or lightheadedness. Other side effects may be observed in patients with diseases such as asthma or diabetes. Patients with asthma may experience shortness of breath or wheezing. This side effect can be minimized with certain β-blocker drugs such as metoprolol (Toprol), but may still occur and should be closely monitored. Diabetic patients, especially those receiving insulin, should closely monitor their blood sugars at home since β-blockers may either increase or decrease blood sugar. In addition, these drugs may interfere with a patient's ability to recognize the symptoms of low blood sugar. Sweating and change in mental status may still occur, but the patient may not experience tremor, rapid heart rate, or anxiety typically observed with low blood sugar in the absence of β-blockers. β-Blockers should not be discontinued abruptly without close medical supervision because of the risk of heart attack or serious heart rhythm disturbances.

The combination of hydralazine and isosorbide, when added to standard ACEI, β-blocker, and diuretic therapy in African-American patients has been shown to improve survival, reduce hospitalizations, and improve quality of life in patients with moderate-to-severe HF. These drugs relax arteries (hydralazine) and veins (isosorbide), improving blood flow, decreasing the work of the heart, and possibly preventing changes in the structure of the heart muscle associated with HF. This drug combination is available as a single fixed combination dosage form (Bidil) or as separate drug entities, which are less costly. A significant disadvantage of the combination is the necessity of administering the drugs 3 times a day. Because most drug therapies for HF are administered once or twice a day, the addition of this combination may challenge the likelihood of successful compliance. The incidence of side effects with this combination is also higher than with most other HF regimens. Headache, dizziness, and gastrointestinal distress increase with dose and are fairly common. Dosage should be gradually increased toward the target maximum dose (hydralazine 75 mg and isosorbide 40 mg 3 times daily) or to a dose which is tolerated by the patient.

There are a number of drugs that should be avoided in patients with HF. Most of these drugs are only available by prescription, and will be known by the physician. These include some drugs used for high blood pressure, diabetes, heart rhythm disturbances, and arthritis. Patients must be aware that some over-the-counter medications have the potential to worsen the symptoms of HF. Most important among these is NSAIDs such as ibuprofen (Motrin), naproxen (Aleve, Naprosyn) and similar drugs for pain and inflammation. Acetaminophen (Tylenol) in appropriate doses is safer. NSAIDs may cause salt and water retention, leading to edema (swelling), worsening shortness of breath, and to a decrease in kidney function. In addition, many herbal products including ginseng, licorice, and St. John wart should be avoided in patients with HF. It is best to consult with the pharmacist or physician before adding any new over-the-counter medication or herbal preparation to the prescribed regimen. Patients with HF are commonly prescribed complicated drug therapy regimens, and have other medical conditions related to heart disease including diabetes, high cholesterol, high blood pressure, or others. Behaviors that improve drug therapy compliance can help reduce the need for hospitalizations. Patients should always keep a list of their current drug therapy regimen with them, especially when visiting health care providers or on admission to the hospital.

Allison Selby
Eyal Herzog
Edgar Argulian
Emad F. Aziz

20

Pathway for the Management of Sleep Apnea in the Cardiac Patient

EPIDEMIOLOGY

Sleep-disordered breathing is a highly prevalent medical condition that is currently estimated to affect 5% to 10% of the general population, regardless of race and ethnicity; almost two-thirds of these are underdiagnosed.[1] More than 80% of patients with moderate-to-severe obstructive sleep apnea (OSA) have not been diagnosed by their health care providers.[2,3] Undiagnosed sleep apnea leads to increased morbidity and mortality, particularly related to increased incidence of cardiovascular events.[4] The cost of untreated OSA is currently estimated to reach $3.4 billion.[5] It is therefore imperative that we identify patient population at high risk for sleep apnea and refer them to the appropriate therapy as early as possible.

SLEEP DISORDERS

OBSTRUCTIVE SLEEP APNEA

OSA is a highly prevalent disorder with an estimated prevalence 3% to 7% in men and 2% to 5% in women.[6] It is characterized by repetitive episodes of airflow cessation (apnea) or reduction (hypopnea) despite persistent thoracic and abdominal respiratory effort, likely due to collapse of the pharyngeal airway that occurs during sleep.[7] This collapse generally occurs posterior to the tongue, uvula, and soft palate. These episodes result in hypoventilation as well as hypoxemia, and provoke awakenings (recurrent arousals) that restore pharyngeal dilator muscle tone and airflow. OSA is generally defined as five or more apneas and/or hypopneas per hour of sleep (Apnea-Hypopnea Index [AHI] > 5) assessed by a cardiorespiratory or full polysomnography (PSG) recording. Obstructive sleep apnea syndrome (OSAS), on the other hand, is defined as an AHI ≥ 5 accompanied by either excessive daytime sleepiness or two or more of the following symptoms such as witnessed apneas, recurrent awakenings, gasping for air, bed partners complaining of excessive snoring, waking unrefreshed, morning headache, daytime fatigue, or impaired concentration or memory.[8] Recurrent episodes throughout the night lead to frequent nocturnal awakenings, resulting in excessive daytime somnolence,[9] which is often the presenting complaint.

CENTRAL SLEEP APNEA

Central sleep apnea (CSA) is common, although less prevalent in the general population than OSA. In a population-based study that included 5804 community-dwelling adults aged 40 years and older, the overall prevalence of CSA on PSG was 0.9%.[10] Approximately half of the CSA cases were associated with Cheyne–Stokes breathing.[11] While the International Classification of Sleep Disorders identifies six different forms of CSA,[12] in general CSA is caused by a loss of ventilatory drive, either due to hyperventilation or hypoventilation leading to cessation of ventilation during sleep. Post-hypocapnia hyperventilation is the underlying pathophysiologic mechanism for central apnea associated with congestive heart failure (HF), high-altitude sickness, and primary CSA. These patients chronically hyperventilate in association with hypocapnia during wake and sleep and demonstrate increased chemoresponsiveness and sleep state instability. CSA due to hypoventilation results from the removal of the wakefulness stimulus to breathe in patients with compromised neuromuscular ventilatory control. Chronic ventilatory failure due to neuromuscular disease or chest wall disease may manifest with central apneas or hypopneas, at sleep onset or during phasic rapid eye movement (REM) sleep. This is typically noted in patients with central nervous system disease, neuromuscular disease, or severe abnormalities in pulmonary mechanics.[13] The apnea episode is 10 seconds or longer in the absence of a respiratory drive, and five or more events occurring in 1 hour are considered abnormal. The diagnostic criteria for CSA depend on the etiology. A diagnosis of primary CSA requires four findings: five or more central apneas/hypopneas per hour of sleep on PSG in the absence of Cheyne–Stokes breathing; patient reports sleepiness, awakening with shortness of breath, witnessed apneas or insomnia; no evidence of daytime or nocturnal hypoventilation; and, finally, absence of a concurrent sleep disorder, medical or neurologic disorder, or substance use disorder than can better explain the patient's symptoms. CSA associated with Cheyne–Stokes respirations, which is typically characterized by an absence of air flow and respiratory effort followed by hyperventilation in a crescendo–decrescendo pattern and most often observed in patients with congestive HF.[14] Furthermore, obstructive and central apnea episodes can occur together in this condition.[15] Diminished upper airway muscle activation at a ventilatory nadir can result in pharyngeal collapse leading to obstruction.

The severity of sleep apnea is quantified using the AHI, which measures the number of episodes/hour. Mild sleep apnea is defined as AHI of 5 to 14 episodes/hour, moderate as 15 to 29, and severe sleep apnea as 30 or more episodes/hour.[16]

CARDIOVASCULAR CONSEQUENCES OF SLEEP APNEA

Prevalence of OSA is noted to be two to three times higher in patients with cardiovascular disease.[17] There is accumulating evidence linking atrial fibrillation,[18–20] hypertension,[21,22] HF,[23,24] and stroke[25] to sleep apnea. It is unclear if these conditions co-exist or if a true causative relationship exists. Prior studies have shown that patients with OSA who were treated conservatively had increased mortality, with most deaths being cardiovascular in origin.[26–28]

There is a bidirectional relationship between OSA and weight gain; up to 80% of patients with sleep apnea are obese, which results in an anatomically small airway leading to recurrent pharyngeal collapse during sleep. However, OSA can also cause or worsen obesity by a number of proposed mechanisms. Frequent nocturnal arousals lead to daytime somnolence, which results in the body craving caffeine and high-calorie sugary foods. These cravings are mediated by the hormone leptin, which is produced by adipose tissue.[29] In addition, patients with OSA have decreased REM sleep, during which the body burns the most calories. There is a significant association between insulin resistance and OSA as well as with atherosclerosis, advocating that the metabolic disturbances may well be a significant link between OSA and cardiovascular disease.[30] Moreover, reports from sleep clinics demonstrated the association between the degree of insulin resistance and severity of OSA.[31] Indeed, those patients with insulin resistance have 5-fold increase in the risk of developing diabetes mellitus, which in turn aggravates obesity.[32]

The prevalence of hypertension in sleep clinics is estimated to be 30% to 50%[33]; likewise, it is estimated that about 50% to 80% of patients with hypertension have OSA.[34,35] Intermittent hypoxemia, sympathetic stimulation, chemoreceptor activation leading to systemic vasoconstriction, and the renin–angiotensin–aldosterone system have been linked to the development of hypertension in OSA.[36] OSA episodes produce surges in systolic and diastolic pressure that keep mean blood pressure (BP) levels elevated at night, resulting in blunted fall in nocturnal BP, or "nondipping phenomena."[37] In many patients, BP remains elevated during the daytime, when breathing is normal. Contributors to this diurnal pattern of hypertension include sympathetic nervous system overactivity and alterations in vascular function and structure caused by oxidant stress and inflammation.[35]

The prevalence of OSA in patients with HF ranges from 12% to 53%, with a higher incidence of Cheyne–Stokes respiration. Recurrent hypoxemia, sympathetic stimulation, and left ventricular (LV) wall stress due to recurrent apnea episodes, over time can lead to LV hypertrophy, dilatation, and systolic dysfunction.[38] OSA in HF has been shown to increase mortality.[39] Thus, a bidirectional relationship may exist between sleep apnea and HF, typically observed by a gradual shift from predominantly obstructive apneas at the beginning of the night to predominantly central apneas toward its end.[40] Salt and fluid retention in HF can contribute to the pathogenesis of OSA and CSA, and effects of the latter can worsen HF. This pathologic relationship may be attributed to marked neurohumoral activation, surges in BP and heart rate (HR), and a greater propensity to lethal arrhythmia induced by CSA.[41,42]

Excessive daytime somnolence is the most common symptom of OSA. Recurrent episodes of nocturnal hypoxemia lead to recurrent arousals. This daytime somnolence frequently results in work-related and motor vehicle accidents. Approximately 25% of patients with untreated OSA report falling asleep while driving.[43]

Cardiac arrhythmias are common in patients with sleep-disordered breathing due to alterations in sympathetic and parasympathetic activity that occurs during periods of hypoxemia.[44,45] Bradycardia, first- to third-degree atrioventricular (AV) conduction block and sinoatrial node block during apneas have been reported in patients with OSA. Becker et al.[46] reported AV-block II–III and/or sinus arrest in 7% of an unselected group of patients with OSA and the prevalence was even higher (20%) in the subgroup with severe OSA. Transmural and intrathoracic pressure gradient changes lead to left atrial enlargement, which has also been linked to the development of atrial fibrillation.[47] The prevalence of atrial fibrillation is significantly higher in patients with OSA than that of the general population. According to the Sleep Heart Study, patients with severe OSA were four times more likely to have atrial fibrillation.[44] Untreated OSA has been shown in several studies to decrease the likelihood of successful rhythm control strategies; likewise, patients who undergo electrical cardioversion and those with untreated OSA are two times more likely to have atrial fibrillation recurrence at 1 year as compared to those who use continuous positive airway pressure (CPAP).[48] Antiarrhythmic drugs have also been shown to be less effective in patients with severe OSA.[49] Although OSA has been shown to increase the risk of atrial fibrillation recurrence after radiofrequency catheter ablation by 40%,[50] its treatment reduces the risk of atrial fibrillation recurrence after catheter ablation.[51]

The higher occurrence of life-threatening ventricular arrhythmias among patients with OSA[52] was suggested to contribute to the abnormal circadian pattern of sudden death in these patients. Gami et al.[53,54] showed a peak in sudden death from cardiac causes during sleeping hours, namely, 10 PM to 6 AM in patients with OSA in contrast to the traditional window of cardiovascular vulnerability which is 6 and 11 AM.

The Busselton Health Study[55] as well as an 18-year follow-up of the Wisconsin Sleep Cohort[56] showed that sleep apnea is an independent risk factor for all-cause mortality. OSA severity, particularly an AHI ≥ 20 as well as the degree of nocturnal hypoxemia have been shown to be directly related to the risk of sudden cardiac death.[54]

Numerous studies linked OSA to an increased risk of myocardial infarction[57,58] which is likely related to the intermittent hypoxemia, systemic vasoconstriction, unpredicted increase in BP, and the resultant changes in intrathoracic and intramural pressures.[59,60] A 7-year prospective study demonstrated that untreated OSA was associated with a 5-fold increase of coronary artery disease (CAD) independent of age, sex, BP, diabetes, or smoking.[61] It has also been suggested that increased oxygen demand and reduced oxygen supply following OSA may trigger an attack of angina pectoris in patients with CAD, who already have reduced coronary flow reserve.[62]

Finally, OSA also appears to be linked to an increased risk of stroke, independent of other cardiovascular risk factors.[63]

Nocturnal fluctuations in BP, nocturnal hypoxemia, reductions in cerebral blood flow, and systemic vasoconstriction appear to contribute to the development of stroke.[64] Habitual snoring and excessive daytime somnolence may also contribute to the risk of developing wake-up stroke.[65]

PATHWAY FOR THE MANAGEMENT OF SLEEP APNEA IN THE CARDIAC PATIENT

Owing to the high incidence of sleep apnea in patients with cardiovascular disease and the increased morbidity and mortality associated with these conditions, we propose a Sleep Apnea Pathway (SAP, **Figure 20.1**) to correctly identify and triage these patients to the appropriate therapy.

STEP A: ASSESSMENT

All patients admitted with diagnosis of atrial fibrillation, syncope, hypertension, and HF should be evaluated for sleep apnea. Those patients with known sleep apnea diagnosis should be initiated on CPAP therapy according to their home setting. Those with suspected sleep apnea based on the following criteria, male gender, body mass index (BMI) > 30, snoring, neck circumference >17 inches, and metabolic disorders such as hyperlipidemia and insulin resistance will be screened by administrating the Berlin Questionnaire (BQ). We advise to perform an echocardiography as well on admission to evaluate heart function, pulmonary pressure, and any valvular disease.

STEP B: DIAGNOSIS

There are a number of tools available to screen for sleep apnea. These questionnaires are the BQ, the Epworth Sleepiness Scale (ESS), STOP, and STOP-Bang. These four questionnaires were compared in a cross-sectional study to determine effectiveness. The BQ, STOP, and STOP-Bang were shown to have the highest sensitivity, whereas the ESS was found to have higher specificity.[66] We have selected the BQ (**Figure 20.2**) as the screening tool for our SAP as it has shown better accuracy and is simpler to classify patients.[67] The BQ has also been shown to be predictive of those patients who are at higher risk for sleep apnea, limiting unnecessary PSG testing in patients who are lower risk and triaging them appropriately to medical management.[68] The BQ includes questions regarding snoring, daytime somnolence, hypertension, and BMI. The patient's family or bed partner is often used to confirm responses.[69]

According to the BQ results, patients will be classified as high- and low-risk patients. High-risk patients are those who score positive in two or more categories, whereas low-risk patients only score positive in one category.

Patients who are deemed a high risk for sleep apnea achieve a score >2 on the BQ. These high-risk patients should then be referred for PSG testing. An AHI of 15 or an AHI of 5 or higher in conjunction with symptoms of daytime somnolence, unrefreshing sleep, waking up choking or gasping for breath, or bed partners confirming snoring or breathing interruptions during sleep warrants treatment. The test will classify patients as being pure OSA or CSA or a mixed picture. Regardless of the diagnosis, all patients should be considered for a treatment trial with CPAP therapy.

TREATMENT

Those patients who score <2 on the BQ are deemed low risk for sleep apnea. They should therefore be deferred to continue medical management of their comorbidities, such as atrial fibrillation,[70] hypertension,[71] syncope,[72] or HF,[73] according to our published pathways.

Although treatment with CPAP is the mainstay of treatment for sleep apnea, education and certain lifestyle modifications in concert with CPAP therapy have shown to be very effective.[74] Patient education program components are listed in **Table 20.1**. Behavioral treatment options include weight loss, exercise, positional therapy, and avoidance of alcohol and sedatives before bedtime; these have shown to decrease the upper airway muscle relaxation that occurs and can precipitate apnea episodes. Side sleeping has also been shown to decrease the upper airway collapse that occurs.[75] A study from Karolinksa Institute in Sweden showed that an average weight loss of 40 lb resulted in a 58% reduction in sleep apnea symptoms and decreased apnea episodes by 21/hour.[76]

OSA treatment using CPAP has been shown to acutely decrease BP and nocturnal sympathetic tone. Several studies have shown that nocturnal CPAP can decrease daytime BP by approximately 2 mm Hg and seems to have the greatest effect in patients with uncontrolled hypertension and severe OSA.[77] Use of CPAP in sleep apnea has been shown to attenuate intrathoracic pressure changes and thus decrease preload, afterload, BP, and HR.[78,79] Kaneko et al.[77] observed that 1 month after initiation of CPAP, the LV ejection fraction increased by 9% in patients with HF. Two observational studies have been performed comparing treated to untreated OSA patients; one study showed a 2-fold higher increase in mortality in the untreated group,[76] whereas the other showed a greater hospitalization-free survival in the treated group.

Treatment of CSA is more controversial; however, CPAP is still often employed to treat this condition. Multiple trials have been performed evaluating the role of CPAP in CSA. Canadian Positive Airway Pressure Trial for Patients With Congestive Heart Failure and Central Sleep Apnea (CANPAP) was a study that included 258 patients. Use of CPAP in this population reduced nocturnal desaturations and showed a modest improvement in LV ejection fraction.[81] However at 2 years, there were no significant differences in outcomes between the treated and untreated groups.

Mixed or complex sleep apnea exhibits signs of OSA; however, on initiation of CPAP therapy, central apneas persist or emerge.[80] Variable positive airway pressure (VPAP) is often used to treat mixed apnea.[82] VPAP normalizes breathing and suppresses CSA and Cheyne–Stokes respirations.

FAILURE OF CONTINUOUS POSITIVE AIRWAY PRESSURE THERAPY

If patients with OSA fail CPAP therapy, then we recommend referral to ear-nose-throat (ENT) specialists for consideration of implantation of the Inspire system (**Figure 20.3**). The Inspire system is an implantable device that senses breathing patterns and maintains airway patency during sleep by delivering stimulation to targeted airway muscles. The system consists of three implanted components including a small generator, breathing sensor lead, and stimulation lead, all controlled with the small handheld Inspire sleep remote. Patients who qualify for the Inspire system

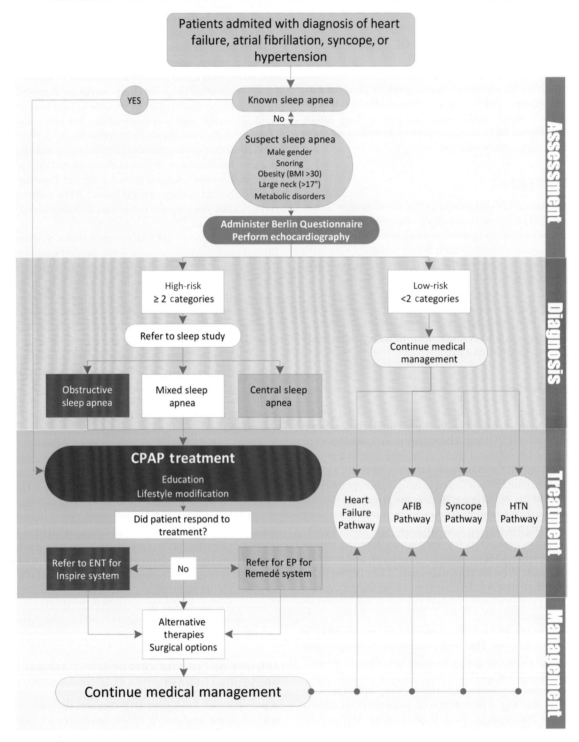

FIGURE 20.1 Pathway for the management of sleep apnea in cardiology. AFIB, atrial fibrillation; BMI, body mass index; CPAP, continuous positive airway pressure; ENT, ear-nose-throat; EP, electrophysiologist; HTN, hypertension.

Berlin Questionnaire

Sleep Evaluation in Primary Care

Please Complete the following:

height _____   age _____

weight _____   male/female _____

Category 1

1. Do you snore?

☐ yes

☐ no

☐ don't know

If you snore:

2. Your snoring is?

☐ slightly louder than breathing

☐ as loud as talking

☐ louder than talking

☐ very loud. Can be heard in adjacent rooms.

3. How often do you snore?

☐ nearly every day

☐ 3-4 times a week

☐ 1-2 times a week

☐ 1-2 times a month

☐ never or nearly never

4. Has your snoring ever bothered other people?

☐ yes

☐ no

5. Has anyone noticed that you quit breathing during your sleep?

☐ nearly every day

☐ 3-4 times a week

☐ 1-2 times a week

☐ 1-2 times a month

☐ never or nearly never

Category 2

6. How often do you feel tired or fatigued after your sleep?

☐ nearly every day

☐ 3-4 times a week

☐ 1-2 times a week

☐ 1-2 times a month

☐ never or nearly never

7. During your waketime, do you feel tired, fatigued or not up to par?

☐ nearly every day

☐ 3-4 times a week

☐ 1-2 times a week

☐ 1-2 times a month

☐ never or nearly never

8. Have you ever nodded off or fallen asleep while driving a vehicle?

☐ yes

☐ no

if yes, how often does it occur?

☐ nearly every day

☐ 3-4 times a week

☐ 1-2 times a week

☐ 1-2 times a month

☐ never or nearly never

Category 3

9. Do you have high blood pressure?

☐ yes

☐ no

☐ don't know

10. BMI > 30 (*See Chart*)

☐ yes

☐ no

Scoring Questions: Any answer within box outline is a positive response.

Scoring categories:

☐ Category 1 is positive with 2 or more positive responses to questions 1-5

☐ Category 2 is positive with 2 or more positive responses to questions 6-8

☐ Category 3 is positive with 1 positive responses to questions 9-10

Final Result: If 2 or more possible categories are positive, you have a high likelihood of sleep apnea.

Name _____

Address _____

_____

FIGURE 20.2 Berlin Questionnaire.

TABLE 20.1	Components of Patient Education Programs

Findings of study, severity of disease
Pathophysiology of sleep apnea
Explanation of natural course and associated disorders
Risk factor identification, explanation of exacerbating factors, and risk factor modifications
Genetic testing when indicated
Treatment options
What to expect from treatment
Outline the patient's role in treatment, address concerns, and set goals
Consequences of untreated disease
Drowsy driving/sleepiness counseling

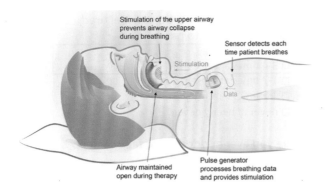

FIGURE 20.3 Inspire system.

must have moderate-to-severe OSA (AHI 20 to 65, with <25% central apnea), be unable to use CPAP, and be free of complete concentric collapse of the palate. Long-term study outcomes in patients using the Inspire system showed a 78% reduction in apnea–hypopnea events from baseline and an 80% reduction in oxygen desaturation levels.[83] In addition, patients had a clinically significant improvement in quality of life, including daytime somnolence that was measured by the ESS. Patients also showed a high adherence rate to therapy and significant improvement in important sleep-related quality-of-life outcome measures that are maintained across a 2-year follow-up period.[84,85]

Patients with CSA who fail CPAP therapy should be referred for consideration to the Remedé system. The system (**Figure 20.4**) is a phrenic nerve stimulator designed to restore the body's normal breathing pattern, which results in better oxygenation and less activation of the sympathetic nervous system. The settings of the device are monitored by the physician and can be changed remotely. Patients who are studied for indication of the Remedé system include those with AHI ≥ 20, Central Apnea Index (CAI) at least 50% of all apneas with at least 30 central apnea events, and Obstructive Apnea Index ≤ 20% of the total AHI. In the pilot study of the Remedé system, performed to evaluate outcomes at 3 and 6 months, CAI decreased by 84%, AHI decreased by 55%, Oxygen Desaturation Index improved by 52%, nocturnal arousals decreased by 35%, and REM by 29%.[86] Data published from the Remedé System Pivotal Trial Study Group showed that a significantly higher proportion of patients in the treatment versus control group achieved a ≥50% AHI reduction, and 91% 12-month freedom from serious adverse events related to the implant procedure, Remedé system, or delivered therapy.[87]

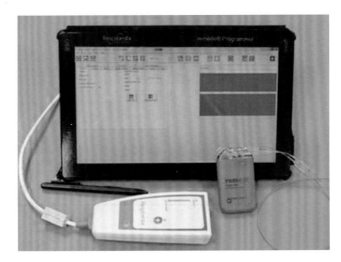

FIGURE 20.4 The Remedé system.

The findings of both the clinical trials of the Inspire system and the Remedé system indicate that by reducing AHI episodes and improving nocturnal oxygen levels, these novel devices may be helpful in reducing cardiovascular morbidity and mortality in those patients who fail CPAP therapy.

ALTERNATIVE AND SURGICAL TREATMENTS FOR THOSE WHO FAIL NOVEL THERAPIES

ORAL DEVICES

There are currently over 100 FDA-approved dental devices that are available to patients to help relieve obstruction in sleep apnea.[88] These devices are designed to hold the lower jaw forward to prevent pharyngeal obstruction during sleep. This treatment is excellent for reducing snoring, although the effect on OSA is sometimes more limited. As a result, dental devices are best used for mild cases of OSA when relief of snoring is the main goal. Failure to tolerate and accept CPAP is another indication for dental devices. Although dental devices are not as effective as CPAP for OSA, some patients prefer a dental device to CPAP. Side effects of dental devices are generally minor, but may include changes to the bite with prolonged use.

SURGICAL OPTIONS

Surgery is an alternative therapy for patients who cannot tolerate or do not improve with nonsurgical treatments such as CPAP or oral devices. Surgery can also be used in combination with other nonsurgical treatments.

There are different types of surgical procedures that can be used in OSA to reshape structures or reposition bone and soft tissue.

1. Uvulopalatopharyngoplasty (UPPP) removes the uvula and excessive tissue in the throat, including the tonsils, if present, to help relieve upper airway obstruction. UPPP is the most common surgical procedure in OSA, but it has variable outcomes. The overall success rate is approximately 50%, with success defined as a 50% reduction in AHI and a post-surgical AHI reduction to less than 20 events/hour.[89] New UPPP variants have been showing more promise in improving OSA outcomes in ongoing clinical trials.

2. Other procedures, such as maxillomandibular advancement (MMA) and tracheotomy,[90] address both the upper and lower pharyngeal airway more globally. These two procedures have been shown to have high success rates and improved PSG outcomes. MMA may have a higher success rate, particularly in people with an abnormal jaw, but it is the most complicated procedure and is typically reserved for patients with severe OSA who have failed prior targeted surgical attempts.[91] In a meta-analysis that included 627 patients undergoing MMA, the overall success rate, which was defined as an AHI <20 events/hour and reduced by at least 50%, was 86%. Cure of OSA, which was defined as an AHI less than five events per hour was achieved in 43% of patients.[92]

All surgical treatments require discussions about the goals of treatment, the expected outcomes, and potential complications.

SUMMARY

Sleep-disordered breathing is a highly prevalent medical condition, particularly in cardiac patients. Utilizing a system evidence-based pathway can identify patients who require treatment and direct them to the appropriate management plan.

REFERENCES

1. Celen YT, Peker Y. Cardiovascular consequences of sleep apnea: I—epidemiology. *Anatol J Cardiol.* 2010;10:75-80.

2. Ravesloot MJ, van Maanen JP, Hilgevoord AA, van Wagensveld BA, de Vries N. Obstructive sleep apnea is underrecognized and underdiagnosed in patients undergoing bariatric surgery. *Eur Arch Otorhinolaryngol.* 2012;269:1865–1871.

3. Young T, Evans L, Finn L, Palta M. Estimation of the clinically diagnosed proportion of sleep apnea syndrome in middle-aged men and women. *Sleep.* 1997;20:705-706.

4. Lurie A. Obstructive sleep apnea in adults: epidemiology, clinical presentation, and treatment options. *Adv Cardiol.* 2011;46:1-42.

5. Kapur VK. Obstructive sleep apnea: diagnosis, epidemiology, and economics. *Respir Care.* 2010;55:1155-1167.

6. Punjabi NM. The epidemiology of adult obstructive sleep apnea. *Proc Am Thorac Soc.* 2008;5:136-143.

7. Brown IG, Bradley TD, Phillipson EA, Zamel N, Hoffstein V. Pharyngeal compliance in snoring subjects with and without obstructive sleep apnea. *Am Rev Respir Dis.* 1985;132:211-215.

8. Park JG, Ramar K, Olson EJ. Updates on definition, consequences, and management of obstructive sleep apnea. *Mayo Clinic Proc.* 2011;86:549-554; quiz 554-555.

9. Kapur VK, Baldwin CM, Resnick HE, Gottlieb DJ, Nieto FJ. Sleepiness in patients with moderate to severe sleep-disordered breathing. *Sleep.* 2005;28:472-477.

10. Donovan LM, Kapur VK. Prevalence and characteristics of central compared to obstructive sleep apnea: analyses from the Sleep Heart Health Study Cohort. *Sleep.* 2016;39:1353-1359.

11. Wisskirchen T, Teschler H. [Central sleep apnea syndrome and Cheyne–Stokes respiration]. *Therapeutische Umschau Revue Therapeutique.* 2000;57:458-462.

12. Ito E, Inoue Y. [The International Classification of Sleep Disorders, third edition. American Academy of Sleep Medicine. Includes bibliographies and index]. *Nihon Rinsho Jpn J Clin Med.* 2015;73:916-923.

13. Mezon BL, West P, Israels J, Kryger M. Sleep breathing abnormalities in kyphoscoliosis. *Am Rev Respir Dis.* 1980;122:617-621.

14. Bitter T, Faber L, Hering D, Langer C, Horstkotte D, Oldenburg O. Sleep-disordered breathing in heart failure with normal left ventricular ejection fraction. *Eur J Heart Failure.* 2009;11:602-608.

15. Ju YE, Finn MB, Sutphen CL, et al. Obstructive sleep apnea decreases central nervous system-derived proteins in the cerebrospinal fluid. *Ann Neurol.* 2016;80:154-159.

16. Manser RL, Rochford P, Pierce RJ, Byrnes GB, Campbell DA. Impact of different criteria for defining hypopneas in the apnea-hypopnea index. *Chest.* 2001;120:909-914.

17. McNicholas WT, Bonsigore MR. Sleep apnoea as an independent risk factor for cardiovascular disease: current evidence, basic mechanisms and research priorities. *Eur Respir J.* 2007;29:156-178.

18. Goldin JM, Naughton MT. Obstructive sleep apnoea induced atrial fibrillation. *Intern Med J.* 2006;36:136-137.

19. Tang RB, Dong JZ, Liu XP, et al. Obstructive sleep apnoea risk profile and the risk of recurrence of atrial fibrillation after catheter ablation. *Europace.* 2009;11:100-105.

20. Zhang L, Hou Y, Po SS. Obstructive sleep apnoea and atrial fibrillation. *Arrhythm Electrophysiol Rev.* 2015;4:14-18.

21. Grote L, Hedner J, Peter JH. Sleep-related breathing disorder is an independent risk factor for uncontrolled hypertension. *J Hypertens.* 2000;18:679-685.

22. Nagai M, Kario K. [Sleep disorder and hypertension]. *Nihon Rinsho Jpn J Clin Med.* 2012;70:1188-1194.

23. Lyons OD, Bradley TD. Heart failure and sleep apnea. *Canadian J Cardiol.* 2015;31:898-908.

24. Yoneyama K, Osada N, Shimozato T, et al. Relationship between sleep-disordered breathing level and acute onset time of congestive heart failure. *Int Heart J.* 2008;49:471-480.

25. Culebras A. Sleep apnea and stroke. *Curr Neurol Neurosci Rep.* 2015;15:503.

26. Somers VK, White DP, Amin R, et al. Sleep apnea and cardiovascular disease: an American Heart Association/american College Of Cardiology Foundation Scientific Statement from the American Heart Association Council for High Blood Pressure Research Professional Education Committee, Council on Clinical Cardiology, Stroke Council, and Council On Cardiovascular Nursing. In collaboration with the National Heart, Lung, and Blood Institute National Center on Sleep Disorders Research (National Institutes of Health). *Circulation.* 2008;118:1080-1111.

27. Stein JH, Stern R, Barnet JH, et al. Relationships between sleep apnea, cardiovascular disease risk factors, and aortic pulse wave velocity over 18 years: the Wisconsin Sleep Cohort. *Sleep Breath.* 2016;20:813-817.

28. Bauters F, Rietzschel ER, Hertegonne KB, Chirinos JA. The link between obstructive sleep apnea and cardiovascular disease. *Curr Atheroscler Rep.* 2016;18:1.

29. Romero-Corral A, Caples SM, Lopez-Jimenez F, Somers VK. Interactions between obesity and obstructive sleep apnea: implications for treatment. *Chest.* 2010;137:711-719.

30. Punjabi NM, Sorkin JD, Katzel LI, Goldberg AP, Schwartz AR, Smith PL. Sleep-disordered breathing and insulin resistance in middle-aged and overweight men. *Am J Respir Crit Care Med.* 2002;165:677-682.

31. Punjabi NM, Shahar E, Redline S, Gottlieb DJ, Givelber R, Resnick HE. Sleep-disordered breathing, glucose intolerance, and insulin resistance: the Sleep Heart Health Study. *Am J Epidemiol.* 2004;160:521-530.

32. Spiegel K, Leproult R, Van Cauter E. Impact of sleep debt on metabolic and endocrine function. *Lancet.* 1999;354:1435-1439.

33. Somers VK, White DP, Amin R, et al. Sleep apnea and cardiovascular disease: an American Heart Association/American College of

Cardiology Foundation Scientific Statement from the American Heart Association Council for High Blood Pressure Research Professional Education Committee, Council on Clinical Cardiology, Stroke Council, and Council on Cardiovascular Nursing. *J Am Coll Cardiol.* 2008;52:686-717.

34. Fletcher EC, DeBehnke RD, Lovoi MS, Gorin AB. Undiagnosed sleep apnea in patients with essential hypertension. *Ann Intern Med.* 1985;103:190-195.

35. Logan AG, Perlikowski SM, Mente A, et al. High prevalence of unrecognized sleep apnoea in drug-resistant hypertension. *J Hypertens.* 2001;19:2271-2277.

36. Dopp JM, Reichmuth KJ, Morgan BJ. Obstructive sleep apnea and hypertension: mechanisms, evaluation, and management. *Curr Hypertens Rep.* 2007;9:529-534.

37. Suzuki M, Guilleminault C, Otsuka K, Shiomi T. Blood pressure "dipping" and "non-dipping" in obstructive sleep apnea syndrome patients. *Sleep.* 1996;19:382-387.

38. van de Borne P, Oren R, Abouassaly C, Anderson E, Somers VK. Effect of Cheyne–Stokes respiration on muscle sympathetic nerve activity in severe congestive heart failure secondary to ischemic or idiopathic dilated cardiomyopathy. *Am J Cardiol.* 1998;81:432-436.

39. Wang H, Parker JD, Newton GE, et al. Influence of obstructive sleep apnea on mortality in patients with heart failure. *J Am Coll Cardiol.* 2007;49:1625-1631.

40. Tkacova R, Niroumand M, Lorenzi-Filho G, Bradley TD. Overnight shift from obstructive to central apneas in patients with heart failure: role of PCO2 and circulatory delay. *Circulation.* 2001;103:238-243.

41. Trinder J, Merson R, Rosenberg JI, Fitzgerald F, Kleiman J, Douglas Bradley T. Pathophysiological interactions of ventilation, arousals, and blood pressure oscillations during cheyne-stokes respiration in patients with heart failure. *Am J Respir Crit Care Med.* 2000;162:808-813.

42. Javaheri S, Corbett WS. Association of low PaCO2 with central sleep apnea and ventricular arrhythmias in ambulatory patients with stable heart failure. *Ann Intern Med.* 1998;128:204-207.

43. Carmona Bernal C, Capote Gil F, Botebol Benhamou G, Garcia Lopez P, Sanchez Armengol A, Castillo Gomez J. [Assessment of excessive day-time sleepiness in professional drivers with suspected obstructive sleep apnea syndrome]. *Archivos de bronconeumologia.* 2000;36:436-440.

44. Mehra R, Benjamin EJ, Shahar E, et al. Association of nocturnal arrhythmias with sleep-disordered breathing: the Sleep Heart Health Study. *Am J Respir Crit Care Med.* 2006;173:910-916.

45. Selim BJ, Koo BB, Qin L, et al. The Association between Nocturnal Cardiac Arrhythmias and Sleep-Disordered Breathing: The DREAM Study. *J Clin Sleep Med.* 2016;12:829-837.

46. Becker H, Brandenburg U, Peter JH, Von Wichert P. Reversal of sinus arrest and atrioventricular conduction block in patients with sleep apnea during nasal continuous positive airway pressure. *Am J Respir Crit Care Med.* 1995;151:215-218.

47. Otto ME, Belohlavek M, Romero-Corral A, et al. Comparison of cardiac structural and functional changes in obese otherwise healthy adults with versus without obstructive sleep apnea. *Am J Cardiol.* 2007;99:1298-1302.

48. Kanagala R, Murali NS, Friedman PA, et al. Obstructive sleep apnea and the recurrence of atrial fibrillation. *Circulation.* 2003;107:2589-2594.

49. Monahan K, Brewster J, Wang L, et al. Relation of the severity of obstructive sleep apnea in response to anti-arrhythmic drugs in patients with atrial fibrillation or atrial flutter. *Am J Cardiol.* 2012;110:369-372.

50. Naruse Y, Tada H, Satoh M, et al. Concomitant obstructive sleep apnea increases the recurrence of atrial fibrillation following radiofrequency catheter ablation of atrial fibrillation: clinical impact of continuous positive airway pressure therapy. *Heart Rhythm* 2013;10:331-337.

51. Fein AS, Shvilkin A, Shah D, et al. Treatment of obstructive sleep apnea reduces the risk of atrial fibrillation recurrence after catheter ablation. *J Am Coll Cardiol.* 2013;62:300-305.

52. Serizawa N, Yumino D, Kajimoto K, et al. Impact of sleep-disordered breathing on life-threatening ventricular arrhythmia in heart failure patients with implantable cardioverter-defibrillator. *J Am Coll Cardiol.* 2008;102:1064-1068.

53. Gami AS, Howard DE, Olson EJ, Somers VK. Day-night pattern of sudden death in obstructive sleep apnea. *N Engl J Med.* 2005;352:1206-1214.

54. Gami AS, Olson EJ, Shen WK, et al. Obstructive sleep apnea and the risk of sudden cardiac death: a longitudinal study of 10,701 adults. *J Am Coll Cardiol.* 2013;62:610-616.

55. Marshall NS, Wong KK, Liu PY, Cullen SR, Knuiman MW, Grunstein RR. Sleep apnea as an independent risk factor for all-cause mortality: the Busselton Health Study. *Sleep.* 2008;31:1079-1085.

56. Young T, Finn L, Peppard PE, et al. Sleep disordered breathing and mortality: eighteen-year follow-up of the Wisconsin sleep cohort. *Sleep.* 2008;31:1071-1078.

57. Zgierska A, Gorecka D, Radzikowska M, et al. [Obstructive sleep apnea and risk factors for coronary artery disease]. *Pneumonologia i alergologia polska.* 2000;68:238-246.

58. Chan HS, Chiu HF, Tse LK, Woo KS. Obstructive sleep apnea presenting with nocturnal angina, heart failure, and near-miss sudden death. *Chest.* 1991;99:1023-1025.

59. De Torres-Alba F, Gemma D, Armada-Romero E, Rey-Blas JR, Lopez-de-Sa E, Lopez-Sendon JL. Obstructive sleep apnea and coronary artery disease: from pathophysiology to clinical implications. *Pulmon Med.* 2013;2013:768064.

60. Glantz H, Thunstrom E, Johansson MC, et al. Obstructive sleep apnea is independently associated with worse diastolic function in coronary artery disease. *Sleep Med.* 2015;16:160-167.

61. Peker Y, Carlson J, Hedner J. Increased incidence of coronary artery disease in sleep apnoea: a long-term follow-up. *Eur Respir J.* 2006;28:596-602.

62. Mooe T, Franklin KA, Wiklund U, Rabben T, Holmstrom K. Sleep-disordered breathing and myocardial ischemia in patients with coronary artery disease. *Chest.* 2000;117:1597-1602.

63. Yaggi HK, Concato J, Kernan WN, Lichtman JH, Brass LM, Mohsenin V. Obstructive sleep apnea as a risk factor for stroke and death. *N Engl J Med.* 2005;353:2034-2041.

64. Stahl SM, Yaggi HK, Taylor S, et al. Infarct location and sleep apnea: evaluating the potential association in acute ischemic stroke. *Sleep Med.* 2015;16:1198-1203.

65. Koo BB, Bravata DM, Tobias LA, et al. Observational Study of Obstructive Sleep Apnea in Wake-Up Stroke: The SLEEP TIGHT Study. *Cerebrovasc Dis.* 2016;41:233-241.

66. Du L, Li Z, Tang X. [Application value of four different questionnaires in the screening of patients with obstructive sleep apnea]. *Zhonghua Yi Xue Za Zhi.* 2015;95(42):3407-10.

67. Tan A, Yin JD, Tan LW, van Dam RM, Cheung YY, Lee CH. Using the Berlin Questionnaire to Predict Obstructive Sleep Apnea in the General Population. *J Clin Sleep Med.* 2016.

68. Sharma SK, Vasudev C, Sinha S, Banga A, Pandey RM, Handa KK. Validation of the modified Berlin questionnaire to identify patients at risk for the obstructive sleep apnoea syndrome. *Indian J Med Res.* 2006;124:281-290.

69. Sagaspe P, Leger D, Taillard J, Bayon V, Chaumet G, Philip P. Might the Berlin Sleep Questionnaire applied to bed partners be used to screen sleep apneic patients? *Sleep Med.* 2010;11:479-483.

70. Herzog E, Aziz E, Bangalore S, Fischer A, Frankenberger O, Steinberg JS. Translation of the RACE pathway for management of atrial fibrillation and atrial flutter into admission forms. *Crit Pathw Cardiol.* 2006;5:15-17.

71. Herzog E, Frankenberger O, Aziz E, et al. A novel pathway for the management of hypertension for hospitalized patients. *Crit Pathw Cardiol.* 2007;6:150-160.

72. Herzog E, Frankenberger O, Pierce W, Steinberg JS. The SELF pathway for the management of syncope. *Crit Pathw Cardiol.* 2006;5: 173-178.

73. Herzog E, Varley C, Kukin M. Pathway for the management of acute heart failure. *Crit Pathw Cardiol.* 2005;4:37-42.

74. Morgenthaler TI, Kapen S, Lee-Chiong T, et al. Practice parameters for the medical therapy of obstructive sleep apnea. *Sleep.* 2006;29:1031-1035.

75. Pevernagie DA, Stanson AW, Sheedy PF 2nd, Daniels BK, Shepard JW Jr. Effects of body position on the upper airway of patients with obstructive sleep apnea. *Am J Respir Crit Care Med.* 1995;152: 179-185.

76. Johansson K, Neovius M, Lagerros YT, et al. Effect of a very low energy diet on moderate and severe obstructive sleep apnoea in obese men: a randomised controlled trial. *BMJ.* 2009;339:b4609.

77. Kaneko Y, Floras JS, Usui K, et al. Cardiovascular effects of continuous positive airway pressure in patients with heart failure and obstructive sleep apnea. *N Engl J Med.* 2003;348:1233-1241.

78. Sin DD, Logan AG, Fitzgerald FS, Liu PP, Bradley TD. Effects of continuous positive airway pressure on cardiovascular outcomes in heart failure patients with and without Cheyne–Stokes respiration. *Circulation.* 2000;102:61-66.

79. Doherty LS, Kiely JL, Swan V, McNicholas WT. Long-term effects of nasal continuous positive airway pressure therapy on cardiovascular outcomes in sleep apnea syndrome. *Chest.* 2005;127: 2076-2084.

80. Gay PC. Complex sleep apnea: it really is a disease. *J Clin Sleep Med.* 2008;4:403-405.

81. Arzt M, Floras JS, Logan AG, et al. Suppression of central sleep apnea by continuous positive airway pressure and transplant-free survival in heart failure: a post hoc analysis of the Canadian Continuous Positive Airway Pressure for Patients with Central Sleep Apnea and Heart Failure Trial (CANPAP). *Circulation.* 2007;115:3173-3180.

82. Vennelle M, White S, Riha RL, Mackay TW, Engleman HM, Douglas NJ. Randomized controlled trial of variable-pressure versus fixed-pressure continuous positive airway pressure (CPAP) treatment for patients with obstructive sleep apnea/hypopnea syndrome (OSAHS). *Sleep.* 2010;33:267-271.

83. Strollo PJ, Jr., Soose RJ, Maurer JT, et al. Upper-airway stimulation for obstructive sleep apnea. *N Engl J Med.* 2014;370:139-149.

84. Strollo PJ Jr, Gillespie MB, Soose RJ, et al. Upper airway stimulation for obstructive sleep apnea: durability of the treatment effect at 18 months. *Sleep.* 2015;38:1593-1598.

85. Soose RJ, Woodson BT, Gillespie MB, et al. Upper airway stimulation for obstructive sleep apnea: self-reported outcomes at 24 months. *J Clin Sleep Med.* 2016;12:43-48.

86. Abraham WT, Jagielski D, Oldenburg O, et al. Phrenic nerve stimulation for the treatment of central sleep apnea. *JACC Heart Fail.* 2015;3:360-369.

87. Costanzo MR, Ponikowski P, Javaheri S, et al. Transvenous neurostimulation for central sleep apnoea: a randomised controlled trial. *Lancet.* 2016;388:974-982.

88. Marklund M, Verbraecken J, Randerath W. Non-CPAP therapies in obstructive sleep apnoea: mandibular advancement device therapy. *Eur Respir J.* 2012;39:1241-1247.

89. Randerath WJ, Verbraecken J, Andreas S, et al. Non-CPAP therapies in obstructive sleep apnoea. *Eur Respir J.* 2011;37:1000-1028.

90. Holty JE, Guilleminault C. Surgical options for the treatment of obstructive sleep apnea. *Med Clin North Am.* 2010;94:479-515.

91. Riley RW, Powell NB, Guilleminault C. Obstructive sleep apnea syndrome: a surgical protocol for dynamic upper airway reconstruction. *J Oral Maxillofacial Surg.* 1993;51:742-747; discussion 748-749.

92. Holty JE, Guilleminault C. Maxillomandibular advancement for the treatment of obstructive sleep apnea: a systematic review and meta-analysis. *Sleep Med Rev.* 2010;14:287-297.

Patient and Family Information for: THE MANAGEMENT OF SLEEP APNEA IN THE CARDIAC PATIENT

Sleep apnea is a very common medical condition that affects 60 million Americans. There are different types of sleep apnea, the most common being obstructive sleep apnea or OSA. OSA is caused by collapse of the upper airway during sleep, leading to obstruction of breathing. Symptoms that suggest that one might have sleep apnea are excessive sleepiness during the day, waking up with headaches, insomnia, and frequent nighttime awakenings. Bed partners may also confirm that there is excessive snoring or periodic episodes of stopping breathing at night. CSA results in a lack of breathing during sleep caused by disrupted signals from the brain to initiate breathing.

Factors that may predispose patients to develop sleep apnea are male gender, obesity, and having a small mouth and throat. Sleep apnea also becomes more common as people age. Sleep apnea is common in patients with high blood pressure (BP), stroke, heart failure (HF), and atrial fibrillation. Undiagnosed and untreated sleep apnea in patients with any of these conditions can result in adverse outcomes. If a physician suspects sleep apnea based on known cardiovascular conditions and the presence of the risk factors previously stated, he may administer the Berlin Questionnaire (BQ) to determine the risk of having sleep apnea.

The BQ is a three-part questionnaire. Section one has five questions that address snoring habits. A bed partner may also be asked to help answer the questions. Section two addresses symptoms of daytime sleepiness. Section three has a question regarding the presence of high BP. The patient will also score a point if he/she is obese and has a BMI of 30 or higher. On the basis of the score, the physician might order a sleep study, also known as PSG testing.

The diagnosis of sleep apnea is confirmed by PSG testing. This is based on how many times per hour the patient stops breathing during the test. If diagnosed with sleep apnea, the physician will likely recommend CPAP for usage at nighttime in conjunction with lifestyle modifications, such as losing weight and avoiding alcohol and sedating medications before sleep. CPAP is a noninvasive method of providing oxygen while asleep. The oxygen is delivered by a face or nasal mask to keep the nasal passages open and to prevent collapse of the airway. Some oral dental devices are also available; however, they are not effective for every patient with sleep apnea.

If the attempt to use CPAP for sleep apnea does not work, there are new and emerging therapies that can be tried depending on the type of sleep apnea the patient has. The Inspire system is a new technology for patients with OSA who fail CPAP therapy. An implanted system, it delivers mild stimulation to important airway muscles to help keep the airway open during sleep. The device is controlled by a small, handheld remote. Patients with central sleep apnea who fail CPAP therapy can be referred for a Remedé system. The Remedé device is placed by a cardiologist in the electrophysiology laboratory. This is a minimally invasive procedure by which the device is placed under the skin and delivers impulses to the muscles that control breathing.

Surgery is also an option for patients who have severe OSA or do not respond or qualify for the abovementioned treatments. UPPP is the most common surgery for OSA and involves removing and repositioning the soft tissues in the throat to help relieve the obstruction that occurs during sleep. These surgeries have been shown to be very effective for some patients in resolving symptoms of sleep apnea. However, it is important that the patient discusses the treatment goals and concerns with the physician to decide what the best treatment option for sleep apnea is.

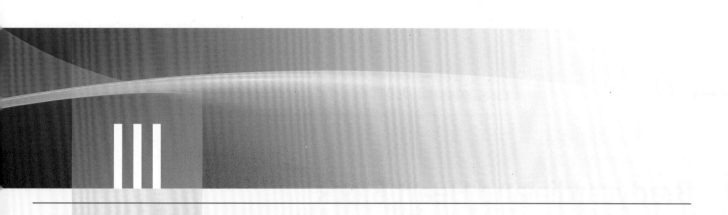

ARRHYTHMIA IN THE CCU

Asaf Danon
Seyed Hamed Hosseini Dehkordi
Eyal Herzog
Arie Militianu
Jorge E. Schliamser

21

Bradycardia and Heart Block

Normal heart rate (HR) is considered to range from 60 to 100 beats per minute (bpm). Therefore, bradycardia refers to an HR of 60 bpm or less. Bradycardia may be associated with symptoms such as weakness, fatigue, syncope or near-syncope, dizziness, shortness of breath with exercise, confusion, and symptoms of heart failure. On occasion, however, bradycardia may be asymptomatic. This occurs especially in otherwise healthy, young, athletic subjects and is usually responsive to exercise. Asymptomatic bradycardia can also happen during sleep secondary to reduced sympathetic and increased parasympathetic tone. These types of asymptomatic, physiologic bradycardias almost never warrant aggressive interventions. However, bradycardia due to extremely slow sinus rate or secondary to conduction block is usually pathologic even in the absence of symptoms because it carries a risk for further adverse cardiovascular outcomes.

The management of bradycardia is dependent on the symptom severity and the reversibility of the cause. A stable patient may be observed while being evaluated, but the unstable patient usually requires treatment with positive chronotropic drugs or temporary pacing until a more permanent solution can be employed.

ANATOMIC CONSIDERATION – SINOATRIAL NODE

Anatomically, the sinoatrial node (SAN) lies in the proximity to the junction of the superior vena cava and the sulcus terminalis, at the high lateral border of the right atrium (RA). Blood supply derives from the SAN branch of the right coronary artery (RCA) in 60% and left circumflex coronary artery (lCx) in 40% of the population. Collateral blood supply is common, which explains the rarity of sinus node infarction.[1] The SAN is densely innervated by both the sympathetic and the parasympathetic (vagus nerve) nervous system. Conduction down to the atria and atrioventricular node (AVN) is through preferential pathways that help in uniform and synchronous activation of the atrial muscle and timely transfer of the generated impulse to the AVN. The main pathways include the anterior internodal tract from which the Bachman bundle separates and courses through the roof of the atria toward the left atrium (LA). The posterior internodal tract ("slow pathway") and the middle internodal tract also preferentially transmit SAN impulses to the AVN.

The AVN is located at the apex of the triangle of Koch in the inferomedial part of the RA and is located anterior and superior to the coronary sinus ostium. It derives its blood supply from a branch of the RCA (in 90% of the population) or the lCx artery.

The bundle of His (HB) connects the distal part of the AVN with the bundle branches. It crosses the membranous interventricular septum to the left side and divides into the right bundle branch (RBB) and the left bundle branch (LBB). Blood supply to the HB is dual, both from the left anterior descending (LAD) coronary artery and posterior descending coronary artery. The RBB and the left anterior fascicle branch of the LBB are supplied mainly by septal branches of the LAD coronary artery. The left posterior fascicle, on the other hand, has dual blood supply, both from the LAD and the RCA.

SINUS RHYTHM

When the SAN is the dominant pacemaker of the heart, the sinus rhythm is present. It is characterized by a P wave that is positive (upright) in the inferior leads, and biphasic in lead V1 (first positive deflection from RA activation is followed by a negative deflection from LA activation). The P wave is negative in lead aVR. Leads V2–6 show positive P waves. The duration of the P wave is generally 120 ms (three small boxes) and its amplitude is <0.25 mV (2.5 small boxes). Larger values may indicate atrial pathology (enlargement) or conduction delay in the atria. The consecutive P waves are identical in morphology and the PR intervals are stable from beat to beat. The SAN has an intrinsic automaticity, but the rate of impulse generation is controlled by the autonomic nervous system. Sympathetic stimulation increases, whereas parasympathetic (vagal) stimulation decreases the SAN firing rate.

SINUS ARRHYTHMIA

Sinus arrhythmia is defined as an irregular sinus rhythm (P-P variation >120 ms), with normal-looking P waves. It is very common and considered to be normal. Differential diagnosis of irregular sinus rate includes wandering atrial pacemaker or frequent premature atrial contractions, both with different P-wave morphologies. Respiratory sinus arrhythmia is the most common type and is related to alteration in the autonomic tone with respiration. Inspiration and expansion of the lung tissue inhibits the parasympathetic tone, thus increasing the sinus rate. This type is usually benign, very common in young individuals but may be associated with obesity and hypertension. In contrast, the effects of respiration on the sinus rate diminish with age and in patients with diabetic neuropathy. Nonrespiratory sinus arrhythmia may be seen in a normal or diseased heart, or may be associated with medications (such as digitalis). Ventriculophasic sinus arrhythmia is typically seen in patients with complete or second-degree heart block. P-P intervals that contain a QRS are shorter in comparison to the following P-P intervals that do not contain a QRS. The mechanism is probably related to increase in stroke volume, which triggers a baroreceptor response and results in widened P-P interval in the following beat.

SINUS NODE DYSFUNCTION

Sinus node dysfunction (SND) is an intrinsic disease of the sinus node and its presentations include the following:

1. Sinus bradycardia (SB), including sinoatrial exit block and sinus pauses
2. Tachycardia-bradycardia syndrome
3. Conversion pauses following termination of atrial arrhythmia
4. Chronotropic incompetence

SB is defined as sinus rate (with normal-appearing P waves) of less than 60 bpm (**Figure 21.1A**). The major causes of SB are depicted in **Table 21.1**. SB may be caused by intrinsic disease of the sinus node or by extrinsic causes, such as medications and metabolic and hormonal changes (see subsequent text).

ETIOLOGY OF SINUS BRADYCARDIA

Increased vagal tone—chronic increase in the parasympathetic tone is typical in trained athletes and during sleep (**Figure 21.1A**). Episodic increase in the vagal tone may occur during vasovagal response. Typically, conduction slowness (prolonged PR interval) and peripheral vascular dilatation also exists in addition to other vagal symptoms (pallor, diaphoresis, nausea), sometimes leading to hypoperfusion of the central nervous system and resultant brief episodes of loss of consciousness. Vagal tone may also be increased by the Valsalva manuever, applying pressure on the carotid body or globe, cough, and acute myocardial infarction (MI), especially of the inferior wall (also known as the Bezold–Jarisch reflex).

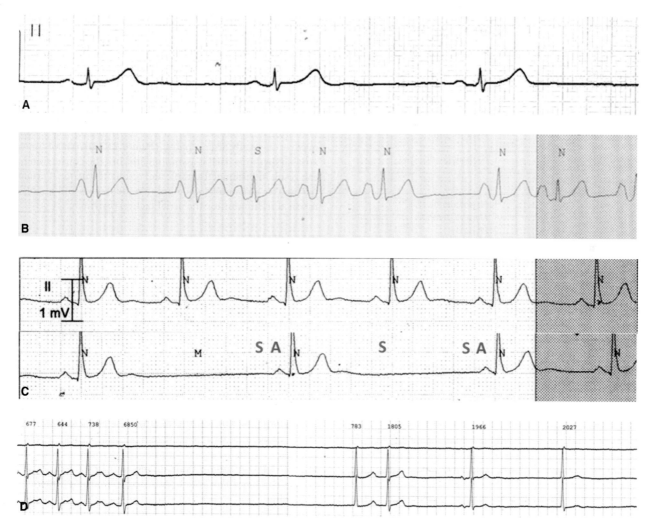

FIGURE 21.1 Sinus node dysfunction. A, Sinus bradycardia of 35 bpm in a young, trained, asymptomatic male. B, Second-degree sinoatrial block, type I (Wenckebach). Note a slight P-P interval prolongation. The pause duration is less than the two preceding P-P intervals. C, Second-degree type II sinoatrial block. The pause duration is exactly twice the regular P-P interval. *S* denotes the expected sinus activity and *A* denotes the atrial activity. D, Conversion pause due to prolonged sinus node recovery time shown in a Holter monitor of a woman with recurrent syncope. Following termination of atrial flutter, a prolonged pause of 6.85 seconds is seen with no P waves, and the first escape beat has no proceeding P wave. Therefore, it is a junctional escape beat.

TABLE 21.1	Major Causes of Sinus Bradycardia
INTRINSIC	**EXTRINSIC**
Idiopathic degeneration (aging)	Autonomical mediated
Ischemia	Neurocardiogenic syncope
Rheumatic fever	Carotid sinus hypersensitivity
Pericarditis	β-Adrenergic blockers
Infiltrative disease	Calcium channel antagonists
Sarcoidosis	Clonidine
Amyloidosis	Digoxin
	Antiarrhythmic agents
Systemic lupus erythematosus	Parasympathetic agents—pyridostigmine, donepezil
Rheumatoid arthritis	Sympatholytic agents—methyldopa, clonidine
Scleroderma	I_f blockers—ivabradine
Myotonic dystrophy	Lithium
Surgical trauma during cardiac surgery	Hepatitis C drugs—sofosbuvir, daclatasavir
Familial disease	Hypothyroidism
Infectious disease	Hypothermia
Chagas disease	Neurologic disorder
Infectious endocarditis	
Lyme disease	Hypokalemia Hyperkalemia Hypoxia Intracranial hypertension

Obstructive sleep apnea may also result in SB and pauses during apneic episodes. A large number of *medications* may cause SB, including sympathetic blockers (beta-blockers, methyldopa, clonidine), parasympathetic agents (digoxin, cholinomimetics), calcium channel antagonists, and antiarrhythmic drugs. Recently, the direct pacemaker-current (I_f) blocker, ivabradine, has been introduced for the treatment of heart failure and inappropriate sinus tachycardia. This medication may also cause SB.

Metabolic derangements that are associated with SB include hypothyroidism and myxedema coma, hypothermia, hypoxia, and hypokalemia. Common *infectious agents* associated with relative SB include *Legionella*, *Salmonella*, and *Trypanosoma cruzi* causing Chagas disease.

SINUS BRADYCARDIA OR PAUSE, SINUS ARREST, AND SINOATRIAL EXIT BLOCK

Sinus pause or arrest results from failure of sinus node impulse generation. It may occur because of intrinsic disease of the SAN, drugs that depress the SAN activity (beta-blockers, anti-arrhythmic

drugs) or from increased vagal tone. Sinoatrial exit block occurs because of the failure to conduct the impulse generated by the SAN to the surrounding atrial tissue. On the surface electrocardiogram (ECG), it is manifested as a pause due to the absence of an expected P wave. The P-P cycle is longer than the P-P interval of the underlying sinus rhythm, but it is always less than two consecutive P-P intervals.

Sinoatrial Exit Block

This arrhythmia results from failure of the impulse generated in the sinus node to depolarize the surrounding atrial tissue. It is usually transient. It can occur because of ischemia or myocarditis, or secondary to medications and excessive vagal tone. With first-degree SA exit block, each SAN impulse is conducted to the atria with a delay. This cannot be diagnosed with surface ECG. **Figure 21.1B** shows an example of second-degree SA exit block of Wenckebach type (Mobitz I). The P-P interval slightly prolongs until a pause occurs. The pause is not a multiplication of the regular P-P interval and its duration is less than the two preceding P-P intervals. An escape from a lower pacemaker (i.e. from the AVN) is often seen, and may result in retrograde conducting P waves with superior axis (negative P waves in II, III, and aVF). In **Figure 21.1C,** expected SAN activity is marked in S, whereas the atrial activity (the P wave) is marked in A. The pause seen is an exact multiplication of the P-P intervals; this is an example of type II second degree SA block.

Conversion Pauses

Following termination of an atrial arrhythmia, the diseased sinus may recover only after a pause (**Figure 21.1D**). Many times the atrial arrhythmia itself is asymptomatic, but the conversion pause can result in prolonged asystole and resultant syncope. Permanent pacemaker placement will eliminate the pauses and enable safe medical treatment for the atrial tachyarrhythmia.

TREATMENT

The treatment of SND depends mainly on symptoms. Asymptomatic SB is common and usually requires no therapy.[2] Symptomatic SND of any type may result in weakness, effort dyspnea, heart failure, and syncope. Here, permanent pacing is required. As a general rule, no oral medication can reliably increase the sinus rate. However, theophylline, a methyl xanthine which is also a phosphodiesterase inhibitor, may increase the sinus rate. It can be tried in patients with contraindications for pacing.[3]

ATRIOVENTRICULAR BLOCK

Atrioventricular block (AVB) is defined as a delay or interruption of impulse conduction from the atria to the ventricles. The conduction disturbance can be transient or permanent. Conduction may be delayed, intermittent, or absent (with or without a lower escape rhythm). The commonly used terminology includes the following:

First-degree AVB—slowed conduction without loss of AV synchrony, manifest in the surface ECG with prolonged PR interval, greater than 200 ms (**Figure 21.2A**). The conduction delay is usually at the level of the AVN. Normally, the PR will shorten during exercise test (due to physiologic shortening of the AV nodal refractory period) and a 1:1 conduction will be seen throughout the exercise despite increased sinus rate. Although no treatment is needed in most of the cases, caution should be taken with administration of negative chronotropic and nodal blocking agents (i.e. beta-blockers, calcium channel antagonists, and anti-arrhythmic drugs).

Second-degree AVB—intermittent loss of AV conduction, often in a regular pattern (e.g. 2:1, 3:2, or higher degrees of block).

- In second-degree AVB type I (referred to as Wenckebach type), the PR interval progressively prolongs from beat to

beat until AVBs occur and result in a dropped beat, which means failure of conduction of an SAN-generated impulse from the atria down to the ventricles. The PR interval following the pause returns to its baseline value and the sequence starts again. **Figure 21.2B** shows a typical example. The top numbers represent the R-R interval, whereas the bottom numbers represent the PR interval. The PR interval in the last conducted beat was 500 ms, and it was shortened to 360 ms after the blocked sinus beat. The pause following the blocked P wave (marked with an asterisk) is shorter than twice the preceding R-R. The QRS is usually

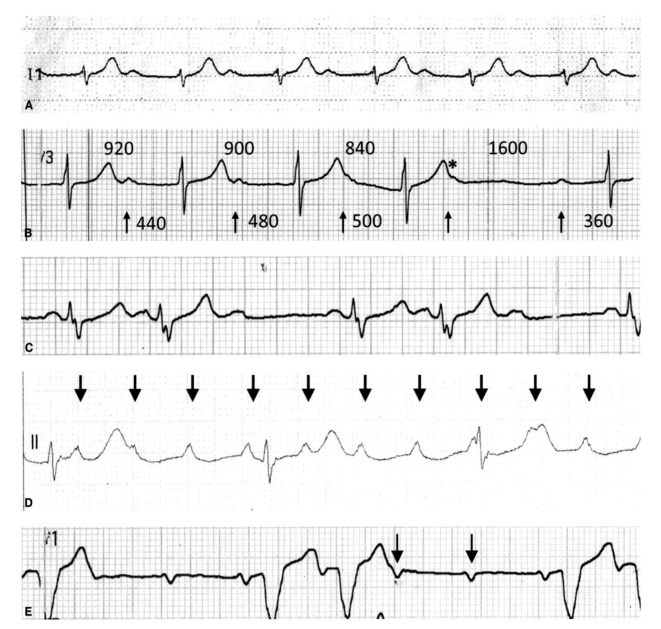

FIGURE 21.2 Types of AV conduction abnormalities. A, First-degree AV block with prolongation of the PR up to 440 ms in an asymptomatic man. B, Second-degree AV block, Mobitz type I (Wenckebach). Progressive PR prolongation is seen (P waves marked with an arrow and the values of the PR are given next to the arrows). Note the decrease in the ΔPR, resulting in a decrease in the RR intervals (denotes above the strip). Following a nonconducting P wave (*), PR shortening is seen and the pause is less than twice the preceding RR. The QRS is narrow, and the conduction delay is most probably at the level of the AV node. C, Second-degree AV block, Mobitz type II. Every third P wave is a block. The PR is fixed. The QRS is wide and the PR is normal (160 ms). The conduction delay is most probably below the level of the AV node. D, Complete AV block with no relationship between the P waves (arrows) and the QRS complexes. E, Advanced AV block with two consecutive blocked P wave (arrows). AV, atrioventricular.

narrow unless the underlying bundle branch block (BBB) is chronically present. The conduction delay is usually at the level of the AVN. Unless symptomatic, with a clear correlation between the ECG finding and the symptoms, this type of conduction abnormalities do not require therapy.

- Second-degree type II block (Mobitz II) is characterized in the surface ECG by a fixed PR interval before and after the blocked sinus beat (**Figure 21.2C**). The QRS is often wide. The conduction block is almost always below the level of the AVN. This type of AVB is usually permanent and often progresses to higher degree or even complete heart block. Implantation of a permanent pacemaker is required, regardless of symptoms.

Third-degree or complete AVB (CAVB)—no conduction is seen from the atria to the ventricles (**Figure 21.2D**). Lower escape rhythm may be seen. The higher the anatomic level of the conduction block, the faster and more stable the escape rhythm. AVB at the level of the AVN will usually give rise to a relatively fast escape rhythm of 40 to 60 bpm with a narrow QRS (unless BBB is chronically present). Lower anatomic level of the block, located at the His-Purkinje bundles, will result in a slow (<40 bpm) escape rhythm, often unstable with a wide QRS complex. As a general rule, the more distal the block, the slower will be the escape pacemaker. Low pacemakers have a rate of 40 bpm or less and are often unreliable, resulting in a very slow rate or asystole and often hemodynamic instability.

AVB should not be confused with other types of AV dissociation, in which there is no conduction from the atria to the ventricle due to other reasons, such as slowing of the sinus and accelerated nodal escape rhythm.

The term *advanced AVB* is referred to as two or more consecutive blocked sinus beats (**Figure 21.2E**).

The causes of AVB are depicted in **Table 21.2**. The main etiologies are discussed here in detail.

PHYSIOLOGIC AND PATHOPHYSIOLOGIC ATRIOVENTRICULAR BLOCK

Increased vagal tone—enhanced vagal tone can normally occur during sleep, in athletes, and as a result of various vagal triggers

TABLE 21.2	Major Causes of Atrioventricular Block
PHYSIOLOGIC AND PATHOPHYSIOLOGIC	**IATROGENIC**
Increased vagal tone	Medications
Fibrosis and sclerosis of the conduction system	β-Blockers, calcium channel antagonists, digitalis, antiarrhythmic medications
Ischemic heart disease	Cardiac surgery
Cardiomyopathy and myocarditis	TAVI or closure of septal defects
Congenital heart disease	Alcohol septal ablation for hypertrophic obstructive cardiomyopathy
Familial forms of AV block	
Other	
Hyperkalemia, infiltrative malignancies and benign tumor, neonatal lupus syndrome, hypothyroidism, trauma, neuromascular diseases	

AV, atrioventricular; TAVI, transcatheter aortic valve implantation.

such as pain, cough, carotid sinus massage, or carotid sinus hypersensitivity. All of these can result in AVB from Mobitz I to even complete AVB.[4] Typically, increased vagal tone results in SB in addition to the conduction abnormality and the QRS is narrow unless BBB is chronically present (**Figure 21.3**).

IDIOPATHIC PROGRESSIVE CARDIAC CONDUCTION DISEASE

Fibrosis and sclerosis of the conduction system accounts for about one-half of cases of AVB. Progressive cardiac conduction defects, referred to as Lenegre or Lev disease, are characterized by progressive impairment of the conduction system:

- The term *Lenegre disease* has been traditionally used to describe a progressive, fibrotic disease of the conduction system in younger individuals. It is frequently associated with slow progression to complete heart block and may be hereditary.

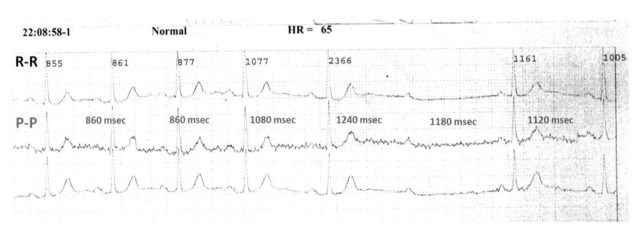

FIGURE 21.3 Vagal AV block. The top numbers (in black) denote the R-R intervals. The numbers in the middle (in red) denote the P-P intervals. Gradual prolongation of the P-P interval is present in addition to the AV block. The patient was asleep during the recording. AV, atrioventricular; HR, heart rate.

- Lev disease refers to sclerosis of the left side of the heart in older patients. Common associated findings include aortic and mitral valve calcifications. Fibrosis of the mitral ring and central fibrous body is common in elderly patients and result in congenital atrioventricular block with a narrow QRS complex. Aortic valve calcifications are commonly associated with fibrosis of the HB and bundle branches. Thus, the QRS complex is usually wide.

ISCHEMIC HEART DISEASE

Both acute and chronic ischemia may result in any degree of AVB. Recognition of the blood supply of the conduction system is important for understanding the mechanism of AVB during ischemia (see the section "Anatomic Consideration"). Up to 20% of patients with acute MI develop conduction abnormalities, but most of these abnormalities are transient.[5] Inferior MI may cause a heightened vagal tone that results in an AVB at the level of the AVN. Prolonged PR, Wenckebach type, and CAVB may be seen, almost always transient and respond to intravenous (IV) atropine. The escape rhythm is of narrow QRS with a rate of 40 to 60 bpm, and thus usually the patients are asymptomatic. In contrast, anterior MI may cause ischemia of the septum, resulting in a slower escape rhythm (<40 bpm) with wider QRS. It is usually seen with an extensive MI due to occlusion of the proximal LAD, and therefore the prognosis is poor. Temporary pacing is often needed.

CARDIOMYOPATHY AND MYOCARDITIS

AVB can be seen in patients with cardiomyopathies, most commonly with infiltrative processes such as amyloidosis and sarcoidosis, and in patients with myocarditis due to a variety of causes including rheumatic fever, Lyme disease, diphtheria, viruses, systemic lupus erythematosus (SLE), toxoplasmosis, bacterial endocarditis, and syphilis. The development of AVB in myocarditis is often a poor prognostic sign.

CONGENITAL HEART DISEASE

Congenital complete heart block may be an isolated lesion or may be associated with other types of congenital heart disease. When isolated, it results from transplacental passage of maternal anti-Ro/SSA and/or anti-La/SSB antibodies in women with SLE. Treatment is indicated mainly in symptomatic patients.

FAMILIAL DISEASE

Familial AV conduction block, characterized by a progression in the degree of block in association with a variable apparent site of block, may be transmitted as an autosomal dominant trait. Genetic mutation may be observed, usually in the *SCN5A* gene, encoding the fast sodium channel. Presentation can occur at any age, but progression of the conduction abnormalities with aging is seen. When presenting at an older age, it is often called hereditary Lenegre disease. It has been proposed that heterozygosity combined with aging leads to a progressive decline in conduction.

AV conduction disturbance can also appear in the setting of inherited arrhythmic syndromes (long QT syndrome type 3, Brugada). In these conditions, ventricular arrhythmias are not uncommon and may result in sudden cardiac death. Therefore, an implantable cardioverter-defibrillator rather than a pacemaker may be required.

MUSCULAR DYSTROPHIES

Muscular dystrophies are often associated with conduction abnormalities. The major syndromes include myotonic dystrophy and Emery–Dreyfuss muscular dystrophy. Muscular symptoms are often easily noticed and aid in diagnosis.

ELECTROLYTE DISTURBANCE

Most commonly seen with hyper- and hypokalemia, the QRS is wide and the treatment is focused on correcting the potassium level. One should keep in mind that primary bradycardia may result in hypotension, acute renal failure, and hyperkalemia, which exacerbates the conduction abnormality. In this setting, pacing is indicated.

IATROGENIC

Cardiac surgery may result in AVB, in particular replacement of calcified aortic and mitral valve and/or closure of ventricular septal defects. CAVB is seen in 5% to 20% of patients undergoing transcatheter aortic valve replacement, especially in patients with prior conduction abnormalities such as right BBB. Alcohol septal ablation for the treatment of hypertrophic obstructive cardiomyopathy is complicated with CAVB in 10% of the cases. AVB might happen during or following catheter ablation of certain arrhythmias, most commonly ablation of AV nodal reentrant tachycardia and focal tachycardias or ablation of accessory pathways located in the septal region. However, the frequency of this complication is low.

MEDICATIONS

A variety of drugs can impair AV conduction, occasionally resulting in AVB. Examples include β-blockers, digitalis, calcium channel antagonists (especially verapamil and, to a lesser extent, diltiazem), amiodarone, and adenosine. The block is usually in the AVN and may be reversible with discontinuation of the drug. In comparison, antiarrhythmic drugs that modulate the sodium channel, such as quinidine, procainamide, flecainide, propafenone, amiodarone, and sotalol can produce block in the more distal His-Purkinje system. Some of these medications (i.e. amiodarone and sotalol) exhibit significant beta-blockade activity and may cause a conduction delay at any level.

Most patients with AVB who are taking drugs that can impair conduction probably have underlying conduction system disease. This was suggested by a study of 169 patients with second- or third-degree AVB associated with medication. Drug discontinuation resulted in resolution of the AVB in 40% of the patients, but half of them recurred even after discontinuation of the drug.[6]

ATRIOVENTRICULAR DISSOCIATION

With AV dissociation, independent activation of the atria and ventricles is seen as a result of absent conduction through the AVN. There is no fixed relationship between the P waves and the QRS complexes, and the PR intervals are variable in a random manner. Assessment of the jugular venous waveform can disclose "cannon" A waves, indicative of contraction of the RA against the closed tricuspid valve. Several conditions may result in AV dissociation (**Figure 21.4**):

- Slowing of the SAN with an escape junctional or ventricular rhythm without retrograde conduction to the AVN may result in AV dissociation. The junctional or ventricular rate is isorhythmic or faster than the sinus rate; thus, the interval between the QRS complexes is similar to or shorter than the PP interval. With isorhythmic AV dissociation, the PR may seem to be very short or the P waves may be buried within the QRS complex and therefore not seen (**Figure 21.4A**). As seen in the figure, the first P wave conducts, whereas the second and the last P waves do not conduct to the ventricle (the PR interval is too short).

- Acceleration or enhanced automaticity of lower or subsidiary pacemakers, such as an accelerated junctional or ventricular rhythm, or with a ventricular tachycardia, and rarely with a junctional tachycardia, may cause AV dissociation. There is a retrograde block of impulse conduction through the AVN (no ventriculoatrial conduction); thus, there is no atrial activation and the sinus node is not suppressed. The RR interval

is shorter than the PP interval. Accelerated idioventricular rhythm (AIVR) is a ventricular rhythm typically seen during reperfusion of cardiac ischemia (typically seen with thrombolysis in the setting of ST-elevation myocardial infarction) (**Figure 21.4B**).

- AVB, type II or III can result in AV dissociation (**Figure 21.4C**).
- Ventricular tachycardia with retrograde ventriculoatrial block (**Figure 21.4D**).

TREATMENT

The degree of the block and the presence or absence of reversible causes determines the treatment. First-degree and second-degree AVB of Wenckebach type usually requires no treatment. For advanced AVB with no reversible cause (second-degree Mobitz II and complete AVB), permanent pacemaker implantation is indicated regardless of symptoms.[7] An exception to that is asymptomatic congenital AVB. These patients usually have a reasonable inotropic response of the escape rhythm on one hand, and high rate of complications if a permanent pacemaker is implanted at a young age.

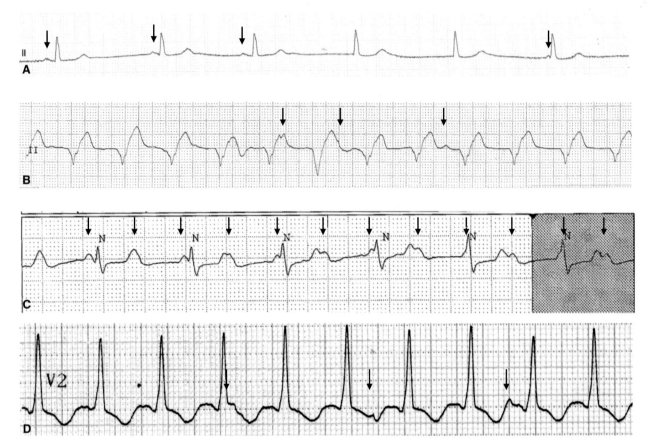

FIGURE 21.4 Atrioventricular dissociation. A, Sinus bradycardia with junctional escape. The sinus and the junctional escape rate are similar. The first P wave conducts to the ventricle, whereas the second and the last P waves do not conduct (the PR interval is too short). The last P wave is buried in the QRS. The third P wave probably does conduct because the PR is normal and the R-R is shorter in comparison to other R-R in the strip. B, Accelerated idioventricular rhythm (AIVR) during reperfusion of an occluded coronary artery. Some P waves are marked with an arrow. C, AV dissociation due to complete AV block. N mark the QRS signal. All R-R intervals are equal, despite alternating relationship between the P wave and the R wave. D, AV dissociation due to ventricular tachycardia (VT). The QRS is relatively narrow because the VT's exit is near the septum. Arrow denotes the dissociated P waves.

MANAGEMENT OF BRADYCARDIA AND HEART BLOCK

Initial assessment should focus on the stability of the patient, including symptoms of bradycardia (see preceding text) and hemodynamic status. **Figure 21.5** depicts the 2015 Advanced Cardiac Life Support (ACLS) bradycardia algorithm. A major modification in this algorithm, which was initially introduced in 2010, is to define the HR for intervention to less than 50 bpm (instead of the previously used formal definition of less than 60 bpm). One should keep in mind that while slow HR of 50 to 60 bpm usually will not cause symptoms and, in fact, may be physiologic, it may be inadequate for certain patients with other comorbidities (such as anemia, sepsis, heart failure). In these cases, holding medications that may lower the HR and increasing HR with anticholinergics or sympathomimetics may be indicated.

Mean blood pressure will often be relatively conserved because of compensatory vasoconstriction. Owing to increased stroke volume and prolonged diastolic time, systolic blood pressure increases while the diastolic blood pressure decreases, resulting in widened pulse pressure. The increased systolic pressure usually requires no treatment. Other patients may have signs and symptoms of hemodynamic compromise such as shock, orthostatic symptoms, oliguria, and confusion. Heart failure symptoms (shortness of breath, orthopnea, and edema) and signs of congestion may appear. Unstable patients should be treated immediately regardless of the diagnosis (SB or AVB). Therapeutic options may include atropine (IV push of 0.5 to 1 mg), sympathomimetics (dopamine or epinephrine infusion), and temporary pacing (**Table 21.3**). However, caution should be exercised if atropine or sympathomimetics are given to a patient with infra-hisian AVB because these medications can increase the sinus rate and aggravate the degree of the block. Patients with asymptomatic bradycardia should be followed up without any immediate intervention. Reversible causes should be sought while a decision regarding placement of a temporary or permanent pacemaker is taken. Important reversible causes include hypothermia, electrolyte disturbance (especially hypokalemia and acidosis), hypoxia, cardiac ischemia, medication use, and overdose.

TEMPORARY PACING

Temporary pacing is indicated in symptomatic bradycardia whenever there is a potentially reversible cause, or when permanent pacing is not available or carries a high risk at that moment (i.e. ongoing infection, risk of bleeding due to drugs, thrombocytopenia, and coagulopathy). If the cause is irreversible and permanent pacing is available, it should be preferred over temporary pacing. However, many unstable patients will require the insertion of a temporary wire to allow safe implantation of a permanent pacemaker.

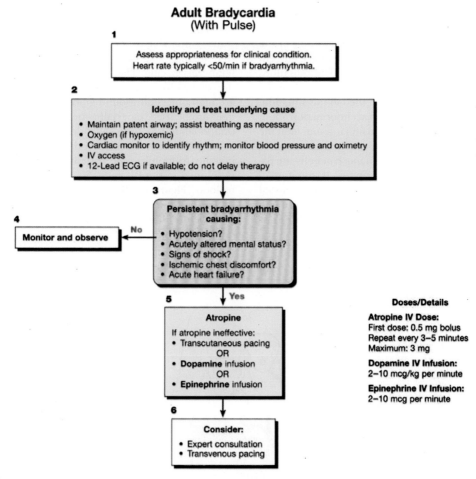

FIGURE 21.5 ACLS adult bradycardia algorithm. ACLS, Advanced Cardiac Life Support; ECG, electrocardiogram; IV, intravenous. (Reproduced from 2015 American Heart Association guidelines for cardiopulmonary resuscitation and emergency cardiovascular care.)

TABLE 21.3	**Medication Used for Bradycardia**		
	MECHANISM OF ACTION	DOSE	SIGNIFICANT SIDE EFFECTS
Atropine	Anticholinergic (ACH-R antagonist)	IV, 0.5–2.0 mg	Tachyarrhythmia, glaucoma, bronchospasm, urinary retention
Isoprenaline	β-Receptor agonist	IV, 1–4 µg/min; IV drip of 15–60 mL/h of 0.4 mg/100 mL NS	Tachycardia, ischemia, hyper- or hypotension, headache
Theophylline	PDE-5 inhibitor	PO, 200 mg bid	Abdominal discomfort, tachycardia, restlessness

ACH-R, acetylcholine receptor; IV, intravenous; NS, normal saline; PDE-5, phosphodiesterase-5.

Temporary pacing may be achieved transcutaneously using external pads, transvenously using an electrode ("wire"), epicardially using an atrial or ventricular epicardial electrode placed during a cardiac surgery, or through an esophageal electrode (mainly for atrial pacing).

TRANSCUTANEOUS PACING

External pads can deliver immediate pacing. Anteroposterior position is the most effective, although anterior-apical can also be tried (**Figure 21.6**). This is reserved for cases with asystole or severe bradycardia and hemodynamic instability and serves only until achieving pacing with other methods. **Figure 21.7A** shows an example of an external pacemaker-defibrillator unit from a specific manufacturer. The arrow indicates the location of the pacing button. In the external monitor-defibrillator, the current is programmed at a high energy (i.e. 80 mA). The pulsations need to be verified, ideally by palpating the radial or femoral pulses. Carotid artery palpation is best avoided in this situation. On occasion, an arterial line can deliver exact information about the blood pressure. Pacing artifacts are usually large and limit the ability to assess capture using the cardiac monitor. The capture should be assessed continuously as a slight movement by the patient or pad movement may result in noncapture. If palpation of the arterial pulse is absent, the pad location needs to be adjusted or the current needs to be increased. Pad malfunction owing to improper contact with the skin (usually due to diaphoresis or

hair over the chest) should be excluded. It should be mentioned that most patients will need some sedation to tolerate the pain involved with pacing, due to cutaneous nerve stimulation and skeletal muscle contractions. The rate of pacing is typically between 60 and 80 bpm. Because of the limitations associated with transcutaneous pacing, this method should be considered only as a temporizing measure for unconscious patients or those in whom sedation can be administered, until either temporary or permanent transvenous pacing can be established.

TRANSVENOUS PACING

Insertion of a temporary wire is best done by an expert physician under fluoroscopy guidance or at the bedside using a pacing wire with an inflatable balloon at the distal end (**Figure 21.7B**). The right jugular or subclavian veins are the optimal access sites for temporary pacing. These sites allow patient mobilization once the pacing wire is secured. However, access-related complications are high unless ultrasound guidance is used. The femoral vein may also be used, especially when done in the cardiac catheterization laboratory for a short duration. Disadvantages of using the femoral vein access include higher risk of infection and inability to mobilize the patient. The temporary wire is often positioned in the RV apex. Some of the wires contain a distal balloon (**Figure 21.7B**), to help advancing the tip of the wire under low-flow conditions. The balloon should be checked for leaks before insertion, inflated once in the vein, and deflated

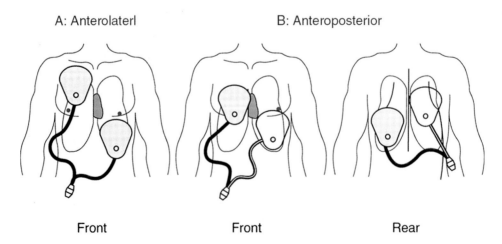

A: Anterolaterl   B: Anteroposterior

Front   Front   Rear

FIGURE 21.6 Pacemaker pads position. A, Apical and lateral. B, Anterior-posterior.

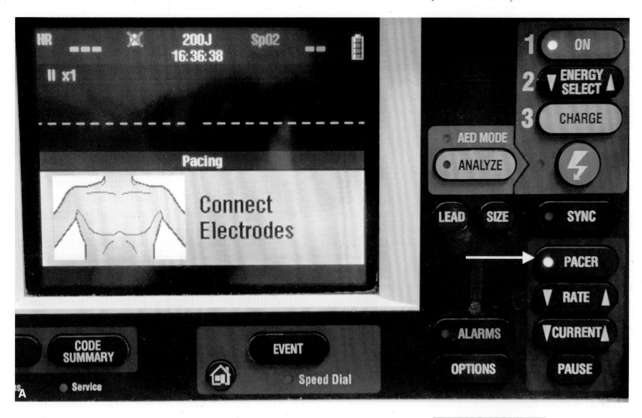

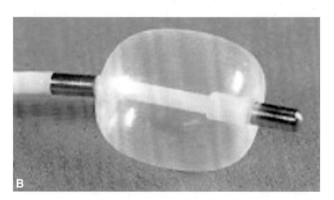

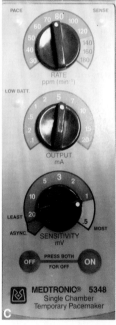

FIGURE 21.7 Temporary pacing units. A, External monitor-defibrillator. The white arrow denotes pacer button. Once pushed, the external pacemaker will pace at the set rate and output (notice green light on the left side of the button). The rate and current buttons are used for setting. Pacing may be started at 60 to 80 bpm with current of 80 mA. The current may be lowered, provided that capture is still manually verified. B, A tip of a temporary wire with distal inflatable balloon. C, Temporary pacing unit. The top button is used to set the rate, the middle button is used to set the output, and the lower button is used to set the sensitivity. The sensitivity is usually set to high (< 1 mV) to avoid pacing immediately after intrinsic activity, unless electrical noise is expected.

after positioning in the RV. The physician caring for paced patients should be familiar with the programming of the temporary pacing unit (**Figure 21.7C**). Once positioned in the RV apex, if there is an intrinsic activity, the sensing light will flash (top left of the pacing unit).

The upper button sets the pacing rate, usually at 60 to 80 bpm. The middle button sets the output delivered. The capture threshold is the minimal amount of output (in mA) required for capture. Threshold test is needed every 8 hours or whenever the patient position is changed (i.e. transferred to an intensive care unit [ICU] bed) (**Figure 21.8**). To test for the threshold, increase the pacing rate 10 to 20 bpm above the intrinsic rate (not less than 60 bpm) and slowly decrease the output till capture is lost (absence of QRS complex following the pacing artifacts). At that point, increasing the output should be done quickly. Output can be programmed to five times the threshold, usually at least 5 mA. This safety margin is required because the temporary electrode's stability is less than those of the permanent leads.

SENSING

This term relates to the ability of the pacemaker to sense the intrinsic electrical activity. To determine an adequate sensing, set the pacemaker rate to 10 to 20 below the intrinsic rate, if possible. Set the sensitivity to the maximal level (**Figure 21.7C**, lower button, indicated by "least"). The sensing light (**Figure 21.7C**, top right) will stop flashing because it will not sense any activity. Slowly decrease the sensitivity threshold until the sensing light flashes. This is the sensing threshold, that is, the minimum intracardiac signal that will be sensed (seen) by the pacemaker and inhibit its activity. The sensitivity should be set to a low value (1 mV, indicated by "most"), not higher than the sensitivity threshold, to prevent pacing on intrinsic activity. However, when external noise is expected (during implantation of the permanent pacemaker with the use of electrocautery), the sensitivity should be programmed to the minimum (high value of 20 mV, depicted in **Figure 21.7C** as "least").

Figure 21.8 shows examples of ECG from paced patients. In **Figure 21.8A**, typical pacing is shown. Each pacing artifact is followed by a QRS. The QRS morphology is typical for RV apical pacing with left BBB pattern and a superior axis (negative QRS in the inferior limb leads). In **Figure 21.8B**, pacemaker intermittent loss of capture is seen. Notice how some of the pacing artifacts (first, third, fifth, ninth, and last) are not followed by a QRS.

The temporary wire is removed once the bradycardia is resolved or a permanent pacemaker is implanted. On occasion, temporary wires perforate the thin RV wall during implantation. It is not uncommon to observe pericardial effusion and tamponade upon removal of a temporary wire which had sealed a perforation, especially in anticoagulated patients.

PERMANENT PACEMAKER

Sinus node dysfunction resulting in bradycardia is an indication for pacemaker implantation mainly when symptomatic. Asymptomatic sinus bradycardia does not carry a risk for syncope or sudden death (2). In contrast, second-degree Mobitz type II, Advanced AV block and CAVB require permanent pacing regardless of symptoms.

Table 21.4 denotes the pacemaker nomenclature endorsed by the NASPE (North-American society of pacing and electrophysiology). The most common pacemaker is coded as DDDR, thus pacing and sensing is available in both atrium and ventricle, the sensing may trigger or inhibit pacing and rate modulation is possible. This type of pacemaker allows for atrio-ventricular synchrony. VDD pacing is a suitable option for patients with a conduction abnormality but a normal sinus function. This pacemaker has one lead which is positioned at the right ventricular apex, with a bipolar sensor located about 15 cm from the distal end of the lead and allows for sensing in the atrium. The nomenclature of this type of pacemaker (VDD) denotes that pacing is possible only in the ventricle (first letter, "V", in the nomenclature). The major advantage of this type of pacemaker is that its single lead allows for AV synchronous pacing. VVI pacemakers can sense and pace the ventricle alone and is used mainly for patients in persistent atrial fibrillation or in patients in sinus rhythm but only infrequent bradycardic

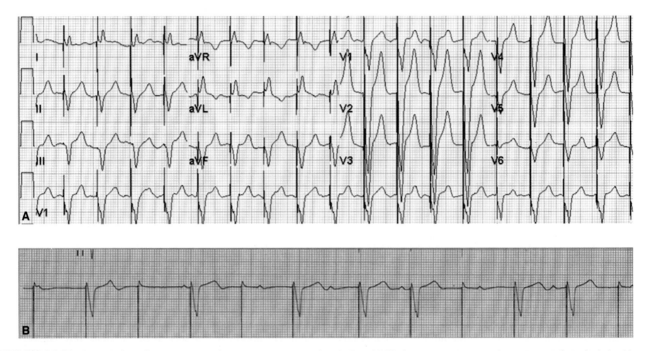

FIGURE 21.8 ECG recordings from patients with a temporary pacemaker. A, Paced ECG showing superior axis (negative in inferior limb leads) and LBBB pattern, typical for an electrode located in the RV apex. B, Pacemaker malfunction. Some of the pacemaker artifact (i.e. first, third, and fifth) are not followed by a QRS, indicating intermittent loss of capture. ECG, electrocardiogram; LBBB, left bundle branch block; RV, right ventricle.

TABLE 21.4	NASPE Generic Code for Pacemakers			
POSITION	I	II	III	IV
Category	Chamber(s) paced	Chamber(s) sensed	Response to sensing	Rate modulation
	O = none	O = none	I = inhibition	O = none
	A = atrium	A = atrium	T = triggered	R = rate modulation
	V = ventricle	V = ventricle	D = dual (I+T)	
	D = dual (A+V)	D = dual (A+V)		

NASPE, North American Society of Pacing and Electrophysiology.

TABLE 21.5	Types of Cardiac Pacemakers and NASPE Codes
CODE	MEANING
A(V)OO	Asynchronous atrial (ventricular) pacemaker without sensing of the patient's atrial (ventricular) rhythm
AA(VV)I	Sensing and pacing in the atrium (ventricle) only
DDD	Multiprogrammable physiologic dual-chamber pacemaker; can sense and pace in the atrium and ventricle
DDI	Dual chamber pacing and sensing in the lower rate only
VDD	Ventricular pacing, dual-chamber sensing with atrial synchronous ventricular pacing

NASPE, North American Society of Pacing and Electrophysiology.

episodes. The last letter in the nomenclature, *I*, denotes that pacing is *inhibited* if the pacemaker senses an intrinsic ventricular activity of the patient. Similarly, AAI pacemaker allows for sensing and pacing in the atrium alone. While it is suitable for patients with sinus node dysfunction and intact AV conduction, it is only infrequently used for fear of later development of a conduction abnormality (**Table 21.5**). The routine management post-pacemaker implantations include prophylactic antibiotic therapy (usually for 24 hours with anti-staphylococcal agents), analgesics, chest X-ray to verify lead position and rule out pneumothorax, and bed restriction (3 hours to overnight, depend in the local policy). Most patients will be discharged within 24 hours, unless their clinical status was not yet stabilize.

REFERENCES

1. Kawashima T, Sasaki H. The morphological significance of the human sinoatrial nodal branch (artery). *Heart Vessels.* 2003;18(4):213.
2. Goldberger GJ, Johnson NP, Gidea C. Significance of asymptomatic bradycardia for subsequent pacemaker implantation and mortality in patients >60 years of age. *Am J Cardiol.* 2011;108:857-861.
3. Alboni P, Menozzi C, Brignole M, et al. Effects of permanent pacemaker and oral theophylline in sick sinus syndrome: the THEOPACE study: a randomized controlled trial. *Circulation.* 1997;96:260-266.
4. Alboni P, Holz A, Brignole M. Vagally mediated atrioventricular block: pathophysiology and diagnosis. *Heart.* 2013;99:904-908.
5. Zimetbaum PZ, Josephson ME. Use of the electrocardiogram in acute myocardial infarction. *N Engl J Med.* 2003;348:933-940.
6. Zeltser D, Justo D, Halkin A, et al. Drug-induced atrioventricular block: prognosis after discontinuation of the culprit drug. *J Am Coll Cardiol.* 2004;44:105-108.
7. Edhag O, Swahn A. Prognosis of patients with complete heart block or arrhythmic syncope who were not treated with artificial pacemakers. *Acta Med Scand.* 1976;200:457-463.

Patient and Family Information for: BRADYCARDIA AND HEART BLOCK

WHAT IS BRADYCARDIA?

Specialized heart cells in the right atrium are called sinus node and are responsible for electrical impulse formation, resulting in a resting HR in most healthy people of 60 to 100 beats per minute. Bradycardia is a slow heart beat (<60 bpm) caused either by abnormal electrical impulse formation (sick sinus syndrome) or by its delayed propagation to the rest of the heart (heart block). During sleep and in well-trained individuals, bradycardia is common and adequate and therefore does not require any treatment.

WHAT CAUSES BRADYCARDIA?

Bradycardia can be caused by the following:

- Changes in the heart that are the result of aging.
- Diseases that damage the heart's electrical system. These include coronary artery disease, heart attack, and infections such as endocarditis and myocarditis.
- Conditions that can slow electrical impulses through the heart. Examples include having a low thyroid hormone level (hypothyroidism) or an electrolyte imbalance, such as too much potassium in the blood.
- Some medicines for treating heart problems or high blood pressure, such as β-blockers, calcium blockers, antiarrhythmic drugs, and digoxin.

WHAT ARE THE SYMPTOMS?

As the HR declines, the heart may not pump enough blood to meet the body's needs. A very slow HR may cause a person to experience the following:

- Feel dizzy, lightheaded
- Feel short of breath and find it harder to exercise
- Feel tired
- Have chest pain or a feeling that the heart is pounding or fluttering (palpitations)
- Feel confused or have trouble concentrating
- Faint, if a slow HR causes a drop in blood pressure

Some people do not have symptoms, or their symptoms are so mild that they think these are just part of getting older. The pulse rate can be assessed by checking it manually with the fingers or with an electronic device such as blood pressure machines and smartphone applications.

If the heart beat is slow or uneven, talk to a doctor.

HOW IS BRADYCARDIA DIAGNOSED?

A doctor may be able to diagnose bradycardia by doing a physical examination, asking questions about past health, and doing an ECG.

An ECG measures the electrical signals that control heart rhythm, so it is the best test for bradycardia. Bradycardia often comes and goes, so a standard ECG done in the doctor's office may not find it. An ECG can identify bradycardia only if the person is actually having it during the test. There may be a need to use a portable (ambulatory) ECG device. This lightweight device is also called a Holter monitor or a cardiac event monitor. The person wears the monitor for a day or more, and it records the heart rhythm while he/she goes about the daily routine. Blood tests may also be necessary to find out whether another problem is causing the slow HR.

HOW IS IT TREATED?

The treatment of a slow heartbeat depends on what is causing it and what are the accompanying symptoms. Sometimes, there is no need for any intervention, especially if the bradycardia is asymptomatic.

If damage to the heart's electrical system causes the heart to beat too slowly, the person will probably need to have a pacemaker. A pacemaker is an electronic device, placed under the chest skin and connected to the heart with electrical wires, which helps correct the slow HR. Older people are most likely to have a type of bradycardia that requires a pacemaker. If another medical problem, such as hypothyroidism or an electrolyte imbalance, is causing a slow HR, treating that problem may cure the bradycardia. If a medicine is causing the heart to beat too slowly, the doctor may adjust the dose or prescribe a different medicine. If the person cannot stop taking that medicine, a pacemaker may be needed. The goal of treatment is to raise the HR so the body gets the blood it needs. If severe bradycardia is not treated, it can lead to serious problems. These may include fainting and injuries from fainting, as well as seizures or even death.

WHAT CAN BE DONE AT HOME FOR BRADYCARDIA?

Bradycardia is often the result of another heart condition, so taking steps to improve heart health will usually improve overall health. The best steps to take are to ensure the following:

- Control cholesterol and blood pressure
- Eat a low-fat, low-salt diet
- Get regular exercise; a doctor can tell what level of exercise is safe
- Stop smoking
- Limit alcohol
- Take medicines as prescribed
- See the doctor for regular follow-up care

People who get pacemakers need to be careful around strong magnetic or electrical fields, such as magnetic resonance imaging machines or magnetic wands used at airports because they may interfere with their functioning. If a pacemaker is placed, the doctor will give information about its type and what precautions are to be taken. Once a cardiac pacemaker is implanted, most patients enjoy a normal life without even noticing its presence.

22

Todd Kobrinski
Emad F. Aziz

Supraventricular Arrhythmias

INTRODUCTION

Of the supraventricular arrhythmias that are encountered in the cardiac care unit (CCU), sinus tachycardia and atrial fibrillation (AF) are most frequently seen owing to their higher incidences among patients with acute myocardial infarction (MI), respiratory failure, sepsis, structural or valvular heart disease, and cardiomyopathy. Because of the distinctness of AF as a clinical entity, it is discussed in conjunction with atrial flutter (AFL) in a separate chapter. This chapter focuses on the general approach to the classification and management of narrow QRS complex tachycardias followed by a description of the common forms of supraventricular tachycardias (SVTs). The algorithms defined in this chapter apply to the most typical clinical scenarios and are not intended to be exhaustive or highly specific.

SVTs are commonly seen in the CCU and in otherwise healthy patients without structural heart disease, with an overall prevalence estimate of 600,000 and annual incidence of 90,000 in the United States alone.[1] They represent a heterogeneous group of tachyarrhythmias that originate in the supraventricular tissue or utilize it as part of a reentrant circuit,[2] and are characterized by a spectrum of electrocardiogram (ECG) findings that are clinically important to understand, identify, and differentiate. SVTs typically present with a regular rate (160–200 bpm) and a narrow QRS complex (<120 milliseconds) on ECG because they follow the normal pathway of atrioventricular (AV) conduction and ventricular activation via the His-Purkinje system. Occasionally, SVTs present with a wide QRS complex (≥120 milliseconds) because of baseline bundle branch blocks, rate-related aberrancy, or conduction via accessory pathways (APs).

Sinus tachycardia, by far the most common SVT, is not a pathologic arrhythmia (with the rare exception of inappropriate sinus tachycardia) but rather is an appropriate cardiac response to a physiologic event. Sinus tachycardia is gradual in onset and recession. The heart rate is regular and classically does not exceed 220 beats per minute (bpm) minus the patient's age. In sinus tachycardia, P waves precede the QRS complex. Sinus tachycardia is virtually always a compensatory response, and it should not be considered the cause of hemodynamic instability. Instead, the underlying precipitant of sinus tachycardia (eg, ischemia, infection, heart failure) must be identified and addressed.

GENERAL APPROACH TO NARROW QRS COMPLEX TACHYCARDIAS

SYMPTOMS AND HEMODYNAMIC IMPACT

SVTs are not usually life threatening to otherwise healthy individuals; however, patients admitted to the CCU who present with narrow QRS complex tachycardias should be thoroughly assessed for clinical signs and symptoms potentially *attributable to* the arrhythmia. These may include hypotension, diminished peripheral pulses and tissue perfusion, shortness of breath, and chest pain. In contrast to patients without organic heart disease, many CCU patients may have ischemic cardiomyopathy, severe valvular stenosis or regurgitation, or reduced left ventricular function. Among such patients, the tachycardia can lead to reduced diastolic filling and decreased cardiac output, which may hasten myocardial ischemia and decompensated heart failure. That said, it is equally important to differentiate these scenarios from those in which the underlying disease is the cause of hemodynamic instability and the precipitant for the SVT. For example, sepsis with vasodilatory shock or acute pulmonary embolism can be a *driver* of the tachyarrhythmia. After careful delineation of these relationships, if the SVT is thought to be the *cause* of hemodynamic instability, expeditious treatment (eg, electrical cardioversion) guided by established Advanced Cardiac Life Support (ACLS) protocol is warranted (**Figure 22.1**).[3]

CLASSIFICATION BASED ON ELECTROCARDIOGRAM FINDINGS

REGULARITY OF THE RHYTHM

A 12-lead ECG is the cornerstone in diagnosing SVT and should be carefully inspected for regularity of QRS complexes. This can be done most accurately using calipers to sequentially compare R-R intervals (**Figure 22.2**) and allows for rapid initial differentiation into two major categories: irregular and regular rhythms (**Figure 22.3**).[4–6] Careful inspection and repeat measurements are usually sufficient to establish regularity; however, irregular SVTs including AF and AFL with variable AV conduction or multifocal atrial tachycardia (MAT) may exhibit very rapid ventricular conduction that can sometimes mask their irregularity. In such instances, the use of heart-rate–slowing maneuvers (ie, increased vagal tone) can be effective in resolving any ambiguity

Adult Tachycardia With a Pulse Algorithm

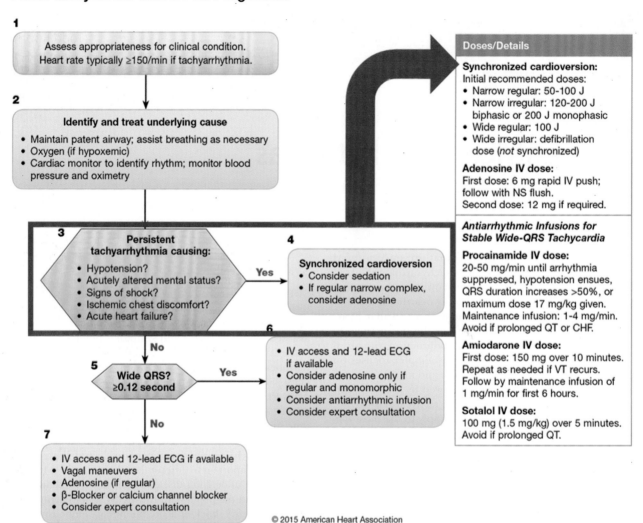

FIGURE 22.1 Algorithm for appropriate use of synchronized electrical cardioversion in the management of unstable patients with persistent narrow QRS complex SVTs. From the American Heart Association (AHA) Advanced Cardiac Life Support (ACLS) algorithm for adults with tachycardia and a pulse.[3]

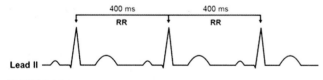

FIGURE 22.2 Determining the regularity of narrow QRS complex SVTs on ECG via measurement of the R-R interval. ECG, electrocardiogram; SVT, supraventricular tachycardia.

(**Table 22.1**). After the regularity has been assessed, the ECG should be analyzed for the presence of P waves and their morphology.

PRESENCE AND MORPHOLOGY OF P WAVES

Identification of P waves and their morphologic patterns are essential for further characterization of regular narrow QRS complex SVTs, as well as their relative origin within the supraventricular conduction system (ie, sinoatrial [SA] node vs atrial vs AV

node). This requires familiarity with P-wave appearance during normal (sinus) conduction on 12-lead ECG, and experience with recognition of oftentimes subtle variations.[7] Cases in which P waves are not well identified might indicate that the activation of the atria and ventricles is occurring almost simultaneously, resulting in a P wave that is buried within or just following the QRS complex. The most common etiologic example of this ECG pattern is atrioventricular nodal reentrant tachycardia (AVNRT), followed less commonly by unifocal atrial tachycardia (AT) and junctional tachycardia (JT). Sinus P waves are positive in the inferior leads (ie, II, III, and aVF) due to normal anterograde conduction, whereas P waves in AVNRT are always negative in the inferior leads (pseudo–S) due to retrograde conduction from the AV node to the atria (**Figure 22.4**). This is similarly seen in atrioventricular reentrant tachycardia (AVRT); however, nonretrograde P waves are sometimes present depending on the location of the AP. The importance of differences in P-wave patterns and timing is not only inherent to AVNRT and AVRT. P waves originating from a different focus (ie, ectopic AT) or

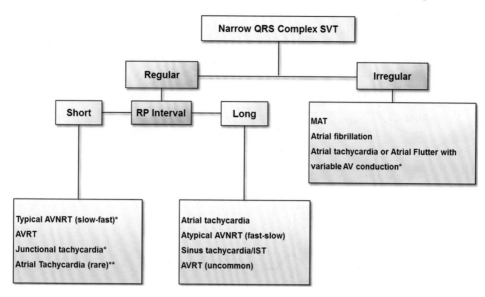

FIGURE 22.3 General approach to classifying narrow QRS complex tachycardias. AV, atrioventricular; AVNRT, atrioventricular nodal reentrant tachycardia; AVRT, atrioventricular reentrant tachycardia; IST, inappropriate sinus tachycardia; MAT, multifocal atrial tachycardia; SVT, supraventricular tachycardia.

TABLE 22.1	Common Methods of Transiently Slowing AV Conduction to Allow for Definitive Diagnosis in the Classification of Narrow QRS Complex Tachycardias		
Modalities that Transiently Slow AV Conduction:	Vagal Maneuvers: • Carotid Massage • Valsalva maneuvers	AV Nodal Medications: • Adenosine • β-blockers (metoprolol) • Nondihydropyridine calcium channel blockers (verapamil, diltiazem)	
Responses of Individual SVTs to Transient Slowing of AV Conduction:	**AVNRT**	**AVRT**	**AT**
Abrupt termination with a P wave after the last QRS complex.	Yes	Yes	Very unlikely
Abrupt termination with a QRS complex.	Yes	Yes	Yes
Some/gradual slowing of the ventricular rate without termination.	No (excludes)	No (excludes)	Common

AT, atrial tachycardia; AV, atrioventricular; AVRT, atrioventricular reentrant tachycardia; AVNRT, atrioventricular nodal reentrant tachycardia; SVT, supraventricular tachycardia.

multiple foci (ie, MAT) in the atria can have variable morphologies and may even mimic sinus P waves (eg, crista terminalis origin). Therefore, comparison of P-wave characteristics with those found on the baseline ECG, as well as onset/termination properties of the tachycardia, is extremely useful in differentiating focal or reentrant tachycardia from sinus tachycardia.

R-P INTERVAL

Following identification of P waves and their morphologies, the next step is examining the relationship of the P wave to the QRS complex. This is done by measuring an RR interval and then the distance from the initial R wave to the next discernable P wave. If the RP interval is less than one-half of the RR interval, the tachycardia is a short-RP tachycardia; otherwise, it is a long-RP tachycardia (**Figure 22.5**). The RP interval alludes to the relative timing of atrial (P) and ventricular (QRS) activation during SVT.

As previously mentioned, atrial and ventricular activation occurs almost simultaneously (P waves buried within/just after

QRS complex) in typical forms of AVNRT and AVRT, which represent the two most common short-RP tachycardias. AVNRT stems from dual-AV nodal physiology, whereas AVRT develops in patients with an extranodal AP that electrically connects the atrium and ventricle. Typical AVRT conducts down the AV node and up the AP resulting in a short-RP interval that may be slightly longer than that of AVNRT. Focal AT typically results in a long-RP tachycardia on ECG (**Figure 22.6A–B**).

ADDITIONAL DIAGNOSTIC MANEUVERS

As part of the systematic approach to identifying and classifying narrow QRS complex SVTs, it is often essential to transiently slow AV conduction to allow for more definitive assessment of regularity, presence of P waves, and RP intervals.[8,9] This is commonly attempted first using bedside vagal maneuvers such as Valsalva and carotid sinus massage, followed by medications (commonly adenosine, sometimes β-blockers and calcium channel blockers [CCBs]) that temporarily block or slow conduction through the AV node.

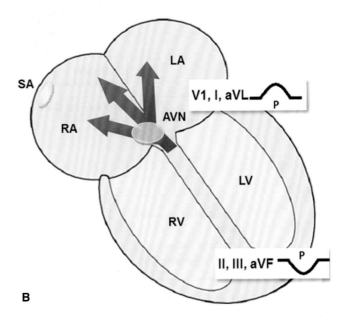

FIGURE 22.4 Differences in P-wave morphology in the inferior leads (II, III, aVF) based on direction of atrial activation. A, In normal antegrade sinus conduction positive P-wave deflections are seen in the inferior leads. B, With AVNRT, the atria are activated in a retrograde direction from the AV node, resulting in P waves that are negative in the inferior leads and positive in V1. AVN, atrioventricular node; LA, left atrium; LV, left ventricle; RA, right atrium; RV, right ventricle; SA, sinoatrial node.

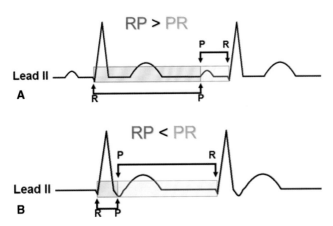

FIGURE 22.5 A, Measurement of the RP (and PR) intervals in ECG lead II. A, Narrow QRS complex tachycardias with RP intervals that are more than one-half of the RR interval (RP > PR) are called *long RP* tachycardias, whereas (B) those with an RP interval that is less than one-half of the RR interval (RP < PR) are known as short RP tachycardias.

Before performing carotid sinus massage, it is crucial to revisit the patient's medical history and physical examination to check for contraindications such as cerebrovascular disease, recent MI, or carotid bruits. Maneuvers should always be performed with the patient in the supine position, and steady pressure should be applied unilaterally for 5 seconds. Bilateral carotid massage should never be performed. It is worthwhile to note that vagal maneuvers are not usually effective in terminating the tachycardia unless the AV node is part of a reentrant circuit (eg, AVNRT, AVRT).

If vagal maneuvers are ineffective, adenosine can be given as a rapid intravenous (IV) bolus followed by saline flush. Patients should be on continuous ECG monitoring during administration

of adenosine to aid in diagnosis and to differentiate between treatment failure and termination with rapid reinitiation of SVT. The initial dose of adenosine is 6 mg, which can be followed by 12 mg if no response is seen. Patients should be forewarned that they are likely to experience side effects such as flushing, chest tightness, and shortness of breath, but these are very short-lasting. Although adenosine has a high tendency to terminate AVNRT and AVRT (AV node is part of the circuit), it is very unlikely to terminate AT or AFL. Nonetheless, it may unmask the underlying arrhythmia for more definitive diagnosis. Of note, adenosine can precipitate transient AF in up to 12% of patients, which poses a potential risk to patients with known Wolff–Parkinson–White (WPW) syndrome.[10] However, ventricular fibrillation (VF) and transient asystole in response to adenosine administration are rare.

Other agents such as IV β-blockers (eg, metoprolol) and CCBs (eg, diltiazem) may be effective in slowing AV conduction for diagnostic purposes, and may even terminate the SVT.[11] **Table 22.1** provides a listing of maneuvers and medications that are utilized diagnostically to transiently slow AV conduction, as well as the respective responsiveness of common SVT subtypes to these therapies.

OVERVIEW AND SAMPLES OF INDIVIDUAL SUPRAVENTRICULAR TACHYCARDIAS

ATRIOVENTRICULAR NODAL REENTRANT TACHYCARDIA

AVNRT is the most frequently encountered of the regular narrow QRS complex tachycardias. The development of AVNRT and inherent behavior of the circuit is dependent on the presence of a particular electrophysiologic (EP) property of the AV node, termed dual-AV node physiology.[12] It is explained by the presence of two pathways with different conduction properties and refractoriness: the *fast pathway*, which conducts more rapidly

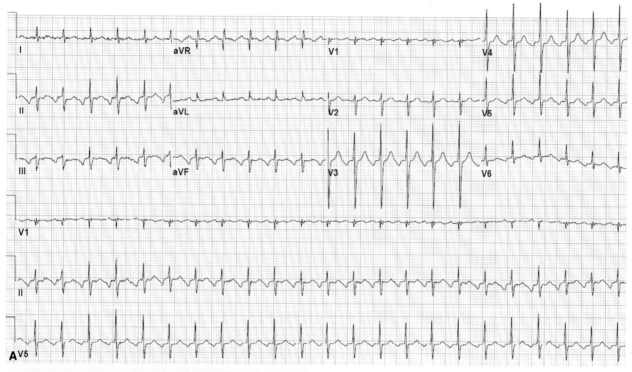

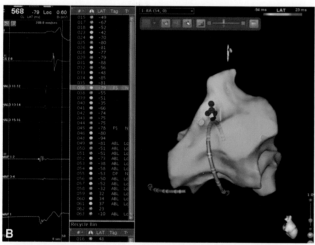

FIGURE 22.6 A, 12-Lead ECG showing narrow QRS complex, *long-RP* tachycardia at a cycle length of 420 ms. Take note of the negative P waves preceding each QRS complex in the inferior leads (II, III, aVF; arrows). This patient subsequently underwent a successful radiofrequency catheter ablation for focal AT. B, CARTO-3 3D electroanatomic map for focal atrial tachycardia originating from the high crista terminalis.

with a longer refractory period, and the *slow pathway*, which conducts more slowly with a somewhat shorter refractory period **(Figure 22.7)**. Normal (anterograde) AV conduction takes place in a forward direction down the *fast pathway*; however, if the *fast pathway* is refractory from a premature atrial complex (PAC), the sinus impulse may conduct over the *slow pathway*. If enough time passes for the *fast pathway* to recover, the impulse can conduct (retrograde) backward up the *fast pathway* and initiate a reentrant circuit that manifests on ECG as a regular tachyarrhythmia at 130 to 250 bpm **(Figure 22.8)**.

P waves are unidentifiable or can be seen just beyond the QRS complex because of the nearly simultaneous activation of the atria and ventricles. The P wave would look like a pseudo-S wave in leads II, III, aVF, and like an r' wave in lead V1, which is the *sine qua non* in the diagnosis.

The rhythm is termed *typical* AVNRT (most common, 90%) if it follows the aforementioned EP properties, whereas in the *atypical* form of AVNRT the impulse travels down the *fast pathway* and up the *slow pathway* (uncommon, 10%) which manifests as a similar ECG finding except that P waves would be further away from the QRS.

As with any SVT, acute treatment of AVNRT should begin with assessment of hemodynamic stability, and patients who are hypotensive should be electrically cardioverted immediately. It is uncommon for AVNRT to cause major hemodynamic instability, and thus vagal maneuvers should be attempted to prolong the refractoriness of AV nodal conduction with a resultant transient anterograde block and termination of the tachycardia. If vagal maneuvers are ineffective, administration of adenosine has been shown to terminate more than 95% of AVNRTs.[13,14] Additional AV nodal agents such as IV (or PO) nondihydropyridine CCBs (ie, diltiazem) or β-blockers are second-line options.

Despite their effectiveness in terminating AVNRT, it is important to keep in mind that the ability of CCBs to slow AV

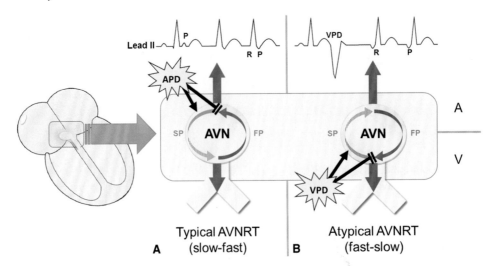

FIGURE 22.7 Mechanisms of atrioventricular nodal reentrant tachycardia (AVNRT), showing each atrioventricular node (bottom) and surface ECG lead (top). Solid arrows indicate conduction over the fast pathway (FP), and striped arrows represent conduction over the slow pathway (SP). A, Typical AVNRT: an APD blocks in the FP and conducts down the SP, followed by retrograde conduction up the FP. Note the nearly simultaneous timing of P waves and QRS complexes during typical AVNRT (RP < PR). Pseudo-S waves at the end of QRS complexes (inferior ECG leads) are a result of the retrograde P′ waves. B, With atypical AVNRT, a VPD blocks at the FP and travels retrograde up the slow pathway, followed by antegrade conduction down the FP. Inverted P′ waves are visible before the onset of the QRS complex in atypical AVNRT (RP > PR). A, atrial; APD, atrial premature depolarization (PAC); AVN, atrioventricular node; AVNRT, atrioventricular nodal reentrant tachycardia; P, P wave; R, R wave; V, ventricular; VPD, ventricular premature depolarization (PVC).

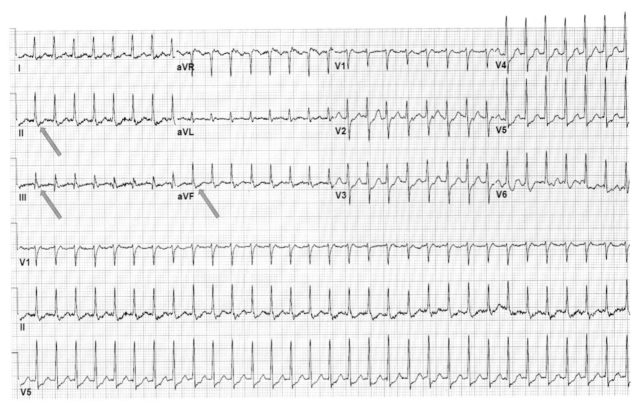

FIGURE 22.8 Typical (slow-fast) atrioventricular nodal reentrant tachycardia on 12-lead ECG. P waves are often not visible because they are buried in the QRS complexes owing to simultaneous activation of the atria and ventricles. In this example, take note of the pseudo S′ waves, which appear at the inferior leads (II, III, aVF) at the end of the QRS complex (*arrows*).

nodal conduction may result in more rapid conduction down an AP in the presence of preexcited AF, leading to VF and sudden cardiac death (SCD). They can also be dangerous for patients with significant systolic heart failure because of their negative inotropic and vasodilatory properties. β-Blockers (ie, metoprolol) are a safer choice in that setting, and amiodarone might be a reasonable third-line option, although robust data on its efficacy is lacking.

ATRIOVENTRICULAR REENTRANT TACHYCARDIA

AVRT is a form of short-RP tachycardia that develops in patients with an AP, a cluster of extranodal tissue that provides an alternative atrio-ventricular electrical connection, which bypasses the AV node and His-Purkinje system. APs can conduct in antegrade, in retrograde, or in both directions. They are described as *manifest* if they conduct antegrade more rapidly than the AV node, demonstrating a characteristic *preexcitation* pattern on resting ECG with slurring of the QRS upstrokes known as *delta* waves, resulting in a broader QRS (>110 ms) and shortened PR interval (less than < 120 ms); *concealed* if they conduct exclusively retrograde; or *latent* if they have the capability to conduct antegrade under certain conditions. When associated with paroxysms of SVT, this pattern is known as WPW syndrome, and the preexcitation pattern on ECG during sinus rhythm signifies early ventricular activation due to rapid anterograde conduction down the *manifest* AP (**Figure 22.9**).

The most common form, *orthodromic* AVRT (95%), results from an impulse (eg, PAC) that blocks at the AP (during refractory period), travels down the AV-node His-Purkinje system to the ventricle, then travels retrograde to the atrium via the AP, and reenters the AV node, continuing the tachycardia (**Figure 22.10**). The RP interval is slightly longer in *orthodromic* AVRT (P wave on top of ST segment) compared with AVNRT (P wave at end of QRS complex), but the difference may be subtle on ECG. *Antidromic* AVRT is a much less common form of AVRT (5%) in which an impulse blocks at the AV node, travels down the AP, and returns retrograde to the atrium via the AV node. This results in a distinctive *wide QRS complex* tachycardia on ECG. It is important to remember that preexcited *antidromic* AVRTs with a *manifest* AP that conducts rapidly from the atrium to the ventricle carry a low (< 1%) but tangible risk of SCD, particularly in the setting of AF, AFL, and AT. This is due to rapidly conducted atrial impulses via the AP to the ventricle, which can cause VF. The risk is most pronounced in the first two decades of life, but can be heightened in patients in the CCU receiving AV nodal blocking agents for rate control (ie, β-blockers, CCBs), which could promote anterograde conduction down the AP.

Acute treatment of AVRT may focus on either the AV node or on the AP. In *orthodromic* or *antidromic* AVRT, the AV nodal conduction is a viable target for maneuvers and medications that delay or block anterograde or retrograde impulses, respectively. As with AVNRT, vagal maneuvers may slow conduction at the AV node and lead to block and termination of the tachycardia. If unsuccessful, antiarrhythmic medications such as IV procainamide, oral flecainide, or propafenone can prolong extranodal tissue refractoriness and block AP conduction. However, these should not be used in patients with structural or ischemic heart disease.[15] Amiodarone is less efficacious than procainamide and may be considered as a last-line option for elderly patients or those refractory to other medications. Owing to its efficacy in delaying extranodal and blocking AP conduction, IV procainamide is considered first line for acute management of *antidromic* AVRT. Predictors of high-risk patients with WPW for SCD are younger males <40 years of age, manifest preexcitation on ECG at all times, multiple APs, and short antegrade effective refractory period of the AP (<240 msec).

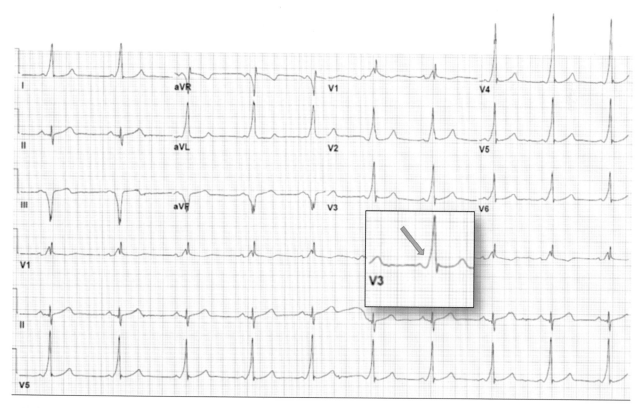

FIGURE 22.9 A 12-lead ECG in sinus rhythm with preexcitation (delta wave). Delta waves on resting ECG are a result of ventricular preexcitation due to concomitant rapid anterograde conducting accessory pathway. Note the characteristic shortened PR interval and broad QRS with slurring of the initial upstroke (*arrow*).

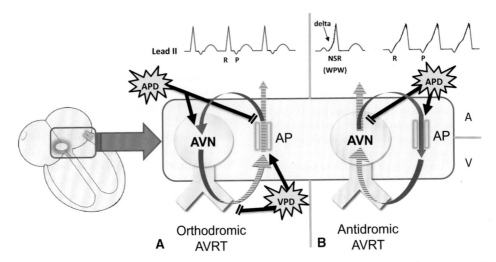

FIGURE 22.10 Mechanisms of atrioventricular nodal reentrant tachycardia (AVRT). A, During orthodromic AVRT, no delta wave is seen because all anterograde conduction is over the AV node (AVN) and His–Purkinje system. Retrograde P waves are seen after each QRS. B, Mechanism of AVRT in patients with the Wolff–Parkinson–White (WPW) syndrome. In sinus rhythm, the slurred QRS upstroke (delta wave) is due to rapid anterograde conduction over the accessory pathway (AP) and early activation of the ventricle (V). During antidromic AVRT, maximal preexcitation results in wide distorted QRS complexes due to V activation exclusively from anterograde conduction over the AP. A, atrium; APD, atrial premature depolarization; AVN, atrioventricular node; NSR, normal sinus rhythm; VPD, ventricular premature depolarization.

ATRIAL TACHYCARDIA

AT is a less common form of SVT that initiates from the atria and (unlike AVNRT or AVRT) does not require that the AV node participates in sustaining the arrhythmia. In other words, the atrial origin *drives* the arrhythmia with an atrial rate that can range from 100 to 250 bpm (**Figure 22.11**). The course of AT is typically benign; however, sicker patients in the CCU may exhibit more incessant forms and be at higher risk for developing tachycardia-induced cardiomyopathy or decompensated heart failure.

ATs can generally be divided into three types (**Figure 22.12**): (1) focal, (2) multifocal, and (3) macro-reentrant. Focal ATs are characterized by centrifugal spread of atrial activation from a small defined area, and are further described in terms of their EP mechanisms including abnormal automaticity, triggered activity, and microreentry.[16,17] MAT is a less understood but not an uncommonly encountered AT in the CCU setting. It is typically seen as secondary to a number of underlying cardiopulmonary conditions, particularly respiratory failure due to chronic obstructive

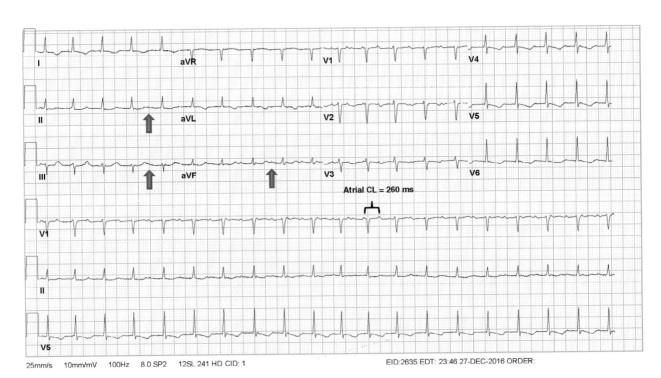

FIGURE 22.11 Atrial tachycardia on 12-lead ECG. Note the upright P waves in the inferior leads (II, III, AVF; arrows) with an atrial cycle length (CL) of 260 ms. ECG, electrocardiogram.

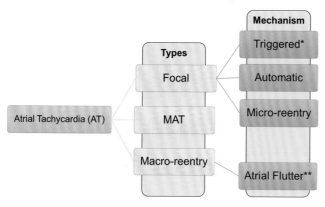

FIGURE 22.12 Classification of AT by type and mechanism. Focal atrial tachycardias (ATs) can commonly occur as a result of early or late afterdepolarizations (triggered activity) or cells with enhanced firing rates compared with normal pacemaker cells (automaticity), or as a result of a small reentrant loop (micro-reentry), which is frequently difficult to locate despite advanced EP mapping software in the lab. Multifocal atrial tachycardia (MAT) is a poorly understood, irregular form of AT characterized by at least 3 different P-wave morphologies. It is often seen as a feature of acute cardiopulmonary illness, especially respiratory failure due to COPD. *Likely etiologic mechanism of a majority of focal ATs. **Atrial flutter discussed in another chapter.

pulmonary disease (COPD). ECG findings should include an irregular tachycardia (ventricular rate ≥100 bpm) with at least three distinct P-wave morphologies and an isoelectric baseline between P waves (**Figure 22.13**). Unfortunately, in the presence of rapid AV nodal conduction, ECG analysis is insensitive for differentiating between ATs.

Thus, to make a definitive diagnosis, it is especially useful to employ vagal maneuvers or adenosine when encountering an AT. Vagal maneuvers usually do not terminate focal ATs, but can result in a transient AV nodal block that allows for clearer delineation of P waves. Similarly, the antiadrenergic and AV nodal blocking properties of adenosine are very effective in differentiating focal from macroreentrant (ie, AFL) ATs, and can provide additional mechanistic information based on resultant termination (eg, triggered AT) or suppression (eg, automatic AT) of the arrhythmia. The importance of a high-quality ECG rhythm strip during adenosine administration cannot be overstated in this scenario. Additional options for acute management of ATs include AV nodal blocking agents for ventricular rate control (ie, IV verapamil or β-blockers), as well as class IC drugs (flecainide, propafenone) with variable

efficacy. In contrast to focal ATs, hospitalized patients with MAT may portend higher morbidity and mortality, and rate- or rhythm-controlling strategies that are typically employed tend to be ineffective. As a mainstay, their predisposing condition should be managed aggressively to offer the best outcomes. Electrical cardioversion is of variable utility depending on the mechanism of AT, and patients with sustained ATs or continued symptoms often benefit (at lower risk) from radiofrequency (RF) catheter ablation as first-line treatment.

INAPPROPRIATE SINUS TACHYCARDIA

In contrast to sinus tachycardia, which is always a normal secondary physiologic response, inappropriate sinus tachycardia (IST) is defined as a sinus tachycardia that cannot be explained by normal physiologic stressors. It is further described by associated symptoms such as weakness, dizziness, and palpitations, which are also not attributable to secondary causes such as thyroid disease, anemia, or drugs. Resting heart rates in patients with IST are typically >100 bpm, with a mean 24-hour heart rate >90 bpm.[18] Etiologies such as neurohormonal dysregulation, sinus node hyperactivity, and dysautonomia have been suggested, but the precise cause is uncertain. There has been some association seen with anxiety disorders, and anxiety can be a trigger. Overall, IST carries a benign prognosis, and no specific recommendations for acute management have been published. For ongoing management, ivabradine was found to reduce the inherent pacemaker activity of the sinus node and has recently been approved by the U.S. Food and Drug Administration for use in patients with concomitant systolic heart failure.[19,20]

JUNCTIONAL TACHYCARDIA

Junctional tachycardia (JT) is seen infrequently in adults, but may be encountered in patients in the CCU following cardiac surgery. The underlying mechanism is abnormal automaticity from a focus at the AV junction.[21] On ECG, JT manifests as a rapid, regular (occasionally irregular), narrow QRS complex tachycardia with ventricular rates ranging from 100 to 220 bpm, and retrograde (in or after the QRS) P waves (**Figure 22.14**). It is not uncommon to misdiagnose other SVTs (ie, AVNRT, AVRT, MAT) because of the often absent P waves and sometimes irregular appearance on ECG. The course of adult patients with JT is essentially benign, and given the low incidence of JT in this population, there is little data regarding diagnosis and management. Nonetheless, IV β-blockers, verapamil, diltiazem, and procainamide may be

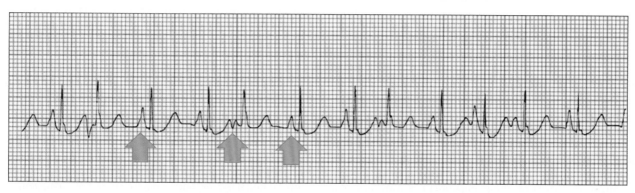

FIGURE 22.13 Multifocal atrial tachycardia (MAT) on a telemetry strip. It is characterized by three distinct P-wave morphologies, with irregular P-to-P intervals, and ventricular rate >100 bpm. MAT is frequently seen during bouts of acute illness, especially respiratory failure due to decompensated COPD.

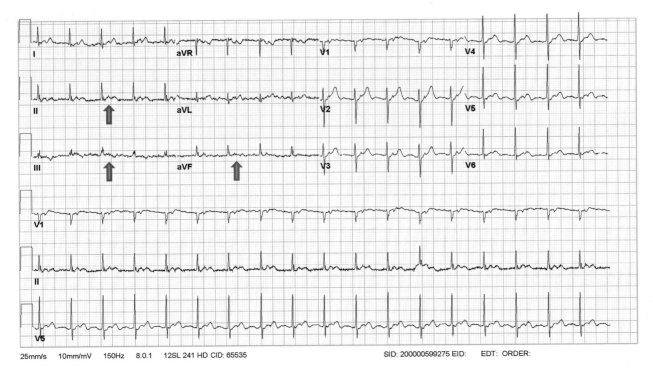

25mm/s   10mm/mV   150Hz   8.0.1   12SL 241 HD CID: 65535   SID: 200000599275 EID: EDT: ORDER:

FIGURE 22.14 Junctional tachycardia (JT) or accelerated junctional rhythm. Note the absence of P waves preceding each QRS complex which appear to be buried in the proceeding T waves (*arrows*).

reasonable in the acute setting. A far more commonly encountered paroxysmal JT in adults is accelerated junctional rhythm. It exhibits a slower ventricular rate (60-100 bpm) than does JT and is frequently seen in the setting of acute MI or digoxin toxicity. Acute management primarily focuses on treating the underlying condition, but there are some data to suggest that β-blockers, verapamil, or adenosine may terminate the arrhythmia.

LONG-TERM MANAGEMENT OF PAROXYSMAL SUPRAVENTRICULAR TACHYCARDIAS

Patients with infrequent episodes of AVNRT that are well tolerated can be managed long term with prophylactic AV nodal blocking medications (eg, PO β-blockers, verapamil, diltiazem). Although antiarrhythmic medications such as flecainide and propafenone are reasonable secondary options in patients without structural or ischemic heart disease, their use in a younger patient is not preferred. Patients with frequent symptomatic episodes, intolerance to medication, or preference of not using long-term medications can undergo curative RF catheter ablation via *slow pathway modification* (**Figure 22.15**) as first-line therapy.[22,23] Technological advances have greatly increased the safety, efficacy, and cost-effectiveness[24] of this approach with success rates of 95% to 99% and less than 1% risk of any complications.

With similarly high success rates, catheter ablation should be strongly considered for long-term management of symptomatic patients with AVRT and WPW syndrome with high-risk features for SCD. Patients who are not inclined to undergo ablation can be given PO class IC (flecainide, propafenone) or class III (amiodarone) agents in the setting of *antidromic* AVRT.

Controversies exist on the management of asymptomatic patients with WPW; this is due to the complexity of the nature

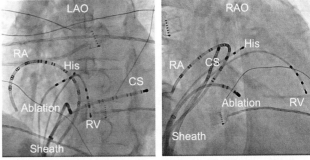

Catheter Positions During Slow-Pathway Modification Ablation

FIGURE 22.15 Catheter positions during slow-pathway modification via radiofrequency ablation for AVNRT. CS, coronary sinus; LAO, left anterior oblique; RA, right atrium; RAO, right anterior oblique; RV, right ventricle ; AVNRT, AV nodal reentrant tachycardia.

of history of asymptomatic WPW. Certainly, the asymptomatic pediatric population is at higher risk of SCD than is the adult asymptomatic population. Intrinsic EP properties of APs, rather than symptoms can quantify this risk and further delineation with an EP study should be encouraged.

Focal ATs can be managed with a rate-control strategy utilizing AV nodal blocking medications such as PO verapamil, diltiazem, or β-blockers. Catheter ablation is a safe and viable option for symptomatic patients or those with incessant ATs, with variable success rates ranging from 70% to 100%.

MAT is most typically seen in patients with advanced lung disease, but can be additionally correlated to structural heart disease and congestive heart failure. Treatment entails a rate-control strategy with AV nodal agents, but remains centered on management of the underlying condition.

SUMMARY

SVTs are commonly encountered in the CCU. Aside from AF, the SVTs most typically seen (in order of frequency) are AVNRT, AVRT, and AT. Narrow QRS complex tachycardias require a systematic approach to differential diagnosis and treatment. Sinus tachycardia is virtually always a compensatory response that requires identification and treatment of the underlying cause. Early identification of patients with hemodynamic compromise due to SVTs with prompt electrical cardioversion is essential. The initial approach to hemodynamically stable patients with SVT should include vagal maneuvers, followed by medications that transiently slow AV conduction and may potentiate termination of the arrhythmia. Long-term management must be individualized and may include PO AV nodal agents and RF catheter ablation.

REFERENCES

1. Orejarena LA, Vidaillet H Jr, DeStefano F, et al. Paroxysmal supraventricular tachycardia in the general population. *J Am Coll Cardiol.* 1998;31(1):150-157.

2. Ganz LI, Friedman PL. Supraventricular tachycardia. *N Engl J Med.* 1995;332:162-173.

3. Neumar RW, Otto CW, Link MS, et al. Part 8: Adult advanced cardiovascular life support: 2010 American Heart Association guidelines for cardiopulmonary resuscitation and emergency cardiovascular care. *Circulation.* 2010;122:S729-S767.

4. Lee KW, Badhwar N, Scheinman MM. Supraventricular tachycardia-I. *Curr Probl Cardiol.* 2008;33(9):467-546.

5. Lee KW, Badhwar N, Scheinman MM. Supraventricular tachycardia-II. *Curr Probl Cardiol.* 2008;33(10):557-622.

6. Blömstrom-Lundqvist C, Scheinman MM, Aliot EM, et al. ACC/AHA/ESC guidelines for the management of patients with supraventricular arrhythmias—executive summary: a report of the American College of Cardiology/American Heart Association Task Force on Practice Guidelines and the European Society of Cardiology Committee for Practice Guidelines (Writing Committee to Develop Guidelines for the Management of Patients With Supraventricular Arrhythmias). Developed in collaboration with NASPE-Heart Rhythm Society. *J Am Coll Cardiol.* 2003;42:1493-1531.

7. Kalbfleisch SJ, el-Atassi R, Calkins H, et al. Differentiation of paroxysmal narrow QRS complex tachycardias using the 12-lead electrocardiogram. *J Am Coll Cardiol.* 1993;21:85-89.

8. Rankin AC, Oldroyd KG, Chong E, et al. Value and limitations of adenosine in the diagnosis and treatment of narrow and broad complex tachycardias. *Br Heart J.* 1989;62:195–203.

9. Ferguson JD, DiMarco JP. Contemporary management of paroxysmal supraventricular tachycardia. *Circulation.* 2003;107: 1096-1099.

10. Strickberger SA, Man KC, Daoud EG, et al. Adenosine-induced atrial arrhythmias: A prospective analysis. *Ann Intern Med.* 1997;127:417-422.

11. DiMarco JP, Miles W, Akhtar M, et al. Adenosine for paroxysmal supraventricular tachycardia: dose ranging and comparison with verapamil. Assessment in placebo-controlled, multicenter trials. *Ann Intern Med.* 1990;113(2):104-110.

12. Anderson RH, Ho SY. The architecture of the sinus node, the atrioventricular conduction axis, and the intermodal atrial myocardium. *J Cardiovasc Electrophysiol.* 1998;9(11):1233-1248.

13. Glatter KA, Cheng J, Dorostkar P, et al. Electrophysiologic effects of adenosine in patients with supraventricular tachycardia. *Circulation.* 1999;99:1034-1040.

14. Cairns CB, Niemann JT. Intravenous adenosine in the emergency department management of paroxysmal supraventricular tachycardia. *Ann Emerg Med.* 1991;20:717-721.

15. Al-Khatib SM, Page RL. Ongoing management of patients with supraventricular tachycardia. *JAMA Cardiol.* December 28, 2016. doi:10.1001/jamacardio.2016.5085.

16. Roberts KC, Kistler PM, Kalman JM. Focal atrial tachycardia 1. *PACE.* 2006;29:643-652.

17. Roberts KC, Kistler PM, Kalman JM. Focal atrial tachycardia 2. *PACE.* 2006;29:769-778.

18. Olshansky B, Sullivan RM. Inappropriate sinus tachycardia. *J Am Coll Cardiol.* 2013;61:793-801.

19. Fox K, Ford I, Steg PG, et al. Ivabradine for patients with stable coronary artery disease and left-ventricular systolic dysfunction (BEAUTIFUL): a randomised, double-blind, placebo-controlled trial. *Lancet.* 2008;372:807-816.

20. Swedberg K, KomajdaM, Böhm M, et al. Ivabradine and outcomes in chronic heart failure (SHIFT): a randomised placebo-controlled study. *Lancet.* 2010;376:875-885.

21. Ruder A, Davis JC, Eldar M, et al. Clinical and electro physiologic characterization of automatic junctional tachycardia in adults. *Circulation.* 1986;73:930–937.

22. Jackman WM, Beckman KJ, McCleland JH, et al. Treatment of supraventricular tachycardia due to atrioventricular nodal reentry by radiofrequency catheter ablation of slow-pathway. *N Engl J Med.* 1992;327(5):313-318.

23. Page RL, Joglar JA, Caldwell MA, et al. 2015 ACC/AHA/HRS Guideline for the Management of Adult Patients With Supraventricular Tachycardia: a report of the American College of Cardiology/American Heart Association Task Force on Clinical Practice Guidelines and the Heart Rhythm Society, *J Am CollCardiol.* 2016;67(13):e27-e115.

24. Cheng CH, Sanders GD, Hlatky MA, et al. Cost-effectiveness of radiofrequency ablation for supraventricular tachycardia. *Ann Intern Med.* 2000;133:864-876.

Patient and Family Information for:
SUPRAVENTRICULAR ARRHYTHMIAS

WHAT IS SUPRAVENTRICULAR TACHYCARDIA?

Supraventricular tachycardia (SVT) is a general term used to classify abnormally fast heartbeats (tachycardias) known as arrhythmias, which originate above (supra-) the ventricles (lower chambers) in the atria (upper chambers) of the heart. The term *paroxysmal* is sometimes used to describe SVTs that start and stop suddenly or intermittently, without warning. Although normal heart rates range from 60 to 100 beats per minute (bpm), heart rates during SVT are usually greater than 130 bpm and may climb above 200 bpm in some instances. The fast heartbeat can last minutes or even hours, and it can happen during rest or with exercise. In a hospital setting, additional stress from the patient's illness(es) may provide a trigger for SVT to occur more frequently. SVT is not a single disease; rather, it encompasses a number of arrhythmias that have different causes and may each require unique treatment strategies. The three most common types of SVT are called atrioventricular nodal reentrant tachycardia (AVNRT), atrioventricular reentrant tachycardia (AVRT), and atrial tachycardia (AT). Atrial fibrillation and atrial flutter with rapid heart rates are also types of SVT and are discussed in detail in a separate chapter.

HOW IS SUPRAVENTRICULAR TACHYCARDIA RECOGNIZED?

Some patients may not experience symptoms during episodes of SVT. If symptoms are present, the patient may have a sensation that his or her heart is beating very rapidly, forcefully, and/or irregularly (also known as palpitations). In addition, the patient may feel tired, dizzy, faint, and, in some instances, pass out because of lack of adequate blood flow to the brain when the heart is beating very rapidly. Patients who also have coronary artery disease or congestive heart failure may also experience symptoms such as difficulty breathing and tightness or pain in the chest. Although symptoms are useful in recognizing arrhythmias, determining specific types of SVT requires careful examination of the 12-lead electrocardiogram (ECG). Because of the intermittent nature of most SVTs, longer-term monitoring is sometimes required. In the hospital or cardiac care unit (CCU) setting, this can be done readily using standard continuous telemonitoring devices worn by many or all patients. A cardiologist may ask the outpatient to wear an external monitoring device for up to one month or may refer him or her to a cardiac electrophysiologist (electrical specialist of the heart), who can implant a longer-lasting device under the skin to provide monitoring for two years or more. On some occasions, a more invasive study called an electrophysiology (EP) study is performed to better pinpoint the exact type of SVT. The procedure is done in a closely monitored laboratory setting using multiple catheters that are introduced into the heart from veins in the legs. Using this minimally invasive technique, abnormal electrical circuits in the heart can be accurately located and mapped.

SINUS TACHYCARDIA VERSUS SUPRAVENTRICULAR TACHYCARDIA

Not to be confused with SVT, sinus tachycardia refers to a fast heart rate, typically 100 to 130 bpm, which originates from and travels through the normal electrical circuits in the heart. It is a normal reaction of the heart to exertion, exercise, and stressors such as anxiety, fever, and pain. It is also commonly associated with various illnesses that directly or indirectly affect the heart such as heart failure, heart attack, infections (e.g., pneumonia), and blood clots in the lungs (pulmonary embolism). Thus, sinus tachycardia is almost always a means by which the body compensates during illness or stress, and it does not require specific treatments aside from managing the underlying stressor. In contrast, SVT is always abnormal (pathologic) and requires treatment.

HOW IS SUPRAVENTRICULAR TACHYCARDIA TREATED?

Paroxysmal SVT most often starts and stops abruptly, but when it occurs, it can result in a spectrum of clinical findings from uncomfortable palpitations to life-threatening hemodynamic instability (low blood pressure) or organ ischemia (low blood flow), requiring urgent intervention. If the patient is unstable, conversion (cardioversion) to normal sinus rhythm can be immediately attempted by applying an electric current (shock) over the chest to the heart. Electrical cardioversion is a generally safe and effective (over 90%) way to quickly restore a normal heart rhythm, and patients are given sedatives and pain medication prior to delivery of the shock if possible. In situations where blood pressure is stable and the patient has a good pulse, doctors may try vagal maneuvers to slow the heart rate and terminate the arrhythmia without medications. Vagal maneuvers affect the nervous system, which then signals the heart to respond by reducing the heart rate. One of these techniques used by doctors is called carotid sinus massage, and is performed by briefly pressing (for 5 to 10 seconds) on a specific area of the neck overlying the carotid arteries that carry blood to the brain. This is done while closely monitoring the patient's ECG and vital signs, as it can cause slowing of the heart rate and may lower the blood pressure. Carotid massage should not be performed by the patient or on patients who have blockages in their carotid arteries. Alternatively, doctors may instruct the patient to try Valsalva maneuvers such as holding a deep breath and straining (as during a bowel movement). Both carotid massage and Valsalva maneuvers can slow the heart rate to better identify the type of SVT or may terminate it completely.

If vagal maneuvers do not work, certain medications can be given orally or intravenously (IV) to try and terminate the SVT. The most commonly used medication is IV adenosine. This medication works by slowing the heart rate and temporarily blocking impulses traveling from the upper to the lower chambers of the heart, which can break the abnormal electrical circuit in the heart and terminate the arrhythmia. After injection, patients often feel brief uncomfortable symptoms such as skin flushing, chest tightness, and shortness of breath, which quickly subside because of adenosine's short duration of action. Other medications that may be used to slow the heart rate or terminate SVT include beta-blockers (e.g., metoprolol), specific calcium channel blockers (e.g., diltiazem, verapamil), and specialized antiarrhythmic medications. If the episodes of SVT are infrequent and patients are not highly symptomatic, daily oral medications to control heart rates during episodes or prevent attacks may be sufficient. In patients with severe symptoms and frequent episodes, an EP study followed by an ablation procedure can be performed to cure the arrhythmia. Like EP studies, ablations are procedures that are done in the EP laboratory and use catheters that are guided into the heart. Catheters are then directed to the specific spots in the heart, from where the SVT is thought to originate, and then tiny controlled burns (called radiofrequency ablation) or extreme cold (cryoablation) is applied to destroy the abnormal electrical circuits that are causing the arrhythmia. In most patients with SVT, the arrhythmia is permanently cured after the ablation procedure.

SUMMARY

Supraventricular arrhythmias are commonly seen in the CCU. Sinus tachycardia should be differentiated from SVT in that it is almost always a normal means by which the body compensates for a stressor such as exercise, fever, or illness. As such, it does not require specific management other than identification and treatment of its underlying cause. In contrast, SVT is always abnormal and can result in a wide range of clinical findings from benign uncomfortable symptoms to ischemia or life-threatening hemodynamic instability. Careful examination of ECG findings can help narrow down specific types of SVT, but pinpointing specific types often requires long-term monitoring because of the intermittent nature of the arrhythmia. Patients who are hemodynamically unstable may require urgent electrical cardioversion to restore normal heart rhythm. After identifying SVT in a stable patient, doctors may attempt vagal maneuvers, followed by IV adenosine in an attempt to slow the heart rate and terminate the arrhythmia. Patients who have severe symptoms or frequent episodes of SVT can have an EP study followed by catheter ablation (radiofrequency or cryoablation) with a high likelihood of permanently curing the arrhythmia. A good basic understanding of the causes and issues related to SVT and its management is important for patients and their families.

Olga Reynbakh
Joshua Aziz
Eyal Herzog
Emad F. Aziz

23

Fundamentals of Atrial Fibrillation and Atrial Flutter

ATRIAL FIBRILLATION

Atrial fibrillation (AF) is the most common arrhythmia in the adult population, with continuously increasing prevalence as the population ages; currently, 6 million adults in the United States are diagnosed with AF. It represents a significant influence on morbidity and mortality rates as well as a large economic and public health burden.[1] AF predisposes to a greater risk of stroke and mortality while impairing quality of life.[2] The estimated cost of treating US citizens with AF is $26 billion a year. It is estimated that by year 2050 the prevalence of AF will be close to 12 million. This assumption is based on increasing mean age of population, obesity epidemic, as well as achievements in treatment of cardiovascular diseases.[3]

Men have a 1.5-fold higher risk for developing AF than women, derived from data adjusted for age and predisposing conditions.[4] Although it seems to be less common in African Americans, lifetime risk of developing AF is higher in men of European descent compared with women of European descent (26% vs 23%). AF is strongly age associated, most commonly presenting at age 80 or above (about 1 in 10) and only 1% of patients with AF are less than the age of 60. Aging of the population is the main underlying factor for rapidly increasing prevalence of AF.[5,6]

ETIOLOGY

Patients with underlying cardiovascular disease often have abnormal atrial size and function. Enlargement of the atrial chamber, fibrosis, fatty or amyloid tissue deposition, and inflammation can contribute to abnormal functionality and electrical remodeling of the atrium leading to pathologic evolution of AF. Some patients have AF occurring under the influence of autonomic nervous system: vagal form (after meals, during sleep) or adrenergic form (exercise induced).

RISK FACTORS

1. Increasing age: especially >80 year old, one in 10 patients above age 80 will develop AF. This represents >1/3 of patients with AF.[7]
2. Male sex: a 1.5-fold higher risk than in females.[8]
3. Tall stature and obesity: these are independently associated with increased incidence of AF.[9] In the Framingham Heart Study, every unit increase in body mass index (BMI) was associated with an approximate 5% increase in risk.
4. Metabolic syndrome[10]: with its components, hypertension (HTN),[8] obesity,[9] diabetes mellitus, hyperlipidemia, are all associated with higher risk of AF.[11] BMI, waist circumference, and sagittal abdominal diameter could similarly predict AF.[12]
5. Valvular heart disease: the most potent association is with mitral stenosis.
6. Myocardial infarction (MI): AF in the setting of acute MI independently predicts stroke and 30-day mortality[13]; can be seen in up to 10% of patients in the early period after acute MI.[8,14]
7. Postsurgical AF: there are heterogeneous patterns of AF after cardiac surgery. The incidence is 20% to 25% in patients undergoing coronary artery bypass grafting and up to 40% after valvular surgery. A substantial minority of AF is short-lived and isolated, with no impact on length of stay; however, recurrent or prolonged AF significantly affects outcomes.[15]
8. Heart failure (HF): there is individual variation of cause–consequence relationship.[16]
9. Obstructive sleep apnea (OSA): predisposes by metabolic and autonomic abnormalities, as well as structural cardiovascular changes.[17] Untreated OSA is associated with much higher risk of development of AF as well as recurrence after AF ablation.[18]
10. Chronic kidney disease.
11. Hyperthyroidism: clinically overt and subclinical, it is associated with higher risk of developing AF.
12. Excessive alcohol consumption, caffeine, cigarette smoking.
13. Excessive physical exertion: athletic lifestyle, especially the one involving endurance activities predisposes to higher risk especially in young patients (due to high vagal tone).
14. Genetic predisposition: parental AF predisposes the offspring by two to three times than in the general population.

PATHOPHYSIOLOGY

The pathophysiology of AF is multifactorial and complex, including genetic and neural system mechanisms. Haissaguerre et al were the first to evaluate and discover pulmonary veins (PVs) as the dominant triggers in the initiation of AF.[19] Focal triggers can lead to reentry in high-frequency rotors, and electrical activation from these rotors may fragment giving fibrillatory conduction.

If this process continues for long periods, there is subsequent atrial remodeling at the cellular level (ion channels) and other triggers raise further perpetuating AF, in particular small and large reentrant wavelets. AF induction may occur in the presence of fibrotic and poorly conducting atria (eg, due to hemodynamic overload, as in HTN or HF); genetic disorders affecting refractory period and/or conduction velocity heterogeneously[20]; or AF itself. By shortening the atrial refractory period, reducing conduction velocity, and provoking contractile and structural remodeling, AF may set the stage for self-perpetuation (ie, "AF begets AF").[21] Structural remodeling of both atria typically happens under the influence of previously mentioned risk factors. This remodeling is mediated by activations of fibroblasts, fibrosis, fatty infiltration, connective tissue deposition, myocyte hypertrophy, necrosis, and inflammatory infiltration. All these processes result in local conduction disturbances and electrical dissociation that leads to micro-reentrant circuits' formation. Genetic mechanisms associated with AF development include abnormalities in potassium or sodium channels, connexin expression or function, and microRNAs[22] (**Figure 23.1**).

CLASSIFICATION

Detecting asymptomatic or minimally symptomatic AF improved with implantable loop recorders (ILRs), pacemakers, and defibrillators.

1. **Lone AF or idiopathic AF:** It used to be defined as patients who have no precipitating cause or associated CV disease. However, the percentage of AF that is considered lone AF decreased from 30% in 1954 to 3% in 2014 based on studies that showed larger proportion of etiologic factors of AF. The term lone AF is generally avoided because it is not fully clear to what extent the workup should be done to consider AF

to be idiopathic and also the term is not useful in making treatment decisions.[23]

2. **Asymptomatic AF** (subclinical): Early recognition of AF at times is difficult owing to its often "silent" nature. For one-third of patients with AF, they are not aware that they are in AF. Recent studies using different monitoring tools, ranging from transtelephonic monitoring to pacemakers, have indicated that the correlation between AF episodes and patient symptoms is very poor: many AF episodes are asymptomatic, whereas many AF-like symptoms are not related to AF episodes.[24] Early detection of the arrhythmia might allow timely introduction of therapies to protect patients from AF complications as well as the possibility of interrupting the progression of AF from a potentially treatable condition to a refractory one. The Asymptomatic Atrial Fibrillation and Stroke Evaluation in Pacemaker Patients and the Atrial Fibrillation Reduction Atrial Pacing Trial (**ASSERT**) monitored patients 65 years or older who had HTN and no prior history of AF and a newly implanted pacemaker or cardioverter defibrillator for development of subclinical atrial tachyarrhythmias (defined as episodes of atrial rate >190 beats per minute [bpm] for more than 6 minutes). At 3 months, 10.1% of the enrolled patients had developed such episodes. Subclinical AF was indeed associated with both an increased risk of clinical AF and ischemic stroke and systemic embolization.[25] More intense and prolonged monitoring is justified in highly symptomatic patients, patients with recurrent syncope, and patients with a potential indication for anticoagulation (especially after cryptogenic stroke).[26]

3. **Paroxysmal AF:** Self-terminating (within 48 hours to 7 days).
4. **Persistent AF:** Continuously present for more than 7 days and up to 1 year.
5. **Long-standing AF:** Continuous AF lasting for ≥1 year.
6. **Permanent AF:** Duration longer than 1 year with failed attempts to restore and maintain sinus rhythm (SR).

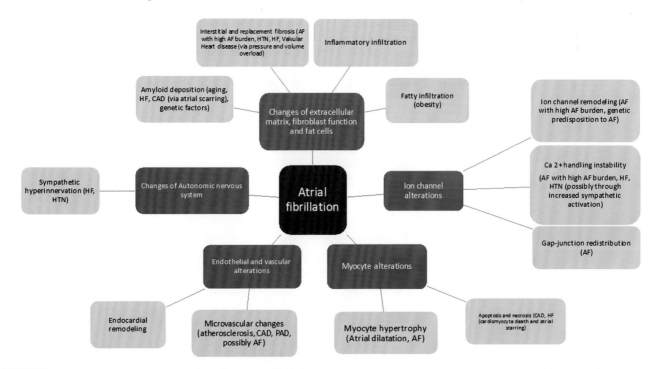

FIGURE 23.1 Key factors in the pathophysiology of atrial fibrillation (AF). CAD, coronary artery disease; HF, heart failure; HTN, hypertension; PAD, peripheral artery disease. Modified from ESC guidelines 2016: management of atrial fibrillation.[22]

ATRIAL FIBRILLATION, A PROGRESSIVE DISEASE

AF is a progressive disease that becomes more difficult to treat with increasing duration. In patients presenting with paroxysmal AF—progression to persistent AF is 10% in 1 year, 25% to 30% in 5 years, and more than 50% in 10 years. In patients with persistent AF lasting more than 1 year, only 40% to 60% remain in SR; and in patients with more than 3 years of duration, only 15% are maintained in SR. Clinical progression, supported by electrical contractile and structural atrial remodeling promotes AF stability and persistence.[21] The HATCH scoring system (based on underlying HTN, age >75 years, history of transient ischemic attack (TIA) or stroke, chronic obstructive pulmonary disease, and HF) was proposed to predict this risk of progression in patients receiving pharmacologic therapy.[27] The clinical outcomes of patients who exhibit progression of AF are worse with respect to hospital admissions and major adverse cardiovascular events. In the Euro Heart survey, patients with AF who had progressed to persistent or permanent AF had higher rates of hospital admissions, TIA, stroke, MI, and death.[28]

WORKING UP ATRIAL FIBRILLATION

Diagnosis

On initial evaluation of the patient who presents with AF, it is important to obtain:

- Key history: Questions such as symptoms, frequency, and duration to establish the AF pattern, initial onset, history of cardiovascular conditions and noncardiovascular conditions that are associated with AF, and assess the risk of complications such as thromboembolism and left ventricular (LV) dysfunction.
- Electrocardiogram (ECG): To establish suspected diagnosis of AF, assess the rate, evaluate for possible conduction abnormalities, ischemic changes, and signs of structural heart disease.
- Echocardiography: To assess ventricular size and function, left atrial (LA) dimensions (left atrium shown to enlarge by about 5 mm in diameter over 1 year in patients with AF, LA enlargement [>55 to 60 mm] associated with failure to maintain SR after successful cardioversion), and to identify any structural disease such as valvular heart disease.

- Transesophageal echocardiography (TEE): To evaluate for presence of thrombus if patient is to undergo cardioversion; although the presence of spontaneous echo contrast (smoke) is not a contraindication for CV, the risk of stroke is increased in the presence of smoke or reduced left atrial appendage (LAA) emptying velocity.[29]
- Blood tests: Thyroid function, kidney function, and electrolytes abnormalities.
- Exercise stress testing or coronary angiogram: In those cases where there is LV dysfunction, ischemic signs are noted or patient has symptoms of ischemia.
- Monitoring: To assess the adequacy of rate control, relate symptoms with AF recurrences, and detect focal induction of bouts of paroxysmal AF. This can be achieved by a Holter monitor, AF auto-trigger monitor, or mobile cardiac outpatient telemetry. They all carry relative diagnosed yield ranging from 5% to 13% in the 24-hour Holter to 45% to 88% in the outpatient telemetry.[30] Previously undiagnosed AF was found in 1.4% of those aged >65 years, suggesting a number needed to screen of 70. These findings encourage the further evaluation of systematic AF screening programs in at-risk populations.[31]
- ILR can be used when the AF burden is relatively small and in asymptomatic patients. They typically have the highest diagnosed yield of more than 80%.[32]

Complications

There are many consequences of AF that lead to disease states. Loss of organized atrial contraction often leads to exercise intolerance and HF.[33] Rapid ventricular rhythm can lead to tachycardia-induced cardiomyopathy and precipitate myocardial ischemia.[4] Certainly, aging and systemic vascular risk factors cause an abnormal atrial tissue substrate, or atrial myopathy, that can result in AF and thromboembolism. AF causes contractile dysfunction and stasis, which further increases the risk of thromboembolism. In addition, over time, the AF causes structural remodeling of the atrium, thereby worsening atrial myopathy and increasing the risk of thromboembolism even further. **Figure 23.2** depicts the recently adapted model of thromboembolic stroke in AF.[34]

AF is associated with increased mortality; 1.5-fold for men and 1.9-fold for women.[35] Other complications are precipitation

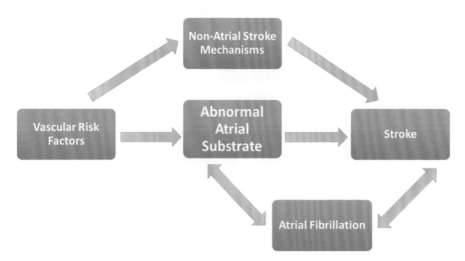

FIGURE 23.2 Recently adapted model of thromboembolic stroke in atrial fibrillation.

of ventricular electrical instability, anti-arrhythmic medication adverse effects, and pro-arrhythmic effects.[36]

ATRIAL FIBRILLATION AND STROKE

One in seven strokes is attributed to AF and it is suspected that subclinical AF is a cause of 1 in 4 ischemic strokes. Risk of death from AF-related stroke is 2-fold higher than that of stroke in patients without AF.[25] Premature atrial contractions,[37] paroxysmal supraventricular tachycardia,[38] ECG-defined LA abnormality,[39] and LA size[40] have been associated with stroke independently of AF. It is widely believed that failure of the fibrillating atrium to contract in patients with AF can lead to atrial stretch and dilatation, in turn promoting stasis and thrombus formation inside the LAA.[41] The LAA arises from the PVs and is an embryologic remnant of the left atrium and consists of a trabeculated 2- to 4-cm–long structure in direct continuity with the left atrium. Thus, its unique shape and anatomy may predispose to in situ thrombus formation.[42]

The individual stroke risk may be estimated using the CHA₂DS₂-VASc (C, congestive HF /LV dysfunction; H, hypertension; A₂, age [≥75 years]; D, diabetes; S₂, stroke/TIA attack; V, vascular disease; A, age 65 to 74 years; and S_c, sex category) classification scheme; classification is based on patient characteristics, with higher scores corresponding to a higher risk for stroke **(Table 23.1).** Thromboprophylaxis is the mainstay of stroke prevention in patients with AF.

ANTICOAGULATION

On the basis of clinical practice guidelines published by the American College of Cardiology, the American Heart Association, the American College of Chest Physicians, and the European Society of Cardiology, patients with AF should generally receive oral anticoagulation (OAC) with vitamin K antagonist (VKA) or novel oral anticoagulants (NOACs) such as apixaban, dabigatran, rivaroxaban, or edoxaban. OAC therapy has shown to prevent the majority of ischemic strokes in patients with AF and can prolong life.[43] VKA is still the only treatment with proven benefit for valvular AF (moderate or severe mitral stenosis or a mechanical valve). For nonvalvular AF, both VKA and NOACs are effective in preventing stroke. There have been multiple recent studies comparing NOACs with warfarin; and large cohort meta-analysis by Ruff et al that included 42,411 patients suggests that NOACS, while offering same level of stroke reduction as warfarin, is associated with greater reduction in mortality, less intracranial bleeding, and more frequent gastrointestinal bleed.[43] According to the 2016 ESC guidelines for the management of AF, NOACs are the preferred anticoagulants (ACs) over VKA for patients with nonvalvular AF.[22]

Antiplatelet therapy is inferior to AC for prevention of stroke and should not be used alone; however, when patients are required to be both on AC and dual oral antiplatelets (DAPTs), the risk of bleeding is increased.

In all patients who require ACs, bleeding risk should be assessed. The most widely used tool is the HAS-BLED score[45] **(Table 23.2).**

The general consensus is that high bleeding score should not avert from using ACs, but the effort should be made to correct identifiable bleeding factors such as (HTN [systolic BP >160], labile international normalized ratio when on VKA, other drugs predisposing to bleeding—DAPTs or NSAIDs, excess alcohol intake [>8 drinks a week]) and potentially modifiable risk factors (anemia, impaired renal function, impaired liver function, and reduced platelet count or function).

Anticoagulation can be risky for some patients and, alternatively, LAA occlusion devices should be considered. Several indications for LAA occlusion may be taken into consideration. Such indications may include stroke reduction: (1) in those with absolute contraindications to OAC, (2) in patients with relative contraindications to OAC, or (3) as an alternative to OAC therapy for those with high fall risk.

Romero et al published data of computed tomography that demonstrated the four most common LAA morphologies: "Cactus"

TABLE 23.1	CHA₂DS₂-VASc Score
RISK FACTOR	**POINTS**
Congestive heart failure (symptoms of HF or evidence of HFrEF)	+1
Hypertension (BP>140/90 or ongoing treatment with anti-HTN drugs)	+1
Age >75	+2
DM (Fasting Glu>125 or HbA1C>6.5 or ongoing treatment)	+1
Previous stroke, TIA, or VTE	+2
Vascular disease (previous MI, PAD, or aortic plaque)	+1
Age 65–74	+1
Female sex	+1

DM, diabetes mellitus; HF, heart failure; HTN, hypertension; MI, myocardial infarction; PAD, peripheral artery disease; TIA, transient ischemic attack; VTE, venous thromboembolism.

TABLE 23.2	HAS-BLED Score
RISK FACTOR	**POINTS**
Hypertension	+1
Abnormal renal function (dialysis, transplant, Cr >2.26 mg/dL or >200 μmol/L)	+1
Abnormal liver function (cirrhosis or bilirubin >2x Normal or AST/ALT/AP >3x Normal)	+1
Stroke history	+1
Prior major bleeding or predisposition to bleeding	+1
Labile INR (unstable/high INRs), time in therapeutic range <60%)	+1
Elderly age >65	+1
Drugs/alcohol use history (≥ 8 drinks/week)	+1

ALT, alanine aminotransferase; AP, alkaline phosphatase; AST, aspartate aminotransferase; INR, international normalized ratio.

has a dominant central lobe with extending secondary lobes. "Windsock" has a dominant lobe larger than the distal portions of the LAA. "Cauliflower" has no dominant lobe, but has more complex characteristics than other morphologies. "Chicken-wing" presents an obvious bend in the proximal or middle part of the dominant lobe, or folding back on itself which can be a secondary lobe or twig[46] (**Figure 23.3**). Three percutaneous devices to facilitate LAA closure have been developed and are in use: Watchman, Amplatzer, and the Lariat suture (**Figure 23.4**). Although the randomized clinical trial PROTECT-AF[47] showed noninferiority of the Watchman device as compared with warfarin therapy for stroke prevention, there are still limited data as to whether the risk of stroke reduction is comparable to OAC and it is therefore recommended to continue OAC for at least 6 weeks after implantation of the Watchman closure device. The Amplatzer plug has been utilized for percutaneous patent foramen ovale closure and has also been adopted as a method for LAA exclusion, although no randomized clinical trial of its use for this indication currently exists. The Lariat device is placed using a combined percutaneous endocardial and epicardial approach, and no OAC therapy is required after Lariat LAA closure.

In case of a TIA, OAC can be resumed 1 day after the event.

In case of a stroke, OAC can be resumed 3 to 12 days after the event, depending on the severity of the stroke.

A controversial question arises when a patient needs OAC and antiplatelet therapy. Two randomized clinical trials are currently testing different antithrombotic combinations for patients on OAC who require stent implantation. The Triple Therapy in Patients on Oral Anticoagulation After Drug Eluting Stent Implantation

(*ISAR-TRIPLE*, clinicaltrials.gov id NCT00776633) trial will address the hypothesis that reducing the length of clopidogrel therapy from 6 months to 6 weeks after implantation of a drug-eluting stent is associated with a reduced net composite of death, MI, definite stent thrombosis, stroke, or major bleeding at 9 months on top of treatment with aspirin and an oral anticoagulant. The Anticoagulation in Stent Intervention (*MUSICA-2*, clinical trials.gov id NCT01141153) trial is investigating the safety and efficacy of a triple antithrombotic regimen of acenocoumarol, low-dose (100 mg/d) aspirin, and clopidogrel versus high-dose (300 mg/d) aspirin and clopidogrel in patients with AF and low-to-moderate risk of stroke (CHADS2 ≤2) referred for percutaneous coronary intervention (PCI).

Currently, it is suggested that patients with AF who are at risk of stroke and who require antiplatelet therapy should minimize the time on triple therapy because of significantly increased risk of bleeding.

TREATMENT

The treatment strategies are subclassified to the acute or new onset of AF and treatment of established AF. **Figure 23.5** illustrates a typical diagram for treatment strategies for acute and chronic AF.

Acute- or New-Onset Atrial Fibrillation

Many patients at presentation require heart rate (HR) control after other possible causes of increased HR are excluded such as infection, pulmonary embolism, and endocrine abnormalities. Agents preferred for acute rate control are β-blockers (BBs) and

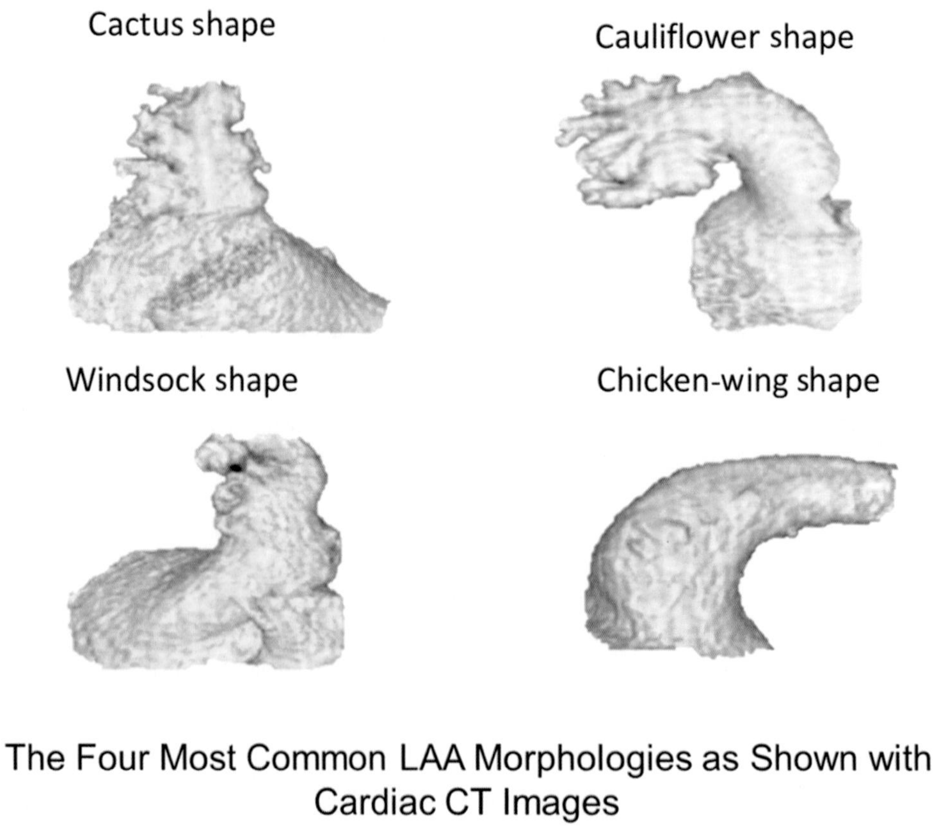

FIGURE 23.3 Left atrial appendage (LAA) morphology as seen by cardiac computed tomography (CT).

The Watchman Closure
(Boston Scientific)

AMPLATZER Amulet Left
Atrial Appendage Occluder
(St. Jude Medical)

The LARIAT Suture
Delivery System
(SentreHeart Inc)

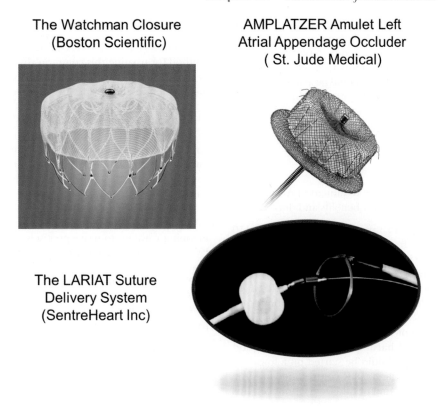

FIGURE 23.4 Available left atrial appendage closure devices.

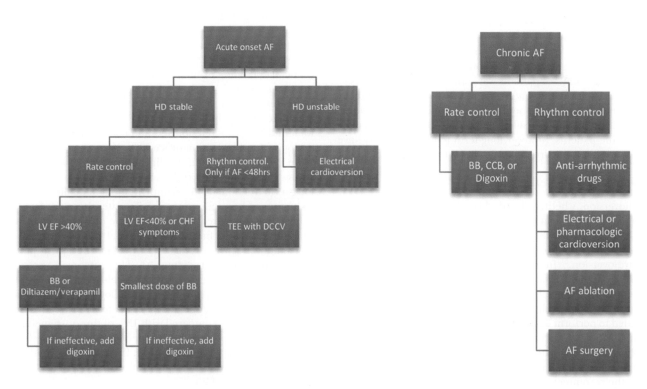

FIGURE 23.5 Treatment strategies for acute and chronic atrial fibrillation (AF). BB, β-blocker; CCB, calcium channel blocker; CHF, congestive heart failure; HD, hemodynamically; LVEF, left ventricular ejection fraction; TEE, transesophageal echocardiography.

non–dihydropyridine calcium channel blockers (ND-CCBs), that is, diltiazem and verapamil given their rapid onset of action. However, the choice of the agent should be based on existing comorbidities. For example, in patients with left ventricular ejection fraction (LVEF) <40%, CCB should be avoided because of its negative inotropic effect and BBs should be used instead. The typical recommended initial controlled HR target should be <110 bpm. Patients who are hemodynamically unstable require immediate direct current cardioversion to restore cardiac output.

Established Atrial Fibrillation Diagnosis

There are two basic strategies for the treatment of AF, rate and rhythm control, and each has its own benefits and drawbacks.

- **Rate control:** Target HR for rate control strategy is <110 bpm at rest. Early data from the RACE and the AFFIRM trials showed that there is no difference in CV events, NYHA class, or hospitalizations[48] between groups of patients with lenient or strict heart rate goals. However, the HR target should still be individually set given that some patients are symptomatic at the HR of 110 bpm. First-line rate control agents are BBs because of their potential beneficial effect on symptoms and lack of harm as well as having a good tolerance profile. Patients should be started on a low dose and uptitrated to achieve target HR control. Second-line agents are ND-CCBs (verapamil or diltiazem); however, this class should be avoided in patients with LVEF <40%. Also, avoid concomitant use with BBs. Digoxin can also be used in combination with BBs or CCBs to achieve better HR control (*ESC 2016 class IB recommendations for AF and class IB for AF with HFrEF*).[49] Amiodarone can be used when combination therapy fails to control HR. The last resort for rate control is the ablate and pace technique, in which AV junctional ablation is performed and a dual chamber of BiV pacemaker is implanted. A study by Queiroga et al showed that ablate and pace is associated with a low overall mortality and, interestingly, 48% of patients were still in SR at 72 months.[50]
- **Rhythm control:** Current 2014 AHA/ACC/HRS guideline for the management of patients with AF consider antiarrhythmic medications as the first-line, long-term treatment for symptomatic patients, however long-term follow-up studies have shown that these drugs can also have pro-arrhythmic effects.

Cardioversion to Normal Rhythm

Cardioversion, whether electrical or pharmacologic, is recommended for symptomatic patients with persistent or long-standing AF. Pretreatment with anti-arrhythmic drugs (AADs), usually class IC or III, is recommended to increase the effectiveness of cardioversion.[51] In a study by Cotiga et al, dofetilide had an unusually high pharmacologic conversion rate, demonstrated an incremental dose response, and was well tolerated and safe in a relatively healthy adult cohort with persistent AF.[52] It is recommended to perform TEE for patients who have had AF for more than 48 hours to exclude LAA thrombi before direct current cardioversion. For patients who were in AF for longer than 48 hours or for an unknown duration and who cannot undergo TEE, the recommendation is to initiate AC for at least 3 weeks before cardioversion and to continue for 4 weeks after CV, unless longer AC is needed because of high stroke risk.

Catheter Ablation for Atrial Fibrillation

Catheter ablation (CA) to cure AF has now evolved as an established method for treating this common rhythm disorder. CA of AF is performed on a daily basis in electrophysiology laboratories in most regions of the world. Cure of AF has had a dramatic impact on quality of life, morbidity, and mortality. The first decade of AF ablation was characterized by new observations and concepts as well as improvement in technology. Most current treatment approaches for AF aim at ablation around the PVs with or without additional ablation lesion lines, a procedure that yields low complication rates and high success rates in both paroxysmal and chronic AF.[53]

Typical pulmonary vein antral isolation (PVAI) of PVs is performed guided by intracardiac echocardiography and a circular mapping catheter to more precisely identify the border of the PV antrum and reduce risk of PV stenosis. PVAI is performed by encircling all PVs based on anatomy, and demonstration of loss of PV potentials and, if possible, inability of signals to go from PV to atrium in the absence of PV potentials.

Figure 23.6A shows intracardiac electrograms (EGMs) from a patient in AF during a PVAI procedure. Note the unorganized atrial activities in the atrium seen on the coronary sinus (CS) catheter, and more organized EGMs seen within the PV circular mapping catheter after isolation of the veins and spontaneous termination of AF to SR. **Figure 23.6B** displays surface ECG in normal rhythm, organized sinus activity seen in the CS catheter, and completely silent (isolated) PV with no activities. In **Figure 23.6C** SR is seen on surface ECG and in the CS, whereas fibrillatory EGMs are seen confined to the PV, confirming complete isolation of the vein with exit block (no external connection to the atrium).

Electroanatomic mapping is typically used during CA to guide in delineating the LA anatomy as well as the anatomy of PVs, and guide the electrophysiologist during the ablation procedure by placing automatic marks at the site of radiofrequency (RF) lesion applications. **Figure 23.6D** represents a CARTO-3 electroanatomic 3D mapping of the left atrium after complete PVAI, the red dots seen mark VisiTags indicating complete circumferential lesion sets around the antra of all PVs. LA voltage map shows complete silence (red color) in the PVs and in the LA posterior wall, indicating good lesion sets and confirming isolation as an endpoint for the ablation procedure.

In recent years, multiple clinical trials have clearly demonstrated the superiority of CA over AAD therapy in terms of long-term freedom from AF, improvement in quality of life, and reduction of hospitalizations.[54,55] To date, there are few small studies that compared CA as a first line of treatment of AAD. The **RAAFT** was the first randomized trial to show the feasibility, safety, and effectiveness of CA as first-line therapy in patients with symptomatic paroxysmal AF. The outcomes assessed in this trial were recurrence of AF, hospitalization, and quality of life at 1-year follow-up. At the end of follow-up, 63% of patients assigned to AAD therapy experienced at least one recurrence of symptomatic AF, as compared with 13% of those assigned to the PVAI treatment arm, accounting for 80% relative risk reduction with CA (P < 0.001). Furthermore, PVAI was associated with a significantly lower rate of hospitalization (9% vs 54%, P < 0.001), and better quality of life.[56]

Presented data from the Medical Antiarrhythmic Treatment or Radiofrequency Ablation in Paroxysmal Atrial Fibrillation

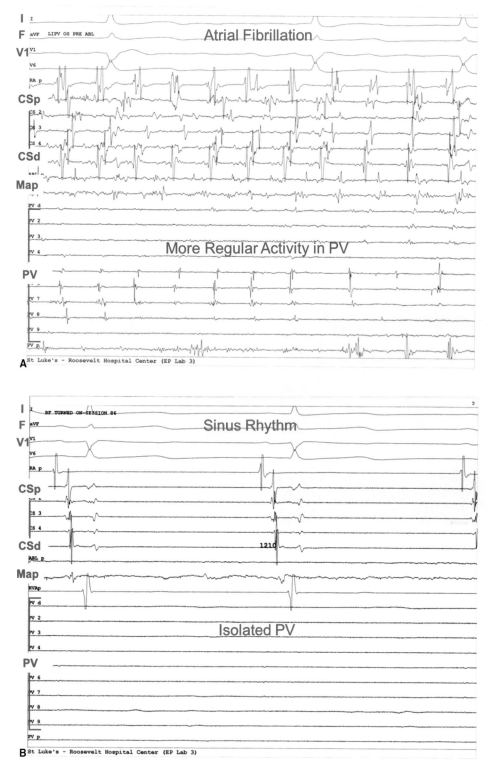

FIGURE 23.6 A, Intracardiac electrograms for a patient in atrial fibrillation. (*Note:* Atrial fibrillation seen in the coronary sinus and more organized activities seen in the pulmonary vein in a patient with atrial fibrillation during electrophysiology study.) B, Same patient after pulmonary vein (PV) antral isolation and conversion to sinus rhythm. (*Note:* Surface ECG shows normal rhythm, organized sinus activity in the coronary sinus, and completely silent [isolated] pulmonary vein with no activities.) CSd, distal coronary sinus catheter; CSp, proximal coronary sinus catheter; LLPV, left lower pulmonary vein; LUPV, left upper pulmonary vein; Map, mapping/ablation catheter; RLPV, right lower pulmonary vein; RUPV, right upper pulmonary vein.

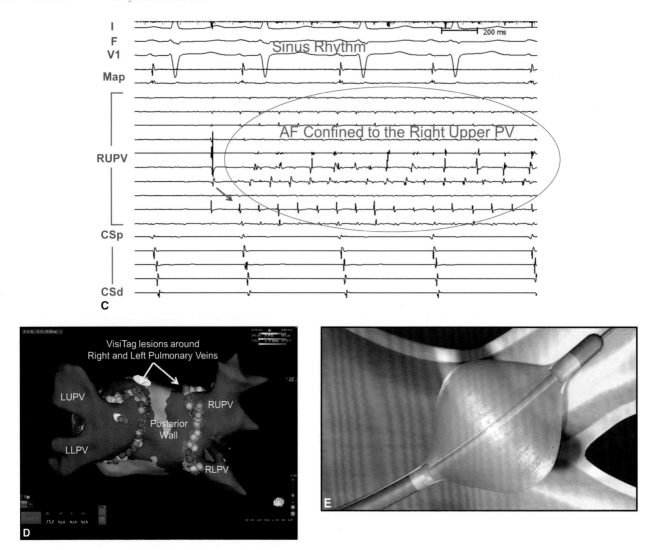

FIGURE 23.6 C, Atrial fibrillation, confined to a PV, while the rest of the heart is in normal sinus rhythm. *Note:* Sinus rhythm is seen on surface ECG and in the coronary sinus, while fibrillatory electrograms are seen confined in the pulmonary vein confirming complete isolation of the vein with exit block (no external connection to the atrium). CSd, distal coronary sinus catheter; CSp, proximal coronary sinus catheter; Map, mapping/ablation catheter; RUPV, right upper pulmonary vein. D, CARTO-3 electroanatomic 3D mapping of the left atrium after PV antral isolation. E, Arctic front balloon catheter for cryoballoon ablation *Note:* Red dots mark VisiTags indicating complete circumferential lesion sets around the antra of all pulmonary veins; also notice left atrial voltage map showing complete silence (red color) in the pulmonary veins and in the left atrial posterior wall. LLPV, left lower pulmonary vein; LUPV, left upper pulmonary vein; RLPV, right lower pulmonary vein; RUPV, right upper pulmonary vein. E, Arctic front balloon catheter for cryoballoon ablation

(**MANTRA-PAF**) trial[57] compared CA with AAD therapy as first-line therapy for symptomatic paroxysmal AF and showed that at 24 months, AF recurred in 15% of patients allocated to CA and in 29% of those receiving AAD, accounting for 48% relative risk reduction (P = 0.004). The corresponding number needed to treat with CA to prevent one episode of recurrent AF was 7. Patients assigned to CA also experienced significantly lower AF burden (P = 0.007) and improved quality of life.

More recently, the RF ablation versus antiarrhythmic drugs as first-line treatment of paroxysmal AF (**RAAFT-2**) trial showed that among patients with paroxysmal AF without previous antiarrhythmic drug treatment, RF ablation compared with antiarrhythmic drugs resulted in a lower rate of recurrent atrial tachyarrhythmias at 24 months.[58]

Finally, data from the CA versus antiarrhythmic drug treatment of persistent AF: a multicenter, randomized, controlled trial (**SARA study**) showed that CA was superior to medical therapy for the maintenance of SR in patients with persistent AF at 12-month follow-up.[59]

In recent years, cryoballoon ablation (**Figure 23.6E**), has gained some favor as an alternative approach to RF ablation for the treatment of symptomatic drug-refractory AF with comparable immediate success and complications.[60] The most recent **FIRE AND ICE** trial showed that while patients treated with cryoballoon as opposed to RF ablation had significantly fewer repeat ablations, direct current cardioversions, all-cause rehospitalizations, and cardiovascular rehospitalizations during the follow-up period, both patient groups had improvement in quality-of-life scores after ablation.[61] The result of this study further establishes the call for ablation as the first-line therapy in younger patients with AF.

AC should be started and continue uninterrupted before the ablation with NOAC or VKA and continued for at least 6 months.[62] Generally it is recommended to continue AAD therapy for 12 weeks after ablation, as there is significant evidence showing prevention of early AF recurrences after ablation when AADs are continued for a few weeks.[63]

CA performed the first time has an efficacy of 60% to 80%, and only a few patients require a second procedure to achieve higher rates of effectiveness. If CA fails to restore rhythm, the patient and the cardiologist can decide between further available options: repeat ablation or hybrid therapy (AAD + ablation).

Outpatient Follow-Up of Patients with AF

Follow-up visits should be focused on assessment of patients' symptoms after initiation of the therapy, possibility of changing the strategy, or stepping to the next available treatment option if the patient is still symptomatic. Assessment of the presence of side effects should take place if the patient is on AAD. Special attention should be devoted to the treatment of comorbidities that could decrease the rate of AF recurrences (such as HF, OSA) as well as monitoring of anticoagulation and assessment for further need of it.

Prognosis

AF associated with increased risk of death independent of embolic stroke, partially because of its comorbidities (HF, coronary artery disease, HTN), but independently AF also increases risk of sudden cardiac death from ventricular arrhythmias.

ATRIAL FLUTTER

Atrial flutter (AFL) is a regular atrial arrhythmia with rates up to 300 bpm, and is typically caused by a macroreentrant (MR) circular activation (reentrant) that revolves around a "large" obstacle, arbitrarily defined as being several centimeters in diameter. Typical AFL,[64] facilitated by the anatomic structure of the right atrium (RA), is the most frequent atrial MR tachycardia; however, owing to the increased incidence of heart surgery with atriotomy and to LA ablation for the treatment of AF, further MR tachycardia can be also seen.

The relationships between AFL and AF are complex. Both arrhythmias frequently occur at various times in the same patient and epidemiologic studies have demonstrated a tendency for patients who initially only present with flutter to develop fibrillation after several years. It is imperative to realize that AFL and AF are expressions of a single arrhythmogenic substrate. The background and diseases associated with AFL are similar to those of AF, including HTN, coronary disease, valvulopathy, chronic obstructive pulmonary disease, myocardiopathy, and 15% to 20% of apparently healthy hearts. In some cases, flutter initiates fibrillation and flutter ablation reduces the incidence of fibrillation.

Typical AFL is an MR arrhythmia due to rotational activation around the RA. The circuit is bounded in front by the tricuspid ring and behind by a mixed anatomic and functional obstacle, formed by the vena cava and crista terminalis.[65] The activation wave goes down via the anterolateral RA and goes up via the septal RA (counterclockwise rotation in left anterior oblique view), necessarily passing between the inferior vena cava (IVC) and the lower tricuspid ring, an area known as the cavotricuspid isthmus (CTI). Cycle length (CL) is typically 200 to 240 ms, with great stability (variations of <20 ms), but under pharmacologic treatment or if there is delayed atrial conduction, the CL can reach 300 ms.

The combination of large valvular and venous orifices together with the functional obstacle in the crista terminalis makes the RA an ideal place for reentry, and this is probably the means by which typical AFL has such a characteristic electrocardiographic and functional image (**Figure 23.7A**). Counterclockwise activation (going down via the anterolateral RA) occurs in 90% of typical flutter, but in 10% there is a reverse or clockwise rotation (going up the anterolateral RA and going down the septal RA).

Typical AFL has a characteristic pattern in leads II, III, and aVF known as "sawtooth pattern." The wave is complex, with a slowly falling segment followed by a negative deflection that changes rapidly to a positive and links with the following cycle (**Figure 23.7B**). The pattern can be difficult to recognize if AV conduction is 2:1, but can be revealed by increasing the degree of block through massaging the carotid sinus or with intravenous adenosine. Clockwise typical AFL produces positive waves in the inferior leads, frequently with a sawtooth pattern, but what is most typical is a negative sawtooth wave, in lead V1.

AV conduction is frequently 2:1 during flutter, even while resting and under conduction-slowing agents; if the flutter rate is slower, conduction can be up to 1:1. However, ventricular rate can also be irregular because of complex block patterns in the AV node.

Indications for treatment are marked by poor tolerance, the poor or adverse response to antiarrhythmic agents, and the possibility of eliminating the circuit via CA. The ablation target is the CTI, being the narrowest part of the circuit, well delimited anatomically, easily accessible, and distant from the AV node.

RF ablation to produce a complete, bidirectional, and persistent CTI block normally requires several RF applications, between the tricuspid edge of the isthmus and the IVC. The use of irrigated-tip ablation catheter that produces deep lesions at lower energies, results in flutter termination (**Figure 23.7C**) and demonstrating bidirectional block across the CTI in 85% to 90% of cases with a complication risk of <1%.[66]

In general, the same guidelines have been adopted regarding anticoagulation therapy as in patients with AF; however, in cases with a high risk of hemorrhage, these standards could be made more flexible. TEE is typically performed before ablation to rule out a thrombus in the left atrium or the LAA and anticoagulation therapy is maintained for 4 weeks after ablation procedure. Once CTI block is obtained, flutter recurs in 5% to 10% of cases, usually within 3 months, and reablation is, in general, technically easier.

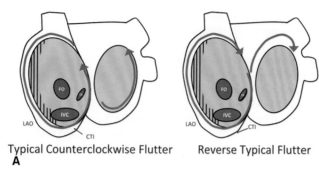

Typical Counterclockwise Flutter   Reverse Typical Flutter
A

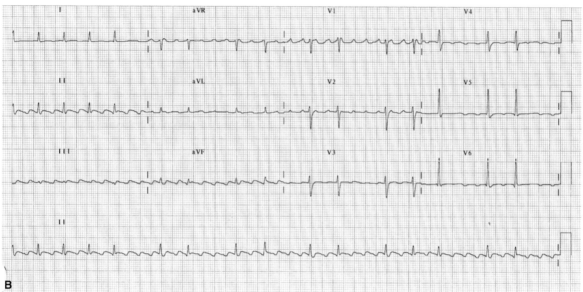

B

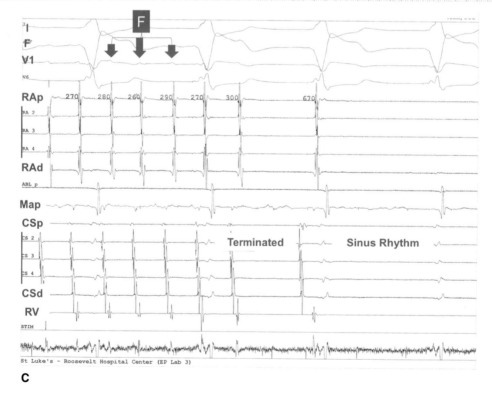

C

FIGURE 23.7 A, Mechanism of typical AFL and reverse typical AFL. B, Typical counterclockwise AFL. (Note the characteristic pattern in leads II, III, and aVF known as "sawtooth pattern." The wave is complex, with a slowly falling segment followed by a negative deflection that changes rapidly to positive to link with the following cycle.) C, Termination counterclockwise AFL during cavotricuspid isthmus (CTI) ablation. Note the beginning of the tracing [F] flutter waves that terminate during the CTI ablation to sinus rhythm. CS, coronary sinus; CSd, distal coronary sinus catheter; CSp, proximal coronary sinus catheter; FO, fossa ovalis; IVC, inferior vena cava; LAO, left anterior oblique; Map, mapping/ablation catheter; Rad, distal right atrium; Rap, proximal right atrium.

REFERENCES

1. Patel NJ, Deshmukh A, Pant S, et al. Contemporary trends of hospitalization for atrial fibrillation in the United States, 2000 through 2010: implications for healthcare planning. *Circulation.* 2014;129(23):2371-2379.

2. Kochhauser S, Joza J, Essebag V, et al. The impact of duration of atrial fibrillation recurrences on measures of health-related quality of life and symptoms. *Pacing Clin Electrophysiol.* 2016;39(2):166-172.

3. Kakkar AK, Joza J, Essebag V, et al. International longitudinal registry of patients with atrial fibrillation at risk of stroke: Global Anticoagulant Registry in the FIELD (GARFIELD). *Am Heart J.* 2012;163(1):13-19 e1.

4. Lloyd-Jones DM, Wang TJ, Leip EP, et al. Lifetime risk for development of atrial fibrillation: the Framingham Heart Study. *Circulation.* 2004;110(9):1042-1046.

5. Wolf PA, Benjamin EJ, Belanger AJ, et al. Secular trends in the prevalence of atrial fibrillation: the Framingham Study. *Am Heart J.* 1996;131(4):790-795.

6. Guo Y, Tian Y, Wang H, et al. Prevalence, incidence, and lifetime risk of atrial fibrillation in China: new insights into the global burden of atrial fibrillation. *Chest.* 2015;147(1):109-119.

7. Haegeli LM, Duru F, Management of patients with atrial fibrillation: specific considerations for the old age. *Cardiol Res Pract,* 2011; 2011:854205.

8. Krahn AD, Manfreda J, Tate RB, et al. The natural history of atrial fibrillation: incidence, risk factors, and prognosis in the Manitoba Follow-Up Study. *Am J Med.* 1995;98(5):476-484.

9. Mahajan R, Lau DH, Brooks AG, et al. Electrophysiological, electro-anatomical, and structural remodeling of the atria as consequences of sustained obesity. *J Am Coll Cardiol.* 2015;66(1):1-11.

10. Nalliah CJ, Sanders P, Kottkamp H, et al. The role of obesity in atrial fibrillation. *Eur Heart J.* 2016;37(20):1565-1572.

11. Nystrom PK, Carlsson AC, Leander K, et al. Obesity, metabolic syndrome and risk of atrial fibrillation: a Swedish, prospective cohort study. *PLoS One.* 2015;10(5):e0127111.

12. Goudis CA, Korantzopoulos P, Ntalas IV, et al. Obesity and atrial fibrillation: a comprehensive review of the pathophysiological mechanisms and links. *J Cardiol.* 2015;66(5):361-369.

13. Wong CK, White HD, Wilcox RG, et al. New atrial fibrillation after acute myocardial infarction independently predicts death: the GUSTO-III experience. *Am Heart J.* 2000;140(6):878-885.

14. Crenshaw BS, Ward SR, Granger CB, et al. Atrial fibrillation in the setting of acute myocardial infarction: the GUSTO-I experience. Global Utilization of Streptokinase and TPA for Occluded Coronary Arteries. *J Am Coll Cardiol.* 1997;30(2):406-413.

15. Tamis-Holland JE, Kowalski M, Rill V, et al. Patterns of atrial fibrillation after coronary artery bypass surgery. *Ann Noninvasive Electrocardiol.* 2006;11(2):139-144.

16. Santhanakrishnan R, Wang N, Larson MG, et al. Atrial fibrillation begets heart failure and vice versa: temporal associations and differences in preserved versus reduced ejection fraction. *Circulation.* 2016;133(5):484-492.

17. Tung P, Anter E, Atrial fibrillation and sleep apnea: considerations for a dual epidemic. *J Atr Fibrillation.* 2016;8(6):1283.

18. Ang R, Earley MJ, The role of catheter ablation in the management of atrial fibrillation. *Clin Med (Lond).* 2016;16(3):267-271.

19. Haissaguerre M, Jaïs P, Shah DC, et al. Catheter ablation of chronic atrial fibrillation targeting the reinitiating triggers. *J Cardiovasc Electrophysiol.* 2000;11(1):2-10.

20. Yang Y, Xia M, Jin Q, et al. Identification of a KCNE2 gain-of-function mutation in patients with familial atrial fibrillation. *Am J Hum Genet.* 2004;75(5):899-905.

21. Wijffels MC, Kirchhof CJ, Dorland R, et al. Atrial fibrillation begets atrial fibrillation: a study in awake chronically instrumented goats. *Circulation.* 1995;92(7):1954-1968.

22. Kirchhof P, Benussi S, Kotecha D, et al. 2016 ESC Guidelines for the management of atrial fibrillation developed in collaboration with EACTS. *Eur J Cardiothorac Surg.* 2016;50(5):e1-e88.

23. Wyse DG, Van Gelder IC, Ellinor PT, et al. Lone atrial fibrillation: does it exist? *J Am Coll Cardiol.* 2014;63(17):1715-1723.

24. Orlov MV, Ghali JK, Araghi-Niknam M, et al. Asymptomatic atrial fibrillation in pacemaker recipients: incidence, progression, and determinants based on the atrial high rate trial. *Pacing Clin Electrophysiol.* 2007;30(3):404-411.

25. Healey JS, Connolly SJ, Gold MR, et al. Subclinical atrial fibrillation and the risk of stroke. *N Engl J Med.* 2012;366(2):120-129.

26. Lewalter T, Boriani G, Relevance of monitoring atrial fibrillation in clinical practice. *Arrhythm Electrophysiol Rev.* 2012;1(1):54-58.

27. Jongnarangsin K, Suwanagool A, Chugh A, et al. Effect of catheter ablation on progression of paroxysmal atrial fibrillation. *J Cardiovasc Electrophysiol.* 2012;23(1):9-14.

28. de Vos CB, Pisters R, Nieuwlaat R, et al. Progression from paroxysmal to persistent atrial fibrillation clinical correlates and prognosis. *J Am Coll Cardiol.* 2010;55(8):725-731.

29. Black IW, Spontaneous echo contrast: where there's smoke there's fire. *Echocardiography.* 2000;17(4):373-382.

30. Rothman SA, Laughlin JC, Seltzer J, et al. The diagnosis of cardiac arrhythmias: a prospective multi-center randomized study comparing mobile cardiac outpatient telemetry versus standard loop event monitoring. *J Cardiovasc Electrophysiol.* 2007;18(3):241-247.

31. Quinn FR, Gladstone D, Screening for undiagnosed atrial fibrillation in the community. *Curr Opin Cardiol.* 2014;29(1):28-35.

32. De Angelis G, Cimon K, Cipriano L, et al. in *Monitoring for atrial fibrillation in discharged stroke and transient ischemic attack patients: a clinical and cost-effectiveness analysis and review of patient preferences 2016*: Ottawa, Ontario, Canada.

33. Steinberg BA, Kim S, Fonarow GC, et al. Drivers of hospitalization for patients with atrial fibrillation: results from the Outcomes Registry for Better Informed Treatment of Atrial Fibrillation (ORBIT-AF). *Am Heart J.* 2014;167(5):735-742 e2.

34. Kamel H, Okin PM, Elkind MS, et al. Atrial fibrillation and mechanisms of stroke: time for a new model. *Stroke.* 2016;47(3):895-900.

35. Benjamin EJ, Wolf PA, D'Agostino RB, et al. Impact of atrial fibrillation on the risk of death: the Framingham Heart Study. *Circulation.* 1998;98(10):946-952.

36. Chen LY, Sotoodehnia N, Bůžková P, et al. Atrial fibrillation and the risk of sudden cardiac death: the atherosclerosis risk in communities study and cardiovascular health study. *JAMA Intern Med.* 2013;173(1):29-35.

37. Larsen BS, Kumarathurai P, Falkenberg J, et al. Excessive atrial ectopy and short atrial runs increase the risk of stroke beyond incident atrial fibrillation. *J Am Coll Cardiol.* 2015;66(3):232-241.

38. Kamel H, Elkind MSV, Bhave PD, et al. Paroxysmal supraventricular tachycardia and the risk of ischemic stroke. *Stroke.* 2013;44(6):1550-1554.

39. Kamel H, Hunter M, Moon YP, et al. Electrocardiographic left atrial abnormality and risk of stroke: Northern Manhattan Study. *Stroke.* 2015;46(11):3208-3212.

40. Benjamin EJ, D'Agostino RB, Belanger AJ, et al. Left atrial size and the risk of stroke and death: the Framingham Heart Study. *Circulation.* 1995;92(4):835-841.

41. Blackshear JL, Odell JA. Appendage obliteration to reduce stroke in cardiac surgical patients with atrial fibrillation. *Ann Thorac Surg.* 1996;61(2):755-759.

42. Cruz-Gonzalez I, Yan BP, Lam YY. Left atrial appendage exclusion: state-of-the-art. *Catheter Cardiovasc Interv.* 2010;75(5):806-813.

43. Ruff CT, Giugliano RP, Hoffman EB, et al. Comparison of the efficacy and safety of new oral anticoagulants with warfarin in patients with atrial fibrillation: a meta-analysis of randomised trials. *Lancet.* 2014;383(9921):955-962.

44. Paciaroni M, Agnelli G, Micheli S, et al. Efficacy and safety of anticoagulant treatment in acute cardioembolic stroke: a meta-analysis of randomized controlled trials. *Stroke.* 2007;38(2):423-430.

45. Pisters R, Lane DA, Nieuwlaat R, et al. A novel user-friendly score (HAS-BLED) to assess 1-year risk of major bleeding in patients with atrial fibrillation: the Euro Heart Survey. *Chest.* 2010;138(5):1093-1100.

46. Romero J, Natale A, Luigi DIB. Left atrial appendage morphology and physiology: "The Missing Piece in the Puzzle". J Cardiovasc Electrophysiol. 2015; 26 (9): 928–933.

47. Reddy VY, Holmes D, Doshi SK, et al. Safety of percutaneous left atrial appendage closure: results from the Watchman Left Atrial Appendage System for Embolic Protection in Patients with AF (PROTECT AF) clinical trial and the continued access registry. *Circulation.* 2011;123(4):417-424.

48. Van Gelder IC, Groenveld HF, Crijns HJGM, et al. Lenient versus strict rate control in patients with atrial fibrillation. *N Engl J Med.* 2010;362(15):1363-1373.

49. Ziff OJ, Kotecha D, Digoxin: The good and the bad. *Trends Cardiovasc Med.* 2016;26(7):585-595.

50. Queiroga A, Marshall HJ, Clune M, et al. Ablate and pace revisited: long term survival and predictors of permanent atrial fibrillation. *Heart.* 2003;89(9):1035-1038.

51. Lafuente-Lafuente C, Mouly S, Longás-Tejero MA, et al. Antiarrhythmic drugs for maintaining sinus rhythm after cardioversion of atrial fibrillation: a systematic review of randomized controlled trials. *Arch Intern Med.* 2006;166(7):719-728.

52. Cotiga D, Arshad A, Aziz E, et al. Acute conversion of persistent atrial fibrillation during dofetilide initiation. *Pacing Clin Electrophysiol.* 2007;30(12):1527-1530.

53. Pappone C, Santinelli V. The who, what, why, and how-to guide for circumferential pulmonary vein ablation. *J Cardiovasc Electrophysiol.* 2004;15(10):1226-1230.

54. Wilber DJ, Pappone C, Neuzil P, et al. Comparison of antiarrhythmic drug therapy and radiofrequency catheter ablation in patients with paroxysmal atrial fibrillation: a randomized controlled trial.*JAMA.* 2010;303(4):333-340.

55. Jais P, Cauchemez B, Macle L, et al. Catheter ablation versus antiarrhythmic drugs for atrial fibrillation: the A4 study. *Circulation.* 2008;118(24):2498-2505.

56. Wazni OM, Marrouche NF, Martin DO, et al. Radiofrequency ablation vs antiarrhythmic drugs as first-line treatment of symptomatic atrial fibrillation: a randomized trial. *JAMA.* 2005;293(21):2634-2640.

57. Jons C, Hansen PS, Johannessen A, et al. The medical antiarrhythmic treatment or radiofrequency ablation in paroxysmal atrial fibrillation (MANTRA-PAF) trial: clinical rationale, study design, and implementation. *Europace.* 2009;11(7):917-9123.

58. Morillo CA, Verma A, Connolly SJ, et al. Radiofrequency ablation vs antiarrhythmic drugs as first-line treatment of paroxysmal atrial fibrillation (RAAFT-2): a randomized trial. *JAMA.* 2014;311(7):692-700.

59. Mont L, Bisbal F, Hernández-Madrid A, et al. Catheter ablation vs. antiarrhythmic drug treatment of persistent atrial fibrillation: a multicentre, randomized, controlled trial (SARA study). *Eur Heart J.* 2014;35(8):501-507.

60. Mandell J, Amico F, Parekh S, et al. Early experience with the cryoablation balloon procedure for the treatment of atrial fibrillation by an experienced radiofrequency catheter ablation center. *J Invasive Cardiol.* 2013;25(6):288-292.

61. Kuck KH, Fürnkranz A, Chun KR, et al. Cryoballoon or radiofrequency ablation for symptomatic paroxysmal atrial fibrillation: reintervention, rehospitalization, and quality-of-life outcomes in the FIRE AND ICE trial. *Eur Heart J.* 2016;37(38):2858-2865.

62. Mardigyan V, Verma A, Birnie D, et al. Anticoagulation management pre- and post atrial fibrillation ablation: a survey of canadian centres. *Can J Cardiol.* 2013;29(2):219-223.

63. Darkner S, Chen X, Hansen J, et al. Recurrence of arrhythmia following short-term oral AMIOdarone after CATheter ablation for atrial fibrillation: a double-blind, randomized, placebo-controlled study (AMIO-CAT trial). *Eur Heart J.* 2014;35(47):3356-3364.

64. Saoudi N, Cosío F, Waldo A, et al. A classification of atrial flutter and regular atrial tachycardia according to electrophysiological mechanisms and anatomical bases: a Statement from a Joint Expert Group from The Working Group of Arrhythmias of the European Society of Cardiology and the North American Society of Pacing and Electrophysiology. *Eur Heart J.* 2001;22(14):1162-1182.

65. Olgin JE, Kalman JM, Fitzpatrick AP, et al. Role of right atrial endocardial structures as barriers to conduction during human type I atrial flutter: activation and entrainment mapping guided by intracardiac echocardiography. *Circulation.* 1995;92(7):1839-1848.

66. Schmieder S, Ndrepepa G, Dong J, et al. Acute and long-term results of radiofrequency ablation of common atrial flutter and the influence of the right atrial isthmus ablation on the occurrence of atrial fibrillation. *Eur Heart J.* 2003;24(10):956-962.

Patient and Family Information for: ATRIAL FIBRILLATION AND ATRIAL FLUTTER

Atrial Fibrillation (AF) is the most common irregular heart rhythm abnormality. It is caused by abnormal electrical signals that cause the heart to beat irregularly and usually very fast.

Symptoms of AF are palpitations (racing heart, skipped beats, and irregular heartbeats), chest tightness, difficulty breathing, and dizziness.

This irregular heart rhythm can be constant or it can come and go. Sometimes it can be provoked by modifiable reasons such as alcohol, caffeine, or an overactive thyroid gland.

AF is classified according to how often the episodes occur and how quickly they terminate.

- Paroxysmal (intermittent): Irregular heart rhythm episodes that reoccur two or more times and stop on their own within 7 days. The heartbeat often normalizes as quickly as within a few seconds or after a few hours.
- Persistent: Irregular heart rhythm episodes that last more than 7 days, or last less than 7 days but necessitates medical therapy or a procedure to restore a normal heart rhythm (cardioversion). Cardioversion is most often done by sending electric shocks to the heart through electrodes placed on the chest.
- Longstanding persistent: Irregular heart rhythm episodes that continue for more than a year. The heart is in a constant state of fibrillation and the condition is considered permanent. In most cases, cardioversion is either ineffective or cannot be attempted.

When the HR stays fast and irregular for a prolonged time, it requires treatment to avoid complications such as stroke or developing a weak heart.

The two main problems with AF is the risk of developing a blood clot and the risk of a fast HR that may weaken the heart.

- A blood clot can develop in the upper chambers of the heart because it is beating out of synchronization. The clot can travel outside of the heart along the blood vessels to the brain and cause a stroke. To decrease this risk, patients need to take anti-coagulants (blood thinners).

- Fast HR can be very uncomfortable for some patients, leading to the symptoms of palpitations. The heart is not pumping the blood effectively in this state. If fast HR persists for a long time, it can cause the heart to become weak. To keep the HR in the normal range, patients are prescribed medications to slow it down.

When a decision is made to attempt to restore regular heart rhythm, several options are available. There are medications called antiarrhythmic medications and they are directed to convert the heart rhythm to a normal rhythm. Another treatment option is called cardioversion and involves applying an electrical shock to the heart.

A unique treatment is called ablation. It is a procedural option that is based on the knowledge that areas of the heart are sending excessive signals and causing the upper chambers of the heart to beat irregularly. The procedure involves applying heat or cold (RF or cryoablation) to destroy small areas that are causing the abnormal heartbeat.

Atrial Flutter (AFL) is another common abnormal heart rhythm. In AFL, the upper chambers (atria) of the heart beat very fast. This results in atrial muscle contractions that are faster and out of synchronization with the lower chambers (ventricles). With AFL, the electrical signal travels along a pathway within the RA. It moves in an organized circular motion, or "circuit," causing the atria to beat faster than do the ventricles. AFL makes a very distinct "sawtooth" pattern on an ECG, a test used to diagnose abnormal heart rhythms. AFL itself is not life threatening. If left untreated, the side effects of AFL can be potentially life threatening. AFL makes it harder for the heart to pump blood effectively. With the blood moving more slowly, it is more likely to form clots. If the clot is pumped out of the heart, it could travel to the brain and lead to a stroke. Ablation procedure is the treatment of choice for AFL, which is performed by inserting a small catheter through the femoral vein and advancing it to the heart till it reaches a specific area called the cavotricuspid isthmus. Delivering RF lesion typically terminates the flutter with a success rate of approximately 85% to 90% and with a complications risk of <1%.

Eyal Herzog
Edgar Argulian
Steven B. Levy
Emad F. Aziz

24

Pathway for the Management of Atrial Fibrillation and Atrial Flutter

Atrial fibrillation (AF) is the most common cardiac rhythm disturbance encountered in clinical practice, and its prevalence is increasing as the population ages.[1,2] Electrocardiographically, AF is characterized by an irregularly irregular ventricular rhythm, with an absence of discrete P-wave activity. Rather, undulating fibrillatory activity (f waves) are seen on the electrocardiogram (ECG) between QRS complexes and T waves. The American College of Cardiology (ACC), the American Heart Association (AHA), and the European Society of Cardiology (ESC) established guidelines for the management of patients with AF.[3,4]

In 2010, the estimated numbers of men and women with AF worldwide were 20.9 million and 12.6 million, respectively, with higher incidence and prevalence rates in developed countries. One in four middle-aged adults in Europe and the United States will develop AF in their lifetime.[4]

The increase in AF prevalence can be attributed to better detection of silent AF,[5-7] alongside increasing age and conditions predisposing to AF.[8]

Atrial flutter (Afl) is less common and is often associated with or preceded by AF or occurs in an isolated pattern. Guidelines for Afl management were included in the ACC/AHA/ESC Guidelines for the Management of Patients with Supraventricular Arrhythmias. The electrocardiographic findings of Afl in its typical counterclockwise form include an atrial deflection with rapid regular undulations that gives rise to a "sawtooth" appearance, mainly in the inferior leads. The atrial rate is usually between 250 and 300 beats/min.

A major limitation of the currently published guidelines for the management of patients with AF and Afl is their complexity, the fact that official guidelines are published separately for each of these arrhythmias, and that they were published several years ago.[3] To address these deficiencies, we have developed a novel pathway for the management of AF and Afl (**Figure 24.1**).

The necessity to develop such a pathway at our institution was compelling, yet typical of the need at many other large medical centers, where it has become increasingly difficult for all house staff to grasp all the subtleties in the management of AF and Afl and to rapidly, efficiently, and accurately implement clinical protocols. It should be emphasized that this pathway is the opinion of our group and may differ somewhat from the published guidelines. The pathway has been designated with the acronym of RACE, which reflects the four main components

in patient management: **R**ate control, **A**nticoagulation therapy, **C**ardioversion, and **E**lectrophysiology/antiarrhythmic medication.

This pathway is an attempt to incorporate, in a user-friendly format, the key concepts of the initial diagnosis and management of these prevalent arrhythmias. This is followed by a comprehensive guideline for therapy using the RACE acronym.

INITIAL ASSESSMENT

All patients should undergo an initial assessment (**Figure 24.2**) on presentation to the emergency department, including a 12-lead ECG, history, and physical examination.

All patients should be immediately assessed for hemodynamic stability. If patients are hemodynamically unstable (low blood pressure, cold extremities, signs of heart failure, depressed mental status), emergency synchronized D/C cardioversion should be considered.

Patients should also be evaluated for acute coronary syndrome if they have suggestive symptoms, ECG changes, and/or elevated cardiac biomarkers. A comprehensive evaluation for acute heart failure is also essential, including an assessment of natriuretic peptide levels when appropriate. Prior studies have demonstrated a strong association between the heart failure syndrome and AF. Acute coronary syndrome and acute heart failure should be treated, respectively, per published guidelines and pathways.[9,10]

Initial laboratory testing should include a comprehensive metabolic panel, complete blood count, magnesium level, thyroid function tests, and coagulation panel if a patient is on warfarin therapy. All patients should have a transthoracic echocardiogram for assessment of left and right ventricular function, valvular disease, and pericardial effusion.

Owing to recent advances in the management of AF, including complexities of medical and nonpharmacologic therapies, early involvement of an arrhythmia service (AF team) should be considered in all patients with AF/Afl.

We have developed a systematic approach to the pathophysiology of AF and Afl (**Figure 24.2**) using acronyms that can easily be remembered by physicians, nurses, and other health care personnel:

a. Non-cardiovascular etiology: **TRAPS**

   T—Thyroid disease

   R—Recreational drug use

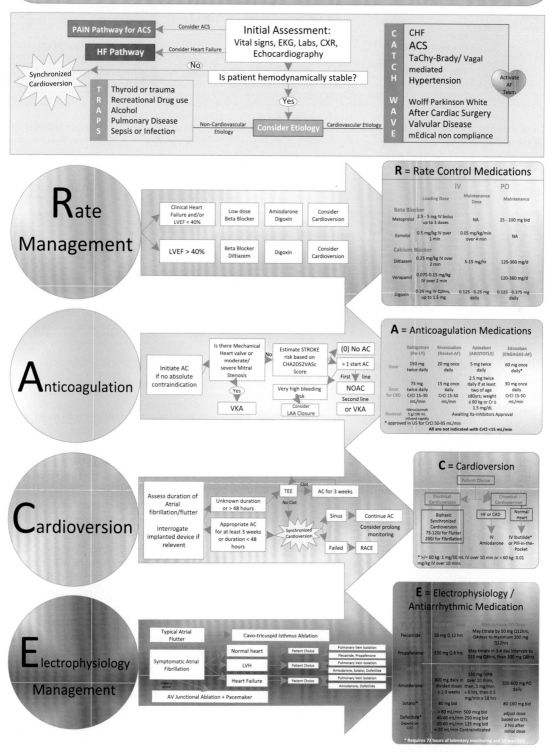

FIGURE 24.1 Pathway for the management of atrial fibrillation and atrial flutter. AC, anticoagulant; ACS, acute coronary syndrome; AF, atrial fibrillation; AV, atrioventricular; CAD, coronary artery disease; CHF, congestive heart failure; CKD, chronic kidney disease; CXR, chest X-ray; ECG, electrocardiogram; HF, heart failure; IV, intravenous; IVPB, intravenous piggyback; LAA, left atrial appendage; LVEF, left ventricular ejection fraction; LVH, left ventricular hypertrophy; NOAC, novel oral anticoagulation; TEE, transesophageal echocardiogram; VKA, vitamin K antagonist.

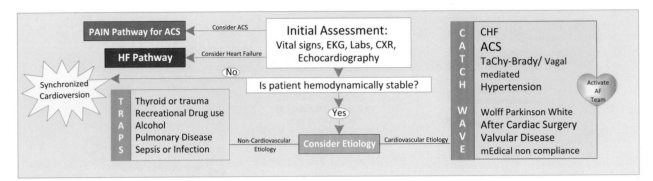

FIGURE 24.2 Initial assessment of patients with atrial fibrillation and atrial flutter. ACS, acute coronary syndrome; AF, atrial fibrillation; CHF, congestive heart failure; CXR, chest X-ray; HF, heart failure.

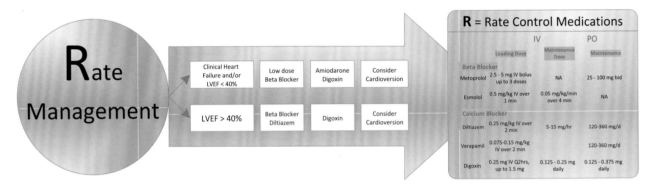

FIGURE 24.3 Rate management in patients with atrial fibrillation and atrial flutter. IV, intravenous; LVEF, left ventricular ejection fraction.

A—Alcohol
P—Pulmonary disease
S—Sepsis/infection
b. Cardiovascular etiology: **CATCH WAVE**
    C—Congestive heart failure
    A—Acute coronary syndrome/acute myocardial infarction (MI)
    TC—TaChy-brady syndrome/vagal mediated
    H—Hypertension
    W—Wolff–Parkinson–White syndrome
    A—After cardiac surgery
    V—Valvular heart disease
    E—mEdical noncompliance

RATE MANAGEMENT

In about 60% to 70% of patients with AF, a rapid ventricular rate is observed, and symptoms are usually present depending on the rapidity of the ventricular response, the length of time the arrhythmia is sustained, and the presence and type of underlying heart disease.[11] Acute ventricular rate control is the primary goal initially because patients' symptoms are chiefly governed by the rapid ventricular rate. In addition, a reduction in ventricular rate in AF results in a longer diastolic filling period and higher ventricular stroke volume. Acute ventricular rate control in AF can be achieved by pharmacotherapy, nonpharmacologic therapy, and early cardioversion to sinus rhythm. In addition, correction of precipitating factors often helps in controlling ventricular rates in addition to enhancing the chances for conversion to sinus rhythm.

We have defined the rate control goal in AF as a resting ventricular rate of less than 110 beats/min.

Atrioventricular (AV) node blocking agents including β-adrenergic blockers, non–dihydropyridine calcium channel blockers, and digoxin are usually effective in controlling ventricular rate in AF and Afl. Intravenous (IV) β-blocker and non–dihydropyridine calcium channel blockers are considered equally effective in rapidly controlling the ventricular rate. The addition of digoxin to the regimen is helpful, but digoxin as a single agent is generally less effective. Magnesium and amiodarone have also been used for acute ventricular rate control in AF. The agent of first choice is usually individualized depending on the clinical situation. β-Blockers are preferable in patients with myocardial ischemia, MI, and hyperthyroidism and in a postoperative state, but should be avoided in patients with bronchial asthma and chronic obstructive pulmonary disease, whereby non–dihydropyridine calcium channels blockers are preferred. β-blockers are preferred in AF during pregnancy. In addition, in AF with Wolff–Parkinson–White syndrome, β-Blockers, calcium channel blockers, and digoxin should be avoided, because these drugs are selective AV node blockers without slowing conduction through the accessory pathway, which can lead to increased transmission of impulses preferentially through the accessory pathway and precipitate ventricular fibrillation. The drug of choice for AF in pre-excitation syndrome is procainamide.

Figure 24.3 outlines our recommendations for rate control medications. It summarizes the IV loading and maintenance dose, as well as the oral dose for recommended medications.

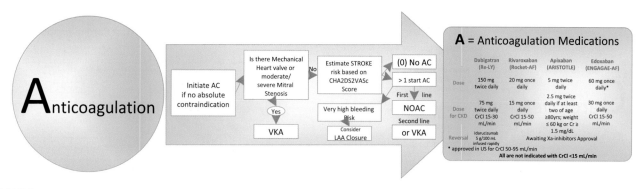

FIGURE 24.4 Anticoagulation in patients with atrial fibrillation and atrial flutter. AC, anticoagulant; LAA, left atrial appendage; NOAC, novel oral anticoagulation; VKA, vitamin K antagonist.

The first-line therapy to slow the ventricular rate in patients with AF and clinical heart failure and/or left ventricular ejection fraction (LVEF) <40% is a low-dose β-blocker.

The second-line therapy includes amiodarone or digoxin. Amiodarone can cause conversion to normal sinus rhythm in some patients and potentially precipitate a cardioembolic event in patients who are not adequately anticoagulated. If all these drugs fail to slow the ventricular rate, we suggest considering cardioversion.

For patients with LVEF >40%, we recommend using a β-blocker or diltiazem and as a second line to use digoxin.

If these agents fail to slow the ventricular rate, cardioversion should be considered.

ANTICOAGULATION

AF is thought to be responsible for approximately 15% to 25% of ischemic strokes.[12,13] The pathophysiology of AF-associated stroke is complex, but it appears to arise as a result of the embolization of a thrombus formed within the dysfunctioning left atrium, especially the left atrial appendage (LAA). Clot formation is more likely to occur under the conditions of stasis accompanying impaired atrial contraction.

Stratification of thromboembolic risk is central to the current recommendation for anticoagulation of patients with AF.

The CHA$_2$DS$_2$-VASc stroke risk stratification score (**Table 23.1**), recommended for use by the 2014 AHA/ACC/HRS Guideline for the Management of Atrial Fibrillation, is an expansion of the CHADS$_2$ score with three additional risk factors including female sex, age of 65 to 74 years, and history of vascular disease, such as prior MI, peripheral arterial disease, and aortic plaque.

The total score of the CHA$_2$DS$_2$-VASc is up to 9 points. On the basis of a strong level of evidence, the recommendation is to provide anticoagulation therapy for CHA$_2$DS$_2$-VASc scores of 2 or higher that indicates high risk for a thrombotic event. A CHA$_2$DS$_2$-VASc score of 1 indicates an intermediate risk of an event, and the clinician may consider offering antithrombotic therapy with either aspirin, an anticoagulant, or no therapy with continued monitoring with an implantable loop recorder for better understanding of the burden of AF. Assessing bleeding risk may assist with the decision process.

Several tools are available to assess the bleeding risk from anticoagulation for AF. The HAS-BLED score (**Table 23.2**) has been validated to predict clinically significant bleeding and has been demonstrated to outperform other scores.

Figure 24.4 outlines our summarized protocol for anticoagulation in the management of AF and Afl.

Our group decided to adopt the ESC definition of valvular AF as a mechanical heart valve or evidence of moderate or severe mitral stenosis. These patients will benefit from anticoagulation with only warfarin.

We recommend estimating the stroke risk based on the CHA$_2$DS$_2$-VASc scores and assessing bleeding risk based on the HAS-BLED score (**Table 23.2**).

Stroke risk of 0 does not require anticoagulation. If the stroke risk is above 1, we recommend assessing the bleeding risk for the purpose of mitigation of the bleeding risk factors.

In patients with a very high risk of bleeding, in patients with bleeding on anticoagulation, and in patients who cannot tolerate long-term anticoagulation therapy, a LAA closure device can be considered.

Otherwise, we recommend anticoagulation and the first-line therapy should be one of the four available novel oral anticoagulation (NOAC) agents. Warfarin should be considered only as a second-line option.

Figure 24.4 outlines the dosing of the currently available NOAC agents.

CARDIOVERSION

The decision to electively cardiovert a patient to and maintain normal sinus rhythm are complex and requires careful consideration of patient-specific factors as well as shared decision making with the patient. Timing the duration of AF and Afl is sometimes difficult if the patient cannot pinpoint the starting time of the arrhythmia. It is well accepted that patients whose arrhythmia is less than 48 hours in duration can safely have a cardioversion performed, and those with arrhythmia over 48 hours may have developed atrial thrombus, which increases the risk of thromboembolic events post cardioversion.

Figure 24.5 outlines our recommendations for cardioversion in patients with AF or Afl. We recommend starting the evaluation of the patient by assessing the duration of AF and Afl.

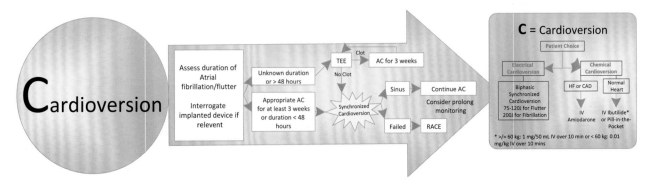

FIGURE 24.5 Cardioversion in patients with atrial fibrillation and atrial flutter. AC, anticoagulant; CAD, coronary artery disease; HF, heart failure; IV, intravenous; TEE, transesophageal echocardiogram.

This assessment can be quite easy if the patient has an implantable device—as the interrogation of the device will reveal the starting time of the arrhythmia.

For patients whose arrhythmia is *firmly established* to be less than 48 hours in duration, or if they have a *documented evidence* of appropriate anticoagulation for at least 3 weeks, a synchronized cardioversion can be safely performed.

When the onset of AF cannot be accurately determined or if AF is longer than 48 hours, anticoagulation should always be administered for at least 3 weeks before attempting cardioversion. Anticoagulation before cardioversion can be shortened if a transesophageal echocardiogram (TEE) is done and indicates the absence of thrombus in the left atrium and the LAA. The TEE-guided approach has been evaluated in the "Assessment of Cardioversion Utilizing Echocardiography (ACUTE) trial."[14,15] With this approach, which we often employ, cardioversion is done immediately when the TEE suggests that there is no evidence of thrombus; anticoagulation is continued for at least 4 weeks or longer depending on the long-term cardioembolic risk.

The consideration to discontinue anticoagulation therapy after 4 weeks can be made when there is no recurrence of AF and there are no stroke risk factors.

Transthoracic electrical cardioversion is more successful than pharmacologic cardioversion, with an overall success rate of 75% to 93%, inversely related to the duration of AF, chest wall impedance, and left atrial size. The success rate for pharmacologic cardioversion in selected patients approaches 70% at best, and there is a risk of proarrhythmia. For this reason, we recommend electrical cardioversion.

Figure 24.5 outlines our recommended options for electrical or chemical cardioversion.

There are two conventional positions for the electrode placement: anterior-lateral and anterior-posterior. Several studies have shown that less energy is required and a higher success rate is achieved with electrodes in the anterior-posterior position. For this reason, we recommend the anterior-posterior location. The energy required for cardioversion of AF is often 200 joules. More energy is required in obese patients and for long-standing AF. The initial energy used depends in part on the waveform of the current delivered by the defibrillation. Biphasic devices have been shown to be more effective and require less energy than monophasic devices.

Although electrical cardioversion is the more widely used technique, chemical cardioversion using class III antiarrhythmic drugs such as ibutilide can certainly be used provided that the patient will be observed for at least 2 hours post cardioversion in a monitored setting. Dofetilide also has been shown to be effective in acute conversion of AF, typically after two doses with a documented conversion rate up to 70%.[16,17]

ELECTROPHYSIOLOGY MANAGEMENT

Over the past decades, various antiarrhythmic drugs and catheter-based procedures have been investigated for maintenance of sinus rhythm in patients with AF. Although the AFFIRM trial showed no significant difference in the outcome of patients using these medications, the long-term outcome of a population-based administrative databases from Quebec, Canada, from 1999 to 2007 in selected patients 66 years or older and followed up for more than 4 years showed rhythm control therapy to be superior in the long term, particularly as the study population got older.[18]

Figure 24.6 presents an abbreviated algorithm for selection of the most appropriate antiarrhythmic drug for maintaining sinus rhythm in selected categories of patients. The figure lists selected doses of our recommended class Ic and class III antiarrhythmic medications.

That being said, several studies have shown that several class IA, IC, and III drugs, as well as class II drugs (β-blockers), are moderately effective in maintaining sinus rhythm; however, they are known to increase adverse events, including proarrhythmia, and some (eg, disopyramide, quinidine, and sotalol) may even increase mortality.[19]

Catheter ablation of AF has become an established therapeutic modality for the treatment of patients with symptomatic AF.

Pulmonary vein (PV) isolation using radiofrequency energy where a wide area or PV antral circumferential ablation strategy or the use of CRYO-ablation poses acute success rates documented in about 85% and long-term freedom from AF that is maintained at follow-up of at least 3 years with rates up to 80% in patients with paroxysmal Afl. Certainly, there are better outcomes when the procedure is performed by experienced operators.[20]

In rare cases when rate and rhythm control are unsuccessful despite maximally tolerated medical therapy and patients continue to be symptomatic because of the rapid Afl, treatment plans should include an electrophysiology (EP) consult to consider AV nodal junction ablation and permanent pacemaker implantation (ablate–pace technique).[21]

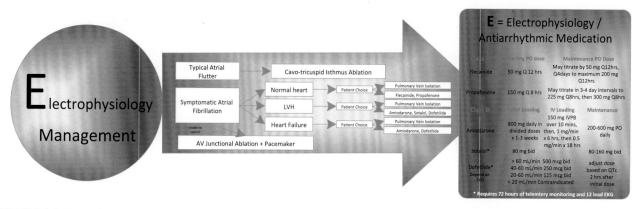

FIGURE 24.6 Electrophysiology management in patients with atrial fibrillation and atrial flutter. AV, atrioventricular; IV, intravenous; LVH, left ventricular hypertrophy.

MANAGEMENT OF ATRIAL FLUTTER

The RACE pathway published in September 2005[1] was the first to include both AF and Afl in a single pathway. Because both arrhythmias will require anticoagulation and rate control medication, the initial assessment and management is similar. However, if the ECG is consistently Afl, we highly recommend consulting the EP team for consideration for Afl ablation, as shown in **Figure 24.6**.

EP studies have shown that Afl results from tachycardia using a reentry circuit. The reentry circuit occupies large areas of the atrium and is referred to as "macroreentrant." The classic type of Afl (typical flutter) is dependent on the cavotricuspid isthmus. Catheter ablation of the cavotricuspid isthmus for isthmus-dependent flutter had been proved to be 95% to 100% successful,[22,23] and is superior to antiarrhythmic therapy.[24]

Our recommendation is to consult the EP team for all patients with Afl for consideration of ablation. If medically treated, Afl resumes in the vast majority of patients within 6 months.[23]

REFERENCES

1. Herzog E, Fischer A, Steinberg JS. The rate control, anticoagulation therapy, and electrophysiology/antiarrhythmic medication pathway for the management of atrial fibrillation and atrial flutter. *Crit Pathways Cardiol.* September 2005;4(3):121-126.

2. Herzog E, Steinberg JS. Management of atrial fibrillation and atrial flutter. In: *Critical Pathway in Cardiovascular Medicine.* Vol 19. 2nd ed. Philadelphia: Lippincott Williams & Wilkins, 2007:181-189.

3. January CT, Wann LS, Alpert JS, et al. AHA/ACC/HRS guideline for the management of patients with atrial fibrillation: executive summary. *JACC.* 2014;64(21):2246-2280.

4. Kirchhof P, Bennussi S, Kotecha, et al. ESC guidelines for the management of atrial fibrillation development in collaboration with EACTS. The task force for management of atrial fibrillation of the European Society of Cardiology (ESC). Endorsed by the European Stroke Organisation (ESO). *Eur Heart J.* 1-90. doi:1093/eurheartj/ehw210.

5. Wang TJ, Larson MG, Levy D, et al. Temporal relations of atrial fibrillation and congestive heart failure and their joint influence on mortality: the Framingham Heart Study. *Circulation.* 2003;107(23):2920-2925.

6. Kishore A, Vail A, Majid A, et al. Detection of atrial fibrillation after ischemic stroke or transient ischemic attack: a systematic review and meta analysis. *Stroke.* 2014;45:520-526.

7. Sanna T, Diener H-C, Passman RS, et al. Cryptogenic stroke and underlying atrial fibrillation. *N Engl J Med.* 2014;370:2478-2486.

8. Schnabel RB, Yin X, Gona P, et al. 50 year trends in atrial fibrillation prevalence, incidence, risk factors, and mortality in the Framingham Heart Study: a cohort study. *Lancet.* 2015;386:154-162.

9. Herzog E, Saint-Jacques H, Rozanski A. The PAIN pathway as a tool to bridge the gap between evidence and management of acute coronary syndrome. *Crit Pathways Cardiol* 2004;3:20-24.

10. Herzog E, Varley C, Kukin, M. Pathway for the management of acute heart failure. *Crit Pathways Cardiol.* 2005;4:37-42.

11. Khan IA, Nair CK, Singh N, et al. Acute ventricular rate control in atrial fibrillation and atrial flutter. *I J Card.* 2004;97:7-13.

12. Hersi A, Wyse DG. Management of atrial fibrillation: *Curr Probl Cardiol.* 2005;30:175-234.

13. Atrial Fibrillation Investigators. Risk factor for stroke and efficacy of antithrombotic therapy in atrial fibrillation: analysis of pooled data from five randomized controlled trials. *Arch Intern Med.* 1994;154:1449-1457.

14. Klein AL, Grimm RA, Black IW, et al. Cardioversion guided by transesophageal echocardiography: the ACUTE pilot study. *Ann Intern Med.* 1997;126: 200-209.

15. Klein AL, Grimm RA, Murray RD, et al. Use of transesophageal echocardiography to guide cardioversion in patients with atrial fibrillation. *N Engl J Med.* 2001;344:1411-1420.

16. Cotiga D, Arshad A, Aziz E, et al. Acute conversion of persistent atrial fibrillation during dofetilide initiation. *Pacing Clin Electrophysiol.* 2007;30(12):1527-1530.

17. Malhotra R, Bilchick KC, DiMarco JP. Usefulness of pharmacologic conversion of atrial fibrillation during dofetilide loading without the need for electrical cardioversion to predict durable response to therapy. *Am J Cardiol.* 2014;113(3):475-479.

18. Ionescu-Ittu R, Abrahamowicz M, Jackevicius CA, et al. Comparative effectiveness of rhythm control vs rate control drug treatment effect on mortality in patients with atrial fibrillation. *Arch Intern Med.* 2012;172(13):997-1004.

19. Lafuente-Lafuente C, Valembois L, Bergmann JF, et al. Antiarrhythmics for maintaining sinus rhythm after cardioversion of atrial fibrillation. *Cochrane Database Syst Rev.* 2015;28(3):CD005049.

20. Ganesan A, Shipp N, Brooks A, et al. Long-term outcomes of catheter ablation of atrial fibrillation: a systematic review and meta-analysis. *J Am Heart Assoc.* 2013;2:e004549.

21. Queiroga A, Marshall H, Clune M, et al. Ablate and pace revisited: long term survival and predictors of permanent atrial fibrillation. *Heart.* 2003;89(9):1035-1038.

22. William S, Weiss C, Ventura R, et al. Catheter ablation of atrial flutter guided by electroanatomic mapping (CARTO): a randomized comparison to the conventional approach. *J Cardiovasc Electrophysiol.* 2000;11:1223-1230.

23. Babaev A, Suma V, Tita C, et al. Recurrence rate of atrial flutter after initial presentation in patients on drug treatment. *Am J Cardiol.* 2003;92:1122-1124.

24. Natale A, Newby KH, Pisano E, et al. Prospective randomized comparison of antiarrhythmic therapy versus first-line radiofrequency ablation in patients with atrial flutter. *J Am Coll Cardial.* 2000;35:1898-1904.

Ankit Chothani
Shawn Lee
Ashish Correa
Davendra Mehta

25

Ventricular Arrhythmia

Ventricular arrhythmias (VAs) refer to a wide variety of tachyarrhythmias, which originate from the left or right ventricle. VA is a spectrum of arrhythmias ranging from premature ventricular contraction to ventricular tachycardia (VT) to ventricular fibrillation (VF). Various forms of VA are commonly seen in both the outpatient and inpatient clinical setting. However, it is prudent to review them while in the cardiac care unit (CCU), because patients with acute and life-threatening VAs will be treated here.

VA can be due to one of the following three mechanisms—Abnormal automaticity, triggered activity, or reentry.

a. **Abnormal automaticity:** Some of the cardiac tissue has the ability to automatically generate electrical impulse through spontaneous depolarization. Abnormal automaticity refers to the automatic firing of electrical impulse by cardiac tissue which, under normal conditions, does not demonstrate automaticity. Example: Right Ventricular Outflow Tachycardia.

b. **Triggered activity:** Triggered activity refers to an electrical impulse which is triggered by preceding impulse. Preceding impulse causes oscillations in the membrane potential of the abnormal cardiac tissue, which are called after-depolarizations. Once the after-depolarization crosses the threshold of depolarization, it creates abnormal electrical impulse. Example: Long QT Syndromes.

c. **Reentry:** This is the most common mechanism for VAs. Reentry refers to propagation of impulse around a circuit that comprises two distinct electrical pathways with distinct electrical properties. As the circuit gets activated, it emits the electrical impulse at fixed cycle length. Example: Ischemic/scar-related VT.

BASIC DEFINITIONS

Table 25.1. describes some of the basic definitions related to VAs.

PREMATURE VENTRICULAR COMPLEXES

Premature ventricular complexes (PVCs) are extremely common in the population, and up to 40 % of people without cardiac disease may have them.[1] PVCs originate from abnormal automaticity foci in the ventricles, which can be due to hypoxia, electrolyte abnormalities, or cardiac pathology. Common areas of these foci include the right ventricular outflow tract (RVOT), left ventricular outflow tract (LVOT), papillary muscle, or diseased cardiac tissue

after a myocardial infarction (MI) or fibrosis. They manifest as isolated widened QRS complexes (>120 ms). Several studies have shown the presence of PVCs to be associated with increased risk of cardiovascular mortality in patients with structural heart disease.[2,3] **Figure 25.1** shows PVCs in a bigeminy pattern.

In the vast majority of patients, PVCs do not produce symptoms, but they can manifest as palpitations and, rarely, lightheadedness or near syncope. Diagnosis of PVCs in the outpatient setting can be made by ambulatory Holter monitor or event monitor, specifically to quantify the burden of PVCs. Whether to treat the PVCs or not depends on the presence of structural heart disease, burden of PVCs, and presence of symptoms. Treatment options for symptomatic patients includes rectifying correctable causes or triggers such as ischemia, alcohol, illicit drugs, or caffeine and also includes workup to check electrolyte levels and thyroid stimulating hormone. For patients with structural heart disease, β-blockers may help reduce the frequency of PVCs. Catheter ablation should be considered for patients with high PVC burden (>10%) that is associated with significant symptoms unresponsive to antiarrhythmic medications and/or left ventricular (LV) dysfunction.[4] PVCs originating from outflow tracts are relatively easily amenable to catheter ablation.

NONSUSTAINED VENTRICULAR TACHYCARDIA

Like PVCs, nonsustained ventricular tachycardia (NSVT) can be seen in a wide range of medical conditions as well as in healthy individuals. NSVT is mostly diagnosed on telemetry, Holter monitors, or event monitors. Typically, NSVT is not associated with hemodynamic compromise. However, it may produce lightheadedness, palpitations, or chest pain when it lasts for more than a few seconds. β-Blockers are recommended for symptomatic NSVT. In some cases, amiodarone can be used to suppress the NSVT in symptomatic patients.

Clinical relevance and prognostic value of NSVT remain the subject of debate in different clinical settings. Studies have shown that patients with significant coronary artery disease, left ventricular ejection fraction (LVEF) < 40%, and NSVT are at increased risk for sudden cardiac death (SCD), if sustained VT can be induced by electrophysiology study. These patients should have an implantable cardioverter defibrillator (ICD) placement (MUSTT trial).[5] However, such an association is absent for the first 48 hours post-MI. In hypertrophic cardiomyopathy patients, NSVT predicts elevated risk of SCD. Placement of defibrillator for primary prevention is justified in these patients.[6]

TABLE 25.1	Basic Definitions of Ventricular Arrythmia
Premature ventricular complexes (PVCs)	Ectopic beats originating from an abnormal automaticity focus. The depolarization of these beats is of ventricular origin and not conducted through the His–Purkinje system; they manifest as isolated wide QRS (>120 ms) complex beats on electrocardiogram (ECG).
Couplet	Two consecutive PVCs
Triplet	Three consecutive PVCs
Ventricular bigeminy	Occurrence of a PVC after every other normal/sinus beat
Ventricular trigeminy	Occurrence of a PVC every third beat
Nonsustained ventricular tachycardia (NSVT)	3 or more consecutive PVCs, at a rate of > 100 beats/min and spontaneously terminates within 30 s, without hemodynamic compromise
Ventricular tachycardia (VT)	Rapid (>100 beats/min), wide QRS complexes (>120 ms) of ventricular origin
Sustained ventricular tachycardia	VT that is greater than 30 s and/or is accompanied by hemodynamic instability and/or symptoms
Monomorphic ventricular tachycardia	VT in which all beats have the same morphology manifesting as uniform widened QRS complexes on ECG. Monomorphic VT originates from a single automaticity focus or reentry circuit within the ventricles
Polymorphic ventricular tachycardia	VT with widened QRS complexes that vary in amplitude and duration on ECG. Polymorphic VT originate from multiple ventricular foci firing together, leading to irregular ventricular depolarizations
Torsades de pointes	Type of polymorphic VT with widened QRS complexes that change in amplitude, giving the appearance of a "twisting pattern." This is usually associated with long QT interval
Ventricular fibrillation	A rapid (typically > 300 beats/min) and irregular rhythm of chaotic electrical activity of ventricular origin, essentially leading to no meaningful cardiac output, and is a rapidly fatal rhythm

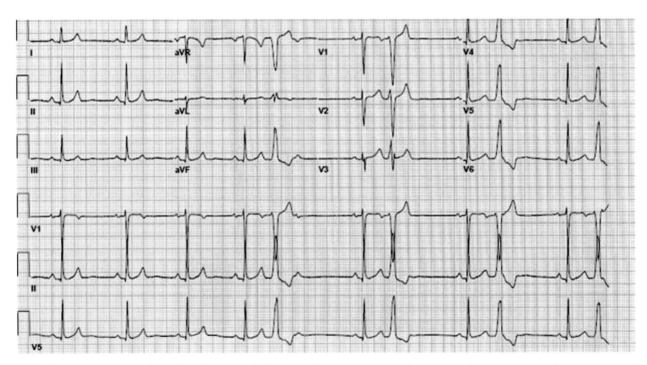

FIGURE 25.1 Normal sinus rhythm followed by ventricular bigeminy. This pattern involves the presence of a premature ventricular complexes (PVC) after every normal sinus beat. aVF; augmented vector foot; aVL; augmented vector left; aVR, augmented vector right.

VENTRICULAR TACHYCARDIA

Sustained VT is characterized by wide complex tachycardia with a rate > 100 beats/min, lasting for more than 30 seconds, or any VT accompanied with hemodynamic compromise. Sustained VT has multiple etiologies-ischemic VT being the most common. Sustained VT can also be seen in patients with structurally normal heart. Refer to **Table 25.2** for details of types and etiologies of VT.

In patients with ischemic heart disease, VT and VF are often the result of scarring and fibrosis secondary to MI. Common nonischemic etiologies include dilated cardiomyopathy, hypertrophic cardiomyopathy, and arrhythmogenic right ventricular cardiomyopathy (ARVC). Infiltrative disorders such as myocarditis, sarcoidosis, and amyloidosis can also cause VT. Finally, electrolyte

abnormalities such as hypokalemia and hypomagnesemia can also precipitate VT.

Along with VF, sustained VT is a cause of sudden cardiac arrest and commonly also of syncope and chest pain in predisposed patients. Occasionally, if sustained VT is slow in rate, patients can be asymptomatic or may only have lightheadedness or dizziness.

One of the most challenging and clinically relevant issues while diagnosing VT from ECG is to distinguish it from supraventricular tachycardia (SVT) with aberrant conduction (**Table 25.3**). Both rhythms have wide QRS complexes (> 120 ms) with rates greater than 100 beats/min. In the emergent setting, recognizing the difference between the two is paramount. When doubt exists, it is safest to assume any wide complex tachycardia is VT, especially in patients with known cardiovascular disease. Presence of underlying structural heart disease is the strongest predictor of VT.[7,8] Previous baseline 12-lead ECG obtained during sinus rhythm may also reveal the etiology of the tachycardia. Fusion or capture beats and atrioventricular (AV) dissociation (**Figure 25.2**) provide the strongest electrocardiographic evidence for differentiating VT from SVT with aberrancy, and are diagnostic of VT. However, in their absence, other clues from the electrocardiogram (ECG) may be required to help with this differentiation. Apart from the aforementioned features, several algorithms have been created for distinguishing VT from SVT with aberrancy, the most notable being Brugada criteria. In any young patient with irregular wide complex tachycardia with rate > 200 beats/min, atrial fibrillation caused by conduction over an accessory pathway should be suspected.

MANAGEMENT OF VENTRICULAR TACHYCARDIA

Pulseless Sustained Ventricular Tachycardia

In any patient with pulseless sustained VT/VF (VT with cardiac arrest), cardiopulmonary resuscitation (CPR) should be initiated immediately. The patient should be treated per Acute Cardiac Life Support (ACLS) protocols. If return of spontaneous circulation is achieved, the patient should be started on chronic VT therapies along with post–cardiac arrest treatment. A detailed discussion of ACLS protocols and post–cardiac arrest treatment is beyond the scope of this chapter.

TABLE 25.2	Types and Etiologies of Ventricular Tachycardia (VT)

Structurally normal heart
- Focal VT
- Fascicular VT

VT due to structural heart disease
- Ischemic VT
- Dilated cardiomyopathy

Inherited channelopathies or genetic causes
- Long QT syndrome
- Brugada syndrome
- Catecholaminergic polymorphic ventricular tachycardia
- Hypertrophic cardiomyopathy
- Arrhythmogenic right ventricular cardiomyopathy (ARVC)

Systemic disease or infiltrative disorders
- Sarcoidosis (cardiac sarcoidosis)
- Rheumatoid arthritis
- Systemic lupus erythematous
- Hemochromatosis
- Amyloidosis
- Myocarditis

Electrolyte abnormalities
- Hypokalemia
- Hypomagnesemia
- Hypocalcemia

Congenital heart disease
- Tetralogy of Fallot
- Mitral valve prolapse

Drugs/medication induced
- IV inotropes
- Digitalis
- Cocaine
- Methamphetamine
- Drugs that prolong the QT interval (class IA and class III antiarrhythmics, methadone, etc.)

Other
- Commotio cordis

TABLE 25.3	Differentiating VT from SVT with Aberrancy

1. History of structural heart disease or coronary artery disease
2. QRS complexes of > 160 ms in absence of any class IC antiarrhythmic
3. True AV dissociation
4. Presence of capture or fusion beats
5. Extreme axis deviation (QRS positive in aVR and negative in I and aVF)
6. Presence of negative or positive concordance (all precordial leads are negative or positive)
7. Presence of these signs:
   a. Rsr′ (left R wave taller than right R wave) pattern or notched downslope of R wave in V1
   b. Notching near the nadir of S wave (i.e., Josephson sign)
   c. R wave > 30 ms in V1 or V2
   d. QRS onset to nadir of S in V1 > 60 ms (i.e. Brugada sign)

AV, atrioventricular; aVF, augmented vector foot; aVR, augmented vector right; SVT, supraventricular tachycardia; VT, ventricular tachycardia.

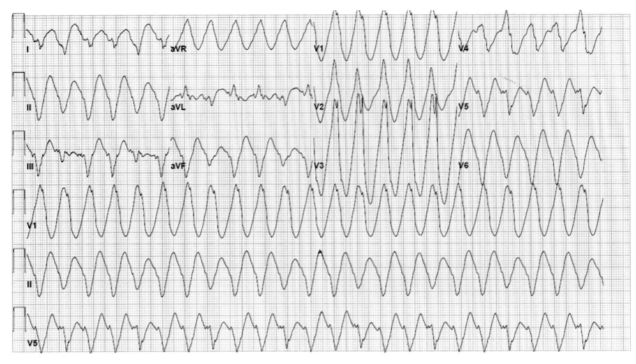

FIGURE 25.2 Sustained ventricular tachycardia (VT) with atrioventricular (AV) dissociation. This figure shows AV dissociation in a sustained VT, wherein the relationship between the P waves and the QRS complexes is completely lost. aVF; augmented vector foot; aVL; augmented vector left; aVR, augmented vector right.

Sustained Monomorphic Ventricular Tachycardia with Pulse

Patients with hemodynamically compromised, unstable VT requires emergent cardioversion or defibrillation. If the patient is stable, he or she can be given antiarrhythmics while being carefully monitored in the critical care unit. Once the acute episode is resolved, workup should be initiated to identify the etiology, along with chronic medical and device therapies (**Table 25.4**). Current guidelines of the American College of Cardiology (ACC)/ American Heart Association (AHA) recommend ICD therapy in patients who are survivors of cardiac arrest or who have had hemodynamically unstable VT for secondary prevention.[9] Sustained monomorphic VT (SMVT) (**Figure 25.3**) is commonly seen with acute myocardial ischemia, chronic ischemic heart disease with LV scar formation as well as in the structurally normal heart. In patients with chronic ischemic heart disease, myocardial cells around the border of the scar act as a substrate for a reentrant circuit, causing monomorphic VT. Idiopathic focal VT is usually a monomorphic VT arising from areas of abnormal automaticity.

All patients with sustained monomorphic VT should have basic workup to assess etiology. Features of instability include chest pain, dyspnea, hemodynamic instability, and altered mental status. Stable patients can be treated with any of three antiarrhythmic medications—lidocaine, amiodarone, or procainamide. Intravenous procainamide is not easily available in the United States. Lidocaine is usually more effective in VT associated with myocardial ischemia or infarction. Amiodarone acts slowly and is the most effective as well as most commonly used out of the three medications. Although IV administration of these medications can be stopped once the acute episode is over, infusion should be continued if there is recurrent SMVT. Intravenous amiodarone can be followed by oral amiodarone to prevent recurrent VT. Other concurrent managements include treatment of the reversible cause—electrolyte imbalance correction or urgent revascularization if myocardial ischemia is present.

Once the acute episode is over, long-term medical therapy should be started, which commonly includes β-blocker with or without antiarrhythmic medication. ICD placement should be considered for secondary prevention. The European Heart Rhythm Association/Heart Rhythm Society (EHRA/HRS) recommends radiofrequency catheter ablation for patients with structural heart disease in the following situations: 1. recurrent VT that is not responding to antiarrhythmic drugs; 2. VT leading to recurrent ICD shocks with no response to or side effects with antiarrhythmic therapy; 3. incessant VT or VT storm not attributable to a reversible cause; 4. a patient who is not a candidate for ICD or refusing ICD.[10]

Surgical therapies for VT can be considered in patients who are undergoing cardiac surgery for another cause (coronary bypass graft placement/valve replacement) and have identifiable substrates such as ventricular aneurysms or large myocardial scars. Surgical approaches that have proven effective include LV aneurysmectomy, encircling endocardial ventriculotomy and subendocardial resection. In some patients with recurrent VT who have failed to respond to antiarrhythmic drugs and catheter ablation, bilateral surgical sympathectomy has been shown to be helpful.

Sustained Polymorphic Ventricular Tachycardia with a Pulse

Polymorphic VTs are classified on the basis of their QT interval. Polymorphic VT with normal QT intervals is most commonly caused by myocardial ischemia after acute MI, severe heart failure, or cardiogenic shock. When feasible, urgent myocardial revascularization should be undertaken. These patients have high

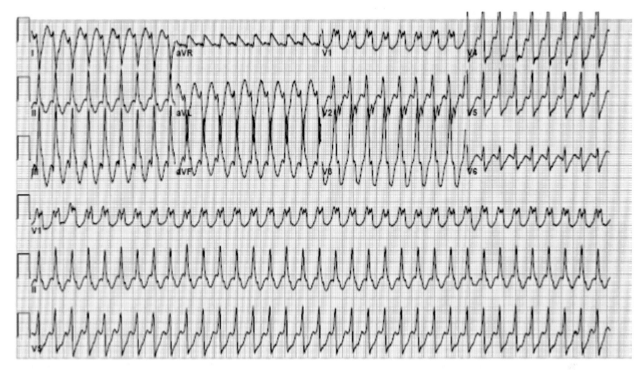

FIGURE 25.3 Sustained monomorphic ventricular tachycardia (SMVT). In SMVT, all beats have the same morphology manifesting as uniform widened QRS complexes on electrocardiogram. aVF; augmented vector foot; aVL; augmented vector left; aVR, augmented vector right.

TABLE 25.4	Acute and Chronic Management of Sustained VT with Pulse
SUSTAINED VT WITH PULSE	
Monomorphic	*Polymorphic*
Unstable: Emergent/urgent cardioversion	**Acute:** Emergent/urgent defibrillation
<ul><li>Supplemental O$_2$</li><li>12-Lead ECG</li><li>Establish IV access</li><li>Initial labs—(electrolyte level, cardiac biomarkers, urine toxicology, magnesium level)</li></ul>	
Stable: Consider one of the following **antiarrhythmic medications**:<ul><li>**Intravenous lidocaine** (1–1.5 mg/kg [typically 75–100 mg] at a rate of 25–50 mg/min; lower doses of 0.5–0.75 mg/kg can be repeated every 5–10 min as needed)</li><li>**Intravenous procainamide** (20–50 mg/min until arrhythmia terminates or a maximum dose of 17 mg/kg is administered)</li><li>**Intravenous amiodarone** (150 mg IV over 10 min, followed by 1 mg/min for the next 6 h; bolus can be repeated if VT recurs)</li></ul>	<ul><li>If in setting of **myocardial ischemia**: consider IV nitroglycerin and urgent revascularization</li><li>**Short QT interval**: can use IV β-blocker or IV amiodarone (150 mg IV over 10 min, followed by 1 mg/min for the next 6 h; bolus can be repeated if VT recurs)</li><li>**Long QT interval**: IV isoproterenol can be used to increase the HR in patients with bradycardia</li><li>**Torsades de Pointes**: IV magnesium should be given even if the magnesium level is normal</li></ul>
Chronic therapies<ul><li>β-Blockers</li><li>ICD implantation</li><li>Antiarrhythmic mediation</li><li>Radiofrequency catheter ablation</li><li>Surgical therapies—sympathetic denervation</li></ul>	

ECG, electrocardiogram; HR, heart tare; ICD, implantable cardioverter defibrillator; VT, ventricular tachycardia.

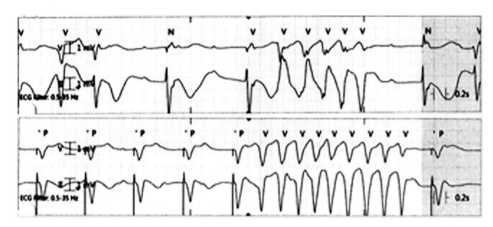

FIGURE 25.4 Torsades de pointes. Both rhythm strips showing electrocardiogram with baseline rhythm having prolonged QT interval and a short burst of polymorphic ventricular tachycardia, that is torsades de pointes. Upper panel: sinus bradycardia with prolonged QT interval. Lower panel: V-paced rhythm with prolonged QT interval.

mortality, especially when VT is associated with heart failure and cardiogenic shock. Antiarrhythmic drugs have limited success in improving their outcome.

Torsades de pointes (TdP) (**Figure 25.4**) is a specific type of polymorphic VT (which has characteristic ECG morphology in which QRS complexes appear to "twist" around the isoelectric line). When in sinus rhythm, an ECG classically shows prolonged QT interval. This can be congenital or acquired. Congenital long QT syndrome is caused by multiple genetic variants. Acquired long QT intervals are secondary to acute myocardial ischemia or drug administration. Medications known to contribute to QT prolongation include several antiarrhythmic drugs (Class III antiarrhythmics), antibiotics (specifically fluoroquinolones and macrolides), antipsychotics, and antihistamines.

There are other types of polymorphic VT without definitive association with QT interval. Bidirectional VT is a rhythm characterized by two distinct wide complex QRS (> 120 ms) morphologies (rate > 100 beats/min) that alternate every beat. Although bidirectional tachycardia is a rare occurrence in general, it is pathognomonic for digoxin toxicity. Catecholaminergic polymorphic ventricular tachycardia (CPVT), also known as familial polymorphic ventricular tachycardia (FPVT), is a congenital disorder caused by mutations in ryanodine receptors or other calcium channel binding proteins in the sarcoplasmic reticulum. It is a rare condition that manifests within the first or second decade of life, presenting as dizziness, syncope, or even sudden death, after exercise or emotional stress. Brugada Syndrome is a rare syndrome that is seen most commonly in South-East Asians. Resting ECGs show right-bundle branch block (RBBB) pattern with ST-elevations in the right precordial leads, specifically in V1 and V2, and have the potential to degenerate into polymorphic VT and even VF.

Most polymorphic VTs are unstable with hemodynamic compromise and require emergent or urgent defibrillation. In the patient with polymorphic VT and normal QT interval, the likely etiology is myocardial ischemia. β-Blockers and IV amiodarone can be used (bolus followed by infusion) to prevent recurrence of the arrhythmia. Urgent coronary angiography and revascularization is necessary to relieve the ischemia.

In the patient with congenital long QT syndrome, β-blockers may be used to reduce the frequency of PVCs and shorten the QT interval. ICD therapy is indicated if patients have recurrent syncope despite β-blocker therapy. Isoproterenol is used in patients with polymorphic VT triggered by sinus pauses or bradycardia. For patients with TdP, IV magnesium is first-line therapy (even in patients with normal serum magnesium) for both termination and prevention of recurrence of this rhythm. If the patient does not respond to intravenous magnesium, temporary intravenous pacing at 100 beats/min may be reasonable to prevent recurrence.

VENTRICULAR FIBRILLATION

VF is a rapid (typically > 300 beats/min) and irregular rhythm of chaotic electrical activity of ventricular origin. VF causes SCD because there is no cardiac output during this rhythm. Typically, this rhythm is seen during the acute phase of MI. VF is further divided into primary VF, which occurs less than 48 hours after a MI, and nonprimary VF, which does not occur in the setting of MI (but typically in the setting of heart failure or recurrent ischemia). Predictors of primary VF include ST-elevation MI (STEMI), early repolarization on baseline ECG during an acute coronary syndrome, hypokalemia, hypotension, large infarcts, male sex, and history of smoking. If not treated immediately, VF is almost universally lethal.

Treatment of VF involves defibrillation and pharmacotherapy. Defibrillation at an initial shock of 120 to 200 joules for biphasic defibrillators and 360 joules for monophasic defibrillators is currently recommended by ACLS guidelines. Pharmacotherapy involves epinephrine, which is to be administered as 1mg IV of 1:10,000 every 3 to 5 minutes. An initial bolus of 300 mg of IV amiodarone diluted in 20 to 30 mL of normal saline, followed by 150 mg IV boluses has been shown to increase the efficacy of electrical defibrillation in out-of-hospital cardiac arrest. Prior to the most recent guidelines regarding ACLS by the AHA, vasopressin was used, but is currently not recommended.[11] Lidocaine has been shown to have no evidence of efficacy in the management of VF. Chronic therapy for VF is similar to sustained VT, which includes ICD implantation for secondary prevention and β-blockers.

VENTRICULAR TACHYCARDIA—SPECIFIC VTS

VENTRICULAR TACHYCARDIA IN THE STRUCTURALLY NORMAL HEART

About 10% of patients with VT do not have any evidence of structural heart disease.[12] In general, these VTs present as monomorphic VT. Although idiopathic VT can originate from any ventricular site, the most frequent sites are RVOT, LVOT and Left ventricular fascicles.

Focal Ventricular Tachycardia

RVOT VT is seen in greater proportion in females compared to males, whereas the distribution of LVOT VT is more equal with respect to gender. They are both seen early in life, sometime between the third and fifth decades. The most likely mechanisms for these rhythms include triggered activity (catecholamine-mediated after-depolarizations). Symptoms include palpitations, dizziness, and, on occasion, syncope. On presentation, these rhythms commonly present as nonsustained repetitive monomorphic VT or paroxysmal exercise-induced VT. Frequent NSVT and high PVC burden can lead to ventricular dysfunction (tachycardia-induced cardiomyopathy) in these patients. On ECG, RVOT VT has a characteristic left bundle branch block morphology with inferior axis, where LVOT VT presents with RBBB morphology with inferior axis.

Idiopathic VTs are associated with good long-term prognosis. The decision to treat depends on the frequency and severity of symptoms, and presence of ventricular dysfunction. Acute termination can be achieved with adenosine and verapamil. RVOT and LVOT VTs respond well to β-blockers, calcium channel blockers, and antiarrhythmic drugs as well. As these patients have no structural heart disease, all antiarrhythmic drugs can be used. However, catheter ablation is preferred management option because it offers a permanent safe cure and has a high success rate, exceeding 90%.

Fascicular Ventricular Tachycardia

Fascicular VT originates from the fascicles in the left ventricle. Although commonly seen in the second to fourth decades of life, frequently patients may recall episodes of palpitations or dizziness at an earlier age. Up to 70% of these patients are males. This rhythm may be precipitated by emotional stress or exercise. Fascicular tachycardias are related to reentry in the His–Purkinje system, most commonly in the left posterior fascicle. At times, the site of origin is a false tendon or a fibromuscular band that extends from the posteroinferior left ventricle wall to the basal septum, which has reportedly been observed on echocardiography.[13] On 12-lead ECG, fascicular VTs have a RBBB-like morphology and relatively short QRS interval (120 ms to 140 ms). Depending on the site of exit in the left ventricle, they are associated with left axis deviation (more commonly) or right axis deviation. Fascicular VT has good long-term prognosis and can be treated medically with β-blockers and calcium channel blockers. They are particularly sensitive to verapamil. Fascicular VT can be confused for SVT because of ECG characteristics and sensitivity to verapamil. Catheter ablation has high success rates (90–95%) and is preferred compared to lifelong medical therapy.

VENTRICULAR TACHYCARDIA IN THE STRUCTURALLY ABNORMAL HEART

Ventricular Tachycardia in Ischemic Heart Disease

This refers to VT that develops in the setting of both acute and chronic ischemic heart disease. Life-threatening VAs, including VT and VF, are infrequent but possible sequelae of acute STEMIs and acute non-ST-elevation MIs (NSTEMI), with an overall lower incidence in NSTEMIs compared to STEMIs. Life-threatening arrhythmias such as symptomatic VT and VF can be the first presentation of acute MI. These are primarily treated by coronary revascularization.

Patients with chronic ischemic heart disease usually have myocardial scarring and present with monomorphic VT. This involves a reentrant circuit involving damaged slow conducting myocardium and increased automaticity in the border zone of myocardial scars. On ECG, VT from old MIs are typically monomorphic, whereas VT in the acute MI presents as polymorphic. Patients who develop VT or VF in the acute MI phase, specifically in the first 24 to 48 hours, do not have an increased risk of sudden death and do not require an implantable cardioverter defibrillator (ICD) for secondary prevention.

For those who develop recurrent VT or VF, and are thus at risk for SCD, the primary treatment is ICD therapy. β-Blockers have anti-ischemic and bradycardic properties and have been shown to reduce SCD, if continued at least 90 days post-MI.[14] Antiarrhythmic medications such as sotalol and amiodarone may be used for recurrent VT and VF despite defibrillator implantation. Catheter ablation has been shown to be highly successful for management of these patients and involves mapping and ablation of areas of slow conduction.

ICDs are indicated for primary and secondary prevention of sudden death in patients with chronic ischemic heart disease. Class IA indications for primary prevention include 1. patients with LVEF < 35% caused by prior MI who are at least 40 days post-MI and are in New York Heart Association (NYHA) Functional Class II or III, 2. patients with LVEF < 30% who are 40 days post-MI and are in NYHA Functional Class I. Class IA recommendation for ICD placement in the patient with ischemic cardiomyopathy for secondary prevention include those who are survivors of cardiac arrest caused by VT/VF.

Ventricular Tachycardia in Dilated Cardiomyopathy

This refers to VT that occurs in the setting of dilated cardiomyopathy (DCM). DCM is the most common cause of heart failure and is among the most common diagnosis that requires hospitalization in North America. The current prevalence of DCM in the United States is roughly 4.7 million, and the 5-year mortality rate in patients with heart failure caused by DCM is 50%.[15]

VT in the patient with dilated cardiomyopathy has been proposed by several different mechanisms: (1) arrhythmogenic substrates may result from myocardial fibrosis, leading to an irritable focus and (2) high catecholamine levels or stretching of myocardial fibers induced by increased LV end-diastolic volume. Acute management of VT in DCM is similar to that of ischemic cardiomyopathy. In addition, β-blockers show similar benefits as they do in ischemic cardiomyopathy. Current guidelines recommend ICD implantation for primary prevention in patients with new diagnosis of nonischemic dilated cardiomyopathy (NIDCM) with NYHA class II–III symptoms and EF <30%; or with at least 3 months of medical therapy in a patient with LVEF <35%.[16] Catheter ablation has been shown to have limited success in patients with VT and NIDCM, but it is particularly successful in a small proportion of these patients when VT is related to bundle branch reentry.

VENTRICULAR TACHYCARDIA RESULTING FROM INHERITED CHANNELOPATHIES OR CONGENITAL CAUSES

This section will focus on several different genetic and congenital causes of VT and their managements. Several of these causes of VT owe their arrhythmogenicity to channelopathies and receptor protein defects.

Long QT Syndrome

Long QT syndrome is a congenital disorder, which is characterized by a prolonged QT interval (greater than 450 ms in adult males and 470 ms in adult females) on baseline ECG. Several different mutations have been identified in patients with genetic long QT syndrome involving several different subunits of potassium and sodium channel proteins. Syncope provoked by being startled, exercise, or swimming in light of previous family history of SCD and an ECG showing prolonged QT may help make this diagnosis. As the QT interval may vary throughout the day, ambulatory ECG monitoring may provide some information to help confirm the diagnosis of long QT syndrome.

As discussed earlier, long QT syndrome can lead to a specific type of VT known as TdP, which is a polymorphic VT with a characteristic twisting pattern around an isoelectric point. TdP in these patients may develop from an adrenergic response precipitated by stress, electrolyte abnormality, or drug administration. Acute management to break TdP involves intravenous administration of magnesium, regardless of serum magnesium levels. β-Blockers and ICD therapy should be used for patients who are survivors of SCD and be considered for patients with a family history of SCD.

Brugada Syndrome

Brugada Syndrome is a rare autosomal dominant disorder that is seen most commonly in the Southeast-Asian male. Mutations in cardiac sodium channels are typically responsible for this condition. Resting ECG shows a right-bundle branch–like pattern with ST-elevations in the right precordial leads. Procainamide has been used as a diagnostic challenge test because it is able to provoke patients who do not have the baseline ECG findings. With Brugada pattern ECGs, ICD therapy is treatment of choice in patients with a history of syncope and aborted sudden death to prevent future SCD. Chronic therapy involving medications such as quinidine and cilostazol have been shown to suppress VAs in these patients, but currently should be used in conjunction with ICD therapy.

Catecholaminergic Polymorphic Ventricular Tachycardia

CPVT is a rare condition that manifests within the first or second decade of life, presenting as dizziness, syncope, or even sudden death, after exercise or emotional stress. Cardiac ryanodine receptor gene and calsequestrin 2 gene mutations induce calcium release, leading to delayed after-depolarizations and triggered activity, which can lead to polymorphic ventricular tachycardia and VF; there are no characteristic baseline ECG findings. Chronic prevention recommendations include avoiding competitive sports and strenuous exercising. All adult patients without any documented VA history should be on a β-blocker. Survivors of cardiac arrest should be on β-blockers and have consideration of an ICD. In the patient who continues to have VAs despite being on a β-blocker and having an ICD, flecainide can be used for further suppression.

Hypertrophic Cardiomyopathy (HCM)

Hypertrophic Cardiomyopathy (HCM) is a relatively common genetic disorder (1 in 500) caused by several mutations involving sarcomere genes, with a multitude of clinical manifestations and hemodynamic abnormalities (LV outflow obstruction, diastolic dysfunction, myocardial ischemia, and mitral regurgitation) that are related to profound hypertrophy and myopathic processes. Signs and symptoms are variable: Some patients are asymptomatic; some may experience dyspnea, palpitations or syncope; and some may experience advanced heart failure symptoms. Current Class I recommendations for treatment of symptoms such as angina or dyspnea include β-blockers and verapamil in patients with obstructive (referring to LV outflow obstruction) or nonobstructive HCM. Phenylephrine can be used for acute hypotension in patients with obstructive HCM who do not respond to fluid administration. Current class I recommendation for patients with severe treatment-refractory symptoms and LVOT obstruction is septal reduction either surgically (myomectomy) or percutaneously (alcohol septal ablation).

This condition may predispose to developing VAs and to SCD in young persons. Patients with a high risk of SCD include those with a previous history of VF, sustained VT or other SCD events, family history of SCD events, unexplained syncope, documented NSVT on Holter monitoring, and maximal LV wall thickness greater than or equal to 30 mm. These patients should be considered for ICD implantation.[2] There is no consensus on the role of electrophysiology testing in risk stratification of asymptomatic HCM patients who do not have any of the aforementioned criteria.

Arrhythmogenic Right Ventricular Cardiomyopathy

ARVC occurs in roughly 1 in 5000 patients and is characterized pathologically by morphologic alterations caused by fibrofatty replacement of the right ventricle. ARVC is known as a cause of VAs developing after strenuous exercise, and 80% of cases are diagnosed before the age of 40. There are no specific findings on ECG, but electrocardiograms may reveal T-wave inversions in leads V1 to V3 in the presence of complete or incomplete RBBB. In addition, epsilon waves (characterized by small amplitude waves after the QRS complexes) have been seen in a large number of ECGs in patients with ARVC. With respect to pharmacologic treatment, β-blockers are reasonable recommendations, which should be added to ICD therapy if the patient has a history of frequent PVCs, NSVT, or sustained VT or VF. Patients with recurrent events should be treated with antiarrhythmic therapy and/or catheter ablation. Radiofrequency ablation in these patients can be attempted with limited success because of multiple arrhythmogenic foci.

Cardiac Sarcoidosis

Cardiac Sarcoidosis is being increasingly recognized as a cause of VTs in young patients. The involvement of cardiac muscle has been noted in 10 to 30% of patients with systemic sarcoidosis. A small proportion of these patients develop AV block and/or VT. Diagnosis is confirmed by the presence of myocardial granulomas in biopsy-proven systemic sarcoidosis. Patients with cardiac sarcoidosis and VT should get ICD. Prophylactic ICDs are indicated for patients with systemic sarcoidosis and large myocardial scar. Therapeutic options for management of recurrent VT in patients with cardiac sarcoidosis include antiarrhythmic drugs and, if need be, catheter ablation. Related to complex arrhythmia substrates, both endocardial and epicardial catheter ablation are often needed and are associated with limited success.

Other Congenital Heart Disorders (Tetralogy of Fallot and Mitral Valve Prolapse)

Tetralogy of Fallot (TOF) is a congenital heart defect classically involving four anatomic abnormalities of the heart (pulmonary stenosis, overriding aorta, ventricular septal defect, and right ventricular hypertrophy.) The prevalence of TOF in the United States is 4 to 5 in 10,000 live births. Pathophysiologically, the severity of symptoms largely depends on the degree of the RVOT obstruction. TOF itself is not responsible for VT; however, repair of the RVOT obstruction may involve scarring and patches that may provide an ideal substrate for reentry. Patients with a QRS longer than 180ms are at higher risk of developing monomorphic VT. Because of the rarity of TOF, there is a lack of strong data for specific drug treatment in VAs in patients with this condition. ICD implantation may be useful in patients with a history of sustained VT or VF. Medical therapy or catheter ablation should be considered for these patients with recurrent VT.[17]

Mitral valve prolapse (MVP) is a valvular disease affecting 2% to 3% of the general population. Proteoglycan accumulation is responsible for leaflet thickening, leading to valvular abnormality. Patients with MVP have a variety of other cardiac complications like atrial fibrillation, congestive heart failure, endocarditis, and, rarely, VAs and sudden cardiac death. The logical explanation for VT in this patient population would be LV dysfunction seen with severe mitral regurgitation. However, multiple sudden cardiac deaths have been reported in MVP patients with mild MR and normal LV function. Etiology in these cases is believed to be caused by VA. VT should be suspected in all patients with MVP who present with presyncope or syncope.

MISCELLANEOUS CAUSES OF VT

Drug-Induced VT

Several drugs may lead to life-threatening VAs. In particular, polymorphic VT and TdP may result from medications that may cause prolongation of the QT interval, leading to acquired long QT syndromes. Antiarrhythmics, macrolide and fluoroquinolone antibiotics, antiprotozoals, antipsychotics, opiates, promotility agents, antihistamines, and toxins such as arsenic are recognized to prolong QT intervals in patients and should be used judiciously in patients with preexisting long QT intervals. Apart from intrinsic properties of the aforementioned medications, electrolyte abnormalities such as hypokalemia and hypomagnesemia should be recognized as potential side effects or from drug–drug interactions.

Commotio Cordis

Translated directly from Latin, meaning "agitation of the heart," commotio cordis refers to VAs caused by chest trauma and has been recognized as a cause of SCD in young athletes. Young males are most affected, and this phenomenon has been reported in sports with physical contact (baseball, hockey, football). There is a 10 - to 30-millisecond window of the cardiac cycle (specifically in the ascending portion of the T wave), in which the heart is particularly vulnerable to mechanical trauma. When applied at the right time, even a small amount of energy can disrupt the normal sinus rhythm into VF. This should be suspected when an athlete collapses following chest trauma even when relatively mild. It is the timing of the trauma with respect to the cardiac cycle rather than force that is important for precipitation of this arrhythmia. Treatment includes immediate initiation of CPR. Availability of automatic external defibrillators on playgrounds will improve survival from commotio cordis.

REFERENCES

1. Kostis JB, McCrone K, Moreyra AE, et al. Premature ventricular complexes in the absence of identifiable heart disease. *Circulation.* 1981;63(6):1351-1356. doi:10.1161/01.CIR.63.6.1351

2. Engel G, Cho S, Ghayoumi A, et al. Prognostic significance of PVCs and resting heart rate. *Ann Noninvasive Electrocardiol.* 2007 Apr;12(2):121-129.

3. Luebbert J, Auberson D, Marchlinski F. Premature ventricular complexes in apparently normal hearts. *Card Electrophysiol Clin.* 2016 Sep;8(3):503-514. doi:10.1016/j.ccep.2016.04.001.

4. Priori SG, Blomstrom-Lundqvist C, Mazzanti A, et al. 2015 ESC guidelines for the management of patients with ventricular arrhythmias and the prevention of sudden cardiac death. *Eur Heart J.* 2015;36(41):2793.

5. Klein HU, Reek S. The MUSTT study: evaluating testing and treatment. *J Interv Card Electrophysiol.* 2000 Jan;4 Suppl1:45-50.

6. Gersh BJ, Maron BJ, Bonow RO, et al. 2011 ACCF/AHA guideline for the diagnosis and treatment of hypertrophic cardiomyopathy. *J Am Coll Cardiol.* 2011;58(25):e212-e260. doi:10.1016/j.jacc.2011.06.011.

7. Page RL, Joglar JA, Caldwell MA, et al. 2015 ACC/AHA/HRS Guideline for the management of adult patients with supraventricular tachycardia: a report of the American College of Cardiology/American Heart Association Task Force on Clinical Practice Guidelines and the Heart Rhythm Society. *J Am Coll Cardiol.* 2016;67:e27-115.

8. Alzand B, Crijns H. Diagnostic criteria of broad QRS complex tachycardia: decades of evolution. *Europace.* 2011;13:465-472.

9. Tracy CM, Epstein AE, Darbar D, et al. 2012 ACCF/AHA/HRS Focused update incorporated into the ACCF/AHA/HRS 2008 guidelines for device-based therapy of cardiac rhythm abnormalities. *J Am Coll Cardiol.* 2013;61(3):e6-e75.

10. Zipes DP, Camm AJ, Borggrefe M, et al. ACC/AHA/ESC 2006 guidelines for management of patients with ventricular arrhythmias and the prevention of sudden cardiac death. *J Am Coll Cardiol.* 2006;48(5):e247.

11. American Heart Association Guidelines for CPR & ECC 2015, Accessible at https://eccguidelines.heart.org/wp-content/uploads/2015/10/ACLS-Cardiac-Arrest-Algorithm.png

12. Badhwar N, Scheinman MM. Idiopathic ventricular tachycardia: diagnosis and management. *Curr Probl Cardiol.* 2007;32:7-43.

13. Thakur RK, Klein GJ, Sivaram et al. Anatomic substrate for idiopathic left ventricular tachycardia. *Circulation.* 1996;93:497-491.

14. Weiss JN, Nadamanee K, Stevenson WG, et al. Ventricular Arrhythmias Ventricular arrhythmias in ischemic heart disease. *Ann Intern Med.* 1991;114(9):784-797. doi:10.7326/0003-4819-114-9-784.

15. Towbin JA, Lorts A. Arrhythmias and dilated cardiomyopathy. *J Am Coll Cardiol.* 2011;57(21):2169-2171. doi:10.1016/j.jacc.2010.11.061

16. Gonzalez-Torrecilla E, Arenal A, Atienza F, et al. Current indications for implantable cardioverter defibrillators in non-ischemic cardiomyopathies and channelopathies. *Rev Recent Clin Trials.* 2015;10:111-127.

17. Folino AF, Daliento L. Arrhythmias after tetrology of fallot repair. *Indian Pacing Electrophysiol J.* 2005 Oct-Dec;5(4):312-324.

Patient and Family Information for:
VENTRICULAR ARRHYTHMIAS

WHAT IS A VENTRICULAR ARRHYTHMIA?

The heart is comprised of four chambers (two upper chambers called the left and right atria and two lower chambers called the left and right ventricles), and a coordinated sequence of electrical activation of these chambers (the atria pump first, followed by filling and pumping of the ventricles) is what allows the heart to effectively pump blood. A normal electrical sequence, also known as normal sinus rhythm, helps to generate adequate blood pressure in the arteries to deliver blood to the rest of the body and the brain. When this electrical sequence is interrupted, an arrhythmia is said to occur. Ventricular arrhythmias (VA) are disturbances of the rhythm of the heart when they originate in the lower chambers—the ventricles.

TYPES OF VENTRICULAR ARRHYTHMIAS

VA can be classified into the following categories:

1. Isolated Premature Ventricular Complexes (PVCs): These are single abnormal extra beats that originate in the ventricles.
2. Ventricular Tachycardia (VT): Refers to a longer sequence of abnormal ventricular beats, which if persistent, may be harmful to patients. VT is defined as more than 3 consecutive PVC. VT can be *nonsustained* if the patient's blood pressure remains stable, and the episode of VT is relatively short in duration (<30 seconds) or *sustained* if the patient is hemodynamically unstable and/or the episode lasts >30 seconds. VTs are typically identified on electrocardiogram (ECG) as having a rate of more than 100 bpm.
3. Ventricular Fibrillation (VF): Ventricular fibrillation happens when the ventricles quiver but do not have an orchestrated contraction, resulting in essentially no meaningful pumping activity. This leads to no circulation of blood within the body and typically leads to death if not treated promptly.

SYMPTOMS

1. Isolated PVCs and nonsustained VT (NSVT) may cause palpitations, and/or dizziness; however, some patients do not feel anything at all.
2. Sustained VT lasts for more than 30 seconds, and many patients may lose consciousness and collapse.
3. VF will lead to collapse of the patient, loss of consciousness, and death if not treated promptly.

CAUSES OF VENTRICULAR ARRHYTHMIA

VAs may occur for a variety of reasons such as structural or inherited, or even on account of other physiologic abnormalities of the body.

1. Structural heart disease:
   a. Coronary Artery Disease (CAD): Many VAs occur in the setting of blocked coronary arteries in the heart after an acute heart attack. When a heart attack occurs, scarring and dead heart tissue cause electrical disruption. This disruption develops by several different mechanisms (explained in the above chapter). VA in the setting of heart attacks may even result in sudden cardiac death.
   b. Cardiomyopathies: This is a general term to describe various diseases of the heart (which may or may not be caused by blockage of the heart vessels such as in CAD). Cardiomyopathy can lead to weakness and/or stiffness of the heart muscle. Diseases that are not caused by CAD include viral infections, thickening of heart tissues, and dilatation of the chambers of the heart.
   c. Infiltrative heart disease: There are some other medical conditions that cause inflammation and scarring of the heart and that can lead to electrical disturbances and cause VAs.
2. VA without structural heart disease: There are some congenital conditions that affect the proteins that mediate the transport of ions (sodium, potassium, and calcium) in heart cells. Improper functioning of these channels causes disruption of electrical activity and increases the chances of VA.
3. Other reversible factors: Most commonly, abnormal levels of ions such as potassium or magnesium in the blood can cause VAs. Lack of oxygen, if severe, has been known to irritate heart muscles and cause arrhythmias. Some medications, if not taken judiciously or combined with other medications, may affect different ions in the blood and lead to predisposition to VAs.

TREATMENT OPTIONS

Treatment of VA is divided into two parts. The first is to acutely treat and terminate the arrhythmia. The second is to prevent further arrhythmias from happening. Three different modalities of treatment currently exist today.

ANTIARRHYTHMIC MEDICATIONS

Antiarrhythmic medications are used to acutely treat rhythm disturbances, but may also be used to help maintain normal heart rhythms. β-blockers can slow down the heart rate and suppress the abnormal ventricular complexes. β-blockers are often used in the setting of a heart attack to help prevent VAs from happening. Traditional antiarrhythmic medications such as Amiodarone can also be used in the setting of VT—both to terminate the VT and to maintain a normal sinus rhythm. It is important to note that many antiarrhythmic medications are associated with the development of new and more severe arrhythmias, so care must be taken when given these medications to patients. Amiodarone is known to cause several side effects involving the liver, lungs, thyroid, and eyes when used chronically.

CATHETER ABLATION OF VENTRICULAR TACHYCARDIA

Patients can sometimes be taken into the electrophysiology lab and have abnormal rhythm pathways essentially destroyed. This is a rather invasive but safe procedure. During catheter ablation, abnormal electrical foci within the heart are identified by electrical stimulation. Heat energy is then delivered by a catheter to ablate/burn abnormal electrical pathways. This procedure can even be used in patients who experience a high enough burden of PVCs.

Depending on the type of disease, ablation may be extremely successful, with reported success rates of up to 95% in preventing recurrence of VAs.

Although they happen infrequently, some rare complications might occur with these procedures that include clot formation at the burn site and/or a collection of blood in the sac that surrounds the heart.

PACING AND ELECTRIC SHOCK

Devices known as implantable cardioverter defibrillators (ICDs) have been shown to reduce the death rate in patients who have experienced VT/VF or in those who are survivors of sudden cardiac death. ICDs can detect VAs and deliver two kinds of therapy that help maintain normal sinus rhythm: antitachycardia pacing (ATP) and electric shock. When a patient has VT, ATP can overdrive the pacing of the heart and slow the heart rate down. When a patient has a sustained VT or experiences VF, ICDs can deliver a shock and terminate the rhythm. This shock is similar to the therapy that is delivered by external defibrillators carried by paramedics and hospitals.

ICDs are placed in patients who have weak hearts after heart attacks, who have previously suffered cardiac arrest, or who are known to have high risks of sudden cardiac death.

Emad F. Aziz
Eyal Herzog

26

The Approach to the Patient with Syncope

Syncope is a syndrome consisting of a relatively short period of temporary and self-limited loss of consciousness caused by transient diminution of blood flow to the brain.[1,2] The term derives from the Greek word *synkoptein*, which means "to cut short,"[3] and is used to classify a common clinical problem. The incidence of self-reported syncope was 6.2 per 1000 person-years in the Framingham study, with a cumulative incidence of 3% to 6% over 10 years.[4,5] In selected patient populations, the lifetime prevalence of syncope could reach almost 50%. In the United States, 1 to 2 million patients are evaluated for syncope annually, making up 3% to 5% of emergency department visits, and 1% to 6% of urgent hospital admissions.[6]

Several guidelines have been published for the diagnostic approach to patients with syncope; however, they do not apply to every clinical situation encountered.[7,8] The European Society of Cardiology[9] and the American College of Cardiology[10] have published detailed documents specifying a classification of the principal causes of syncope (**Table 26.1**). However, given the vast differential diagnosis, the varied therapies for patients presenting with syncope and the lack of consensus guidelines, a structured approach to the management of these patients was needed. To address this issue, we developed a standardized pathway which is comprehensive, yet simple, and provides guidelines for the management of all patients presenting with syncope[11] (**Figure 26.1**).

INITIAL ASSESSMENT OF A PATIENT WITH SYNCOPE

The initial assessment of a patient with syncope includes a meticulous and comprehensive medical history; incorporating eyewitness accounts can help determine the cause of syncope (**Table 26.2**).[7] Important questions to be asked in assessing patients with syncope are listed in **Table 26.3**. Orthostatic hypotension and autonomic dysfunction can be identified by measuring blood pressure and pulse rate in the upper and lower extremities in the supine and upright positions. A 12-lead electrocardiogram (ECG) and basic laboratory tests, including a basic metabolic panel and complete blood count, should be performed in all patients with syncope.

DEFINITION OF TRUE SYNCOPE

We use the acronym **SELF-1** which reflects the four criteria that should be met for an event to be considered true syncope. These criteria include

S—**S**hort period, self-limited, spontaneous recovery
E—**E**arly-rapid onset

L—**L**oss of consciousness—transient
F—**F**ull recovery—fall
Patients who did not lose consciousness are defined as "not true syncope."

CLASSIFICATION OF SYNCOPE WHEN THERE IS A CERTAIN OR SUSPECTED DIAGNOSIS

These are certain disorders causing true syncope with a transient loss of consciousness:

1. *Reflex syncope:* Reflex syncope is a neurally mediated reflex syndrome[12] in the absence of structural heart disease. It refers to a reflex that, when triggered, gives rise to vasodilatation and bradycardia. These triggers include fear, pain, instrumentation, blood phobias, prolonged standing, crowded warm places, nausea, vomiting, and abdominal pain.

2. *Orthostatic hypotension syncope:* In orthostatic hypotension syncope, syncope occurs with assumption of an upright position. It can occur after starting of medications that can lead to hypotension, or can be due to an autonomic neuropathy.[13] Volume depletion is an important cause of orthostatic hypotension.

3. *Cardiovascular disease:* Structural heart disease can cause syncope when circulatory demands outweigh the impaired ability of the heart to increase its output. Cardiac arrhythmia can cause a decrease in cardiac output, which usually occurs irrespective of circulatory demands.

RISK STRATIFICATION FOR ADMISSION

One of the main dilemmas that face emergency department physicians is whether to admit patients to the hospital or to refer them for an outpatient evaluation. Many risk assessment scores have been developed. These include the San Francisco Syncope Rule (SFSR),[14] the *Osservatorio Epidemiologico della Sincopenel Lazio* (OESIL),[15] and the Evaluation of Guidelines in Syncope Study (EGSYS).[16] In all of these risk scores, there is a consensus to admit patients with abnormal ECG, hypotension, heart failure, and anemia. In our standardized SELF pathway,[11] we use the **SELF-2** criteria to evaluate the need for admission. These criteria include

S—**S**tructural heart disease
E—abnormal **E**CG
L—atrial f**L**utter
F—atrial **F**ibrillation

TABLE 26.1	Classification of the Principle Causes of Syncope (Adapted from the European Society of Cardiology guidelines[9])

Reflex (neurally mediated) syncope
- Vasovagal:
  - Mediated by emotional distress: fear, pain, instrumentation, blood phobia
  - Mediated by orthostatic stress
- Situational:
  - Cough, sneeze
  - Gastrointestinal stimulation (swallow, defecation, visceral pain)
  - Micturition (post micturition)
  - Post exercise
  - Postprandial
- Carotid sinus syncope

Syncope due to orthostatic hypotension
- Primary autonomic failure:
  - Pure autonomic failure, Parkinson disease with autonomic failure, dementia
- Secondary autonomic failure:
  - Diabetes, amyloidosis, uremia, spinal cord injuries
- Drug-induced orthostatic hypotension:
  - Alcohol, vasodilators, diuretics, phenothiazine, antidepressants
- Volume depletion:
  - Hemorrhage, diarrhea, vomiting

Cardiac syncope (cardiovascular)
- Arrhythmia as primary cause:
  - Bradycardia:
    - Sinus node dysfunction (including bradycardia/tachycardia syndrome)
    - AV conduction system disease
    - Implanted device malfunction
  - Tachycardia:
    - Supraventricular
    - Ventricular (idiopathic, secondary to structural heart disease or to channelopathies)
  - Drug-induced bradycardia and tachyarrhythmias
- Structural disease:
  - Cardiac: cardiac valvular disease, acute myocardial infarction/ischemia
  - Hypertrophic cardiomyopathy, cardiac masses (atrial myxoma, tumors)
  - Pericardial disease/tamponade, congenital anomalies of coronary arteries, prosthetic valve dysfunction
- Others: pulmonary embolus, acute aortic dissection, pulmonary hypertension

AV, atrioventricular.

Admitted patients should be monitored for a minimum of 24 hours, which could potentially reveal bradyarrhythmias or tachyarrhythmias. The management of bradyarrhythmias may include an electrophysiologic testing with or without subsequent pacemaker implantation. Tachyarrhythmias include ventricular tachycardia, supraventricular tachycardia, atrial fibrillation, and atrial flutter. The treatment for these patients may include radiofrequency ablation or a device therapy with a pacemaker or an implantable cardioverter defibrillator (ICD). We recommend that all patients with a diagnosis of cardiac syncope be evaluated by an electrophysiologist during their hospitalization.

MANAGEMENT OF CARDIAC SYNCOPE

The major goal of the evaluation of syncope in patients with heart disease is to identify a potentially life-threatening diagnosis, particularly arrhythmias. Workup and management of these patients can include medical therapy, stress testing with cardiac imaging, cardiac catheterization, and possible revascularization with a percutaneous coronary intervention or cardiac surgery.

DIAGNOSTIC TOOLS THAT AID IN THE MANAGEMENT OF CARDIAC SYNCOPE

Electrocardiogram

Electrocardiography is essential in the workup of patients with unexplained syncope; however, it may only reveal a direct cause in 5% of patients. Abnormal ECGs include the following findings: sinus bradycardia resulting from sinus node dysfunction or atrioventricular (AV) block resulting from AV node or His-Purkinje system dysfunction, pre-excitation patterns, a long/short QT-interval, Brugada syndrome, and characteristic ECG features of arrhythmogenic right ventricular dysplasia. Patients with unexplained bradycardia (heart rate of < 50 beats/min) should be evaluated for potential medical causes, specifically hypovolemia, hypoxia, acidosis, hypoglycemia, and hypothermia. Mild hyperkalemia when combined with a low *glomerular filtration rate* can also potentiate cardiac syncope in the elderly.[17] Hypothyroidism should also be considered in this age group.

Marked bradycardia can be the result of many medications such as β-blockers, calcium channel blockers, and digoxin, particularly in the presence of renal disease; this should be assessed and managed promptly. Lyme disease can be an unusual cause of heart block and needs to be considered in a patient from an endemic area. Finally, heart block can be a manifestation of myocardial infarction (MI), and patients with acute anterior wall MI and Mobitz type-II second-degree AV block, have a class IIa indication for a temporary transvenous pacing. This is in contrast to patients with inferior wall MI, where heart block can be a manifestation of the Bezold–Jarisch reflex (*this is a cardiovascular decompressor reflex involving a marked increase in vagal efferent discharge to the heart, elicited by stimulation of chemoreceptors, primarily in the left ventricle*). It causes a slowing of the heart beat and dilatation of the peripheral blood vessels with resultant lowering of the blood pressure. In patients with inferior wall MI, the heart block usually has a narrow escape rhythm and it usually resolves within a few days.

Echocardiography

Echocardiography should be performed in all patients with true syncope because it can identify patients with critical aortic stenosis, aortic dissection, severe pulmonary hypertension, acute pulmonary embolism, left atrial myxoma, and pericardial tamponade—situations that can lead to obstruction of flow in

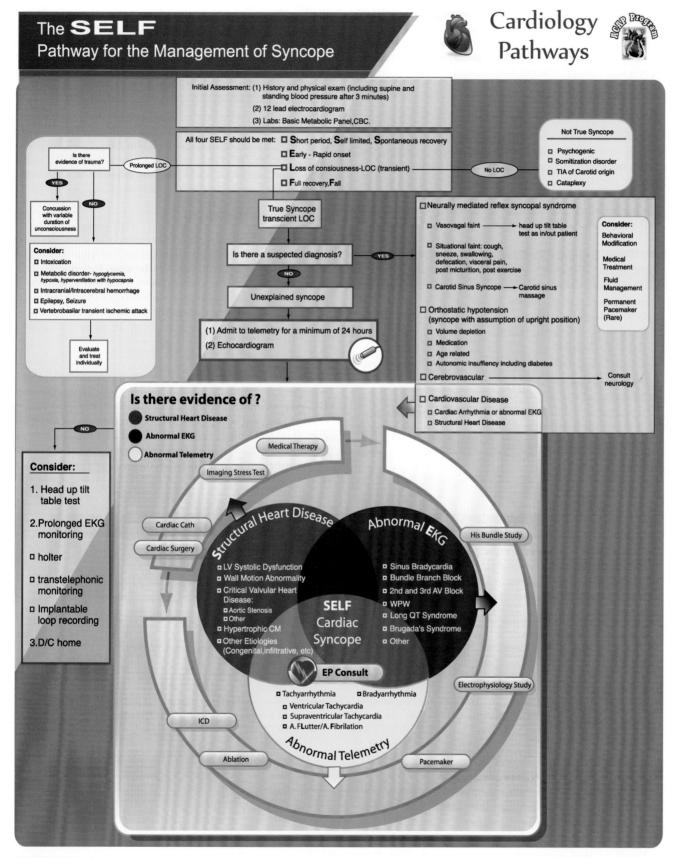

FIGURE 26.1 The SELF pathway for the management of syncope. CBC, complete blood count; ECG, electrocardiogram; EP, electrophysiologic; ICD. implantable cardioverter defibrillator; TIA, transient ischemic attack; WPW, Wolff–Parkinson–White.

the heart and cause syncope.[18] These patients tend to be seriously ill and may require a lengthy intensive care stay. Echocardiography is considered the gold standard diagnostic tool for the finding of hypertrophic cardiomyopathy, segmental wall motion abnormalities suggestive of ischemic heart disease, and left ventricular systolic dysfunction.

Holter Monitoring

Holter monitoring enables correlation of symptoms with episodes of bradycardia; diagnostic clues are obtained in 50% to 70% of patients with bradycardia suspected on clinical grounds. However, events can be missed if symptoms do not occur in the 24- to 48-hour monitoring period. Holter monitoring can reveal sinus pauses, sinus arrest, second- or third-degree AV block, or severe sinus bradycardia with symptoms. Nocturnal asymptomatic

TABLE 26.2	Initial Assessment of a Patient with Syncope

For every patient presenting with syncope:
   Detailed history
   Comprehensive physical examination
   Standard 12-lead ECG
   Basic labs (including basic metabolic panel, complete blood count)

For all admitted patients (when appropriate):
   Echocardiogram
   In-hospital 24-h telemetry monitoring (out-of-hospital telemetry may be applicable where available)
   Neurologic evaluation

ECG, electrocardiogram.

bradycardia and pauses are not uncommon in the normal heart and are probably nondiagnostic. First-degree AV block or Mobitz type I AV block may be noted while patients are asleep owing to a high vagal tone. A long-monitored strip should be obtained because a 2:1 AV block is unlikely to persist. The other forms of AV block (Mobitz I or II) should then become apparent. Monitoring while the patient performs some form of exertion (eg, arm exercise, standing, and walking) may also help demonstrate the level of block. A block at the level of the AV node should improve with the adrenergic stimulation, but a block below the AV node in the His-Purkinje system may worsen as AV nodal conduction improves and increases the frequency of inputs to the His-Purkinje system.

Cardiac Event Monitoring

Cardiac event monitors, particularly those with auto-triggering capability, are widely used in the diagnosis of symptomatic and asymptomatic bradycardia and can be worn for up to 30 days. These devices can detect sinus pauses, sinus arrest, second- or third-degree AV block, or severe sinus bradycardia with symptoms[19]; however, their diagnostic yield for syncope and presyncope is only 6% to 25%.[20,21]

Exercise Testing

A subnormal increase in heart rate after exercise (*chronotropic incompetence*) can be useful in diagnosing sick sinus syndrome. However, sensitivity and specificity are unclear and the results obtained may not be reproducible.[22] Exercise-induced AV block, even if asymptomatic, can be significant and suggests disease of the His-Purkinje system. Identifying symptoms due to sinus bradycardia can be difficult; nonetheless, exercise testing can

TABLE 26.3	Important Questions That Can Be Asked in Assessing Patients with Syncope

Questions about situations before syncope
- Position (supine, sitting, or standing)
- Activity (rest, change in posture, during or after exercise, during or immediately after urination, defecation, cough, or swallowing)
- Predisposing factors (crowded or warm places, prolonged standing, postprandial period) and precipitating events (fear, intense pain, neck movements)

Questions about onset of syncope
- Nausea, vomiting, abdominal discomfort, feeling of cold, sweating, pain in neck or shoulders, blurred vision, dizziness
- Trauma

Questions for eyewitness
- Way of falling (slumping forward, backward, or kneeling over), skin color (pallor, cyanosis, flushing), duration of loss of consciousness, breathing pattern (snoring), movements (seizure-like) and their duration, onset of movement in relation to fall, tongue biting

Questions after the episode
- Nausea, vomiting, sweating, feeling of cold, confusion, muscle aches, skin color, injury, chest pain, palpitations, urinary or fecal incontinence

Questions about past family and medical history
- Family history of sudden death, congenital arrhythmogenic heart disease or fainting
- Previous cardiac disease (coronary artery disease, heart failure)
- Neurologic history (epilepsy, narcolepsy)
- Metabolic disorders (diabetes, hypo or hyperthyroidism)
- Medication (antihypertensive, antianginal, antiarrhythmic, diuretics, and QT prolonging agents)
- In instance of recurrent syncope, information on recurrences such as the time from the first syncopal episode and on the number of spells

be useful to help determine sinus node dysfunction as the cause of symptoms.

Electrophysiologic Testing

Electrophysiology testing is recommended when symptoms cannot be correlated clearly with a syncopal event and when significant bradyarrhythmias are suspected but cannot be diagnosed by noninvasive modalities. Sinus node dysfunction (*diagnosed as sinus node recovery time more than 1600 to 2000 milliseconds and/or corrected sinus node recovery time over 525 milliseconds*) serve only as an adjunct to clinical and noninvasive parameters because these tests are based on assumptions that limit their validity and clinical utility. There is little utility for electrophysiology testing in already-documented second- and third-degree AV block. Testing can be useful in patients with AV block and no clear symptom association; in patients with symptoms of bradycardia in whom AV block is suspected but not documented; and when the site of AV block cannot be determined reliably by surface tracings. His-ventricle interval of over *100 milliseconds* in a patient with bradycardia, even in the absence of symptoms, is a high-risk finding. Asymptomatic patients with Mobitz II AV block may benefit from this test to localize the site of block and to guide therapy. Overall, the role of electrophysiologic testing for bradycardia is limited, owing to low sensitivity and specificity. Positive findings may not be the reason for patient symptoms.[23]

MANAGEMENT OF PATIENTS WITH UNEXPLAINED SYNCOPE BUT WITH NO EVIDENCE OF CARDIAC ETIOLOGY

In the absence of underlying heart disease, syncope is not associated with excess mortality. Our recommendation for these patients is for early discharge, with consideration of head-up tilt-table testing and prolonged ECG monitoring (including Holter monitoring, trans-telephonic monitoring, and implantable loop recording).

OUTPATIENT DIAGNOSTIC TOOLS

Tilt-Table Testing

Tilt-table testing is used to evaluate the adequacy of the autonomic system, especially when there is suspicion of neurocardiogenic syncope.[24] The test can be performed either using head-upright tilting, which causes dependent venous pooling and thereby provokes the autonomic response, or by using adenosine to facilitate the induction of vasovagal syncope. However, this test is limited by its poor sensitivity and the lack of uniformity.

Implantable Loop Monitor

Implantable loop recorders (ILRs) are subcutaneous monitoring devices that are typically implanted in the left parasternal or pectoral region and used for the detection of cardiac arrhythmias (**Figure 26.2**). The monitor has a loop memory and a battery life of 3 to 4 years. The current versions store an ECG that includes tracings recorded up to 40 minutes before and 2 minutes after activation by the patient and up to 7 hours of abnormal rhythm. If the patient activates the device when his consciousness returns, the probability of demonstrating a correlation between the ECG signals and the syncope is high. Krahn et al.[25] were among the first to describe a high diagnostic yield of the ILR

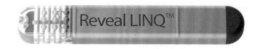

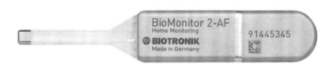

FIGURE 26.2 Example of commercially available implantable loop recorder; Reveal (Medtronic), Biomonitor II (Biotronik).

in 16 patients with recurrent syncope. Extensive investigations including electrophysiology studies, treadmill testing, 48-hour ambulatory monitoring, and tilt-table testing failed to obtain a definite diagnosis in these patients. In 94% of the cases, recurrent syncope had occurred after implantation of the device revealing an arrhythmogenic cause in 60%. Consequently, in 40% of these patients, no arrhythmias were detected. In all patients with an arrhythmogenic cause, successful therapy was implemented. The Place of Reveal in the Care Pathway and Treatment of Patients with Unexplained Recurrent Syncope (*PICTURE*) registry,[26] a prospective, multicenter, observational study that followed up 570 patients with recurrent unexplained presyncope or syncope who received an ILR, showed that these patients were evaluated on average by three different specialists and underwent a median of 13 nondiagnostic tests (ranges between 9 and 20). Within the first year, syncope recurred in a third of the patients; the ILR provided a diagnosis in 78% of the patients, most commonly a cardiac etiology. In addition, the remote capability of these loops has revolutionized management for patients with syncope, as the patient is monitored continuously 24 hours a day, 7 days a week, and any abnormality is automatically transmitted through the Internet to the caring physician who then can take an action for management (**Figure 26.3**).

Figure 26.3 demonstrates a long pause in a young patient who was mistakenly diagnosed as having seizure for a long time. A long sinus pause of 12 seconds is seen and was transmitted by the ILR.

Clinical validation of the SELF pathway from a database of 3100 patients who were followed up longitudinally at our institution showed that this novel pathway is comprehensive, yet simple and provides effective risk stratification for patients presenting to the hospital with unexplained syncope and even with patients who could be missed by the standard risk stratification scores.[27] Also, implementing this pathway predicts the short- and long-term outcomes for those patients.[28]

CONCLUSION

In summary, having a standardized protocol for the management of patients with unexplained syncope should begin with a thorough medical history and a detailed physical examination including basic laboratory testing. High-risk patients (meeting SELF-2 criteria) should be admitted for at least 24-hour monitoring and echocardiography evaluation. Low-risk patients do not require hospital admission and they can be evaluated as outpatients with tilt-table testing or with a prolonged monitoring including ILR.

ECG Detail: *Pause (ID# 18)*, 15-Nov-2016

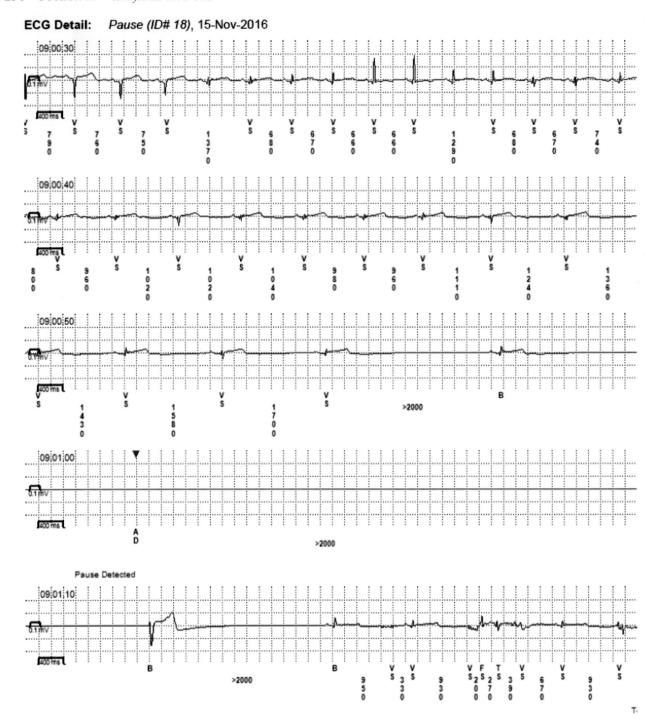

FIGURE 26.3 A long pause in a young patient who was mistakenly diagnosed with seizure for a long time. A long sinus pause of 12 seconds is seen and was transmitted by the implanted loop recorder.

REFERENCES

1. Brignole M, Alboni P, Benditt DG, et al. Guidelines on management (diagnosis and treatment) of syncope-update 2004. Executive Summary. *Eur Heart J.* 2004;25(22):2054-2072.

2. Brignole M, Alboni P, Benditt DG, et al. [Guidelines on management (diagnosis and treatment) of syncope. Update 2004. Executive summary]. *Rev Esp Cardiol.* 2005;58(2):175-193.

3. Soteriades ES, Evans JC, Larson MG, et al. Incidence and prognosis of syncope. *N Engl J Med.* 2002;347(12):878-885.

4. Savage DD, Corwin L, McGee DL, et al. Epidemiologic features of isolated syncope: the Framingham study. *Stroke.* 1985;16(4):626-629.

5. Chen L, Chen MH, Larson MG, et al. Risk factors for syncope in a community-based sample (the Framingham heart study). *Am J Cardiol.* 2000;85(10):1189-1193.

6. Shen WK, Decker WW, Smars PA, et al. Syncope Evaluation in the Emergency Department Study (SEEDS): a multidisciplinary approach to syncope management. *Circulation.* 2004;110(24):3636-3645.

7. Linzer M, Yang EH, Estes NA, 3rd, et al. Diagnosing syncope. Part 1: Value of history, physical examination, and electrocardiography. Clinical Efficacy Assessment Project of the American College of Physicians. *Ann Intern Med.* 1997;126(12):989-996.

8. Linzer M, Yang EH, Estes NA, 3rd, et al. Diagnosing syncope. Part 2: Unexplained syncope. Clinical Efficacy Assessment Project of the American College of Physicians. *Ann Intern Med.* 1997;127(1):76-86.

9. Moya A, Sutton R, Ammirati F, et al. The task force for the diagnosis and management of syncope of the european society of cardiology (ESC). Guidelines for the diagnosis and management of syncope (version 2009). *Eur Heart J.* 2009;30:2631-2671.

10. Strickberger SA, Benson DW, Biaggioni I, et al. AHA/ACCF scientific statement on the evaluation of syncope: from the American Heart Association Councils on Clinical Cardiology, Cardiovascular Nursing, Cardiovascular Disease in the Young, and Stroke, and the Quality of Care and Outcomes Research Interdisciplinary Working Group; and the American College of Cardiology Foundation In Collaboration with the Heart Rhythm Society. *J Am Coll Cardiol.* 2006;47(2):473-484.

11. Herzog E, Frankenberger O, Pierce W, et al. The SELF pathway for the management of syncope. *Crit Pathways Cardiol.* 2006;5(3):173-178.

12. Sheldon R, Rose S, Connolly S, et al. Diagnostic criteria for vasovagal syncope based on a quantitative history. *Eur Heart J.* 2006;27(3):344-350.

13. Pont M, Froment R. Essential orthostatic hypotension persisting for 25 years; syncope during defecation and post-syncopal obnubilation. *Lyon Med.* 1950;183(50):389-390.

14. Quinn JV, Stiell IG, McDermott DA, et al. Derivation of the San Francisco Syncope Rule to predict patients with short-term serious outcomes. *Ann Emerg Med.* 2004;43(2):224-232.

15. Ammirati F, Colivicchi F, Minardi G, et al. The management of syncope in the hospital: the OESIL study (Osservatorio Epidemiologico della Sincope nel Lazio). *G Ital Cardiol.* 1999;29(5):533-539.

16. Del Rosso A, Ungar A, Maggi R, et al. Clinical predictors of cardiac syncope at initial evaluation in patients referred urgently to a general hospital: The EGSYS score. *Heart.* 2008;94(12):1620-1626.

17. Aziz EF, Javed F, Korniyenko A, et al. Mild hyperkalemia and low eGFR a tedious recipe for cardiac disaster in the elderly: an unusual reversible cause of syncope and heart block. *Heart Int.* 2011;6(2):e12.

18. Recchia D, Barzilai B. Echocardiography in the evaluation of patients with syncope. *J Gen Intern Med.* 1995;10(12):649-655.

19. Sivakumaran S, Krahn AD, Klein GJ, et al. A prospective randomized comparison of loop recorders versus Holter monitors in patients with syncope or presyncope. *Am J Med.* 2003;115(1):1-5.

20. Fogel RI, Evans JJ, Prystowsky EN. Utility and cost of event recorders in the diagnosis of palpitations, presyncope, and syncope. *Am J Cardiol.* 1997;79(2):207-208.

21. Zimetbaum P, Kim KY, Ho KK, et al. Utility of patient-activated cardiac event recorders in general clinical practice. *Am J Cardiol.* 1997;79(3):371-372.

22. Kosinski D, Grubb BP, Karas BJ, et al. Exercise-induced neurocardiogenic syncope: Clinical data, pathophysiological aspects, and potential role of tilt table testing. *Europace.* 2000;2(1):77-82.

23. DiMarco JP. Value and limitations of electrophysical testing for syncope. *Cardiol Clin.* 1997;15(2):219-232.

24. Benditt DG, Ferguson DW, Grubb BP, et al. Tilt table testing for assessing syncope. American College of Cardiology. *J Am Coll Cardiol.* 1996;28(1):263-275.

25. Krahn AD, Klein GJ, Yee R, et al. Use of an extended monitoring strategy in patients with problematic syncope. Reveal Investigators. *Circulation.* 1999;99(3):406-410.

26. Edvardsson N, Frykman V, van Mechelen R, et al. Use of an implantable loop recorder to increase the diagnostic yield in unexplained syncope: results from the PICTURE registry. *Europace.* 2011;13(2):262-269.

27. Aziz EF, Pamidimukala CK, Park T, et al. A novel SELF-pathway for management of patients presenting with unexplained-syncope appropriately identify high risk patients as validated by the OESIL score. *Cardiovasc Qual Outcomes.* 2012;5:A225.

28. Aziz EF, Pamidimukala C, Bastawrose J, et al. Short and long term outcomes of patients admitted with unexplained syncope using a simple novel SELF-pathway. *Cardiovasc Qual Outcomes.* 2012;5:A52.

Patient and Family Information for: THE APPROACH TO THE PATIENT WITH SYNCOPE

Syncope (sin-co-pee) is a medical term used to describe a temporary loss of consciousness that is caused by a sudden lack of blood flow to the brain. Syncope is commonly called fainting or "passing out." If an individual is about to faint, he or she will feel dizzy, lightheaded, or nauseated and his field of vision may "white out" or "black out." The skin may be cold and clammy. After fainting, an individual may be unconscious for a short time, but will eventually return to his baseline. Syncope can occur in otherwise healthy people and affects all age groups, but it is more common among the elderly. It can occur in many situations, such as standing up fast, working or playing hard especially in hot weather, breathing too fast (called hyperventilating), being upset, during long standing, during coughing, urinating, or all other situations that get in the way of the flow of oxygen to the brain.

There are several types of syncope. Vasovagal syncope usually has an easily identifiable triggering event such as emotional stress, trauma, pain, the sight of blood, or prolonged standing. Carotid sinus syncope is a medical term used for a situation in which there is pressure on the carotid artery in the neck and this may occur after turning the head, while shaving, or even when wearing a tight collar. Situational syncope is the term used when syncope occurs with urination, defecation, coughing, or as a result of gastrointestinal stimulation. Syncope is not usually a primary sign of a neurologic disorder, but it may indicate an increased risk for some neurologic disorders such as Parkinson disease, diabetic neuropathy, and other types of neuropathy. Certain medicines can cause fainting, including diuretics, calcium channel blockers, angiotensin-converting enzyme inhibitors, nitrates, antipsychotic medications, antihistamines, levodopa, and narcotics. Alcohol, cocaine, and marijuana can also cause fainting.

INITIAL EVALUATION OF A PATIENT WITH SYNCOPE

A doctor would like to know what exactly happened when the person fainted and all the details about how he or she felt. Symptoms vary from patient to patient; however, the most common symptoms are light headedness, dizziness, and nausea. Some people will feel very hot and clammy, sweaty, and will complain of visual and hearing disturbances. Information about current medications and preexisting medical conditions such as diabetes, heart disease, or psychiatric illness can help pinpoint the cause of syncope. There are certain tests and procedures that might be ordered to help guide management. These tests might lead the physician to a definitive diagnosis and would guide treatment.

PHYSICAL EXAMINATION AND LABORATORY TESTING

The doctor will compare the heart rate and blood pressure while the patient is lying down with the heart rate and blood pressure in a standing position. The doctor will listen to the heart beats for abnormal sounds that can be present in conditions such as narrowing of the aortic valve. The doctor will listen for *bruit* in the sides of the neck to rule out narrowing of the neck arteries (called carotid arteries). The doctor may firmly massage the carotid artery while the heart rate is closely monitored with an ECG. The heart's response to this maneuver can give clues to the cause of the syncope.

Laboratory tests may identify low red blood cell count (*anemia*) or other abnormalities including thyroid abnormalities and electrolyte imbalances (sodium, potassium, glucose, and magnesium).

ADDITIONAL DIAGNOSTIC TESTS

ELECTROCARDIOGRAM

An ECG will be performed on arrival. Sticky pads will be placed on the chest, arms, and legs, and will be connected to a recording device with long, thin cables. This is not a painful procedure and there is no risk involved. The ECG provides a picture of the electrical activity throughout the heart muscle. A normal ECG does not necessarily mean that syncope is not caused by a heart rhythm problem. Heart rhythm problems are often brief, intermittent, and may not be present at the moment when the ECG is performed.

TILT-TABLE TESTING

Tilt-table testing is a noninvasive test performed to diagnose recurrent or unexplained light headedness or fainting spells. The test can define whether a patient has a condition called vasovagal syncope, in which there is malfunction of nerves that causes the heart to slow down and the blood pressure to drop with a change in position. The test takes about an hour to complete, and in preparation for it the patient would be asked not to eat or drink for 5 hours before the test including holding the medications. The patient will be asked to lie down on a special flat table. A nurse will insert an intravenous line in a vein in the arm. ECG electrodes will be attached to the chest to monitor the heart rate and the rhythm during the procedure. A blood pressure cuff will be placed on the arm. Safety straps will secure the patient to the table. After obtaining the blood pressure and ECG while lying on the table, the table will be tilted to a 60-degree angle. The patient will be standing on a footboard at the bottom of the table. The blood pressure and ECG will be monitored as the patient remains tilted up for 20 to 30 minutes. The patient will be instructed to tell the nurse if any symptoms, such as feeling sweaty, nauseous, lightheaded, or cold and clammy, are experienced. If the blood pressure starts to fall, the patient will be returned to the flat position. A doctor will be in the room during the entire procedure. If no symptoms are experienced, the table will be lowered to the flat position and the test will be terminated. On occasion, a short-acting medication may be given intravenously to assist in the test. The patient may need to rest for several minutes after the test before going home. A nurse will stay with the patient until the conditions for discharge are met.

ELECTROPHYSIOLOGY STUDY

An electrophysiology study is an invasive procedure performed in the hospital setting. Sedative medications are given before the procedure, but the patient may stay awake during the procedure. The physician uses a local anesthetic to numb a small area over the blood vessels (veins), usually in the groin, and then threads small catheters (thin electrical wires) through the blood vessels into the heart using X-ray (fluoroscopic) guidance. Once in the heart, precise measurements of the heart's electrical function can be obtained. This procedure typically lasts 60 to 90 minutes.

IMPLANTABLE LOOP RECORDER

With ILR, the heart rate and rhythm can be monitored for a long time. The device has a memory and a battery that can last between 3 and 4 years. The ILR is implanted under the skin, usually in the upper left chest area. It stores events automatically according to programmed criteria, or it can be activated by the patient. The ILR may be useful if symptoms are sporadic and an arrhythmia is suspected, and other forms of testing were negative or inconclusive.

THERAPIES

PERMANENT PACEMAKER

A pacemaker is a small device, the size of a silver dollar, which is implanted under the skin just below the collarbone. The device is connected to wires threaded into the heart muscle, where they emit impulses that help regulate the heartbeat. Pacemakers are occasionally recommended if the syncope is caused by a very slow heartbeat, carotid sinus hypersensitivity, or by heart block. A pacemaker battery typically lasts 8 to 12 years and would require replacement after that time period with a simple procedure.

IMPLANTABLE CARDIOVERTER DEFIBRILLATOR

Certain dangerous conditions arise when irregular heartbeats originate from the lower chamber of the heart (ventricles), particularly in patients with a very weak heart. These patients may benefit from an ICD. Similar to a pacemaker, the ICD is typically implanted under the skin just below the collarbone. The device is connected to wires threaded into the heart muscle. However, in addition to its pacemaker capability, the ICD has the ability to detect fatal arrhythmias and deliver a high-energy electrical shock to the heart, which in turn will terminate the arrhythmia and return the heart to normal rhythm.

Emad F. Aziz
Nektarios Souvaliotis

27

Basic Approach to Pacemaker and ICD Interrogation

INTRODUCTION

Cardiovascular implantable electronic device (CIED) is a term that encompasses pacemakers (PPM) for bradyarrhythmia treatment, implantable cardioverter defibrillators (ICD) for tachyarrhythmia management, and cardiac resynchronization therapy (CRT) devices for systolic dysfunction with conduction delays.[1] Cardiac arrhythmias have an estimated prevalence of 14.4 million patients in the United States, and they account for approximately 40,700 deaths annually.[2] As the indications for device placement continue to expand, these devices have evolved from a treatment of last resort to a first-line therapy to an increasing number of patients.[3] Approximately 1.6 million patients in the United States and Europe receive a PPM or ICD each year. Therefore, it is imperative that all physicians understand the operational basics of these devices and be able to retrieve and manage essential data when needed particularly in the critical care hospital setting.

A summary of the most updated pacing and defibrillator indications are seen in **Figures 27.1 and 27.2**.

EVALUATION OF CIED ON ADMISSION AND REASON FOR CONSULTATION

When called for a device evaluation consultation, it is imperative to identify the reason for the consult. This may include the evaluation for device functionality such as appropriate pacing and sensing, particularly if there is any question of device malfunction, or to identify arrhythmias like atrial fibrillation or ventricular tachycardia, or to rule out device-delivered therapy like antitachycardia therapy or firing. Device interrogation could also be appropriate after surgery, especially if device parameters were changed or cautery was used close to the device site.

IDENTIFICATION OF THE DEVICE MAKER

The first step is to identify the manufacturer of the device and the type of the device in order to utilize the proper programmer for the interrogation. Most patients carry a device identification card with them (**Figure 27.3**). If the card is not available, searching the

patients' electronic medical records or manufacturers' patient registries can be of help. **Table 27.1** has the phone numbers for major device companies.

In those instances where none of the above are available, or if the patient is incoherent or intubated, one can identify the device from the CaRDIA-X algorithm (**Figure 27.4**) published by Jacob et al.[4] or the CRMD Finder app (**Figure 27.5**), which is based on the same source. This guide is unique as it utilizes a stepwise algorithm including device-specific radiopaque alphanumeric codes (ANC), device type (ICD, pacemaker, or ILR), the shape of the device, and the battery as well as the device leads. Currently in the United States, five major device manufacturers can be identified: Medtronic, St. Jude Medical, Boston Scientific, Biotronik, and Sorin.

Once the device maker is identified, one should examine the x-ray for the following:

1. Identify device type: ILR, pacemaker, or ICD
2. If ILR, identify either Medtronic Linq, Transoma, or Biotronik (BioMonitor–II)
3. Identify if the device is a single, dual-chamber, or biventricular one
4. Epicardial leads or arrays
5. Recognize any further potential malfunctions like lead fractures, conductor externalization (Riata leads), dislodgment, twiddler syndrome, or any abandoned leads

After identifying the device manufacturer, the next step is to use the appropriate programmer and link it to the device by placing the wand at the device site. **Figure 27.6** illustrates the programmers of the five major device companies in the United States.

ANALYZING THE PATIENTS' RHYTHM

1. Obtain presenting rhythm strip:
   a. After the summary screen has been displayed, press the "25 mm" button on the programmer to print a presenting rhythm strip.
   b. Press the "0 mm" button to stop printing.
   c. This step will identify if the patient is (atrial, ventricular, or biventricular) paced.

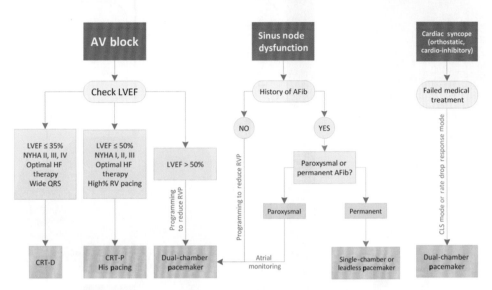

FIGURE 27.1 Class I pacing indications according to the published guidelines. AFib: atrial fibrillation; CLS: closed-loop system; HF: heart failure; LVEF: left ventricular ejection fraction; NYHA: New York Heart Association Class; RVP: right ventricular pacing.

2. Obtain underlying rhythm strip:
   a. In this step, one must go to the Temporary Pacing Parameters screen. The Temporary Parameters screen allows you to change any and all pacing parameters in a temporary setting—without affecting any permanent settings.
   b. Suggested Settings to view intrinsic rhythm: Mode: DDI; Rate: 30 bpm (if tolerated by patient); AV Delay: 300 ms (400 ms, if allowed); "DDI will allow backup ventricular pacing if needed, and allow you to see heart block by separating Atrial and Ventricular pacing function—and AV Delays greater than 300 ms. You must assess patient's ability to tolerate lower rate change prior to running test."
   c. Run paper (press the 25-mm button) to document underlying rhythm. Press the "0 mm" button to stop printing.

INTERROGATION AND REPORTING

After placing the wand over the device, interrogation will either automatically begin or need to be initiated by pressing the interrogate button, depending on the programmer. At the end of the chapter, the appendix depicts examples from the initial page of each programmer with description of their most important functions.

BATTERY LIFE

Most device manufacturer will have a battery management screen that displays a battery "gauge," voltage graph, voltage, and/or estimated longevity (**Figure 27.7**). There are few abbreviations that one needs to be familiar with when evaluating a battery status; ***ERI*** (elective replacement indicator), ***RRT*** (recommended replacement time), ***EOS*** (end of service), and ***EOL*** (end of life). The general rule of thumb is that *ERI* is about three months before reaching *EOL*.

What to Do When ERI is Reached?

In Brady Devices (Pacemakers)

- Use all the available data, voltage, battery impedance, longevity predictors.
- Manufacturers can give accurate predictions with access to telemetry data.
- Look at follow-up intervals as ERI approaches; consider use of remote monitoring and consider changes at ERI (VVI).
- Have access to technical data; be aware of safety margins and errors in prediction.

In Tachy Devices (Defibrillators)

- Use remote monitoring to manage battery Middle of Life 2 (MOL2) → ERI period.
- Ensure patient is familiar with alarms/vibrations indicating ERI.
- Check advisories for changes in ERI point of some devices.
- Longer charge time usually indicates battery depletion; a charge time in excess of 20 seconds is abnormal.

SENSING TESTING

The ability of a pacemaker lead to sense an intrinsic electrical signal of the chamber that it is placed in is measured in millivolts (mV). The programmed sensitivity setting indicates the minimum intracardiac signal that will be sensed (seen) by the pacemaker to initiate the pacemaker response (inhibited or triggered). It is important to evaluate the trend of sensing of the chamber overtime rather than the actual sensed value of the (P) or (R) waves (**Figure 27.8**). There are certain conditions that can affect the sensing of a lead, such as dislodgment, chronic fibrosis at the lead tip, metabolic changes, and myocardial infarction.

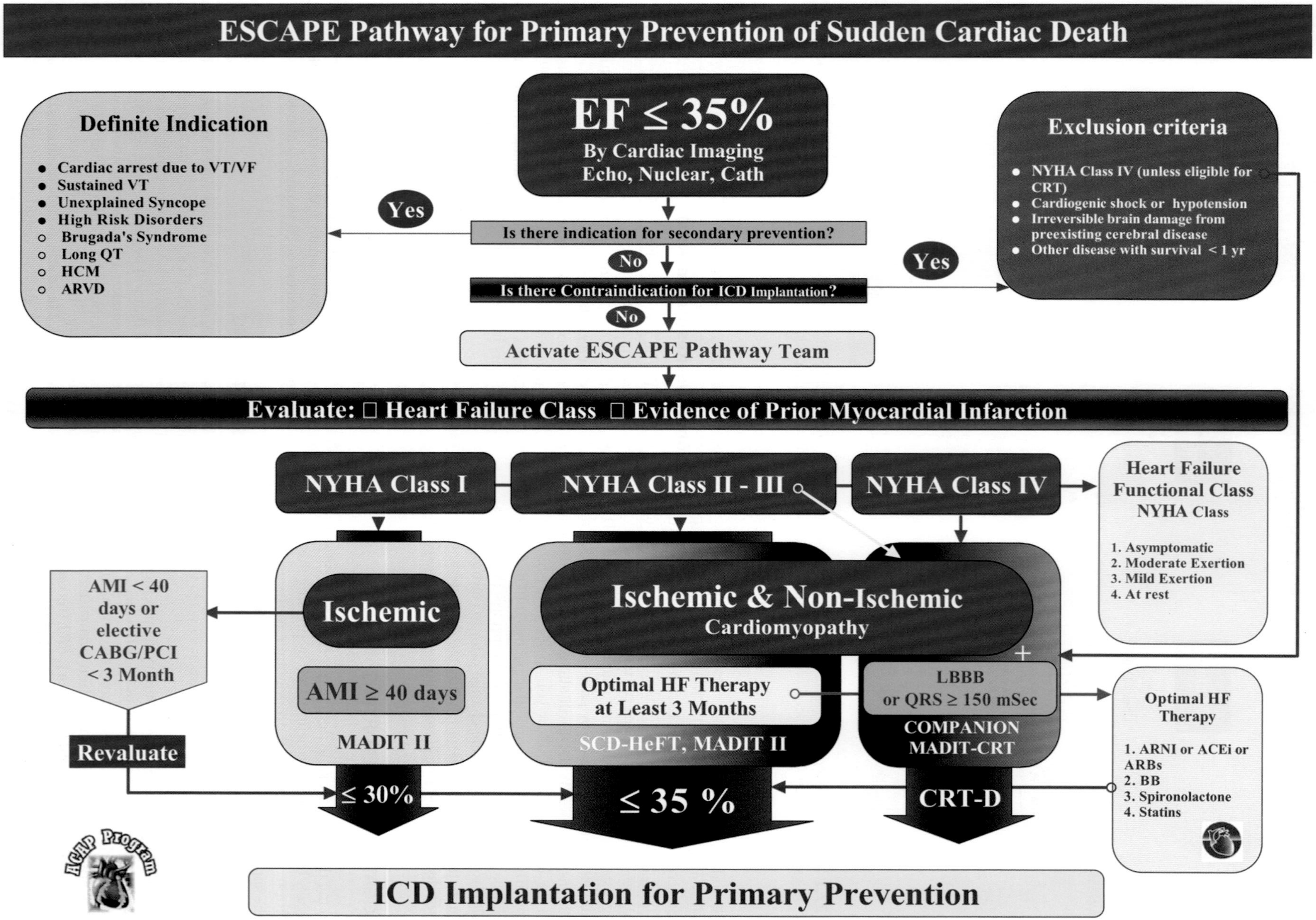

ESCAPE Pathway for Primary Prevention of Sudden Cardiac Death

Definite Indication

- Cardiac arrest due to VT/VF
- Sustained VT
- Unexplained Syncope
- High Risk Disorders
- Brugada's Syndrome
○ Long QT
○ HCM
○ ARVD

EF ≤ 35%
By Cardiac Imaging
Echo, Nuclear, Cath

Yes →

Is there indication for secondary prevention? — **No** →

Is there Contraindication for ICD Implantation? — **No** →

Activate ESCAPE Pathway Team

Yes →

Exclusion criteria

- NYHA Class IV (unless eligible for CRT)
- Cardiogenic shock or hypotension
- Irreversible brain damage from preexisting cerebral disease
- Other disease with survival < 1 yr

Evaluate: □ Heart Failure Class □ Evidence of Prior Myocardial Infarction

NYHA Class I

Ischemic

AMI ≥ 40 days

MADIT II

≤ 30%

AMI < 40 days or elective CABG/PCI < 3 Month

Revaluate

NYHA Class II – III

Ischemic & Non-Ischemic
Cardiomyopathy

Optimal HF Therapy at Least 3 Months

SCD-HeFT, MADIT II

≤ 35 %

NYHA Class IV

+

LBBB or QRS ≥ 150 mSec

COMPANION MADIT-CRT

CRT-D

Heart Failure Functional Class
NYHA Class

1. Asymptomatic
2. Moderate Exertion
3. Mild Exertion
4. At rest

Optimal HF Therapy

1. ARNI or ACEi or ARBs
2. BB
3. Spironolactone
4. Statins

ICD Implantation for Primary Prevention

FIGURE 27.2 The ESCAPE pathway for prevention of sudden cardiac death.

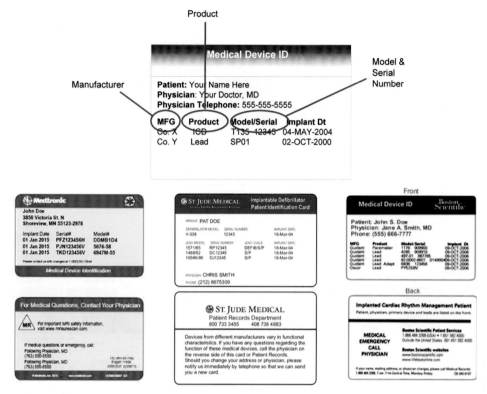

FIGURE 27.3 Patient identification cards examples from different manufacturers.

TABLE 27.1	Contact Number for Major Device Companies
COMPANY	**CONTACT NUMBER**
Biotronik	(800) 547-0394
Boston Scientific (Cameron, CPI, Guidant)	(800) CARDIAC
Medtronic (Vitatron)	(800) MEDTRONic
Sorin (ELA)	(877) 663-7674
St. Jude Medical (Pacesetter, Telectronics, Ventritex)	(800) SHOCKVF

We Recommend

- To evaluate the sensing of a chamber, adjust the Brady parameters if necessary to maintain proper device performance. (For pacemakers, the sensed P and R waves should be at least twice the sensitivity setting.)
- Suggested settings: Mode: DDI; Rate: 30 bpm; AV Delay: 300 ms (400 ms if allowed)

    "DDI will allow backup ventricular pacing if needed, and allow you to see heart block by separating Atrial and Ventricular pacing function—and AV Delays greater than 300 ms. DDI is not available on some older pacemakers. Use DDD or VVI on these devices as appropriate."

It is very important to test the sensing of the device to avoid potential problems that could result from undersensing or oversensing.

- **Undersensing** occurs when the pacemaker fails to sense native cardiac activity, which results in asynchronous pacing. This could be due to increased stimulation threshold at electrode site (exit block), poor lead contact, new bundle branch block, or programming problems.
- **Oversensing** occurs when electrical signal are inappropriately recognized as native cardiac activity and pacing is inhibited. These inappropriate signals may be large P or T waves, skeletal muscle activity, or lead contact problems.

LEAD IMPEDANCE TESTING

Lead impedance describes the sum of all resistance to current flow. It is a function of the characteristics of the conductor (wire), the electrode (tip), and the myocardium; thus, checking the lead impedances gives us information about the lead integrity. Normal lead impedance ranges from 300 to 1000 ohms (some leads have higher impedances by design). Similar to sensing amplitude, the steadiness of lead impedances overtime is more important than the number obtained (**Figure 27.8**). Lead impedance values can change as a result of lead fractures or insulation breakage.

- *Low-impedance* conditions, mainly insulation break exposing the lead wire to body fluids, which have low resistance, allows current to drain through the insulation break to the path of

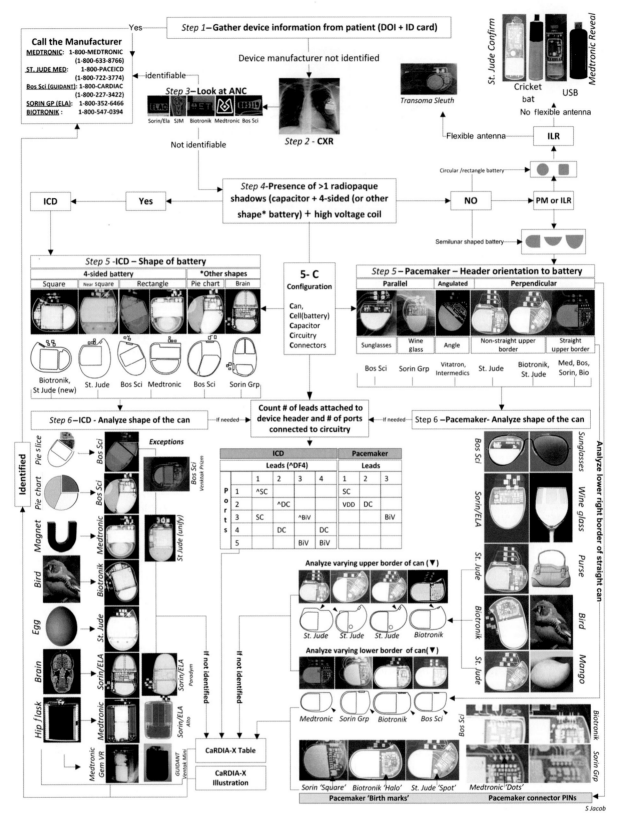

FIGURE 27.4 CaRDIA-X algorithm. (From Jacob S, Shahzad MA, Maheshwari R, et al. Cardiac rhythm device identification algorithm using X-Rays: CaRDIA-X. *Heart Rhythm.* 2011;8(6):915-922.)

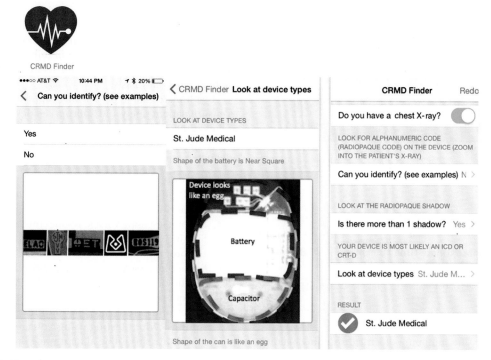

FIGURE 27.5 CRMD Finder app.

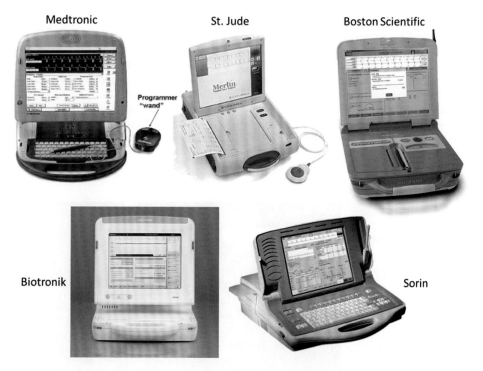

FIGURE 27.6 The programmers of the 5 major device manufacturers: Medtronic, St. Jude Medical, Boston Scientific, Biotronik, and Sorin.

least resistance, leading to potential loss of capture and more rapid battery depletion.

- *High-impedance* conditions, mainly due to fractured conductor, are a result of not enough current flow from the device battery to the tissues. Other reason for high impedance is the lead not having properly seated in the pacemaker header.

All devices perform automatic lead impedances in the course of the initial device interrogation. However, ICDs require you to test the pacing leads separately from the shocking lead impedance. Should you need to test impedance manually, look for the appropriate tabs on the Impedance screen to select which leads you are testing (ie, RA, RV, LV, and shocking lead impedance).

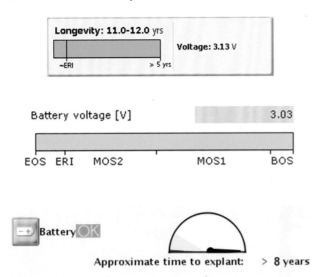

FIGURE 27.7 Examples of battery status, graphs, and gauges.

THRESHOLD (CAPTURE) TESTING

Capture threshold is the minimum electrical stimulus needed to consistently capture the myocardium. There are few factors that affect pacing thresholds. First, lead maturation as a result of the fibrotic capsule that develops around the tip of the lead can cause a slight rise in the threshold. Second, the newer leads that are steroid eluted reduce the inflammatory process and allow the leads to maintain low chronic thresholds.

Myocardial capture is a function of amplitude, which is the strength of the impulse expressed in volts as it must be large enough to depolarize the heart and the pulse width, which is the duration of the current flow expressed in milliseconds. This is done using the strength–duration curve,[5] which illustrates the relationship of amplitude and pulse width as seen in **Figure 27.9**;

any combination of pulse width and voltage on or above the curve will result in capture.

By accurately determining capture thresholds, we can assure adequate safety margins, keeping in mind that thresholds may differ in acute or chronic pacing systems and could slightly fluctuate on a daily basis.

The ultimate goal in performing capture threshold testing is to ensure patient safety and appropriate device performance as well as extend the service life of the battery if possible. A common output value is ≤2.5 V, but we should always maintain an adequate safety margin.

- To perform threshold testing, find the appropriate tab and adjust Brady parameters if necessary to maintain proper device performance.
  - Perform test using Voltage Testing criteria (fixed Pulse Width). Starting voltage should be approximately three-fourths of the programmed Amplitude setting.
  - Some older pacemakers will require Pulse Width testing (as the only option). Starting Pulse Width should be the current setting.
  - Thresholds are related to Amplitude and Pulse Width settings. When testing using Voltage, the programmed amplitude should be at least twice the measured threshold. When using Pulse Width, the programmed pulse width should be at least three times the measured threshold. The exception is when the auto capture is programmed ON.
- Useful tricks to performing Threshold testing:
  i. Always test at a rate of at least 10 bpm above the patient's intrinsic rate—this helps to prevent fusion and makes loss of threshold seem as a pause related to a change in rate.
  ii. When starting out, *always run paper during the entire test* (press the 25 button under the screen). This will make it easier for you to verify loss.

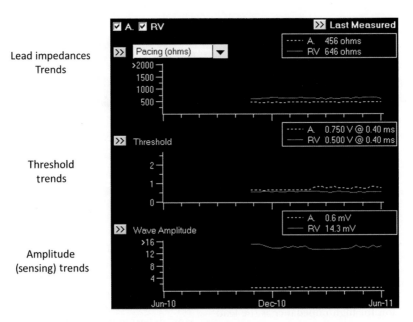

FIGURE 27.8 Example of a Medtronic device sensing, thresholds, and lead impedance trends.

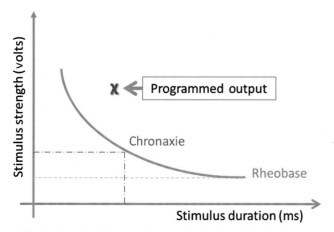

- The rheobase is the least voltage needed to depolarize the heart at infinite pulse duration.
- The chronaxie is the shortest pulse duration required to depolarize the heart at a voltage twice the rheobase.
- (X) is the programmed output equal 2x chronaxie.

FIGURE 27.9 The strength–duration curve.

iii. Atrial Thresholds:
1. The safest way to test Atrial Thresholds for any patient is in DDD mode. This will ensure ventricular support if the patient has any form of block—and for patients with intrinsic conduction, assist by adding another visual clue when Atrial capture is lost.
2. If patient has intact intrinsic conduction, one can test it in two ways:
   a. Atrial Thresholds in DDD mode will result in an Ap/Vs response at the paced atrial rate. Capture is verified by paced P waves and by QRS response. Loss of capture will result in a slight pause in rate (the difference between the intrinsic PR and the AV Delay), a loss of P wave capture, and will be immediately followed by a paced ventricular response (you will transition from a narrow upright QRS to a wide-paced QRS). *Suggested Settings: Mode: DDD, Rate: at least 10 bpm above intrinsic rate, AV Delay: max allowed (300 or 400 ms).*
   b. Atrial Thresholds in AAI mode will result in a ventricular response on the surface EGM at the paced atrial rate. Capture is verified by paced P waves and by QRS response. Loss of capture will result in a pause in rate as well as a loss in P wave capture. *Suggested Settings: Mode: AAI, Rate: at least 10 bpm above intrinsic rate.*
3. For patients with block, performing atrial thresholds in DDD mode is required to provide support for ventricular function. Here, capture is verified by loss of P waves only. Loss of capture will result in ventricular-only pacing. *Suggested Settings: Mode: DDD, Rate: 10 bpm max above intrinsic rate, AV Delay: 150 ms or greater. Increasing the AV Delay separates the P waves from the paced QRS, allowing the P waves to be seen easier. Keep the rate as low as possible when testing in this manner to allow the most space between paced QRSs.*

SPECIAL TESTING AND PARAMETERS FOR BRADYCARDIA THERAPY DEVICES

Pacemaker programming is very complex; however, for simplicity, medical personal should be at least familiar with the most common pacing modes. The North American Society of Pacing and Electrophysiology (NASPE) and British Pacing and Electrophysiology Group (BPEG) published as a joint effort the pacemaker code. This joint project is known as the *NBG pacemaker code*. The NBG was initially published in 1983 and was last revised in 2002.[6] It describes the five-letter code for operation of implantable pacemakers and defibrillators (**Figure 27.10**).

Main Pacing Modes

- The *AAI or AAIR* is an atrial demand pacing (atrium paced, atrium sensed, and pacemaker inhibited in response to sensed atrial beat) and is appropriate for patients with sinus node dysfunction who have intact AV nodal function. Patients with symptomatic sinus bradycardia or sinus pauses, but with an intact ability to accelerate their heart rate with exertion, can be programmed in an AAI mode. Those who cannot adequately accelerate their heart rate should have rate-responsive capability available.
- The *VOO* pacemaker is asynchronous ventricular pacemaker; there are no adaptive rate control or antitachyarrhythmia functions.
- The *VVI or VVIR* pacemaker is a ventricular "demand" pacemaker with electrogram-waveform telemetry; there are no adaptive rate control or antitachyarrhythmia functions. Those who cannot adequately accelerate their heart rate should have rate-responsive capability available. The new leadless pacemaker (*Micra*) is VVI pacemakers.
- The *VDD* pacemaker is used for AV nodal dysfunction with intact and appropriate sinus node behavior.
- The **DDD** *or* **DDDR** pacemaker is a multiprogrammable "physiologic" dual-chamber pacemaker; there are no adaptive rate control or antitachyarrhythmia functions. Those who cannot adequately accelerate their heart rate should have rate-responsive capability available.
- The **DDI** pacer is used for a patient with a dual-chamber pacemaker that has episodes of paroxysmal atrial fibrillation. DDI prevents high ventricular rates. Some DDD pacemakers are programmed to enter the DDI mode when high atrial rates occur.

One of the most important aspects of checking the pacemaker function is to evaluate for percentage of pacing. BLOCK-HF trial[7] showed that the increased RV pacing can lead to RV-pacing-induced cardiomyopathy. Likewise, in patients with biventricular pacemakers, less than 90% pacing is considered inadequate. Investigations should be done to find the cause of less biventricular pacing (eg, higher LV thresholds than the programmed parameter, high frequency of PVCs, atrial fibrillation with rapid ventricular rates) and to correct it.

Important Programmable Features

Mode switching: This is the algorithm that identifies the presence of atrial tachyarrhythmias and switch the device to a nontracking mode (VVI, DVI, or DDI), allowing the pacing rate to be driven by the programmed lower-rate limit or sensor-indicated rate.

Generic Pacemaker Code (NBG): NASPE/BPEG

Position	I	II	III	IV	V
Function	Pacing chamber	Sensing chamber	Response(s) to sensing	Rate modulation	Multisite pacing
Specific Designations	O=none A=Atrium V=Ventricle D=Dual (A+V)	O=none A=Atrium V=Ventricle D=Dual (A+V)	O=none T=Triggered I=Inhibited D=Dual (T+I)	O=none R=Rate modulation	O=none A=Atrium V=Ventricle D=Dual (A+V)

- The first two positions of this code (Chamber Paced and Sensed) are relatively straightforward.
- The third position could be confusing. The most frequently used programs are the DDD (dual-chamber pacing and sensing both triggered and inhibited mode), VVI (for single-chamber, ventricular pacing in the inhibited mode), VDD (ventricular pacing with atrial tracking), and DDI (dual-chamber pacing and sensing, but inhibited mode only).
- The third position is described as follows:
  - D (Dual): In DDD pacemakers, atrial pacing is in the inhibited mode (the pacing device will emit an atrial pulse if the atrium does not contract). In DDD and VDD pacemakers, once an atrial event has occurred (whether paced or native) the device will ensure that an atrial event follows.
  - I (Inhibited): The device will pulse to the appropriate chamber unless it detects intrinsic electrical activity. In the DDI program, AV synchrony is provided only when the atrial chamber is paced. If on the other hand intrinsic atrial activity is present, then no AV synchrony is provided by the pacemaker.
  - T (Triggered): Triggered mode is only used when the device is being tested. The pacing device will emit a pulse only in response to a sensed event.
- The fourth position, rate modulation, increases the patient's heart rate in response to "patient exercise." A number of mechanisms (vibration, respiration, and pressure) are used to detect "patient exercise." As the exercise wanes, the sensor indicated rate returns to the programmed mode.
- The fifth position describes multisite pacing functionality. Atrial multisite pacing is being investigated as way to prevent atrial fibrillation. Ventricular multisite pacing is a treatment for pacing a patient with dilated cardiomyopathy.

FIGURE 27.10 The North American Society of Pacing and Electrophysiology (NASPE) and British Pacing and Electrophysiology Group (BPEG) published as a joint effort the pacemaker code. This joint project is known as the NBG pacemaker code. The NBG was initially published in 1983 and was last revised in 2002. It describes the five-letter code for operation of implantable pacemakers and defibrillators.

Minimizing ventricular pacing: Managed ventricular pacing (MVP)[8] from Medtronic and its likeness *ventricular pace suppression* (VPS) from Biotronik, *SafeR* pacing[9] from Sorin, *ventricular intrinsic preference* (VIP)[10] from St. Jude Medical, and *Rhythmiq* from Boston Scientific all have an atrial-based pacing mode that significantly reduces unnecessary right ventricular pacing by primarily operating in an AAI(R) pacing mode while providing the safety of a dual-chamber backup mode if necessary.

Rate-adaptive pacing: This refers to an increase in the pacing rate in response to a combination of sensors including association of an activity sensor giving a rapid response for short-duration exercise, a metabolic sensor, or minute ventilation sensor, to improve exercise capacity, particularly in patients with chronotropic incompetence.

SPECIAL TESTING AND PARAMETERS FOR TACHYCARDIA THERAPY DEVICES

Appropriate ICD programming is crucial to deliver critical therapy to true arrhythmia (VT/VF) and to avoid unnecessary shock or inappropriate shocks. Multiple trials have been conducted with this aim in mind, namely, *PainFree I,*[11] *PainFree II,*[12] *PREPARE,*[13] *ShockLess,*[14] and *MADIT-RIT*[15] all of which showed that along

with delivery of painless therapies and optimal programming, the use of discrimination algorithms play an important role in specifically reducing inappropriate shocks.

Tiered-therapy ICDs have 2 to 3 zones defined by the longest RR interval in each zone. The primary determinants of the boundaries of therapy zones are programming of specific therapies and SVT discrimination. The lower boundary between sinus and VT zone is programmed at approximately 180 to 188 bpm in primary prevention patients and at 30 to 60 ms greater than the cycle length of the slowest observed VT (150–160 bpm in most trials) in secondary prevention patients. Programming in the VT zone is focused on preventing therapy for SVT and nonsustained VT. We routinely program three zones in primary prevention patients, using the slowest VT zone for monitoring only at 160 to 166 bpm. In secondary prevention patients, the slower VT zone is programmed with three to four sequences of ramp/burst ATP compared with 1-burst ATP followed by shocks in the faster VT zone. The following are the SVT discriminators:

- *Onset:* Sudden onset is usually indicative of ventricular tachycardia.
- *Stability:* Wobbly R-R interval is indicative of atrial fibrillation.

- *Morphology:* Comparing the morphology of the tachycardia to an acquired template in sinus rhythm can help in discriminating supraventricular versus ventricular arrhythmias.
- *A/V counter:* More (V) than (A) is indicative of ventricular tachycardia.

ARRHYTHMIA REPORTING

One of the most important aspects in device interrogation is reporting on any documented arrhythmia on the device such as atrial fibrillation, ventricular tachycardia, supraventricular tachycardia, or pacemaker-mediated tachycardia.

When reporting these arrhythmias, it is essential to report the number of episodes and their length and the percentage of mode switching. Greater than five and a half hours of atrial fibrillation has been associated with stroke, and these patients should be recommended for anticoagulation. Most devices will have a printed log of events for all arrhythmias and therapies and a report if the delivered therapies (whether ATP or ICD shocks) were appropriate or inappropriate.

In special situations, particularly cases with lead failure causing oversensing resulting in multiple inappropriate ICD firing, placing a magnet over the device will suspend all tachy therapies.

NEW ON THE HORIZON FOR PACING CARDIAC DEVICES

Leadless pacemakers: About 93% smaller than other modern-day pacemakers, the recent FDA-approved Micra pacemaker (Medtronic, Minneapolis, MN) (**Figure 27.11**) is the world's smallest pacemaker, yet it offers a complete set of features. The proprietary hybrid battery chemistry provides improved longevity, reliability, and predictable performance. It is MRI SureScan, which allows the patient to be safely scanned using either a 1.5-T or a 3-T full-body MRI. Currently, the device has a 99.2% implant success rate. About 96% of patients experienced no major complications at 6 months. The device has a 51% lower complication rate than traditional pacing systems, with no dislodgements or systemic infections.[16]

SonR-Closed-Loop Optimization: The new Sorin SonR tip atrial lead is a bipolar sugar-coated lead that picks up vibrations that reflect global contractility and not just local cardiac wall movements. The embedded sensor is a micro-accelerometer that detects cardiac muscle vibrations that reflect the first heart sound and are correlated with LV dP/dt_{max}. The SonR tip lead performs automated V-V and A-V optimization at rest and during exercise. The recently published RESPOND-CRT trial[17] showed 30% reduction of all-cause mortality or heart failure hospitalization at 24-month follow-up (**Figure 27.12**).

WiSE-CRT system: The WiSE-CRT system (EBR Systems, Sunnyvale, CA) uses a multicomponent strategy to provide leadless cardiac resynchronization. A tiny (9.1 mm × 2.7 mm, 0.05 cm³) receiver electrode composed of polyester-covered titanium is implanted endocardially in the LV. A subcutaneous

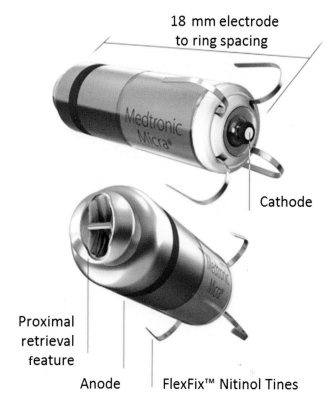

FIGURE 27.11 Leadless pacemaker Micra (Medtronic, Minneapolis, Minnesota).

pulse generator is placed in the left lateral thorax and generates ultrasound pulses, which are converted to electrical pacing stimuli by the endocardial seed (**Figure 27.13**). All patients in the WiSE-CRT study had a traditional pacemaker or defibrillator; the subcutaneous WiSE-CRT pulse generator detected the RV pacing pulse from the standard system, which triggered endocardial LV pacing. In the initial trial, patients with failed coronary sinus lead placement, nonresponse to CRT, or need for an upgrade to CRT were enrolled. Data from small studies demonstrated significant QRS narrowing, absolute EF improvements of 5%, and improvements in composite clinical scores at 6 months.[18] The initial WiSE-CRT study was stopped for safety reasons. Following delivery system redesign, early data from 14 patients demonstrated no implant-related adverse events.

CONCLUSION

Implantable devices are an essential part of medical management for a large number of cardiac patients. Basic knowledge is needed to perform a complete and thorough device evaluation.

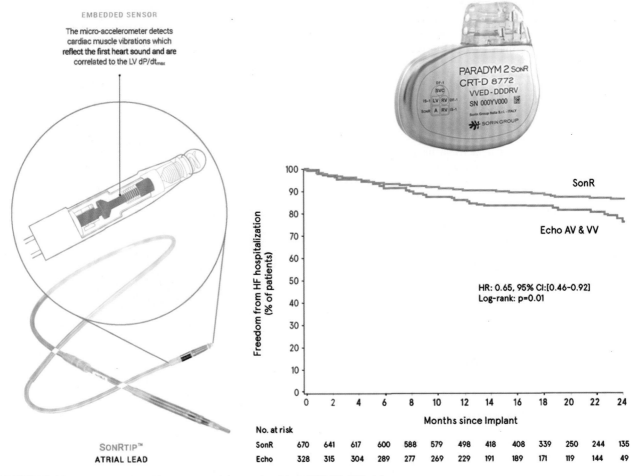

FIGURE 27.12 SonR tip atrial lead from Sorin, and the results of the RESPOND-CRT trial.

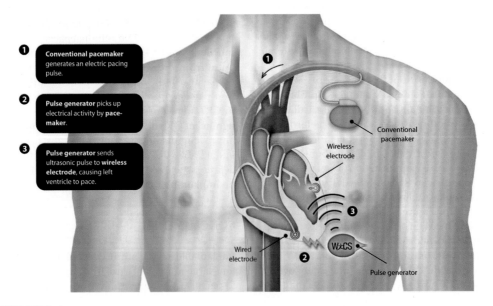

FIGURE 27.13 WiSE-CRT System.

APPENDIX: LIMITED KEY GUIDE OF THE FIVE MAJOR DEVICE MANUFACTURER PROGRAMMERS

1. Medtronic CareLink Programmer (**Figure 27.14**)
2. Boston Scientific ZOOM LATITUDE Programming System (**Figure 27.15**)

3. St. Jude Medical Merlin Programmer (**Figure 27.16**)
4. Biotronik Renaamic Programmer (**Figure 27.17**)
5. Sorin Orchestra Plus Programmer (**Figure 27.18**)

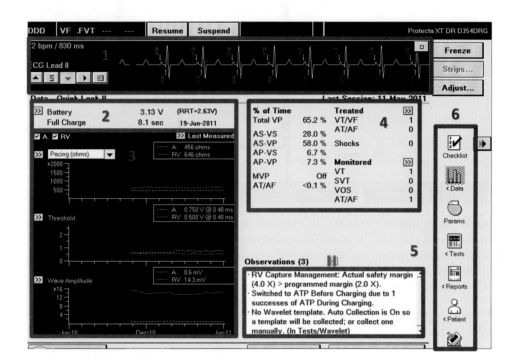

The initial screen of the Medtronic CareLink Programmer shows six main sections as marked in the figure.

1. Surface ECG
2. Battery management showing battery voltage as well as the marker for RRT
3. Trending section: This shows the trends overtime for measured amplitudes (sensing), thresholds, and lead impedances
4. Overview window for device statistics: This includes, percentage pacing over time, total atrial pacing (AP), and total ventricular pacing (VP). This section also shows the number of episodes of any arrhythmias including ventricular tachycardia/fibrillation (VT/VF), atrial tachycardia/fibrillation (AT/AF), and therapies if applicable for ICDs (shocks)
5. Observations window: This shows a short summary of most observation like fluid status (OptiVol), any thresholds issues (capture), or therapies
6. The sidebar set menu: This has a list of icons that help during the device interrogation, including checklist, statistical data, device setparameters, tests, reports and patient

FIGURE 27.14 Medtronic CareLink Programmer.

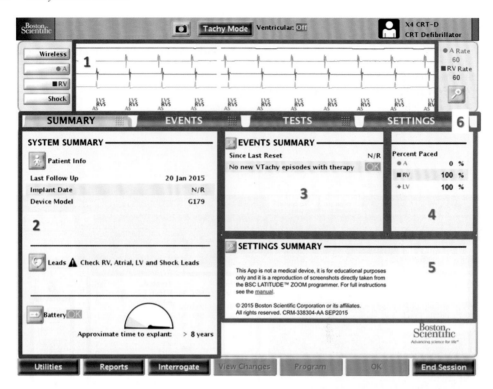

The initial screen of the Boston Scientific ZOOM LATITUDE Programming System shows six main sections as marked in the figure.

1. Surface ECG and intracardiac markers from the device leads (atrial, ventricular)
2. System summary window: This includes three sections, namely, patient information, leads notifications, and battery gauge showing indication of battery longevity with estimation for the time to explant
3. Events summary: This section shows the number of episodes of any arrhythmias, including ventricular tachycardia/fibrillation (VT/VF), atrial tachycardia/fibrillation (AT/AF), and therapies if applicable for ICDs (shocks)
4. Percentage paced: Total atrial pacing (AP) and total ventricular pacing (VP)
5. Setting summary: Device parameters setting
6. The upper ribbon tabs: These four tabs can take you directly to summary, events, tests, and device programmed settings. Reports printing can be selected by the button "reports" at the bottom of the screen

FIGURE 27.15 Boston Scientific ZOOM LATITUDE Programming System.

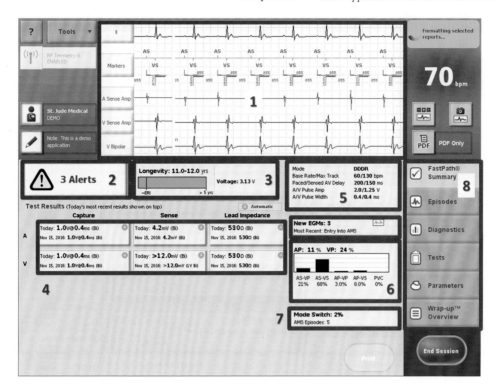

The initial screen of the St. Jude Medical Merlin Programmer shows eight main sections as marked in the figure.

1. Surface ECG and intracardiac markers from the device leads (atrial, ventricular)
2. Alerts windows: For any abnormalities, including lead issues, arrhythmia, or ICD therapy if applicable
3. Battery management window: This shows battery voltage as well as a graph depicting the estimated longevity
4. Daily test results summary window: This shows capturing thresholds, sensing amplitude, and lead impedances from most recent test check
5. Device setting summary
6. Percentage paced: Total atrial pacing (AP) and total ventricular pacing (VP)
7. Mode switching: This describes a percentage of automatic mode switching that occurs due to atrial arrhythmia. Mode-switching algorithms are designed to alleviate symptoms related to tracking of atrial arrhythmias
8. The sidebar set menu: This has a list of icons that help during the device interrogation, including FastPath summary, episodes, diagnostics, tests, parameters, and wrap-up overview from which reports are selected for printing

FIGURE 27.16 St. Jude Medical Merlin programmer.

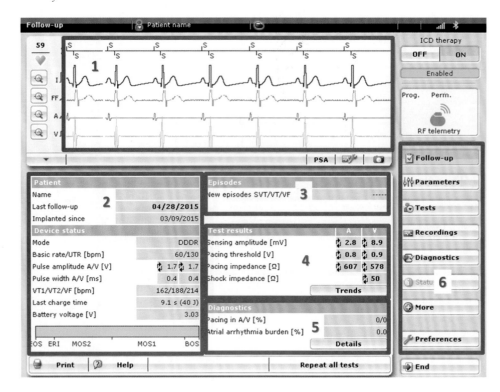

The initial screen of the Biotronik Renamic Programmer shows six main sections as marked in the figure.

1. Surface ECG and intracardiac markers from the device leads (atrial, ventricular)
2. Patient information, device parameters, and battery management window
3. Episodes windows: For any arrhythmia episodes SVT/VT/VF
4. Daily test results summary window: This shows capturing thresholds, sensing amplitude, and lead impedances from most recent test check
5. Diagnostics: Total percentage pacing for atrial pacing (A) and ventricular pacing (V) as well as atrial arrhythmia burden percentage
6. The sidebar set menu: This has a list of icons that help during the device interrogation, including follow-up, parameters, tests, recordings, diagnostics, and preferences. Reports printing can be selected by a button at the right lower part of the screen

FIGURE 27.17 Biotronik Renamic programmer.

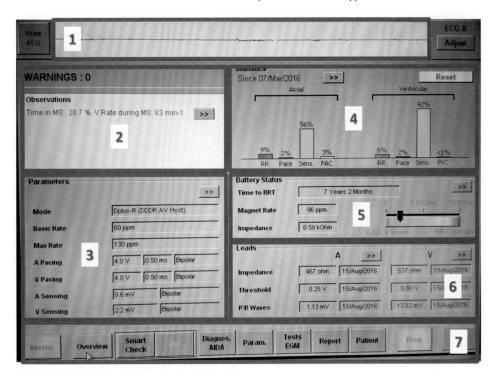

The initial screen of the Sorin Orchestra Plus programmer shows seven main sections as marked in the figure.

1. Surface ECG and intracardiac markers from the device leads (atrial, ventricular)

2. Warnings and observations: This section also shows the number of episodes of any arrhythmias, including ventricular tachycardia/fibrillation (VT/VF), atrial tachycardia/fibrillation (AT/AF), and therapies if applicable for ICDs (shocks)

3. Device parameters and setting

4. Statistics: This shows the total percentage pacing for atrial pacing (A) and ventricular pacing (V) as well as atrial arrhythmia burden percentage

5. Battery management: This shows battery voltage and time to RRT

6. Leads: daily test results summary window: This shows capturing thresholds, sensing amplitude, and lead impedances from most recent test check

7. The lower bar menu: This has a list of buttons that help during the device interrogation, including interrogate, overview, smart check, diagnostics, parameters, tests, and reports

FIGURE 27.18 Sorin Orchestra Plus programmer.

REFERENCES

1. Roger VL, Go AS, Lloyd-Jones DM, et al. Heart disease and stroke statistics—2011 update: a report from the American Heart Association. *Circulation.* 2011;123(4):e18-e209.

2. Moss AJ, Zareba W, Jackson Hall W, et al. Prophylactic implantation of a defibrillator in patients with myocardial infarction and reduced ejection fraction. *N Engl J Med.* 2002;346(12):877-883.

3. Epstein AE, Epstein AE, Darbar D, et al. 2012 ACCF/AHA/HRS focused update incorporated into the ACCF/AHA/HRS 2008 guidelines for device-based therapy of cardiac rhythm abnormalities: a report of the American College of Cardiology Foundation/American Heart Association Task Force on Practice Guidelines and the Heart Rhythm Society. *Circulation.* 2013;127(3):e283-352.

4. Jacob S, Shahzad MA, Maheshwari R, et al. Cardiac rhythm device identification algorithm using X-Rays: CaRDIA-X. *Heart Rhythm.* 2011;8(6):915-922.

5. Coates S, Thwaites B. The strength-duration curve and its importance in pacing efficiency: a study of 325 pacing leads in 229 patients. *Pacing Clin Electrophysiol.* 2000;23(8):1273-1277.

6. Bernstein AD, Daubert JC, Fletcher RD, et al. The revised NASPE/BPEG generic code for antibradycardia, adaptive-rate, and multisite pacing. North American Society of Pacing and Electrophysiology/British Pacing and Electrophysiology Group. *Pacing Clin Electrophysiol.* 2002;25(2):260-264.

7. St John Sutton M, Plappert T, Adamson PB, et al. Left ventricular reverse remodeling with biventricular versus right ventricular pacing in patients with atrioventricular block and heart failure in the Block HF trial. *Circ Heart Fail.* 2015;8(3):510-518.

8. Sweeney MO, Ellenbogen KA, Miller EH, et al. The Managed Ventricular pacing versus VVI 40 Pacing (MVP) Trial: clinical background, rationale, design, and implementation. *J Cardiovasc Electrophysiol.* 2006;17(12):1295-1298.

9. Davy JM, Hoffmann E, Frey A, et al. Near elimination of ventricular pacing in SafeR mode compared to DDD modes: a randomized study of 422 patients. *Pacing Clin Electrophysiol.* 2012;35(4):392-402.

10. Yadav R, Jaswal A, Chennapragada S, et al. Effectiveness of Ventricular Intrinsic Preference (VIP) and Ventricular AutoCapture (VAC) algorithms in pacemaker patients: results of the validate study. *J Arrhythm.* 2016;32(1):29-35.

11. Wathen MS, Sweeney MO, DeGroot PJ, et al. Shock reduction using antitachycardia pacing for spontaneous rapid ventricular tachycardia in patients with coronary artery disease. *Circulation.* 2001;104(7):796-801.

12. Wathen MS, DeGroot PJ, Sweeney MO, et al. Prospective randomized multicenter trial of empirical antitachycardia pacing versus shocks for spontaneous rapid ventricular tachycardia in patients with implantable cardioverter-defibrillators: Pacing Fast Ventricular Tachycardia Reduces Shock Therapies (PainFREE Rx II) trial results. *Circulation.* 2004;110(17):2591-2596.

13. Wilkoff BL, Williamson BD, Stern RS, et al. Strategic programming of detection and therapy parameters in implantable cardioverter-defibrillators reduces shocks in primary prevention patients: results from the PREPARE (Primary Prevention Parameters Evaluation) study. *J Am Coll Cardiol.* 2008;52(7):541-550.

14. Silver MT, Sterns LD, Piccini JP, et al. Feedback to providers improves evidence-based implantable cardioverter-defibrillator programming and reduces shocks. *Heart Rhythm.* 2015;12(3):545-553.

15. Kobe J, Eckardt L, Nitschmann S. [ICD programming: multicenter automatic defibrillator implantation trial—reduce inappropriate therapy (MADIT-RIT)]. *Internist (Berl).* 2013;54(8):1023-1026.

16. Reynolds D, Duray GZ, Omar R, et al. A leadless intracardiac transcatheter pacing system. *N Engl J Med.* 2016;374(6):533-541.

17. Brugada J, Delnoy PP, Brachmann J, et al. Contractility sensor-guided optimization of cardiac resynchronization therapy: results from the RESPOND-CRT trial. *Eur Heart J.* 2017;38(10):730-738.

18. Auricchio A, Delnoy PP, Regoli F, et al. First-in-man implantation of leadless ultrasound-based cardiac stimulation pacing system: novel endocardial left ventricular resynchronization therapy in heart failure patients. *Europace.* 2013;15(8):1191-1197.

Emad F. Aziz
Eyal Herzog

28

Strategies for the Prevention of Sudden Cardiac Death

INTRODUCTION

Sudden cardiac death (SCD), also known as sudden cardiac arrest, is a major health problem worldwide.[1] According to the American Heart Association (AHA) Statistical Data from 2015, each year 326,000 people experience EMS-assessed out-of-hospital cardiac arrests in the United States and approximately 60% of out-of-hospital cardiac arrests are treated by EMS personnel.[2–3] It is usually defined as the cessation of cardiac mechanical activity, as confirmed by the absence of signs of circulation. Cardiac arrest is traditionally categorized as being of cardiac or noncardiac origin. A dynamic triggering factor usually interacts with an underlying heart disease, either genetically determined or acquired, and the final outcome is the development of lethal tachyarrhythmias or, less frequently, bradycardia.[4]

There is no comprehensible consensus on the definition of SCD, which is witnessed in only two-thirds of cases. Because the duration of symptoms preceding the terminal event usually defines the sudden nature of death, the World Health Organization defines SCD as unexpected death within 1 hour of symptom onset if witnessed or within 24 hours of the person having been observed alive and symptom free if unwitnessed.[5] Exclusion of noncardiac causes, such as pulmonary embolus or drug overdose, is also critical because sudden cardiac arrhythmias may be the final common pathway in these disease states as well.

According to Framingham Heart Study, during a 20-year follow-up, 13% of the deceased have died of sudden death.[6] In more than 80% of cases, sudden death is caused by coronary disease.[7] The mechanism of sudden death is ventricular fibrillation (VF) in 65% to 85%, ventricular tachycardia (VT) in 7% to 10%, and electromechanical dissociation in 20% to 30%.

RISK FACTORS

About 80% of individuals who suffer SCD have coronary heart disease; the epidemiology of SCD to a great extent parallels that of coronary heart disease. On the basis of recent published data, the following variables have been associated with patients at higher risk of SCD: (1) syncope at the time of the first documented episode of arrhythmia, (2) NYHA class III or IV, (3) VT/VF occurring early after myocardial infarction (3 days to 2 months),

and (4) history of previous myocardial infarction.[8] Other factors such as age, hypertension, left ventricular hypertrophy, intraventricular conduction block, elevated serum cholesterol, glucose intolerance, decreased vital capacity, smoking, relative weight, and heart rate are also postulated in identifying individuals at risk for SCD.[9–11] Even family history of myocardial infarction has been reported to be associated with the risk of primary cardiac arrest.[12] Another entity of patients at highest risk for early SCD are those with hereditary ion channel or myocardial defects, such as a long or short QT syndrome, hypertrophic cardiomyopathy, and arrhythmogenic right ventricular dysplasia (ARVD).

PATHOPHYSIOLOGY OF ARRHYTHMIA

The most common electric sequence of events in SCD is degeneration of VT (abnormal acceleration of ventricular rate) into VF, during which disorganized contractions of the ventricles fail to eject blood effectively, often followed by asystole or pulseless electrical activity.[7] Polymorphic VT or torsade de pointes may be the initial arrhythmia in patients with genetic or acquired forms of structural heart disease.[13] Bradyarrhythmias or electromechanical dissociation may be the primary electrical event in advanced heart failure or in the elderly patients.[14–15] Among patients with implantable cardioverter-defibrillators (ICDs), arrhythmic death accounts for 20% to 35% of deaths, and electromechanical dissociation after shock is a frequent cause of death. Asystole may be the first rhythm observed in the field, but this may be a marker of the duration of arrest because coarse VF ultimately degenerates into asystole.

MANAGEMENT

RISK STRATIFICATION

Current parameters for risk stratification of patients with CAD for SCD include medical history (presence of nonsustained VT or syncope), ejection fraction (EF), electrocardiogram (QRS duration, QT interval, QT dispersion), signal-averaged electrocardiogram, heart rate variability, and baroreflex sensitivity. However, the sensitivity and specificity of these parameters have not yet been studied in detail in large patient populations. The single major parameter associated with higher incidence and studied in many clinical trials is the left ventricular ejection fraction (LVEF). At present, only left ventricular (LV) dysfunction with reduced EF reliably defines "high risk" for SCD in patients with ischemic and nonischemic cardiomyopathy. The heart failure functional class and history of prior MI or CAD are also important prognostic risk factors along with sudden specific definite indications.[16]

PREVENTION

Prevention of sudden death means detection of high-risk patients and application of medical treatment in order to postpone it. The high risk of development of SCD is majorly attributed to fatal ventricular arrhythmias. Electrophysiologic anomalies in cells lead to development of ventricular ectopic activity or ventricular arrhythmias, which comes to the end with fibrillation and eventually death if not terminated in time. Because survival rates for out-of-hospital cardiac arrests are extremely low, ranging from 2% to 25% in the United States,[17] secondary prevention strategies only addresses a small portion of patient population at risk of SCD. The accumulated data have allowed guidelines to be formulated, which allow us to predict with more certainty patients at risk for SCD and address the challenge to identify patients at risk before the first event as primary prevention. However, applying those guidelines in practice requires systems to structure the environment in which care is delivered so that "doing the right thing" becomes automatic.[18] This requires tools that simplify and provide focus by embedding the recommendations for evidence-based care into the care itself.

PHARMACOLOGIC THERAPY

β-Blockers

Of the different drugs that have been evaluated, only β-blockers have reduced sudden death in the myocardial infarction survivor.[19] The BHAT study showed that β-blockade with propranolol reduced all-cause mortality by 25% especially in patients with diminished LV function and/or ventricular arrhythmias.[20] A randomized trial of nearly 46,000 patients showed that, in the acute MI setting, early administration of high-dose β-blocker drugs orally has been shown to prevent VF.[21] In the Metoprolol CR/XL Randomized Intervention Trial in Congestive Heart Failure (MERIT-HF) trial, 3,991 patients with NYHA class II-IV heart failure and EF ≤ 40% were randomized to long-acting metoprolol with a dose-escalation protocol.[22] At 1-year follow-up, overall mortality was lower in the treated group compared with placebo (7.2% vs. 11% per patient-years of follow-up). There was also a 41% relative risk reduction in sudden death with long-acting metoprolol. These data provide unequivocal benefit of β-blockade in acute MI, post-MI, and congestive heart failure for prevention of mortality and SCD.

Antiarrhythmic Drugs

The sine qua non for efficacy of common antiarrhythmic drugs in prevention against SCD based on well-designed, placebo-controlled clinical trials have shown no added benefit.[19–23] Class I drugs (mexiletine, flecainide), calcium antagonists, and class III drugs (d-sotalol, dofetilide) all failed to reduce, or even increased, the incidence of SCD after a myocardial infarction.[24] Amiodarone

has also been shown to have no definitive effect on mortality in patients after MI in preventing SCD, as manifested in the Sudden Cardiac Death in Heart Failure Trial (SCD-HeFT).[25]

Statins

The role of the statins has been well studied in the patients with CAD and has been shown to be extremely beneficial in reducing mortality but whether they play any significant role in preventing SCD remains controversial. A Multicenter Automatic Defibrillator Implantation Trial (MADIT II) substudy[26] demonstrated that, among patients treated with ICDs, those with background statin therapy had a lower rate of ventricular tachyarrhythmias. This finding was intriguing because it was unclear whether this observation was due to reductions in coronary events, decreased inflammation, unique antiarrhythmic properties, or unidentified confounders. Recently, the Cholesterol Lowering and Arrhythmia Recurrences After Internal Defibrillator Implantation (CLARIDI) study demonstrated that intensive lipid-lowering therapy using 80 mg of atorvastatin led to a 40% relative risk reduction (from 38% to 21%) in VT/VF recurrence in ICD patients during a 12-month follow-up. Yet, there are no definite guidelines supporting addition of statins as adjuvant therapy for prevention of SCD beyond conventional indications.

THE ROLE OF ICD DEVICES IN PRIMARY AND SECONDARY PREVENTION AGAINST SCD

Multiple prospective randomized multicenter clinical trials have documented improved survival with ICD therapy in high-risk patients with LV dysfunction due to either prior myocardial infarction or nonischemic cardiomyopathy. On a background of optimal medical therapy (with or without antiarrhythmic drug therapy), ICD therapy has been associated with a 23% to 55% mortality reduction due almost exclusively to a reduction in SCD. Superiority of an ICD over antiarrhythmic drug therapy for secondary prevention against SCD (predominantly amiodarone) was primarily noticed in the Antiarrhythmic Versus Implantable Defibrillator (AVID) trial.[27] The AVID trial enrolled 1,016 patients resuscitated from an episode of VT (if associated with hemodynamic collapse, cardiac symptoms, or occurring in the setting of an EF ≤ 40%) or VF. Patients were randomized to receive either medical therapy alone or in conjunction with an antiarrhythmic drug, which was most commonly amiodarone. The trial was stopped prematurely when a survival benefit was noted in patients receiving ICDs compared with those treated with sotalol or amiodarone. The unadjusted survival rates for the ICD versus drug groups were 89% versus 82% at 1 year, 82% versus 75% at 2 years, and 75% versus 65% at 3 years. The major effect of the ICD was to prevent arrhythmic death (4.7% vs. 10.8% in patients treated with an antiarrhythmic drug). Results consistent with the AVID study were also reported from the CIDS[28] and the CASH[29] studies.

MADIT TRIAL

To test the efficacy of ICDs in prevention of SCD, the MADIT trial randomized 196 patients with ischemic cardiomyopathy,[30] EF ≤35%, a documented episode of nonsustained VT (NSVT), and inducible VT on electrophysiology study to ICD (n = 95) versus conventional medical therapy (n = 101). After a mean follow-up of 27 months, the relative risk reduction for all-cause mortality in the patients receiving ICDs was 54% ($P = 0.009$), thus showing the benefit of prophylactic ICD placement in a high-risk population.

MADIT II TRIAL

However, to make an impact on the overall population at risk for sudden death, high-risk patients need to be identified before an episode of VT or VF (primary prevention). The MADIT II study highlighted the possibility of preventing sudden death in patients with coronary artery disease (CAD). According to this trial, patients with a previous MI and low LVEF (≤30%) on optimal medical therapy were randomized to receive either an ICD or no ICD. Patients implanted with an ICD had a mortality rate of 14.2% versus 19.8% in the conventional therapy group ($P = 0.016$), with a 31% relative risk reduction in mortality during a follow-up period of 20 months. The survival benefit was entirely due to a reduction in the incidence of SCD and became apparent at 9 months after device implantation. This trial was novel in that there was no requirement for invasive electrophysiologic testing of prior ventricular arrhythmias. This trial expanded on the findings of MADIT I, which showed the superiority of ICD therapy in patients with CAD with an EF of 35% or less.

SCD-HEFT TRIAL

The significant role of ICD therapy in primary prevention against SCD in both ischemic and nonischemic cardiomyopathy patients was further clarified by the Sudden Cardiac Death in Heart Failure Trial (SCD-HeFT).[31] This trial enrolled 2,521 patients with New York Heart Association[32] class II or III CHF and an EF of ≤35%. Patients were randomized to receive optimal medical therapy alone (847 patients), optimal medical therapy along with amiodarone (845 patients), or optimal medical therapy along with a conservatively programmed, shock-only, single-lead ICD (829 patients). Placebo and amiodarone were administered in a double-blind fashion. The primary end point of the study was all-cause mortality with mean follow-up of 3.8 years. A 23% reduction in mortality ($P = 0.007$) was observed with the ICD; the benefit of ICD was similar in both ischemic (hazard ratio, 0.79; $P = 0.05$) and nonischemic cardiomyopathy (hazard ratio, 0.73; $P = 0.06$). In contrast, mortality was similar in patients either on medical therapy alone or when combined with amiodarone. The benefit of ICD therapy was comparable for ischemic and nonischemic cardiomyopathy.

DEFINITE TRIAL

The Defibrillators in Non-Ischemic Cardiomyopathy Treatment Evaluation (DEFINITE) trial was the MADIT II counterpart. This trial included 458 patients with nonischemic dilated cardiomyopathy, EF ≤35%, nonsustained VT or premature ventricular contractions, and NYHA class I, II, or III who were randomly divided to standard medical therapy or ICD.[33] At a 2-year follow-up, there was a trend in mortality reduction with ICD (7.9% vs. 14.1%; hazard ratio = 0.65, $P = 0.08$). The largest benefit was seen in NYHA Class III patients (hazard ratio = 0.37). In part on the basis of the results of this trial, the Centers for Medicare & Medical Services expanded coverage for ICD implementation to patients with nonischemic cardiomyopathy for more than 9 months in duration who have NYHA class III or IV heart failure and EF ≤35%.

TIMING OF ICD IMPLANTATION

CABG PATCH TRIAL

In the CABG Patch study, 900 patients with LVEF of <36% and abnormal signal-averaged ECG who were undergoing elective coronary bypass surgery were randomized to ICD or no antiarrhythmic therapy.[34] This trail showed no difference in survival between the two groups at an average of 32-month follow-up. Of note, 88 patients enrolled were not randomized because they were deemed too unstable at the time of surgery for ICD placement. Additionally, EFs of these patients were not assessed postoperatively. Nevertheless, results suggest that revascularization should be performed when feasible and SCD risk stratification should be performed after revascularization.

DINAMIT TRIAL

In this randomized, open-label trial comparing ICD therapy to optimal medical therapy, 674 high-risk patients (defined by an EF <35%) were enrolled 6 to 40 days after myocardial infarction.[35–36] The primary end point was death from any cause; death from arrhythmia was a secondary end point. During a mean follow-up of 30 months, there was no difference in overall mortality between two treatment groups. A reduction in arrhythmia was balanced by an increase in overall mortality (cardiac but nonarrhythmogenic) in the ICD group. The reason for this surprising finding is unclear but may be related to impaired cardiac autonomic function early after MI. The benefits of ICD therapy for prevention of SCD may not become evident until years after myocardial infarction and may not have been captured in the mean 30-month follow-up of DINAMIT Trial. Current guidelines therefore recommend deferring ICD implantation for at least 40 days following MI.

Aggressive treatment of myocardial ischemia, including revascularization, is the main treatment in these patients, and early implantation of ICD does not reduce overall mortality after early MI (the DINAMIT study). Implantation of ICD should be deferred in these cases as is currently recommended, with reassessment of LV function after 40 days to determine whether ICD is still required for primary prevention of SCD (if LVEF <35%), although in some individual circumstances it may be considered (eg, in patients with recurrent, sustained arrhythmias).

CARDIAC RESYNCHRONIZATION THERAPY

Cardiac resynchronization therapy (CRT), or biventricular pacing, can improve cardiac pump function in advanced heart failure by simultaneous activation of the left and right ventricles in those with underlying or pacing-induced bundle branch block. CRT[37] is approved in the United States for EF ≤ 35%, evidence of dyssynchrony, and class III–IV heart failure despite optimal medical therapy. A brief review of the clinical data supporting their current use follows.

COMPANION TRIAL

CRT with either a pacemaker or a pacemaker-defibrillator has been shown to be very beneficial in the COMPANION trial,[38] which randomized patients with class III or IV heart failure, normal sinus rhythm, LVEF <35%, LV end diastolic volume > 60 mm, and QRS interval > 120 milliseconds. In this trial CRT with a pacemaker decreased the risk of the primary end point (hazard ratio, 0.81; $P = 0.014$), as did CRT with a pacemaker-defibrillator (hazard ratio, 0.80; $P <$ 0.01). The risk of the combined end point of death or hospitalization for heart failure was reduced by 34% in the pacemaker group ($P <$ 0.002) and by 40% in the pacemaker-defibrillator group ($P < 0.001$). A pacemaker reduced the risk of the secondary end point of death from any cause by 24% ($P = 0.059$), and a pacemaker-defibrillator reduced the risk by 36% ($P = 0.003$).

CARE-CHF TRIAL

The Cardiac Resynchronization in Heart Failure Study (CARE-HF) trial was a nonblinded European trial, which enrolled patients with class III or IV heart failure, LVEF <35%, LV end diastolic volume >30 mm, QRS interval >150 milliseconds, or QRS >120 milliseconds with echocardiographic parameters of dyssynchrony.[39] This trial confirmed earlier trials that the benefits of CRT are in addition to those achieved with standard pharmacologic therapy in patients with moderate-to-severe heart failure due to LV systolic dysfunction with evidence of cardiac dyssynchrony. CARE-HF is the first study to show benefit with CRT with respect to survival and the first to show benefit and continued improvement for a period of over 2 years.

MADIT-CRT

In a large randomized study of NYHA Class I and II patients, the primary endpoint showed that CRT-D were associated with 34% relative reduction in the risk of all-cause mortality or first heart failure event; in addition, there were 41% relative reduction of heart failure events compared with ICD patients. One-year follow-up confirmed an improvement of 11% in LVEF compared with 3% improvement for ICD patients.[40] The trial showed the best benefit were for patients with left bundle branch block or with non–left bundle branch with QRS > 150 msec, which led to an update in the guidelines that was published in 2012.[42]

A GENERALIZED SIMPLE SYSTEMATIC APPROACH TOWARD PREVENTION OF SCD (ESCAPE PATHWAY)

Multiple pathways have been developed in recent past to address these complex issues faced in the management of SCD; however, most of them lack simplicity, and practicality of implementation, which in turn affect their overall outcome and patient care. Here, we describe the ESCAPE pathway,[41] which is a simple novel pathway for primary and secondary prevention of sudden cardiac arrest aiming to increase physician awareness and incorporate a tool for appropriate referral for ICD evaluation (**Figure 28.1**).

STEP A: INITIAL EVALUATION OF PATIENTS

The initial and foremost thing to observe while assessing for the prevention against SCD is the EF. The ACC/AHA/ESC 2006 guidelines for management of patients with ventricular arrhythmias and the prevention of SCD criteria include patients with either ischemic or nonischemic cardiomyopathy with EF ≤ 35%, or NYHA class II or III heart failure.

On the basis of the initial evaluation of the patients with EF ≤ 35%, they can be divided into three subgroups: (A) patients with a clear indication for secondary cardiac arrest prevention, (B) patients who have a contraindication to ICD or have no proven benefit from ICDs for SCD prevention as per clinical data available

to date, and (C) patients who neither have any indication for ICD placement at this time as a part of secondary prevention of SCD nor have any contraindication.

Group A involves the following patients (**Figure 28.2**):

- Survivors of sudden cardiac arrest due to VT/VF
- Those with a previous documented episode of hemodynamically destabilizing sustained VT
- Those with unexplained syncope in the setting of underlying structural heart disease
- Those with high-risk short or long QT syndrome (LQTS or SQTS)
- Those with high-risk Brugada syndrome
- Those with high-risk hypertrophic cardiomyopathy
- Those with arrhythmogenic right ventricular dysplagia (ARVD)

This group of patient population on presentation should be referred directly for ICD implantation for secondary prevention against SCD.

Group B involves patients with a contraindication for ICD implantation and include the following (**Figure 28.3**):

- NYHA class IV patients (unless QRS ≤ 120 milliseconds who are eligible for CRT)
- Those with cardiogenic shock or hypotension
- Those with irreversible brain damage from preexisting cerebral disease
- Those with other disease (eg, cancer, uremia, liver failure), associated with a likelihood of survival of less than 1 year

Group C patients need further work-up to decide whether or when they should get ICDs and should enter into step B.

STEP B: EVALUATION OF HEART FAILURE CLASSES

To determine the best course of therapy, these patients require assessment of the stage of heart failure according to the NYHA classification (**Figure 28.4**).[42–43]

- Class I: No limitation of physical activity. Ordinary physical activity does not cause undue fatigue, palpitation, or dyspnea (shortness of breath).
- Class II: Slight limitation of physical activity. Comfortable at rest, but ordinary physical activity results in fatigue, palpitation, or dyspnea.
- Class III: Marked limitation of physical activity. Comfortable at rest, but less-than-ordinary activity causes fatigue, palpitation, or dyspnea.
- Class IV: Unable to carry out any physical activity without discomfort. Symptoms of cardiac insufficiency at rest. If any physical activity is undertaken, discomfort is increased.

STEP C: EVALUATION OF CAD OR PRIOR MI IN NYHA CLASS I PATIENT

Evaluation for any evidence of prior MI or CAD requiring intervention is further necessary (**Figure 28.5**).

- Patients with NYHA class I heart failure whose EF is lower or equal to 30% and who are at least 40 days post-MI should be referred for an ICD implantation according to MADIT II trial.
- Patients with low EF and are ≤40 days post-MI should be managed medically for their heart failure at present.[44] If repeat imaging at 40 days confirms EF ≤ 30% (or ≤35% in

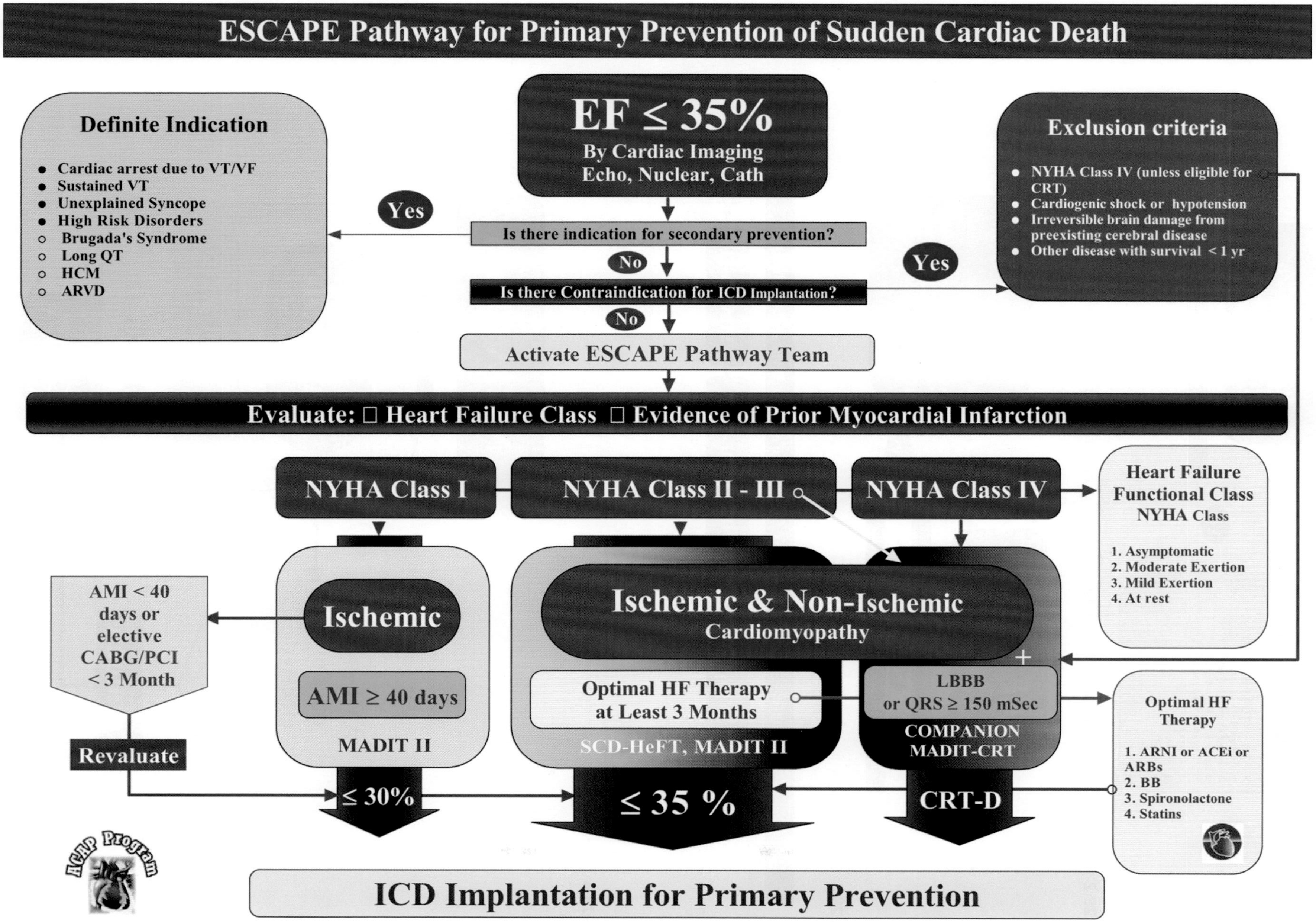

FIGURE 28.1 The ESCAPE pathway for prevention of sudden cardiac death.

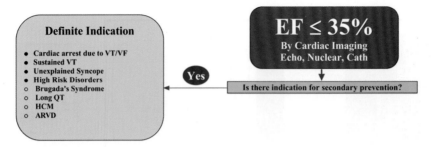

FIGURE 28.2 Indications for ICD implantation as secondary prevention of sudden cardiac death.

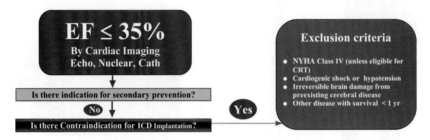

FIGURE 28.3 Contraindication for ICD implantation.

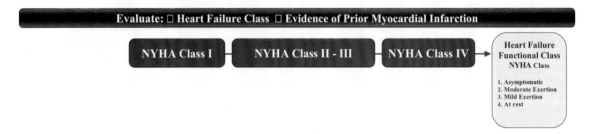

FIGURE 28.4 Evaluation of New York Heart Association classes.

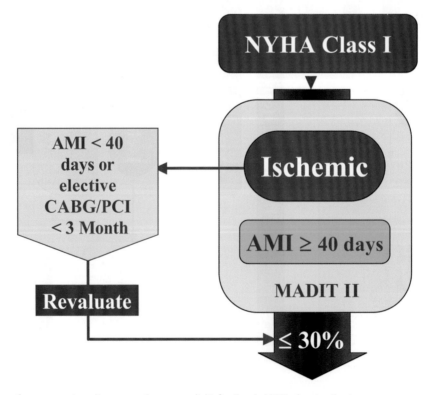

FIGURE 28.5 Evaluation of coronary artery disease or prior myocardial infarction in NYHA class I patients.

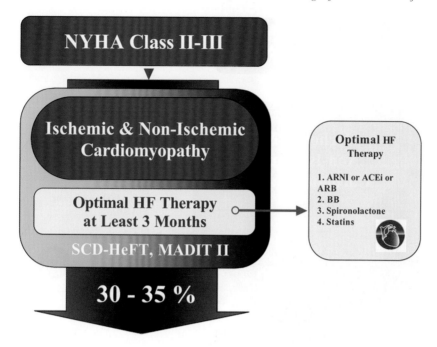

FIGURE 28.6 Primary prevention of sudden cardiac death in NYHA class II–III patients with low ejection fraction.

patients with class II or III NYHA class CHF), these patients should be referred for an ICD implantation.

- Patients with low EF who underwent elective revascularization either by percutaneous intervention or coronary bypass surgery in ≤3 months should be managed medically with optimal therapy for heart failure and if repeated imaging at 3 months confirms EF ≤ 30% (or ≤35% in patients with class II or III NYHA class CHF), these patients should be referred for an ICD implantation.

STEP D: PRIMARY PREVENTION OF SCD IN NYHA CLASS II–III PATIENTS WITH LOW EF

According to the ACC/AHA/HFSA Focused Update on New Pharmacological Therapy for Heart Failure: An Update of the 2016 ACCF/AHA Guideline for the Management of Heart Failure[43] (**Figure 28.6**),

- Angiotensin-converting enzyme (ACE) inhibitors are recommended for routine administration to symptomatic and asymptomatic patients with LVEF ≤40% (strength of evidence = A).
- β-Blockers shown to be effective in clinical trials of patients with HF are recommended for patients with an LVEF ≤ 40% (strength of evidence = A).
- Angiotensin-receptor blockers (ARBs) are recommended for routine administration to symptomatic and asymptomatic patients with an LVEF ≤40% who are intolerant to ACE inhibitors

for reasons other than hyperkalemia or renal insufficiency (strength of evidence = A).

- Angiotensin-receptor/neprilysin inhibitor (ARNI), Valsartan/sacubitril may be used instead of an ACE inhibitor or an ARB in people with heart failure and a reduced LVEF (strength of evidence = A).
- Administration of an aldosterone antagonist should be considered in patients following an acute MI, with clinical HF signs and symptoms and an LVEF ≤40%. Patients should be on standard therapy, including an ACE inhibitor (or ARB) and a β-blocker (strength of evidence = A).

If repeated imaging at 3 months confirms EF ≤35% and still in NYHA class II to III, these patients will be referred for an ICD implantation.

STEP E: PRIMARY PREVENTION OF SCD IN NYHA CLASS III AND IV HEART FAILURE PATIENTS WITH LEFT BUNDLE BRANCH BLOCK OR NON–LEFT BUNDLE WITH PROLONGED QRS (≥150 MILLISECONDS)

Patients with left bundle branch block or non–left bundle with QRS ≥150 milliseconds and in NYHA class (II, III, and IV) according to COMPANION, CARE-HF, and MADIT-CRT trials will be referred for CRT with an ICD (CRT-D), whereas patients with NYHA class IV but QRS > 120 milliseconds should be treated with optimal medical therapy (**Figure 28.7**).[19]

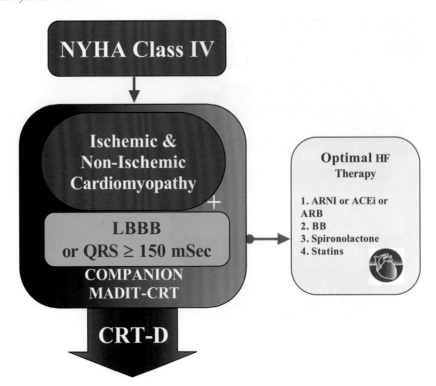

FIGURE 28.7 Primary prevention of sudden cardiac death in NYHA class III–IV heart failure patients with left bundle branch block (LBBB) or non-LBBB with prolonged QRS ≥150 ms.

CONCLUSION

Over the last three decades, revolutionary advances in the understanding and treatment of SCD have been accomplished. Structural and electrical mechanisms of terminal arrhythmias have been elucidated. Over two-dozen genetic mutations and polymorphisms have been identified, which in turn have increased our understanding of ion channel structure and function. At the same time, randomized trials that demonstrated harm from antiarrhythmic drugs have curtailed the use of such drugs alone in the prevention of SCD. The ICD was developed and has proven to be a highly effective therapy in the prevention of SCD to date. However, most cases of SCD occur in patients without these high-risk features, and the biggest challenge still remains: to accurately identify patients at risk for SCD for primary prevention.

REFERENCES

1. Mozaffarian D, Benjamin, EJ, et al. Heart disease and stroke statistics–2015 update: a report from the American Heart Association. *Circulation.* 2015 Jan 27;17:e205-e214.

2. Myerburg RJ, Kessler KM, Castellanos A. Sudden cardiac death: epidemiology, transient risk, and intervention assessment. *Ann Intern Med.* 1993;119:1187-1197.

3. Chugh SS, Jui J, Gunson K, et al. Current burden of sudden cardiac death: multiple source surveillance versus retrospective death certificate-based review in a large U.S. community. *J Am Coll Cardiol.* 2004;44:1268–1275

4. Stevenson WG, Stevenson LW, Middlekauff HR, Saxon LA. Sudden death prevention in patients with advanced ventricular dysfunction. *Circulation.* 1993;88:2953-2961.

5. Chugh SS, Jui J, Gunson K, et al. Current burden of sudden cardiac death: multiple source surveillance versus retrospective death certificate-based review in a large U.S. community. *J Am Coll Cardiol.* 2004;44:1268-1275.

6. Topalov V, Radisic B, Kovacevic D. [Sudden cardiac death]. *Med Pregl.* 1999;52:179-183.

7. Zipes DP, Wellens HJ. Sudden cardiac death. *Circulation.* 1998;98:2334-2351.

8. Brugada P, Talajic M, Smeets J, Mulleneers R, Wellens HJ. The value of the clinical history to assess prognosis of patients with ventricular tachycardia or ventricular fibrillation after myocardial infarction. *Eur Heart J.* 1989;10:747-752.

9. Burke AP, Farb A, Malcom GT, Liang YH, Smialek J, Virmani R. Coronary risk factors and plaque morphology in men with coronary disease who died suddenly. *N Engl J Med.* 1997;336:1276-1282.

10. Albert CM, McGovern BA, Newell JB, Ruskin JN. Sex differences in cardiac arrest survivors. *Circulation.* 1996;93:1170-1176.

11. Escobedo LG, Zack MM. Comparison of sudden and nonsudden coronary deaths in the United States. *Circulation.* 1996;93:2033-2036.

12. Friedlander Y, Siscovick DS, Weinmann S, et al. Family history as a risk factor for primary cardiac arrest. *Circulation.* 1998;97:155-160.

13. Huikuri H. Abnormal dynamics of ventricular repolarization: a new insight into the mechanisms of life-threatening ventricular arrhythmias. *Eur Heart J.* 1997;18:893-895.

14. Luu M, Stevenson WG, Stevenson LW, Baron K, Walden J. Diverse mechanisms of unexpected cardiac arrest in advanced heart failure. *Circulation.* 1989;80:1675-1680.

15. Pratt CM, Greenway PS, Schoenfeld MH, Hibben ML, Reiffel JA. Exploration of the precision of classifying sudden cardiac death: implications for the interpretation of clinical trials. *Circulation.* 1996;93:519-524.

16. Choudhury L, Mahrholdt H, Wagner A, et al. Myocardial scarring in asymptomatic or mildly symptomatic patients with hypertrophic cardiomyopathy. *J Am Coll Cardiol.* 2002;40:2156-2164.

17. Eisenberg MS, Horwood BT, Cummins RO, Reynolds-Haertle R, Hearne TR. Cardiac arrest and resuscitation: a tale of 29 cities. *Ann Emerg Med.* 1990;19:179-186.

18. Cannon CP, Hand MH, Bahr R, et al. Critical pathways for management of patients with acute coronary syndromes: an assessment by the National Heart Attack Alert Program. *Am Heart J.* 2002;143:777-789.

19. The cardiac arrhythmia suppression trial. *N Engl J Med.* 1989;321:1754-1756.

20. Lampert R, Ickovics JR, Viscoli CJ, Horwitz RI, Lee FA. Effects of propranolol on recovery of heart rate variability following acute myocardial infarction and relation to outcome in the Beta-Blocker Heart Attack Trial. *Am J Cardiol.* 2003;91:137-142.

21. Chen ZM, Pan HC, Chen YP, et al. Early intravenous then oral metoprolol in 45,852 patients with acute myocardial infarction: randomised placebo-controlled trial. *Lancet.* 2005;366:1622-1632.

22. Effect of metoprolol CR/XL in chronic heart failure: Metoprolol CR/XL Randomised Intervention Trial in Congestive Heart Failure (MERIT-HF). *Lancet.* 1999;353:2001-2007.

23. Effect of the antiarrhythmic agent moricizine on survival after myocardial infarction. The Cardiac Arrhythmia Suppression Trial II Investigators. *N Engl J Med.* 1992;327:227-233.

24. Waldo AL, Camm AJ, deRuyter H, et al. Effect of d-sotalol on mortality in patients with left ventricular dysfunction after recent and remote myocardial infarction. The SWORD Investigators. Survival With Oral d-Sotalol. *Lancet.* 1996;348:7-12.

25. Julian DG, Camm AJ, Frangin G, et al. Randomised trial of effect of amiodarone on mortality in patients with left-ventricular dysfunction after recent myocardial infarction: EMIAT. European Myocardial Infarct Amiodarone Trial Investigators. *Lancet.* 1997;349:667-674.

26. Moss AJ, Zareba W, Hall WJ, et al. Prophylactic implantation of a defibrillator in patients with myocardial infarction and reduced ejection fraction. *N Engl J Med.* 2002;346:877-883.

27. A comparison of antiarrhythmic-drug therapy with implantable defibrillators in patients resuscitated from near-fatal ventricular arrhythmias: the Antiarrhythmics versus Implantable Defibrillators (AVID) Investigators. *N Engl J Med.* 1997;337:1576-1583.

28. Connolly SJ, Gent M, Roberts RS, et al. Canadian Implantable Defibrillator Study (CIDS): study design and organization. CIDS Co-Investigators. *Am J Cardiol.* 1993;72:103F-8F.

29. Kuck KH, Cappato R, Siebels J, Ruppel R. Randomized comparison of antiarrhythmic drug therapy with implantable defibrillators in patients resuscitated from cardiac arrest: the Cardiac Arrest Study Hamburg (CASH). *Circulation.* 2000;102:748-754.

30. Farre J. [Implantable automatic defibrillator after MADIT and EMIAT]. *Rev Esp Cardiol.* 1996;49:709-713.

31. Bardy GH, Lee KL, Mark DB, et al. Amiodarone or an implantable cardioverter-defibrillator for congestive heart failure. *N Engl J Med.* 2005;352:225-237.

32. Barshop BA, Nyhan WL, Naviaux RK, McGowan KA, Friedlander M, Haas RH. Kearns-Sayre syndrome presenting as 2-oxoadipic aciduria. *Mol Genet Metab.* 2000;69:64-68.

33. Ellenbogen KA, Levine JH, Berger RD, et al. Are implantable cardioverter defibrillator shocks a surrogate for sudden cardiac death in patients with nonischemic cardiomyopathy? *Circulation.* 2006;113:776-782.

34. Bigger JT, Jr. Prophylactic use of implanted cardiac defibrillators in patients at high risk for ventricular arrhythmias after coronary-artery bypass graft surgery. Coronary Artery Bypass Graft (CABG) Patch Trial Investigators. *N Engl J Med.* 1997;337:1569-1575.

35. Hohnloser SH, Kuck KH, Dorian P, et al. Prophylactic use of an implantable cardioverter-defibrillator after acute myocardial infarction. *N Engl J Med.* 2004;351:2481-2488.

36. Hohnloser SH, Crijns HJ, van Eickels M, et al. Effect of dronedarone on cardiovascular events in atrial fibrillation. *N Engl J Med.* 2009;360:668-678.

37. New CRT technology boosts care for heart failure patients. Cardiac resynchronization therapy can provide better rhythm control and better communication with the doctor to help lower your risks. *Heart Advis.* 2008;11:10.

38. Bristow MR, Saxon LA, Boehmer J, et al. Cardiac-resynchronization therapy with or without an implantable defibrillator in advanced chronic heart failure. *N Engl J Med.* 2004;350:2140-2150.

39. Cleland JG, Daubert JC, Erdmann E, et al. The CARE-HF study (CArdiac REsynchronisation in Heart Failure study): rationale, design and end-points. *Eur J Heart Fail.* 2001;3:481-489.

40. Moss AJ, Hall WJ, Cannom DS, et al. Cardiac-resynchronization therapy for the prevention of heart-failure events. *N Engl J Med.* 2009;361:1329-1338.

41. Herzog E, Aziz EF, Kukin M, Steinberg JS, Mittal S. Novel pathway for sudden cardiac death prevention. *Crit Pathw Cardiol.* 2009;8:1-6.

42. Tracy CM, Epstein AE, Darbar D, et al. 2012 ACCF/AHA/HRS Focused Update of the 2008 Guidelines for Device-Based Therapy of Cardiac Rhythm Abnormalities. *J Am Coll Cardiol.* October 2, 2012;60(14):1297-1313.

43. Yancy CW, Jessup M, Bozkurt B, Butler J, Casey DE Jr, Colvin MM, et al. 2016 ACC/AHA/HFSA Focused Update on New Pharmacological Therapy for Heart Failure: An Update of the 2013 ACCF/AHA Guideline for the Management of Heart Failure: A Report of the American College of Cardiology/American Heart Association Task Force on Clinical Practice Guidelines and the Heart Failure Society of America. *J Am Coll Cardiol.* 2016 Sep 27;68(13):1476-1488.

44. Herzog E, Varley C, Kukin M. Pathway for the management of acute heart failure. *Crit Pathw Cardiol* 2005;4:37-42.

Eyal Herzog
Lee Herzog
Emad F. Aziz

29

Cardiopulmonary Resuscitation and Cardiocerebral Resuscitation Using Therapeutic Hypothermia

DEFINING SUDDEN CARDIAC ARREST

Cardiac arrest is defined as the cessation of cardiac mechanical activity, as confirmed by the absence of signs of circulation. Cardiac arrest is traditionally categorized as being of cardiac or noncardiac origin. An arrest is presumed to be of cardiac origin unless it is known or likely to have been caused by trauma, submersion, drug overdose, asphyxia, exsanguination, or any other noncardiac cause as best determined by rescuers.[1]

It is challenging to define what "unexpected" or "sudden" death is. Current practice defines sudden cardiac death as unexpected death without an obvious noncardiac cause that occurs within 1 hour of symptom onset (witnessed) or within 24 hours of last being observed in normal health (unwitnessed).[2]

EPIDEMIOLOGY OF OUT-OF-HOSPITAL CARDIAC ARREST

Based on the American Heart Association (AHA) Statistical Data from 2015[1]

- Each year, 326,000 people experience emergency medical services (EMS)–assessed out-of-hospital cardiac arrests in the United States.
- Approximately 60% of out-of-hospital cardiac arrests are treated by EMS personnel.[3]
- Twenty-five percent of those with EMS-treated out-of-hospital cardiac arrest have no symptoms before the onset of arrest.[4]
- Among EMS-treated out-of-hospital cardiac arrests, 23% have an initial rhythm of ventricular fibrillation (VF) or ventricular tachycardia (VT) or are shockable by an automated external defibrillator (AED).[5]
- The incidence of cardiac arrest with an initial rhythm of VF is decreasing over time; however, the incidence of cardiac arrest is not decreasing.[6]
- The median age for out-of-hospital cardiac arrest is 66 years.[7]
- Cardiac arrest is witnessed by a bystander in 38.7% of cases, by an EMS provider in 10.9% of cases, and is unwitnessed in 50.4% of cases.[7]

- In the Cardiac Arrest Registry to Enhance Survival (CARES) registry, 31,127 out-of-hospital cardiac arrests were treated in 2013. Survival to hospital discharge was 10.6%, and survival with good neurologic function (Cerebral Performance Category 1 or 2) was 8.3%. For bystander witnessed arrest with a shockable rhythm, survival to hospital discharge was 33.0%.[7]
- According to the CARES registry, in 2013 the majority of out-of-hospital cardiac arrests occurred at a home or residence (69.5%).[7]
- A family history of cardiac arrest in a first-degree relative is associated with a 2-fold increase in risk of cardiac arrest.[8,9]

EPIDEMIOLOGY OF IN-HOSPITAL CARDIAC ARREST

Based on the AHA Statistical Data from 2015[1]:

- Each year, 209,000 people are treated for in-hospital cardiac arrest in the United States.[10]
- According to the Get With The Guidelines (GWTG)-Resuscitation database from 2014, 25.5% of adults who experienced in-hospital cardiac arrest with any first recorded rhythm in 2013 survived to discharge.[1]
- In the United Kingdom National Cardiac Arrest Audit database between 2011 and 2013, the overall unadjusted survival rate was 18.4%. Survival was 49% when the initial rhythm was shockable and 10.5% when the initial rhythm was not shockable.[11]

CARDIOPULMONARY RESUSCITATION
GUIDELINE EVOLUTION

The initial attempts to treat cardiac arrest focused on chest compressions. Closed chest defibrillation and closed chest cardiac massage were first described in the 1960s.

In the initial publication, some patients were treated with chest compression without positive pressure. However, with time, ventilation gradually became an essential pillar of cardiopulmonary resuscitation.

Given the prevalence and lethality of cardiac arrest, the AHA disseminated cardiopulmonary resuscitation (CPR) and emergency cardiovascular care (ECC) information to health care professionals and the lay public in the 1970s.

The International Liaison Committee on Resuscitation (ILCOR) was formed in 1993. In 1999, the AHA hosted the first ILCOR conference to evaluate resuscitation science and develop common resuscitation guidelines. Since 2000, researchers from the ILCOR member councils have evaluated and reported their International Consensus on CPR and ECC Science With Treatment Recommendations(CoSTR) in 5-year cycles.[12]

HIGHLIGHTS OF THE 2015 AMERICAN HEART ASSOCIATION GUIDELINES UPDATED FOR CARDIOPULMONARY RESUSCITATION AND EMERGENCY CARDIOVASCULAR CARE

BASIC LIFE SUPPORT

Systems of Care

The 2015 AHA Updated Guidelines highlighted a new perspective on systems of care, differentiating in-hospital cardiac arrests (IHCAs) from out-of-hospital cardiac arrests (OHCAs).[13]

The care for all post–cardiac arrest patients, regardless of the location of the arrests, converges in the hospital, generally in an intensive care unit (ICU) where post–cardiac arrest care is provided. The systems of care before that convergence are very different for the two settings. Patients who have an OHCA depend on their community for support. Lay rescuers must recognize the arrest, call for help, initiate CPR, and provide defibrillation (ie, public-access defibrillation [PAD]) until EMS assumes responsibility and transports the patient to an emergency department (ED) and/or cardiac catheterization lab. The patient is ultimately transferred to a critical care unit for continued care.

In contrast, patients who have an IHCA depend on a system of appropriate surveillance (ie, rapid response or early warning system) to prevent cardiac arrest. If cardiac arrest occurs, patients depend on the smooth interaction of the institution's various services and a multidisciplinary team of professional providers, including physicians, nurses, and respiratory therapists, among others.

Community Lay Rescuer Automated External Defibrillator Programs

It is recommended that PAD programs for patients with OHCA be implemented in public locations where there is a relatively high likelihood of witnessed cardiac arrest (eg, airports, casinos, sports facilities).

There is clear and consistent evidence of improved survival from cardiac arrest when a bystander performs CPR and rapidly uses an AED. Thus, immediate access to a defibrillator is a primary component of the system of care. The implementation of a PAD program requires 4 essential components: (1) a planned and practiced response, which, ideally, includes identification of locations and neighborhoods where there is high risk of cardiac arrest, placement of AEDs in those areas, and ensuring that bystanders are aware of the location of the AEDs, and, typically, oversight by an HCP; (2) training of anticipated rescuers in CPR and use of the AED; (3) an integrated link with the local EMS system; and (4) a program of ongoing quality improvement.

Figure 29.1 outlines the 2015 guidelines recommendations for the initial approach to a patient who is unresponsive.

Chest Compressions

Untrained lay rescuers should provide compression-only (hands-only) CPR, with or without dispatcher guidance, for adult victims of cardiac arrest. The rescuer should continue compression-only CPR until the arrival of an AED or rescuers with additional training. All lay rescuers should, at a minimum, provide chest compressions for victims of cardiac arrest. In addition, if the trained lay rescuer is able to perform rescue breaths, he or she should add rescue breaths in a ratio of 30 compressions to 2 breaths. The rescuer should continue CPR until an AED arrives and is ready for use, EMS providers take over care of the victim, or the victim starts to move.

Chest Compression Rate

In most studies, more compressions are associated with higher survival rates, and fewer compressions with lower survival rates.

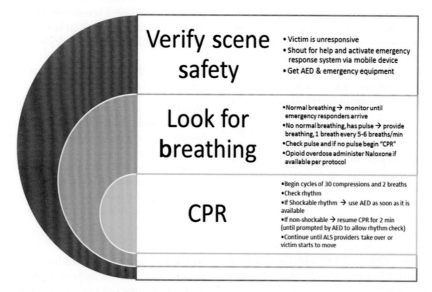

FIGURE 29.1 Updated 2015 guidelines recommendation for unresponsive patient management. AED, automated external defibrillator; ALS, advanced life support.

New to the 2015 Guidelines Update are upper limits of recommended compression rate and compression depth, based on preliminary data suggesting that excessive compression rate and depth adversely affect outcomes.

For the critical outcome of survival to hospital discharge, evidence exists from two observational studies[14,15] representing 13 469 adult patients. They compared chest compression rates of greater than 140/min, 120 to 139/min, less than 80/min, and 80 to 99/min with the control rate of 100 to 119/min. When compared with the control chest compression rate of 100 to 119/min, there was a 4% decrease in survival to hospital discharge with compression rates of greater than 140/min, a 2% decrease in survival to hospital discharge with compression rates of 120 to 139/min, a 1% decrease in survival to hospital discharge with compression rates of less than 80/min, and a 2% decrease in survival to hospital discharge with compression rates of 80 to 99/min.

The study showed that chest compression depth declined with increasing chest compression rate. The relationship of reduced compression depth at different compression rates was as follows: for a compression rate of 100 to 119/min, 35% of compressions had a depth of less than 3.8 cm; for a compression rate of 120 to 139/min, 50% of compressions had a depth of less than 3.8 cm; and for a compression rate of 140/min or greater, 70% of the compressions had a depth of < 3.8 cm.

TREATMENT RECOMMENDATIONS

The 2015 guidelines recommend a manual chest compression rate of 100 to 120/min.

Chest Compression Depth

During manual CPR, rescuers should perform chest compressions to a depth of at least 2 inches (5 cm) for an average adult, while avoiding excessive chest compression depths (> 2.4 inches [6 cm]).

The reason for emphasis on accurate chest compression depth is the following: compressions create blood flow primarily by increasing intrathoracic pressure and directly compressing the heart, which in turn results in critical blood flow and oxygen delivery to the heart and brain. Rescuers often do not compress the chest deeply enough despite the recommendation to "push hard." Although a compression depth of at least 2 inches (5 cm) is recommended, the 2015 Guidelines Update, as previously noted, incorporates new evidence about the potential for an upper threshold of compression depth (> 2.4 inches [6 cm]) beyond which complications may occur. Compression depth may be difficult to judge without use of feedback devices, and identification of upper limits of compression depth may be challenging.

For the critical outcome of survival to hospital discharge, 3 observational studies[16–18] suggest that survival may improve with increasing compression depth. In the largest study (9,136 patients), a covariate-adjusted spline analysis showed a maximum survival at a mean depth of 4.0 to 5.5 cm (1.6 to 2.2 inches), with a peak at 4.6 cm (1.8 inches).[18]

Another important study showed injuries were reported in 63% with compression depth of more than 6 cm (more than 2.4 inches) and 31% with compression depth of less than 6 cm. Injuries were reported in 28%, 27%, and 49% with compression depths of < 5 cm (< 2 inches), 5 to 6 cm (2 to 2.4 inches), and > 6 cm (> 2.4 inches), respectively.[19]

TREATMENT RECOMMENDATIONS

The 2015 guidelines recommend a chest compression depth of approximately 5 cm (2 inches) while avoiding excessive chest compression depths (> 6 cm [> 2.4 inches] in an average adult) during manual CPR.

Compression–Ventilation Ratio

The critical outcome of survival with favorable neurologic outcome at discharge was studied in two observational studies.[20,21] Of the 1,711 patients included, those who were treated under the 2005 guidelines with a compression–ventilation ratio of 30:2 had slightly higher survival than those patients treated under the 2000 guidelines with a compression–ventilation ratio of 15:2 (8.9% vs. 6.5%; RR 1.37 [0.98–1.91]).

The critical outcome of survival to hospital discharge was tested in 4 observational studies.[20–23] Of the 4,183 patients included, those who were treated under the 2005 guidelines with a compression–ventilation ratio of 30:2 had slightly higher survival than those patients treated under the 2000 guidelines with a compression–ventilation ratio of 15:2 (11.0% vs. 7.0%; RR 1.75 [1.32–2.04]).

For the critical outcome of survival to 30 days, 1 observational study[24] found that patients treated under the 2005 guidelines had slightly higher survival than those patients treated under the 2000 guidelines (16.0% vs. 8.3%; RR 1.92 [1.28–2.87]).

For the critical outcome of any return of spontaneous circulation (ROSC), 2 observational studies[20,21] found that patients treated under the 2005 guidelines had a ROSC more often than those patients treated under the 2000 guidelines (38.7% vs. 30.0%; RR 1.30 [1.14–1.49]).

Treatment Recommendation

The 2015 guidelines suggest a compression–ventilation ratio of 30:2 compared with any other compression–ventilation ratio in patients in cardiac arrest.

Ventilation During Cardiopulmonary Resuscitation with Advanced Airway

The 2015 guidelines suggest that it may be reasonable for the provider to deliver 1 breath every 6 seconds (10 breaths per minute) while continuous chest compressions are being performed (ie, during CPR with an advanced airway).

Bystander Naloxone in Opioid-Associated Life-Threatening Emergencies

New for the 2015 guidelines is that for patients with known or suspected opioid addiction who are unresponsive with no normal breathing but a pulse, it is reasonable for appropriately trained lay rescuers and basic life support (BLS) providers to administer intramuscular (IM) or intranasal (IN) naloxone in addition to providing standard BLS care.

In 2014, the naloxone autoinjector was approved by the US Food and Drug Administration for use by lay rescuers and HCPs.[3]

Shock First Versus Cardiopulmonary Resuscitation First

Numerous studies have addressed the question of whether a benefit is conferred by providing a specified period (typically 1½ to 3 minutes) of chest compressions before shock delivery, as compared to delivering a shock as soon as the AED can be readied. No difference in outcome has been shown.

For witnessed adult cardiac arrest when an AED is immediately available, it is reasonable that the defibrillator be used as soon as possible. For adults with unmonitored cardiac arrest or for whom an AED is not immediately available, it is reasonable that CPR be initiated while the defibrillator equipment is being retrieved and applied and that defibrillation, if indicated, be attempted as soon as the device is ready for use.

CPR should be provided while the AED pads are applied and until the AED is ready to analyze the rhythm.

Chest Recoil

On the basis of the 2015 guidelines, it is reasonable for rescuers to avoid leaning on the chest between compressions, to allow full chest wall recoil for adults in cardiac arrest.

Figure 29.2 summarizes the new 2015 guidelines recommendations for a high-quality CPR.

ADVANCED LIFE SUPPORT

Mechanical Cardiopulmonary Resuscitation Devices

The 2015 updated guidelines recommend against the routine use of automated mechanical chest compression devices to replace manual chest compressions.[24]

For the critical outcome of survival to 1 year, 1 RCT[25] using the Lund University Cardiac Arrest System (LUCAS) device showed no benefit or harm when compared with manual chest compressions (survival 5.4% vs. 6.2%; RR, 0.87; 95% CI, 0.68–1.11).

For the critical outcome of survival to 180 days, 1 RCT[26] using a LUCAS device enrolling 2,589 OHCA patients showed no benefit or harm when compared with manual chest compressions when quality of chest compressions in the manual arm was not measured (survival 8.5% vs. 8.1%; RR, 1.06; 95% CI, 0.81–1.41).

Drugs During Cardiopulmonary Resuscitation

Epinephrine Versus Vasopressin

A single RCT[27] (*n* = 336) compared multiple doses of single-dose epinephrine (SDE) with multiple doses of standard-dose vasopressin in the ED after OHCA.

For the critical outcome of survival to discharge with favorable neurologic outcome (cerebral performance category [CPC] 1 or 2), there was no advantage with vasopressin (RR, 0.68; 95% CI, 0.25–1.82; *P* = 0.44).

For the important outcome of ROSC, there was no observed advantage with vasopressin (RR, 0.93; 95% CI, 0.66–1.31; *P* = 0.67).

The 2015 guidelines suggest vasopressin should not be used instead of epinephrine in cardiac arrest.[24]

Epinephrine Versus Vasopressin in Combination with Epinephrine

For the critical outcome of survival to hospital discharge with CPC of 1 or 2, 3 RCTs[28–30] (*n* = 2,402) comparing SDE with vasopressin and epinephrine combination therapy showed no superiority with vasopressin and epinephrine combination (RR, 1.32; 95% CI, 0.88–1.98).

For the important outcome of ROSC, 6 RCTs[28–33] showed no ROSC advantage with vasopressin and epinephrine combination therapy (RR, 0.96; 95% CI, 0.89–1.04; *P* = 0.31).

The 2015 guidelines suggest against adding vasopressin to SDE during cardiac arrest.

Single-Dose Epinephrine Versus High-Dose Epinephrine

In adult patients in cardiac arrest in any setting, high-dose epinephrine (HDE) (at least 0.2 mg/kg or 5 mg bolus dose) was compared with SDE (1 mg bolus dose).

For the critical outcome of survival to hospital discharge with CPC 1 or 2, 2 RCTs comparing SDE with HDE[34,35] (*n* = 1,920) did not show advantage with HDE (RR, 1.2; 95% CI, 0.74–1.96).

For the critical outcome of survival to hospital discharge, 5 RCTs comparing SDE with HDE (*n* = 2,859) did not show any survival to discharge advantage with HDE (RR, 0.97; 95% CI, 0.71–1.32).

The 2015 guidelines recommend against the routine use of HDE in cardiac arrest (weak recommendation, low-quality evidence).

Timing of Administration of Epinephrine

IN-HOSPITAL CARDIAC ARREST

For IHCA, for the critical outcome of survival to hospital discharge, one observational study[36] in 25,095 IHCA patients with a nonshockable rhythm showed an improved outcome with early administration of epinephrine. Compared to the reference interval of 1 to 3 minutes, adjusted OR for survival to discharge was 0.91 (95% CI, 0.82–1.00) when epinephrine was given after 4 to 6 minutes, 0.74 (95% CI, 0.63–0.88) when given after 7 to 9 minutes, and 0.63 (95% CI, 0.52–0.76) when given at more than 9 minutes after onset of arrest.

For IHCA, for the critical outcome of neurologically favorable survival at hospital discharge, an improved outcome was observed from early administration of epinephrine: compared with the reference interval of 1 to 3 minutes, adjusted OR was 0.93 (95% CI, 0.82–1.06) when epinephrine was given after 4 to 7 minutes, 0.77 (95% CI, 0.62–0.95) when given after 7 to 9 minutes, and 0.68 (95% CI, 0.53–0.86) when given at more than 9 minutes after onset of arrest.

For IHCA, for the important outcome of ROSC, an improved outcome from early administration of epinephrine: adjusted OR compared with reference interval of 1 to 3 minutes of 0.90 (95% CI, 0.85–0.94) when given after 4 to 7 minutes, 0.81 (95% CI,

---

Perform Chest Compressions at a rate of 100-120/min
Compress to a depth of at least 2 inches (5 cm)
Allow for full recoil after each compression
Minimize pauses in compressions
Ventilate adequately (2 breaths after 30 compressions, each breath delivered over 1 second, each causing chest rise)

FIGURE 29.2 2015 guidelines recommendation for high-quality CPR.

0.74–0.89) when given after 7 to 9 minutes, and 0.70 (95% CI, 0.61–0.75) when given after 9 minutes.

For the critical outcome of neurologically favorable survival at hospital discharge (assessed with CPC 1 or 2), 4 observational studies[37–40], involving more than 262,556 OHCAs, showed variable benefit from early administration of epinephrine.

For the important outcome of ROSC, there was very-low-quality evidence (downgraded for risk of bias, indirectness, and imprecision) from 4 observational studies,[38,41–43] of more than 210,000 OHCAs, showing an association with improved outcome and early administration of adrenaline. One study[42] showed increased ROSC for patients receiving the first vasopressor dose early (<10 vs. >10 minutes after EMS call): OR, 1.91 (95% CI, 1.01–3.63).

The 2015 guidelines recommendations for cardiac arrest with an initial nonshockable rhythm are that if epinephrine is to be administered, it should be given as soon as possible after the onset of the arrest.

Antiarrhythmic Drugs for Cardiac Arrest

Antiarrhythmic drugs can be used during cardiac arrest for refractory ventricular dysrhythmias. Refractory VF/pVT is defined differently in many trials but generally refers to failure to terminate VF/pVT with 3 stacked shocks, or with the first shock.

For the important outcome of ROSC, 1 RCT, involving 504 OHCA patients, showed higher ROSC with administration of amiodarone (300 mg after 1 mg of adrenaline) compared with no drug (64% vs. 41%; *P* = 0.03; RR, 1.55; 95% CI, 1.31–1.85).[44]

The 2015 guidelines recommendations for antiarrhythmia drugs for cardiac arrest suggest the use of amiodarone in adult patients with refractory VF/pVT to improve rates of ROSC.

The guidelines also suggest the use of lidocaine or nifekalant (a Class III antiarrhythmic drug) as an alternative to amiodarone in adult patients with refractory VF/pVT.

The 2015 guidelines recommend against the routine use of magnesium in adult patients.

CARDIOCEREBRAL RESUSCITATION

Brief History of Therapeutic Hypothermia

The use of therapeutic hypothermia (TH) to mitigate various types of injury, in particular, posthypoxic injury to the brain, has been studied since the late 1930s.[45] Interest was initially kindled by reports of survival after prolonged exposure to cold, or submersion in ice-cold water, indicating a possible protective effect of low temperature on hypoxic injuries.[46]

Use of hypothermia after cardiac arrest was first described in the late 1950s[47,48], but proof that hypothermia could improve outcome in these patients remained elusive.[49,50] At the time it was thought that protective effects of TH were purely a result of hypothermia-induced lowering of metabolism; therefore, it was presumed that very low temperatures (25–28°C) were needed to provide significant neuroprotection.

This perception changed in the late 1980s, when animal studies demonstrated that significant protective effects also occurred with mild hypothermia (30–34°C), with far fewer side effects, and that a variety of destructive mechanisms were moderated by

hypothermia rather than just reductions in brain metabolism.[49] In the late 1990s, a number of small nonrandomized, clinical trials provided better evidence for the efficacy of TH.[51–54] This led to the initiation of 2 landmark multicenter RCTs to test TH treatment, the results of which were published side by side in 2002.[55,56] Both reported clear and significant improvements in outcome in cardiac arrest patients treated with therapeutic cooling.

The largest study, performed in 11 centers in Europe, enrolled 275 patients with witnessed cardiac arrest and an initial rhythm of VF or pulseless VT. The authors observed a 15.8% absolute (35.1% relative) improvement in outcome in the hypothermia group (*P* < 0.01).[55] The other RCT enrolled 77 patients across 4 centers in Australia, reporting an absolute improvement of 22.3% (relative improvement of 43.7%) in patients with witnessed VT/VF treated with hypothermia compared with controls (*P* < 0.05).[56] A meta-analysis calculated that 1 additional case of good neurologic outcome would be gained for every 6 patients treated with TH.[57] Guidelines from various medical societies such as the AHA, European Resuscitation Council (ERC), and Neurocritical Care Society (NCS) began recommending cooling after cardiac arrest.[58,59]

A larger RCT, the Therapeutic Temperature Management (TTM) study, compared temperature management at 33.0°C to maintaining a core temperature of 36.0°C.[60] The study enrolled 939 patients with witnessed cardiac arrest regardless of initial rhythm, including those with persistent hypoxia and hypotension who had been excluded from previous studies, with predefined subgroup analyses to correct for various risk factors. The results of this study were negative.[60] Rates of survival with good neurologic outcome were 46.5% in the 33°C group versus 47.8% in the 36°C group (*P* = 0.78). The rate of survival with excellent outcome (no neurologic residual) was 41.6% versus 39.4%, whereas survival with mild neurologic impairment was 4.9% versus 8.4%.[60] The authors concluded that maintaining core temperature at 36°C has equally good outcomes as cooling to 33°C.

Pathways for the Management of Survivors of Out of and In-Hospital Cardiac Arrest

At our institution, similar to many tertiary medical centers, algorithms for the management of patients post–cardiac arrest have been developed.

Our first algorithm was published in 2010.[61] We continue to update it, as new scientific information and updated guidelines are published.[62]

The term *therapeutic hypothermia* has now been replaced with *targeted temperature management* (TTM).

Our 2015 updated TTM pathway is shown in **Figure 29.3A**. The pathway is divided into three steps.

- Step I. From the field through the ED into the cardiac catheterization laboratory and to the critical care unit.
- Step II. Induced hypothermia protocol in the critical care unit.
- Step III. The management following the rewarming phase, including the recommendation for out-of-hospital therapy and the ethical decision to define goals of care.

STEP I

Presentation to the emergency department, proceeding to the cardiac catheterization laboratory and to the critical care unit. Upon arrival of a survivor of OHCA at the ED, the initial assessment (**Fig. 29.3B**) includes vital signs, physical examination, and neurologic examination with Glasgow coma score. Immediate 12-lead ECG is obtained and laboratory testing performed.

Initial laboratory testing includes complete blood count (CBC) with differential, basic metabolic panel, cardiac marker (troponin, CPK, CPK-MB), B-type natriuretic peptide (BNP), prothrombin time (PT), partial thromboplastin time (PTT), international normalized ratio (INR), lipid profile, phosphorus, calcium, magnesium, lactate, ß-HCG (for women), TSH, and toxicology screening. We recommend a head CT without contrast only if it is clinically indicated and will not delay transfer to the cardiac catheterization laboratory.

The patient is stabilized in the ED, where antiarrhythmic and vasopressor therapy may be administered, in addition to ventilator support.

The ED physician receives the emergency medical services (EMS) report of the primary rhythm and duration of cardiopulmonary resuscitation (CPR). This reported arrhythmia is the key decision point in our pathway.

The prognostically important distinction is between patients with documented VF or sustained VT who had a restoration of spontaneous circulation (ROSC) in <30 minutes and patients with reported asystole or pulseless electrical activity (PEA) (**Figure 29.3C**).

1. If the initial rhythm was VF or VT with an ROSC of ≤30 minutes, the cardiac arrest team is activated, and the patient will proceed to the cardiac catheterization laboratory (**Figure 29.3D**).
2. If the initial reported arrhythmia was PEA or asystole, the next step will depend on the ECG performed in the ED. If the ECG performed in the ED is suggestive of priority acute coronary syndrome (ACS), including ST elevation myocardial infarction (STEMI), left bundle branch block, or acute posterior wall MI, the MI team should be activated, and the care is similar to those patients with reported VF or VT arrest.
3. If priority ECG findings are not seen but the etiology of the arrest is most likely due to primary cardiac disease, the cardiology fellow will admit the patient to the cardiac care unit. We recommend an emergency echocardiogram.
4. If the etiology is likely noncardiac, the patient will be admitted to the medical ICU.

The cardiac arrest team includes the following 10 people.

The traditional (acute coronary syndrome) ACS-MI team comprises the following members:

1. Interventional cardiologist on-call team leader
2. Coronary care unit (CCU) director
3. Cardiology fellow on-call
4. Interventional cardiology fellow on-call
5. Cath lab nurse on-call
6. Cath lab technician on-call
7. CCU nurse manager on-call

In addition, the following personnel form the team:

8. The neurologist on-call
9. The critical care attending on-call
10. The medical resident screener

The MI team is activated by a single page to the central call center by the ED physician.

STEPS IN THE EMERGENCY DEPARTMENT

1. Decision to initiate induced hypothermia is made jointly by the ED physician and the cardiology or critical care physician. It is very important to review the hospital center's inclusion and exclusion criteria and decide whether the patient is a candidate for the TH protocol (**Figure 29.3E**).
2. The physician places an order to initiate hypothermia protocol.

Our goal is to transfer the patient to the percutaneous coronary intervention (PCI) center as soon as possible with a target door-to-balloon time of <90 minutes.

The management of the patient at this point is according to our Priority risk, Advanced risk, Intermediate risk, and Negative/low risk (PAIN) pathway following the priority ACS algorithm.[63]

Following cardiac catheterization, several steps occur while the patient is still in the catheterization laboratory:

1. The femoral arterial sheath can be maintained as an arterial catheter, which may be necessary to obtain blood pressure readings and arterial blood gas analyses.
2. The intravascular hypothermia catheter is inserted under strict aseptic technique (if it was not done earlier).

All patients are then transferred from the catheterization laboratory to the CCU where invasive hypothermia is initiated.

STEP II

Induced TH protocol in the critical care unit. The clinicians review the case and confirm the appropriateness of induced hypothermia (**Figure 29.3E**).

In summary, we recommend induced hypothermia for patients >18 years of age, who sustained a cardiac arrest and remain in coma. The patient must be comatose, not following commands or demonstrating purposeful movements. Patients excluded from the hypothermia protocol include patients who are awake, suffered prolonged ischemic times, experience refractory shock, demonstrate multiorgan failure, or have severe underlying illnesses, including terminal illnesses and do-not-resuscitate (DNR) status.

The hypothermia protocol is divided into three phases, as seen in **Figure 29.3F**:

Phase 1: Cooling phase for the first 24 hours
Phase 2: Rewarming phase
Phase 3: Maintenance phase

Phase 1: Cooling phase for the first 24 hours. We recommend 24 hours of the cooling therapy at a temperature goal of 33°C.

As will be discussed later in this chapter, the dose of the temperature management is controversial, and some centers cool patients to 36°C.

Endovascular catheters are an effective method of inducing TH (if a core cooling method is chosen). The catheters are usually inserted into the inferior vena cava through the femoral vein.

Continuous core temperature monitoring is required and generally accomplished using a temperature probe in the bladder (urinary catheter) or the rectum.

Monitoring of clinical condition and potential complications during the cooling phase.

As there are many physiologic effects of hypothermia, we recommend continuous monitoring and hourly documentation of vital signs; core temperature; cardiac rhythm; hemodynamic, respiratory, neurology status; and urine output. Common hemodynamic changes observed with cooling include hypertension,

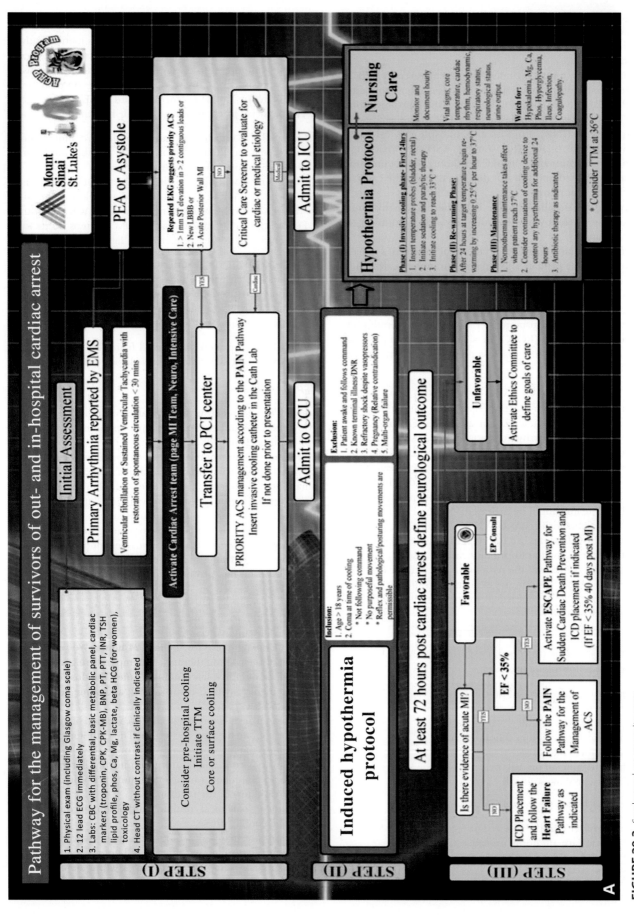

FIGURE 29.3 See legend on opposite page.

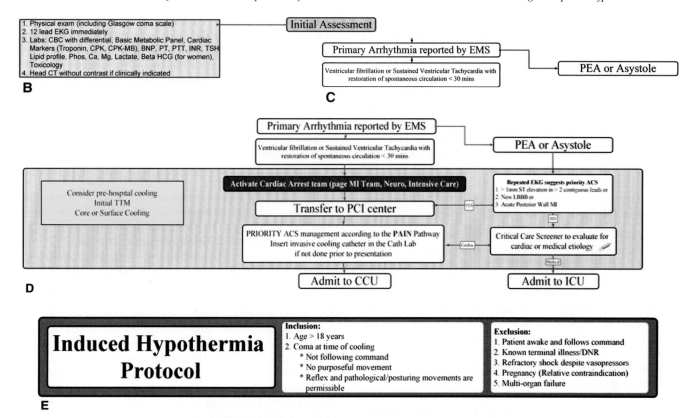

B

1. Physical exam (including Glasgow coma scale)
2. 12 lead EKG immediately
3. Labs: CBC with differential, Basic Metabolic Panel, Cardiac
   Markers (Troponin, CPK, CPK-MB), BNP, PT, PTT, INR, TSH
   Lipid profile, Phos, Ca, Mg, Lactate, Beta HCG (for women),
   Toxicology
4. Head CT without contrast if clinically indicated

Initial Assessment

Primary Arrhythmia reported by EMS

Ventricular fibrillation or Sustained Ventricular Tachycardia with
restoration of spontaneous circulation < 30 mins

PEA or Asystole

C

D

Primary Arrhythmia reported by EMS

Ventricular fibrillation or Sustained Ventricular Tachycardia with
restoration of spontaneous circulation < 30 mins

PEA or Asystole

Consider pre-hospital cooling
Initial TTM
Core or Surface Cooling

Activate Cardiac Arrest team (page MI Team, Neuro, Intensive Care)

Repeated EKG suggests priority ACS
1. > 1mm ST elevation in > 2 contiguous leads or
2. New LBBB or
3. Acute Posterior Wall MI

Transfer to PCI center — YES

PRIORITY ACS management according to the **PAIN** Pathway
Insert invasive cooling catheter in the Cath Lab
if not done prior to presentation — Cardiac

NO

Critical Care Screener to evaluate for
cardiac or medical etiology

Medical

Admit to CCU

Admit to ICU

E

Induced Hypothermia Protocol

Inclusion:
1. Age > 18 years
2. Coma at time of cooling
   * Not following command
   * No purposeful movement
   * Reflex and pathological/posturing movements are
     permissible

Exclusion:
1. Patient awake and follows command
2. Known terminal illness/DNR
3. Refractory shock despite vasopressors
4. Pregnancy (Relative contraindication)
5. Multi-organ failure

F

Hypothermia Protocol

Phase (I) Invasive cooling phase- First 24hrs
1. Insert temperature probes (bladder, rectal)
2. Initiate sedation and paralytic therapy
3. Initiate cooling to reach 33°C*

Phase (II) Re-warming Phase:
After 24 hours at target temperature begin rewarming by increasing 0.25°C per hour to 37°C

Phase (III) Maintenance
1. Normothermia maintenance takes affect
   when patient reach 37°C
2. Consider continuation of cooling device to
   control any hyperthermia for additional 24
   hours
3. Antibiotic therapy as indicated.

Nursing Care

Monitor and
document hourly

Vital signs, core
temperature, cardiac
rhythm, hemodynamic,
respiratory status,
neurological status,
urine output.

Watch for:
Hypokalemia, Mg, Ca,
Phos, Hyperglycemia,
Ileus, Infection,
Coagulopathy.

* Consider TTM at 36°C

G

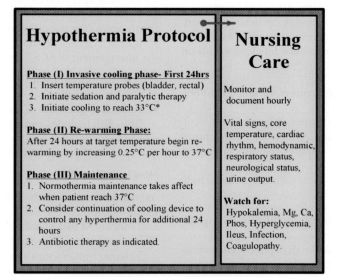

At least 72 hours post cardiac arrest define neurological outcome

STEP (III)

Is there evidence of acute MI? — Favorable

Unfavorable

Activate Ethics Committee to
define goals of care

NO

ICD Placement
and follow the
Heart Failure
Pathway as
indicated

YES

EF < 35%

EP Consult

NO

Follow the PAIN
Pathway for the
Management of
ACS

YES

Activate ESCAPE Pathway for
Sudden Cardiac Death Prevention and
ICD placement if indicated
(If EF < 35% 40 days post MI)

FIGURE 29.3 A, Pathway for management
of survivors of out-of- and in-hospital cardiac
arrest. B, Initial assessment of patients who
survive an out-of-hospital cardiac arrest. C,
Identification of the primary arrhythmia that
led to the cardiac arrest. D, Activation of the
cardiac arrest team, transfer to percutaneous
coronary intervention (PCI) center, and transfer to
the critical care unit. E, Inclusion and exclusion
criteria for patients who are candidates for the
therapeutic hypothermia protocol. F, Induced
therapeutic hypothermia protocol. G, Management of the post–rewarming phase including
the recommendation for out-of-hospital therapy
and the ethical decision to define goal of care.

decreased cardiac output, and increased systemic vascular resistance. The hypertension and the increased systemic vascular resistance are believed to result from the cold-induced vasoconstriction.

Serum electrolyte imbalance is common during the cooling phase and results from the cooling-induced intracellular shifts of potassium, magnesium, calcium, and phosphate, leading to low levels of all these electrolytes. During the rewarming phase, these electrolytes shift back to the extracellular space.

Our protocol therefore recommends measurements of the basic metabolic panel every 4 hours for a total of 48 hours, measuring electrolytes (calcium, magnesium, and phosphate) PT, PTT, and INR, and a CBC every 12 hours up to 48 hours.

Additional possible side effects of cooling to be monitored include the following:

1. *Coagulopathy.* Coagulopathy is generally not significant with careful temperature monitoring and avoiding temperature of <33°C. If active bleeding occurs during the cooling phase, evaluation of coagulation factors and platelets should be performed and deficiencies corrected.
2. *Hyperglycemia.* Hypothermia suppresses insulin release and causes insulin resistance. Our insulin infusion protocol for the management of hyperglycemia in critical care unit is used.[64]
3. *Infection.* Infection is usually multifactorial, including emergency intubation and intravenous catheter insertion and aspiration pneumonia at the time of arrest.

    Furthermore, the hypothermia itself can suppress white blood cell production and impairs neutrophil and macrophage function. All measures to reduce ventilator-associated pneumonia are employed, including elevating the head of the bed.
4. *Shivering.* Our protocol aims to prevent shivering by administration of sedation and neuromuscular blocking agents on induction of hypothermia.

Phase 2: Rewarming phase. After 24 hours of the target temperature, the rewarming phase starts.

Controlled rewarming is a very important phase of this protocol.

Rewarming should be slow; at a rate of 0.25°C per hour, which we recommend, it typically requires 16 hours to rewarm to 37°C.

Potential complications during the rewarming phase include the following:

1. Hypotension—owing to peripheral vasodilation during the rewarming phase.
2. Electrolyte imbalance—increased levels of potassium, magnesium, calcium, and phosphate caused by intracellular shifting of these ions back to the serum during the rewarming phase.

Phase 3: Maintenance of normothermia phase. The maintenance phase is the last phase of the TH protocol.

Normothermia maintenance takes effect when the patient's temperature reaches 37°C.

We recommend continuation of the cooling device to maintain a temperature of 37°C and avoidance of fever that can potentially worsen a cerebral injury.

The duration of the additional maintenance phase is usually between 24 and 48 hours.

STEP III

The management following hypothermia and rewarming depends on the neurologic prognosis (**Figure 29.3G**).

At least 72 hours after cardiac arrest, the neurologic examination is performed by the neurology team. The neurologic examination may be affected by the hypothermia protocol, including requirements for sedation and therapeutic paralysis, so the formulation of a neurologic prognosis may be delayed. In general, we defer neurologic prognostication until 6 days postarrest in patients undergoing hypothermia protocol.

Pathways for the patients will divide depending on whether the patient has a favorable neurologic prognosis or an unfavorable neurologic prognosis. An unfavorable neurologic prognosis would be defined as expectation of a persistent coma or vegetative state, or severe disability.

If the prognosis appears unfavorable, we recommend activating the ethics committee to meet with the family and clinicians to define the goals of care. From our experience, in most instances, life support is limited or withdrawn in such patients.

If the neurologic prognosis appears favorable, then the key question regarding further therapy is based on whether the cardiac arrest was because of MI.

If there is no evidence of acute MI (negative cardiac markers), then we recommend electrophysiology service consultation for consideration of implantable cardioverter defibrillator (ICD) placement and treatment of heart failure based on our heart failure pathway.[65]

If acute MI is confirmed by positive cardiac markers, we advise care based on the LV ejection fraction (LVEF) as it is defined by echocardiography or other imaging modalities. If LVEF ≤35%, we recommend activation of the ESCAPE pathway for sudden cardiac death prevention[66] and to consider ICD placement if EF ≤35% at 40 days post-MI. Also, we recommend managing heart failure according to our heart failure pathway.[65]

If EF >35%, we recommend following our PAIN pathway for the management of ACS,[63] including the following:

- Lifestyle modification
- Cardiac rehabilitation
- Secondary prevention medication (dual oral antiplatelet, ß-blocker, high-dose statin, ACE inhibitor/ARB)

Unresolved Practical Questions Regarding TTM

How Low Should We Go?

As mentioned earlier, the TTM study compared temperature management at 33°C to maintaining a core temperature of 36°C[60] and concluded that maintaining core temperature at 36°C has outcomes that are as good as cooling to 33°C.

This observation seems to contradict the findings of all previous studies and may have been a result of selection bias.

Our group hypothesizes that a potential difference in outcome based on degree of cooling will depend on the severity of brain injury.

Our group opinion regarding this difference in outcome depending on the selection of patients for TTM appears in **Figure 29.4**.

As seen in this figure, we can divide patients who survive cardiac arrest into 5 groups based on the degree of their postarrest brain injury.

1. Very severe brain injury
2. Severe brain injury
3. Moderate brain injury
4. Mild brain injury
5. Very minimal brain injury

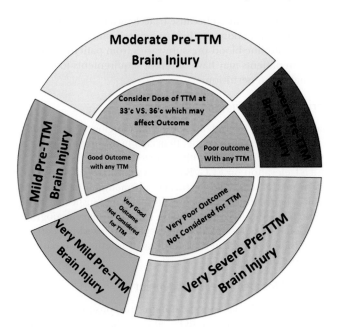

FIGURE 29.4 Degree of postarrest brain injury and proposed decision for Therapeutic Temperature Management (TTM).

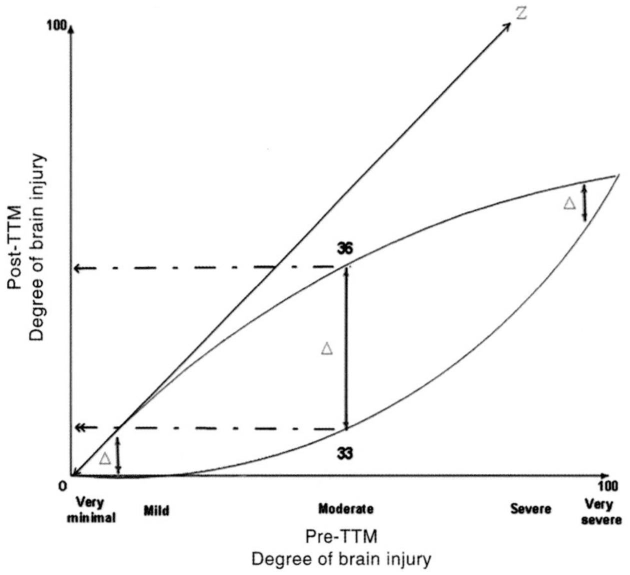

FIGURE 29.5 Applying Bayes' theorem to the relationship between post-TTM degree of brain injury and pre-TTM degree of brain injury. TTM, therapeutic temperature management.

Patients who fall into the first or the last category are unlikely to be considered for TTM in any health care system (as seen in the lower half of the figure).

- Patients who fall into groups 2, 3, and 4 are expected to have variable outcome.
- Patients in group 2, with severe brain injury, are expected to have poor outcome with any TTM.
- Patients in group 4 with mild brain injury are expected to have a good outcome with any TTM.

However, for patients in group 3, with moderate brain injury, the dose of TTM may affect outcome.

Our hypothesis is derived by applying Baye's theorem to the relationship between post-TTM degree of brain injury and pre-TTM degree of brain injury.

Our hypothesis is seen in **Figure 29.5**.

In this figure, we have plotted the pre-TTM degree of brain injury on the x-axis, with score of 0 to 100 and the post-TTM degree of brain injury on the y-axis with score of 0 to 100, where a score of 0 mean no brain injury, and a score of 100 means irreversible brain injury.

As outlined earlier, we have five groups of patients based on their severity of brain injury:

- Very minimal, mild, moderate, severe, and very severe.
- The equivocal line (Z) represents where the pretreatment group brain injury is exactly the same as the posttreatment group brain injury.
- The other two lines represent the different temperature doses of 33°C and 36°C.
- It is the delta (Δ) between these lines that defines whether the therapy has potential benefits.

On the left end of this figure, the delta is very small for patients with very minimal or mild brain injury.

This is the same case for patients with severe or very severe brain injury where the delta between the two doses of therapy is very small.

However, for patients with moderate brain injury, the delta is quite large. In our hypothesized algorithm, there is a potential to reduce the post-TTM degree of brain injury from a high to a low score.

On the basis of this hypothesis, our group suggests that the dose of temperature management should be 33°C because it is difficult prognostically to determine moderate brain injury level.

We have to remember that this is only a hypothesis and larger studies enrolling solely patients with moderate brain injury should be conducted.

Our group believes that the Achilles heel of the field of TTM is our current limitations in the prognostication of postarrest brain injury.

Endovascular Versus Surface Cooling

Technologies can be broadly divided into invasive (core cooling) and noninvasive (surface cooling) methods.[67]

There is no evidence for a difference in outcome based on cooling method.

The advantages of invasive cooling over surface cooling are:

1. Greater speed of hypothermia/normothermia induction when core cooling is used; however, it is unclear whether more rapid induction improves outcome.
2. Fewer and smaller temperature fluctuations in the maintenance phase.
3. Continuous central temperature measurement in some types of endovascular catheter is possible.
4. No risk of surface cooling–induced skin lesions.
5. Ease of accessibility to patient, that is, no need to cover large areas of the skin to achieve cooling.

6. Less medication may be needed to control shivering because there is more effective shivering suppression with skin counterwarming (ie, the entire surface area can be warmed using warm air, leading to a significantly diminished shivering response).[49,68,69]

The advantages of surface cooling over invasive cooling are as follows:

1. Ease of use; can be applied by nurses without the need for a physician to be present.
2. No invasive procedure required; therefore, no risk of mechanical complications.
3. Can be started immediately, without waiting for catheter insertion procedure, so potentially less delay in initiation of cooling.
4. No risk of catheter-induced thrombus formation.
5. Can be more easily applied outside the ICU setting.

A study by Deye and coworkers compared endovascular to surface cooling in a prospective, multicenter RCT.[70] The authors enrolled 400 patients; 203 were treated with endovascular cooling (using Zoll femoral Icy catheters) and 197 with external cooling (ice packs, fans, and a homemade tent). The main findings were as follows: significantly shorter time to target temperature (33°C), greater stability of temperature (defined as time within target ±1°C) in the maintenance phase, and reduced nursing workload (10 vs. 38 minutes, $P < 0.001$) in the endovascular group; more minor side effects in the endovascular group ($P = 0.009$); a nonsignificant trend toward more favorable outcome at 28 days (36.0% vs. 28.4%, OR 1.41 [0.93–2.16], $P = 0.107$; for shockable rhythm 53.7% vs. 37.1%, OR 1.97 [0.99–3.9], $P = 0.269$) and at 90 days (34.6% vs. 26.0%, OR 1.51 [0.96–2.35], $p = 0.07$) in the endovascular group; and fewer cases of severe overshoot (below 30°C) in the endovascular group ($n = 0$ vs. $n = 3$).[70] Strict fever control was maintained for a minimum of 3 days following rewarming in both groups.

This study had some limitations, especially the fact that newer and more powerful surface cooling devices such as the Arctic Sun system were not used and surface cooling was accomplished using fairly basic tools and devices.

We believe that the cooling method should be determined by institutional protocol.

Highlights from the 2015 Guidelines Recommendation for Post–Cardiac Arrest Care

Out-of-Hospital Cooling

Based on the 2015 guidelines: The routine prehospital cooling of patients with rapid infusion of cold IV fluids after ROSC is not recommended.[24]

Hemodynamic Goals After Resuscitation

It may be reasonable to avoid and immediately correct hypotension (systolic blood pressure < 90 mm Hg, mean arterial pressure < 65 mm Hg) during post–cardiac arrest care.[24]

Why: Studies of patients after cardiac arrest have found that a systolic blood pressure of < 90 mm Hg or a mean arterial pressure of < 65 mm Hg is associated with higher mortality and diminished functional recovery, whereas systolic arterial pressures of > 100 mm Hg are associated with better recovery. Although higher pressures appear superior, specific systolic or mean arterial pressure targets could not be identified because trials typically studied a bundle of many interventions, including hemodynamic control. Also, because baseline blood pressure varies from patient to patient, different patients may have different requirements to maintain optimal organ perfusion.

Early Coronary Angiography

Based on the 2015 guidelines: Coronary angiography should be performed emergently (rather than later in the hospital stay or not at all) for OHCA patients with suspected cardiac etiology of arrest and ST elevation on ECG. Emergency coronary angiography is reasonable for select (eg, electrically or hemodynamically unstable) adult patients who are comatose after OHCA of suspected cardiac origin but without ST elevation on ECG. Coronary angiography is reasonable in post–cardiac arrest patients for whom coronary angiography is indicated, regardless of whether the patient is comatose or awake.[24]

Targeted Temperature Management

All comatose (ie, lacking meaningful response to verbal commands) adult patients with ROSC after cardiac arrest should have TTM, with a target temperature between 32°C and 36°C selected and achieved, then maintained constantly for at least 24 hours.[24]

Continuing Temperature Management Beyond 24 Hours

Actively preventing fever in comatose patients after TTM is reasonable. In observational studies, fever after rewarming from TTM is associated with worsened neurologic injury, although studies are conflicting. Because preventing fever after TTM is relatively benign and fever may be associated with harm, preventing fever is suggested.[24]

Prognostication After Cardiac Arrest

The earliest time to prognosticate a poor neurologic outcome using clinical examination in patients not treated with TTM is 72 hours after cardiac arrest, but this time can be even longer after cardiac arrest if the residual effect of sedation or paralysis is suspected to confound the clinical examination.[24]

Why: Clinical findings, electrophysiologic modalities, imaging modalities, and blood markers are all useful for predicting neurologic outcome in comatose patients, but each finding, test, and marker is affected differently by sedation and neuromuscular blockade. In addition, the comatose brain may be more sensitive to medications, and medications may take longer to metabolize after cardiac arrest. No single physical finding or test can predict neurologic recovery after cardiac arrest with 100% certainty. Multiple modalities of testing and examination used together to predict outcome after the effects of hypothermia and medications have been allowed to resolve are most likely to provide accurate prediction of outcome.

Organ Donation

All patients who are resuscitated from cardiac arrest but who subsequently progress to death or brain death should be evaluated as potential organ donors. Patients who do not achieve ROSC and who would otherwise have resuscitation terminated may be considered potential kidney or liver donors in settings where rapid organ recovery programs exist.[24]

Why: No difference has been reported in immediate or long-term function of organs from donors who reach brain death after cardiac arrest when compared with donors who reach brain death from other causes. Organs transplanted from these donors have success rates comparable to organs recovered from similar donors with other conditions.

REFERENCES

1. Mozaffarian D, Benjamin EJ, et al. Heart disease and stroke statistics—2015 update: a report from the American Heart Association. *Circulation.* 2015 Jan 27;17:e205-e214.

2. Fishman GI, Chugh SS, Dimarco JP, et al. Sudden cardiac death prediction and prevention: report from a National Heart, Lung, and Blood Institute and Heart Rhythm Society Workshop. *Circulation.* 2010;122:2335-2348.

3. Chugh SS, Jui J, Gunson K, et al. Current burden of sudden cardiac death: multiple source surveillance versus retrospective death certificate-based review in a large U.S. community. *J Am Coll Cardiol.* 2004;44:1268-1275.

4. Muller D, Agrawal R, Arntz HR. How sudden is sudden cardiac death? *Circulation.* 2006;114:1146-1150.

5. Nichol G, Thomas E, Callaway CW, et al. Regional variation in out-of-hospital cardiac arrest incidence and outcome [published correction appears in *JAMA.* 2008;300:1763]. *JAMA.* 2008;300:1423-1431.

6. Cobb LA, Fahrenbruch CE, Olsufka M, Copass MK. Changing incidence of out-of-hospital ventricular fibrillation, 1980–2000. *JAMA.* 2002;288:3008-3013.

7. Centers for Disease Control and Prevention. 2013 Cardiac Arrest Registry to Enhance Survival (CARES) National Summary Report. https://mycares.net/sitepages/uploads/2014/2013CARESNationalSummaryReport.pdf. Accessed July 15, 2014.

8. Maron BJ, Doerer JJ, Haas TS, Tierney DM, Mueller FO. Sudden deaths in young competitive athletes: analysis of 1866 deaths in the United States, 1980–2006. *Circulation.* 2009;119:1085-1092.

9. Harmon KG, Asif IM, Klossner D, Drezner JA. Incidence of sudden cardiac death in National Collegiate Athletic Association athletes. *Circulation.* 2011;123:1594-1600.

10. Merchant RM, Yang L, Becker LB, et al. Incidence of treated cardiac arrest in hospitalized patients in the United States. *Crit Care Med.* 2011;39:2401-2406.

11. Nolan JP, Soar J, Smith GB, et al. Incidence and outcome of in-hospital cardiac arrest in the United Kingdom National Cardiac Arrest Audit. *Resuscitation.* 2014;85:987-992.

12. Hazinski MF, Nolan JP, Aickin R, et al. Part 1: Executive summary. 2015 international consensus on cardiopulmonary resuscitation and emergency cardiovascular care science with treatment recommendations. *Circulation.* 2015;132(suppl 1):S2-S39.

13. Travers AH, Perkins GD, Berg RA, et al. Part 3: Adult basic life support and automated external defibrillation. 2015 international consensus on cardiopulmonary resuscitation and emergency cardiovascular care science with treatment recommendations. *Circulation.* 2015;132(suppl 1):S51-S83.

14. Idris AH, Guffey D, Aufderheide TP, et al. Resuscitation outcomes consortium investigators. Chest compression rates and survival following out-of-hospital cardiac arrest. *Crit Care Med.* 2015;45:840-848.

15. Idris AH, Guffey D, Aufderheide TP, et al. Resuscitation outcomes consortium (ROC) investigators. Relationship between chest compression rates and outcomes from cardiac arrest. *Circulation.* 2012;125:3004-3012.

16. Vadeboncoeur T, Stolz U, Panchal A, et al. Chest compression depth and survival in out-of-hospital cardiac arrest. *Resuscitation.* 2014;85:182-188.

17. Stiell IG, Brown SP, Christenson J, et al. Resuscitation outcomes consortium (ROC) investigators. What is the role of chest compression depth during out-of-hospital cardiac arrest resuscitation? *Crit Care Med.* 2012;40:1192-1198.

18. Stiell IG, Brown SP, Nichol G, et al. Resuscitation outcomes consortium investigators. What is the optimal chest compression depth during outof-hospital cardiac arrest resuscitation of adult patients? *Circulation.* 2014;130:1962-1970.

19. Hellevuo H, Sainio M, Nevalainen R, et al. Deeper chest compression—more complications for cardiac arrest patients? *Resuscitation.* 2013;84:760-765.

20. Hinchey PR, Myers JB, Lewis R, et al. Improved outof-hospital cardiac arrest survival after the sequential implementation of 2005 AHA guidelines for compressions, ventilations, and induced hypothermia: the Wake County experience. *Ann Emerg Med.* 2010;56:348-357.

21. Olasveengen TM, Vik E, Kuzovlev A, et al. Effect of implementation of new resuscitation guidelines on quality of cardiopulmonary resuscitation and survival. *Resuscitation.* 2009;80:407-411.

22. Sayre MR, Cantrell SA, White LJ, et al. Impact of the 2005 American Heart Association cardiopulmonary resuscitation and emergency cardiovascular care guidelines on out-of-hospital cardiac arrest survival. *Prehosp Emerg Care.* 2009;13:469-477.

23. Steinmetz J, Barnung S, Nielsen SL, et al. Improved survival after an out-of-hospital cardiac arrest using new guidelines. *Acta Anaesthesiol Scand.* 2008;52:908-913.

24. Callaway CW, Soar J, Aibiki M, et al. Part 4: Advanced life support: 2015 international consensus on cardiopulmonary resuscitation and emergency cardiovascular care science with treatment recommendations. *Circulation.* 2015 Oct 20;132(16 Suppl 1):S84-S145.

25. Perkins GD, Lall R, Quinn T, et al. PARAMEDIC trial collaborators. Mechanical versus manual chest compression for out-of-hospital cardiac arrest (PARAMEDIC): a pragmatic, cluster randomised controlled trial. *Lancet.* 2015;385:947-955.

26. Rubertsson S, Lindgren E, Smekal D, et al. Mechanical chest compressions and simultaneous defibrillation vs conventional cardiopulmonary resuscitation in out-ofhospital cardiac arrest: the LINC randomized trial. *JAMA.* 2014;311:53-61.

27. Mukoyama T, Kinoshita K, Nagao K, Tanjoh K. Reduced effectiveness of vasopressin in repeated doses for patients undergoing prolonged cardiopulmonary resuscitation. *Resuscitation.* 2009;80:755-761.

28. Gueugniaud PY, David JS, Chanzy E, et al. Vasopressin and epinephrine vs. epinephrine alone in cardiopulmonary resuscitation. *N Engl J Med.* 2008;359:21-30.

29. Ong ME, Tiah L, Leong BS, et al. A randomized, double-blind, multi-centre trial comparing vasopressin and adrenaline in patients with cardiac arrest presenting to or in the Emergency Department. *Resuscitation.* 2012;83:953-960.

30. Wenzel V, Krismer AC, Arntz HR, et al. A comparison of vasopressin and epinephrine for out-of-hospital cardiopulmonary resuscitation. *N Engl J Med.* 2004 Jan 8;350(2):105-113.

31. Ducros L, Vicaut E, Soleil C, et al. Effect of the addition of vasopressin or vasopressin plus nitroglycerin to epinephrine on arterial blood pressure during cardiopulmonary resuscitation in humans. *J Emerg Med.* 2011 Nov;41(5):453-459.

32. Lindner KH, Dirks B, Strohmenger HU, et al. Randomised comparison of epinephrine and vasopressin in patients with out-of-hospital ventricular fibrillation. *Lancet.* 1997;349:535-537.

33. Callaway CW, Hostler D, Doshi AA, et al. Usefulness of vasopressin administered with epinephrine during out-of-hospital cardiac arrest. *Am J Cardiol.* 2006;98:1316-1321.

34. Callaham M, Madsen CD, Barton CW, et al. A randomized clinical trial of high-dose epinephrine and nonepinephrine vs standard-dose epinephrine in prehospital cardiac arrest. *JAMA.* 1992;268:2667-2672.

35. Gueugniaud PY, Mols P, Goldstein P, et al. A comparison of repeated high doses and repeated standard does of epinephrine for cardiac arrest outside the hospital. European Epinephrine Study Group. *N Engl J Med.*1998;339:1595-1601.

36. Donnino MW, Salciccioli JD, Howell MD, et al. Time to administration of epinephrine and outcome after in-hospital cardiac arrest with non-shockable rhythms: retrospective analysis of large in-hospital data registry. *BMJ.* 2014 May 20;348:g3028.

37. Dumas F, Bougouin W, Geri G, et al. Is epinephrine during cardiac arrest associated with worse outcomes in resuscitated patients? *J Am Coll Cardiol.* 2014;64:2360-2367.

38. Goto Y, Maeda T, Goto Y. Effects of prehospital epinephrine during outof-hospital cardiac arrest with initial non-shockable rhythm: an observational cohort study. *Crit Care.* 2013;17:R188.

39. Hayashi Y, Iwami T, Kitamura T, et al. Impact of early intravenous epinephrine administration on outcomes following out-of-hospital cardiac arrest. *Circ J.* 2012;76:1639-1645.

40. Nakahara S, Tomio J, Nishida M, et al. Association between timing of epinephrine administration and intact neurologic survival following out-of-hospital cardiac arrest in Japan: a population-based prospective observational study. *Acad Emerg Med.* 2012;19:782-792.

41. Stiell IG, Hebert PC, Weitzman BN, et al. High-dose epinephrine in adult cardiac arrest. *N Engl J Med.* 1992;327:1045-1050.

42. Koscik C, Pinawin A, McGovern H, et al. Rapid epinephrine administration improves early outcomes in out-of-hospital cardiac arrest. *Resuscitation.* 2013;84:915-920.

43. Cantrell CL Jr, Hubble MW, Richards ME. Impact of delayed and infrequent administration of vasopressors on return of spontaneous circulation during out-of-hospital cardiac arrest. *Prehosp Emerg Care.* 2013;17:15-22.

44. Kudenchuk PJ, Cobb LA, Copass MK, et al. Amiodarone for resuscitation after out-of-hospital cardiac arrest due to ventricular fibrillation. *N Engl J Med.* 1999;341:871-878.

45. Britton SW. Extreme hypothermia in various animals and in man: with notes on the detection of life and the possibility of recovery in cases of apparent death from exposure to cold. *Can Med Assoc J.* 1930;22:257-261.

46. Polderman KH, Varon J. How low should we go? Hypothermia or strict normothermia after cardiac arrest? *Circulation.* 2015;131:669-675.

47. William GR Jr, Spencer FC. The clinical use of hypothermia following cardiac arrest. *Ann Surg.* 1958;148:462-428.

48. Benson DW, Williams GR Jr., Spencer FC, et al. The use of hypothermia after cardiac arrest. *Anesth Analg.* 1959;38:423-428.

49. Polderman KH. Mechanisms of action, physiological effects, and complications of hypothermia. *Crit Care Med.* 2009;37(7 Suppl):S186-S202.

50. Polderman KH. Induced hypothermia and fever control for prevention and treatment of neurological injuries. *Lancet.* 2008;371:1955-1969.

51. Bernard SA, Jones BM, Horne MK. Clinical trial of induced hypothermia in comatose survivors of out-of-hospital cardiac arrest. *Ann Emerg Med.* 1997;30:146-153.

52. Yanagawa Y, Ishihara S, Norio H, et al. Preliminary clinical outcome study of mild resuscitative hypothermia after out-of-hospital cardiopulmonary arrest. *Resuscitation.* 1998;39:61-66.

53. Nagao K, Hayashi N, Kanmatsuse K, et al. Cardiopulmonary cerebral resuscitation using emergency cardiopulmonary bypass, coronary reperfusion therapy and mild hypothermia in patients with cardiac arrest outside the hospital. *J Am Coll Cardiol.* 2000;36:776-783.

54. Zeiner A, Holzer M, Sterz F, et al. Mild resuscitative hypothermia to improve neurological outcome after cardiac arrest: a clinical feasibility trial. *Stroke.* 2000;31:86-94.

55. Hypothermia after Cardiac Arrest Study Group. Mild therapeutic hypothermia to improve the neurologic outcome after cardiac arrest. *N Engl J Med.* 2002;346:549-556.

56. Bernard SA, Gray TW, Buist MD, et al. Treatment of comatose survivors of out-of-hospital cardiac arrest with induced hypothermia. *N Engl J Med.* 2002;346:557-563.

57. Holzer M, Bernard SA, Hachimi-Idrissi S, et al. Hypothermia for neuroprotection after cardiac arrest: systematic review and individual patient data meta-analysis. *Crit Care Med.* 2005;33:414-418.

58. Peberdy MA, Callaway CW, Neumar RW, et al. American Heart Association. Part 9: Post-cardiac arrest care: 2010 American Heart Association guidelines for cardiopulmonary resuscitation and emergency cardiovascular care. *Circulation.* 2010;122(18 Suppl 3):S768-S786.

59. Rittenberger JC, Polderman KH, Smith WS, et al. Emergency neurological life support: resuscitation following cardiac arrest. *Neurocrit Care.* 2012;17(Suppl 1):S21-S28.

60. Nielsen N, Wetterslev J, Cronberg T, et al. TTM Trial Investigators. Targeted temperature management at 33°C versus 36°C after cardiac arrest. *N Engl J Med.* 2013;369:2197-2206.

61. Herzog E, Shapiro J, Aziz EF, et al. Pathway for the management of survivors of out-of-hospital cardiac arrest. *Crit Pathw Cardiol.* 2010 Jun;9(2):49-54.

62. Herzog, E. Pathway for the management of survivors of out-of-hospital cardiac arrest, including therapeutic hypothermia. In: Herzog E, editor. *The Cardiac Care Unit Survival Guide.* Philadelphia, PA: Wolters Kluwer/Lippincott Williams & Wilkins Health; 2012; 20, pp. 212-219.

63. Herzog E, Saint-Jacques H, Rozanski A. The PAIN pathway as a tool to bridge the gap between evidence and management of acute coronary syndrome. *Crit Pathw Cardiol.* 2004 Mar;3(1):20-24.

64. Herzog E, Aziz E, Croitor S, et al. Pathway for the management of hyperglycemia in critical care units. *Crit Pathw Cardiol.* 2006 Jun;5(2):114-120.

65. Herzog E, Varley C, Kukin M. Pathway for the management of acute heart failure. *Crit Pathw Cardiol.* 2005 Mar;4(1):37-42.

66. Herzog E, Aziz EF, Kukin M, et al. Novel pathway for sudden cardiac death prevention. *Crit Pathw Cardiol.* 2009 Mar;8(1):1-6.

67. Polderman, K. How to stay cool in the intensive care unit? Endovascular versus surface cooling. *Circulation.* 2015 Jul 21;132(3):152-157.

68. Polderman KH, Herold I. Therapeutic hypothermia and controlled normothermia in the intensive care unit: practical considerations, side effects, and cooling methods. *Crit Care Med.* 2009;37:1101-1120.

69. van Zanten AR, Polderman KH. Blowing hot and cold? Skin counter warming to prevent shivering during therapeutic cooling. *Crit Care Med.* 2009;37:2106-2108.

70. Deye N, Cariou A, Girardie P, et al. Endovascular versus external targeted temperature management for patients with out-of-hospital cardiac arrest: a randomized, controlled study. *Circulation.* 2015;132:182-193.

Emad F. Aziz
Joshua Aziz
May Bakir

30

Principles of Antiarrhythmic Drug Therapy

INTRODUCTION

Ion channels in cardiac cells that generate the action potential are the basis for most arrhythmias. Thus, it is critical to know their function in order to understand the mechanisms of most arrhythmias and their treatment.[1]

The action potential is a representation of the changes in voltage of a single cardiac cell plotted over time.

There are five phases of the normal action potential (Figure 30.1)[2]:

1. **Phase (4):** is the resting potential, which is stable at –90 mV in working myocardial cells. It is principally permeable to potassium ions.
2. **Phase (0):** is the rapid depolarization where there is a rapid increase in sodium permeability that forces the membrane potential into the positive range.
3. **Phase (1):** is the initial repolarization phase of the action potential, which is the result of a rapid decline in the sodium permeability and increase in potassium and chloride ions permeability.
4. **Phase (2):** is the plateau phase of the action potential, which is the result of a balance of residual inward sodium and calcium currents and outward components of current carried by potassium ions.
5. **Phase (3):** is the phase of rapid repolarization, which is the result of a sustained increase in potassium permeability.

The pacemaker cells in the sinoatrial (SA) and atrioventricular (AV) nodes have significantly different action potential from the myocardial cells (**Figure 30.2**). Typically, phase (4) is resting at –50 mV and undergoes a slow depolarization that merges into phase (0). This is the effect of hyperpolarization-activated current, I_F. Depolarization is much slower as a result of calcium ion carriers.

The sciences of ion channels are well correlated with the shape of the action potential, and this correlation is depicted in **Table 30.1**.

Spontaneous depolarization of the SA node activates the neighboring atrial myocardium through electrotonic interactions. Elevation of the atrial membrane potential from its resting level to more positive values activates voltage-dependent Na^+ channels, giving rise to the peak Na^+ current (I_{Na}), which further depolarizes the membrane potential and produces the upstroke of the atrial action potential (AP). Subsequent activation of L-type Ca^{2+} channels produces a small influx of Ca^{2+} into the cell ($I_{Ca,L}$), which

triggers a much larger Ca^{2+} release from the intracellular stores of the sarcoplasmic reticulum (SR) through the cardiac ryanodine receptor channels (RyR2), a process termed Ca^{2+}-induced Ca^{2+} release.[3] The Ca^{2+} released into the cytosol (Ca^{2+} transient) binds to the contractile machinery and initiates contraction, thereby linking electrical excitation and mechanical contraction (excitation–contraction coupling). The Ca^{2+} transient also feeds back to the L-type Ca^{2+} channels, causing Ca^{2+}-dependent inactivation to prevent excessive Ca^{2+} influx.[4] Relaxation of the atrial myocytes occurs as Ca^{2+} is extruded from the cell via both the electrogenic Na^+–Ca^{2+} exchanger (NCX1; giving rise to I_{NCX}) and plasmalemmal Ca^{2+}-ATPase, and is resequestered into the SR via the SR Ca^{2+}-ATPase (SERCA2a). The latter is controlled by the inhibitory proteins phospholamban (PLN) and sarcolipin.[5] The depolarizing Na^+ and Ca^{2+} currents are countered by repolarizing currents, predominantly carrying K^+ ions. The transient outward K^+ current (I_{to}) produces a rapid repolarization immediately following the AP upstroke. A concerted effort of delayed rectifier K^+ currents with slow, rapid, and ultrarapid kinetics (I_{Ks}, I_{Kr}, and I_{Kur}, respectively) and the Na^+–K^+ ATPase current (I_{NaK}) control AP duration (APD).

There is a change in the APD across the myocardium from endocardium to epicardium, with the action potential being the longest in the midmyocardial areas.[6] This dispersion can also be responsible for certain reentrant arrhythmias.

The average duration of the ventricular action potential is reflected in the QT interval on the surface electrocardiogram (ECG). It is this relationship that identifies the factors that produce QT-interval prolongation and the arrhythmias that are related to it, such as *torsade de pointes*.

Action potentials may be initiated within cells or groups of cells that have the property of automaticity. Diastolic depolarization during phase (4) of the AP is the basis of the automaticity in the SA and AV nodes. Abnormal automaticity may take other forms, such as early afterdepolarizations (EADs) and delayed afterdepolarizations (DADs), which are examples of triggered activity because they are dependent on the preceding action potential.[7] Action potential prolongation is essential for EADs, with a net membrane current shift from outward to inward that, in consequence, produces oscillations of the membrane potential that may reach threshold; an example of this is torsade de pointes in long QT.[8] EADs can be abolished by interventions that return the APD toward normal or block the sodium current (I_{Na}) and calcium current (I_{Ca}). This can be achieved by increasing the heart rate with pacing or isoproterenol infusion;

333

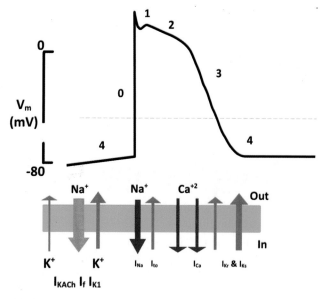

FIGURE 30.1 Action potential of cardiac cell depicting phases and ion movement across cell membrane. Downward arrows mark inward current; upward arrows mark outward current.

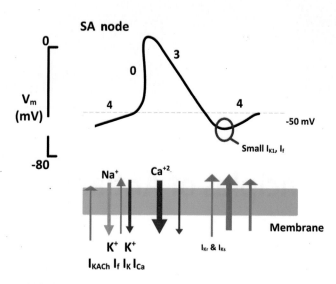

FIGURE 30.2 Action potential of cardiac pacemaker cells (SAN) depicting phases and ions movement across cell membrane. Downward arrows mark inward current; upward arrows mark outward current.

TABLE 30.1	Membrane Currents Controlling the Action Potential		
ACTION POTENTIAL PHASE	**CURRENT**	**DESCRIPTION**	**ACTIVATION MECHANISM**
Phase (4)	I_{K1}	Inward rectifier	Depolarization
Phase (0)	I_{Na}	Sodium current	Depolarization
Phase (1)	$I_{to,f}$	Transient outward, fast	Depolarization
	$I_{to,s}$	Transient outward, slow	Depolarization
	I_{Kur}	Delayed rectifier, ultrarapid	Depolarization
Phase (2)	I_{CaL}	Calcium current, L-type	Depolarization
	I_{Na}	Sodium current, late	Depolarization
Phase (3)	I_{Kr}	Delayed rectifier, rapid	Depolarization
	I_{Ks}	Delayed rectifier, slow	Depolarization
	I_{K1}	Inward rectifier	Depolarization
Multiple Phases	I_B	Background current	Metabolism, stretch
	I_{KATP}	ADP activated K^+ current	ADP/ATP
	Na-K, NCX	Pump currents	Ionic concentrations

or by blocking the I_{Na} and I_{Ca} with class IC and class IV antiarrythmics, respectively.

On the other hand, DADs are characteristics of conditions that lead to Ca^{2+} overload. Ca^{2+} antagonists can block these. An example of DAD-mediated arrhythmias are the tachyarrhythmias that occur with digitalis toxicity. Characteristics of the modulation of EADs and DADs are depicted in (**Figure 30.3**).

CLASSIFICATION OF ANTIARRHYTHMIC DRUGS

For the past two decades, antiarrhythmic drugs have been differentiated according to the well-known classification system developed by Vaughan Williams[9] and subsequently modified by Harrison.[10] The original system includes four major groups of antiarrhythmic

drugs: classes I, II, III, and IV. **Table 30.2** summarizes all the pharmacodynamic and pharmacokinetic properties of these drugs.

VAUGHAN WILLIAMS CLASS I: SODIUM CHANNEL BLOCKADE

Class I antiarrhythmic drugs block the rapid inward sodium channel during phase 0 of the action potential, slowing the rate of depolarization. The Hodgkin and Huxley[11] model describes these channels as existing in one of three states (open, closed, and inactivated), giving a different affinity for each drug.[12] These characteristics explain the feature of use dependence of drugs in this class, whereby block increases with increasing rate of stimulation, that is to say, with increased stimulation more sodium channels are in an open or inactivated state. Drugs that have

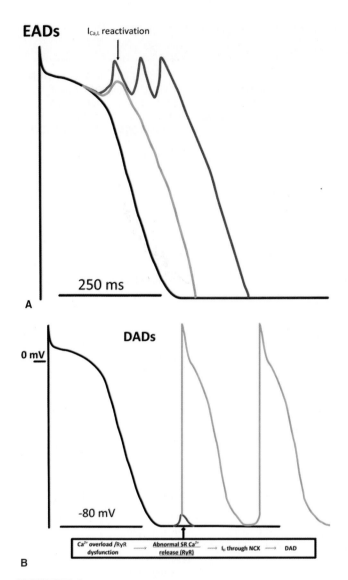

FIGURE 30.3 A, Early afterdepolarizations (EADs) are due to progressive prolongation of the action potential that results in oscillations at the plateau level of membrane potential. B, Delayed afterdepolarizations (DADs) are due to progressive prolongation of the action potential that results in oscillations during phase 4 of membrane potential.

greater affinity for their receptor when the sodium channel is open or inactivated bind more readily at faster stimulation rates. Drugs also show different rates for association or dissociation from their receptor, which is the basis for the subclassification refinement for class I drugs to (IA, IB, and IC).

Drugs with class IA action (eg, quinidine, procainamide, and disopyramide) prolong the depolarization and the refractoriness of myocardial cells in addition to blocking the rapid inward sodium channels. Thus, they may increase QRS duration and QT intervals. Class IB drugs (eg, lidocaine and mexilitine) shorten the action potential, but produce a minimum inhibition of the inward sodium channels, thus having a minimal effect on the QRS and QT durations. Drugs with class IC action (eg, flecainide and propafenone) are important sodium channel blockers that slow its conduction velocity and could thus increase the QRS duration more than any of the other class I drugs.

Class IA

These drugs have an intermediate rate of association and dissociation from sodium channels. In addition to blocking the sodium channels, they also decrease automaticity and excitability in the atria, ventricles, and Purkinje fibers because of the blockade of the rapidly activating potassium channel I_{Kr}.[13]

Quinidine

Quinidine depresses conduction and excitability, slows repolarization, and lengthens the AP duration. Because of its I_{kr} channel blockade, it reduces the maximum reentry frequency and thus slows tachycardia. It also possesses an α-adrenergic blocking property that promotes vasodilation and, in turn, causes a reflex increase in the SA node rate. It also has a greater potassium channel blockade than procainamide; thus, these drugs should be avoided in patients with heart failure because of their proarrhythmic and negative inotropic effect. In addition, quinidine decreases the potassium current during phase 1 of the action potential by blocking the I_{to} current. This effect may prevent the heterogeneity in membrane potentials during phase 2, which is believed to underlie the ST-segment elevation in the right precordial leads and initiation of ventricular fibrillation seen in Brugada syndrome.[14] This characteristic has been postulated in some studies for the management of electrical storm in Brugada syndrome patients.[15–17] Quinidine is predominantly metabolized by the P450 enzyme CYP3A4, and thus requires a lower dosage in patients with liver dysfunction. Importantly, it reduces the renal clearance of digoxin and may lead to digoxin toxicity.[18,19] Metabolism of quinidine is inhibited by cimetidine and increased by phenytoin, phenobarbital, and rifampin. The main side effects of quinidine include hypotension, thrombocytopenia, hepatitis, and cinchonism, whose symptoms include tinnitus, blurred vision, headaches, and dizziness.[20] It also can worsen symptoms in patients with myasthenia gravis.[21]

Disopyramide

In addition to its class IA characteristics, it exerts marked cardiac antimuscarinic effects leading to sinus node suppression as well as slow AV nodal conduction. Because of this anticholinergic effect, this drug can cause urinary retention, dry mouth, blurred vision, and closed-angle glaucoma and should thus be avoided in patients with glaucoma and men with symptomatic prostatic hyperplasia. For the past few years, disopyramide has emerged as an important drug in the management of patients with obstructive hypertrophic cardiomyopathy,[22–24] which may be its only use nowadays. It is eliminated by both renal and hepatic routes. It should be titrated up gradually from low doses because of its characteristics of saturable protein binding that can lead to disproportionally increased levels of the free drug.
Dosage: 150 mg every 8 hours up to 1 gm/day.

Procainamide

It is a derivative of the local anesthetic agent procaine, and its active metabolite N-acetylprocainamide (NAPA) is the reason for its I_{kr} blockade. It is indicated for acute conversion of ventricular and atrial dysrhythmias, and although it is less effective in suppressing abnormal ectopic pacemaker activity, it has more effective Na+ channel blockers in depolarized cells. Procainamide given intravenously in a maximal dose of 10 mg/kg body weight

TABLE 30.2	Vaughan Williams Antiarrhythmic Drugs Pharmacodynamics and Pharmacokinetic Properties						
DRUG	EFFECT ON ION CURRENTS, CHANNELS	ECG CHANGES	ELIMINATION	BIOAVAILABILITY (%)	TIME TO PEAK PLASMA CONCENTRATION (HR)	USUAL INITIAL DOSE	MODIFICATION OF DOSE IF RENAL (RD), HEPATIC (HD) DYSFUNCTION
Procainamide	I_{Na}, I_{Kr}	↑ QT	Hepatic (40–70%) Renal (30–60%)	100	1	500 mg q6h	q6h ↓ RD
Quinidine	I_{Na}, I_{Kr}, I_{to}	↑ QT	Hepatic (50–90%) Renal (10–30%)	70	1.5–3	200 mg q6h	↓ HD
Disopyramide	I_{Na}, I_{Kr}	↑ QT	Hepatic (20–30%) Renal (40–50%)	80–90	1–2	100 mg q6h	↓ RD ↓ HD
Lidocaine	I_{Na}		Hepatic			Load (75–225 mg followed by 1–4 mg/min IV)	↓ HD ↓ CHF
Mexiletine	I_{Na}		Hepatic	90	2–4	200 mg q8h	q8h↓ HD ↓ CHF
Propafenone	I_{Na}, βB	↑ PR, ↑ QRS	Hepatic	10–50	2–3	150 mg q8h	
Flecainide	I_{Na}	↑ PR, ↑ QRS	Hepatic (70%) Renal (30%)	90–95	2	50–100 mg q12h	↓ RD ↓ HD
Amiodarone	I_{Kr}, I_{Ks}, IK$_{Ach}$, Ca, I_{Na}, βB	↑ PR, ↑ QRS ↑ QT	Hepatic	50	3–7 (onset of action may take weeks)	400 mg q12h × 7 days, followed by 200 mg daily	
Dronedarone	I_{Kr}, I_{Ks}, IK$_{Ach}$, Ca, I_{Na}, βB	↑ PR, ↑ QT	Hepatic	4–15	3–6	400 mg q12h	Avoid in Acute HF
Dofetilide	I_{Kr}	↑ QT	Renal	90	2–3	500 mcg q12h	↓ RD
Sotalol	I_{kr}, βB	↑ QT	Renal	90	2.5–4		↓ RD
Ibutilide	I_{Kr}	↑ QT	Hepatic			1 mg IV over 10 min	Increase risk of torsades in CHF
Vernakalant	$I_{Kur,}$ HERG, I_{KAch}	↑ QRS ↑ QT	Hepatic			3 mg/kg IV over 10 min followed by 2 mg/kg	

over a 5-minute period during sinus rhythm produced complete anterograde block in the accessory pathway.[25] The usual effective concentration of procainamide is 4 to 8 mcg/mL and NAPA 7 to 15 mcg/mL.[26] Because of its Variable hepatic metabolism in relation to NAPA, monitoring of both procainamide and NAPA levels is needed during initiation of the drug or up titration of dosage because each component reaches steady-state levels at different times. The QT interval should be monitored during initiation to assess the risk of torsade de pointes. Procainamide can cause a drug-induced lupus-like syndrome that appears in about 20% of patients, with positive antinuclear antibodies in all patients, these symptoms range from arthralgia, arthritis, fever, and malar rash

to pleural and cardiac effusions. It is also associated with the development of agranulocytosis.[27] It certainly has negative inotropic properties that may lead to hypotension with rapid IV infusion, and it is thus contraindicated in patients with heart failure.
Dosage: Acute: 17 mg/kg at 20 mg/min (50 mg/min, if urgent). Infusion: 1–4 mg/min (depends on renal function).

Class IB

These drugs block fast sodium channels, decreasing V_{max}, the rate of depolarization during phase 0 of the action potential. They are typically used in treatment of ventricular tachycardia because they have no significant effect on atrial tissue. Both lidocaine and mexiletine are metabolized in the liver by the P450 enzyme CYP2D6; thus drugs that inhibit this enzyme (ie, amiodarone, quinidine, citalopram, cimetidine) can increase their plasma levels and the risks of toxicity.

Lidocaine

It is indicated in acute management and treatment of ventricular arrhythmia and is administered intravenously only to treat arrhythmias associated with myocardial infarction.[28] It is rapidly acting exclusively on Na⁺ channels and may slightly shorten action potential duration and effective refractory period of normal conducting tissues, thus prolonging diastole and extending the time to recovery. However, some studies have suggested a facilitation of subnodal block in patient with abnormal conduction[29]; thus, when it is used as a local anesthetic, it should be given with caution in patients with heart block.[30] Lidocaine can cause sinus node standstill, in addition to causing neurologic system toxicity, which can be manifested by paresthesias, tremor, nausea, lightheadedness, hearing disturbances, slurred speech, and convulsions.
Dosage: 1.0–1.5 mg/kg IV push over 1–2 min; repeat every 5–10 min with 0.5–0.75 mg/kg, as needed, until 3 mg/kg total dose. Typical maintenance dose: 1.0 to 4.0 mg/min.

Mexilitine

It is an overall analog of lidocaine and can be safely used in patients with severe systolic dysfunction. It has an approximately 90% bioavailability, with only 1% of total body content within the plasma. Side effects of mexilitine include severe gastritis, tremor, blurred vision, nausea, dysphoria, dizziness, and agranulocytosis.
Dosage: 200 mg every 8 hours; consider lower dose in renal dysfunction patients.

Class IC

Flecainide and propafenone slow conduction velocity and V_{max} by blockade of sodium channels, with slow association/dissociation channel kinetics, resulting in marked use-dependent characteristics. Both prolong the PR and QRS durations, although flecainide can slightly increase the QT interval. The concomitant use of a β-blocker or nondihydropyridine calcium channel antagonist is generally recommended to prevent rapid atrioventricular conduction in the event of atrial flutter. Both can be effective at maintaining sinus rhythm with recurrence rates of 31% to 70%, as seen in the RAFT trial.[31]

Flecainide

It slows conduction in all cardiac tissue, has negative inotropic effect, and is shown to block the delayed rectifier potassium channels.[32] It is used primarily in patients with supraventricular tachycardia and atrial fibrillation (AF). It should be avoided in patients with coronary artery disease, reduced ventricular function, and ventricular arrhythmia, as seen in clinical trials, including the Cardiac Arrhythmia Suppression Trial (CAST)[33] and the Cardiac Arrest Study Hamburg (CASH).[34]

Flecainide can cause sinus node dysfunction and can increase pacing thresholds as well as increased levels of digoxin.
Dosage: 100 to 200 mg every 12 hours.

Propafenone

It blocks both open and inactivated sodium channels; in addition, it blocks both voltage-dependent calcium currents and potassium currents such that the action potential duration is essentially unchanged.[35] It has β-blocking properties that are particularly obvious in patients who poorly metabolize propafenone to 5-hydroxy propafenone. It is metabolized in the liver by enzyme CYP2D6 and thus increases the levels of digoxin, metoprolol, and warfarin.
Dosage: 450–900 mg every 8 hours.

Pill-in-the-Pocket

Class IC medication has been tested for safety and efficacy to be used in the emergency room with patients who have recent-onset atrial fibrillation; treatment was successful in 94% of the episodes occurring during the 15 months' follow-up, with conversion occurring over the mean of two hours.[36] The major concern of this approach was the possibility of ventricular tachyarrhythmias that ranged up to 5%. The pill-in-the-pocket approach should be considered an outpatient self-administration of single oral loading dose only in patients with lone AF and normal hearts, after being initially used in an in-hospital monitor setting that proved to have a safe response to single-dose therapy[37] with reported conversion rates of 70% to 80%.[38]
Dosage: depending on patient weight < 70 kg: immediate-release propafenone 450 mg once and flecainide 200 mg once, for weight ≥ 70 kg: 600 mg once and 300 mg once, respectively.

VAUGHAN WILLIAMS CLASS II: β-RECEPTOR BLOCKADE

This class of medications include those that selectively block receptors in cardiac tissue (β_1) or nonselectively including receptors in the lung and the blood vessel (β_2). Their predominant actions include a reduction in automaticity in cardiac tissue and conduction through the AV node. B_1 selective drugs like metoprolol, bisoprolol, and atenolol are better rate control drugs particularly in patients with heart failure.[39] Nonselective drugs that block both β_1 and β_2 receptors include propranolol, nadolol, and carvedilol, which, in addition, block α_1-adrenergic receptor, making it a great drug for rate control in patients with heart failure and hypertension.[40]

VAUGHAN WILLIAMS CLASS III: POTASSIUM BLOCKADE

Medications in this class block potassium channels, resulting in prolongation of the action potential. This group includes amiodarone, dronadarone, sotalol, ibutilide, and dofetilide. Vernakalant is a new agent that blocks potassium channels selectively in the atrial tissue.

Agents that block the rapidly activating inward rectifying potassium channels (I_{kr}) display reverse use dependence, wherein block is greater at slower heart rate. Therefore, drugs that block I_{kr} result in delays in repolarization and QT prolongation predominantly at slower heart rate (eg, dofetilide).

Amiodarone

It is the most commonly used antiarrhythmic drugs by far because it exerts effects across all Vaughan Williams classes. It increases the action potential duration and the refractory period via potassium channel blockade in a use-dependent manner, and noncompetitive inhibition of α- and β-receptors.[41] It increases the refractory period in all cardiac tissues, and decreases automaticity by slowing phase 4 depolarization. Although it might increase QT interval, torsade de pointes very rarely occurs (<1%).[42]

Amiodarone possesses class I effects by blocking activated sodium channels[43,44] and also blocks L-type calcium channels. Amiodarone and dofetilide are second-line agents for patients without heart disease but are first-line agents for patients with heart failure. When given intravenously, it can cause hypotension that is related to the solvents polysorbate 80 and benzyl alcohol.[45] The iodine moiety in amiodarone is responsible for hypothyroid or hyperthyroid status. Iodine released from amiodarone in its metabolism directly inhibits thyroid function and hormone synthesis, producing a state of hypothyroidism.[46] Hyperthyroidism can occur in up to 10% of patients with two forms described.[47] Type-I hyperthyroidism, occurs in populations with an underlying thyroid pathology such as autonomous nodular goiter or Graves' disease. In these patients, there is accelerated thyroid hormone synthesis secondary to the iodide load from the amiodarone therapy (the Jod-Basedow phenomenon). In type-II hyperthyroidism, there is an inflammatory thyroiditis with release of stored thyroid hormone.[48,49]

Amiodarone-induced pneumonitis may develop after several months or years, with cumulative prevalence estimated between 1% and 15%, depending on daily dose.[50] In addition, amiodarone may cause optic neuritis (0.1–2%), skin discoloration (4–9%), peripheral neuropathy (0.3%),[51] and hepatitis (0.6%), although an increase in transaminases can occur without it to hepatic toxic effect.[41]

It has a large volume of distribution, as a result of accumulation in fatty tissue and in the liver, lung, and spleen. Elimination is by excretion into bile, with a slow but valuable elimination rate and a half-life ranging between 13 and 103 days.[52]

There is a strong correlation between amiodarone and warfarin potentiation; thus, the warfarin dose should be reduced with close monitoring of the international normalized ratio. Other examples of drug-drug interactions are those documented with digoxin, risk of rhabdomyolysis when given in combination with statins and prolongation of the QT interval when given with fluoroquinolone and macrolides.[41]

Dosage:

An oral dosing protocol
- 15 mg/kg/day × 1 week (~400 mg TID)
- 10 mg/kg/day × 2 weeks (~400 mg BID)
- 5 mg/kg/day (~400 mg QD)
- Eventually reduce to 100–200 mg daily

General IV load
- All arrhythmia: Monitor heart rate and blood pressure
  - 150 mg over 10 minutes
  - 1 mg/min × 6 hours
  - 0.5 mg/min × 18 hours or longer

- Ventricular fibrillation
  - 300 mg IVP; may repeat w/150 mg IVP
- Ventricular tachycardia
  - 150 mg over 10 min; repeat as needed to a total of 2.2 gm in 24 hours

For chronic use, the prescriber should consider at least twice yearly assessment of pulmonary, hepatic, eye, and thyroid function during amiodarone therapy.

Dronedarone

Dronedarone is, like amiodarone, a benzofuranyl compound with iodine removed and a methane sulfonyl group added. Removing iodine from the molecule was intended to eliminate or reduce iodine-related organ toxicity. Dronedarone retains many of amiodarone's electrophysiologic effects. It is a multi-channel blocker with effects on the rapid and slow components of the delayed rectifier potassium channels (I_{Kr} and I_{Ks}), slow L-type calcium currents, (I_{Ca-L}), the inward sodium current (I_{Na}), and the inward rectifier potassium current (I_{K1}). It also inhibits the acetylcholine receptor–dependent K^+ current (I_{K-Ach})[53] and the pacemaker current (I_f) and is a noncompetitive α- and β-adrenergic antagonist,[54] thus reducing sinus rate and prolonging AV nodal conduction and refractoriness.[53] Dronedarone has been shown to prevent atrial fibrillation/flutter (AF/AFl) recurrences in several multicenter trials.[55,56] In addition to its rhythm control properties, dronedarone has rate control properties and slows the ventricular response during AF. In patients with decompensated heart failure, dronedarone treatment increased mortality and cardiovascular hospitalizations.[57] Results of the PALLAS trial suggested that dronedarone should not be used in the long-term treatment of patients with permanent AF.[58] As a result, the usage of dronedarone has fallen out of favor.[59] In our opinion, its use is limited only to cases when other medications are contraindicated, as in patients with atrial tachycardia who have underlying pulmonary disease. It is metabolized by CYP3A4 and thus subject to interactions with drugs that inhibit this enzyme such as verapamil, diltiazem ketoconazole, as well as macrolides, which could increase dronedarone levels and in turn worsen bradycardia or AV conduction block. It can increase digoxin levels by interacting with P-glycoprotein.[60]

Dosage: 400 mg every 12 hours.

Dofetilide

The most potent drug in this class,[61] it works by blocking the fast component of the delayed rectified potassium current, I_{kr}. Thus, it is indicated for chemical cardioversion as well as maintenance of sinus rhythm in patients with AF/AFl.[62] No negative inotropic effects are associated with this drug, and it could be used in patients with heart failure.[63] The EMERALD trial[61] showed that a full dose of dofetilide (500 mcg twice daily) was superior to low-dose dofetilide (250 mcg twice daily), low-dose sotalol (80 mg twice daily), and placebo.

The risk for torsade de pointes at doses of 250 to 500 mcg twice daily was less than 1% but as high as 2.9% in the DIAMOND-MI trial[64] and 3.3% in DIAMOND-CHF.[65] For this reason, the FDA recommends that dofetilide therapy be initiated in the hospital over a period of 3 days. It is excreted mainly by the kidneys (80%) through both glomerular filtration and cationic renal (active tubular) secretion, which is inhibited by cimetidine, ketoconazole, trimethoprim, prochlorperazine, and megestrol. Dofetilide carries a black box warning. Verapamil has a relative contraindication because it increases peak plasma level of dofetilide by 42% and was shown in the DIAMOND trial to increase the risk of torsade de pointes. Thiazide diuretics also have a block box warning in view of the risk of hypokalemia because they were shown to increase dofetilide AUC by 27% and further increased the QTc over time by 197%. In addition, any other drug that prolongs the QT interval or promotes hypokalemia or hypomagnesemia should be avoided with dofetilide.

As previously mentioned, the FDA recommends that dofetilide therapy be initiated in the hospital over a period of 3 days and prescribed and dispensed by certified personnel. Generally, three half-lives should be used after stopping a previous antiarrhythmic before starting dofetilide. However, in the case of amiodarone, a waiting period of 3 months should be allowed (or until amiodarone concentration < 0.3 mcg/mL is reached).

Dosage is determined on the basis of renal function, calculated by creatinine clearance.
Dosage:

> 60 mL/min	500 mcg twice daily
40–60 mL/min	250 mcg twice daily
20–39 mL/min	125 mcg twice daily
< 20 mL/min	contraindicated (or if QTc is >440 msec)

If the QTc increases by more than 15% after the drug initiation, dofetilide dose is to be decreased by 50%; while, if the QTc exceeds 500 msec after the second dose, dofetilide should be stopped entirely.

Sotalol

It is prepared as a mixture of d- and l-isomers, of which the l-isomer is responsible for β-blockade. Both isomers block the rapid component of the delayed potassium rectifier channel (I_{Kr}). The initial d-Sotalol drug was found to have a higher mortality in patients with a history of myocardial infarction, as seen in the SWORD trial[66]; however, the racemic mixture of d- and l-isomers does not increase mortality.[67]

It prolongs the action potential by prolonging the repolarization by blockade of I_{Kr} channels, in both atrial and ventricular tissue. As a result of both β-blockade and potassium channel blockades, there is an overall slowing of the heart rate, AV node conduction, conduction across accessory bypass tracts,[68] and increase in AV nodal refractory period.[69] Class III effects are seen at more than 160 mg daily; at dosages of up to 640 mg/d, the QT interval is increased by 40 to 100 msec and the corrected QT interval by 10 to 40 msec.[70] Sotalol carries a dose-related proarrhythmic risk of torsade de pointes, which increases in the setting of bradycardia, female gender, history of heart failure, or preexisting QT prolongation. Sotalol is excreted by the kidneys, and thus caution is indicated in patients with renal dysfunction. Antacids should be avoided within 2 hours because they may reduce peak serum concentrations and area under the plasma concentration curve. For a creatinine clearance of 30 to 59 mL/min, sotalol should be administered at an interval of 24 hours, starting at a low dose of 80 mg. Because of its β-blocking effect, sotalol should be used with caution in asthmatic patients, or in patients with other drugs that affect AV conduction.

Dosage: 80–320 mg orally twice daily can also be administered intravenously at 75 mg IV over 5 hours.

Precautions:
- Do not initiate if QTc > 450 msec
- Accepted QTc < 500 msec the for first 3 days to keep the risk of torsades de pointes under 2%.
- QTc < 520 msec could be accepted thereafter.
- Dosage greater than 320 mg/day may be lead to a substantial increase in the incidence of torsades de pointes (as high as 11% in patients whose corrected QT interval exceeds 550 ms).

Ibutilide

Ibutilide has antiarrhythmic effects through blockade of the rapid component of the delayed rectified potassium current, I_{Kr}, as well as enhancing the slow inward sodium current; therefore, it prolongs the action potential duration and the QT interval in proportion to its plasma concentration.[71] There is no significant effect on the heart rate, the PR interval, or QRS duration and no significant change in the cardiac output or the blood pressure. When administered as a 1 mg dose followed by a second dose of 0.5 or 1 mg, ibutilide converted 47% of patients compared with 2% of placebo.[71] The overall risk for torsade de pointes is about 5%,[72] and thus the patient should be monitored for 4 hours after administration of the drug. If ibutilide fails to convert, it may at least enhance the response to electrical cardioversion. Because it is extensively metabolized by first pass, it must be given intravenously. It can be administered to patients receiving digoxin, calcium channel blockers, or β-blockers without interaction; however, the risk of proarrhythmia may increase.
Dosage: 1 mg (0.01 mg/kg < 60 kg) over 10 min; repeat, if needed, after 10 min. In our practice, we preload the patient with magnesium to keep the magnesium level above >2.

Vernakalant

Vernakalant is an atrial-selective, multiple ion channel blocker that is approved in Europe for the treatment of AF; however, the FDA judged that additional information was necessary for approval. Vernakalant blocks the rapidly activating delayed rectifier potassium channel I_{Kur}, which is present in higher density in the atria, making it relatively atrial selective. It also blocks other potassium currents (I_{to}, hERG, and I_{KAch}) and exhibits rate- and voltage-dependent blockade of the fast inward sodium current I_{Na}. Vernakalant has, therefore, a much greater effect in fibrillating atria than in the ventricle and is less likely to be proarrhythmic.

In the ACT II trial[73] that was performed in patients with new-onset atrial fibrillation or flutter after cardiac surgery, 47% converted to sinus rhythm opted for infusions of Vernakalant, compared with 14% who received placebo with median time to conversion of 12 minutes. In a recently published controlled randomized trial, Vernakalant was found to have significant advantages: it achieved conversion to a normal sinus rhythm within an average of 10 minutes, compared to ibutilide with an average of 26 minutes. Approximately 90 minutes after treatment began, 69% of Vernakalant-treated patients were in sinus rhythm, compared to 43% of patients treated with ibutilide.[74] Most studies were performed on patients with recent-onset atrial fibrillation <7 days, and the conversion rate changed from 45% to 61% within the first 10 to 15 minutes after intravenous administration with the most commonly used regimen (2 mg/kg bolus followed by 3 mg/kg 30 minutes later if AF continued).[73,75]

Vernakalant is hepatically metabolized by CYP2D6; it is not clear what effect abnormal liver function has on the metabolism of the drug. Differences in renal function, age, sex, race, blood pressure, and heart failure status have not been shown to affect the pharmacokinetics of Vernakalant.[76] The new European guidelines added IV Vernakalant as a first-line treatment for chemical cardioversion for recent-onset atrial fibrillation in patients with coronary artery disease, moderate heart failure, and left ventricular hypertrophy.[77]

VAUGHAN WILLIAMS CLASS IV: CALCIUM CHANNEL BLOCKADE

Diltiazem and verapamil block the L-type calcium channels, resulting in the relaxation of arterial smooth muscle and vasodilation, and decreased contractility in cardiac myocytes. These drugs also slow AV nodal conduction and increase AV nodal refractoriness. Verapamil also blocks sodium channels, but this is not believed to be a clinically important effect. They are both well absorbed from the gastrointestinal tract and undergo significant first pass effects in the liver, giving a bioavailability of 20% for verapamil and about 40% of diltiazem. They are metabolized in the liver by CYP3 A4; levels can thus be increased in the presence of inhibitors of this P450 enzyme such as ketoconazole and human immunodeficiency virus antiviral agents.

OTHER ANTIARRHYTHMIC DRUGS

Ranolazine

Ranolazine has antianginal properties and is currently approved for use in chronic angina. It reduces myocardial ischemia by its effects on the late inward Na current (I_{NaL}). Ranolazine inhibits peak I_{Na} in the atrium but not the ventricle. This effect results in reduced atrial excitability and a rate-dependent increase in postrepolarization atrial refractoriness. Ranolazine has variable systemic availability after oral administration because of its extensive first pass metabolism in the gut and liver. Metabolism is mainly via CYP3A4 and, to a lesser extent, CYP2D6. The terminal elimination half-life is 7 hours. The recommended dosage in patients with angina is 500 to 1000 mg twice daily. Ranolazine results in a 2- to 6-ms mean increase in the QTc interval, but drug-induced polymorphic ventricular tachycardia has not been observed. The MERLIN-TIMI 36 trial showed significant decreases in the frequency of nonsustained ventricular and supraventricular tachycardia and in the trend toward less frequent new-onset atrial fibrillation.

Pearls

Greater caution should be used when treating women with antiarrhythmic drugs that prolong repolarization, especially when additional risk factors for developing torsade de pointes are present (**Table 30.3**). Patient synchronic class I a or class III drugs should have regular follow-up so that electrocardiogram can be checked for conduction changes or prolongation of the QT interval. Periodic monitoring of laboratory data is also important, including electrolytes, creatinine, and liver enzymes as appropriate for the particular antiarrhythmic agent. Both sotalol and dofetilide are renally excreted, and their use should be carefully monitored in patients with renal disease.

TABLE 30.3	Risk factors for Developing Drug-induced Torsade De Pointes
Congenital long QT	
Female gender	
Electrolyte abnormalities (hypokalemia, hypomagnesemia, hypocalcemia)	
Diuretic use	
Bradycardia	
Cardiac hypertrophy	
Myocardial fibrosis	
Congestive heart failure	
Renal and liver insufficiency	
Co-administration of drugs blocking P450 isoenzyme CYP3A4	
High doses or rapid intravenous infusion of the drug	
Baseline electrocardiographic abnormalities	
Prolonged QT, T wave lability	

REFERENCES

1. Whalley DW, Wendt DJ, Grant AO. Basic concepts in cellular cardiac electrophysiology: Part I: Ion channels, membrane currents, and the action potential. *Pacing Clin Electrophysiol.* 1995;18(8):1556-1574.
2. Hoshiko T, Sperelakis N. Components of the cardiac action potential. *Am J Physiol.* 1962;203:258-260.
3. Bers DM, Calcium cycling and signaling in cardiac myocytes. *Annu Rev Physiol.* 2008;70:23-49.
4. Sun H, Leblanc N, Nattel S. Mechanisms of inactivation of L-type calcium channels in human atrial myocytes. *Am J Physiol.* 1997;272(4 Pt 2):H1625-H1635.
5. Xie LH, Shanmugam M, Park JY, et al. Ablation of sarcolipin results in atrial remodeling. *Am J Physiol Cell Physiol.* 2012;302(12):C1762-C1771.
6. Ashraf A, Nygren A. Cardiac action potential wavefront tracking using optical mapping. *Conf Proc IEEE Eng Med Biol Soc.* 2009;2009:1766-1769.
7. Asakura K, Cha CY, Yamaoka H, et al. EAD and DAD mechanisms analyzed by developing a new human ventricular cell model. *Prog Biophys Mol Biol.* 2014;116(1):11-24.
8. Cranefield PF, Aronson RS. Torsade de pointes and other pause-induced ventricular tachycardias: the short-long-short sequence and early afterdepolarizations. *Pacing Clin Electrophysiol.* 1988;11(6 Pt 1):670-678.
9. Cobbe SM, Clinical usefulness of the Vaughan Williams classification system. *Eur Heart J.* 1987;8(Suppl A):65-69.
10. Harrison DC, Current classification of antiarrhythmic drugs as a guide to their rational clinical use. *Drugs.* 1986;31(2):93-95.
11. Hodgkin AL, Huxley AF. A quantitative description of membrane current and its application to conduction and excitation in nerve. 1952. *Bull Math Biol.* 1990;52(1-2):25-71; discussion 5-23.
12. Hondeghem L, Katzung BG. Test of a model of antiarrhythmic drug action. Effects of quinidine and lidocaine on myocardial conduction. *Circulation.* 1980;61(6):1217-1224.

13. Yao JA, Trybulski EJ, Tseng GN. Quinidine preferentially blocks the slow delayed rectifier potassium channel in the rested state. *J Pharmacol Exp Ther.* 1996;279(2):856-864.

14. Antzelevitch C, The Brugada syndrome. *J Cardiovasc Electrophysiol.* 1998;9(5):513-516.

15. Mok NS, Chan NY, Chiu AC. Successful use of quinidine in treatment of electrical storm in Brugada syndrome. *Pacing Clin Electrophysiol.* 2004;27(6 Pt 1):821-823.

16. Bettiol K, Gianfranchi L, Scarfò S, et al. Successful treatment of electrical storm with oral quinidine in Brugada syndrome. *Ital Heart J.* 2005;6(7):601-602.

17. Mizusawa Y, Sakurada H, Nishizaki M, et al. Effects of low-dose quinidine on ventricular tachyarrhythmias in patients with Brugada syndrome: low-dose quinidine therapy as an adjunctive treatment. *J Cardiovasc Pharmacol.* 2006;47(3):359-364.

18. Walker AM, Cody RJ, Greenblatt DJ, et al. Drug toxicity in patients receiving digoxin and quinidine. *Am Heart J.* 1983;105(6):1025-1028.

19. Ujhelyi MR. Spotlight article: quinidine enhances digitalis toxicity at therapeutic serum digoxin levels. (Mordel A, Halkin H, Zulty I, Almog S, Ezra D. *Clin Pharm Ther.* 1993;53:457-462). *Heart Lung.* 1993;22(6):560-562.

20. Wolf LR, Otten EJ, Spadafora MP. Cinchonism: two case reports and review of acute quinine toxicity and treatment. *J Emerg Med.* 1992;10(3):295-301.

21. Stoffer SS, Chandler JH. Quinidine-induced exacerbation of myasthenia gravis in patient with Graves' disease. *Arch Intern Med.* 1980;140(2):283-284.

22. Sherrid M, Delia E, Dwyer E. Oral disopyramide therapy for obstructive hypertrophic cardiomyopathy. *Am J Cardiol.* 1988;62(16):1085-1088.

23. Sherrid MV, Barac I, McKenna WJ, et al. Multicenter study of the efficacy and safety of disopyramide in obstructive hypertrophic cardiomyopathy. *J Am Coll Cardiol.* 2005;45(8):1251-1258.

24. Sherrid MV, Arabadjian M. A primer of disopyramide treatment of obstructive hypertrophic cardiomyopathy. *Prog Cardiovasc Dis.* 2012;54(6):483-492.

25. Antzelevitch C, The Brugada syndrome: ionic basis and arrhythmia mechanisms. *J Cardiovasc Electrophysiol.* 2001;12(2):268-272.

26. Roden DM, Reele SB, Higgins SB,et al. Antiarrhythmic efficacy, pharmacokinetics and safety of N-acetylprocainamide in human subjects: comparison with procainamide. *Am J Cardiol.* 1980;46(3):463-468.

27. Ellrodt AG, Murata GH, Riedinger MS, et al. Severe neutropenia associated with sustained-release procainamide. *Ann Intern Med.* 1984;100(2):197-201.

28. Wyman MG, Lalka D, Hammersmith L, et al. Multiple bolus technique for lidocaine administration during the first hours of an acute myocardial infarction. *Am J Cardiol.* 1978;41(2):313-317.

29. Gupta PK, Lichstein E, Chadda KD. Lidocaine-induced heart block in patients with bundle branch block. *Am J Cardiol.* 1974;33(4):487-492.

30. Aravindakshan V, Kuo CS, Gettes LS. Effect of lidocaine on escape rate in patients with complete atrioventricular block. A. Distal His bundle block. *Am J Cardiol.* 1977;40(2):177-183.

31. Pritchett EL, Page RL, Carlson M, et al. Efficacy and safety of sustained-release propafenone (propafenone SR) for patients with atrial fibrillation. *Am J Cardiol.* 2003;92(8):941-946.

32. Follmer CH, Colatsky TJ. Block of delayed rectifier potassium current, IK, by flecainide and E-4031 in cat ventricular myocytes. *Circulation.* 1990;82(1):289-293.

33. Preliminary report: effect of encainide and flecainide on mortality in a randomized trial of arrhythmia suppression after myocardial infarction. The Cardiac Arrhythmia Suppression Trial (CAST) Investigators. *N Engl J Med.* 1989;321(6):406-412.

34. Kuck KH, Cappato R, Siebels J, et al. Randomized comparison of antiarrhythmic drug therapy with implantable defibrillators in patients resuscitated from cardiac arrest: the Cardiac Arrest Study Hamburg (CASH). *Circulation.* 2000;102(7):748-754.

35. Grant AO, Propafenone: an effective agent for the management of supraventricular arrhythmias. *J Cardiovasc Electrophysiol.* 1996;7(4):353-364.

36. Alboni P, Botto GL, Baldi N, et al. Outpatient treatment of recent-onset atrial fibrillation with the "pill-in-the-pocket" approach. *N Engl J Med.* 2004;351(23):2384-2391.

37. Anusionwu O, Wali A. 'Pill-in-the-pocket' treatment for recent-onset atrial fibrillation. *Heart.* 2010;96(19):1605; author reply 1605-1606.

38. Reiffel JA, Cardioversion for atrial fibrillation: treatment options and advances. *Pacing Clin Electrophysiol.* 2009;32(8):1073-1084.

39. Effect of metoprolol CR/XL in chronic heart failure: metoprolol CR/XL Randomised Intervention Trial in Congestive Heart Failure (MERIT-HF). *Lancet.* 1999;353(9169):2001-2007.

40. Packer M, Bristow MR, Cohn JN, et al. The effect of carvedilol on morbidity and mortality in patients with chronic heart failure. U.S. Carvedilol Heart Failure Study Group. *N Engl J Med.* 1996;334(21):1349-1355.

41. Vassallo P, Trohman RG. Prescribing amiodarone: an evidence-based review of clinical indications. *JAMA.* 2007;298(11):1312-1322.

42. Vorperian VR, Havighurst TC, Miller S, et al. Adverse effects of low dose amiodarone: a meta-analysis. *J Am Coll Cardiol.* 1997;30(3):791-798.

43. Mason JW, Hondeghem LM, Katzung BG. Amiodarone blocks inactivated cardiac sodium channels. *Pflugers Arch.* 1983;396(1):79-81.

44. Mason JW, Amiodarone. *N Engl J Med.* 1987;316(8):455-466.

45. Cushing DJ, Kowey PR, Cooper WD, et al. PM101: A cyclodextrin-based intravenous formulation of amiodarone devoid of adverse hemodynamic effects. *Eur J Pharmacol.* 2009;607(1-3):167-172.

46. Amico JA, Richardson V, Alpert B, et al. Clinical and chemical assessment of thyroid function during therapy with amiodarone. *Arch Intern Med.* 1984;144(3):487-490.

47. Klein I, Danzi S. Thyroid disease and the heart. *Curr Probl Cardiol.* 2016;41(2):65-92.

48. Bogazzi F, Bartalena L, Tomisti L, et al. Glucocorticoid response in amiodarone-induced thyrotoxicosis resulting from destructive thyroiditis is predicted by thyroid volume and serum free thyroid hormone concentrations. *J Clin Endocrinol Metab.* 2007;92(2):556-562.

49. Tomisti L, Urbani C, Rossi G, et al. The presence of anti-thyroglobulin (TgAb) and/or anti-thyroperoxidase antibodies (TPOAb) does not exclude the diagnosis of type 2 amiodarone-induced thyrotoxicosis. *J Endocrinol Invest.* 2016;39(5):585-591.

50. Morady F, Sauve MJ, Malone P, et al. Long-term efficacy and toxicity of high-dose amiodarone therapy for ventricular tachycardia or ventricular fibrillation. *Am J Cardiol.* 1983;52(8):975-979.

51. Charness ME, Morady F, Scheinman MM. Frequent neurologic toxicity associated with amiodarone therapy. *Neurology.* 1984;34(5):669-671.

52. Holt DW, Tucker GT, Jackson PR, et al. Amiodarone pharmacokinetics. *Br J Clin Pract Suppl.* 1986;44:109-114.

53. Wegener FT, Ehrlich JR, Hohnloser SH. Dronedarone: an emerging agent with rhythm- and rate-controlling effects. *J Cardiovasc Electrophysiol.* 2006;17(Suppl 2): S17-S20.

54. Chatelain P, Meysmans L, Matteazzi JR, et al. Interaction of the antiarrhythmic agents SR 33589 and amiodarone with the beta-adrenoceptor and adenylate cyclase in rat heart. *Br J Pharmacol.* 1995;116(3):1949-1956.

55. Hohnloser SH, Connolly SJ, Crijns HJ, et al. Rationale and design of ATHENA: a placebo-controlled, double-blind, parallel arm trial to assess the efficacy of dronedarone 400 mg bid for the prevention of cardiovascular hospitalization or death from any cause in patients with atrial fibrillation/atrial flutter. *J Cardiovasc Electrophysiol.* 2008;19(1):69-73.

56. Pikto-Pietkiewicz W. The effect of dronedarone on the frequency of cardiovascular events in patients with atrial fibrillation—ATHENA studies. *Kardiol Pol.* 2009;67(4):455-456.

57. Hohnloser SH, Crijns HJGM, van Eickels M, et al. Dronedarone in patients with congestive heart failure: insights from ATHENA. *Eur Heart J.* 2010;31(14):1717-1721.

58. Kirchhof P, Nitschmann S. Dronedarone in high-risk patients with atrial fibrillation: PALLAS study. *Internist (Berl).* 2012;53(10):1248-1250.

59. Iannone P, Haupt E, Flego G, et al. Dronedarone for atrial fibrillation: the limited reliability of clinical practice guidelines. *JAMA Intern Med.* 2014;174(4):625-629.

60. Vallakati A, Chandra PA, Pednekar M, et al. Dronedarone-induced digoxin toxicity: new drug, new interactions. *Am J Ther.* 2013;20(6):e717-e719.

61. Boriani G, Biffi M, Bacchi L, et al. A randomised cross-over study on the haemodynamic effects of oral dofetilide compared with oral sotalol in patients with ischaemic heart disease and sustained ventricular tachycardia. *Eur J Clin Pharmacol.* 2002;58(3):165-169.

62. Singh S, Zoble RG, Yellen L, et al. Efficacy and safety of oral dofetilide in converting to and maintaining sinus rhythm in patients with chronic atrial fibrillation or atrial flutter: the symptomatic atrial fibrillation investigative research on dofetilide (SAFIRE-D) study. *Circulation.* 2000;102(19):2385-2390.

63. Pedersen OD, Bagger H, Keller N, et al. Efficacy of dofetilide in the treatment of atrial fibrillation-flutter in patients with reduced left ventricular function: a Danish investigations of arrhythmia and mortality on dofetilide (diamond) substudy. *Circulation.* 2001;104(3):292-296.

64. Olesen RM, Bloch Thomsen PE, Saermark K, et al. Statistical analysis of the DIAMOND MI study by the multipole method. *Physiol Meas.* 2005;26(5):591-598.

65. Pedersen OD, Brendorp B, Køber L, Torp-pedersen C. Prevalence, prognostic significance, and treatment of atrial fibrillation in congestive heart failure with particular reference to the DIAMOND-CHF study. Congest Heart Fail. 2003;9(6):333-40.

66. Waldo AL, Camm AJ, deRuyter H, et al. Effect of d-sotalol on mortality in patients with left ventricular dysfunction after recent and remote myocardial infarction. The SWORD Investigators. Survival With Oral d-Sotalol. *Lancet.* 1996;348(9019):7-12.

67. Julian DG, Prescott RJ, Jackson FS, et al. Controlled trial of sotalol for one year after myocardial infarction. *Lancet.* 1982;1(8282):1142-1147.

68. Kunze KP, Schluter M, Kuck KH. Sotalol in patients with Wolff-Parkinson-White syndrome. *Circulation.* 1987;75(5):1050-1057.

69. Kopelman HA, Woosley RL, Lee JT, et al. Electrophysiologic effects of intravenous and oral sotalol for sustained ventricular tachycardia secondary to coronary artery disease. *Am J Cardiol.* 1988;61(13):1006-1011.

70. Hohnloser SH, Woosley RL. Sotalol. *N Engl J Med.* 1994;331(1):31-38.

71. Murray KT, Ibutilide. *Circulation.* 1998;97(5):493-497.

72. Kowey PR, VanderLugt JT, Luderer JR. Safety and risk/benefit analysis of ibutilide for acute conversion of atrial fibrillation/flutter. *Am J Cardiol.* 1996;78(8A):46-52.

73. Kowey PR, Dorian P, Mitchell LB, et al. Vernakalant hydrochloride for the rapid conversion of atrial fibrillation after cardiac surgery: a randomized, double-blind, placebo-controlled trial. *Circ Arrhythm Electrophysiol.* 2009;2(6):652-659.

74. Simon A, Niederdoeckl J, Skyllouriotis E, et al. Vernakalant is superior to ibutilide for achieving sinus rhythm in patients with recent-onset atrial fibrillation: a randomized controlled trial at the emergency department. *Europace.* 2016;19(2):233–240.

75. Pratt CM, Roy D, Torp-Pedersen C, et al. Usefulness of vernakalant hydrochloride injection for rapid conversion of atrial fibrillation. *Am J Cardiol.* 2010;106(9):1277-1283.

76. Mao Z, Wheeler JJ, Townsend R, et al. Population pharmacokinetic-pharmacodynamic analysis of vernakalant hydrochloride injection (RSD1235) in atrial fibrillation or atrial flutter. *J Pharmacokinet Pharmacodyn.* 2011;38(5):541-562.

77. Kirchhof P, Benussi S, Kotecha D, et al. 2016 ESC Guidelines for the management of atrial fibrillation developed in collaboration with EACTS: The Task Force for the management of atrial fibrillation of the European Society of Cardiology (ESC) developed with the special contribution of the European Heart Rhythm Association (EHRA) of the ESC endorsed by the European Stroke Organisation (ESO). *Eur Heart J.* 2016;37(38):2893–2962.

Patient and Family Information for: PRINCIPLES OF ANTIARRHYTHMIC DRUG THERAPY

Antiarrhythmic drugs are medicines that are used to treat abnormal heart rhythms resulting from irregular electrical activity of the heart. Antiarrhythmics correct irregular heartbeats and slow down hearts that beat too fast. Normally, the heart beats at a steady, even pace. The pace is controlled by electrical signals that begin in one part of the heart and quickly spread through the whole heart. If something goes wrong with this control system, the result may be an irregular heartbeat, or an arrhythmia. Antiarrhythmic drugs control these irregular heartbeats. If the heart is beating too fast, these drugs will slow it down. By correcting these problems, antiarrhythmic drugs help the heart work more efficiently. These medications only control abnormal heart rhythms, not cure them, and therefore you may have to take them for life. There are many different types of antiarrhythmic drugs, and your doctor will decide what class and medication is best for you. We will explain the purpose and how to use the most commonly used medications here.

Antiarrhythmic medicines are split into four categories:

- **Class I antiarrhythmic** medicines are sodium channel blockers, which slow electrical conduction in the heart.
  - **Flecainide**: Take this medication by mouth with or without food, usually twice daily.
    - Supraventricular tachycardia: 100 to 200 mg/day every 12 hours
    - Paroxysmal atrial fibrillation: 50 to 300 mg/day taken 2 to 3 times daily
    - Should not be used in people with liver impairment
  - **Propafenone**: Generally needs to be started in a hospital setting to ensure ECG monitoring of the patient.
    - There are many different dosages of propafenone, depending on clinical presentation of the arrhythmia. The treatment is generally begun with relatively high dosages (450–900 mg/day), decreasing to near 300 mg/day.
    - This medicine works best when there is a constant amount in the blood. To help keep the amount constant, do not miss any doses. Also, it is best to take each dose at evenly spaced times day and night. For example, if you are to take 3 doses a day, doses should be spaced about 8 hours apart.
    - If you miss a dose of this medicine, take it as soon as possible. However, if it is almost time for your next dose, skip the missed dose and go back to your regular dosing schedule. Do not double doses.
  - These two drugs can be used as a "pill-in-the-pocket" method for use with single dosage in patients with lone AF episodes. This method can be utilized only in patients with normally structured hearts, with initial dose delivered in a hospital setting.
- **Class II antiarrhythmic** medicines are β-blockers, which work by blocking the impulses that may cause an irregular heart rhythm and by interfering with hormonal influences (such as adrenaline) on the heart's cells. By doing this, they also reduce blood pressure and heart rate.
  - **Metoprolol**: A β-blocker that works by blocking the effects of epinephrine, causing the heart to pump more slowly and with less force.
    - Metoprolol tartrate (short-acting) dosage: 50 to 200 mg taken every 12 hours.
    - Toprol XL (long-acting) dosage: 50 to 200 mg taken once daily
- **Class III antiarrhythmic** medicines slow the electrical impulses in the heart by blocking the heart's potassium channels.
  - **Amiodarone**: Most commonly used antiarrhythmic medication.
    - Maintenance dose: 100 to 200 mg daily
    - Avoid eating grapefruit or drinking grapefruit juice while using this medication unless your doctor instructs you otherwise. Grapefruit can increase the amount of this medication in your bloodstream.
    - Nausea, vomiting, constipation, loss of appetite, shaking, or tiredness may occur.
    - Tell your doctor right away if you have any of the following serious side effects: easy bruising/bleeding, loss of coordination, tingling/numbness of the hands or feet, uncontrolled movements, new or worsening symptoms of heart failure (such as ankle/leg swelling, increased tiredness, increased shortness of breath when lying down).
    - Amiodarone may rarely cause thyroid problems. Either low thyroid function or overactive thyroid function may occur. Tell your doctor right away if you develop any symptoms of low or overactive thyroid, including cold or heat intolerance, unexplained weight loss/gain, thinning hair, unusual sweating, nervousness, irritability, restlessness, or lump/growth in the front of the neck (goiter).
    - Amiodarone has many interactions with medications, so be sure to discuss all the medications you are taking with your doctor.
    - Many patients who are prescribed amiodarone are also on the blood thinner coumadin, also known as warfarin. The blood levels of coumadin are higher when used with amiodarone, and therefore the dose of coumadin will need to be adjusted.
    - Digoxin dose will also most likely need to be lowered to prevent levels of digoxin in the blood from being too high.
    - Muscle breakdown can happen when taking amiodarone with cholesterol medications.
    - Amiodarone can cause other electrical disturbances within the heart when taken with certain antibiotics, so be sure to inform any primary care provider before taking any additional medication when treating an infection.
  - **Sotalol**: Maintaining a normal heartbeat in patients who have AF or AFl.
    - Dosage: take one tablet 80 to 320 mg every 12 hours.
    - Patients who begin taking or restart sotalol should be observed in a hospital or similar setting in which heart and kidney function monitoring may be performed for

at least 3 days after starting sotalol. Close monitoring of your heart or kidney function may also be needed if your dose is changed.

- Sotalol may sometimes cause a new or worsened irregular heartbeat (prolonged QT interval), which could be life threatening. Talk with your doctor if you have prolonged QT interval or kidney problems.
- Sotalol has many drug and herbal interactions, so be sure to go over everything you are taking and have recently taken with your health care provider before starting sotalol.
- **Dofetilide**: Used for the maintenance of sinus rhythm in individuals prone to the occurrence of AF and AFl arrhythmias, and for chemical cardioversion to sinus rhythm from AF and AFl.
  - There is risk of fatal heart rhythm when starting this medication, and therefore it must be initiated in a hospital setting where heart and kidney monitoring can occur for 3 days.

- If you have been taking amiodarone, it should be stopped for 3 months before starting dofetilide.
- There is a very specific dosing regimen when initiating dofetilide, which will be carried out by a trained professional in the hospital. The home dose is 500 mcg twice daily.
- **Class IV antiarrhythmic** medicines slow the electrical impulses in the heart by blocking the calcium channels in the heart.
  - **Diltiazem**: This medication is used to treat high blood pressure and chest pain as well as heart rhythm problems. Diltiazem affects the movement of calcium ions within heart tissue that occur during each heartbeat. This helps to relax the muscles of the heart and also open up blood vessels around the heart. It is known as a calcium channel blocker.
    - Diltiazem should not be used if you have heart failure.
    - Extended release tablets dosage: 180 to 480 mg daily.

Steven B. Levy
Kimberly M. Sarosky
Eyal Herzog

31

Modern Anticoagulation Therapy

BACKGROUND

Atrial fibrillation (AF) is among the most common sustained cardiac tachyarrhythmia in hospitalized patients.[1] The lifetime rate of developing AF in individuals 40 years and older is approximately 25%; with an estimated 16 million Americans with AF by 2050. There is about a 5-fold increased risk in developing an acute ischemic stroke in patients with AF.[1] In a meta-analysis, the rate of ischemic stroke in patients managed for AF with adjusted-dose warfarin reduced by 66% and antiplatelet agents by 22%.[2] To that end, adjusted-dose warfarin has traditionally been the gold standard in those with AF who are at risk for stroke.

Warfarin, however, is a complicated anticoagulant to manage, with a diverse mechanism of action profile on the clotting cascade.[3] Therefore, to improve the effectiveness of antithrombotic therapy in AF and reduce the relative risks of bleeding, newer modern anticoagulants have been developed with more direct-acting mechanisms on the clotting cascade that yield a more predictable anticoagulant effect.[3] As such, the purpose of this chapter is to provide clinicians with an overview of the evolving field of anticoagulation therapy as it pertains to AF, particularly when cardiac valves are not involved, such as mechanical valve repairs and replacements.

As research advances and the understanding of the incidence and etiologies of AF evolves in the context of valvular conditions, we recognize that at the time this chapter was developed, there were established differences in the worldwide definition of nonvalvular atrial fibrillation (NVAF) that only recently emerged.[4,5] The American College of Cardiology (ACC), American Heart Association (AHA), and the Heart Rhythm Society (HRS) definition of NVAF can be summarized by the presence of AF in the absence of rheumatic mitral valve stenosis, a mechanical or bioprosthetic heart valve, or a mitral valve repair.[4] In contrast, the 2016 consensus of the European Society of Cardiology (ECS), European Heart Rhythm Association, and European Stroke Organisation removed the term "nonvalvular" AF, but rather references the specific underlying contributory clinical conditions.[5] Such scenarios may include AF secondary to structural heart disease, mitral stenosis, or prosthetic heart valves, suggesting the need for being more specific when selecting an anticoagulant or estimating stroke risk. For the purposes of this chapter, we refer to the ACC/AHA/HRS definition of NVAF.

The United States Food and Drug Administration (US FDA) has approved traditional and modern anticoagulants for the prevention of stroke and systemic embolism in patients with NVAF, thromboprophylaxis postoperatively in orthopedic and other procedures, as well as in treatment and in risk reduction of recurrent venous thromboembolism, such as deep vein thrombosis and pulmonary embolism. The scope of this chapter is a focus on the use of anticoagulants for AF with an emphasis on NVAF. The goal is to provide a decision analysis of anticoagulant drug selection and use based on clinical pharmacology, evidence, and patient characteristics.

ESTABLISH STROKE AND BLEEDING RISK

CHA$_2$DS$_2$-VASc SCORE

In addition to the shared decision making between clinician and patient, selecting the appropriate antithrombotic therapy for NVAF is often based on assessing the risk of thromboembolic stroke and bleeding.[4] The CHA$_2$DS$_2$-VASc stroke risk stratification score (**Table 31.1**), recommended for use by the 2014 AHA/ACC/HRS Guideline for the Management of Atrial Fibrillation, is an expansion of the CHADS$_2$ score with three additional risk factors including female sex, age of 65 to 74 years, and history of vascular disease, such as prior myocardial infarction, peripheral arterial disease, and aortic plaque.[4] Therefore, the CHA$_2$DS$_2$-VASc score is said to be a more accurate predictor of stroke risk in patients with a CHADS$_2$ score of 0 or 1 and thus improving guidance on the need for anticoagulant therapy.

The total score of the CHA$_2$DS$_2$-VASc is up to 9 points. On the basis of a strong level of evidence, the recommendation is to provide anticoagulation therapy for CHA$_2$DS$_2$-VASc scores of 2 or higher that indicate high risk for a thrombotic event. A CHA$_2$DS$_2$-VASc score of 1 indicates an intermediate risk of an event and thus the clinician may consider offering antithrombotic therapy with either aspirin, an anticoagulant, or no therapy with continued monitoring. Assessing bleeding risk may assist with the decision process.

When the decision is to initiate anticoagulation therapy, several considerations need to be evaluated. Warfarin remains the gold-standard anticoagulant method for AF due to a mechanical or bioprosthetic heart valve.[4] The intensity of warfarin anticoagulation

TABLE 31.1	CHA₂DS₂-VASc and HAS-BLED Risk Stratification Tools		

CHA$_2$DS$_2$-VASc		HAS-BLED	
CONDITION	**POINTS**	**CONDITION**	**POINTS**
Chronic heart failure	1	Hypertension (ie, uncontrolled)	1
Hypertension	1	Abnormal renal/liver function	1 or 2
Age ≥ 75 y	2	Stroke	1
Diabetes mellitus	1	Bleeding tendency or predisposition	1
Stroke/TIA or thromboembolism, prior	2	Labile INR	1
Vascular disease (MI, PAD, or aortic plaque)	1	Age (eg, >65 y)	1
Age 65–74 y	1	Drugs (eg, concomitant aspirin or NSAIDs) or alcohol	1 or 2
Sex category (female)	1		
Total possible score	9	Total possible score	9

INR, international normalized ratio; MI, myocardial infarction; NSAIDs, non-steroidal anti-inflammatory drugs; PAD, peripheral arterial disease; TIA, transient ischemic attack.

to a target international normalized ratio (INR) of 2.5 (range 2 to 3) is recommended for mechanical aortic valves without risks for thromboembolism (eg, CHA$_2$DS$_2$-VASc = 0), bioprosthetic aortic or mitral valves, and mitral valve stenosis or regurgitation. On the other hand, a target INR of 3 (range 2.5 to 3.5) is recommended for mechanical aortic valves with risks for thromboembolism (eg, CHA$_2$DS$_2$-VASc ≥ 2) and mechanical mitral valves.[6] When introducing warfarin, a parenteral anticoagulant with complete anticoagulant activity using either unfractionated heparin (UFH) as a continuous infusion with a steady-state target-activated partial thromboplastin time (aPTT) 1.5 to 2 times the upper limit of the "normal" range or a low-molecular-weight heparin (LMWH), such as enoxaparin, is recommended concomitantly with warfarin until the INR is at target on two separate samples 24 hours apart after at least 5 days of overlap.[3] The timing in which therapeutic INR is achieved is dependent on the half-lives of vitamin-K–dependent clotting factors II, VII, IX, and X. On average, a therapeutic INR is achieved by day 5, which is based on complete depletion of factor II, which has the longest half-life of approximately 48 to 64 hours.[7]

For NVAF with a CHA$_2$DS$_2$-VASc score of 2 or greater, oral anticoagulation therapy with either warfarin to a target INR 2 to 3 or a novel oral anticoagulant (NOAC) is recommended.[4] The NOAC agents include dabigatran, which elicits its anticoagulant effect by directly inhibiting thrombin activity, similar to argatroban; and apixaban, edoxaban, and rivaroxaban that inhibit factor Xa (FXa) activity similar to that of LMWHs.[8–11]

HAS-BLED

Several tools are available to assess the risk of bleeding from anticoagulation for AF. The HAS-BLED score (**Table 31.1**) has been validated to predict clinically significant bleeding and has been demonstrated to outperform the HEMORR(2)HAGES and ATRIA (**An T**icoagulation and **R**isk factors **I**n **A**trial fibrillation) assessment tools that are more complicated to complete.[12,13]

The components of the HAS-BLED tool include modifiable and nonmodifiable risk factors such as hypertension, abnormal renal and/or liver function, stroke, bleeding tendencies, labile INR, age (eg, older than 65 years), and drug (eg, aspirin, P2Y$_{12}$ antiplatelet agents, nonsteroidal anti-inflammatory drugs [NSAIDs]) or alcohol use that increases the risk of bleeding. The highest possible HAS-BLED score is 9, whereby a score of 0 suggests a low risk of bleeding, 1 to 2 an intermediate risk of bleeding, and 3 or higher indicating a high risk of bleeding. In patients with a high risk of bleeding, improvements of modifiable risk factors, such as blood pressure control and avoidance of alcohol, may assist in determining anticoagulation selection during follow-up.

Although the clinical utility of these scoring systems requires additional evidence,[4] their results are useful in identifying those at a high risk of bleeding and may aid in the decision-making process between the clinician and patient. To illustrate a thought process for clinically evaluating stroke and bleeding risks, **Figure 31.1** illustrates a decision pathway that incorporates the CHA$_2$DS$_2$-VASc in the context of the HAS-BLED score. For example, an intermediate risk of stroke (eg, CHA$_2$DS$_2$-VASc score of 1) may result in one of three therapeutic options including no antithrombotic therapy, aspirin, or oral anticoagulation therapy. To help guide the clinician and patient in this scenario, using the HAS-BLED scoring system may lead to a more conservative approach from the standpoint of bleeding risk, such as selecting no antithrombotic therapy or aspirin. On the other hand, a high risk of stroke (eg, CHA$_2$DS$_2$-VASc score of 2 or greater) and a high risk of bleeding (eg, HAS-BLED score greater of 3 or equal) is a therapeutic challenge often encountered that requires careful consideration of the risks and benefits. One approach may be to address modifiable bleeding risk factors during routine follow-up while selecting an anticoagulant with complete reversibility.

Once the decision has been confirmed to initiate anticoagulation therapy in the cardiac intensive care unit, patient characteristics need to be considered for selecting an agent(s).

Anticoagulation Pathway for Atrial Fibrillation in the Cardiac Intensive Care Unit

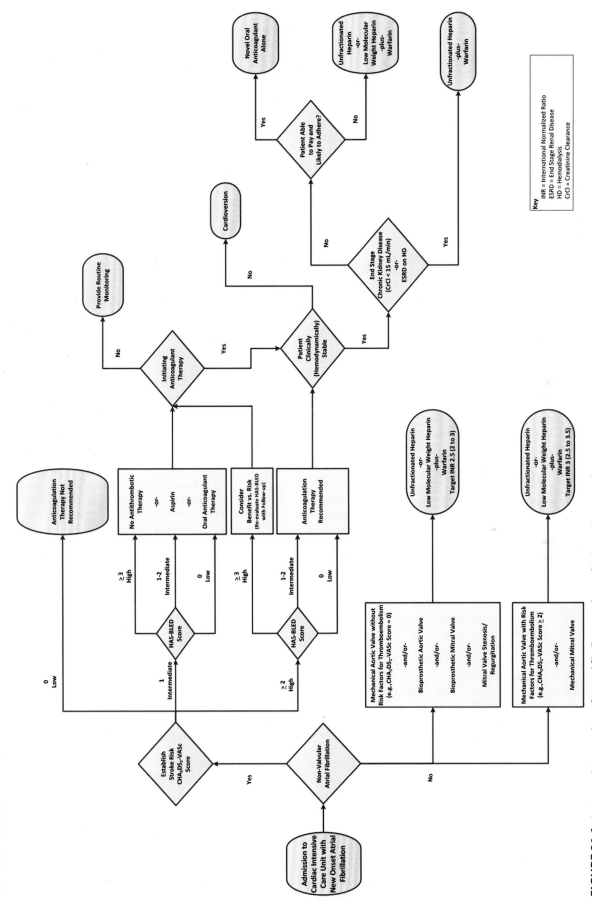

FIGURE 31.1 Anticoagulation pathway for atrial fibrillation in the cardiac intensive care unit.

ANTICOAGULANT DECISION BASED ON PATIENT CHARACTERISTICS

HEMODYNAMICALLY UNSTABLE REQUIRING CARDIOVERSION

Details surrounding patient selection criteria for and procedures involved with synchronized direct current electrical cardioversion are not discussed in this section because the technique extends beyond the scope of this chapter. For the hemodynamically unstable patient, it is important to first rule out AF as, indeed, the primary problem and not a compensatory response of another underlying condition, such as sepsis or hemorrhage.

Synchronized direct current electrical cardioversion is preferred for hemodynamically unstable patients presenting with new-onset AF greater than 48 hours for restoration of normal sinus rhythm, but does carry a risk for cardioembolic events, particularly during the first 72 hours after the procedure.[4] Anticoagulation should be initiated immediately following the procedure and continued for at least 4 weeks with life-long anticoagulation dependent upon the CHA$_2$DS$_2$-VASc score.[4,5] Following cardioversion in hemodynamically unstable patients with AF or atrial flutter less than 48 hours, the decision to provide anticoagulation is dependent upon the patient's CHA$_2$DS$_2$-VASc score.

Warfarin has traditionally been the preferred agent for anticoagulation in combination with either UFH or an LMWH until a therapeutic INR is achieved in this setting; however, growing evidence supports the use of NOACs in this population.[4,5] Selecting the specific anticoagulant therapy is discussed in further detail based on specific patient characteristics.

HEMODYNAMICALLY STABLE WITH ELECTIVE CARDIOVERSION

In a nonurgent setting for those who are hemodynamically stable with AF greater than 48 hours or unknown duration, transesophageal echocardiography (TEE) should be performed to exclude the left atrial thrombus for elective cardioversion.[4,5] When a thrombus is present, anticoagulation should be initiated for 3 weeks and a repeat TEE should be completed to verify resolution to proceed with cardioversion.[4,5] In the absence of a thrombus, the patient should proceed with immediate anticoagulation with UFH, starting with a weight-based bolus, followed by continuous infusion to attain target-aPTT, or weight-based LMWH, or a NOAC. The results of a recent trial utilizing data from the Finnish CardioVersion (FinCV) study demonstrated that peri-procedural anticoagulation reduced the risk for thromboembolic complications (TEC) by 82% and the CHA$_2$DS$_2$-VASc score provided a strong predictor for TEC post cardioversion in those without anticoagulation.[14] Following cardioversion, anticoagulation should be continued for a period of 4 weeks and life-long therapy is guided by the CHA$_2$DS$_2$-VASc score. Both warfarin and NOACs have been used for anticoagulation in this population of patients. To further consider anticoagulant selection, patient-specific factors including renal function needs to be considered.

CHRONIC KIDNEY DISEASE OR END-STAGE RENAL DISEASE ON HEMODIALYSIS

In the setting of stage 5 chronic kidney disease (CKD), defined as a creatinine clearance (CrCl) less than 15 mL/min or end-stage

renal disease (ESRD) requiring hemodialysis, the NOACs have minimal data to support the use in NVAF. This is because all of these agents are, to some extent, renally excreted and thus pose an increased risk for accumulation and bleeding.[15] CKD itself poses an increased risk for bleeding as well as thromboembolism.[5] In addition, with a moderate reduction in renal function, when the CrCl calculated by the Cockcroft–Gault equation is less than 50 mL/min, NOACs have been demonstrated to differ from one another in their relative risk for major bleeding.[15] **Table 31.2** compares the differences in dosing with renal impairment for anticoagulants. LMWH as an alternative to NOAC is also not preferred in this patient population because the use is relatively contraindicated in CrCl less than 15 mL/min.

Warfarin therefore remains the oral anticoagulant option for patients with CKD stage 5 (CrCl < 15 mL/min) or ESRD requiring hemodialysis or renal replacement therapy. To achieve therapeutic INR, warfarin must be initiated with an infusion of UFH until therapeutic INR is achieved, as previously described.

HEMODYNAMICALLY STABLE WITH ADEQUATE RENAL FUNCTION

All anticoagulants are potential options for the hemodynamically stable patient with adequate renal function (defined as those with up to CKD stage 3 with CrCl > 30 mL/min). Therefore, the decision to select an anticoagulant is multifactorial. Factors to consider for anticoagulant selection are baseline risk assessment for bleeding and thromboembolic events, potential for drug interactions, patient medication adherence, compliance with provider follow-up, cost, and drug tolerability. **Table 31.2** provides an overview of the anticoagulant options for NVAF. UFH or an LMWH transitioning to warfarin has traditionally been the gold-standard anticoagulation regimen. The time in therapeutic range for target INR is an important consideration for those on warfarin because there is a direct correlation with the annual risk for stroke or systemic embolism when frequently above or below the target range.

The NOACs include the direct thrombin inhibitor, dabigatran, and FXa inhibitors apixaban, edoxaban, and rivaroxaban. Their primary difference from that of warfarin is the rapid onset of action, which eliminates the need for bridging with UFH or an LMWH and the elimination of required laboratory monitoring for therapeutic efficacy. However, there are notable differences between each of the NOACs, which should be taken into consideration when selecting the optimal agent.

NOAC DOSING COMPARISON

Dabigatran etexilate is a prodrug that is rapidly converted into its active form dabigatran independently of the cytochrome P-450 (CYP) pathway. The lack of direct involvement with the CYP pathway is attractive to patients who may be on multiple medications, because this minimizes the risk for drug interactions, which are extensively hepatically metabolized by this means. The adverse effect of dyspepsia (5% to 10%) seen in the RE-LY (**R**andomized **E**valuation of **L**ong-Term Anticoagulation Therap**Y**) trial is attributed to its formulation with tartaric acid,[8] thereby making it a pH-dependent environment for absorption within the gastrointestinal tract. Thus, the medication should not be crushed or chewed and the contents of the capsule cannot be opened for administration down feeding tubes because this will increase the

TABLE 31.2 Clinical Pharmacology Overview of Anticoagulants for Nonvalvular Atrial Fibrillation

	DABIGATRAN DIRECT THROMBIN INHIBITOR	APIXABAN FACTOR XA INHIBITOR	EDOXABAN FACTOR XA INHIBITOR	RIVAROXABAN FACTOR XA INHIBITOR	DALTEPARIN FACTOR XA INHIBITOR	ENOXAPARIN FACTOR XA INHIBITOR	WARFARIN VITAMIN K ANTAGONIST	UNFRACTIONATED HEPARIN
Dosing for stroke and systemic embolism prevention in nonvalvular atrial fibrillation	150 mg PO twice daily	5 mg PO twice daily	60 mg PO once daily (for patients with CrCl 51–95 mL/min)	20 mg PO once daily with evening meal	100 units/kg (actual body weight) SubQ every 12 h	1 mg/kg (actual body weight) SubQ every 12 h (Consider unfractionated heparin or anti-FXa monitoring when actual body weight exceeds 190 kg)	Initial (usual): 5 mg PO daily (Consider lower initial dose in patients with hepatic disease, CHF, malnutrition, age > 65 y, clinical hyperthyroidism, those at high risk of bleeding and those taking medications that can increase INR such as amiodarone, metronidazole, TMP/SMX, erythromycin, azole antifungals, and fluoroquinolones)	Bolus optional, if given 60 units/kg (max 4000 units) Initial infusion: 12 units/kg/h (max 1000 units/h), then titrate to institution-specific protocol based on aPTT
Onset of action for complete therapeutic effect	0.5–2 h	3–4 h	1–3 h	2–4 h	1–2 h	3–5 h	5–7 d	20–30 min
Protein binding (%)	35	78	55	92–95	Not applicable	Not applicable	Not applicable	Not applicable
Renal dose adjustments	CrCl 15–30 mL/min: 75 mg PO twice daily CrCl < 15 mL/min or on dialysis: avoid use	CrCl < 15 mL/min or on dialysis: no data Any two of the following: age ≥ 80, weight ≤ 60 kg, serum creatinine ≥ 1.5 mg/dL then use: 2.5 mg PO twice daily	CrCl > 95 mL/min or <15 mL/min: avoid use CrCl 15–50 mL/min, body weight < 60 kg, or if on P-gp inhibitor: 30 mg PO once daily	CrCl 15–50 mL/min: 15 mg PO once daily CrCl ≤ 15: avoid use	CrCl < 30 mL/min: monitor anti-FXa levels to determine dose, consider unfractionated heparin alternative Dialysis: avoid use	CrCl < 30 mL/min: 1 mg/kg (actual body weight) SubQ once daily Dialysis: avoid use	Not applicable	Severe renal impairment: half-life and elimination may be prolonged
Hepatic impairment	Mild: no dosage adjustments Moderate–severe: not recommended	Mild: no dosage adjustments Moderate: use caution adjustments Severe: not recommended	Mild: no dosage adjustments Moderate–severe: not recommended	Mild: no dosage adjustments Moderate–severe: not recommended	Dosage adjustments unknown, use caution or consider unfractionated heparin	Dosage adjustments unknown, use caution or consider unfractionated heparin	Consider lower initial dose and monitor PT/INR	Cirrhosis: half-life and elimination may be prolonged

(continued)

TABLE 31.2   Clinical Pharmacology Overview of Anticoagulants for Nonvalvular Atrial Fibrillation (continued)

	DABIGATRAN DIRECT THROMBIN INHIBITOR	APIXABAN FACTOR XA INHIBITOR	EDOXABAN FACTOR XA INHIBITOR	RIVAROXABAN FACTOR XA INHIBITOR	DALTEPARIN FACTOR XA INHIBITOR	ENOXAPARIN FACTOR XA INHIBITOR	WARFARIN VITAMIN K ANTAGONIST	UNFRACTIONATED HEPARIN
Routine laboratory monitoring (considerations)	Not routinely recommended (aPTT, ECT)	Not routinely recommended (anti-FXa, PT/INR)	Not routinely recommended (anti-FXa, PT/INR)	Not routinely recommended (anti-FXa, PT/INR)	Not routinely recommended (anti-FXa)	Not routinely recommended (anti-FXa)	PT/INR	aPTT (anti-FXa)
Half-life	14 h (up to 34 h with severe renal impairment)	12 h (prolonged with renal impairment)	10–14 h Elderly: relatively unchanged (prolonged with renal impairment)	5–9 h Elderly: 11–13 h (prolonged with renal impairment)	3–5 h	4.5–7 h	20–60 h mean: 40 h (highly variable among individuals)	1.5–2.5 h
Metabolism and transport	P-gp	CYP3A4 and P-gp	Minimal CYP3A4 (primarily unchanged in urine)	CYP3A4 and P-gp	Not applicable	Not applicable	CYP2C9 (primary pathway), 2C19, 2C8, 2C18, 1A2, 3A4	Complex metabolism
Removed by dialysis	Yes (62%–68%)	No	No	No	No	No	No	No
Box warnings	Discontinuation in patients without adequate continuous anticoagulation increases risk of stroke Spinal/epidural hematoma: may occur with neuraxial anesthesia or undergoing spinal puncture; consider benefits and risks, and monitor for neurologic impairment	Discontinuation in patients without adequate continuous anticoagulation increases risk of stroke	Reduced efficacy in nonvalvular atrial fibrillation patients with CrCl ≥ 95 mL/min Premature discontinuation increases the risk of ischemic events Spinal/epidural hematoma: may occur with neuraxial anesthesia or undergoing spinal puncture; consider benefits and risks, and monitor for neurologic impairment	Discontinuation places patients at an increased risk of thrombotic events Spinal/epidural hematoma: may occur with neuraxial anesthesia or undergoing spinal puncture; consider benefits and risks, and monitor for neurologic impairment	Spinal/epidural hematoma: may occur with neuraxial anesthesia or undergoing spinal puncture; consider benefits and risks, and monitor for neurologic impairment	Spinal/epidural hematoma: may occur with neuraxial anesthesia or undergoing spinal puncture; consider benefits and risks, and monitor for neurologic impairment	Can cause major or fatal bleeding Perform regular monitoring of INR in all treated patients Drugs, dietary changes, and other factors affect INR levels Instruct patients about prevention measures to minimize risk of bleeding and to report signs and symptoms of bleeding	None

anti-Fxa, antifactor Xa activity; aPTT, activated partial thromboplastin time; CrCl, creatinine clearance; ECT, ecarin clotting time; INR, international normalized ratio; kg, kilograms; P-gp, P-glycoprotein (transport); PO, per oral; PT, prothrombin time; SubQ, subcutaneously.

risk of bleeding. Taking dabigatran with food delays the onset of action up to 2 hours. It is suggested that patients requiring acid-suppressive therapy for peptic ulcer disease and individuals with total or subtotal gastrectomy as well as gastric bypass surgery should avoid this anticoagulant or use it with caution.[16]

Despite its twice-daily dosing being an issue for medication compliance, apixaban has demonstrated superiority to warfarin in NVAF. In ARISTOTLE, patients with a CHA_2DS_2-VASc score greater than 1, apixaban is associated with a lower annual incidence of stroke or systemic embolism (1.27% vs 1.60%) while having a decreased rate of lower major bleeding (2.13% vs 3.09%) than warfarin.[9] Apixaban tablets may be chewed or crushed for ease of administration down feeding tubes and are administered without regard to meals.

Edoxaban is not yet incorporated into the ACC/AHA/HRS guidelines for AF because the publication of its utility versus warfarin in NVAF in ENGAGE AF-TIMI 48 was published after the cutoff for inclusion into the most recent guidelines.[4] However, a class I, level A recommendation in the ESC guidelines for AF yields preference to edoxaban along with the other NOACs over vitamin K antagonists (VKAs) such as warfarin.[5] Edoxaban may be administered independent of meals, but may have some benefit when administered with food, because bioavailability has been shown to increase from 6% to 22%.[16] Presently, there is no existing data on the effects of bioavailability if this medication is chewed or crushed to administer down a feeding tube.

Rivaroxaban must be administered with food because bioavailability is significantly increased from 66% to greater than 80%.[16] As with apixaban, rivaroxaban may be chewed or crushed for ease of administration down feeding tubes. The pharmacokinetic profile of this medication along with dabigatran is not affected by extremes in body weight.

Medication adherence may be a concern with both dabigatran and apixaban because they are both administered twice daily. Edoxaban and rivaroxaban may be more suitable for patients who are at risk for issues with adherence because they are administered once daily. All NOACs have shorter half-lives than their counterpart warfarin. Thus, the importance of not missing doses should be strongly emphasized during patient education because of the increased risk for embolic events.

HEPATIC AND RENAL IMPAIRMENT AND OTHER DOSAGE CONSIDERATIONS

Unlike rivaroxaban and dabigatran, apixaban is minimally excreted by the kidneys and predominantly through multiple nonrenal mechanisms including fecal and hepatic. This provides an advantage of apixaban over dabigatran, edoxaban, and rivaroxaban, with the potential for its use with moderate hepatic dysfunction. All NOACs require renal dose adjustments and should not be used in patients with an estimated CrCl < 15 mL/min depending on the individual agent.

In the ENGAGE AF-TIMI 48 study, NVAF patients with CrCl > 95 mL/min had an increased rate of ischemic stroke with edoxaban 60 mg once daily compared with patients treated with warfarin.[10] Although uncommon for the majority of patients with NVAF, this anticoagulant is recommended for use only for those with a CrCl less than 95 mL/min. Apixaban and dabigatran should be used with caution in patients at and older than 80 years of age. With respect to lower extremes of weight, apixaban and edoxaban require dosage adjustment in patients less than 60 kg.

DRUG INTERACTIONS

There are two primary considerations for drug interactions with the NOACs: CYP450 isoenzyme metabolism, specifically CYP3A4, and P-glycoprotein (P-gp) transport. Each of these mechanisms may take the form of either inhibiting or inducing drug metabolism. Inhibition may increase NOAC exposure leading to toxicities, such as major or minor bleeding events. Induction may decrease NOAC exposure leading to insufficient NOAC exposure, resulting in thrombotic events.

The CYP3A4 isoenzyme is involved in the metabolism of all NOACs, with the exception of dabigatran. Despite this advantage, many medications commonly metabolized by CYP3A4 are also involved with P-gp transport for elimination, which must be considered with concomitant use of dabigatran. Common CYP3A4 and P-gp inhibitors include erythromycin, clarithromycin, grapefruits and grapefruit juice, and protease inhibitors. Common inducers include barbiturates, phenytoin, rifampin, and carbamazepine. Additional monitoring is recommended when these agents are concomitantly administered.

CONVERTING FROM ONE ANTICOAGULATION REGIMEN TO ANOTHER

Throughout the course of an inpatient hospitalization, it may be necessary to convert between different anticoagulation regimens for NVAF. This may be particularly relevant for the patient admitted to the intensive care unit, where there may be acute changes in hemodynamics and organ function. **Table 31.3** outlines the specific details on transitioning between anticoagulation regimens.

NOAC MONITORING

Routine laboratory monitoring is not required for the novel oral anticoagulants.

The aPTT test provides an approximation of dabigatran's anticoagulant effect.

Anti-FXa activity with apixaban and rivaroxaban can be used to determine the degree of anticoagulation. Signs and symptoms of bleeding should be part of a daily routine and managed accordingly if bleeding should occur.

ACTIVE BLEEDING AND REVERSING ANTICOAGULANTS

In the emergent need for surgery or urgent need for a procedure that might result in clinically significant bleeding, there may be a requirement for reversing the anticoagulant effects. In addition, bleeding is a heterogeneous phenomenon with management that requires individualized treatment approaches.[17] **Figure 31.2** illustrates a decision pathway for addressing bleeding while on anticoagulants, and **Tables 31.4 to 31.6** provide information on reversal strategies for anticoagulants used when treating AF. The use of a reversal agent is probably not warranted in most cases when active bleeding is responding to supportive care, attempting to accelerate the time to an elective procedure, a response to high drug serum concentrations, or elevated laboratory parameters.[4]

The source of bleeding has to be appropriately identified, managed, and treated such that rapid reversal of anticoagulation will not necessarily solve the underlying bleeding.[4] Thus, once bleeding is identified, the first priority is to locate the source and discontinue

TABLE 31.3	**Converting Novel Oral and Other Anticoagulants**			
	APIXABAN (ELIQUIS) FACTOR XA INHIBITOR	**EDOXABAN (SAVAYSA) FACTOR XA INHIBITOR**	**RIVAROXABAN (XARELTO) FACTOR XA INHIBITOR**	**DABIGATRAN (PRADAXA) DIRECT THROMBIN INHIBITOR**
Warfarin to NOAC	Discontinue warfarin, initiate when INR < 2	Discontinue warfarin, initiate when INR ≤ 2.5	Discontinue warfarin, initiate when INR < 3	Discontinue warfarin, initiate when INR < 2
NOAC to warfarin	Start parenteral anticoagulant plus warfarin at next time of apixaban dose Discontinue parenteral anticoagulant when INR is within therapeutic range	(Oral option): reduce edoxaban dose in half and begin warfarin concomitantly. Measure INR at least weekly and just before edoxaban dose. Once INR stable ≥ 2, discontinue edoxaban (Parenteral option): Start parenteral anticoagulant and warfarin at time of next dose	Initiate warfarin and a parenteral anticoagulant 24 h after discontinuation of rivaroxaban	CrCl > 50 mL/min: Initiate warfarin 3 d before discontinuation of dabigatran CrCl 31–50 mL/min: initiate warfarin 2 d before discontinuation of dabigatran CrCl 15–30 mL/min: initiate warfarin 1 d before discontinuation of dabigatran
NOAC to non-warfarin oral anticoagulants	Discontinue apixaban, start new agent at time of next scheduled apixaban dose	Discontinue edoxaban, start new agent at time of next scheduled edoxaban dose	Initiate the new agent 24 h after discontinuing rivaroxaban	Discontinue dabigatran, start new agent at time of next scheduled edoxaban dose
Non-warfarin oral anticoagulants to NOAC	Discontinue current agent, start apixaban at time of next scheduled dose	Discontinue current agent, start edoxaban at time of next scheduled dose	Discontinue current agent, initiate rivaroxaban within 2 h of the next scheduled dose	Discontinue current agent, initiate dabigatran within 2 h of the next scheduled dose
LMWH to NOAC	Discontinue LMWH, start apixaban at time of next scheduled dose	Discontinue LMWH, start edoxaban at time of next scheduled dose	Discontinue the LMWH, initiate rivaroxaban within 2 h of next dose	Discontinue the LMWH, initiate dabigatran within 2 h of next dose
NOAC to LMWH	Discontinue apixaban, start LMWH at time of next dose	Discontinue edoxaban, start LMWH at time of next dose	Discontinue rivaroxaban, start LMWH at time of next dose	Discontinue dabigatran, start LMWH at time of next dose

CrCl, creatinine clearance; INR, international normalized ratio; LMWH, low-molecular-weight heparin; NOAC, novel oral anticoagulant.

the anticoagulant agent. The clinical stability of the patient should serve as a guide for the next steps. For example, significant blood loss causing hypovolemic shock from a gastrointestinal bleed may require volume administered with blood transfusions. In addition, directly reversing the anticoagulant effect may also aid in restoring the bleeding diathesis. On the other hand, an intracranial hemorrhage generally requires less volume, but directly reversing the anticoagulant effect may be preferred. Volume restoration during hemorrhage, for example, with crystalloids, colloids, and/or blood transfusion protocols is beyond the scope of this chapter, but an overview of anticoagulant reversal agents is provided.

Reversal agents and strategies discussed include idarucizumab for dabigatran, andexanet alfa (andexanet) for anti-FXa NOACs and LMWHs, prothrombin complex concentrates (PCCs) with vitamin K for warfarin, and protamine sulfate for UFH. Andexanet is currently in later phases of premarketing clinical trials. An additional agent, ciraparantag, is in very early stages of development with a broader spectrum of anticoagulants potentially reversed by this agent.

IDARUCIZUMAB FOR DABIGATRAN REVERSAL

Idarucizumab is a monoclonal antibody fragment that binds dabigatran with a 350-fold or so higher affinity to that of thrombin.[18]

As a result, idarucizumab adheres to thrombin-bound dabigatran and neutralizes its activity. Currently, idarucizumab is approved by the US FDA for the reversal of the anticoagulant effects of dabigatran, needed for emergency surgery/urgent procedures or in life-threatening or uncontrollable bleeding.

The RE-VERSE AD trial examined the safety and reversal capacity of idarucizumab on dabigatran in patients who had a serious bleeding event or required reversal for an urgent procedure.[18] Serious bleeding was defined as overt, uncontrollable, or life-threatening bleeding that was judged by the treating clinician to require a reversal agent, and an urgent procedure was defined as requiring surgery or other invasive procedures that could not be delayed for at least 8 hours and for which normal hemostasis was required.[18] Idarucizumab was administered as a 5-g dose divided into two separate bolus infusions of 2.5 g in 50 mL within 15 minutes of one another. The results demonstrated rapid and complete reversal effects of dabigatran in 88% to 98% of patients.[18]

Idarucizumab is not without potential side effects that may include direct effects of the agent such as anaphylaxis, other hypersensitivity reactions, and serious reactions with hereditary fructose intolerance because sorbitol is a component of the preparation. A prothrombotic effect of dabigatran reversal by idarucizumab leading to thrombosis may also occur once the

Pathway for Active Bleeding with Anticoagulation

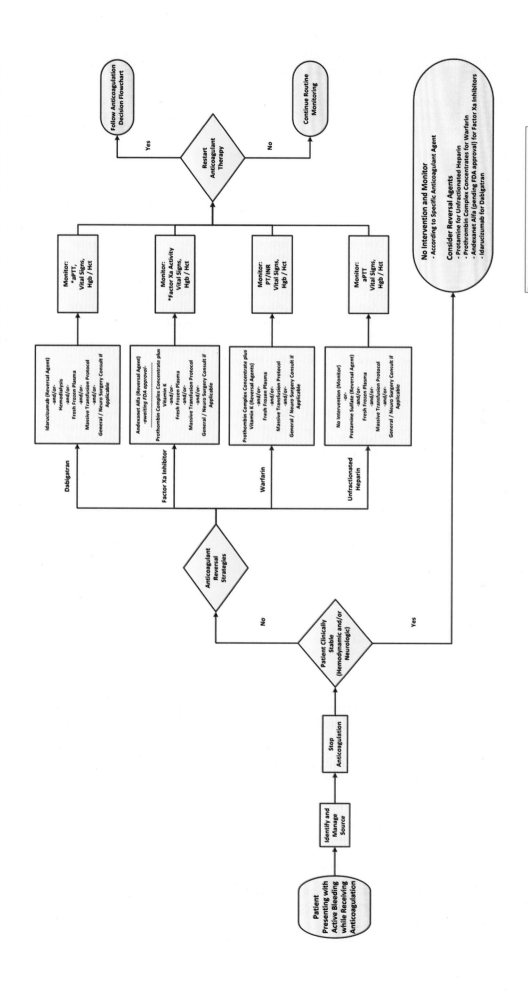

FIGURE 31.2 Pathway for active bleeding with anticoagulation.

TABLE 31.4	Reversal Strategies for Anticoagulants						
	APIXABAN FACTOR XA INHIBITOR	**EDOXABAN FACTOR XA INHIBITOR**	**RIVAROXABAN FACTOR XA INHIBITOR**	**ENOXAPARIN FACTOR XA INHIBITOR**	**DABIGATRAN DIRECT THROMBIN INHIBITOR**	**WARFARIN VITAMIN K ANTAGONIST**	**UNFRACTIONATED HEPARIN**
Reversal agents	Prothrombin complex concentrate, 4-factor	Prothrombin complex concentrate, 4-factor	Prothrombin complex concentrate, 4-factor	Prothrombin complex concentrate, 4-factor	Idarucizumab	Prothrombin complex concentrate, 4-factor-plus-vitamin K[c]	Protamine sulfate
Alternative reversal agents	Andexanet alfa[a] (pending US FDA approval)	Andexanet alfa[a] (pending US FDA approval)	Andexanet alfa[a] (pending US FDA approval)	Protamine sulfate[b] Andexanet alfa[a] (pending US FDA approval)	None	Fresh frozen plasma-plus-vitamin K[c]	None
Reversal dosing	Andexanet alfa[a] 400 mg IV bolus over 15–30 min, then 480 mg IV infusion over 2 h (if apixaban last dose > 7 h)	Andexanet alfa[a] 800 mg IV bolus over 15–30 min, then 960 mg IV infusion over 2 h (if edoxaban last dose ≤ 7 h or unknown time)	Andexanet alfa[a] Low dose: 400 mg IV bolus over 15–30 min, then 480 mg IV infusion over 2 h; or High dose: 800 mg IV bolus over 15–30 min, then 960 mg IV infusion over 2 h Higher dose used if rivaroxaban last dose ≤ 7 h or unknown time	Andexanet alfa[a] 800 mg IV bolus over 15–30 min, then 960 mg IV infusion over 2 h if ≤7 h since last dose or unknown time	5 mg (2 × 2.5 g vials) as a slow IV push or infusion	PCC 4-factor: INR 2–3.9: 25 units/kg, max 2500 units INR 4–6: 35 units/kg, max 3500 untis INR > 6: PCC 50 units/kg, max 5000 units vitamin K[c] 10 mg infused IV over 30 min when used with PCC	Each 1 mg protamine reverses 100 units of heparin Maximum dose: 50 mg IV An additional 50% of the initial dose may be needed
Hemodialysis removal	No	No	No	20%	Yes 62%–68%	No	Partial
Activated charcoal	Consider use if appropriate	Consider use if appropriate	Consider use if appropriate	Not recommended	Consider use if appropriate	Not recommended	Not recommended

INR, international normalized ratio; IV, intravenous; PCC, prothrombin complex concentrate.
Prothrombin complex concentrate, 4-factor use is off-label for reversing apixaban, edoxaban, rivaroxaban, and enoxaparin.
[a]Andexanet alfa is not yet approved by the United States Food and Drug Administration, doses adapted from the ANNEXA-4 interim analysis study.
[b]Evidence does not support complete reversal of the anticoagulant effect. Use clinical judgment and consider other treatment options.

TABLE 31.5	Reversal of Warfarin for Elevated INR and/or Bleeding
INR < 5 without significant bleeding	Lower or hold next dose, then resume at lower dose when INR is therapeutic
INR between 5 and 9 without significant bleeding	Hold warfarin until INR is in therapeutic range, then resume at a lower dose May consider PO vitamin K 2.5 mg
INR > 9 without significant bleeding	Hold warfarin and give PO vitamin K 2.5–5 mg, expect INR reversal in 24–48 h
Significant bleeding with any INR	Hold warfarin Administer prothrombin complex concentrate (PCC) 25–50 units/kg-or-FFP 15 mL/kg (1 unit = 200–250 mL) plus vitamin K IV[a] 10 mg over 30 min depending on clinical situation Note: Expect INR reversal with vitamin K within 12–48 h, FFP within 1–4 h, and PCC within 15 min PCC preferred option in patients with TBI and/or ICH

[a]Evidence does not support complete reversal of the anticoagulant effect. Use clinical judgment and consider other treatment options.
FFP, fresh frozen plasma; ICH, intracranial hemorrhage; INR, international normalized ratio; IV, intravenously; PCC, prothrombin complex concentrate;
PO, per oral; TBI, traumatic brain injury.

TABLE 31.6	Protamine Sulfate Dosing for Low-Molecular-Weight and Unfractionated Heparins
TIME SINCE LAST LMWH DOSE	**PROTAMINE DOSE FOR EACH: DALTEPARIN 100 UNITS OR ENOXAPARIN 1 MG**
<8 h	1 mg (or 50 mg fixed dose)
8–12 h	0.5 mg (or 25 mg fixed dose)
>12 h	Not likely useful (consider 25 mg fixed dose)
TIME SINCE LAST HEPARIN DOSE	**PROTAMINE DOSE FOR EACH 100 UNITS OF HEPARIN**
Immediate	1 mg (or 25 mg fixed dose)
30 min	0.5 mg (or 10 mg fixed dose)
>2 h	0.25 mg (or 10 mg fixed dose)
Consider a second protamine dose (50% of first dose) if prolonged aPTT continues	

aPTT, activated partial thromboplastin time; LMWH, low-molecular-weight heparin.

anticoagulant effects have been reversed, for example, in those with a high CHA_2DS_2-VASc score. In some patients, a delayed increase in dabigatran serum concentrations, such as 12 to 24 hours after idarucizumab administration, may reflect an increase in clotting time markers possibly due to intravascular redistribution of dabatran.[18] It is unknown whether additional doses of idarucizumab would be effective and safe in such scenarios.[18]

Because the cost of each dose of idarucizumab is currently in the several thousands of US dollars, it may be fiscally prudent for hospitals and health systems to create multidisciplinary policies, procedures, and standardized protocols. Components of such consensus documents may include selecting appropriate clinical scenarios for use, monitoring parameters and frequencies, procurement quantities, and location of refrigerator storage within the institution to avoid waste.

ANDEXANET ALFA FOR FACTOR XA INHIBITOR REVERSAL

Not yet approved by the US FDA, andexanet alfa (andexanet) is a recombinant modified human FXa decoy protein that reverses the inhibitory effects of anti-FXa agents.[19] These counteractive effects of FXa inhibition by NOACs and LMWHs restore FXa activity and therefore the potential for clot formation.

The ANNEXA-4 trial is actively evaluating the activity of andexanet in patients with acute major bleeding within 18 hours of the administration of an FXa inhibitor, including apixaban, edoxaban, rivaroxaban, and enoxaparin.[19] Andexanet was administered by an initial bolus infusion over 15 to 30 minutes followed by a 2-hour infusion to maintain activity against the anti-FXa agent. Doses were relatively lower for patients who had taken apixaban or rivaroxaban more than 7 hours before the administration of andexanet and higher for patients who had taken enoxaparin, edoxaban, or rivaroxaban 7 hours or less before the administration of the bolus dose or at an unknown time. Clinical monitoring parameters for efficacy endpoints included changes in anti-FXa activity and hemostasis within a 12-hour period.[19] The most updated preliminary analysis of this ongoing trial demonstrated 79% of patients with relatively effective hemostasis after receiving the bolus and 2-hour infusion of andexanet. There were no reported serious side effects attributed directly to andexanet; however, thrombotic events occurred in 18% of patients.[19]

Additional data from the ongoing ANNEXA-4 trials, as well as from controlled trials, are needed to determine the safety of thrombotic event frequency compared with what is expected.[19] Further research is necessary to understand how this antidote will be used in clinical practice.

PROTHROMBIN COMPLEX CONCENTRATES WITH VITAMIN K FOR WARFARIN REVERSAL

The traditional approach to treat bleeding associated with warfarin is to administer fresh frozen plasma (FFP). However, there are significant drawbacks with using FFP. All clotting factors are included in FFP, derived from human plasma, which often contains numerous antibodies. This increases the risk of infusion-related reactions, with the most severe consequence being transfusion-related acute lung injury. In addition, an extensive volume (15 mL/kg per unit) is required for reversal, which may be a limiting factor for volume-restricted patients with poor cardiovascular status. FFP also possesses its own intrinsic INR ranging from 1.5 to 1.7, owing to the presence of all clotting factors.

PCC is a concentrated form of factors II, VII, IX, and X and proteins C and S, which specifically targets all mechanisms involved with warfarin and includes those involved with NOACs. This product requires a higher degree of purity for processing compared with FFP, which dramatically lessens the likelihood of transfusion-related complications. The major advantages of PCC is that reversal requires much smaller volumes (1 to 2 mL/kg per unit), which can be infused over a shorter period of time.

Vitamin K may be administered as an individual agent in the setting of INR elevations with warfarin without significant bleeding. When administered as a single agent as intravenous or po, it is extremely slow to reverse the effects of INR, which will not be evident until approximately 24 to 48 hours after administration.

Over time, concentrated vitamin-K–dependent clotting factors have been used until recently with the introduction of 4-factor (4F)-PCC with vitamin K. In a multicenter, open-label, randomized, plasma-controlled noninferiority clinical trial using FFP versus 4F-PCC in patients with acute bleeding associated with VKA therapy for the achievement of effective hemostasis within 24 hours was evaluated. Superiority was also examined through reduction of INR to ≤1.3 within 30 minutes of the completed infusion.[20] Effective hemostasis was defined as cessation of bleeding within 4 hours of the end of the infusion and no additional coagulation intervention required within 24 hours. Within 24 hours, hemostasis was achieved in 72.4% of those receiving 4F-PCC versus 65.4% receiving FFP, demonstrating noninferiority.[20] There was no statistically significant difference detected for mortality or length of stay between 4F-PCC and FFP. Serious adverse events associated with reversal of VKAs with 4F-PCC were reported in 31% of patients, of which only 10 were deemed directly related to treatment.[20] When compared with FFP, rates of serious adverse events appeared similar; however, no clinical trial has been powered to specifically evaluate differences in safety.

Tables 31.4 and 31.5 outline the specific information regarding the dosing for FFP, PCC, and vitamin K for anticoagulation reversal.

PROTAMINE FOR REVERSAL OF HEPARINS

Particularly relevant to those patients requiring bridging with UFH when initiating therapy with warfarin, protamine will provide an effective means for stopping acute bleeding. There is no role for the use of protamine for reversal of NOACs. Protamine provides complete reversal of anticoagulant effects from UFH and partial reversal with LMWH, enoxaparin and dalteparin. See **Table 31.6** for dosing recommendations for protamine, which is based on administration times for each anticoagulant. Protamine should be administered slowly, with a maximum dose of 50 mg over 10 minutes to minimize the adverse effect of hypotension. If outcomes are promising from the future reversal agent in the pipeline, ciraparantag may end up replacing protamine for these agents, noting its broad effect upon reversal of anticoagulants.

REINITIATING ANTICOAGULATION POST BLEEDING

When bleeding occurs, especially from the gastrointestinal or urinary tracts, the presence of an underlying occult lesion should always be considered.[3] Once hemostasis is achieved, the decision whether and when to reinitiate anticoagulation therapy after reversing the anticoagulant effects for a severe bleeding episode may be necessary and should be considered on an individualized basis.[4] The ongoing use of the $CHADS_2$-DS_2-VASc and HAS-BLED systems together may provide guidance in this particular decision-making process. In patients for whom anticoagulation therapy is needed after hospitalization for a gastrointestinal bleed, reinitiating anticoagulation within 90 days of the event demonstrated positive outcomes on thrombotic events and death.[21,22]

PERIOPERATIVE BRIDGING FOR SURGERY AND PROCEDURES

When chronic anticoagulation therapy is required, such as in AF, adequate anticoagulation before and after surgery or an invasive procedure may be needed, particularly when the risk of thromboembolism is high. The concept of anticoagulant "bridging" is essentially administering a short-acting anticoagulant (eg, UFH or LMWH) during the time when a long-acting warfarin is being withheld before the surgery, then continued after the surgery or procedure until the long-acting anticoagulant is again within the target therapeutic range.[23] Because the NOACs have a faster offset of action compared with warfarin and a rapid onset of action, bridging with UFH or an LMWH may not be necessary, unless the patient is not able to take oral therapy such as with gastric resection or postoperative ileus.[23]

Not all procedures require anticoagulants to be held, for example, minor dental and skin procedures, cataract extraction, and selected cardiac device implantation.[23] The NOACs need to generally be held for 1 to 4 days before the procedure, with the interruption interval depending on the specific agent, patient's renal function, and type of bleeding risk of the procedure.[24] **Table 31.7** provides recommendations by the manufacturers and from clinical trials for the timing of discontinuing anticoagulants before surgery or procedures. Postoperative resumption of NOACs should take into account their rapid onset of action (1 to 3 hours postingestion), and can be restarted approximately 24 hours after low-bleed risk and 48 to 72 hours after high-bleed risk procedures.[24] With urgent surgery, there is no evidence suggesting higher bleeding rates with NOACs as compared with patients treated with warfarin.[24]

The BRIDGE investigators conducted a randomized, double-blind, placebo-controlled trial to determine whether foregoing anticoagulant bridge therapy in patients with AF treated with warfarin is noninferior to bridging with the LMWH dalteparin and superior with respect to major bleeding.[25] The mean $CHADS_2$ score was 2.3 (CHA_2DS_2-VASc score was not used for risk stratification at the time of the trial) with only about one-third with a score of 3 or higher, suggesting a relatively lower risk of thrombosis. It is important to point out that patients at high risk for thrombosis, such as those with CHA_2DS_2-VASc scores 2 or greater, and/or those requiring higher intensity warfarin, for example, with mechanical mitral valves may still require perioperative bridge therapy because these scenarios were excluded in the study.[25] In addition, surgical procedures associated with high risks of thrombosis, such as carotid endarterectomy, major cancer surgery, cardiac surgery, or neurosurgery were excluded from the trial. The results of this trial, demonstrated in patients with AF on warfarin therapy, that LMWH perioperative bridge therapy did not prevent thromboembolic events, but did increase the risk of major bleeding.

It therefore may be reasonable to forego bridging warfarin with UFH or an LMWH in patients at relatively low thromboembolic risk and undergoing procedures to avoid clinically significant bleeding. Using this approach, the patient would therefore discontinue warfarin usually until the INR decreases to below 1.5 (approximately 5 days) before the procedure without being additionally anticoagulated. The perioperative treatment plan should therefore be designed in collaboration with the operating clinician and the patient.

ANTIPLATELET THERAPIES WITH ATRIAL FIBRILLATION

The Stroke Prevention in Atrial Fibrillation-1 (SPAF-1) trial from the early 1990s is the only trial among eight or so evaluated in a meta-analysis to show the benefit of aspirin alone in preventing stroke among patients with AF.[4] The dose seemingly effective was aspirin 325 mg once daily. Aspirin was not effective in those older than 75 years of age, did not prevent severe stroke, and has not been studied in low-risk populations.[4]

Clopidogrel 75 mg once daily plus aspirin 75 to 100 mg once daily was evaluated for stroke prevention in the *A*trial *F*ibrillation *C*lopidogrel *T*rial With *I*rbesartan for Prevention of *V*ascular *E*vents (ACTIVE-W) trial and terminated early because in patients with a mean $CHADS_2$ score of 2, the combination of antiplatelet agents was inferior to warfarin (target INR 2 to 3).[4] The ACTIVE-A trial compared clopidogrel plus aspirin versus aspirin alone and demonstrated superiority in stroke

TABLE 31.7	Periprocedural Bridging: Anticoagulation Interruption for Surgery and Procedures						
	APIXABAN FACTOR XA INHIBITOR	EDOXABAN FACTOR XA INHIBITOR	RIVAROXABAN FACTOR XA INHIBITOR	ENOXAPARIN FACTOR XA INHIBITOR	DABIGATRAN DIRECT THROMBIN INHIBITOR	WARFARIN VITAMIN K ANTAGONIST	UNFRACTIONATED HEPARIN
Procedures to not withhold anticoagulation	Not all procedures require anticoagulation to be held. Examples include minor dental procedures (such as cleaning, scaling, extraction), minor skin procedures, cataract extraction, selected cardiac device implantation, and routine endoscopy. Design a plan with the clinician performing the procedure and the patient.						
Elective low risk surgery and procedures	Discontinue apixaban at least 24 h before elective procedure	Discontinue edoxaban at least 24 h before invasive or surgical procedures. Risk of bleeding should be considered against the urgency of intervention if surgery cannot be delayed	Discontinue rivaroxaban at least 24 h before the procedure	Discontinue 12–18 h before the procedure	CrCl $\geq$ 50 mL/min Discontinue dabigatran 1–2 d before elective procedure CrCl < 50 mL/min Discontinue dabigatran 3–5 d before elective procedure	Discontinue until desired INR is reached (usual target < 1.5, acheived over 4–5 d)	Discontinue 6–12 h before procedure
Elective moderate to high-risk surgery and procedures	Discontinue apixaban at least 48 h before elective procedure	Discontinue edoxaban at least 24 h before invasive or surgical procedures. Risk of bleeding should be considered against the urgency of intervention if surgery cannot be delayed	Consider longer times based on clinical judgment	Discontinue 12–18 h before the procedure	Consider longer times for major surgery, spinal puncture, or spinal or epidural catheter or port placement	Discontinue until desired INR is reached (usual target < 1.5, acheived over 4–5 d)	Discontinue 6–12 h before procedure

CrCl, creatinine clearance; INR, international normalized ratio.

prevention of the combination antiplatelet therapy to aspirin alone; however, the benefits were diminished by the increases in severe bleeding rates.

The AVERROES study was a direct comparison between aspirin and the FXa inhibitor apixaban.[4,26] This double-blind study of 5,599 patients deemed unsuitable for warfarin therapy were randomized to apixaban 5 mg twice daily (2.5 mg twice daily for those who had two of the following three: age $\geq$ 80 years, weight $\leq$ 60 kg, serum creatinine $\geq$ 1.5 mg/dL) or to aspirin 81 or 325 mg once daily. The trial was prematurely terminated owing to the observed superiority of apixaban over aspirin for the occurrence of any stroke or systemic embolism. Major bleeding rates were similar between apixaban and aspirin.

With respect to triple antithrombotic therapy with concomitant dual antiplatelet agents and NOACs, there is a paucity of literature for evaluation. Several landmark trials that studied NOACs for stroke prophylaxis with NVAF excluded the combination of aspirin with a P2Y$_{12}$ inhibitor (eg, clopidogrel, prasugrel, ticagrelor).[8–11,26] Therefore, an important remaining unanswered question is in patients with AF requiring anticoagulation and at the same time dual antiplatelet therapy with aspirin and a P2Y$_{12}$ inhibitor for coronary intervention such as stenting.

The SAFE-A study that compares 1-month versus 6-month P2Y$_{12}$ inhibitor therapy in combination with aspirin and apixaban, in patients with AF who undergo drug-eluding stent implantation, is currently under way.[27] The primary outcome will be the incidence of all bleeding complications occurring within 12 months. Ultimately, this study will provide data that may guide the optimal management of triple antithrombotic therapy.

Additional medications that have antiplatelet properties should be used with caution when taken concomitantly with NOACs. Such agents include NSAIDs, such as naproxen, ibuprofen, celecoxib, diclofenac, and meloxicam. In addition, selective serotonin reuptake inhibitors (SSRIs) commonly used as antidepressants, such as paroxetine, fluoxetine, sertraline, citalopram, and escitalopram, and serotonin norepinephrine reuptake inhibitors (SNRIs) commonly used as antidepressants and neurogenic pain analgesics, such as duloxetine and venlafaxine, should be used with caution.

ABILITY TO PAY AND LIKELY TO ADHERE TO THERAPY

Perhaps the greatest risk factor for thrombotic events with AF is the inability to take the prescribed anticoagulant on a daily basis.[4]

This is particularly important with NOACs because the duration of action is shorter than that of warfarin, so missing even one dose of a NOAC increases the risk of thrombosis.

The reasons for nonadherence to a drug therapy regimen are multifaceted and highly individualized. Barriers that cause patients not to take their medication as prescribed may include the health literacy of the patient and/or caregiver, emotional state and acceptance of the need for chronic daily medications, side effects and intolerances, and the inability to obtain the drug because of cost or other reasons. Discontinuing a NOAC should not occur without proper anticoagulant coverage, such as with warfarin and/or LMWH for patients who will still require treatment.[4] During the transitions of care when patients are admitted to and discharged from the hospital and/or patient care units, it is critical to accurately reconcile the medication regimen, including anticoagulant therapy to avoid thromboembolic events from omission errors. Prescribers are encouraged to discuss outpatient prescription drug coverage and the patient's intentions and ability to continue the oral anticoagulant therapy upon hospital discharge.

REFERENCES

1. You JJ, Singer, DE, Howard PA, et al. Antithrombotic therapy for atrial fibrillation: Antithrombotic Therapy and Prevention of Thrombosis, 9th ed: American College of Chest Physicians Evidence-Based Clinical Practice Guidelines. *Chest.* 2012;141:e531S-e575S.

2. Hart RG, Pearce LA, Aguilar MI. Meta-analysis: antithrombotic therapy to prevent stroke in patients who have nonvalvular atrial fibrillation. *Ann Intern Med.* 2007;146:857-867.

3. Ageno W, Gallus AS, Wittkowsky A, et al. Oral anticoagulant therapy: Antithrombotic Therapy and Prevention of Thrombosis, 9th ed: American College of Chest Physicians Evidence-Based Clinical Practice Guidelines. *Chest.* 2012;141:e44S-e88S.

4. January CT, Wann LS, Alpert JS, et al. 2014 AHA/ACC/HRS guideline for the management of patients with atrial fibrillation: executive summary. *JACC.* 2014;64(21):2246–2280.

5. Kirchhof P, Benussi S, Kotecha D, et al. 2016 ESC Guidelines for the management of atrial fibrillation development in collaboration with EACTS. The Task Force for the management of atrial fibrillation of the European Society of Cardiology (ESC). Endorsed by the European Stroke Organisation (ESO). *Eur Heart J.* 2016;37:2893-2962. doi:10.1093/eurheartj/ehw210.

6. Whitlock RP, Sun JC, Fremes SE, et al. Antithrombotic and thrombolytic therapy for valvular disease: Antithrombotic Therapy and Prevention of Thrombosis, 9th ed: American College of Chest Physicians Evidence-Based Clinical Practice Guidelines. *Chest.* 2012;141:e567S-e600S.

7. Nutescu EA, Shapiro NL, Chevalier A, et al. A pharmacological overview of current and emerging anticoagulants. *Cleve Clin J Med.* 2005;72(Suppl 1):S2-S6.

8. Connolly SJ, Ezekowitz MD, Yusuf S, et al; RE-LY Steering Committee and Investigators. Dabigatran versus warfarin in patients with atrial fibrillation. *N Engl J Med.* 2009;361:1139-1151.

9. Granger CB, Alexander JH, McMurray JV, et al; ARISTOTLE Committees and Investigators. Apixaban versus warfarin in patients with atrial fibrillation. *N Engl J Med.* 2011;365:981-992.

10. Giugliano RP, Ruff CY, Braunwald E, et al; ENGAGE AF-TIMI 48 Investigators. Edoxaban versus warfarin in patients with atrial fibrillation. *N Engl J Med.* 2013;369:2093-2104.

11. Patel MR, Mahaffey KW, Garg J, et al; ROCKET AF Investigators. Rivaroxaban versus warfarin in nonvalvular atrial fibrillation. *N Engl J Med.* 2011;365:883-891.

12. Apostolakis S, Lane D, Gao Y, Buller H, Lip GY. Performance of the HEMORR2HAGES, ATRIA and HAS-BLED bleeding risk prediction scores in anticoagulated patients with atrial fibrillation: The AMADEUS study. *J Am Coll Cardiol.* 2012;60:861-867.

13. Roldan V, Martin F, Fernandez H, et al. Predictive value of the HAS-BLED and ATRIA bleeding scores for the risk of serious bleeding in a "real-world" population with atrial fibrillation receiving anticoagulant therapy. *Chest.* 2013;143(1):179-184.

14. Gronberg T, Harika J, Nuotio I, et al. Anticoagulation, CHA2DS2VASc score, and thromboembolic risk of cardioversion of acute atrial fibrillation (from the FinCV study). *Am J Cardiol.* 2016;117:1294-1298.

15. Lau Y, Proietti M, Guiducci E, et al. Atrial fibrillation and thromboembolism in patients with chronic kidney disease. *J Am CollCardiol.* 2016;68(13):1452-1464.

16. Schaefer JK, McBane RD, Wysokinski WE. How to choose appropriate direct oral anticoagulant for patient with nonvalvular atrial fibrillation. *Ann Hematol.* 2016;95:437-449.

17. Ageno W, Büller HR, Falanga A, et al. Managing reversal of direct oral anticoagulants in emergency situations. Anticoagulation Education Task Force White Paper. *Thromb Haemost.* 2016;116:1003-1010. doi:10.1160/TH16-05-0363.

18. Pollack CV, Reilly PA, Eikelboom J, et al. Idarucizumab for dabigatran reversal (RE-VERSE AD). *N Engl J Med.* 2015;373:511-520.

19. Connolly SJ, Milling TJ, Eikelboom JW, et al. Andexanet alfa for acute major bleeding associated with factor Xa inhibitors (ANNEXA-4 study). *N Engl J Med.* 2016;375:1131-1141. doi:10.1056/NEJMoa1607887. http://www.NEJM.org/doi/full/10.1056/NEJMoa1607887. Published August 30, 2016. Accessed July 11, 2017.

20. Sarode RS, Milling TJ, Refaai MA, et al. Efficacy and safety of a 4-factor prothrombin complex concentrate in patients on vitamin K antagonists presenting with major bleeding: a randomized, plasma-controlled, phase IIIb study. *Circulation.* 2013;128:1234-1243.

21. Staerk L, Lip GYH, Olesen JB, et al. Stroke and recurrent haemorrhage associated with antithrombotic treatment after gastrointestinal bleeding in patients with atrial fibrillation: nationwide cohort study. *BMJ.* 2015;351:h5876.

22. Witt DM, Delate T, Garcia, DA, et al. Risk of thromboembolism, recurrent hemorrhage, and death after warfarin therapy interruption for gastrointestinal tract bleeding. *Arch Intern Med.* 2012;172(19):1484-1491.

23. Spyropoulos AC, Douketis JD. How I treat anticoagulated patients undergoing an elective procedure or surgery. *Blood.* 2012;120(15):2954-2962.

24. Bell BR, Spyropoulos AC, Douketis JD. Perioperative management of the direct oral anticoagulants: a case-based review. *Hematol Oncol Clin North Am.* 2016;30:1073-1084.

25. Douketis JD, Spyropoulos AC, Kaatz S, et al. Perioperative bridging anticoagulation in patients with atrial fibrillation. *N Engl J Med.* 2015;373:823-833.

26. Connolly SJ, Eikelboom J, Joyner C, et al; AVERROES Steering Committee and Investigators. Apixaban in patients with atrial fibrillation. *N Engl J Med.* 2011;364:806-817.

27. Hoshi T, Sato A, Nogami A, et al. Rationale and design of the SAFE-A study: SAFety and Effectiveness trial of Apixaban use in association with dual antiplatelet therapy in patients with atrial fibrillation undergoing percutaneous coronary intervention [published online ahead of print July 18, 2016]. *J Cardiol.* 2017;69:648-651. doi:10.1016/j.jjcc.2016.06.007.

Patient and Family Information for: MODERN ANTICOAGULATION THERAPY

ATRIAL FIBRILLATION

AF is an irregular heart beat that increases the risk of forming a blood clot in the heart. If the blood clot travels from the heart, it can cause a stroke. Anticoagulants are medications that lower the chances of having a stroke by thinning the blood and therefore helping to prevent clots from forming.

A patient who stops taking the prescribed anticoagulant may have an increased risk of forming a clot in the heart and bloodstream. Do not stop taking the prescribed anticoagulant without talking to the doctor who prescribed it. Missing even one dose may increase the chances of forming a blood clot. In case the anticoagulant medicine has to be stopped, be sure to tell the doctor.

TAKING ANTICOAGULANT MEDICATIONS

Take medication exactly as prescribed by the doctor. If the instructions are not clear, ask the doctor or pharmacist to explain.

- Do not change the dose or stop taking the anticoagulant unless the doctor says so.
- The doctor will tell how much medicine to take and when to take it.
- The doctor may change the dose if needed.

SIDE EFFECTS

All medications have the potential to cause side effects, and anticoagulants are no exception. There is a difference between an allergic reaction and a side effect. Allergic reactions are types of side effects, for example, a rash, which usually means the patient never takes the medicine again. Side effects, for example, bleeding or an upset stomach, due to an anticoagulant are usually dealt with simply by stopping the medication or changing to another similar alternative. It is important to report any side effects the patient may think he or she is having and to get medical help right away if the patient thinks he or she is bleeding. It is important to learn the signs or symptoms of bleeding.

Anticoagulants can cause bleeding in the brain that can be serious and can cause internal bleeding, which on rare occasions lead to death. This is because anticoagulants are blood thinner medications that reduce blood clotting. While on anticoagulants, the patient is likely to bruise more easily and it may take longer for the bleeding to stop. Do not stop taking the anticoagulant without notifying the doctor on noticing bruising.

SIGNS AND SYMPTOMS OF BLEEDING

Examples of unexpected bleeding or bleeding that lasts a long time may include the following:

- Unusual bleeding from the gums
- Nose bleeds that happen often

- Menstrual bleeding that is heavier than normal or vaginal bleeding
- Bleeding that is severe or cannot be controlled
- Red, pink, or brown urine
- Bright red or black tarry stools
- Coughing up blood or blood clots
- Vomiting blood or the vomit looks like "coffee grounds"
- Headaches and feeling dizzy or weak
- Pain, swelling, or new drainage at wound sites

DRUG INTERACTIONS

There is a chance that while on anticoagulants the patient may have a higher likelihood of bleeding if he or she takes other medicines that cause bleeding. These medications may include aspirin or aspirin-containing products, clopidogrel (Plavix), prasugrel (Effient), ticagrelor (Brilinta), NSAIDs, SSRIs, SNRIs, or any other medicines to prevent or treat blood clots. Inform the doctor about taking any of these medicines and ask the doctor or pharmacist if unsure whether the medicine is one among those listed earlier. Also ask the doctor or pharmacist before taking any new medications, over-the-counter medications, vitamins, or herbal supplements.

SPINAL OR EPIDURAL BLOOD CLOTS

People who take a blood thinner medicine and have an injection into their spinal and epidural area or have a spinal puncture have a risk of forming a blood clot that can cause long-term or permanent loss of the ability to move.

It is important to recognize the signs and symptoms of spinal or epidural blood clots if receiving spinal anesthesia or a spinal puncture. Tell the doctor immediately in case of back pain, tingling, numbness, muscle weakness (especially in the legs and feet), and loss of control of the bowels or bladder (incontinence).

Do not take an anticoagulant, without first talking to the doctor, under the following conditions:

- If the patient has certain types of abnormal bleeding
- If the patient is allergic to the prescribed medication or any of the ingredients; a pharmacist can help identify these ingredients

What to tell the doctor before taking an anticoagulant medication: Inform the doctor about the following:

- Bleeding problems
- Liver or kidney problems
- Any other medical condition
- Being pregnant or planning to become pregnant
- Breastfeeding or plan to breastfeed

Tell the doctor about all the medicines the patient takes, including prescription and nonprescription medicines, vitamins, and herbal supplements.

Also inform all the doctors and dentists about taking an anticoagulant medication.

They should talk to the doctor who prescribed the anticoagulant before the patient has any surgery and medical or dental procedure.

How to take anticoagulant medications:

- Take the medication exactly as prescribed by the doctor.
- Do not change the dose or stop taking the anticoagulant unless the doctor says so.

- The doctor will tell how much anticoagulant to take and when to take it.
- The doctor may change the dose if needed.

How to store anticoagulant medication:

- Anticoagulant medications should be stored at room temperature between 68°F to 77°F (20°C to 25°C).
- Be sure to keep all medicines out of the reach of children.

IV

AORTIC, PERICARDIAL, AND VALVULAR DISEASE IN THE CCU

32

Alan F. Vainrib
Muhamed Saric

Acute Aortic Syndrome

INTRODUCTION

Acute aortic syndrome (AAS) represents a spectrum of life-threatening conditions with similar clinical presentation and the need for urgent management. It includes classic acute aortic dissection (CAAD), intramural hematoma (IMH), and penetrating aortic ulcer (PAU). Although not included in the original definition of AAS, traumatic aortic rupture (TAR) and aortic aneurysm rupture have also been considered to be part of the AAS spectrum.

AAS is characterized by disruption of the media layer of the aorta and typically presents with acute chest pain. The term "acute aortic syndrome" was first coined in 2001 by the Spanish cardiologists Vilacosta and San Román, who described AAS as a spectrum of interlinked lesions[1] with the intent to increase awareness and to speed up diagnosis and appropriate treatment (**Figure 32.1**).

Although the incidence of AAS is lower than that of acute coronary syndrome (ACS), AAS carries a higher mortality, and is therefore a critical component of the differential diagnosis of chest pain in the Cardiac Care Unit (CCU). Overall incidence of AASs is 2 to 4 cases per 100,000 individuals. Because AAS is rare, the International Registry of Acute Aortic Dissection (IRAD) was created in 1996 as a way to combine data acquired from multiple top institutions in Europe, North America, and Asia.[2] The 2010 intersocietal guidelines for the diagnosis and management of patients with thoracic aortic disease proposed a standard approach to the diagnosis and treatment of AAS.[3]

Although clinical history and physical examination are important, imaging is essential in the diagnosis of AAS. Transesophageal echocardiography (TEE), computed tomography (CT), and magnetic resonance imaging (MRI) are the preferred imaging modalities and angiography is rarely needed.

CLASSIFICATION OF ACUTE AORTIC SYNDROMES

Historically, CAAD was the first recognized form of AAS. The classification schemes used for the classic aortic dissection were subsequently extended to include IMH and PAU.

AASs are classified on the basis of the location and extent of involvement of the aorta. Two systems have been proposed, the DeBakey and the Stanford systems (**Figure 32.2**). The DeBakey system, which was proposed in 1965 by the Lebanese-American surgeon Michael Ellis DeBakey, divided aortic dissection into three types based on the anatomic location. Type I originates in the ascending aorta and propagates beyond the aortic arch, type II is limited to the ascending aorta only, and type III is limited to the descending aorta.[4]

The Stanford system, which was created by researchers at Stanford University in 1970, divides aortic dissections into two types. Type A includes any dissection that involves the ascending aorta, whereas type B dissections are limited to the descending thoracic aorta.[5] The Stanford classification appears to have wider acceptance and is now used for all three AAS types: CAAD, IMH, and PAU.

INTRAMURAL HEMATOMA

IMH is defined by crescentic or circumferential thickening of the media layer of the aortic wall. IMH is likely due to a ruptured vasa vasorum resulting in intramural bleeding but without a detectable intimal tear. It was first described in 1920 by the German pathologist Ernst Kruckenberg, who is also well known for his description of the so-called Kruckenberg tumors (transperitoneal ovarian metastases from stomach and colon cancers). On TEE, CT, or MRI, IMH is typically visualized as a crescentic or concentric thickening of the aortic wall > 5 mm (**Figure 32.3**).

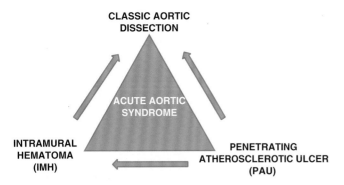

FIGURE 32.1 Acute aortic syndrome. The acute aortic syndrome triad first described by Vilacosta and San Román. Arrows signify possible progression of aortic lesions (penetrating aortic ulcer to IMH, penetrating aortic ulcer to classic dissection, IMH to classic dissection). IMH, intramural hematoma.

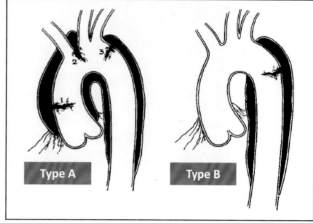

DE BAKEY CLASSIFICATION

Type I   Type II   Type III

J. Thorac. Cardiovasc. Surg. **1965;** 49:130-149.

STANFORD CLASSIFICATION

Type A   Type B

Ann Thorac Surg. **1970** Sep;10(3):237-47.

FIGURE 32.2 DeBakey and Stanford classifications. Left: DeBakey classification of aortic dissection. Type I includes the ascending and descending aorta, type II includes the ascending aorta only, and type III includes the descending thoracic aorta only. (DeBakey ME, Henly WS, Cooley DA, et al. Surgical management of dissecting aneurysms of the aorta. *J Thorac Cardiovasc Surg.* 1965;49:130-149.) Right: Stanford classification. Type A aortic dissection involves the ascending thoracic aorta, and type B involves the descending thoracic aorta only. All three AAS conditions; CAAD, IMH, and PAU use the Stanford classification. CAAD, classic acute aortic dissection; IMH, intramural hematoma; PAU, penetrating aortic ulcer. (Daily PO, Trueblood HW, Stinson EB, et al. Management of acute aortic dissections. *Ann Thorac Surg.* 1970;10[3]:237-247.)

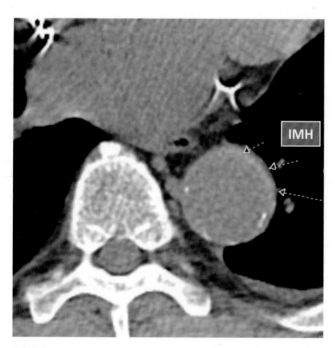

IMH

FIGURE 32.3 Intramural hematoma: CT. CT of the chest shows the descending thoracic aorta. The crescentic-shaped lesion on the patient's left signifies an IMH (dashed arrows). CT, computed tomography; IMH, intramural hematoma.

The natural history of IMH often includes progression to CAAD, which accounts for its high morbidity and mortality.

Etiology and Pathophysiology

IMH may account for up to 6% to 30% of all AAS, with a higher reported prevalence among the Korean and Japanese populations as compared with Western subjects.[6] It is unclear whether this is a true discrepancy in prevalence versus a reflection of differing classification, evaluation, or treatment practices. Often, IMH is diagnosed as such even though very small intimal tears indicative of limited aortic dissection may be present but missed by modern imaging modalities. This may overestimate the true prevalence of IMH as opposed to CAAD.

The characteristic feature of IMH is its location in the portion of the media closer to the adventitia, as opposed to CAAD which is typically located in the media closer to the intima. Although the most cited hypothesis of the pathophysiologic mechanism of IMH is rupture of the vasa vasorum, there is very little corroborating clinical or experimental evidence. Owing to the low incidence of IMH and the close association with CAAD, a definitive etiology still remains unclear.[7]

Clinical Manifestations

According to the IRAD experience, IMH typically presents with the symptoms of severe chest and back pain, similar to CAAD. However, IMH is less likely to present with manifestations of severe aortic regurgitation and pulse deficits.[6] IMH is rarely stable. It may either progress to CAAD or regress spontaneously, and therefore serial imaging is crucial. Stanford type B lesions in the descending aorta are more common than type A lesions in the ascending aorta (60% vs 35% of all IMH, respectively). Cardiogenic shock may be present in 14% of patients, more typically with type A IMH.[8] Pericardial effusion and tamponade may also be present, which are also more common in type A IMH. When compared with CAAD, type A IMH has a significantly higher risk of rupture (26% vs 8%, respectively).[9] A widened mediastinum may be present on chest X-ray; however, this is neither sensitive nor specific to IMH.

Diagnosis

As with all types of AAS, rapid diagnosis is paramount in IMH. TEE, CT, and MRI are the preferred diagnostic tools. CT is often

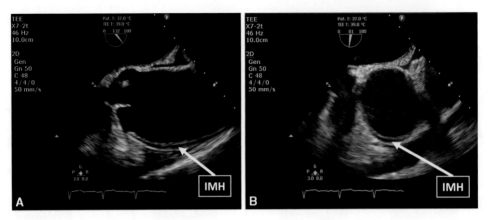

FIGURE 32.4 Intramural hematoma: TEE. Two-dimensional (2D) TEE of the ascending thoracic aorta in the long-axis (A) and short-axis (B) views. Yellow arrows point to a crescentic thickening of the anterior portion of the ascending thoracic aortic wall, consistent with a type A IMH. IMH, intramural hematoma; TEE, transesophageal echocardiography.

chosen because of widespread availability, rapid acquisition, and its ability to diagnose other causes of acute chest pain such as trauma and pulmonary embolism.

Classically, absence of an intimal flap or tear differentiates IMH from CAAD. Often, IMH can be identified even on non–contrast-enhanced CT. On contrast CT scans, a crescentic or circular area of high attenuation that does not enhance with contrast is present. Similar findings are seen on MRI, which has the advantage of not requiring iodinated contrast.

On TEE, IMH is diagnosed if there is regional thickening of the aortic wall > 5 mm in a crescentic or circumferential pattern without an intimal flap or tear (**Figure 32.4A, B**). Limitations of TEE in diagnosing IMH arise from the TEE's inability to visualize all portions of the aorta including the area around the origin of the brachiocephalic artery and all but the most proximal portions of the abdominal aorta. TEE is very useful in diagnosing complications of IMH, such as pericardial effusion or aortic regurgitation.

Small intimal tears may be missed by any modern imaging technique, challenging the diagnosis of classic IMH.

Management and Prognosis

The prognosis of IMH is somewhat better than that of CAAD. As in all AAS, the main determinant of prognosis is its aortic location. According to the IRAD registry, the mortality of type A IMH is approximately 27%, compared with 4% in type B IMH. Invasively managed patients with type A IMH typically fare better than medically managed patients. Invasive options include open surgical repair and percutaneous thoracic endovascular aortic repair. Medical management typically consists of heart rate (HR), blood pressure, and pain control. Surgical mortality for IMH is similar to that for other forms of AAS.

Type B IMH is often managed medically. Approximately 50% of type B patients may improve with medical management alone, 15% will remain stable, and 35% may progress to aneurysm formation, CAAD, or focal aortic rupture (pseudoaneurysm).[10]

Intramural Hematoma in Pregnancy

Although there are no specific guidelines in pregnancy for patients with IMH, pregnancy is considered a risk factor for the development of aortic pathology, especially in Marfan syndrome.

As with other forms of AAS, expedited delivery via caesarian section is considered reasonable for pregnant patients with acute IMH, if possible.

CLASSIC ACUTE AORTIC DISSECTION

CAAD is the most common form of AAS.[2] It occurs in approximately 66% to 75% of all AAS. The overall incidence of CAAD is low, estimated at 0.5 to 4.0 cases per 100,000 per year, and is thought to affect men more than women in a 2:1 ratio.

Risk factors for CAAD include connective tissue disorders such as Marfan (fibrillin gene), Loeys–Dietz (transforming growth factor β receptor 1 and 2 genes), Ehlers–Danlos type 4 (collagen gene), and Turner syndrome (X monosomy), as well as the aortopathy associated with bicuspid aortic valve (*NOTCH1* gene). In addition, hypertension is a significant risk factor and is more prevalent among older patients. Last, aortic instrumentation or surgery, as well as cardiac catheterization, are rare but reported causes of aortic dissection.

CAAD was first described in 1555 by Andreas Vesalius (1514–1564) who reported traumatic abdominal aortic aneurysm in a man who fell off a horse.[11] Intimal tear, the hallmark of CAAD, was first described by Daniel Sennert (1572–1637), a German anatomist and published in 1650 posthumously.[12] A very famous description of CAAD was by the British royal physician Frank Nichols (1699–1778) who provided the first unmistakable account of CAAD (deemed a "Transverse fissure of the aortic trunk") in his autopsy of King George II, who died in 1760 while straining in the lavatory. Successful surgical repair of descending aortic dissection was not reported until 1955, by Michael Debakey (1908–2008) and his colleagues, and ascending dissection until 1962 by Frank Spencer and Hu Blake.[13,14]

Etiology and Pathophysiology

CAAD is characterized by an intimal tear, which leads to abnormal blood flow from the aortic lumen into the media (**Figure 32.5**). Consequently, there is a longitudinal separation of the media layers by the blood flow, which tears an intimomedial flap from the remainder of the aortic wall (**Figure 32.6A–C**). This flap separates the abnormal false lumen from the true aortic lumen. Intimal tears typically occur at the locations within the aorta

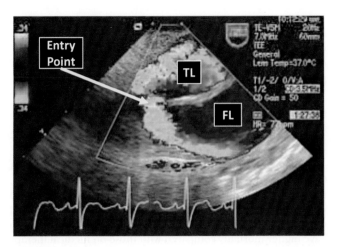

FIGURE 32.5 Classic acute aortic dissection: entry point on TEE. Two-dimensional (2D) TEE with color Doppler of the aortic arch in the upper esophageal view. Yellow arrow points to the entry point of flow from the true lumen to the false lumen, characteristic of CAAD. CAAD, classic acute aortic dissection; FL, false lumen; TEE, transesophageal echocardiography; TL, true lumen.

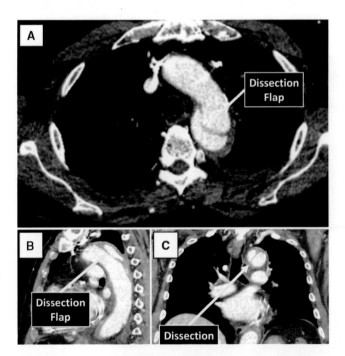

FIGURE 32.6 Classic acute aortic dissection: CT. Multidetector row CT with intravenous iodinated contrast in the axial view (A), sagittal view (B), and the coronal view (C). Yellow arrows point to dissection flap at the junction of the aortic arch and descending thoracic aorta, consistent with CAAD. CAAD, classic acute aortic dissection; CT, computed tomography.

with the highest shear stress. These are at the right side of the ascending aorta immediately distal to the ostium of the right coronary artery (type A dissections) and immediately distal to the ostium of the subclavian artery adjacent to the insertion of the ligamentum arteriosus (type B dissections).

Complications such as aortic regurgitation and pericardial tamponade can occur; and, over time, chronic changes such as false lumen thrombosis and aneurysm are common.

Clinical Manifestations

The typical symptom of acute aortic dissection is "aortic pain" similar to other forms of AAS. Acute, severe, tearing chest pain is the hallmark symptom of CAAD. Pain limited to the chest is typical of type A CAAD, and pain in the back is more often the symptom of type B CAAD. One study found older patients are less likely to abrupt onset of pain as compared with younger patients.[15]

Pulse deficit, present in up to 33% of patients according to the IRAD study, reflects impaired or absent blood flow to peripheral vessels. This is manifested by weak carotid, brachial, or femoral pulses on physical examination.

Other physical examination findings of CAAD include diastolic murmur or aortic regurgitation, hypotension related to either tamponade or aortic rupture, focal neurologic deficits reflecting propagation of the dissection toward involvement of carotid or cerebral arteries, and syncope.

Electrocardiogram (ECG) may be useful in distinguishing the chest pain of AAS from ACSs; unlike ACS, uncomplicated CAAD does not present with ischemic ECG changes. However, if the aortic dissection leads to coronary ischemia through involvement of coronary ostia (type A), the ECG will be less helpful with differentiation of symptoms.

Chest X-ray (CXR) imaging occasionally shows widening of the mediastinum, a nonspecific finding seen with other syndromes such as mediastinal hematoma. Other CXR findings are double aortic knob (40% of patients), tracheal displacement to the right, and enlargement of the cardiac silhouette.

Serum biomarkers such as D-dimer are often elevated in CAAD, but this is a nonspecific finding. In contrast, a normal D-dimer level may help exclude the diagnosis of CAAD. Investigational biomarkers such as elastin degradation products, calponin, fibrinogen, fibrillin, and smooth muscle myosin heavy chain are currently being evaluated.

Diagnosis

As with other forms of AAS, the 2010 intersocietal guidelines for the diagnosis and management of patients with thoracic aortic disease provide a useful decision tool to help guide diagnostic and management strategies for CAAD with a special emphasis on a combination of clinical risk assessment and rapid imaging.

CT with intravenous iodinated contrast is often the diagnostic modality of choice for CAAD because of its superb spatial resolution, rapid acquisition times, widespread availability, and its ability to diagnose other causes of acute chest pain such as trauma and pulmonary embolism. The reported sensitivity of CT for CAAD is 87% to 94% and specificity is 92% to 100%. CT features of CAAD are intimal tear, dissection flap with a true and false lumen, dilatation of the aorta, and pericardial effusion.

TEE is especially useful in the diagnosis of CAAD when a CT with contrast cannot be performed, such as in hemodynamically unstable patients or in patients in whom the risk of iodinated intravenous contrast is high such as renal insufficiency or severe allergy. The reported sensitivity of TEE is 98% and specificity is 63% to 93%. Findings on TEE are a dissection flap separating the true and false lumen, site of intimal tear represented by flow from the true lumen into the false lumen on color Doppler (**Figure 32.7**). Spectral Doppler may help corroborate the diagnosis by demonstrating "to and fro" flow into and out of the false lumen.

The true lumen is identified by its expansion with systole and contraction in diastole. The true lumen is often smaller than the false lumen. In early stages, the false lumen may be echo free or may contain spontaneous echo contrast (also known as "smoke") due to stasis of blood flow. In later, more chronic stages, the false lumen may be partly or completely obliterated by thrombus formation.

Complications of CAAD may be seen on echocardiography such as aortic regurgitation, pericardial effusion/tamponade, and wall motion abnormalities indicative of ischemia if there is coronary ostial involvement.

It is important not to confuse the intimomedial flap of CAAD with either artifacts or surrounding vascular structures. Linear reverberation artifacts in the ascending aorta should not be mistaken for type A aortic dissection. Typically, reverberation artifacts are located twice as deep as the anterior aortic wall. In addition, a dilated azygos vein adjacent to the descending thoracic aorta may give an illusion of a type B dissection. Color or spectral Doppler imaging in both instances may help distinguish true aortic dissection from its masqueraders (**Figure 32.8**).

Although on transthoracic echocardiography (TTE) aortic dissection can occasionally be seen, TTE should only be used as a screening tool owing to lack of sufficient sensitivity and specificity.

MRI and aortography also may reveal aortic dissection; however, they are reserved for specific situations. MRI may be used when the patient cannot receive iodinated contrast for CT nor undergo TEE. Aortography is of limited use and is typically performed during invasive endovascular therapeutic procedures.

Management and Prognosis

Type A CAAD is a true medical emergency, requiring immediate surgical repair because the mortality increases by the hour. Approximately 90% of medically managed patients with type A CAAD die within 3 months of presentation. On the other hand, the prognosis is more favorable for patients with type B CAAD in whom medical management is often preferred over surgical repair because surgically managed patients have been shown to have higher mortality compared with those on medical therapy alone. Medical therapy generally consists of tight blood pressure control and β-blockade. Surgical management of type A CAAD typically consists of excision of the intimal tear if possible and obliteration of entry into the false lumen, as well as implantation of a graft to replace the ascending aorta.[16] Surgical therapy for type B is more complicated because of the presence of many spinal artery branches, and therefore has a risk of paraplegia. Nevertheless, surgical therapy of type B dissection is often

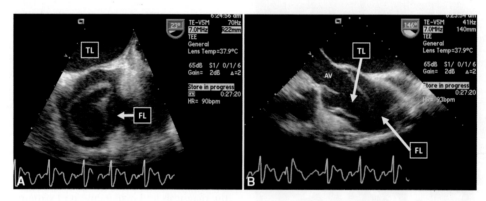

FIGURE 32.7 Classic acute aortic dissection: dissection flap on TEE. Two-dimensional (2D) TEE of the ascending thoracic aorta in short axis (A) and long axis (B) demonstrating CAAD. In this case, the dissection flap is circumferential with a 360° separation of the true and false lumens. CAAD, classic acute aortic dissection; FL, false lumen; TEE, transesophageal echocardiography; TL, true lumen.

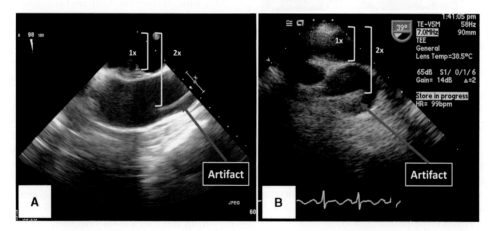

FIGURE 32.8 Reverberation artifact masquerading as type A dissection on TEE. Two-dimensional (2D) TEE of the ascending thoracic aorta in a long-axis view (A) and a short-axis view (B). Red arrows point to linear reverberation artifact. Note that the reverberation artifact is located twice as deep (2×) as the anterior aortic wall, characteristic of reverberation artifacts. TEE, transesophageal echocardiography.

necessary when there is aortic branch ischemia and end-organ damage. Endovascular graft therapy to treat type B CAAD has shown promise (**Figure 32.9**).[17]

It is important to identify risk factors for higher mortality in type A CAAD such as advanced age, prior cardiac surgery, hypotension or shock, pulse deficit, cardiac tamponade, and ischemic ECG changes.

Classic Acute Aortic Dissection in Pregnancy

The 2010 intersocietal guidelines for the diagnosis and management of patients with thoracic aortic disease recommends expedited fetal delivery via caesarian section for patients with CAAD during pregnancy given the high mortality of the disease (class IIa recommendation). The diagnostic imaging modality of choice is MRI without gadolinium to avoid exposing the mother and fetus to ionizing radiation.[18] TEE is an option and is considered safe in pregnancy; however, caution must be used when providing procedural sedation because the medications typically administered (midazolam and fentanyl) may be teratogenic, especially in the first trimester. In these cases, topical anesthesia with viscous lidocaine is crucial. There have been reports recommending monitoring fetal HR and uterine tone during TEE.[19]

PENETRATING AORTIC ULCER

PAU represents the process by which an atherosclerotic plaque erodes and penetrates through the elastic lamina into the media layer of the aorta, causing ulceration (**Figure 32.10**). PAU may further erode through the adventitia leading to either focal (pseudoaneurysm) or complete aortic rupture (**Figure 32.11**). Thrombus occasionally forms within PAU. In addition, PAU may lead to either IMH or aortic dissection, which is why PAU is characterized as an AAS.

Etiology and Pathophysiology

PAU accounts for 2% to 11% of all AASs.[20,21] It was first described in 1986 by Anthony Stanson and colleagues.[22] Patients with PAU typically are older (>70 years old) and have risk factors for atherosclerosis including hypertension, smoking, and hyperlipidemia.

The natural history of PAU is not well described. PAU may cause remodeling of the aortic wall and aneurysm formation, contained rupture through the aortic wall and attendant pseudoaneurysm formation, complete aortic rupture with mediastinal or pleural hemorrhage, or progression to IMH and CAAD.

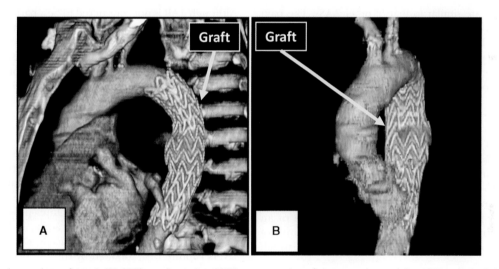

FIGURE 32.9 Endovascular graft repair: 3D CT. Three-dimensional (3D) reconstruction of contrast-enhanced chest CT in a sagittal view (A) and coronal view with surrounding structures removed (B) demonstrating an endovascular stent graft located between the junction of the aortic arch and descending thoracic aorta, extending to the distal descending thoracic aorta. CT, computed tomography.

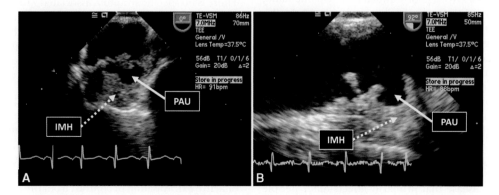

FIGURE 32.10 Penetrating aortic ulcer: TEE. Two-dimensional (2D) TEE of the descending thoracic aorta in the midesophageal short-axis view (A) and long-axis view (B). Yellow arrows point to demonstrating severe atherosclerotic plaque and PAU; yellow dashed arrows point to an area with developing IMH. IMH, intramural hematoma; PAU, penetrating aortic ulcer; TEE, transesophageal echocardiography.

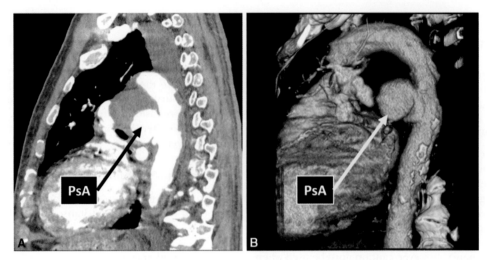

FIGURE 32.11 Penetrating aortic ulcer with rupture/pseudoaneurysm visualized by contrast-enchanced 2D (A) and 3D CT (B). Arrows point to PAU with aortic rupture and pseudoaneurysm of anterior portion of the proximal descending thoracic aorta. CT, computed tomography; PsA, pseudoaneurysm.

Clinical Manifestations

Symptoms of PAU are similar to that of other AASs. The pain associated with PAU is variable, and dependent on the location of the ulceration. Type A PAU typically presents with chest pain and type B PAU is more likely to present with back pain. Unlike IMH or CAAD, there have been reports of PAU as an incidental finding in asymptomatic patients.

Diagnosis

The diagnosis of PAU is primarily made by CT, TEE, and MRI. Aortography is not typically used for PAU because of lack of direct visualization of the aortic wall. All three techniques are able to image atherosclerotic changes, ulceration, and complications such as pseudoaneurysm, rupture, and mediastinal and pleural hemorrhage. Identification of an ulcer crater distinguishes PAU from IMH. PAU lesions are typically focal as opposed to those of CAAD and IMH, which are more extensive.

Management and Prognosis

The natural history of PAU is poorly understood. On one hand, PAU is considered to be a surgical emergency with risk similar to or worse than other forms of AAS. On the other, reports have described the progression of PAU as slow, with a low prevalence of life-threatening complications.[23] There is therefore equipoise regarding the optimal medical versus surgical treatment strategies. Nevertheless, surgical management of PAU with aortic grafting is considered appropriate in the presence of aortic rupture, persistent or recurrent pain, hemodynamic instability, or rapidly expanding aortic diameter.

Penetrating Aortic Ulcer in Pregnancy

Because PAU is a disease that primarily affects older people (>70 years of age), it is highly unlikely that it will occur during pregnancy. There is therefore no available guideline to direct optimal management.

TRAUMATIC AORTIC RUPTURE

Although TAR is not considered to be a part of the original AAS triad, it is a life-threatening aortic emergency with only a 15% to 20% survival.[24] TAR is typically caused by deceleration injuries sustained in motor vehicle accidents (MVAs) and falls greater than 3 m.[25] It is the second leading cause of death after blunt trauma, occurring in approximately 1.5% to 1.9% cases.[26]

Etiology and Pathophysiology

The most common site of injury in TAR is at the aortic isthmus, immediately distal to the left subclavian artery at the site of the ductus arteriosus. This location is considered to be the most vulnerable to torsional and shear forces because it is thought to be a transition zone between the semi-mobile aortic arch and the fixed descending thoracic aorta. Other possible sites of injury are the transverse arch, ascending aorta, and descending aorta proximal to the diaphragm.[27] Typically, the intima and medial layers rupture first, followed by rupture of the adventitia after an unpredictable interval of time.[28] Multiple tears may occur.

Clinical Manifestations

There is no specific symptom associated with TAR. Chest pain in the patient with trauma should, however, raise suspicion, especially in the presence of the "seat belt sign" (seat belt imprint on the surface of the skin). Pulse deficit and murmur of aortic regurgitation may be present. CXR may show a widened mediastinum, obscured aortic knob, and left hemothorax.

Diagnosis

TAR is best diagnosed using either contrast-enhanced CT or TEE because both modalities have high diagnostic sensitivity and specificity (**Figure 32.12**). Findings seen on CT include intimal flap, periaortic hematoma, luminal filling defects, pseudoaneurysm, or active extravasation of contrast from the aorta. It is important to distinguish TAR from a ductus arteriosus diverticulum, which is helped by the improved special and temporal resolution of modern multidetector row CT scanners. However, TEE may be

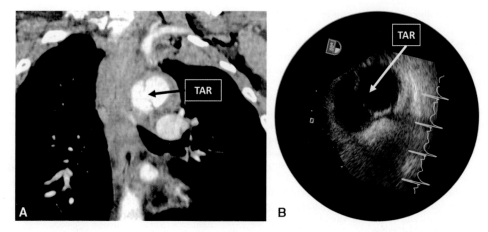

FIGURE 32.12 Traumatic aortic rupture. CT of the chest with iodinated contrast, coronal view (A), and TEE upper esophageal view (B) of the aortic arch. Arrows point to traumatic aortic rupture. Note that the TEE image was rotated to align with the CT image. CT, computed tomography; TAR, traumatic aortic rupture; TEE, transesophageal echocardiography.

more specific in differentiating ductus arteriosus diverticula from TAR. Another very useful advantage of TEE is its portability, with the ability to be performed at the bedside of hemodynamically unstable patients, a common scenario in TAR. The main limitation of TEE is an apparent "blind spot" at the distal ascending aorta and proximal aortic arch caused by bronchial shadowing. Aortography, the former gold standard, may be performed; however, it is invasive and can result in worsening of the aortic rupture in as many as 10% of patients and is therefore not the preferred diagnostic modality.

Management and Prognosis

Emergent surgical therapy is the standard of care for TAR. As with AAS, medical therapy consists of very close blood pressure and HR control. Hemodynamically unstable patients should be operated on immediately. Surgical options comprise open repair with prosthetic grafts, and endovascularly delivered fabric-covered stents. Endovascular repair has been shown to have decreased overall mortality compared with surgical repair and is recommended when possible. The overall survival of TAR is approximately 10% to 18%. Survival to emergency room care greatly improves the odds of long-term survival, and survival to surgical therapy improves the odds even more, to approximately 70% to 90%.[29]

Traumatic Aortic Rupture in Pregnancy

Although there are no specific guidelines for the management of TAR in pregnancy, expedited delivery via caesarian section with emergent aortic surgery is a reasonable therapeutic approach given the high mortality both to the mother and fetus.

REFERENCES

1. Vilacosta I, San Román JA. Acute aortic syndrome. *Heart.* 2001;85:365-368.
2. Hagan PG, Nienaber CA, Isselbacher EM, et al. The International Registry of Acute Aortic Dissection (IRAD): new insights into an old disease. *JAMA.* 2000;283:897-903.
3. Hiratzka LF, Bakris GL, Beckman JA, et al. 2010 ACCF/AHA/AATS/ACR/ASA/SCA/SCAI/SIR/STS/SVM Guidelines for the diagnosis and management of patients with thoracic aortic disease. A Report of the American College of Cardiology Foundation/American Heart Association Task Force on Practice Guidelines, American Association for Thoracic Surgery, American College of Radiology, American Stroke Association, Society of Cardiovascular Anesthesiologists, Society for Cardiovascular Angiography and Interventions, Society of Interventional Radiology, Society of Thoracic Surgeons, and Society for Vascular Medicine. *J Am Coll Cardiol.* 2010;55:e27-e129.
4. DeBakey ME, Henly WS, Cooley DA, Morris GC Jr, Crawford ES, Beall AC Jr. Surgical management of dissecting aneurysms of the aorta. *J Thorac Cardiovasc Surg.* 1965;49:130-149.
5. Daily PO, Trueblood HW, Stinson EB, Wuerflein RD, Shumway NE. Management of acute aortic dissections. *Ann Thorac Surg.* 1970;10(3):237-247.
6. Harris KM, Braverman AC, Eagle KA, et al. Acute aortic intramural hematoma: an analysis from the International Registry of Acute Aortic Dissection. *Circulation.* 2012;126:S91-S96.
7. Goldberg JB, Kim JB, Sundt TM. Current understandings and approach to the management of aortic intramural hematomas. *Semin Thorac Cardiovasc Surg.* 2014;26:123-131.
8. Moizumi Y, Komatsu T, Motoyoshi N, Tabayashi K. Clinical features and long-term outcome of type A and type B intramural hematoma of the aorta. *J Thorac Cardiovasc Surg.* 2004;127:421-427.
9. Tittle SL, Lynch RJ, Cole PE, et al. Midterm follow-up of penetrating ulcer and intramural hematoma of the aorta. *J Thorac Cardiovasc Surg.* 2002;123:1051-1059.
10. Mussa FF, Horton JD, Moridzadeh R, Nicholson J, Trimarchi S, Eagle KA. Acute aortic dissection and intramural hematoma: a systematic review. *JAMA.* 2016;316:754-763.
11. O'Malley CD. Andreas Vesalius 1514-1564: In Memoriam. *Med Hist.* 1964;8:299-308.
12. Sennertus D. Cap. 42. *Op Omn Lib.* 1650;5:306-315.
13. De Bakey ME, Cooley DA, Creech O Jr. Surgical considerations of dissecting aneurysm of the aorta. *Ann Surg.* 1955;142:586-610; discussion 611-612.
14. Spencer FC, Blake H. A report of the successful surgical treatment of aortic regurgitation from a dissecting aortic aneurysm in a patient with the Marfan syndrome. *J Thorac Cardiovasc Surg.* 1962;44:238-245.
15. Pape LA, Awais M, Woznicki EM, et al. Presentation, diagnosis, and outcomes of acute aortic dissection: 17-year trends from the International Registry of Acute Aortic Dissection. *J Am Coll Cardiol.* 2015;66:350-358.

16. Braverman AC. Acute aortic dissection: clinician update. *Circulation.* 2010;122:184-188.

17. Nienaber CA, Kische S, Rousseau H, et al. Endovascular repair of type B aortic dissection: long-term results of the randomized investigation of stent grafts in aortic dissection trial. *Circ Cardiovasc Interv.* 2013;6:407-416.

18. Hiratzka LF, Bakris GL, Beckman JA, et al. 2010 ACCF/AHA/AATS/ACR/ASA/SCA/SCAI/SIR/STS/SVM guidelines for the diagnosis and management of patients with thoracic aortic disease: executive summary. A report of the American College of Cardiology Foundation/American Heart Association Task Force on Practice Guidelines, American Association for Thoracic Surgery, American College of Radiology, American Stroke Association, Society of Cardiovascular Anesthesiologists, Society for Cardiovascular Angiography and Interventions, Society of Interventional Radiology, Society of Thoracic Surgeons, and Society for Vascular Medicine. *Catheter Cardiovasc Interv.* 2010;76:E43-E86.

19. Stoddard MF, Longaker RA, Vuocolo LM, Dawkins PR. Transesophageal echocardiography in the pregnant patient. *Am Heart J.* 1992;124:785-787.

20. Hirst AE Jr, Johns VJ Jr, Kime SW Jr. Dissecting aneurysm of the aorta: a review of 505 cases. *Medicine.* 1958;37:217-279.

21. Eggebrecht H, Plicht B, Kahlert P, Erbel R. Intramural hematoma and penetrating ulcers: indications to endovascular treatment. *Eur J Vasc Endovasc Surg.* 2009;38:659-665.

22. Stanson AW, Kazmier FJ, Hollier LH, et al. Penetrating atherosclerotic ulcers of the thoracic aorta: natural history and clinicopathologic correlations. *Ann Vasc Surg.* 1986;1:15-23.

23. Hayashi H, Matsuoka Y, Sakamoto I, et al. Penetrating atherosclerotic ulcer of the aorta: imaging features and disease concept. *Radiographics.* 2000;20:995-1005.

24. Fabian TC, Richardson JD, Croce MA, et al. Prospective study of blunt aortic injury: multicenter trial of the American Association for the Surgery of Trauma. *J Trauma.* 1997;42:374-380; discussion 380-383.

25. Sanchez-Ross M, Anis A, Walia J, et al. Aortic rupture: comparison of three imaging modalities. *Emerg Radiol.* 2006;13:31-33.

26. Dyer DS, Moore EE, Ilke DN, et al. Thoracic aortic injury: how predictive is mechanism and is chest computed tomography a reliable screening tool? A prospective study of 1,561 patients. *J Trauma.* 2000;48:673-682; discussion 682-683.

27. Sevitt S. The mechanisms of traumatic rupture of the thoracic aorta. *Br J Surg.* 1977;64:166-173.

28. Nikolic S, Atanasijevic T, Mihailovic Z, Babic D, Popovic-Loncar T. Mechanisms of aortic blunt rupture in fatally injured front-seat passengers in frontal car collisions: an autopsy study. *Am J Forensic Med Pathol.* 2006;27:292-295.

29. Smith RS, Chang FC. Traumatic rupture of the aorta: still a lethal injury. *Am J Surg.* 1986;152:660-663.

Patient and Family Information for:
ACUTE AORTIC SYNDROME

GENERAL CONCEPTS OF ACUTE AORTIC SYNDROME

WHAT IS THE ILLNESS?

AAS refers to four related diseases of the large vessel that leaves the heart, called the aorta. These are CAAD, IMH, PAU, and TAR. These conditions involve damage to the wall of the aorta and require prompt care because they are associated with a high chance of dying unless treated rapidly.

HOW WILL THE PATIENT BE TREATED?

Once the diagnosis of AAS is established by CT, TEE, or MRI, the disease is typically treated with mediations that lower blood pressure and HR. The doctor will determine the type of AAS (type A or type B) based on the location of involvement in the aorta. A cardiothoracic surgeon may be consulted, who will assess the need for surgery. Surgery is often needed as soon as possible.

WHAT IF THE PATIENT IS PREGNANT OR THINKING OF BECOMING PREGNANT?

Given the high mortality of AAS and the frequent need for emergency cardiac surgery, the doctor may recommend expedited delivery. If at risk of AAS because of genetic conditions that may affect the aorta, the patient should consult the doctor to assess the risk if she is thinking about becoming pregnant.

INTRAMURAL HEMATOMA

WHAT IS THE ILLNESS?

IMH is described as bleeding into the wall of the aorta due to breakage of the internal blood vessels of the aorta. Symptoms of IMH are sudden severe chest or back pain. IMH is best diagnosed by imaging the aorta using CT, TEE, or MRI. On experiencing symptoms suggestive of IMH, the patient or a family member should seek medical care immediately because the risk of dying from this condition increases by the hour.

HOW WILL THE PATIENT BE TREATED?

Once the diagnosis of IMH is established, medications will be given to reduce the blood pressure and HR. A cardiothoracic surgeon may be consulted, who will assess the need for surgery. Surgery will often involve either replacement of the diseased portions of the aorta or placement of special type of stent within the aorta that will help contain the bleeding and prevent the aorta from bursting.

WHAT IF THE PATIENT IS PREGNANT OR THINKING OF BECOMING PREGNANT?

IMH carries a high risk of mortality, and often requires emergency surgery. The doctor will tailor the medications for IMH to include only those with minimal risk to the baby. If the pregnant patient or family member requires emergency surgery, expedited delivery is prudent. Rapid consultation with an obstetrician is crucial. If the person has a condition that puts her at risk for IMH such as Marfan syndrome or other genetic disorders of the aorta, consult the doctor to assess the risk if thinking about becoming pregnant.

CLASSIC ACUTE AORTIC DISSECTION

WHAT IS THE ILLNESS?

CAAD is the most common type of AAS. It is caused by a tear of the inner layer of the aorta, called the intima. This tear can then propagate, leading to separation of the layers of the aorta. There are hereditary disorders such as Marfan syndrome and bicuspid aortic valve that may put the person or a family member at risk of CAAD because of weakening of the aortic wall.

Symptoms typically experienced are severe "tearing" chest or back pain that occurs at rest. If the person or a family member experiences such symptoms, seek medical care immediately.

CAAD will be diagnosed using CT, TEE, or MRI, which are widely available and can be performed and interpreted rapidly.

HOW WILL THE PATIENT BE TREATED?

As with other types of AAS, the doctor will prescribe medications that lower blood pressure and HR. A cardiothoracic surgeon may be consulted immediately, who will assess the need for surgery. The location of the dissection is a crucial component in deciding what the best treatment is. Surgical options are open heart surgery or placement of a tube called stent. The cardiothoracic surgeon will assess which procedure is the most appropriate.

WHAT IF THE PATIENT IS PREGNANT OR THINKING OF BECOMING PREGNANT?

As with other types of AAS, CAAD is often a surgical emergency. As such, consultation with an obstetrician and expedited delivery may be recommended. If the patient or a family member has a disorder that involves the aorta, consult the obstetrician before deciding to conceive.

PENATRATING AORTIC ULCER

WHAT IS THE ILLNESS?

Atherosclerosis or hardening of the arteries is a disease in which cholesterol and fat build up within the walls of the blood vessels called arteries. PAU is caused when a very severe plaque breaks through the aorta, causing a hole, or ulceration. Risk factors for PAU include advanced age, high blood pressure, high cholesterol, and smoking. Symptoms include chest and back pain, although some patients may have no symptoms.

Along with other forms of AAS, PAU is diagnosed by CT, TEE, or MRI.

HOW WILL THE PATIENT BE TREATED?

The doctor may recommend close monitoring with imaging studies, medications, or surgery.

WHAT IF THE PATIENT IS PREGNANT OR THINKING OF BECOMING PREGNANT?

PAU is typically a disease that affects older people (more than 70 years of age). It is highly unlikely that it will occur during pregnancy.

TRAUMATIC AORTIC RUPTURE

WHAT IS THE ILLNESS?

TAR describes tearing of the aorta after a chest injury. It most commonly occurs after MVAs and bad falls.

TAR is a very dangerous condition and requires prompt medical attention. A mark across the skin of the chest due to a seat belt often is present when TAR is caused by an MVA. TAR is diagnosed using CT and TEE.

HOW WILL THE PATIENT BE TREATED?

Emergency surgery is the standard of care for TAR. The doctor may prescribe medications to lower HR and blood pressure if necessary; however, a cardiothoracic surgeon may be consulted as soon as possible. Treatment typically requires open heart surgery.

WHAT IF THE PATIENT IS PREGNANT OR THINKING OF BECOMING PREGNANT?

Because TAR is a surgical emergency, consultation with an obstetrician for early delivery is crucial.

The surgeon may recommend delivery by cesarean section at the time of surgery to repair the broken aorta.

Edgar Argulian
Eyal Herzog

33

Pericardial Effusion and Tamponade

INTRODUCTION

Pericardial effusion is a relatively common finding in high-risk patients evaluated in the acute setting.[1] It should be considered in differential diagnosis for a variety of clinical presentations including chest pain, shortness of breath, and hypotension.[1] Pericardial effusion can be directly causal for patients' complaints (like in patients with pericardial tamponade) or be an incidental finding still carrying a prognostic significance (like in patients with pulmonary hypertension). The general approach to pericardial effusion once it is recognized includes establishing the cause of pericardial disease and assessing its hemodynamic significance.

RECOGNIZING THE PRESENCE OF PERICARDIAL EFFUSION

Pericardial effusion can be recognized on the basis of clinical suspicion or it can be an incidental finding on chest or cardiac imaging.[2] The following clinical settings may indicate the need to specifically evaluate for the presence of pericardial effusion[3]:

1. Cardiac arrest with pulseless electrical activity or asystole
2. Chest discomfort and/or any signs of hemodynamic instability in chest trauma, recent cardiac surgery, or percutaneous cardiac intervention
3. Any of the following when otherwise unexplained: chest pain, fever, dyspnea, and elevated cardiac biomarkers
4. Physical and electrocardiographic findings attributable to pericardial disease; the latter includes tachycardia, low voltage, and electrical alternans (**Figure 33.1**)
5. Enlarged cardiac silhouette or pleural effusions on chest X-ray
6. Any patient with ascending aortic dissection, severe pulmonary hypertension, renal failure, use of some medications, rheumatic diseases, malignancy, or other systemic conditions when pericardial effusion is thought to contribute to presentation or have prognostic significance[3]

Echocardiography is the most commonly used modality to diagnose pericardial effusion: owing to its accuracy and portably, it can be easily used in any health care setting including bedside in an acutely ill patient. Other modalities (such as computed tomography [CT] scan or cardiac magnetic resonance) can be occasionally used to diagnose pericardial effusion, especially when echocardiographic examination is limited or nondiagnostic.[4]

ESTABLISHING THE CAUSE OF PERICARDIAL EFFUSION

There is a long list of possible causes for pericardial effusion (**Table 33.1**), but a limited number of etiologies account for the majority of diagnoses.[5] A structured approach helps establish the cause of pericardial effusion in most cases.[6] A very aggressive approach, as is used in some studies, has a high diagnostic yield but low clinical relevance, especially for small effusions.[7,8] Routine sampling of pericardial fluid for diagnostic purposes is unnecessary.[3] History and physical examination often provide clues to the etiology of pericardial effusion. For example, the pericardium can be involved in patients with active systemic malignancy, and malignant effusion should be strongly considered in these patients. Active or recent infection, radiation therapy, rheumatic disease, and recent acute coronary syndrome, cardiac surgery, or percutaneous cardiac procedure, all provide relevant clues to etiology. A typical clinical presentation, physical findings, and electrocardiographic changes commonly confirm the diagnosis of acute idiopathic pericarditis.[9] In one study, the presence of "inflammatory" signs (characteristic chest pain, pericardial friction rub, fever, and/or diffuse ST-segment elevation) in patients with pericardial effusion was strongly associated with acute idiopathic pericarditis.[10]

We use a parsimonious stepwise approach to laboratory testing and imaging in patients with pericardial effusion at our institution (**Figure 33.2**).[6] Transthoracic echocardiography is the standard test in establishing the presence of pericardial effusion, quantifying the size of the effusion and assessing its hemodynamic impact. The initial tier of testing includes complete blood count, complete metabolic panel, coagulation studies, inflammatory markers (erythrocyte sedimentation rate, C-reactive protein), cardiac biomarkers, thyroid stimulating hormone level, and chest X-ray. In appropriate clinical settings, human immunodeficiency virus (HIV) testing, autoantibodies, and blood cultures are obtained. Advanced chest imaging (CT scan, positron emission tomography, and magnetic resonance imaging) can be helpful in certain clinical situations, especially

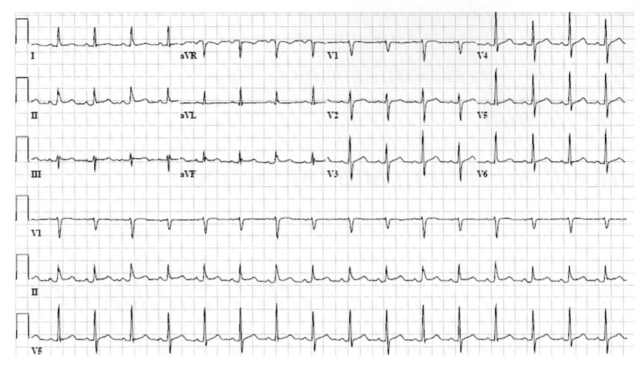

FIGURE 33.1 Electrocardiogram in a patient with large pericardial effusion. Electrical alternans is evident in multiple leads including V1and V5. ECG, electrocardiogram.

TABLE 33.1	Causes of Pericardial Effusion
Aortic dissection	
Endocrine (hypothyroidism)	
Idiopathic	
Infectious (including viral, tuberculous, and purulent pericarditis)	
Medications	
Neoplastic (typically secondary)	
Perimyocardial infarction and postcardiotomy syndrome	
Pulmonary hypertension and right-sided heart failure	
Radiation	
Renal failure	
Rheumatic/autoimmune diseases	
Traumatic (chest injury, procedure, surgery)	

when malignancy is suspected. Besides, CT scan and cardiac magnetic resonance can be used as adjunct imaging modalities for assessing pericardial effusion in some patients.[4] They offer precise effusion localization, quantification, and tissue characterization, which are especially important for loculated and complex effusions. Tuberculosis testing should also be considered in the right epidemiologic and clinical settings. Viral cultures have little clinical significance and should not be routinely obtained, but they may be useful in some patients (eg, cytomegalovirus infection

in transplant patients).[3] Transesophageal echocardiography can diagnose loculated effusion when transthoracic echocardiography is limited (eg, postoperative patients) and regional tamponade is considered. Our structured approach has yielded diagnosis by noninvasive targeted testing in 68% of patients, based on a retrospective review.[6]

Simple clinical assessment has also been shown to assist in establishing the diagnosis: large effusion without "inflammatory" signs or clinical signs of tamponade (jugular venous distension, hypotension, and/or pulsus paradoxus) commonly signifies chronic idiopathic pericardial effusion (likelihood ratio = 20, *P* < .001), whereas large effusions with clinical signs of tamponade and without "inflammatory" signs should raise the suspicion for malignancy (likelihood ratio = 2.9, *P* < .001).[10]

Pericardial effusion sampling for diagnostic purposes and occasionally for pericardial biopsy should be considered in the following settings:

1. Concern for purulent and tuberculous pericarditis
2. Clinical suspicion of neoplastic pericardial effusion
3. Moderate-to-large pericardial effusion in patients with advanced HIV and/or immune suppression
4. Moderate-to-large or progressive pericardial effusion in patients who are not responding to initial therapy or when the tiered workup is inconclusive

Pericardial fluid analysis can include Gram and acid-fast bacilli stains and cultures, polymerase chain reaction, tuberculosis-specific testing (eg, adenosine deaminase, lysozyme, and gamma-interferon), tumor markers, and cytology.[3] Contrary to common practice and unlike pleural effusion workup, cell count, lactate dehydrogenase, and protein and glucose levels have not been shown to be particularly useful in differential diagnosis and

Comprehensive history and physical examination, medical chart review, ECG, Transthoracic echocardiography

Complete blood count, complete metabolic panel, coagulation studies, inflammatory markers , cardiac biomarkers, thyroid stimulating hormone level, and chest X-ray

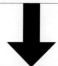

Human immunodeficiency virus (HIV) testing, autoantibodies, blood cultures, viral testing, tuberculosis testing, advanced chest imaging, transesophageal echocardiography

**Pericardial fluid sampling
Pericardial biopsy
?Pericardioscopy**

FIGURE 33.2 Parsimonious stepwise approach to laboratory testing and imaging in patients with pericardial effusion. This systematic approach allows establishing diagnosis noninvasively in the majority of patients with moderate-to-large pericardial effusion. Question mark indicates optional and controversial.

management of patients with pericardial effusion.[11] Pericardioscopy allows a targeted pericardial biopsy and it can potentially increase the diagnostic accuracy of sampling (eg, neoplastic pericardial effusion).

ASSESSING HEMODYNAMIC SIGNIFICANCE OF PERICARDIAL EFFUSION

When evaluating the hemodynamic impact of pericardial effusion one should take into account the acuity of presentation. Acute accumulation of fluid (within minutes to hours) rapidly exceeds the pericardial stretch limit and commonly presents as cardiogenic shock.[12] This dramatic presentation is called acute or surgical tamponade and it requires immediate intervention. Chamber perforation during a percutaneous procedure is a good example of acute tamponade. Blunt chest trauma and ascending aortic dissection resulting in blood accumulation within the pericardium require prompt surgical intervention, and percutaneous pericardial effusion drainage is relatively contraindicated. When pericardial fluid accumulates slowly (within days to weeks), a large amount of fluid can be present without dramatic lowering

of the cardiac output.[12] This can lead to subacute or medical tamponade, which requires careful assessment of both clinical and imaging data to establish the need for pericardial effusion drainage.[13] The following discussion elaborates the assessment for subacute (medical) tamponade.

HISTORY AND PHYSICAL EXAMINATION

Although many refer to pericardial tamponade as a "clinical diagnosis," the existing evidence suggests that subacute tamponade is a difficult diagnosis to make on mere clinical grounds.[13] Dyspnea is the cardinal symptom of subacute pericardial tamponade, but it is nonspecific. Other symptoms such as fever, cough, and chest pain can occur and typically reflect the underlying cause (ie, pericarditis) rather than pericardial fluid accumulation. Clinical findings of pericardial tamponade include tachycardia, jugular venous distension, pulsus paradoxus, and diminished heart sounds; and all lack both sensitivity and specificity.[14] Tachycardia is common in hospitalized patients for many reasons and it could be blunted by medications such as β-blockers. In a systematic review, the jugular venous distension had a pooled sensitivity of 76% for pericardial tamponade.[14] Assessment of jugular venous distension is limited by the experience of the observer; it can be difficult in some patients, even for experienced clinicians. Besides, jugular venous distension is associated with other conditions causing shortness of breath such as pulmonary hypertension and congestive heart failure. Although patients with acute (surgical) tamponade rapidly progress to cardiogenic shock, hypotension is rather uncommon in patients with subacute tamponade who accumulate pericardial effusion within days to weeks. On the contrary, many patients are hypertensive because of the high levels of circulating catecholamines in response to hemodynamic stress. In studies of pericardial tamponade, the mean systolic blood pressure ranged from 127 to 144 mm Hg.[15] According to a recent review, hypertensive tamponade is seen in 27% to 43% of patients.[15] Systolic blood pressure commonly decreases in these patients after pericardial effusion drainage, and treating the hypertensive response without draining the effusion can be dangerous.

PULSUS PARADOXUS

Pulsus paradoxus is considered the cornerstone of the clinical diagnosis of pericardial tamponade.[12] Under normal conditions, the decrease in blood pressure is <10 mm Hg, and it is explained by phasic variation in the filling of the right- and left-sided cardiac chambers related to intrathoracic pressure changes with respiration. With tamponade, the accumulating pericardial effusion restricts cardiac filling and makes the respiratory variation in the right and left ventricular filling more pronounced and interdependent.[12] Pulsus paradoxus is measured by manual sphygmomanometer as the difference between intermittent and persistent Korotkoff sounds during normal respiration, not with deep breathing (**Figure 33.3**).[14] A wide variation in the incidence of pulsus paradoxus has been reported in patients with pericardial tamponade, ranging from 12% to 75%.[16] In patients with "low-pressure" tamponade, the incidence of pulsus paradoxus was reported as only 7%.[17] Besides limited sensitivity for pericardial tamponade, pulsus paradoxus is not very specific. A myriad of conditions have been reported to be associated with

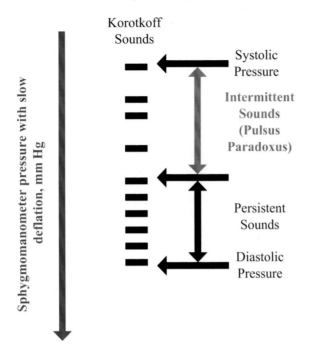

FIGURE 33.3 Assessing for pulsus paradoxus. Pulsus paradoxus is measured by manual sphygmomanometer as the difference between intermittent and persistent Korotkoff sounds during normal respiration.

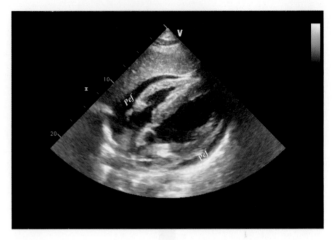

FIGURE 33.4 Pericardial effusion as seen with the ultrasound examination. Pericardial effusion (*Pef*) is easily recognized during ultrasound examination as an echo-free space around the heart.

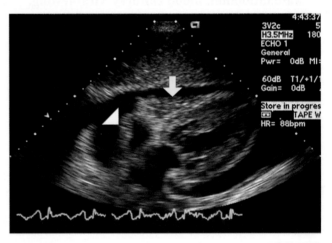

FIGURE 33.5 Chamber collapse with pericardial tamponade as seen with the ultrasound examination. There is evidence of right atrial collapse (arrowhead) as well as right ventricular compression by pericardial fluid (arrow).

pulsus paradoxus; a short list includes asthma, right ventricular infarction, severe hypovolemia, constrictive pericarditis, restrictive cardiomyopathy, pneumothorax, chronic obstructive lung disease, and pulmonary embolism.[13] Some of these conditions can also cause jugular venous distension and tachycardia, common associated findings of pericardial tamponade.

INVASIVE AND IMAGING DATA

Before the widespread use of echocardiography, invasive data using cardiac catheterization were commonly obtained to confirm the diagnosis of tamponade. Cardiac catheterization in tamponade demonstrates equilibration of diastolic intracardiac pressures and respiratory variation in right- and left-sided cardiac pressures corresponding to pulsus paradoxus.

Echocardiography is currently the cornerstone of hemodynamic evaluation of pericardial effusion.[4] Pericardial effusion is easily recognized during ultrasound examination as an echo-free space around the heart (**Figure 33.4**). Normally, intrapericardial pressure is lower than the central venous pressure. As pericardial fluid accumulates, the intrapericardial pressure equilibrates first with the right-sided filling pressures and then left-sided filling pressures.[14] During tamponade, intrapericardial pressure temporarily exceeds intracavitary pressure in various chambers during the cardiac cycle and results in chamber collapse (**Figure 33.5**).[4] Certain pitfalls should be kept in mind when interpreting echocardiographic findings. Transient buckling of the right atrium is commonly seen in patients with pericardial effusion and it is not specific. A more sustained collapse of the right atrium lasting at least one-third of the cardiac cycle appears to be more specific for pericardial tamponade.[18] Right ventricular early diastolic collapse is a less sensitive finding but has a high specificity. Left-sided chamber collapse is much less sensitive but highly specific

for tamponade. Importantly, a study by Merce et al showed that 34% of patients with pericardial effusion but without clinical features of pericardial tamponade had at least one chamber collapse on echocardiography.[19] Therefore, in patients with pericardial effusion who have chamber collapse, one should carefully document respiratory flow variation across valves as a sign of ventricular interdependence (**Figure 33.6**) and interrogate the inferior vena cava size and collapsibility as a sign of elevated right-sided filling pressures.[20] The presence of respiratory variation in the inflow velocities is defined by consensus as >30% across the mitral valve and >60% for the tricuspid valve.[4] These echocardiographic signs, when present, increase the specificity of diagnosis. Finally, the size of the pericardial effusion seems to be an important but frequently underappreciated part of the echocardiographic assessment. In one study of hospitalized patients with pericardial effusion, the size of the effusion was the only independent predictor of adverse in-hospital outcomes in a multivariate model, but not chamber collapse or inferior vena cava plethora.[21]

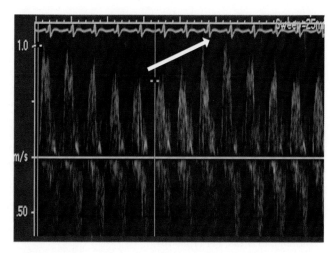

FIGURE 33.6 Doppler echocardiography in pericardial tamponade. Respiratory variation in the mitral inflow velocities (arrow) is seen.

The diagnosis of pericardial tamponade may be particularly difficult in patients with pulmonary hypertension and right ventricular failure because they commonly accumulate pericardial effusion. Pericardial effusion in these patients is a marker of adverse outcomes. Common clinical findings of pericardial tamponade such as tachycardia and jugular venous distension may not be helpful in differential diagnosis for shortness of breath and progressive right-sided heart failure. Collapse of the left-sided cardiac chambers has been described as an important echocardiographic clue to the presence of pericardial tamponade in these settings.[22] Conversely, more common findings of tamponade such as right atrial and ventricular collapse can be masked by elevated right-sided filling pressures. Poor outcomes have been reported with routine draining of pericardial effusion in these patients.

INTEGRATIVE APPROACH TO PERICARDIAL DRAINAGE

The diagnosis of subacute pericardial tamponade can be challenging because most patients are not hypotensive and can actually be hypertensive. An integrative approach that includes careful consideration of both clinical and imaging data helps clinicians assess the hemodynamic impact of pericardial effusion and the need for drainage.[13] The decision making should include the following factors:

1. Presence and timeline for symptoms (commonly dyspnea)
2. Supportive physical findings (jugular venous distension, tachycardia, and pulsus paradoxus)
3. Etiology of pericardial effusion and response to initial treatment
4. Size of pericardial effusion
5. Evidence of chamber collapse on echocardiography
6. Supporting signs for pericardial tamponade on echocardiography (respiratory variation in velocities and flows, engorgement of the inferior vena cava)

Percutaneous pericardiocentesis guided by echocardiography is the intervention of choice in many cases when pericardial drainage is desired. Emergency pericardiocentesis in acute (surgical) tamponade can be lifesaving. A study summarizing the 21-year experience from Mayo Clinic showed that echo-guided approach is rapid, safe, and effective with a major complication rate of 1.2%.[23] Extended catheter drainage has been used in certain scenarios, including neoplastic pericardial effusion when intrapericardial treatment is also occasionally employed. Stepwise drainage of pericardial effusion is reasonable in very large effusions and patients with pulmonary hypertension to avoid acute right ventricular dilation ("decompression syndrome").[3] Surgical drainage is generally preferred in traumatic pericardial effusion, aortic dissection, small effusions, recurrent effusions, and purulent pericarditis. In loculated (typically postsurgical) effusions, surgical approach or video-assisted thoracoscopic pericardiectomy can be used. Pericardial biopsy, when necessary, can be done using surgical procedure or pericardioscopy. Postdrainage echocardiography is important in assessing the efficacy of the procedure, possible complications and fluid reaccumulation, and diagnosing constriction physiology.[3]

SUPPORTIVE CARE

Promptly instituted treatment for presumed etiology of pericardial effusion (ie, anti-inflammatory therapy in acute pericarditis) can result in improvement and defer the need for pericardial drainage. The response should be monitored by serial echocardiographic examinations. Endotracheal intubation with positive pressure ventilation requires great caution because it can markedly reduce cardiac preload and result in rapid hemodynamic deterioration.[24] Fluid resuscitation should also be used cautiously. In a hemodynamic study by Sagrista-Sauleda et al, 49 patients with pericardial tamponade were given 500 mL of intravenous normal saline before pericardiocentesis.[25] Increase in cardiac index > 10% from baseline was observed in 47% of patients. The improvement in cardiac index was modest, and only patients with systolic blood pressure < 100 mm Hg got the benefit. Actually, 31% of patients experienced a decrease in the cardiac output as the result of volume expansion. Intravenous saline infusion also consistently caused a significant increase in intrapericardial pressure, right atrial pressure, and left ventricular end-diastolic pressure.[25]

CONCLUSIONS

Pericardial disease is relatively common in acute settings and it requires prompt diagnosis. A structured approach to differential diagnosis of pericardial effusion and hemodynamic assessment is necessary in managing patients with pericardial effusion and suspected pericardial tamponade.

REFERENCES

1. Arntfield RT, Millington SJ. Point of care cardiac ultrasound applications in the emergency department and intensive care unit—a review. *Curr Cardiol Rev.* 2012;8(2):98-108.
2. Argulian E, Halpern DG, Aziz EF, Uretsky S, Chaudhry F, Herzog E. Novel "CHASER" pathway for the management of pericardial disease. *Crit Pathw Cardiol.* 2011;10(2):57-63.
3. Adler Y, Charron P. The 2015 ESC Guidelines on the diagnosis and management of pericardial diseases. *Eur Heart J.* 2015;36(42):2873-2874.
4. Klein AL, Abbara S, Agler DA, et al. American Society of Echocardiography clinical recommendations for multimodality

cardiovascular imaging of patients with pericardial disease: endorsed by the Society for Cardiovascular Magnetic Resonance and Society of Cardiovascular Computed Tomography. *J Am Soc Echocardiogr.* 2013;26(9):965-1012.e15.

5. Halpern DG, Argulian E, Briasoulis A, Chaudhry F, Aziz EF, Herzog E. A novel pericardial effusion scoring index to guide decision for drainage. *Crit Pathw Cardiol.* 2012;11(2):85-88.

6. Agarwal V, El Hayek G, Chavez P, Po JR, Herzog E, Argulian E. A structured, parsimonious approach to establish the cause of moderate-to-large pericardial effusion. *Am J Cardiol.* 2014;114(3):479-482.

7. Corey GR, Campbell PT, Van Trigt P, et al. Etiology of large pericardial effusions. *Am J Med.* 1993;95(2):209-213.

8. Levy PY, Corey R, Berger P, et al. Etiologic diagnosis of 204 pericardial effusions. *Medicine (Baltimore).* 2003;82(6):385-391.

9. Zayas R, Anguita M, Torres F, et al. Incidence of specific etiology and role of methods for specific etiologic diagnosis of primary acute pericarditis. *Am J Cardiol.* 1995;75(5):378-382.

10. Sagrista-Sauleda J, Merce J, Permanyer-Miralda G, Soler-Soler J. Clinical clues to the causes of large pericardial effusions. *Am J Med.* 2000;109(2):95-101.

11. Ben-Horin S, Bank I, Shinfeld A, Kachel E, Guetta V, Livneh A. Diagnostic value of the biochemical composition of pericardial effusions in patients undergoing pericardiocentesis. *Am J Cardiol.* 2007;99(9):1294-1297.

12. Spodick DH. Acute cardiac tamponade. *N Engl J Med.* 2003;349(7):684-690.

13. Argulian E, Messerli F. Misconceptions and facts about pericardial effusion and tamponade. *Am J Med.* 2013;126(10):858-861.

14. Roy CL, Minor MA, Brookhart MA, Choudhry NK. Does this patient with a pericardial effusion have cardiac tamponade? *JAMA.* 2007;297(16):1810-1818.

15. Argulian E, Herzog E, Halpern DG, Messerli FH. Paradoxical hypertension with cardiac tamponade. *Am J Cardiol.* 2012;110(7):1066-1069.

16. Spodick DH. Acute pericarditis: current concepts and practice. *JAMA.* 2003;289(9):1150-1153.

17. Sagrista-Sauleda J, Angel J, Sambola A, Alguersuari J, Permanyer-Miralda G, Soler-Soler J. Low-pressure cardiac tamponade: clinical and hemodynamic profile. *Circulation.* 2006;114(9):945-952.

18. Gillam LD, Guyer DE, Gibson TC, King ME, Marshall JE, Weyman AE. Hydrodynamic compression of the right atrium: a new echocardiographic sign of cardiac tamponade. *Circulation.* 1983;68(2):294-301.

19. Merce J, Sagrista-Sauleda J, Permanyer-Miralda G, Soler-Soler J. Should pericardial drainage be performed routinely in patients who have a large pericardial effusion without tamponade? *Am J Med.* 1998;105(2):106-109.

20. Merce J, Sagrista-Sauleda J, Permanyer-Miralda G, Evangelista A, Soler-Soler J. Correlation between clinical and Doppler echocardiographic findings in patients with moderate and large pericardial effusion: implications for the diagnosis of cardiac tamponade. *Am Heart J.* 1999;138(4 Pt 1):759-764.

21. Eisenberg MJ, Oken K, Guerrero S, Saniei MA, Schiller NB. Prognostic value of echocardiography in hospitalized patients with pericardial effusion. *Am J Cardiol.* 1992;70(9):934-939.

22. Frey MJ, Berko B, Palevsky H, Hirshfeld JW Jr, Herrmann HC. Recognition of cardiac tamponade in the presence of severe pulmonary hypertension. *Ann Intern Med.* 1989;111(7):615-617.

23. Tsang TS, Enriquez-Sarano M, Freeman WK, et al. Consecutive 1127 therapeutic echocardiographically guided pericardiocenteses: clinical profile, practice patterns, and outcomes spanning 21 years. *Mayo Clin Proc.* 2002;77(5):429-436.

24. Little WC, Freeman GL. Pericardial disease. *Circulation.* 2006;113(12):1622-1632.

25. Sagrista-Sauleda J, Angel J, Sambola A, Permanyer-Miralda G. Hemodynamic effects of volume expansion in patients with cardiac tamponade. *Circulation.* 2008;117(12):1545-1549.

Patient and Family Information for: PERICARDIAL EFFUSION AND TAMPONADE

Pericardial effusion refers to fluid accumulation in the double-membrane pericardial sack which surrounds the heart. Normally, there is a little amount of fluid that allows the heart to expand and receive blood. Abnormal fluid or blood accumulation in the pericardial sack can occasionally compress the heart and impair normal filling of heart chambers and therefore normal heart functioning. This is referred to as "tamponade," a potentially life-threatening condition. Pericardial effusion can develop suddenly, for example, during a cardiac procedure when even a small amount of accumulated blood around the heart can cause compression; immediate intervention is necessary in that case to relieve the compression. Sometimes pericardial fluid accumulates slowly, over days and weeks as a result of infection, cancer spread, renal failure, or some other causes. In those cases, the symptoms are less dramatic but commonly include shortness of breath. Other symptoms may include tiredness, chest pain, and fever. Certain findings on physical examination and changes on electrocardiogram and chest X-ray can be suggestive of pericardial effusion. Ultrasound of the heart (also called echocardiogram) is the most commonly used diagnostic test to establish the presence of pericardial effusion and to assess the degree of heart compression. To establish the cause of pericardial effusion, the physician will typically order certain diagnostic tests which may include blood tests and occasionally advanced imaging tests (such as CT scan). Draining the pericardial fluid can be considered in some patients for two reasons: (1) establishing the diagnosis if the other tests are inconclusive and (2) relieving compression of the heart. It is performed either by a needle or surgery. During the former, a needle is introduced into the pericardial sack commonly under the guidance of ultrasound or X-ray. The physician may decide to leave a tube (called a "drain") in the pericardial sack for several days to avoid re-accumulation. The tube can be pulled out easily once the amount of drainage from the pericardial sack decreases significantly.

Eyal Herzog
Dan G. Halpern
Emad F. Aziz
Edgar Argulian

34

Pathway for the Management of Pericardial Disease

Pericardial disease is a broad term that describes a wide range of pathologies. The clinical aspects of pericardial disease encompass acute pericarditis, pericardial tamponade, pericardial effusion, constrictive pericarditis, and effusive–constrictive pericarditis. These disorders differ not only in clinical presentation but also in the timeline of disease development; for example, pericardial tamponade is commonly an acute, life-threatening event, whereas constrictive pericarditis is a chronic process developing over months to years. Therefore, pericardial disease management is challenging for most clinicians. The evidence base in the field is relatively scarce compared with other disease entities in cardiology. The European Society of Cardiology released in 2015 its updated guidelines for the diagnosis and management of pericardial diseases.[1] Currently, there are no guidelines from American cardiology societies to help clinicians in managing pericardial disease. In this chapter we outline a unified, stepwise, pathway-based approach for the management of pericardial disease (**Figure 34.1**).[2]

THE ADVANCED CARDIAC ADMISSION PROGRAM

The "Advanced Cardiac Admission Program (ACAP)" was launched in New York, in 2004. It consists of a series of projects that have been developed to bridge the gap between published guidelines and implementation during "real-world" patient care. The pericardial disease management pathway is the ninth project of the ACAP program.[2]

HOW TO USE THE PATHWAY

ENTERING THE PATHWAY

Despite the broad range of pericardial pathologies, there are a limited number of clinical presentations that would make a clinician suspect pericardial disease (**Figure 34.2**). We assigned each clinical presentation a certain pathway, which starts with patients' complaints and continues along the lines of further workup, diagnosis, and management. Typical clinical presentations in patients with pericardial disease include chest pain, hypotension/arrest, dyspnea, and right-predominant heart failure. Incidental finding of pericardial effusion during imaging study is also

a common clinical scenario. **Figure 34.2** outlines the entry points into the pericardial disease management pathway. The timeline of symptom development is a continuum ranging from acute, immediate presentation to subacute and chronic symptoms. The recent European guideline[1] classified inflammatory pericardial syndromes as follows:

A. Acute pericarditis: new-onset pericarditis
B. Recurrent pericarditis: recurrence of symptoms after being symptom-free for 4 to 6 weeks
C. Incessant pericarditis: symptoms over 4 to 6 weeks
D. Chronic pericarditis: symptoms over 3 months

A systematic approach to patients with suspected pericardial disease starts with the chief presenting complaint and is followed by a history taking, physical examination, electrocardiogram (ECG), and echocardiography. Further diagnostic testing is tailored to the initial findings.

The following are the five entry points:

1. Chest Pain

Acute pericarditis should be considered in the differential diagnosis of any patient presenting with chest pain along with other etiologies. The chest pain algorithm of the pathway is outlined in **Figure 34.3**. The diagnosis of acute pericarditis relies on the following four cardinal features: characteristic chest pain which is pleuritic and positional, friction rub on physical examination, characteristic evolving ECG changes (**Table 34.1**), and pericardial effusion demonstrated by echocardiography.[3–5] Presence of at least two of these features is usually diagnostic of acute pericarditis. Most cases of acute pericarditis in the Western world are idiopathic or viral, but other causes should also be considered.[6] Initial testing in all patients with acute pericarditis should include tier 1 testing (**Figure 34.3**).[7] Positive cardiac biomarkers indicate myocardial involvement and carry a worse prognosis. Inflammatory markers such as C-reactive protein can be followed sequentially to monitor disease progression and response to treatment. Typical treatment includes nonsteroidal anti-inflammatory agents at full doses for 7 to 10 days.[1] We recommend the following doses: ibuprofen 600 to 800 mg every 6 to 8 hours for 7 to 10 days or aspirin 800 mg every 6 to 8 hours for 7 to 10 days. In post–myocardial infarction pericarditis, aspirin is preferred. In patients without contraindications, colchicines at a dose of 1 to 2 mg first day followed by

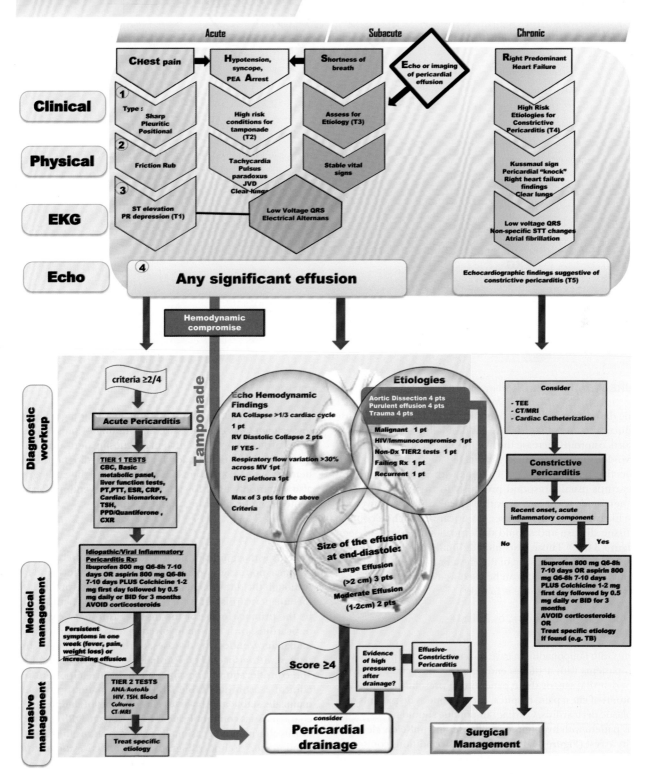

FIGURE 34.1 Novel "CHASER" pathway for the management of pericardial disease. The figure outlines a unified, stepwise pathway-based approach to pericardial disease management. ANA, antinuclear antibody; CBC, complete blood count; CRP, C-reactive protein; CT, computed tomography; CXR, chest X-ray; ESR, erythrocyte sedimentation rate; HIV, human immunodeficiency virus; IVC, inferior vena cava; JVD, jugular vein distension; MRI, magnetic resonance imaging; MV, mitral valve; PEA, pulseless electrical activity; PPD, purified protein derivative; PT, prothrombin time; PTT, partial thromboplastin time; RA, right atrium; RV, right ventricle; TB, tuberculosis; TEE, transesophageal echocardiography; TSH, thyroid-stimulating hormone. T1: Table 34.1, T2: Table 34.2, T3: Table 34.3, T4: Table 34.4, T5: Table 34.5

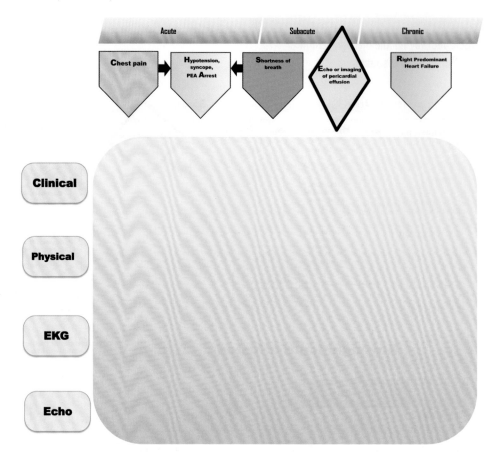

FIGURE 34.2 Entry points into the pericardial disease pathway. The entry points based on the initial clinical presentation form the "CHASER" acronym.

0.5 mg daily or twice daily for 3 months should be given because it reduces the rate of recurrence substantially.[5,8]

Corticosteroids increase the likelihood of relapse and should be avoided unless specifically indicated (eg, in patients with connective tissue disease).[5,9] Patients with idiopathic or viral pericarditis usually respond promptly to treatment. Patients with persistent symptoms or with atypical clinical features are more likely to have other causes of pericarditis such as connective tissue disease and should undergo tier 2 testing, as seen in **Figure 34.3**.[10] Those tests include imaging studies such as computed tomography scan of the chest or magnetic resonance imaging.[1] Corticosteroids can be used as a last resort for those patients if no specific cause is found.[1]

2. Hypotension, Syncope, or Pulseless Electrical Activity Arrest

Patients with tamponade can have an acute, dramatic presentation as do patients with acute ascending aortic dissection involving the pericardial sac, or these patients can present with subacute symptoms of chest pain, dyspnea, and syncope as do patients with neoplastic pericarditis. Cardiac tamponade should be suspected in any patient with hypotension, collapse, and pulseless electrical activity arrest (**Figure 34.4**), and high-risk conditions commonly associated with tamponade should be specifically thought of (**Table 34.2**).[11] These include blunt chest trauma, recent procedure/intervention (eg, electrophysiology procedures and coronary interventions), chest surgery, and aortic dissection. Neoplastic pericardial effusion, tuberculous pericarditis, and, uncommonly, idiopathic pericarditis can progress to tamponade. Physical examination findings should focus on pulsus paradoxus, jugular

vein pressure, and lung auscultation. ECG findings may include low-voltage QRS complex size and finding of pulsus alternans. Echocardiography is essential in diagnosing pericardial effusion and confirming tamponade by the echocardiographic signs of hemodynamic compromise (**Figure 34.5**). Echocardiography is also commonly used for guiding the intervention. Pericardiocentesis can be lifesaving in these patients.

3. Dyspnea

Patients with significant pericardial effusion often present with dyspnea, poor exercise tolerance, chest discomfort, and fatigue. Although the differential diagnosis of dyspnea is broad, it should include pericardial effusion (**Figure 34.6**). The pericardium can be the primary focus for the disease, as in most cases of acute pericarditis, or it can be involved in a systemic process such as malignancy, endocrine diseases, or rheumatic diseases. In every patient with suspected pericardial disease, a systematic approach and consideration of possible etiologies are important parts of clinical reasoning (**Table 34.3**). These patients are hemodynamically stable and have no clinical signs of tamponade. ECG characteristics commonly include low-voltage QRS complex size. Pulsus alternans is occasionally seen with large effusions without tamponade.[11] Echocardiography is an effective and inexpensive tool in diagnosing pericardial effusion.

4. Incidental Finding of Pericardial Effusion

Sometimes, pericardial effusion is found as an incidental finding in patients worked up for other causes. Although it is important to search systematically for possible etiologies of pericardial disease in

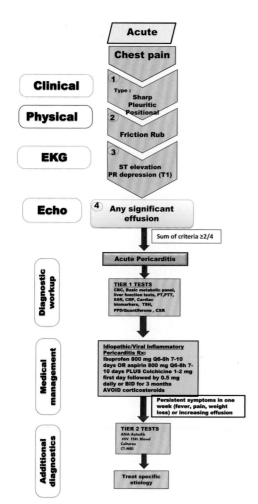

FIGURE 34.3 Evaluation of chest pain in patient with possible acute pericarditis. A stepwise algorithm outlines evaluation and management of chest pain patients suspected to have acute pericarditis. ANA, antinuclear antibody; CBC, complete blood count; CRP, C-reactive protein; CT, computed tomography; CXR, chest X-ray; ESR, erythrocyte sedimentation rate; MRI, magnetic resonance imaging; PPD, purified protein derivative; PT, prothrombin time; PTT, partial thromboplastin time; TSH, thyroid-stimulating hormone. T1: Table 34.1

TABLE 34.1	ECG Features of Acute Pericarditis

Stage 1: diffuse ST-segment elevation and PR-segment depression
Stage 2: normalization of ST-segment changes
Stage 3: diffuse T-wave inversion
Stage 4: normalization of T-wave changes

ECG, electrocardiogram.

each individual patient (**Table 34.3**), a substantial number of these cases remain unexplained.[12,13] In patients with moderate-to-large effusion, tier 1 and tier 2 testing seem reasonable.[12] If a specific cause is found, it should be addressed. In patients with no obvious clue to the cause of the effusion and no evidence of hemodynamic compromise, elevated inflammatory markers suggest acute idiopathic pericarditis and trial of nonsteroidal anti-inflammatory agents is justified. If inflammatory markers are within normal limits and there is no evidence of hemodynamic compromise, idiopathic pericardial effusion is high on the list of differential diagnoses.[12] Some patients with pericardial effusion have elevated right-sided pressures after pericardial drainage and they might have effusive–constrictive pericarditis.[14]

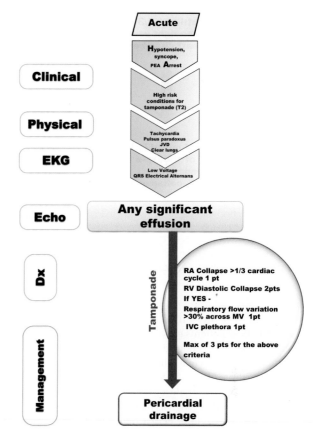

FIGURE 34.4 Approach to a patient with hypotension, syncope, or PEA arrest with possible pericardial tamponade. Initial clinical evaluation of patients suspected to have cardiac tamponade is outlined in the figure. JVD, jugular vein distension; MV, mitral valve; PEA, pulseless electrical activity; RA, right atrial; RV, right ventricular. T2: Table 34.2

TABLE 34.2	High-Risk Conditions for Tamponade

Advanced renal failure
Aortic dissection
Chest trauma
Connective tissue disease
Malignancy
Purulent infection
Recent acute coronary syndrome
Surgery/intervention
Suspected tuberculosis

5. Right-Sided Heart Failure

Patients with constrictive pericarditis typically present with right-predominant heart failure (**Figure 34.7**). Careful review of medical history for high-risk conditions associated with constrictive pericarditis is necessary (**Table 34.4**).[15] Peripheral edema, hepatomegaly, jugular venous distension, and ascites are prominent findings on physical examination. The lungs are typically clear, although pleural effusion may be present. ECG findings, especially repolarization abnormalities, are nonspecific. Atrial fibrillation is present in over one-fifth of patients.[16]

Collapse of the right atrium > 1/3 of the cardiac cycle
Diastolic collapse of the right ventricle
Collapse of the left heart chambers

Respiratory variation of mitral inflow velocity >30%
Respiratory variation of tricuspid inflow velocity >60%
Ventricular interdependence
IVC plethora and < 50% collapse in inspiration

FIGURE 34.5 Echocardiographic signs of hemodynamic compromise. The findings of heart chamber collapse are presented in order of decreasing sensitivity and increasing specificity. Confirmatory signs include respiratory variation across the atrioventricular valves, ventricular interdependence, and IVC plethora. IVC, inferior vena cava.

Echocardiography is essential in patients suspected to have constriction; these patients typically have normal left ventricular ejection fraction. Other echocardiographic findings include biatrial enlargement and restrictive filling pattern on the mitral inflow Doppler recording (**Table 34.5**).[14] Further studies to confirm the diagnosis and differentiate it from restrictive cardiomyopathy include imaging studies (such as magnetic resonance imaging) and cardiac catheterization. Pericardial thickness as measured by transesophageal echocardiography may be helpful in making the diagnosis.[17] Early stages of pericardial constriction due to idiopathic pericarditis may have an inflammatory component and may respond to anti-inflammatory therapy.[18] Surgical therapy is otherwise the standard of care.

PERICARDIAL EFFUSION SCORE

Acute cardiac tamponade necessitates immediate pericardiocentesis. The decision to drain the pericardium in patients with slowly accumulating and subacute tamponade is often challenging. We proposed a score approach to decision making in clinically stable patients with pericardial effusion, as outlined in **Figure 34.8**. The score is composed of the following three major parameters: the etiology of the effusion, the size of the effusion, and the echocardiographic assessment of hemodynamic parameters. Etiologic factors favoring drainage of the effusion include traumatic effusion, aortic dissection, and purulent effusion. These effusions typically require surgical drainage as opposed to pericardiocentesis.[1] In malignant effusions, drainage should be considered to relieve symptoms and confirm neoplastic involvement of the pericardium.[19] Pericardial effusion in patients with advanced human immunodeficiency virus and immunosuppression, as well as unexplained and progressive effusion should also be considered for drainage because some of the neoplastic and infectious causes in these patients are treatable.[20,21] The size of the pericardial effusion as assessed by echocardiography at the end of a diastole is a very important variable.[22] It should be viewed in the context of disease progression (the rate of fluid accumulation).

Chronic large effusions present for more than 3 months are less likely to cause hemodynamic compromise as opposed to recent effusion (<1 month).[14] Echocardiographic signs of hemodynamic compromise provide important evidence in favor of drainage because they may indicate early or impending tamponade. Of note, right atrial collapse is the earliest sign of hemodynamic compromise but has a low specificity if only buckling is present. Right atrial collapse lasting more than one-third of the cardiac cycle seems to be both specific and sensitive.[23] Right ventricular diastolic collapse is a specific sign of hemodynamic compromise but is less sensitive than right atrial collapse.[24] In patients with

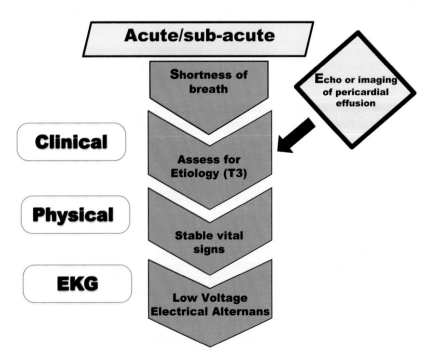

FIGURE 34.6 Approach to a patient with dyspnea and possible pericardial effusion. Initial clinical evaluation of patients suspected to have pericardial effusion is outlined in the figure. Some patients are diagnosed with incidental pericardial effusion during imaging study done for other indications. T3: Table 34.3

TABLE 34.3	Causes of Pericardial Disease

Endocrine
Hemopericardium (trauma, procedure, aortic dissection)
Idiopathic
Infectious (including viral, tuberculosis, and purulent)
Medications
Neoplastic
Perimyocardial infarction
Postcardiotomy syndrome
Radiation
Renal failure
Rheumatic/autoimmune diseases

TABLE 34.4	High-Risk Conditions for Constrictive Pericarditis

Cardiac surgery
Connective tissue disease
HIV infection
Previous pericarditis
Radiation therapy to the chest
Tuberculosis

HIV, human immunodeficiency virus.

TABLE 34.5	Echocardiographic Findings of Constrictive Pericarditis

Normal left ventricular ejection fraction
Normal left ventricular wall thickness
Thickened pericardium (>2 mm) and/or pericardial calcifications
Restrictive filling pattern (E>>A wave, high E-wave velocity, short E-wave deceleration time)
Respiratory flow variations across atrioventricular valves
Displacement of interventricular septum
Rapid flow propagation (>100 cm/s)
Normal tissue Doppler findings (E′ > 8 cm/s)
Expiratory hepatic veins flow reversal

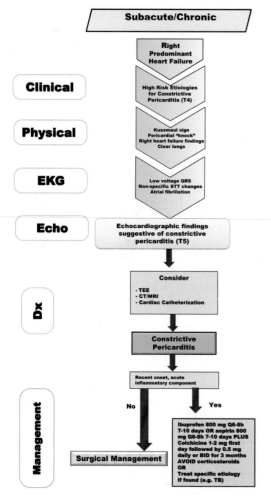

FIGURE 34.7 Evaluation of right-predominant heart failure in a patient with possible constrictive pericarditis. A stepwise algorithm outlines evaluation and management of patients with right-predominant heart failure suspected to have constrictive pericarditis. CT, computed tomography; MRI, magnetic resonance imaging; TB, tuberculosis; TEE, transesophageal echocardiography. T4: Table 34.4, T5: Table 34.5

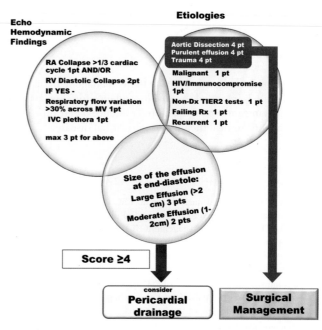

FIGURE 34.8 Pericardial effusion score. The pericardial effusion score, which has three components (etiology of the effusion, effusion size, and echocardiographic evidence of hemodynamic compromise), helps guide clinical decision making in clinically stable patients with pericardial effusion. HIV, human immunodeficiency virus; IVC, inferior vena cava; MV, mitral valve; RA, right atrial; RV, right ventricular.

significant pulmonary hypertension and right ventricular hypertrophy, the sensitivity of this finding is even lower. Left-sided chamber collapse is a late finding in tamponade, and therefore lacks sensitivity.[25] Confirmatory findings should be specifically looked for once a chamber collapse is present. These include respiratory variation in flow velocity across the atrioventricular valves (the mitral and the tricuspid valves), implying ventricular

interdependence and engorgement of the inferior vena cava with reduced respiratory collapse. Any chamber collapse combined with a confirmatory finding has a very high sensitivity and specificity for tamponade.[26] In general, a score of 4 or more provides strong evidence in favor of draining the effusion. It should not be viewed as an absolute indication for drainage but rather as a qualitative measure to support decision making. Importantly, the score may change over time as the variables change. Patients with a borderline score may need frequent reassessment in terms of effusion size progression and echocardiographic evidence of hemodynamic compromise.

We conducted a case–control study in consecutive hospitalized patients with moderate-to-large pericardial effusion who had no evidence of hemodynamic compromise upon admission. Patients with pericardial effusion drained for diagnostic and/or therapeutic purpose served as cases, and patients who were not drained served as controls. Our conclusion was that the pericardial effusion scoring index obtained at the initial presentation in patients without immediate hemodynamic compromise showed a high accuracy in identifying patients who required pericardial effusion drainage downstream.[27]

PERICARDIAL DRAINAGE

In patients who need pericardial drainage, echocardiographically guided pericardiocentesis appears to be safe.[28] Depending on the pericardial fluid accumulation pattern, parasternal, subxiphoid, and apical approaches are all acceptable. As mentioned, the surgical drainage of pericardial effusion is more appropriate in certain patient groups such as in patients with aortic dissection, traumatic hemopericardium, purulent pericarditis, and loculated effusions.[1]

CONCLUSIONS

A stepwise, pathway-based approach to the management of pericardial disease is intended to provide guidance for clinicians in decision making and a patient-tailored evidence-based approach to medical and surgical therapy for pericardial disease.

REFERENCES

1. Adler Y, Charron P, Imazio M, et al. ESC Guidelines for the diagnosis and management of pericardial diseases: the Task Force for the Diagnosis and Management of Pericardial Diseases of the European Society of Cardiology (ESC). Endorsed by: the European Association for Cardio-Thoracic Surgery (EACTS). *Eur Heart J.* 2015;36(42):2921-2964.
2. Argulian E, Halpern DG, Aziz EF, Uretsky S, Chaudhry F, Herzog E. Novel "CHASER" pathway for the management of pericardial disease. *Crit Pathw Cardiol.* 2011;10:57-63.
3. Troughton RW, Asher CR, Klein AL. Pericarditis. *Lancet.* 2004;363:717-727.
4. Spodick DH. Acute pericarditis: current concepts and practice. *JAMA.* 2003;289:1150-1153.
5. Imazio M, Bobbio M, Cecchi E, et al. Colchicine in addition to conventional therapy for acute pericarditis: results of the COlchicine for acute PEricarditis (COPE) trial. *Circulation.* 2005;112:2012-2016.
6. Zayas R, Anguita M, Torres F, et al. Incidence of specific etiology and role of methods for specific etiologic diagnosis of primary acute pericarditis. *Am J Cardiol.* 1995;75:378-382.
7. Permanyer-Miralda G. Acute pericardial disease: approach to the aetiologic diagnosis. *Heart.* 2004;90:252-254.

8. Imazio M, Bobbio M, Cecchi E, et al. Colchicine as first-choice therapy for recurrent pericarditis: results of the CORE (COlchicine for REcurrent pericarditis) trial. *Arch Intern Med.* 2005;165:1987-1991.
9. Lange RA, Hillis LD. Clinical practice. Acute pericarditis. *N Engl J Med.* 2004;351:2195-2202.
10. Imazio M, Demichelis B, Parrini I, et al. Day-hospital treatment of acute pericarditis: a management program for outpatient therapy. *J Am Coll Cardiol.* 2004;43:1042-1046.
11. Spodick DH. Acute cardiac tamponade. *N Engl J Med.* 2003;349:684-690.
12. Sagrista-Sauleda J, Merce J, Permanyer-Miralda G, Soler-Soler J. Clinical clues to the causes of large pericardial effusions. *Am J Med.* 2000;109:95-101.
13. Levy PY, Corey R, Berger P, et al. Etiologic diagnosis of 204 pericardial effusions. *Medicine (Baltimore).* 2003;82:385-391.
14. Little WC, Freeman GL. Pericardial disease. *Circulation.* 2006;113:1622-1632.
15. Ling LH, Oh JK, Schaff HV, et al. Constrictive pericarditis in the modern era: evolving clinical spectrum and impact on outcome after pericardiectomy. *Circulation.* 1999;100:1380-1386.
16. Talreja DR, Edwards WD, Danielson GK, et al. Constrictive pericarditis in 26 patients with histologically normal pericardial thickness. *Circulation.* 2003;108:1852-1857.
17. Ling LH, Oh JK, Tei C, et al. Pericardial thickness measured with transesophageal echocardiography: feasibility and potential clinical usefulness. *J Am Coll Cardiol.* 1997;29:1317-1323.
18. Haley JH, Tajik AJ, Danielson GK, Schaff HV, Mulvagh SL, Oh JK. Transient constrictive pericarditis: causes and natural history. *J Am Coll Cardiol.* 2004;43:271-275.
19. Maisch B, Ristic A, Pankuweit S. Evaluation and management of pericardial effusion in patients with neoplastic disease. *Prog Cardiovasc Dis.* 2010;53:157-163.
20. Chen Y, Brennessel D, Walters J, Johnson M, Rosner F, Raza M. Human immunodeficiency virus associated pericardial effusion: report of 40 cases and review of the literature. *Am Heart J.* 1999;137:516-521.
21. Gowda RM, Khan IA, Mehta NJ, Gowda MR, Sacchi TJ, Vasavada BC. Cardiac tamponade in patients with human immunodeficiency virus disease. *Angiology.* 2003;54:469-474.
22. Eisenberg MJ, Oken K, Guerrero S, Saniei MA, Schiller NB. Prognostic value of echocardiography in hospitalized patients with pericardial effusion. *Am J Cardiol.* 1992;70:934-939.
23. Gillam LD, Guyer DE, Gibson TC, King ME, Marshall JE, Weyman AE. Hydrodynamic compression of the right atrium: a new echocardiographic sign of cardiac tamponade. *Circulation.* 1983;68:294-301.
24. Leimgruber PP, Klopfenstein HS, Wann LS, Brooks HL. The hemodynamic derangement associated with right ventricular diastolic collapse in cardiac tamponade: an experimental echocardiographic study. *Circulation.* 1983;68:612-620.
25. Fusman B, Schwinger ME, Charney R, Ausubel K, Cohen MV. Isolated collapse of left-sided heart chambers in cardiac tamponade: demonstration by two-dimensional echocardiography. *Am Heart J.* 1991;121:613-616.
26. Merce J, Sagrista-Sauleda J, Permanyer-Miralda G, Evangelista A, Soler-Soler J. Correlation between clinical and Doppler echocardiographic findings in patients with moderate and large pericardial effusion: implications for the diagnosis of cardiac tamponade. *Am Heart J.* 1999;138:759-764.
27. Halpern DG, Argulian E, Briasoulis A, Chaudhry F, Aziz EF, Herzog E. A novel pericardial effusion scoring index to guide decision for drainage. *Crit Pathw Cardiol.* 2012;11(2):85-88.
28. Tsang TS, Freeman WK, Sinak LJ, Seward JB. Echocardiographically guided pericardiocentesis: evolution and state-of-the-art technique. *Mayo Clin Proc.* 1998;73:647-652.

Gustavo S. Guandalini
Alan F. Vainrib
Muhamed Saric

35

Aortic Valvular Disease in the Cardiac Care Unit

INTRODUCTION

The aortic valve normally consists of three semilunar leaflets. It is designed to allow unrestricted blood flow from the left ventricle into the ascending aorta during systole and to prevent backflow during diastole. A pathologic state is established whenever each of these two functions is compromised: either aortic stenosis (AS) or aortic regurgitation (AR).

In AS, blood cannot flow freely out of the left ventricle during systole; in AR, the blood flows back into the left ventricle during diastole. AS or AR can be primary causes of severe illness, or they can exacerbate concomitant diseases in critically ill patients presenting to cardiac care units (CCUs).

Because there is no effective medical therapy for these conditions, severe AS and AR ultimately require surgical or transcatheter aortic valve replacement (TAVR) to achieve clinical stability and alter their natural progression. Rapid diagnosis and supportive medical therapy are necessary until definitive treatment can be provided.

With the introduction of TAVR, a true revolution has occurred. Patients with severe AS who were previously deemed too high risk to undergo surgery are now able to be treated safely and effectively. In the early days of TAVR, the procedure was done under general anesthesia and required postprocedural care with CCU observation. However, there has been a general trend to replace general anesthesia with moderate sedation, and CCU care is often shortened or even unnecessary.[1]

AORTIC STENOSIS

ETIOLOGY AND PATHOPHYSIOLOGY

In the adult CCU, the most common etiology of AS is calcific degeneration (**Figure 35.1**) of a previously normal trileaflet aortic valve (TAV) or a congenitally bicuspid aortic valve (BAV). Calcific TAV stenosis is typically encountered among the elderly and calcific BAV stenosis in middle-aged patients. It is estimated that moderate or severe AS is present in 0.4% of all Americans, and in 2.8% of people 75 years of age or older.[2]

Once thought to be the result of passive wear and tear, AS of a TAV is now understood to be a manifestation of generalized atherosclerosis, an active proliferative and inflammatory process.[3,4]

Thus, this form of AS and atherosclerosis share risk factors such as smoking, hyperlipidemia, and hypertension.[5,6] In addition, disorders of calcium phosphate metabolism such as end-stage renal disease and Paget disease, as well as mediastinal radiation treatment, increase the risk for development of AS.[7]

BAV is the most common congenital heart defect, occurring in approximately 1% to 2% of all live births.[8] BAV may evolve into

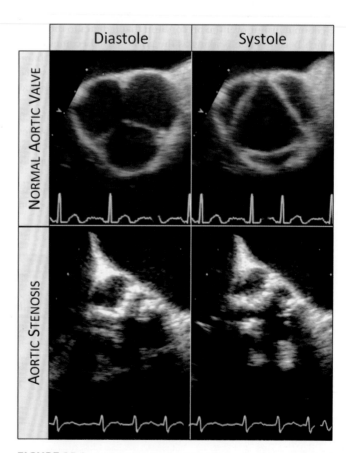

FIGURE 35.1 Aortic stenosis on echocardiography. Transesophageal echocardiogram (TEE) showing normal valve anatomy and a severely stenotic aortic valve, both in diastole and systole. Note how calcified and narrowed the stenotic valve appears.

AS or AR and may be associated with diseases of the aorta such as aortic aneurysm, aortic dissection, and coarctation.[9]

The most important physiologic adaptation to the pressure overload from AS is left ventricular hypertrophy (LVH). This leads to concentric hypertrophy, a process in which the left ventricular (LV) chamber becomes smaller and its wall thicker; such changes decrease the wall stress and preserve left ventricular ejection fraction (LVEF) for very long periods. When LVEF starts to decrease, the underlying mechanism is an afterload-LVH mismatch (insufficient hypertrophy for the degree of AS) rather than true cardiomyopathy.

CLINICAL PRESENTATION

The classic triad of symptomatic severe AS consists of angina, syncope, and dyspnea from heart failure. AS is usually asymptomatic unless severe. The importance of recognizing the symptomatic stage of AS, as established by the seminal work by Ross and Braunwald, is the rapid rise in mortality once symptoms develop.[10] Following a latent asymptomatic period, patients who progress to severe symptomatic AS experience over 50% mortality in the next 2 to 3 years if no intervention is pursued.[11]

DIAGNOSIS

Although physical examination may establish the diagnosis, it is often unable to precisely grade AS severity. The typical findings in auscultation of AS include a systolic crescendo–decrescendo ejection murmur over the precordium that radiates to the neck, which becomes late peaking as the aortic valve becomes more stenotic. The prolonged ejection time leads to a single or, paradoxically, split second heart sound (S2), with occasional absence of S2 in severe cases.[12] Carotid upstroke is typically weak and delayed (*pulsus parvus et tardus*).

Electrocardiogram (ECG) often meets criteria for LVH and left atrial enlargement. Although chest X-ray (CXR) rarely provides direct evidence of AS, it occasionally shows aortic valve calcifications. In addition, pulmonary venous congestion is frequently seen in decompensated patients.

The primary means of diagnosing and grading AS is echocardiography, and aortic valve area (AVA) is the primary criterion

of AS. When there is normal flow across the aortic valve, the magnitude of the peak and mean systolic gradient across the aortic valve is inversely related to AVA (**Table 35.1**). Additional echocardiographic findings in patients with significant AS include LVH, left atrial enlargement, and typically preserved LVEF.

A low transvalvular gradient (mean gradient ≤30 mm Hg) does not exclude severe AS. In patients with low transaortic volume flow rate, peak and mean systolic gradients do not accurately reflect severity of AS. Low flow may occur for two separate reasons: (1) low stroke volume in the setting of small hypertrophied left ventricle with preserved LVEF and (2) low stroke volume in the setting of LV systolic dysfunction and low LVEF. Low flow is typically defined as a low LV stroke volume index of <35 mL/m².

In patients with low-flow, low-gradient severe AS with normal LVEF, echocardiography demonstrates small LV chamber size, abnormal diastolic filling, and increased LV relative wall thickness. In contrast, in patients with systolic dysfunction and depressed LVEF, low transvalvular gradients are found for two reasons: either afterload-hypertrophy mismatch or concomitant cardiomyopathy (such as ischemic heart disease). Differentiating between these two groups is extremely important because the patients in the first group will benefit from aortic valve surgery, whereas those in the second group may not (**Figure 35.2**).[13]

To differentiate between these two groups, various LV and aortic valve parameters are assessed at rest and following intravenous infusion of increasing amounts of dobutamine starting at 5 μg/kg/min and escalating up to 20 μg/kg/min.[14] These parameters are usually measured by echocardiography (modified dobutamine stress echocardiogram). However, these parameters may also be evaluated during cardiac catheterization.

In patients with low-gradient AS with reduced LVEF, changes in the following three parameters are measured during dobutamine stress testing: LV stroke volume, AVA, and mean gradient. If the stroke volume increases ≤20%, the patient likely has severe cardiomyopathy and is usually not a candidate for aortic valve surgery. On the other hand, if the stroke volume increases more than 20%, two scenarios are possible: (1) AVA remains essentially the same but the mean gradient increases above 30 mm Hg and (2) AVA increases by 0.2 cm² or more but the gradient remains essentially unchanged. In the first scenario, patients have true severe AS and will benefit from aortic valve surgery.

TABLE 35.1	**Aortic Valve Stenosis Criteria in Patient With Preserved Transvalvular Flow**			
	NONSTENOTIC AORTIC VALVE	**MILD AS**	**MODERATE AS**	**SEVERE AS**
Valve area (cm²)	2.0–4.0	>1.5	1.0–1.5	<1.0
Valve area index (cm²/m²)				<0.6
Peak velocity (m/s)	<2.5	2.5–3.0	3.1–4.0	>4.0
Peak gradient (mm Hg)	<25	25–36	37–64	>64
Mean gradient (mm Hg)		<25	25–40	>40
ACC/AHA stage	A (at risk)	B (progressive)		C (asymptomatic) D (symptomatic)

ACC, American College of Cardiology; AHA, American Heart Association.

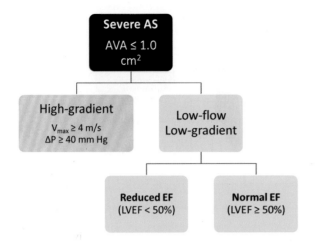

FIGURE 35.2 Three forms of AS. Flowsheet showing three different categories of severe aortic stenosis. Hemodynamic parameters (peak velocity and mean gradient) discriminate high-gradient from low-gradient severe AS. In low-gradient severe AS with reduced EF, dobutamine stress echocardiography is used to confirm true severe AS. In low-gradient severe AS with normal EF, low stroke volume, LV size and abnormal LV parameters are commonly present. AS, aortic stenosis; EF, ejection fraction; LV, left ventricular; LVEF, left ventricular ejection fraction.

In the second scenario, patients have pseudosevere AS due to LV cardiomyopathy; they are unlikely to benefit from aortic valve surgery (**Figure 35.3**).

Cardiac catheterization is usually unnecessary because echocardiography is the gold standard for diagnosis and quantification of AS. However, because coronary artery disease is common in patients with AS, coronary angiography is usually performed before surgical or percutaneous AVR. In this setting, aortic valve gradients may be evaluated using invasive hemodynamic measurements.

When comparing aortic gradients obtained by cardiac catheterization, it is the mean but not the peak aortic gradient that correlates with echocardiography. Cardiac catheterization and echocardiography measure two separate peak gradients (**Figure 35.4**).

On catheterization, the so-called peak-to-peak (P2P) gradient is measured, which represents the pressure difference between the peak LV systolic pressure and the peak aortic systolic pressure. These two peaks do not occur simultaneously and are thus nonphysiologic; the more severe the AS, the greater the time difference between the two pressure peaks.

On echocardiography, the peak instantaneous pressure gradient (PIG) is measured instead; it represents the pressure difference between LV systolic and aortic pressure at the same time point. P2P is typically lower than PIG, largely due to the pressure recovery phenomenon (kinetic energy converted to potential energy in the ascending aorta).[15]

MEDICAL THERAPY

There are no proven medical therapies for prevention or treatment of AS, and routine antibiotic prophylaxis of bacterial endocarditis in patients with AS is no longer recommended.[16]

Usually, patients with severe AS present to the CCU with clinical signs of heart failure. Pharmacologic therapy including diuretics, angiotensin-converting enzyme (ACE) inhibitors, and digitalis may be used with caution. Although intravenous vasodilators used to be contraindicated in patients with severe AS, intravenous nitroprusside has been demonstrated to relieve symptoms of heart failure in patients with severe AS and severely reduced LV systolic function.[17] In that study, intravenous nitroprusside was started at a mean dose of 14 ± 10 µg/min, and the dose was increased to a mean of 103 ± 67 µg/min at 6 hours and 128 ± 96 µg/min at 24 hours.

Patients with severe AS may also present with other critical illnesses, such as septic shock. Management of these patients can

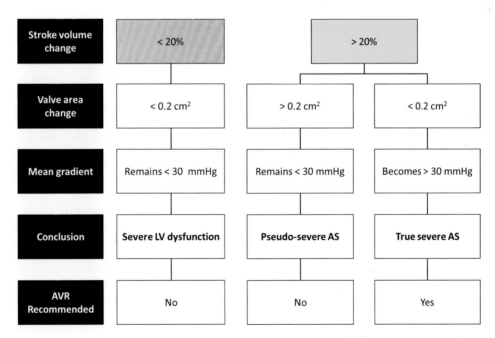

FIGURE 35.3 Dobutamine stress testing for severe low-gradient aortic stenosis with diminished LVEF. AS, aortic stenosis; AVR, aortic valve replacement.

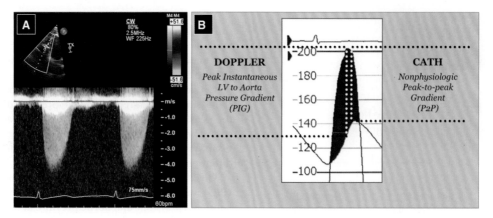

FIGURE 35.4 Aortic stenosis: echocardiography versus catheterization. Comparison between echocardiographic measurement of systolic aortic valve pressure gradient by peak velocity (A) and peak-to-peak gradient measured by cardiac catheterization (B). With simultaneous left ventricular and aortic pressure tracing, it becomes apparent that peak-to-peak gradient underestimates true maximum pressure gradient. Note the very high ventricular pressure in systole, and the delayed low-pressure peak in the aortic root (the hemodynamic basis for *pulsus parvus et tardus*). LV, left ventricular; PIG, peak instantaneous pressure gradient.

TABLE 35.2	Major Indications for Aortic Valve Replacement in Patients With Aortic Stenosis			
SYMPTOMS	**RECOMMENDATION FOR AORTIC VALVE REPLACEMENT**	**ACC/AHA STAGE**	**COR**	**LOE**
Symptomatic	Symptomatic high-gradient severe AS (by history or exercise testing)	D1	I	B
	Symptomatic low-flow/low-gradient severe AS with reduced EF (confirmed by dobutamine stress echocardiography)	D2	IIa	B
	Symptomatic low-flow/low-gradient severe AS with preserved EF (if valve obstruction is considered the cause of symptoms)	D3	IIa	B
	Severe AS undergoing other cardiac surgery	C or D	I	B
Asymptomatic	Asymptomatic high-gradient severe AS with LV dysfunction (EF <50%)	C	I	B
	Asymptomatic high-gradient very severe AS ($V_{max} \geq 5$ m/s) and low surgical risk	C	IIa	B

ACC, American College of Cardiology; AHA, American Heart Association; AS, aortic stenosis; COR, class of recommendation; EF, ejection fraction; LOE, level of evidence; LV, left ventricular; V_{max}, peak velocity.

For a complete list, refer to the 2014 AHA/ACC Valvular Heart Disease Guideline. Note the lower class of recommendation for symptomatic patients with low-flow severe AS, both with reduced and preserved EF.

be extremely challenging owing to the narrow balance between preload and afterload. Hemodynamic compromise is common. Hypotension from severe sepsis or septic shock may initiate a spiral of death, in which low aortic pressure leads to low coronary perfusion, with further ventricular impairment that fails to pump blood against a severely stenotic valve. This negative feedback rapidly leads to cardiac arrest and should be promptly recognized so that vasopressors are administered before such cascade takes place.

SURGICAL AND PERCUTANEOUS INTERVENTIONAL THERAPY

AS is a mechanical problem that requires a mechanical intervention. AVR is the preferred therapeutic choice in patients with AS to improve symptoms and increase survival. Major indications for AVR are listed in **Table 35.2**.

Surgical aortic valve replacement (SAVR) is the standard approach, indicated for patients with acceptable surgical risk who

meet indications for AVR.[13] The technical aspects are beyond the scope of this chapter, but clinicians should be familiar with the decision process when choosing a surgical prosthesis. In addition to the appropriate size, such that there is no postoperative patient–prosthesis mismatch, the valve material has significant implications for the patient. Although a bioprosthesis is considered to be less durable than a mechanical valve, it offers the advantage of not requiring systemic anticoagulation. As such, in patients who are older or who have a contraindication for anticoagulation, a bioprosthetic implant is preferred. Conversely, in younger patients who have no contraindications for anticoagulation, a mechanical valve is reasonable. Above all, this should be a shared decision process between the surgeon and the patient.

Percutaneous interventions for AS include aortic valve balloon valvuloplasty and TAVR. Balloon valvuloplasty is an effective form of therapy for congenital AS. However, balloon valvuloplasty in calcific TAV or BAV AS is rather ineffective (valve area seldom increases above 1.0 cm² and there is a high rate of restenosis) and has significant morbidity and mortality.

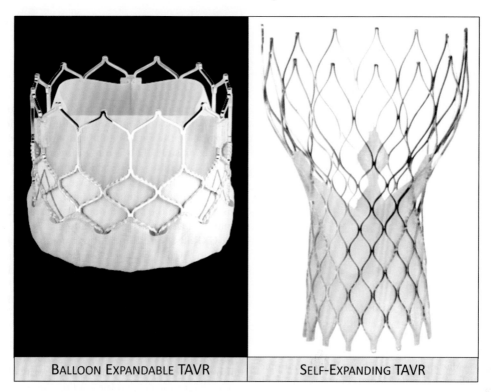

| BALLOON EXPANDABLE TAVR | SELF-EXPANDING TAVR |

FIGURE 35.5 Transcatheter aortic valve replacement valves. Two major types of transcatheter implantable aortic valves. The balloon-expandable valve has a short and straight frame (left), whereas the self-expandable valve is longer and hourglass-shaped (right). These different metallic frames facilitate identification in routine chest radiography. TAVR, transcatheter aortic valve replacement. (Images available at the manufacturer's websites: www.tavrbyedwards.com and www.corevalve.com, respectively.)

Currently, typical indications for balloon valvuloplasty in calcific AS include short-term relief of AS in patients undergoing noncardiac surgery (such as hip replacement), in those with terminal illness (such as cancer), or as a temporizing measure in patients who are rapidly decompensating from severe AS in whom durable interventions are being entertained.

TAVR has changed the landscape of therapy for AS, allowing for patients who were previously too ill for surgery to receive lifesaving therapy. Since the first percutaneous replacement was performed by Alain Cribier in 2002, there have been over 200,000 TAVR procedures performed worldwide.[18] TAVR is now approved in patients with symptomatic severe AS who are inoperable, or are either high or intermediate risk for SAVR.

TAVR was considered experimental until 2010, when the first randomized trial showed a markedly improved survival in patients who were not surgical candidates.[19] These findings were subsequently confirmed in head-to-head trials comparing TAVR with SAVR in high-risk and intermediate-risk surgical patients.[20] In addition, TAVR is currently being investigated in low-risk patients.

Consequently, concerns regarding durability of transcatheter valves in comparison with surgical valves emerged, highlighted by the limited reliable data available on TAVR durability beyond five years.[21] Still, factors like lower rates of patient-prosthesis valve mismatch in TAVR compared with SAVR[22] might skew the durability data in favor of transcatheter prosthesis. There are currently two approved device types in the United States, a balloon-expandable (Edwards Sapien family of TAVR valves) and a self-expandable valve (Medtronic CoreValve family of TAVR valves), both of which been updated with new design features to reduce paravalvular AR (**Figure 35.5**).

POST-TRANSCATHETER AORTIC VALVE REPLACEMENT COMPLICATIONS

Patients who undergo TAVR are usually cared for in the CCU postprocedurally, so it is important to be familiar with the most common complications such as vascular access complications, neurologic events, conduction abnormalities, coronary artery obstruction, low cardiac output, annular rupture, and paravalvular AR.

Besides femoral access bleeding and vascular complications from the large sheaths used, patients should be closely monitored for neurologic changes given the risk of stroke from the large-profile devices advanced through the arterial system and crushing the calcified native valve.

Patients are also monitored for conduction abnormalities, specifically complete heart block from extrinsic compression of the conductions system following valve deployment. These patients routinely receive temporary venous pacemaker placement preprocedurally. Persistent heart block requiring permanent pacemaker is more common in patients with preexisting conduction system disease, especially right bundle branch block. Need for permanent pacing was previously more commonly seen in the self-expandable valve. However, with the latest generation of TAVR valve, the rate of permanent pacemaker implantation is similar between self-expanding and balloon-expandable TAVR valves.[23]

Periprocedural complications, usually diagnosed before transfer to CCU for monitoring, include coronary artery obstruction, low cardiac output, annular rupture, and paravalvular AR. Late complications include leaflet thrombosis, valvular degeneration, and infective endocarditis.

IMPACT OF SEVERE AORTIC STENOSIS ON PREGNANCY

Patients with calcific AS are seldom of child-bearing age. In patients of child-bearing age, AS is usually caused by noncalcific congenital abnormalities (such as unicuspid aortic valve). Young patients with moderate-to-severe AS should be advised against conception until AS is relieved. Those who nonetheless become pregnant may or may not develop severe symptoms. Pregnant patients with AS and mild symptoms may be managed conservatively during pregnancy with bed rest, oxygen, and β-blockers. Pregnant patients with severe symptoms may need percutaneous or surgical intervention. These procedures carry significant risk to both the mother and the unborn child.[24]

AORTIC REGURGITATION

ETIOLOGY AND PATHOPHYSIOLOGY

AR may be caused by disorders of the aortic root or the aortic valve leaflets. BAV, ascending aortic aneurysm, aortic dissection, and endocarditis are common causes of AR. Conditions predisposing the patient to aortopathies and AR include hypertension and connective tissue disorders (such as Marfan syndrome, Ehlers–Danlos syndrome, and ankylosing spondylitis). In less developed countries, rheumatic heart disease and tertiary syphilis remain important causes of AR.

In AR, the blood flows back into the ventricle through the aortic valve during diastole, joining the systemic volume that entered the left ventricle through the mitral valve. During the subsequent systole, both volumes leave the aortic valve together; the systemic volume continues into the aorta and its branches, whereas the regurgitant volume flows back into the ventricle. The cycle then repeats itself. Subsequent pathophysiology depends on whether AR is chronic or acute.

In chronic AR, the left ventricle progressively enlarges to accommodate the combined systemic stroke volume and the regurgitant volume. This remodeling often prevents significant elevation of left heart pressures. It may take years, if not decades, for patients with chronic AR to develop congestive heart failure owing to progressive LV systolic dysfunction. This adaptation contrasts with acute AR, in which there is sudden volume overload of a nondilated left ventricle, marked elevation of LV and left atrial pressures, life-threatening pulmonary edema, and even cardiogenic shock.

Patients with severe AR, whether acute or chronic, typically present to the CCU with signs and symptoms of heart failure. Although severe acute AR represents only a minority of AR cases, its often fulminant and life-threatening course necessitates CCU admission. The rest of the section on AR is devoted to severe acute AR.

CLINICAL PRESENTATION

The most common etiologies of severe acute AR are chest trauma, bacterial endocarditis, and dissection of the ascending aorta (Stanford type A aortic dissection). Less commonly, severe acute AR may result following balloon valvuloplasty for severe AS.

Patients with severe acute AR frequently present with fulminant pulmonary edema and cardiogenic shock. Patients with endocarditis will also have general signs and symptoms of a systemic bacterial illness. Patients with acute type A aortic dissection usually complain of severe chest pain, often in the setting of uncontrolled systemic hypertension.

DIAGNOSIS

In severe acute AR, there may be few or no auscultatory findings of AR; the diastolic murmur is often soft, short, or even absent because of the rapid equilibration of aortic and LV pressures during diastole. This is due to the acute nature of the disease, which precludes increased compliance of the left ventricle. Therefore, the rapid rise in LV end-diastolic pressure limits the total regurgitant volume, explaining the underwhelming diastolic murmur and the lack of wide pulse pressure. There is, however, marked tachycardia and S3 gallop.

CXR in severe acute AR frequently reveals pulmonary congestion. ECG may show tachycardia; there may also be signs of myocardial ischemia (owing to high myocardial demand caused by very elevated LV pressures or when acute aortic dissection extends into the coronary artery ostia). When endocarditis leads to periaortic valve abscess, ECG may demonstrate varying degrees of atrioventricular conduction block.

Transthoracic and transesophageal echocardiography are the primary means of evaluating AR. Echocardiography may establish the etiology, mechanism, and severity of AR (**Figure 35.6**). The diagnostic criteria for grading the severity of AR are listed in **Table 35.3**.

MEDICAL THERAPY

Severe acute AR is a life-threatening medical emergency that necessitates highest levels of CCU care. Diuretic therapy, positive end-expiratory pressure, and supplemental oxygen administration with endotracheal intubation are used to treat pulmonary edema. Afterload reduction may be achieved with the use of intravenous vasodilators (such as nitroprusside). Disease-specific therapies, if available, should also be administered (such as antibiotic therapy for endocarditis).

SURGICAL AND PERCUTANEOUS INTERVENTIONAL THERAPY

In severe acute AR, aortic valve surgery should be performed as soon as possible, especially in cases of type A aortic dissection and infective endocarditis. The standard procedure of choice is surgical AVR. At present, there is no approved percutaneous option for patients with pure AR.

Aortic valve sparing surgeries may be an alternative to surgical AVR in specialized centers. This surgery, known as the David procedure (after Tirone David, the Brazilian surgeon who conceived and first performed this technique), involves ascending aorta repair with a vascular graft, followed by coronary artery reimplantation, reconstruction of the aortic root, and reimplantation of the aortic valve.[25] This technique is better suited for young patients with genetic syndromes associated with aortic root dilatation, and it is still not employed universally.

In-hospital and long-term survival is significantly improved in patients who promptly undergo SAVR or repair.[26] However, such intervention might be prohibitive in patients with severe embolic strokes or comorbid conditions that diminish the prospect of reasonable recovery.

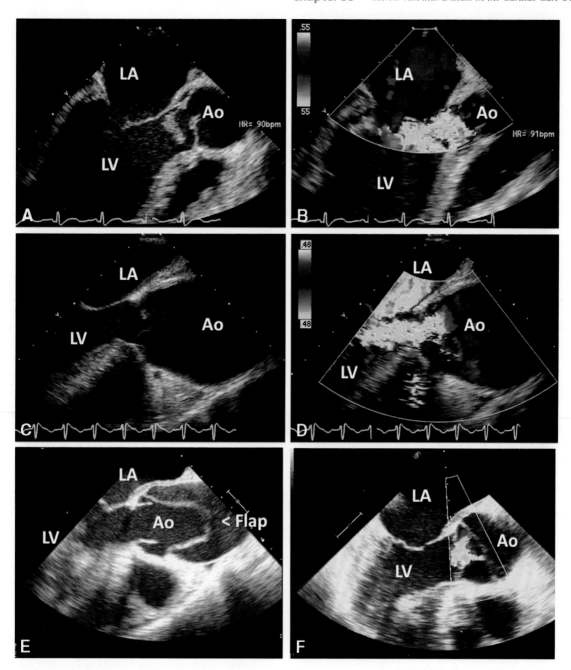

FIGURE 35.6 Aortic regurgitation on echocardiography. Causes of severe aortic regurgitation include aortic valve endocarditis (A and B), ascending aortic aneurysm (C and D), and type A aortic dissection (E and F). Ao, ascending aorta; LA, left atrium; LV, left ventricle.

Despite the excitement about transcatheter therapies in severe AS, use of TAVR in severe AR has been reported only anecdotally. A stenotic calcific aortic valve forms a solid structure for anchoring in transcatheter replacement, whereas a regurgitant aortic valve—often associated with a dilated aortic root—poses a great challenge in holding a transcatheter valve. Still, TAVR may represent a last resort in patients who present with severe symptomatic AR who are not surgical candidates.

Registry data from self-expanding TAVR (which have a larger anchoring profile than balloon-expandable valves) in patients with predominant AR show significantly increased mortality when compared with patients undergoing TAVR for severe AS (around 20%), particularly in patients in whom valvular calcification was absent.[27,28]

Furthermore, intra-aortic balloon pump (IABP) is absolutely contraindicated when significant AR is present. Diastolic counterpulsations—which are the hallmarks of IABP function—worsen AR. This, in turn, decreases effective stroke volume and cardiac output, worsening cardiogenic shock. In addition, it increases LV end-diastolic pressure and myocardial oxygen consumption, worsening pulmonary edema and myocardial ischemia. Therefore, in conditions that usually require IABP for medical stabilization (such as cardiogenic shock and refractory ischemia), use of counterpulsation is prohibitive with moderate or severe AR.

TABLE 35.3	**Grades of Aortic Regurgitation**			
	MILD AR	**MODERATE AR**	**MODERATE–SEVERE AR**	**SEVERE AR**
Grade	1+	2+	3+	4+
Regurgitant orifice area (cm^2)	<0.1	0.10–0.19	0.20–0.29	>0.3
Regurgitant fraction	<30%	30%–39%	40%–49%	>50%
Regurgitant volume (mL)	30	30–44	45–59	>60
Vena contracta (cm)	<0.3	0.3–0.6	>0.6	
ACC/AHA Stage		B (progressive)		C (asymptomatic) D (symptomatic)

ACC, American College of Cardiology; AHA, American Heart Association; AR, aortic regurgitation.
Note that stage A denotes a nonregurgitant aortic valve, which is at risk for aortic regurgitation (such as bicuspid aortic valve or ascending aortic aneurysm).

IMPACT ON PREGNANCY

The hemodynamic changes associated with pregnancy (increased cardiac output from increased heart rate and stroke volume) are more likely to decompensate patients with stenotic valvular diseases compared with those with insufficient valves, given the mechanical obstruction to blood flow in such conditions. Conversely, regurgitant lesions are better tolerated in pregnancy, and AR is generally tolerated unless it is severe.

Severe AR, whether acute or chronic, is one of the valvular heart lesions that may be associated with high maternal and/or fetal risk during pregnancy. Pregnant women with AR who have New York Heart Association functional class III to IV symptoms, severe pulmonary hypertension (pulmonary pressure >75% of systemic pressures), and/or LV systolic dysfunction are at particular risk for maternal and fetal complications. The same is true for pregnant women having Marfan syndrome with or without AR.[24]

REFERENCES

1. Frohlich GM, Lansky AJ, Webb J, et al. Local versus general anesthesia for transcatheter aortic valve implantation (TAVR)—systematic review and meta-analysis. *BMC Med.* 2014;12:41.

2. Nkomo VT, Gardin JM, Skelton TN, Gottdiener JS, Scott CG, Enriquez-Sarano M. Burden of valvular heart diseases: a population-based study. *Lancet.* 2006;368(9540):1005-1011.

3. Dweck MR, Jones C, Joshi NV, et al. Assessment of valvular calcification and inflammation by positron emission tomography in patients with aortic stenosis. *Circulation.* 2012;125(1):76-86.

4. Thanassoulis G, Massaro JM, Cury R, et al. Associations of long-term and early adult atherosclerosis risk factors with aortic and mitral valve calcium. *J Am Coll Cardiol.* 2010;55(22):2491-2498.

5. Stewart BF, Siscovick D, Lind BK, et al. Clinical factors associated with calcific aortic valve disease. Cardiovascular Health Study. *J Am Coll Cardiol.* 1997;29(3):630-634.

6. Smith JG, Luk K, Schulz CA, et al. Association of low-density lipoprotein cholesterol-related genetic variants with aortic valve calcium and incident aortic stenosis. *JAMA.* 2014;312(17):1764-1771.

7. Saric M, Kronzon I. Aortic stenosis in the elderly. *Am J Geriatr Cardiol.* 2000;9(6):321-330.

8. Saric M, Kronzon I. Congenital heart disease in adults. In: Lang RM, Vannan MA, Khanderia BK, eds. *Dynamic Echocardiography: A Case-Based Approach.* St Louis, MO: Springer; Saunders, an imprint of Elsevier, Inc; 2010:438-439.

9. Saric M, Kronzon I. Aortic dissection. In: Lang RM, Vannan MA, Khanderia BK, eds. *Dynamic Echocardiography: A Case-Based Approach.* St Louis, MO: Springer; Saunders, an imprint of Elsevier, Inc; 2010:171-175.

10. Ross J Jr, Braunwald E. Aortic stenosis. *Circulation.* 1968;38 (1 Suppl):61-67.

11. Kelly TA, Rothbart RM, Cooper CM, Kaiser DL, Smucker ML, Gibson RS. Comparison of outcome of asymptomatic to symptomatic patients older than 20 years of age with valvular aortic stenosis. *Am J Cardiol.* 1988;61(1):123-130.

12. Selzer A, Lombard JT. Clinical findings in adult aortic stenosis—then and now. *Eur Heart J.* 1988;9(Suppl E):53-55.

13. Nishimura RA, Otto CM, Bonow RO, et al. 2014 AHA/ACC guideline for the management of patients with valvular heart disease: executive summary: a report of the American College of Cardiology/American Heart Association Task Force on Practice Guidelines. *J Am Coll Cardiol.* 2014;63(22):2438-2488.

14. de Filippi CR, Willett DL, Brickner ME, et al. Usefulness of dobutamine echocardiography in distinguishing severe from nonsevere valvular aortic stenosis in patients with depressed left ventricular function and low transvalvular gradients. *Am J Cardiol.* 1995;75(2):191-194.

15. Heinrich RS, Fontaine AA, Grimes RY, et al. Experimental analysis of fluid mechanical energy losses in aortic valve stenosis: importance of pressure recovery. *Ann Biomed Eng.* 1996;24(6):685-694.

16. Wilson W, Taubert KA, Gewitz M, et al. Prevention of infective endocarditis: guidelines from the American Heart Association: a guideline from the American Heart Association Rheumatic Fever, Endocarditis, and Kawasaki Disease Committee, Council on Cardiovascular Disease in the Young, and the Council on Clinical Cardiology, Council on Cardiovascular Surgery and Anesthesia, and the Quality of Care and Outcomes Research Interdisciplinary Working Group. *Circulation.* 2007;116(15):1736-1754.

17. Khot UN, Novaro GM, Popović ZB, et al. Nitroprusside in critically ill patients with left ventricular dysfunction and aortic stenosis. *N Engl J Med.* 2003;348(18):1756-1763.

18. Cribier A, Eltchaninoff H, Bash A, et al. Percutaneous transcatheter implantation of an aortic valve prosthesis for calcific aortic stenosis: first human case description. *Circulation.* 2002;106(24):3006-3008.

19. Leon MB, Smith CR, Mack M, et al. Transcatheter aortic-valve implantation for aortic stenosis in patients who cannot undergo surgery. *N Engl J Med.* 2010;363(17):1597-1607.

20. Leon MB, Smith CR, Mack MJ, et al. Transcatheter or surgical aortic-valve replacement in intermediate-risk patients. *N Engl J Med.* 2016;374(17):1609-1620.

21. Arsalan M, Walther T. Durability of prostheses for transcatheter aortic valve implantation. *Nat Rev Cardiol.* 2016;13(6):360-367.

22. Finkelstein A, Schwartz AL, Uretzky G, et al. Hemodynamic performance and outcome of percutaneous versus surgical stentless bioprostheses for aortic stenosis with anticipated patient–prosthesis mismatch. *J Thorac Cardiovasc Surg.* 2014;147(6):1892-1899.

23. De Torres-Alba F, Kaleschke G, Diller GP, et al. Changes in the pacemaker rate after transition from Edwards SAPIEN XT to SAPIEN 3transcatheter aortic valve implantation: the critical role of valve implantation height. *JACC Cardiovasc Interv.* 2016;9(8):805-813.

24. Warnes CA, Williams RG, Bashore TM, et al. ACC/AHA 2008 Guidelines for the Management of Adults with Congenital Heart Disease: a report of the American College of Cardiology/American Heart Association Task Force on Practice Guidelines (writing committee to develop guidelines on the management of adults with congenital heart disease). *Circulation.* 2008;118(23):e714-e833.

25. David TE. Aortic valve sparing in different aortic valve and aortic root conditions. *J Am Coll Cardiol.* 2016;68(6):654-664.

26. Lalani T, Cabell CH, Benjamin DK, et al. Analysis of the impact of early surgery on in-hospital mortality of native valve endocarditis: use of propensity score and instrumental variable methods to adjust for treatment-selection bias. *Circulation.* 2010;121(8):1005-1013.

27. Roy DA, Schaefer U, Guetta V, et al. Transcatheter aortic valve implantation for pure severe native aortic valve regurgitation. *J Am Coll Cardiol.* 2013;61(15):1577-1584.

28. Testa L, Latib A, Rossi ML, et al. CoreValve implantation for severe aortic regurgitation: a multicentre registry. *EuroIntervention.* 2014;10(6):739-745.

Patient and Family Information for: AORTIC VALVULAR DISEASE IN THE CARDIAC CARE UNIT

GENERAL CONCEPTS OF AORTIC VALVULAR DISEASE

The heart is a muscular organ whose primary function is to pump blood in our body. To accomplish this goal, several valves are present in its different chambers to prevent backflow. The aortic valve is a valve composed of three thin leaflets, separating the aorta—the largest artery in the body from which all the blood pumped out of the heart flows—and the left ventricle—the chamber that pumps blood out of the heart to the rest of the body. When the aortic valve becomes too narrowed, doctors call it aortic stenosis. When it becomes leaky, it is called aortic insufficiency.

AORTIC STENOSIS

WHAT IS THE ILLNESS?

If the aortic valve becomes too narrow, pumping blood out of the heart becomes difficult. When patients feel symptoms from this valve narrowing (called stenosis), they usually report episodes of passing out, chest pain with exertion, and shortness of breath. Usually the cause of AS is wear and tear over many years, making it harder and less flexible with aging (the reason these patients are usually elderly). However, some patients are born with malfunctioning valves, and in these cases they develop valve narrowing at a younger age.

HOW WILL THE PATIENT BE TREATED?

There are no medicines that fix AS, so an invasive procedure is usually indicated in symptomatic patients. The standard procedure is to replace the valve with a prosthesis. In some patients this is done through open heart surgery, and in others the valve is replaced through catheters.

In patients with severe AS, the disease may progress rapidly and even cause death if not treated in time. Therefore, once diagnosed, planning for receiving a new valve should be undertaken.

WHAT IF THE PATIENT IS PREGNANT OR THINKING OF BECOMING PREGNANT?

If there is severe narrowing of the aortic valve, pregnancy may need to be delayed until the narrowing is relieved—usually through the use of balloon catheter inserted through the groin, threaded to the heart, and blown up inside the valve to make it larger. If already pregnant and there are symptoms (such as shortness of breath or chest pain), the patient may need to take certain medications that are effective for her but not harmful to the child. If the symptoms during pregnancy are severe, the balloon catheter treatment or even open heart surgery may be needed. These procedures carry significant risk to both the mother and the unborn child.

AORTIC REGURGITATION

WHAT IS THE ILLNESS?

AR is the medical term to describe a leaky aortic valve, allowing blood to backflow into the heart after it is pumped to the aorta. When this happens, there is extra work for the heart to pump blood forward, and this backflow may cause breathing problems from water buildup in the lungs and other parts of the body.

One of the most common causes of AR in the United States is a dilated aorta, where the valve sits. When this artery becomes too big, the valve leaflets become too far apart from each other and blood leaks back into the heart. This enlargement may happen from wear and tear in older patients, or from a loose buildup in patients born with genetic predisposition to aortic enlargement.

Another common cause for AR is infection in the valve, causing destruction of the leaflets and, consequently, leakage. Wear and tear of the valve leaflets may also cause AR, not only in older patients but also in young patients born with a malfunctioning valve. Finally, in patients born outside of the United States, long-standing syphilis and rheumatic fever may also lead to AR.

HOW WILL THE PATIENT BE TREATED?

In patients who develop AR in a short period of time, such that the heart does not have enough time to accommodate the leakage, quick medical stabilization in an intensive care unit is necessary. However, the ultimate treatment requires valve replacement with prosthesis.

Similar to AS, a severely leaky valve of AR may be replaced through open heart surgery. However, in contrast to AS, a severely leaky valve of AR cannot be replaced using catheters in most patients.

If the AR developed slowly, the heart eventually will become large and weak trying to accommodate the backflow of blood. However, in cases of rapidly developing severe AR, the disease may cause imminent death unless appropriate medicines and, eventually, surgery for valve replacement are employed.

WHAT IF THE PATIENT IS PREGNANT OR THINKING OF BECOMING PREGNANT?

Severe leakage of the aortic valve may not be well tolerated during pregnancy and the condition may harm the unborn child. Women with severe leakage who are considering pregnancy may need to delay it until the condition is treated. If already pregnant, significant heart problems may be experienced during the pregnancy.

Ahmadreza Moradi
Karan Sud
Jacqueline Danik

36

Mitral Valve Disease in the Cardiac Care Unit

INTRODUCTION

Severe mitral valve disease due to mitral stenosis or mitral regurgitation can lead to clinical decompensation requiring the care of a patient in the cardiac care unit setting. The backdrop of such decompensation may be chronic valve disease on which acute injury is superimposed.

MITRAL VALVE STENOSIS

ETIOLOGY AND PATHOPHYSIOLOGY OF MITRAL STENOSIS

The mitral valve is a left atrioventricular valve or bicuspid valve that lies in the annulus between the left atrium and the left ventricle. A competent mitral valve requires the coordination of all the components of the mitral valve: the valve leaflets, the chordal attachments, the annulus, the papillary muscles, and the supporting ventricular walls into which the apparatus inserts. Failure or malfunction of any component of the mitral valve apparatus with failure to open results in stenosis with difficulty of left atrial emptying into the left ventricle.

Mitral stenosis (MS) results in delayed emptying of blood from the left atrium (LA) into the left ventricle (LV) during diastole. This can result in elevated pressures in the left atrium, pulmonary vasculature and eventually the right side of the heart, leading to pulmonary hypertension.

The Euro Heart Study Survey was specifically designed to study the management of patients with valvular heart disease and prospectively included 5001 patients from 92 centers in 25 European countries.[1,2] This survey does not represent the general population, but rather the type of valve disease seen in a European referral population for treatment of heart disease. The most common valvular etiology was degenerative disease, representing 63% of all cases of native heart disease (likely representing an aging population), with a mean age of >50 years among patients with aortic and mitral valve disease, followed by rheumatic heart disease (RHD) in 22% of all patients,[2] representing the distribution in industrialized countries.

The incidence of RHD has decreased in industrialized countries over the past 60 years, but still exists in elderly patients who were exposed to acute rheumatic fever during childhood.

The incidence remains lowest in America and Western Europe ($\leq$10 per 100,000 of the population per year), higher in Eastern Europe (>10 per 100,000), and approximated to have an incidence of 13 cases per 100,000 per year in sub-Saharan Africa.[3]

RHD is usually a consequence of rheumatic fever, caused by group A β-hemolytic streptococci. As streptococcal proteins share antigenic properties with certain connective tissue proteins in the human host, the immune response that is mounted against the streptococci can lead to progressive and delayed valve damage. RHD causes mitral commissural adhesion; thickened, calcified, immobile mitral valve leaflets; and fibrosis, thickening, shortening, fusion, and calcification of the chordae tendineae (**Figures 36.1 and 36.2**). The male to female ratio for RHD is approximately 1:2. RHD remains prevalent in developing countries. Approximately 60% of patients with acute rheumatic fever will develop RHD.[3]

Etiologies, aside from degenerative valvular disease and RHD, include infective endocarditis, inflammatory disease, and congenital heart disease. These account for less than 10% of all cases of valvular heart disease.[1]

The normal mitral valve area in an adult measures approximately 4 to 6 cm^2. Patients may become symptomatic with shortness of breath as the valve area decreases over time. The diastolic gradient across the valve may increase, resulting in LA enlargement. Often, patients may have an acute event such as development of a rapid atrial arrhythmia (such as atrial fibrillation [AF]) that precipitates heart failure and decompensation of the patient requiring intensive medical care. Often, AF in the setting of MS is a highly prothrombotic state, marked by stasis of blood in the LA and left atrial appendage where thrombus can form. This puts the patient at risk for systemic thromboembolism.

Medical and interventional approaches to the management of patients with valvular MS depend on accurate diagnosis of the cause and stage of the disease process.

CLINICAL PRESENTATION OF MITRAL STENOSIS

Patients with severe MS can have elevated LA and pulmonary pressure causing dyspnea and other signs and symptoms of congestive heart failure. The severity of symptoms is related to the transmitral gradient in diastole.[4-6] In turn, the magnitude of the mitral gradient is the result of interplay between the mitral valve area and the blood flow. Doubling the blood flow will

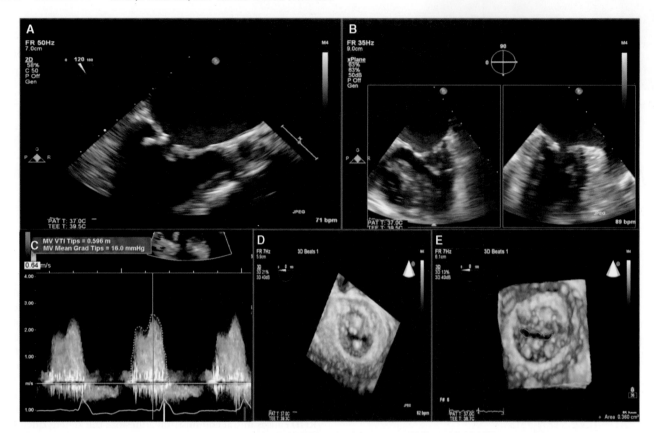

FIGURE 36.1 Severe mitral stenosis. A, A midesophageal view of the mitral valve via transesophageal echocardiogram (TEE). The mitral valve is thickened and shows restrictive leaflet motion. B, A biplane view on TEE of the mitral valve, again showing restricted leaflet motion. C, Demonstrates transmitral mean gradients are 16 mm Hg, consistent with very severe mitral stenosis. D and E, 3D images of severe mitral stenosis with severely restricted mitral valve motion. By planimetry, the mitral valve area was calculated to be about 0.4 cm^2.

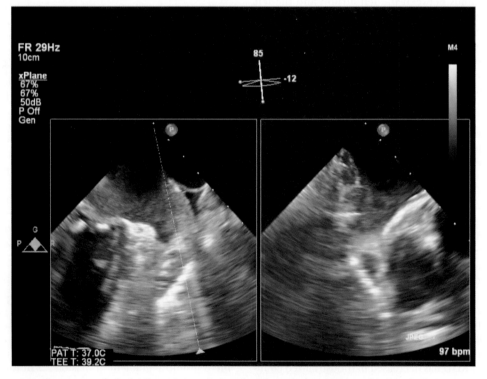

FIGURE 36.2 Severe mitral stenosis with fresh left atrial thrombus in the left atrial appendage, visible on a biplane view acquired by TEE in the midesophgeal view. Smoke is also visible in the dilated left atrium consistent with a low-flow state.

quadruple the gradient. The heart's compensatory mechanisms such as left atrial enlargement may fail in the setting of rapid heart rates induced by exercise, pregnancy, hyperthyroid crisis, fever, or tachyarrhythmia (ie, AF).

DIAGNOSIS

Classic auscultatory findings of MS include loud first heart sound (S1), an opening snap (OS) after the second heart sound (S2), and a diastolic rumble. The duration of the S2–OS interval is inversely related to the severity of MS (a shorter interval suggests more severe MS). In patients with normal sinus rhythm, there is also an end-diastolic ("presystolic") accentuation of the rumble.

The electrocardiogram may demonstrate signs of LA enlargement characterized by wide, saddle-shaped P-wave in leads I and II (so-called P mitrale) as well as late, deep P-wave inversion in lead V1. AF is frequently present and there may be signs of right ventricular hypertrophy.

A transthoracic echocardiogram (TTE) is indicated in patients with signs and symptoms of MS. By TTE one can establish the diagnosis, determine the morphology of the mitral valve (to determine suitability for mitral commissurotomy), quantify hemodynamic severity (mean pressure gradient, mitral valve area, and pulmonary artery pressure), and assess concomitant valvular lesions.

Chest X-ray usually demonstrates LA enlargement with straightening of the left cardiac silhouette. Right ventricular enlargement, signs of pulmonary venous congestion, and mitral valve calcification are frequently observed.

Cardiac catheterization is not necessary for the diagnosis of MS in most instances because hemodynamic data can be acquired from a careful TTE, performed when the heart rates and blood pressures have been optimized, and there is optimal time for diastolic filling of the left ventricle.

GRADING OF MITRAL STENOSIS

The 2009 guidelines from the American Society of Echocardiography defined mitral stenosis with mean gradients of <5 mm Hg, MVA of >1.5 cm^2 as being mild mitral stenosis; mean gradient of 5 to 10 mm Hg, MVA 1.0 to 1.5 cm^2 as moderate stenosis; mean gradient of >10 mm Hg, MVA < 1.0 cm^2 as severe mitral stenosis.[7] The 2014 American Heart Association/American College of Cardiology (AHA/ACC) guideline for the management of patients with valvular heart disease took this even further, applying grading of valvular disease as stages across a clinical continuum: stage A for patients at risk of MS; stage B as patients with progressive MS with mitral valve area > 1.5 cm^2, possible mild to moderate left atrial enlargement; stage C as asymptomatic severe MS, with MVA ≤ 1.5 cm^2, often severe left atrial enlargement and elevated pulmonary artery pressures; stage D as symptomatic severe MS, with MVA ≤ 1.5 cm^2, severe left atrial enlargement, pulmonary hypertension, exertional dyspnea, and decreased exercise tolerance (**Table 36.1**).[5]

The mean pressure gradient is highly dependent on the transvalvular flow and diastolic filling period and may vary greatly with change in heart rate. The diastolic pressure half-time depends on the degree of mitral obstruction and the compliance of the LV and LA and other measures of mitral valve area. Medical optimization and reevaluation in an intensive care setting may be necessary for a patient who presents with acute decompensation.

TABLE 36.1	Stages of MS Per the ACC/AHA Guidelines[5]			
STAGE/DEFINITION	**VALVE ANATOMY**	**VALVE HEMODYNAMICS**	**HEMODYNAMIC CONSEQUENCES**	**SYMPTOMS**
Stage A: at risk of MS	Mild valve doming during diastole	Normal transmitral flow velocity	None	None
Stage B: progressive MS	Rheumatic valve changes with commissural fusion and diastolic doming of the mitral valve leaflets Planimetered MVA > 1.5 cm^2	Increased transmittal flow velocities MVA > 1.5 cm^2 Diastolic pressure half-time < 150 ms	Mild-to-moderate LA enlargement Normal pulmonary pressure at rest	None
Stage C: asymptomatic severe MS	Rheumatic valve changes with commissural fusion and diastolic doming of the mitral valve leaflets Planimetered MVA ≤ 1.5 cm^2 MVA ≤ 1.0 cm^2 with very severe MS	MVA ≤ 1.5 cm^2 (MVA ≤ 1.0 cm^2 with very severe MS) Diastolic pressure half-time ≥ 150 ms Diastolic pressure half-time ≥ 220 ms with very severe MS	Severe LA enlargement Elevated PASP > 30 mm Hg	None
Stage D: symptomatic severe MS	Rheumatic valve changes with commissural fusion and diastolic doming of the mitral valve leaflets Planimetered MVA ≤ 1.5 cm^2	MVA ≤ 1.5 cm^2 MVA ≤ 1.0 cm^2 with very severe MS Diastolic pressure half-time ≥ 150 ms Diastolic pressure half-time > 220 ms with very severe MS	Severe LA enlargement Elevated PASP > 30 mm Hg	Decreased exercise tolerance Exertional dyspnea

The transmitral mean pressure gradient should be obtained to further determine the hemodynamic effect of the MS and is usually >5 to 10 mm Hg in severe MS; however, due to the variability of the mean pressure gradient with heart rate and forward flow, it has not been included in the criteria for severity.

LA, left atrial; LV, left ventricular; MS, mitral stenosis; ms, milliseconds; MVA, mitral valve area; PASP, pulmonary artery systolic pressure.

MEDICAL THERAPY FOR MITRAL STENOSIS

Patients with MS often present to the cardiac care unit (CCU) with clinical signs of heart failure, frequently in the setting of AF. Optimizing medical therapy can alleviate symptoms and prevent systemic thromboembolism. Congestion secondary to heart failure (HF) may need intravenous diuretic therapy. Heart rate control with β-blockers, certain calcium channel blockers (such as verapamil and diltiazem), and digitalis can be beneficial in patients with MS and AF to control rapid ventricular response and to allow greater time for diastolic filling of the LV.

Anticoagulation is indicated in patients with MS who present with AF, whether it is paroxysmal, persistent, or permanent. This is particularly true in a patient with a prior embolic event who is at higher risk for a repeat thromboembolic event and certainly if the patient is diagnosed with a left atrial thrombus. Intravenous heparin may be indicated with bridging to a vitamin K antagonist such as warfarin. There is as of yet insufficient large-scale data to attest to the efficacy of non–vitamin K oral anticoagulants in preventing thromboembolism in valvular AF.

PERCUTANEOUS INTERVENTION FOR MITRAL STENOSIS

In the absence of LA thrombus or moderate-to-severe MR and favorable valve morphology, percutaneous mitral balloon commissurotomy is recommended for the following: (1) symptomatic patients with severe MS; (2) symptomatic patients with mitral valve area > 1.5 cm² if there is evidence of hemodynamically significant MS based on pulmonary artery wedge pressure > 25 mm Hg or mean mitral valve gradient > 15 mm Hg during exercise; (3) asymptomatic patients with very severe MS (mitral valve area ≤ 1.0 cm², stage C); (4) asymptomatic patients with severe MS with new onset of AF. Percutaneous mitral balloon commissurotomy is also indicated in symptomatic patients (New York Heart Association [NYHA] class III to IV) with severe MS with suboptimal valve anatomy and are high-risk candidates for surgery.

Transthoracic echocardiography can help detect whether the valve has structural characteristics favorable for percutaneous mitral balloon commissurotomy. The Wilkins score captures the degree of leaflet deformity, scoring leaflet mobility, degree of thickening of the subvalvular chordal apparatus, leaflet thickening, and leaflet calcification on a score of 1 to 4. A summed score of 8 or less predicts a more favorable outcome with valvuloplasty than those with a higher score, although a high score does not preclude valvuloplasty (**Table 36.2**).[8]

Transesophageal echocardiography (TEE) should be performed on patients considered for percutaneous mitral balloon commissurotomy to better define the leaflet anatomy and to perform direct planimetry of the mitral valve. Three-dimensional (3D) imaging can be used to optimize the plane at which direct planimetry is performed. Detailed views of the LA and left atrial appendage can be obtained to assess for concomitant left atrial thrombus.

SURGICAL INTERVENTION FOR MITRAL STENOSIS

If percutaneous intervention is unavailable or the valve morphology is unfavorable for balloon valvuloplasty, appropriate patients are referred for surgical intervention.

As per the 2014 AHA guidelines, patients with very severe MS (MVA ≤ 1.0 cm²), who are symptomatic (stage D), and have morphology unfavorable for percutaneous mitral balloon commissurotomy should be considered for mitral valve repair or replacement.[5]

If a patient with *severe* (mitral valve area ≤ 1.5 cm²) or *moderate* (mitral valve area 1.6 to 2.0 cm²) MS is undergoing a cardiac surgery for other operative indications (eg, aortic valve disease, coronary artery disease [CAD], tricuspid regurgitation [TR], aortic aneurysm), *concomitant* mitral valve surgery is recommended.

Mitral valve surgery and excision of the left atrial appendage may be considered for patients with severe MS who have had recurrent embolic events while receiving adequate anticoagulation.

PROGNOSIS OF MITRAL STENOSIS

AF, LA thrombus formation, and systemic thromboembolism (such as ischemic stroke) are important contributors to morbidity and mortality of MS.

TABLE 36.2	The Wilkins Score/Mitral Valvuloplasty Score[8]			
GRADE	**MOBILITY**	**SUBVALVULAR THICKENING**	**THICKENING**	**CALCIFICATION**
1	Highly mobile valve with only leaflet tips restricted	Minimal thickening just below the mitral leaflets	Leaflets near normal in thickness (4–5 mm)	Single area of increased echo brightness
2	Leaflet mid and base portions have normal mobility	Thickening of chordal structures extending up to one-third of the chordal length	Mid leaflets normal, considering thickening of margins (5–8 mm)	Scattered areas of brightness confined to leaflet margins
3	Valve continues to move forward in diastole, mainly from the base	Thickening extending to the distal third of the chords	Thickening extending through the entire leaflet (5–8 mm)	Brightness extending into the mid portion of the leaflets
4	No or minimal forward movement of the leaflets in diastole	Extensive thickening and shortening of all chordal structures extending down to the papillary muscles	Considerable thickening of all leaflet tissue (>8–10 mm)	Extensive brightness throughout much of the leaflet tissue

Mitral valve score = leaflet mobility + valve thickening + calcification + subvalvular thickening. Each item is graded from 1 to 4 to yield a score from 4 to 16. A score of 8 or less predicts a more favorable outcome than those with a higher score, but higher scores do not preclude mitral valvuloplasty.

IMPACT ON PREGNANCY

Often pregnancy is the first time that a patient with rheumatic MS becomes symptomatic due to a physiologic increase in intravascular volume, cardiac output, and heart rate. Percutaneous mitral balloon commissurotomy can be performed during pregnancy, but diagnosis and treatment before pregnancy is ideal.

MITRAL REGURGITATION

ETIOLOGY AND PATHOPHYSIOLOGY

Mitral regurgitation (MR), also known as mitral insufficiency or mitral incompetence, is one of the most common acquired valvular heart diseases. MR is a disorder where the mitral valve does not close properly during the systolic phase. Its onset may be acute or chronic, and the etiology can stem from any process that disturbs the architecture of the mitral valve apparatus.

Failure of any component of the mitral valve apparatus can result in failure of leaflet coaptation and regurgitation of blood during systole into the LA rather than being ejected out of the left ventricular outflow tract, across to the aortic valve into the systemic circulation to perfuse important organs.

Defining the etiology of MR is important because it influences the management and prognosis of such patients. Diseases that are primarily structural in origin are managed differently than those with primarily functional MR.

In MR, blood exits the LV both antegrade—through the left ventricular outflow tract (systemic stroke volume)—and retrograde—through the mitral valve (regurgitant volume). During diastole, the regurgitant volume meets in the LA with the systemic volume returning through the pulmonary veins. The combined volume then enters the LV through the mitral valve. This process leads to volume overload of the left heart.

CLINICAL PRESENTATION

In chronic MR, there is progressive enlargement of the LA and the LV to accommodate the combined systemic stroke volume and regurgitant volume. This remodeling often prevents significant elevation of left heart pressures; consequently, it may take years, if not decades, for the patient to develop congestive heart failure (due to progressive left ventricular systolic dysfunction) and AF (due to left atrial enlargement). In contrast, acute-on-chronic or acute MR can present with flash pulmonary edema requiring intensive care support and urgent intervention.

CHRONIC MITRAL REGURGITATION (PRIMARY VS SECONDARY)

In primary MR, a problem with one of the components of the valve, including the leaflets, chordae tendinae, or papillary muscles, causes valve incompetence and regurgitation of blood from LV to LA during the systolic phase. Common causes of primary MR include mitral prolapse, due to myxomatous degeneration in a younger population or problems such as fibroelastic deficiency disease in older population, infective endocarditis or myxomatous degeneration. Other etiologies for primary MR include connective tissue disorder, rheumatic heart disease, cleft mitral valve, and radiation heart disease.

In contrast, *secondary (functional)* MR occurs where the mitral valve is normal but the supporting structures for the valve are abnormal. An abnormal or dilated LV can cause papillary muscle displacement and leaflet tethering. Annular displacement or dilatation as well as wall motion abnormalities due to myocardial ischemia or infarction can prevent leaflet coaptation. With secondary MR, restoration of mitral competence is not by itself curative.

ACUTE MITRAL REGURGITATION

It is estimated that there are approximately 2.5 million patients with moderate-to-severe or severe MR in the United States at present. Although acute MR represents only a minority of these cases, every health care professional working in the CCU setting should become proficient in diagnosing and managing this often life-threatening form of MR. In acute MR, there is sudden volume overload of nondilated left heart chambers leading to marked elevation of left atrial pressures, life-threatening pulmonary edema, and eventually cardiogenic shock.

The leading causes of acute MR are bacterial endocarditis (**Figures 36.3, 36.4, and 36.7**), papillary muscle rupture (traumatic or following myocardial infarction; **Figure 36.5**), and chordal rupture in the setting of preexisting myxomatous valve degeneration (**Figure 36.6**) and mitral valve prolapse.

Irrespective of the cause, patients with severe, acute MR frequently present with fulminant pulmonary edema and cardiogenic shock. Patients with endocarditis will present with general signs and symptoms of a systemic bacterial illness. Nontraumatic papillary muscle rupture is a mechanical complication that usually occurs 3 to 5 days after acute myocardial infarction (**Figure 36.5**).

Posteromedial papillary muscle (which usually has solitary blood supply from either the right coronary or the left circumflex artery) ruptures more frequently than the anterolateral one (which is usually supplied by both the left anterior descending and circumflex arteries).

SEVERITY OF MITRAL VALVE REGURGITATION

In addition to defining etiologic and anatomic mechanisms of MR, assessment of its severity and its hemodynamic impact on risk stratification determine the timing of intervention. The recent American College of Cardiology/American Heart Association (ACC/AHA) guidelines to help grade the severity of MR are summarized in **Table 36.3**.

DIAGNOSIS

In any patient with *chronic primary MR*, TTE is indicated for baseline structural and functional evaluation of the heart. The mitral valve apparatus and leaflets can be visualized in detail, with color Doppler evaluation and hemodynamic assessment of MR.

Severe primary MR may be marked by a central jet of MR that is >40% LA or a holosystolic eccentric jet of MR, a vena contracta ≥ 0.7 cm, a regurgitant volume ≥ 60 mL or an effective regurgitant orifice (ERO) ≥ 0.4 cm^{2}.[5] TEE is also a helpful tool in primary MR to establish anatomic structures and guide valvular repair.

In any patient with chronic secondary MR, TTE is indicated to evaluate the extent and location of wall motion abnormalities and to assess global LV function, severity of MR, and magnitude of pulmonary hypertension. Severe secondary MR may be marked by an ERO ≥ 0.2 cm^{2}, as adverse outcomes are associated with

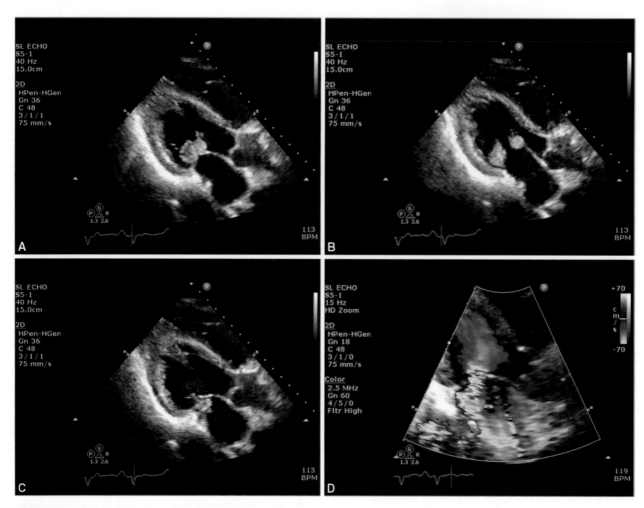

FIGURE 36.3 Large bileaflet mitral valve endocarditis with severe mitral regurgitation seen in the parasternal long-axis view on transthoracic echocardiogram TTE). A–C, Large mobile vegetations on both the anterior and posterior mitral valve leaflets, disrupting coaptation of the mitral valve and prolapsing into the left atrium. D, Resulting severe jet of eccentric mitral regurgitation.

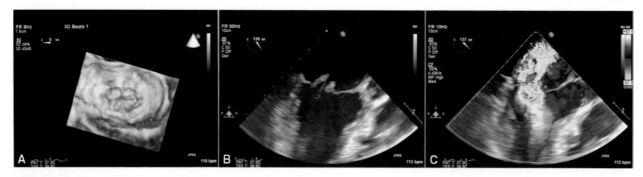

FIGURE 36.4 Bileaflet mitral valve endocarditis as seen on transesophageal echocardiogram (TEE). A TEE was obtained of the bileaflet vegetations seen in transthoracic echocardiogram in Figure 36.3. A, A 3D view of the mitral valve obtained on TEE in the midesophageal view, where the prolapse of the vegetations into the left atrium is visible at the coaptation plane. B, A 2D view of the mitral valve on TEE. C, Color Doppler of severe jet of eccentric mitral regurgitation.

a smaller calculated ERO as compared to primary MR, regurgitant volume ≥ 30 mL. The MR will likely progress due to associated progression of LV dysfunction and adverse remodeling. There is often underestimation of the ERO by 2D echo-derived flow convergence due to the often crescentic shape of the regurgitant orifice in secondary MR.[5]

In *severe acute MR*, there may be few or no auscultatory findings of MR per se; the systolic murmur is often soft, short, or even absent because there is rapid equilibration of left ventricular and left atrial pressures during systole. Other frequent findings include tachycardia and S3 gallop. Chest X-ray (CXR) in severe, acute MR routinely shows signs of

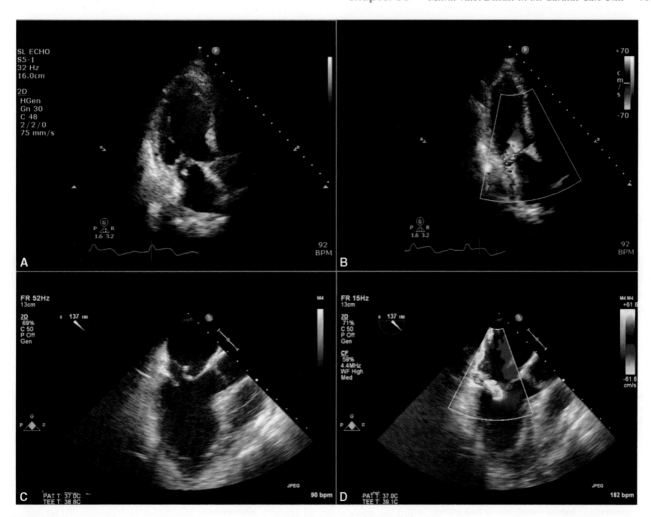

FIGURE 36.5 Flail mitral valve with papillary muscle rupture from inferior myocardial infarction (MI). A, A transthoracic echo image of the mitral valve in the apical five-chamber view. A density can be seen prolapsing into the left atrium, which was confirmed to be a papillary muscle during cardiac surgery. B, The same view with eccentric severe mitral regurgitation. C and D, Transesophageal echo images in the midesophageal view where the prolapse of the ruptured papillary muscle is evident.

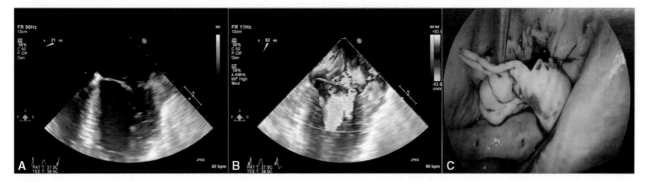

FIGURE 36.6 A and B, Midesophageal views on TEE. A myxomatous mitral valve can be seen with severe mitral regurgitation and flail posterior mitral valve (primarily P2). C, The flail leaflet as seen in the operating room during mitral valve surgery.

pulmonary congestion. ECG may show tachycardia; there may also be signs of myocardial infarction when acute MR is caused by papillary muscle rupture. Transthoracic and transesophageal echocardiography are the primary means of evaluating MR. Echocardiography can establish the etiology, mechanism, and severity of MR.

ECHOCARDIOGRAPHY FINDINGS

Echocardiography has several important roles in MR: (1) Evaluation of the etiology of MR; (2) Grading the severity of MR; (3) Assessment of its impact on overall cardiac function, especially left ventricular function; (4) Guidance for further management, including timing of surgical intervention. TTE is the modality of choice for evaluation

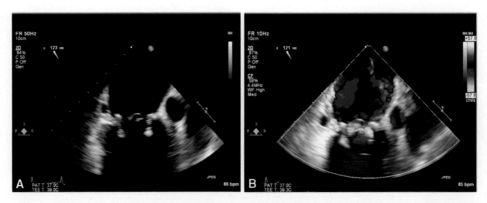

FIGURE 36.7 A, A transesophageal echo at the midesophageal position where a bioprosthetic mitral valve has a soft tissue echo density. This was prosthetic valve endocarditis. B, Associated moderate eccentric paravalvular mitral regurgitation that resulted from destruction of the valve.

TABLE 36.3	Stages of MR Per the ACC/AHA Guidelines[5]			
STAGE/ DEFINITION	**VALVE ANATOMY**	**VALVE HEMODYNAMICS**[a]	**HEMODYNAMIC CONSEQUENCES**	**SYMPTOMS**
Stage A: at risk of MR	Mild mitral valve prolapse with normal coaptation Mild valve thickening and leaflet restriction	No MR jet or small central jet area < 20% LA on Doppler Small vena contracta < 0.3 cm	None	None
Stage B: progressive MR	Severe mitral valve prolapse with normal coaptation Rheumatic valve changes with leaflet restriction and loss of central coaptation Prior IE	Central jet MR 20%–40% LA or late systolic eccentric jet MR Vena contracta < 0.7 cm Regurgitant volume < 60 mL Regurgitant fraction < 50% ERO < 0.40 cm² Angiographic grade 1–2+	Mild LA enlargement No LV enlargement Normal pulmonary pressure	None
Stage C: asymptomatic severe MR	Severe mitral valve prolapse with loss of coaptation or flail leaflet Rheumatic valve changes with leaflet restriction and loss of central coaptation Prior IE Thickening of leaflets with radiation heart disease	Central jet MR > 40% LA or holosystolic eccentric jet MR Vena contracta ≥ 0.7 cm Regurgitant volume ≥ 60 mL Regurgitant fraction ≥ 50% ERO ≥ 0.40 cm² Angiographic grade 3–4+	Moderate or severe LA enlargement LV enlargement Pulmonary hypertension may be present at rest or with exercise C1: LVEF > 60% and LVESD < 40 mm C2: LVEF ≤ 60% and LVESD ≥ 40 mm	None
Stage D: symptomatic severe MR	Severe mitral valve prolapse with loss of coaptation or flail leaflet Rheumatic valve changes with leaflet restriction and loss of central coaptation Prior IE Thickening of leaflets with radiation heart disease	Central jet MR > 40% LA or holosystolic eccentric jet MR Vena contracta ≥ 0.7 cm Regurgitant volume ≥ 60 mL Regurgitant fraction ≥ 50% ERO ≥ 0.40 cm² Angiographic grade 3–4+	Moderate or severe LA enlargement LV enlargement Pulmonary hypertension present	Decreased exercise tolerance Exertional dyspnea

[a]Several valve hemodynamic criteria are provided for assessment of MR severity, but not all criteria for each category are present in each patient. Categorization of MR severity as mild, moderate, or severe depends on data quality and integration of these parameters in conjunction with other clinical evidence.

ERO, effective regurgitant orifice; IE, infective endocarditis; LA, left atrium/atrial; LV, left ventricular; LVEF, left ventricular ejection fraction; LVESD, left ventricular end-systolic dimension; MR, mitral regurgitation.

and follow-up of MR and global cardiac function. TEE plays an important role when differences exist between clinical assessment and TTE findings, or when mitral valve surgery is needed. Defining the etiology of MR is important because this influences management and prognosis of such patients. Diseases that are primarily structural in origin are managed differently as compared with functional MR.

TREATMENT

There are different treatment options based on the MR type. As described earlier, *chronic primary MR* is mainly due to a dysfunctional valve. A prolonged and severe chronic primary MR will cause subsequent volume overload, myocardial damage, HF, and eventual death. Hence, correction of the MR in this group is "curative" and every effort should be made to repair the valve.

However, if it is the *chronic secondary type*, MR is secondary to myocardial disease (ie, ischemic, nonischemic, and idiopathic myocardial diseases; severe LV dysfunction, etc.). Hence, mitral valve repair by itself is not curative. Thus, efforts should be focused on treatment of the causes of chronic secondary MR such as revascularization or treating other underlying medical conditions as well as management of HF (ie, standard guideline-directed medical therapy for HF [including ACE inhibitors, ARBs, β-blockers, and/or aldosterone antagonists as indicated], and cardiac resynchronization therapy with biventricular pacing for symptomatic patients who meet the indications for device therapy). Mitral valve surgery could be considered in patients with severe and chronic secondary MR who are undergoing other cardiac surgery like coronary artery bypass grafting (CABG) or aortic valve replacement (AVR), as well as severely symptomatic patients with persistent symptoms despite optimal guideline-directed medical therapy for HF.

Severe acute MR is a life-threatening medical emergency that requires the highest level of care in the CCU. Acute events such as an ST elevation myocardial infarction can lead to disruption of normal mitral valve anatomy, such as rupture of a mitral valve papillary muscle. Such a mechanical complication leads to an incompetent mitral valve, severe MR, heart failure, and possibly requirement of intubation to provide respiratory support and intravenous medications to provide intensive medical therapy.

Endotracheal intubation, oxygen administration, and diuretic therapy are used to treat pulmonary edema. Afterload reduction may be achieved with the use of intravenous vasodilators (such as nitroprusside). Disease-specific therapies, if available, should also be administered (such as coronary revascularization and anti-ischemic medical therapy).

CARPENTIER'S SURGICAL CLASSIFICATION OF MITRAL VALVE PATHOLOGY

Carpentier's surgical classification of mitral valve pathology merits discussion as one works with cardiac surgery colleagues to characterize the mitral valve. Carpentier divided MR into three categories based on the opening and closing motions of both leaflets:

A. Type I, annular dilatation: Type I MR occurs despite normal leaflet motion. This can be due to annular dilatation seen in dilated cardiomyopathy.
B. Type II, excessive leaflet motion: Type II regurgitation refers to MR that occurs because of leaflet prolapse. This may be due to simple elongation of the leaflets, with prolapse into the LA.
C. Type IIIa refers to valvular and subvalvular thickening that can restrict mitral leaflet motion. Mitral annular calcification and thickening of the subvalvular apparatus are seen with increasing age, or as the sequelae of RHD.
D. Type IIIb, restricted leaflet motion: When leaflet motion is restricted, with displacement of the papillary muscles, this is referred to as Type IIIb MR. The most common culprit is dilated cardiomyopathy, where enlargement of left ventricular chamber is accompanied by elongation of papillary muscles

and their displacement toward the apex, relative to the mitral valve leaflets.

PERCUTANEOUS INTERVENTIONAL THERAPY AND MITRAL VALVE SURGERY

Severe acute MR often requires percutaneous insertion of the intra-aortic balloon pump (IABP), which is threaded through the femoral artery into the descending thoracic aorta with its tip just distal to the origin of the left subclavian artery. Significant coexisting aortic regurgitation is a contraindication for IABP insertion. IABP and the medical therapies described in Chapters 17 and 19 are usually only palliative.

The patient may require urgent surgery to repair or replace the mitral valve. For the first time, the 2014 ACC/AHA Guidelines incorporated percutaneous mitral valve repair into their recommendations.[5] Transcatheter mitral valve repair may be considered for severely symptomatic patients (NYHA Class III/IV) with chronic severe primary MR (stage D), who have a reasonable life expectancy but a prohibitive surgical risk because of severe comorbidities. The anatomy of the mitral valve, however, has to lend itself to a mitral valve clip.

IMPACT ON PREGNANCY

Severe MR, whether acute or chronic, is one of the valvular heart lesions that may be associated with high maternal and/or fetal risk during pregnancy. Pregnant women with MR who have NYHA functional class III–IV symptoms, severe pulmonary hypertension (pulmonary pressure > 75% of systemic pressures), and/or LV systolic dysfunction are at particular risk for maternal and fetal complications.

REFERENCES

1. Iung B, Baron G, Butchart EG, et al. A prospective survey of patients with valvular heart disease in Europe: the Euro Heart Survey on valvular heart disease. *Eur Heart J.* 2003;24:1231-1243.
2. Iung B, Baron G, Tornos P, Gohlke-Bärwolf C, Butchart EG, Vahanian A. Valvular heart disease in the community: a European experience. *Curr Probl Cardiol.* 2007;32:609-661.
3. Carapetis JR, Steer AC, Mulholland EK, Weber M. The global burden of group A streptococcal diseases. *Lancet Infect Dis.* 2005;5:685-694.
4. Carpentier A, Deloche A, Dauptain J, et al. A new reconstructive operation for correction of mitral and tricuspid insufficiency. *J Thorac Cardiovasc Surg.* 1971;61:1-13.
5. Nishimura RA, Otto CM, Bonow RO, et al. 2014 AHA/ACC guideline for the management of patients with valvular heart disease: a report of the American College of Cardiology/American Heart Association Task Force on Practice Guidelines. *Circulation.* 2014;129:e521-e643.
6. Stuge O, Liddicoat J. Emerging opportunities for cardiac surgeons within structural heart disease. *J Thorac Cardiovasc Surg.* 2006;132:1258-1261.
7. Baumgartner H, Hung J, Bermejo J, et al. Echocardiographic assessment of valve stenosis: EAE/ASE recommendations for clinical practice. *J Am Soc Echocardiogr.* 2009;22:1-23; quiz 101-102.
8. Wilkins GT, Weyman AE, Abascal VM, Block PC, Palacios IF. Percutaneous balloon dilatation of the mitral valve: an analysis of echocardiographic variables related to outcome and the mechanism of dilatation. *Br Heart J.* 1988;60:299-308.

Patient and Family Information for: MITRAL VALVE DISEASE IN THE CARDIAC CARE UNIT

GENERAL CONCEPTS OF MITRAL VALVE DISEASE

The mitral valve is an important valve through which blood flows from the left atrium (LA) into the left ventricle (LV). The LV is the main heart pump for the body. Mitral stenosis (MS) occurs when the valve does not open well, impeding blood flow. Mitral regurgitation (MR) occurs when the valve does not close well, resulting in backflow of blood into the LA.

MITRAL STENOSIS

WHAT IS MY ILLNESS?

If the mitral valve becomes too narrow, it takes a long time for blood to empty from the LA into the LV. There can be many reasons for this including simply advancing age and degeneration of the mitral valve. If you have had rheumatic fever as a child, that may result in thickening of the mitral valve later in life.

HOW WILL I BE TREATED?

Mild MS may be treated with medications to keep your heart rate from beating too rapidly because this gives time for blood to drain from the LA into the LV. If MS becomes severe, and you have symptoms such as severe shortness of breath or heart failure, you may be referred for mitral balloon commissurotomy (also referred to as a mitral valvuloplasty). In this procedure, a balloon on a catheter is used to open up the mitral valve further through your leg in the cardiac catheterization laboratory. If your MS cannot be treated with mitral balloon commissurotomy, you may be referred for mitral valve surgery performed by a cardiac surgeon.

WHAT IF I AM PREGNANT OR THINKING OF BECOMING PREGNANT?

If you have mild MS, you may be able to work with your physician during your pregnancy. If, however, you have severe MS, the degree of volume overload that you experience during pregnancy may put you in danger of developing severe shortness of breath and heart failure. Management of your MS and seeing your cardiologist is prudent and you may have to delay pregnancy until the narrowing of your mitral valve is relieved.

MITRAL REGURGITATION

WHAT IS MY ILLNESS?

MR describes a leaky mitral valve that results in backflow of blood from the LV into the LA. In primary MR, there is a problem with the mitral valve. Common causes of primary MR include mitral prolapse due to myxomatous degeneration in a younger population or problems such as fibroelastic deficiency disease in older population, infective endocarditis, or myxomatous degeneration. Secondary MR occurs when the mitral valve is normal but its supporting structures are abnormal. Sudden MR can occur from complications of bacterial endocarditis, papillary muscle rupture (eg, after a heart attack), or chordal rupture from preexisting valve degeneration. In acute MR, there is sudden volume overload of nondilated left heart chambers leading to marked elevation of left atrial pressures, life-threatening pulmonary edema, and possibly even shock.

HOW WILL I BE TREATED?

In patients who develop MR over a short period of time, such that the heart does not have enough time to accommodate the leakage, medical stabilization in an intensive care setting may be necessary. Mitral valve surgery may be needed to repair or replace the mitral valve. New therapies are on the horizon for specific types of mitral valve disease such as percutaneous mitral valve clips.

WHAT IF I AM PREGNANT OR THINKING OF BECOMING PREGNANT?

Severe leakage of the mitral valve may not be well tolerated during pregnancy. Women with severe leakage who are considering pregnancy may wish to delay it until the condition is treated, and until a long discussion occurs with a cardiologist as to their options.

37

Avinoam Shiran

Tricuspid and Pulmonic Valvular Disease in the Cardiac Care Unit

The tricuspid valve (TV) used to be called "the forgotten valve." In recent years, the prevalence of TV disease and, in particular, tricuspid regurgitation (TR) has become apparent. Moderate or severe TR is present in 15% of patients referred to echocardiography, and it is strongly associated with heart failure and death.[1] This chapter focuses on TR, which is by far the most common lesion of right-sided valvular heart disease in the cardiac care unit (CCU) setting. In addition, we briefly discuss the pulmonic valve.

TRICUSPID REGURGITATION

ETIOLOGY AND PATHOPHYSIOLOGY

TR is most often functional, secondary to pulmonary hypertension (PHT), right ventricular (RV) remodeling, and tricuspid annular (TA) dilatation.[2]

PHT (usually >50 mm Hg) may be secondary to left heart failure, cor pulmonale, or pulmonary vascular disease. It results in elevated RV pressure, which may cause RV remodeling (both dilatation and distortion of the normal RV shape) and RV failure. RV remodeling causes papillary muscle displacement (similar to functional mitral regurgitation) and TA dilatation, TV leaflet tethering, and malcoaptation resulting in TR. TR in turn causes RV volume overload, which combined with pressure overload causes further RV remodeling and TR progression, resulting heart failure, and if left unchecked, death. RV pressure and volume overload may also be caused by pulmonic valve disease.

TA dilatation may also be caused by right atrial dilatation secondary to atrial fibrillation, even in the absence of PHT. Worsening PHT and permanent atrial fibrillation are the most common cause of TR progression.[3]

Several disease processes directly affect the TV and may cause primary TR (**Table 37.1**). TV endocarditis is most often seen in IV drug abuse patients and may lead to destruction and perforation of the valve leaflets and chordal rupture, as well as septic pulmonary emboli. TR is common in rheumatic heart disease (prevalent now mainly in developing countries), especially in patients with mitral valve disease, and may appear years after successful mitral valve surgery (**Figure 37.1**).[2] In rheumatic patients TR is often functional, but may also be due to rheumatic involvement of the TV leaflets with leaflet thickening, restriction, and shortening. In Ebstein anomaly, the abnormal TV is displaced toward the RV

apex, resulting in atrialization of the RV with a small dysfunctional RV, large right atrium (RA), and TR. In carcinoid syndrome, fibrous plaques may cause thickening and significant shortening of the TV leaflets resulting in severe TR.

Pacemaker and implantable cardioverter-defibrillator (ICD) leads are increasingly identified as a cause of TR, due to leaflet perforation, interference with TV closure, or with the subvalve apparatus (**Figure 37.2**).

CLINICAL PRESENTATION

Patients with severe TR may be asymptomatic, especially when PHT and RV dysfunction are absent. With cor pulmonale or heart failure, dyspnea and fatigue are usually present. In the CCU setting, TR is most often seen in the setting of acute decompensated heart failure with dominant right heart failure, volume overload, peripheral edema, and ascites. Right upper abdominal pain may be present secondary to a congested liver.

TR may sometimes complicate RV infarction. Such patients can present with a low-output state, hypotension, and right heart failure that can be resistant to inotropic therapy.[4]

In patients with right-sided endocarditis and TR, right heart failure may be absent initially if pulmonary pressure is normal, but may appear later as the RV eventually fails.

DIAGNOSIS

The clinical findings in severe TR are usually pathognomonic. Giant V waves are usually present in the jugular venous pulse, and are best seen in the sitting position. The liver may be distended, tender, and, most importantly, pulsatile. A right ventricular heave can be felt in the left parasternal area. When placing two hands, one on the left parasternal area and the other on the liver, a "seesaw" motion can be felt. In systole, the RV partially empties into the jugular and hepatic veins through the incompetent TV, producing a parasternal descent with jugular V waves and hepatic expansion. During diastole, the systemic veins empty into the RA and RV, producing RV parasternal lift and liver contraction. A left parasternal holosystolic murmur can sometimes be heard, which is typically augmented by inspiration (Carvallo sign).

Transthoracic echocardiography is key in the diagnostic workup of TR. In functional severe TR, there is usually RV dilatation,

407

TA dilatation (>3.5 cm) and malcoaptation of the leaflets. Large TV vegetation and leaflet destruction are usually seen with TV endocarditis and TR. Color flow Doppler usually shows a large jet in the RA, with systolic flow reversal in the hepatic veins. In patients with wide-open TR, estimation of pulmonary artery systolic pressure using the TR jet velocity is inaccurate, due to equalization of systolic pressures in the RA and RV and difficulty in estimating RA pressure accurately. Spectral continuous-wave Doppler typically shows a low-velocity triangular TR flow (**Figure 37.1D**).

MEDICAL THERAPY

Patients with acute decompensated heart failure and secondary severe functional TR may respond well to heart failure therapy aimed to reduce PHT and eliminate volume overload. TR may regress considerably in such patients due to reverse remodeling of the RV and the TA. Diuretics, angiotensin-converting enzyme inhibitors, and resynchronization therapy, when indicated, can reverse TR in patients with left ventricular failure. In patients with pulmonary arterial hypertension (PAH), RV failure, and functional TR, successful PAH therapy has been associated with improvement in TR severity and better outcome.[5]

Prolonged antibiotic therapy is indicated in TV endocarditis, but severe TR will usually not regress with medical treatment.

SURGICAL THERAPY

In patients with functional TR undergoing left heart surgery, and in particular mitral valve surgery, concomitant TV surgery

TABLE 37.1	Etiology of Tricuspid Regurgitation

Secondary (functional)

Primary

    Infective endocarditis (IV drug abuse)
    Rheumatic
    Pacemaker/ICD leads
    Congenital (Ebstein anomaly)
    Carcinoid
    Myxomatous (prolapse, ruptured chords)
    Trauma (blunt or penetrating)
    Repeated endomyocardial biopsies in heart transplants
    Prosthetic valve failure

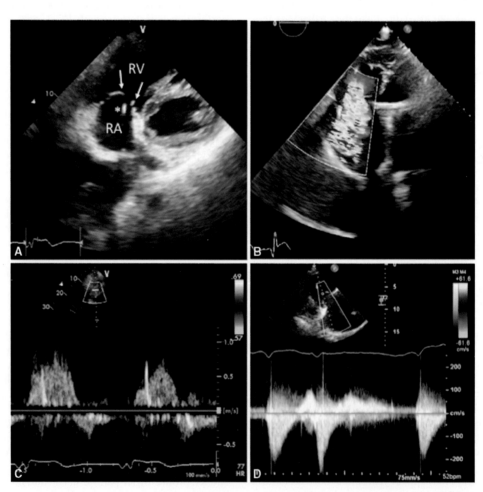

FIGURE 37.1 Tricuspid regurgitation. A, A 67-year-old woman with rheumatic heart disease and heart failure after mitral and aortic valve replacement. Parasternal short-axis view. TV leaflets *(arrows)* are thickened and restricted with severe malcoaptation. B, Modified four-chamber view showing severe TR on color Doppler. C, Pulsed wave Doppler of the hepatic veins (subcostal view) showing systolic flow reversal. D, Continuous wave Doppler (RV inflow view) showing a dense, triangular, low-velocity jet. RA, right atrium; RV, right ventricle; *, pacemaker electrode.

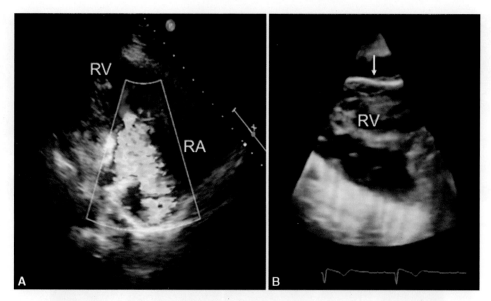

FIGURE 37.2 Tricuspid regurgitation after permanent pacemaker implantation. A, Severe symptomatic TR in a 48-year-old woman who had a pace-maker implantation with an RV lead after mitral valve replacement. RV inflow view. B, Transgastric 3D TEE showing the pacemaker electrode lodged in the subvalve apparatus. At surgery, the pacemaker electrode was found piercing and displacing the papillary muscle. TR resolved after repositioning of the electrode and TV annuloplasty. RA, right atrium; RV, right ventricle; arrow, pacemaker electrode; TEE, transesophageal echocardiography.

should always be considered.[2] TR may persist and even progress years after mitral valve replacement, especially in patients with rheumatic heart disease. In such patients, concomitant TV repair with a ring annuloplasty should be considered when there is more than mild TR, with a dilated TA ($\geq$3.5 cm) or with permanent atrial fibrillation.

TV surgery is more challenging with isolated TR, and surgical outcome in these patients used to be poor. In symptomatic patients with isolated severe TR, surgery (repair or replacement with a bioprosthetic valve) should be considered early when significant PHT is absent and RV function is still preserved.[6]

TV surgery is indicated in TV endocarditis and uncontrolled infection (persistent bacteremia despite antibiotic therapy >7 to 10 days or resistant organisms such as fungi). In such cases, all the infected tissue should be thoroughly excised, and the valve should be repaired, if possible. When the pulmonary pressure is normal, patients can tolerate severe TR after valve excision for several months or years, but eventually the RV will usually fail. IV drug addicts undergoing TV replacement are at high risk for recurrent endocarditis of the prosthetic valve if not successfully rehabilitated.

TRICUSPID STENOSIS

Tricuspid stenosis (TS) is rarely seen in the CCU. The etiology is almost always rheumatic, usually in conjunction with TR, mitral valve disease, and sometimes aortic valve disease as well. Patients may present with effort intolerance and fatigue due to a low-output state, but typically without dyspnea despite the accompanying mitral valve disease. In severe long-standing cases, cardiac cirrhosis may also be present. On physical examination, neck veins are distended, the liver congested, and ascites, splenomegaly, and peripheral edema are usually present as well. Echocardiography

typically shows thickened TV leaflets with restricted opening and turbulent diastolic flow on color flow Doppler (**Figure 37.3**). In significant TS, mean Doppler TV gradient is $\geq$5 mm Hg.[7] The RA and inferior vena cava are dilated, and inspiratory collapse of the inferior vena cava absent.

Sodium restriction and diuretics may reduce volume overload and improve liver function. In selected patients without significant TR, balloon valvuloplasty can be beneficial. In patients with significant symptomatic TS, TV commissurotomy or replacement with a bioprosthetic valve may be necessary, usually with concomitant mitral or aortic valve surgery.

PULMONIC STENOSIS

Pulmonic stenosis (PS) is rarely seen in the CCU setup. The etiology is usually congenital, and PS is usually mild in adults. Mild PS does not progress with time, but moderate PS can progress to severe PS in 20% of the patients due to calcification of the valve. Rarely, PS may be caused by carcinoid plaque deposition, with or without pulmonic regurgitation. Severe PS causes RV pressure overload and may result in effort intolerance, RV failure, and functional TR. On auscultation, a pulmonic systolic ejection murmur is heard in the second left intercostal space. When the valve is pliable, an ejection click can be heard as well. P2 may be diminished when the valve is dysplastic or calcified.

The pulmonic valve (PV) can be visualized on echocardiography using the parasternal short-axis view or parasternal RV outflow view, or the subcostal short-axis view. When PS is caused by commissural fusion, the valve leaflets appear thin and systolic doming may be evident (**Figure 37.4**). With dysplastic valves, the leaflets are thickened and may calcify with time. The PV gradient can be estimated using continuous wave Doppler. Severe PS is

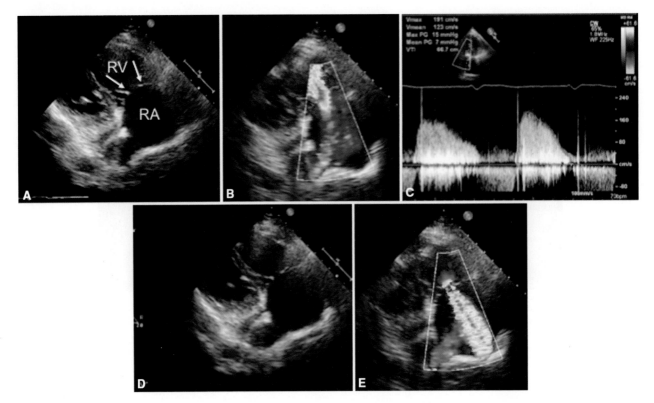

FIGURE 37.3 Tricuspid stenosis and regurgitation. A 47-year-old man with rheumatic TV disease, moderate TS, and severe TR. The patient had concomitant mitral and aortic disease. A, RV inflow view diastolic frame showing thickened restricted TV leaflets (arrows). B, Diastolic color Doppler frame showing a turbulent RV inflow. C, Continuous wave Doppler showing a mean diastolic tricuspid gradient of 7 mm Hg. D, RV inflow, systolic frame, showing severe malcoaptation of the TV leaflets. E, Color Doppler, systolic frame, showing severe TR. RA, right atrium; RV, right ventricle.

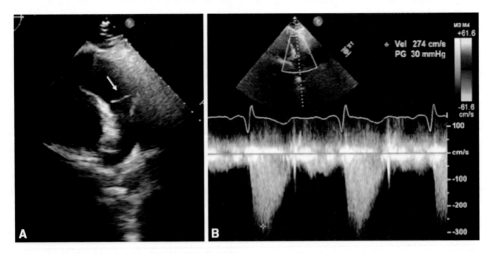

FIGURE 37.4 Pulmonic stenosis. A, Short-axis view, showing nonthickened pulmonic valve leaflets (arrow). B, Continuous wave Doppler showing increased pulmonic flow velocity and a peak pulmonic gradient of 30 mm Hg, corresponding to mild pulmonic stenosis. In this case, estimated peak systolic RV pressure, using TR velocity, was 43 mm Hg but pulmonary artery pressure was normal (43 − 30 = 13 mm Hg).

defined as maximal PV jet velocity > 4 m/sec (peak gradient > 64 mm Hg).[7] When trying to estimate systolic pulmonary artery pressure in patients with PS, using TR velocity and the Bernoulli equation, one must remember to subtract the pulmonic gradient from the RV estimated systolic pressure.

In young patients with symptomatic or severe PS and a pliable PV, balloon valvuloplasty may be beneficial. Percutaneous transcatheter PV implantation is indicated in patients with symptomatic PS (<65% expected exercise capacity) and maximal PV jet velocity > 3.5 m/sec, or in asymptomatic patients with

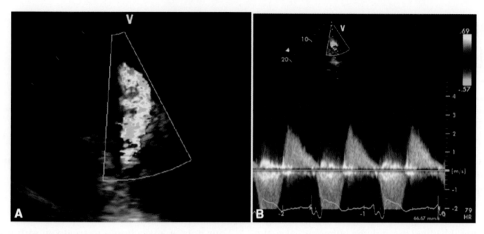

FIGURE 37.5 Pulmonic regurgitation. A 23-year-old patient with severe pulmonic regurgitation (PR) after repair of tetralogy of Fallot. A, Color Doppler short-axis view showing a wide PR jet. B, Continuous wave Doppler showing a dense diastolic signal with steep deceleration and a triangular shape. Moderate pulmonic stenosis was present in this case as well.

peak jet velocity > 4 m/sec or RV systolic pressure greater than two-thirds of systemic systolic pressure.

PULMONIC REGURGITATION

Pulmonic regurgitation (PR) is usually caused by PHT and secondary dilatation of the PV annulus or pulmonary artery and is usually nonsevere. Infective endocarditis can cause PR but it rarely affects the PV. Rarely PR can be caused by carcinoid plaques. Severe PR in adults is usually due to congenital heart disease, and seen mainly in patients with repaired tetralogy of Fallot or after PV valvuloplasty. Severe PR is usually well tolerated unless PHT is also present, which may then lead to RV failure and TR. On auscultation, a typical Graham Steell high-pitched decrescendo murmur is heard in the left 2 to 4 intercostal space in patients with concomitant PHT. Unlike in aortic regurgitation, the pulse pressure is not widened in PR. When pulmonary pressure is normal, the murmur is low pitched. The PR murmur is accentuated during inspiration, and the second heart sound may be widely split due to delayed RV emptying.

Echocardiography may show RV dilatation and diastolic flattening of the interventricular septum in patients with severe PR and RV volume overload. Color flow Doppler shows the regurgitant jet, which is wide in severe AR (**Figure 37.5**). Continuous wave Doppler of the PR jet can be used to estimate pulmonary artery diastolic pressure using the end diastolic PR velocity, similar to the way the TR jet is used to estimate pulmonary artery systolic pressure. With severe PR, the continuous wave diastolic Doppler signal is dense, with a steep deceleration reaching the baseline before the end of diastole.

Percutaneous transcatheter PV implantation is indicated in patients with severe symptomatic PR, progressive RV dilatation or dysfunction, or with progressive TR.

REFERENCES

1. Nath J, Foster E, Heidenreich PA. Impact of tricuspid regurgitation on long-term survival. *J Am Coll Cardiol.* 2004;43:405-409.

2. Shiran A, Sagie A. Tricuspid regurgitation in mitral valve disease. Incidence, prognostic implications, mechanism, and management. *J Am Coll Cardiol.* 2009;53:401-408.

3. Shiran A, Najjar R, Adawi S, Aronson D. Risk factors for progression of functional tricuspid regurgitation. *Am J Cardiol.* 2014;113:995-1000.

4. Dhainaut JF, Ghannad E, Villemant D, et al. Role of tricuspid regurgitation and left ventricular damage in the treatment of right ventricular infarction-induced low cardiac output syndrome. *Am J Cardiol.* 1990;66(3):289-295.

5. Medvedofsky D, Aronson D, Gomberg-Maitland M, et al. Tricuspid regurgitation progression and regression in pulmonary arterial hypertension: implications for right ventricular and tricuspid valve apparatus geometry and patients outcome [published online ahead of print February 11, 2016]. *Eur Heart J Cardiovasc Imaging.* 2017;18(1):86-94. doi:10.1093/ehjci/jew010.

6. Nishimura RA, Otto CM, Bonow RO, et al. 2014 AHA/ACC guideline for the management of patients with valvular heart disease: executive summary: a report of the American College of Cardiology/American Heart Association Task Force on Practice Guidelines. *Circulation.* 2014;129:2440-2492.

7. Baumgartner H, Hung J, Bermejo J, et al. Echocardiographic assessment of valve stenosis: EAE/ASE recommendations for clinical practice. *Eur J Echocardiogr.* 2009;10:1–25.

Patient and Family Information for: TRICUSPID AND PULMONIC VALVULAR DISEASE IN THE CARDIAC CARE UNIT

There are two valves on the right side of the heart. The tricuspid valve (TV) is located between the two chambers in the right heart—the right atrium, which receives unoxygenated blood from the veins in the body, and the right ventricle. The right atrium delivers the blood through the tricuspid valve to the right ventricle, which pumps the blood through the pulmonic valve, the second valve in the right heart, to the lungs. In the CCU, tricuspid regurgitation (TR), a leaky tricuspid valve, is the most common of all right heart valves conditions. We focus, therefore, on TR.

TRICUSPID REGURGITATION

WHAT IS MY ILLNESS?

One of your heart valves, the tricuspid valve (TV) is leaking. This condition is called "tricuspid regurgitation" or sometimes "tricuspid insufficiency." This causes blood from the right heart pumping chamber, the right ventricle, to leak back into the right atrium and from there to the veins in your body, instead of going forward to the lungs.

Because of the leak, you may notice that the veins in your neck are dilated and pulsating with the heartbeat. You may also have a painful liver from the blood flowing back to it, under the rib cage on your right side. Your legs may be swollen from excess salt and water in your body.

The most common cause of your condition is failure of the left side of your heart, which overloads the right side of the heart as well. Any condition that causes high pressure in the arteries of your lungs may cause overload of your right heart and TR. Another possible cause of TR is infection of the valve with germs from your bloodstream, which can damage the valves and cause it to leak. These germs can get into your bloodstream if you shoot drugs.

HOW WILL I BE TREATED?

Your doctors may choose to treat you with medications such as diuretics. These drugs can remove excess fluids from your body through the kidneys, which will cause the right ventricle to get smaller and the TR to reduce. Other heart failure medications and medications to lower the pressure in the lung arteries may help as well. If you have infection of the valve, you will be treated with antibiotics delivered through your veins.

Your doctors may decide to refer you to a surgeon for an open heart surgery to treat your leaky TV and other dysfunctional heart valves, if necessary. In this case, your valve may be repaired or replaced, usually with a bioprosthesis. A bioprosthetic valve is made from either pig or cow tissue. Unlike a metal prosthesis, it does not require medications to prevent clotting of the valve, but it may last for a shorter period. Nevertheless, a bioprosthetic TV usually lasts for 15 years and even more.

In any case, complete abstinence from illicit drugs is mandatory to prevent reinfection of your valve, which could be fatal.

WHAT IF I AM PREGNANT OR THINKING OF BECOMING PREGNANT?

If you have a leaky TV and normal pressure in your lung arteries, and you have good function of your left and right ventricles, then most likely your pregnancy will be well tolerated. Otherwise, you need to consult with your doctor about the risk for you and your baby during pregnancy.

Ankit Chothani
Eyal Herzog
Edgar Argulian

38

Infective Endocarditis

Infective endocarditis (IE) refers to the infection of the endocardium or heart endothelium, which may include heart valve endocardium or mural wall endocardium. In the United States, 10 to 15 new cases of IE per 100,000 persons are reported annually.[1] There has been a steady increase in the incidence of IE over the last decade. Despite the recent advances in medical and surgical therapies, IE continues to be a life-threatening disease. A recent study reports 15% to 20% in-hospital mortality and about 40% 1-year mortality for patients diagnosed with IE.[2] Up to 20% to 50% patients have cardioembolic complications like stroke.[3]

ETIOLOGY

RISK FACTORS

Table 38.1 summarizes the common risk factors associated with IE. In general, preexisting native valve disease or prosthetic material can serve as a nidus for bacterial seeding. Conditions predisposing to transient bacteremia (like hemodialysis, poor dentition) and causing immune suppression (like diabetes mellitus) are also important identifiable risk factors. Patients with a prosthetic valve or prosthetic material, congenital heart disease, previous history of IE, and cardiac transplantation valvulopathy are at the highest risk of developing IE. As per current guidelines, routine antibiotic prophylaxis is recommended only for this subgroup of patients.

MICROBIOLOGY

Staphylococcus aureus is the most common organism isolated from blood cultures of patients with IE. It is the most common cause of acute IE, nosocomial endocarditis, and endocarditis associated with intravenous drug abuse. Other common bacteria include *Streptococcus viridans* and coagulase-negative Staphylococci (usually found in normal skin flora). Enterococci and *Streptococcus bovis* are usually associated with genitourinary and intestinal source, respectively. Gram-negative bacilli, HACEK organisms (*Haemophilus aphrophilus*, *Actinobacillus actinomycetemcomitans*, *Cardiobacterium hominis*, *Eikenella corrodens*, and *Kingella kingae*), fungi, and polymicrobial infection account for a small number of IE cases. Occasionally, no organisms can be isolated in patients with established IE (culture-negative endocarditis).[7,8]

PATHOPHYSIOLOGY

The pathogenesis of endocarditis involves three steps.[9] First is transient bacteremia, which can be spontaneous, associated with invasive procedures that break mucosal or skin integrity, or caused by noncardiac infection. Next, the bacteria adhere to the endocardium. Bacterial deposition is facilitated by preexisting valve disease and platelet aggregates on the damaged endothelial surface and/or foreign/prosthetic material. Highly virulent bacteria (such as *Staphylococcus aureus*) have the ability to infect structurally normal valves. The third step involves bacterial proliferation and inflammation resulting in vegetation formation, valve destruction, and spread into the surrounding cardiac tissue. The latter can result in intracardiac fistula and abscess formation. Vegetations are typically friable resulting in embolization causing tissue infarction as well as metastatic infection. Ongoing intravascular infection also results in a high burden of circulating immune complexes that produce immunologic phenomena of IE (such as glomerulonephritis).

CLASSIFICATION

Based on clinical presentation, native valve endocarditis can be divided into acute and subacute IE.

Acute IE classically refers to rapidly progressive IE with acute clinical presentation. Distant metastatic infection is common. It is typically caused by highly virulent organisms such as *Staphylococcus aureus*. Acute IE can be fatal in days to weeks despite appropriate medical therapy.

Subacute IE usually has an indolent course, extending over weeks to months. It is typically caused by organisms with lower virulence like streptococci. Distant metastatic infection is less common.

Prosthetic valve endocarditis (PVE) and cardiovascular implantable electronic device (CIED) endocarditis are divided into early and late.[6]

Early PVE refers to endocarditis within the first 60 days of the prosthetic valve or CIED implantation. The prosthetic material and tissue–suture interface are not endothelialized during this timeframe. They can get infected during implantation or get seeded during any transient bacteremia.

Late PVE refers to endocarditis more than 60 days after the prosthetic valve implantation. Late infection occurs as a result of hematogenous bacterial spread with pathogenesis resembling that of native valve endocarditis.

TABLE 38.1	Risk Factors of Infective Endocarditis
Patient-Related Factors	
Age	Highest incidence for age > 60 years
Male gender[4]	2- to 3-fold higher prevalence in men
Comorbid Conditions	
Acquired valvular disease	Rheumatic heart disease (most commonly mitral valve), degenerative valve disease (aortic valve sclerosis or stenosis), mitral annular calcification, prior IE
Congenital heart disease	Mitral valve prolapse, bicuspid aortic valve, ventricular septal defect, tetralogy of Fallot
Prosthetic valves	Mechanical valves (especially in first 3 months of implantation), bioprosthetic valves
Cardiovascular implantable electronic device (CIED)[5,6]	Device/lead infection and endocarditis
Intravascular devices	Intravascular catheters and probes can cause bacteremia
Diabetes mellitus	Higher risk of IE and poor response to treatment
End-stage renal disease requiring hemodialysis	Calcific valvular disease, immune impairment, transient bacteremia with intravenous access
HIV infection	Higher risk of IE, occasionally unusual organisms like Salmonella
Others	
Intravenous drugs abuse	Common cause of right-sided IE (tricuspid valve) but can also cause left-sided IE
Poor dentition	IE caused by oral flora

IE, infective endocarditis.

Health care associated IE (nosocomial IE) refers to IE diagnosed 48 hours after admission to hospital, with no signs of IE on presentation to the hospital, or associated with any procedure within last 4 weeks.

CLINICAL FEATURES

Symptoms

Fever is the most common symptom seen in > 90% of the patients. It can be low grade in the beginning of acute IE or in subacute IE. Other symptoms include chills, night sweats, weight loss, malaise, myalgia, abdominal pain, cough, shortness of breath, and pleuritic chest pain.

Signs

New cardiac murmur is the most common sign present in endocarditis. Cardiac murmurs are heard because blood regurgitates through a damaged or perforated valve.

Vascular lesions of IE typically present as petechiae on skin or mucosal surfaces and should be specifically looked for. Subungual, dark linear streaks (splinter hemorrhages) can be seen, likely representing an embolic phenomenon. Janeway lesions are nontender, erythematous macules on palms or soles. Histologically, they are microabscesses with neutrophil infiltration due to embolism.

Osler nodes are tender, subcutaneous, violaceous nodules on distal finger and toe pads.
Roth spots are exudative, edematous hemorrhagic lesions of the retina with a pale center.
Splenomegaly can be seen in patients with subacute IE.

The source of bacteremia should be identified and eradicated if possible. This includes careful dental examination and diagnosis of ongoing periodontal disease.

ELECTROCARDIOGRAM (ECG) AND LABORATORY STUDIES

New conduction abnormalities (like atrioventricular block, bundle branch block, or complete heart block) can be seen on ECG due to bacterial invasion and involvement of the paravalvular area.[10] Uncommonly, coronary embolic phenomena can manifest as acute myocardial ischemia.

Routine laboratory findings are nonspecific for endocarditis but reflect an ongoing inflammation. These include leukocytosis, anemia, elevated erythrocyte sedimentation rate (ESR) and C-reactive protein (CRP), hypergammaglobulinemia, hypocomplementemia, and positive rheumatoid factor. Glomerular damage due to circulating immune complexes results in microscopic hematuria and proteinuria; occasionally, full-blown glomerulonephritis can be seen.

Noncardiac imaging studies such as X-rays, CT scans, and MRI can be useful in evaluating embolic phenomena due to IE (including strokes, abdominal organ infarcts, septic lung emboli, etc.) as well as exploring metastatic infection sites.

DIAGNOSIS

It is imperative to make an early diagnosis of IE because delayed initiation of treatment is associated with higher mortality and risk of embolic complications including stroke.[11] IE should be suspected in any patient with fever, bacteremia, and/or endocarditis risk factors.

In all patients suspected for IE, three sets of blood cultures should be drawn from different venipuncture sites with at least 1 hour between the first and the last sets. Transthoracic echocardiogram (TTE) should also be done as soon as possible to assess for the presence of vegetations, valvular regurgitation, and other complications of IE (**Figure 38.1**). Transesophageal echocardiogram (TEE) has a higher sensitivity for IE and its complications compared to TTE. It is recommended in all patients with suboptimal TTE images and in high-risk patients, even if TTE is negative. These include (but are not limited to) patients with suspected paravalvular involvement, prosthetic heart valves, CIED, and *Staphylococcus aureus* bacteremia without known source (**Figure 38.2**).[3,7,12] Other cardiac imaging modalities for diagnosing IE (such as cardiac CT scan and nuclear techniques) are evolving and are supplemental at this stage.

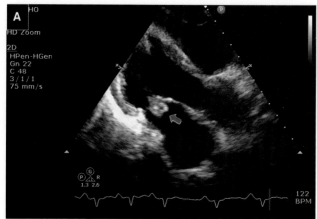

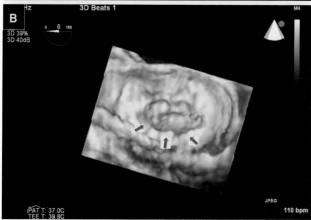

FIGURE 38.1 A, Large vegetation (arrow) present on the mitral valve as seen on transthoracic echocardiogram. B, Three-dimensional transesophageal echocardiographic image of the same vegetation (arrows).

MODIFIED DUKE CRITERIA

Modified Duke Criteria (see **Tables 38.2 and 38.3**)[13] use clinical, microbiologic, radiologic, and echocardiographic factors to stratify patients into definite IE, possible IE, and rejected categories. Current American Heart Association/ American College of Cardiology (AHA/ACC) guidelines for IE support using Modified Duke Criteria in all patients with suspected IE.[7] These criteria have been extensively validated for left-sided native valve endocarditis. They likely have lower sensitivity for right-sided IE, prosthetic valve endocarditis, and CIED endocarditis.

Complications of IE are common and have been shown to increase morbidity and mortality. **Table 38.4** summarizes potential IE complications.

MANAGEMENT

Management of IE can be broadly divided into antimicrobial therapy and surgical therapy. However, given the complexity of this disease a multispecialty management approach is needed, which includes infectious disease specialist, cardiologist, cardiac surgeon, and cardiac anesthesiologist (if surgical therapy is planned).

TABLE 38.2	Modified Duke Criteria

Definite Infective Endocarditis

- Pathologic criteria:
  - Microorganisms demonstrated by culture or histologic examination of a vegetation that has embolized, or an intracardiac abscess specimen;
  - Pathologic lesions: vegetation or intracardiac abscess confirmed by histologic examination showing active endocarditis

- Clinical criteria:
  - 2 major criteria; or
  - 1 major criterion and 3 minor criteria; or
  - 5 minor criteria

Possible Infective Endocarditis

- 1 major criterion and 1 minor criterion; or 3 minor criteria

Rejected

- Firm alternative diagnosis;
- Resolution of IE syndrome with antibiotic therapy for <4 days;
- No pathologic evidence of IE at surgery or autopsy with antibiotic therapy for <4 days;
- Criteria for possible IE are not met.

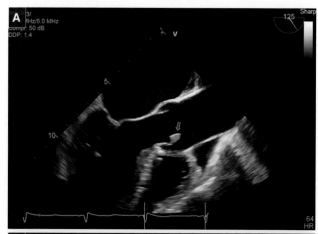

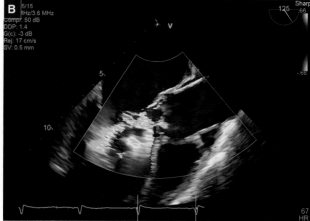

FIGURE 38.2 A, Small round vegetation (arrow) present on aortic valve as seen on transesophageal echocardiogram. B, Color Doppler imaging shows an eccentric aortic regurgitation jet due to aortic valve damage.

TABLE 38.3	Definition of Major and Minor Criteria

Major Criteria

Blood culture positive for IE
- Typical microorganisms consistent with IE from 2 separate blood cultures (*Streptococcus viridans, Streptococcus bovis*, HACEK group, *Staphylococcus aureus*, or community-acquired enterococci) or
- Persistently positive blood cultures defined as follows:
  - At least 2 positive cultures of blood samples drawn > 12 hours apart or
  - All 3 or a majority of ≥4 separate cultures of blood (with first and last sample drawn at least 1 hour apart)
  - Single positive blood culture for *Coxiella burnetii* or anti–phase I IgG antibody titer ≥ 1:800

Evidence of endocardial involvement
Echocardiogram positive for IE, which is defined as follows:
- Oscillating intracardiac mass on valve or supporting structures, in the path of regurgitant jets, or on implanted material in the absence of an alternative anatomic explanation; or
- Abscess; or
- New partial dehiscence of prosthetic valve; or
- New valvular regurgitation.

Minor Criteria

Predisposition, predisposing heart condition, or intravenous drug use

Fever (temperature > 38°C)

Vascular phenomena: major arterial emboli, septic pulmonary infarcts, mycotic aneurysm, intracranial hemorrhage, conjunctival hemorrhages, Janeway lesions

Immunologic phenomena: glomerulonephritis, Osler nodes, Roth spots, rheumatoid factor

Microbiologic evidence: positive blood culture but does not meet a major criterion as noted above or serologic evidence of active infection with organism consistent with IE.

IE, infective endocarditis.

TABLE 38.4	Complications Related to Infective Endocarditis

Cardiac	CNS
• Heart failure	• Embolic stroke
• Conduction abnormalities	• Mycotic aneurysm
• Perivalvular abscess	• Intracranial hemorrhage
• Pericarditis	• Cerebral abscess
• Intracardiac fistulas	• Meningitis
• Coronary embolization	

Pulmonary	Renal
• Pulmonary embolism	• Glomerulonephritis
	• Renal infarction

Musculoskeletal and Others	Complications Related to Therapy
• Limb ischemia	• Ototoxicity or nephrotoxicity from aminoglycoside antibiotics
• Septic arthritis	• Drug fever
• Splenic infarct	• Intravenous catheter thrombosis

CNS, central nervous system.

ANTIMICROBIAL THERAPY

General Principles

It is essential that blood cultures are obtained before initiating antimicrobial therapy. Antimicrobial therapy should always be parenteral, bactericidal, and prolonged to ensure bacterial eradication. Synergistic antimicrobial agents should be used to increase the efficacy. In most cases, especially in patients who are clinically unstable, empirical, broad-spectrum antimicrobial regimen is recommended. Specific antimicrobial therapy should be substituted once the specific pathogen has been isolated from blood cultures. It is reasonable to obtain at least two sets of blood cultures every 24 to 48 hours until bloodstream infection has cleared to assess the response to the antimicrobial therapy. Duration of the therapy is usually up to 6 weeks. These days are counted from the first negative blood culture. Temporary discontinuation of anticoagulation is recommended for patients with IE, especially if complications like embolic stroke occur. It is also important to monitor patients' renal function and liver function during the treatment because antibiotic dosage needs to be adjusted according to creatinine clearance and hepatic impairment. Patients can finish their therapy as outpatients provided they are able to manage the intravenous access and follow up diligently.

Specific antimicrobial regimens have been suggested by recent 2015 American Heart Association (AHA)/Infectious Disease Society of America (IDSA) statement on IE management.[7] **Tables 38.5 and 38.6** show the recommended antibiotics regimen for the most common bacterial species—*Streptococcus viridans* or *Streptococcus bovis*, and *Staphylococcus aureus*. Antibiotic therapy should be adjusted as necessary based on bacterial susceptibility.

HACEK organisms are gram-negative fastidious bacilli that grow very slowly on standard blood culture media.[3] Patients with HACEK endocarditis should be treated with intravenous ceftriaxone, ampicillin, or ciprofloxacin for 4 weeks.

Fungal endocarditis is rare and most commonly due to *Candida* or *Aspergillus* species. Current guidelines recommend two-phase antimicrobial treatment with surgical management. The first phase involves intravenous antifungal therapy for 6 weeks followed by the second long-term suppressive period with oral antifungal medications.

SURGICAL THERAPY

The basic principle of surgical therapy is to debride infected and nonviable tissue, as well as to reconstruct the involved cardiac area and restore the competency of the damaged valve. Although randomized control data are limited, single-center observational studies show the decrease in in-hospital mortality and embolic complications with early surgery in selected patients with IE.

Early surgery (during initial hospitalization) is indicated in IE patients with signs or symptoms of heart failure due to valve dysfunction, endocarditis caused by highly resistant organisms such as fungi, and intracardiac complications of IE causing abscess or heart block. Persistent bacteremia despite appropriate antimicrobial treatment is also an indication for surgery. Surgery

TABLE 38.5		**Antibiotic Regimen for Native Valve Endocarditis**[7]		
REGIMEN	**MEDICINE**	**DOSAGE**	**DURATION**	**COMMENT**
Streptococcus viridans or *Streptococcus bovis* (Highly Penicillin-Susceptible Organisms)				
1	Penicillin G or	12–18 million units IV/day in 4 or 6 equally divided doses	4 weeks	
	Ceftriaxone	2 g/day IV/IM in 1 dose		
2	Penicillin G or	12–18 million units IV/day in 6 equally divided doses	2 weeks	
	Ceftriaxone plus	2 g/day IV/IM in 1 dose		
	Gentamicin	3 mg/kg/day IV/IM in 1 dose		
3	Vancomycin	Consider loading dose Load: 15–25 mg/kg or 25–30 mg/kg (severe infection) Maintenance: 15–20 mg/kg q8–12h (infuse each 1 g over at least 1 hour to avoid infusion-related red man syndrome)	4 weeks	Patient unable to tolerate ceftriaxone or penicillin Use actual body weight for dosing. Target trough Concentrations (before the 4th dose): >10 mg/L: always optimal to prevent resistance 15–20 mg/L: for IE dosing adjustment based on trough Nephrotoxicity and ototoxicity are rare without a concomitant offending agent.
Staphylococcus aureus				
1	Nafcillin or oxacillin	12 g/day IV in 4 or 6 equally divided in doses	6 weeks	Methicillin sensitive
2	Cefazolin	6 g/day IV in 3 equally divided doses	6 weeks	For nonanaphylactic penciling allergy
3	Vancomycin	Consider loading dose Load: 15–25 mg/kg or 25–30 mg/kg (severe infection) Maintenance: 15–20 mg/kg q8–12h (infuse each 1 g over at least 1 hour to avoid infusion related red man syndrome)	6 weeks	Methicillin resistant Use actual body weight for dosing. Target trough Concentrations (before the 4th dose): >10 mg/L: always optimal to prevent resistance 15–20 mg/L: for IE Dosing adjustment based on trough Nephrotoxicity and ototoxicity are rare without a concomitant offending agent.

is considered with recurrent embolic events and persistent vegetations despite antimicrobial therapy and in patients with large mobile vegetations.[12,14]

Right-sided endocarditis carries better prognosis with antimicrobial therapy compared with left-sided endocarditis, but can also require surgical intervention. Valve replacement should be avoided in intravenous drug users given the risk of subsequent device infection with continued intravenous drug use. Valve repair rather than replacement should be performed when feasible for right-sided endocarditis.[7]

CIED endocarditis: In patients with CIED endocarditis, retained hardware (generator and leads) can lead to higher rate of infection relapse. Complete device and lead removal are recommended for all patients with definite CIED infection, as evidenced by valvular and/or lead endocarditis. Any patient with occult staphylococcal bacteremia or with persistent occult gram-negative bacteremia despite appropriate antibiotic therapy should also be considered for device explant. Current AHA/Heart Rhythm Society (HRS) guidelines recommend at least 14 days of antibiotics before reimplantation. Reimplantation of CIED should be done on the contralateral side.[6]

INFECTIVE ENDOCARDITIS PROPHYLAXIS

Revised 2007 AHA guidelines[15] recommend IE prophylaxis for patients with cardiac conditions associated with the highest risk of adverse events: patients with a prosthetic valve (including bioprosthetic valves); patients with previous history of IE; patients with unrepaired cyanotic congenital heart disease (including patients who underwent palliative procedures); patients with repaired congenital heart disease with residual defect at the site of prosthetic material; patients with completely repaired congenital heart disease with prosthetic material (first 6 months after the procedure); and cardiac transplant recipients with valvular disease.

Antibiotic prophylaxis is recommended only for dental procedures that involve manipulation of the gingival tissues, periapical region of teeth, or perforation of oral mucosa as well as procedures on respiratory tract or infected skin, skin structures, or musculoskeletal tissue. Antibiotic prophylaxis is not recommended for genitourinary or gastrointestinal tract procedures unless there is an ongoing infection. Recommended prophylaxis regimens are listed in **Table 38.7**.

TABLE 38.6	Antibiotic Regimen for Prosthetic Valve Endocarditis[7]			
REGIMEN	MEDICINE	DOSAGE	DURATION	COMMENT
Streptococcus viridans or *Streptococcus bovis* (Highly Penicillin-Susceptible Organisms)				
1	Penicillin G or	24 million units IV/day in 4–6 equally divided doses	6 weeks	
	Ceftriaxone With or without	2 g/day IV/IM in 1 dose		
	Gentamicin	3 mg/kg/day IV/IM in 1 dose	2 weeks	
2	Vancomycin	Same as above	6 weeks	Patients unable to tolerate ceftriaxone or penicillin
Staphylococcus aureus				
1	Nafcillin plus	12 g/day IV in 6 equally divided doses	≥6 weeks	Methicillin sensitive
	Rifampin plus	900 mg/day IV in 3 equally divided dose		
	Gentamicin	3 mg/kg/day IV/IM in 2–3 equally divided doses	2 weeks	
2	Vancomycin plus	Same as above	≥6 weeks	Methicillin resistant
	Rifampin plus	900 mg/day IV in 3 equally divided dose		
	Gentamicin	3 mg/kg/day IV/IM in 2–3 equally divided doses	2 weeks	

TABLE 38.7	Infective Endocarditis Prophylaxis Regimen[15]	
SITUATION	MEDICATION	DOSE (SINGLE DOSE 30 TO 60 MIN BEFORE PROCEDURE)
Oral	Amoxicillin	2 g po
Unable to take oral medication	Ampicillin or	2 g IM/IV
	Cefazolin or ceftriaxone	1 g IM/IV
Allergic to penicillin—oral	Cephalexin or	2 g po
	Clindamycin or	600 mg po
	Azithromycin or clarithromycin	500 mg po
Allergic to penicillin—not able to take oral medication	Cefazolin or ceftriaxone or	1 g IM/IV
	Clindamycin	600 mg IM/IV

REFERENCES

1. Pant S, Patel NJ, Deshmukh A, et al. Trends in infective endocarditis incidence, microbiology, and valve replacement in the United States from 2000 to 2011. *J Am Coll Cardiol.* 2015;65(19):2070-2076.

2. Fedeli U, Schievano E, Buonfrate D, Pellizzer G, Spolaore P. Increasing incidence and mortality of infective endocarditis: a population-based study through a record-linkage system. *BMC Infect Dis.* 2011;11:48.

3. Habib G, Lancellotti P, Antunes MJ, et al. 2015 ESC Guidelines for the management of infective endocarditis. The Task Force for the Management of Infective Endocarditis of the European Society of Cardiology (ESC). Endorsed by: European Association for Cardio-Thoracic Surgery (EACTS), the European Association of Nuclear Medicine (EANM). *Eur Heart J.* 2015;36(44):3075-3128.

4. Hill EE, Herijgers P, Claus P, Vanderschueren S, Herregods MC, Peetermans WE. Infective endocarditis: changing epidemiology and predictors of 6-month mortality: a prospective cohort study. *Eur Heart J.* 2007;28(2):196-203.

5. Baddour LM, Cha YM, Wilson WR. Clinical practice. Infections of cardiovascular implantable electronic devices. *N Engl J Med.* 2012;367(9):842-849.

6. Baddour LM, Epstein AE, Erickson CC. Update on cardiovascular implantable electronic device infections and their management: a scientific statement from the American Heart Association. *Circulation.* 2010;121(3):458-477.

7. Baddour LM, Wilson WR, Bayer AS. Infective endocarditis in adults: diagnosis, antimicrobial therapy, and management of complications: a scientific statement for healthcare professionals from the American Heart Association. *Circulation.* 2015;132(15):1435-1486.

8. Murdoch DR, Corey GR, Hoen B, et al. Clinical presentation, etiology, and outcome of infective endocarditis in the 21st century: the International Collaboration on Endocarditis-Prospective Cohort Study. *Arch Intern Med.* 2009;169(5):463-473.

9. Werdan K, Dietz S, Löffler B. Mechanisms of infective endocarditis: pathogen–host interaction and risk states. *Nat Rev Cardiol.* 2014;11:35-50.

10. Cahill TJ, Prendergast BD. Infective endocarditis. *Lancet.* 2016;387:882-893.

11. Dickerman SA, Abrutyn E, Barsic B, et al. The relationship between the initiation of antimicrobial therapy and the incidence of stroke in infective endocarditis: an analysis from the ICE Prospective Cohort Study (ICE-PCS). *Am Heart J.* 2007;154:1086-1094.

12. Nishimura RA, Otto CM, Bonow RO. 2014 AHA/ACC guideline for the management of patients with valvular heart disease. *J Am Coll Cardiol.* 2014;63:e57-185

13. Li JS, Sexton DJ, Mick N. Proposed modifications to the Duke criteria for the diagnosis of infective endocarditis. *Clin Infect Dis.* 2000;30(4):633-638.

14. Lauridsen TK, Park L, Tong SY, et al. Echocardiographic findings predict in-hospital and 1-year mortality in left-sided native valve *Staphylococcus aureus* endocarditis: analysis from the International Collaboration on Endocarditis-Prospective Echo Cohort Study. *Circ Cardiovas Imaging.* 2015;8(7):e003397.

15. Wilson W, Taubert KA, Gewitz M, et al. Prevention of infective endocarditis: guidelines from the American Heart Association: a guideline from the American Heart Association Rheumatic Fever, Endocarditis, and Kawasaki Disease Committee, Council on Cardiovascular Disease in the Young, and the Council on Clinical Cardiology, Council on Cardiovascular Surgery and Anesthesia, and the Quality of Care and Outcomes Research Interdisciplinary Working Group. *Circulation.* 2007;116:1736-1754.

Patient and Family Information
for: INFECTIVE ENDOCARDITIS

Infective endocarditis (IE) refers to infection of the inner lining of the heart or heart valves. IE, if not diagnosed and treated early, could lead to death and/or grave complications.

CAUSES AND RISK FACTORS

The highest incidence of IE has been noted in individuals over 60 years of age. IE is more common in patients with preexisting heart valve disease or structural heart disease. These could be congenital (present since birth) or acquired during the lifetime. Diabetes, HIV, or any low-immunity state decrease the body's ability to fight infection and are associated with increased IE risk. Poor dental hygiene, external catheters, frequent dialysis, and intravenous drug abuse can directly introduce bacteria to bloodstream, which can result in heart valve infection. At last, bacteria can easily attach to any foreign material in the body, like a prosthetic valve or pacemaker lead, and cause infection.

HOW DOES INFECTIVE ENDOCARDITIS DEVELOP?

Bacterial invasion to the bloodstream due to various reason, is usually the first step of the IE. Next, bacteria get attached to the damaged heart tissue, prosthetic valve, or pacemaker lead. Some aggressive strains of bacteria can infect structurally normal heart valves as well. Finally, bacteria grow and cause damage to the surrounding heart tissue. Bacterial growth leads to development of vegetation, an infected tissue attached to the inner lining of the heart, heart valves, or foreign material (like a pacemaker lead). Further spread of the infection can lead to heart tissue destruction and pus accumulation (abscess).

SIGNS AND SYMPTOMS

Most common symptoms include fever, chills, night sweats, weight loss, shortness of breath, fatigue, or chest pain. The physician can hear a heart murmur due to blood leakage through the damaged valves. Vegetations that have developed due to IE can break off and obstruct the blood supply to other organs; stroke is a well-known complication of IE.

DIAGNOSIS

Blood culture and ultrasound imaging of the heart (echocardiogram) are the two most important tests for diagnosis of IE. Several blood cultures are collected from the patient and repeated after treatment is started to document clearance of the infection. Echocardiogram should be done as soon as possible if IE is suspected. Other imaging studies like CT scan or MRI of the head, chest, or abdomen may also be necessary to rule out other organ involvement or distant spread of infection.

COMPLICATIONS

Heart valve malfunction, congestive heart failure, and abscess formation are known complications of IE. IE can also cause a stroke. Infection can spread outside the heart causing pus collection in different organs including the spine.

TREATMENT

IE management usually needs a multi-pronged approach with the help of infectious disease specialists, cardiologists, and cardiac surgeons. Proper antibiotic therapy and surgery in appropriate cases are the key for successful management of IE. Antibiotics should be started early but typically after the blood cultures are drawn. The antibiotic therapy is tailored to specific bacterial species cultured from the blood. Any primary source of infection and infected foreign material should be identified and treated. The antibiotic therapy is usually prolonged and intravenous.

Many patients with IE are considered for early surgical intervention. These include but are not limited to patients with heart valve damage causing heart failure or heart abscess formation. Damaged valves may need to be replaced during the surgery. Cardiac surgery is usually a high-risk procedure in this situation but provides the best chance for recovery. The infected pacemaker and leads should be removed.

PROPHYLAXIS

Prophylactic antibiotics are recommended for patients who are at the highest risk of developing IE, including patients with prior IE, some types of congenital heart disease, patients with a prosthetic heart valve, and heart transplant patients with valve disease. Only certain procedures require antibiotic prophylaxis (such as invasive dental procedures or procedures on infected skin). Typically, the prophylaxis consists of a single dose of oral antibiotic given 30 to 60 minutes before the procedure.

39

Chetan Huded
Samir Kapadia

Percutaneous Therapy for Valvular Heart Disease

INTRODUCTION

Patients with both acute and chronic presentations of severe valvular heart disease are frequently encountered in the intensive care setting due to heart failure and cardiogenic shock. In these patients, medical therapy can reduce symptoms of congestion and optimize their hemodynamic state, but an interventional or surgical approach to correct the valvular lesion is often required for a durable solution. Many intensive care patients are poor candidates for open heart surgery due to comorbidities. Some high-risk patients who are not surgical candidates may benefit from percutaneous interventions. Over the past decade, percutaneous interventions for valvular heart disease have rapidly expanded such that many patients can be successfully treated without an open surgical approach. Additionally, a minority of stable patients who undergo percutaneous valvular therapies on an elective basis will require intensive care in the immediate postprocedure period for monitoring and treatment of procedural complications. For these reasons, the practice of modern critical care cardiology requires an in-depth understanding of percutaneous therapies for valvular heart disease.

BALLOON AORTIC VALVULOPLASTY

Severe aortic stenosis (AS), defined as an aortic valve area < 1.0 cm^2 with mean aortic valve gradient > 40 mm Hg and peak aortic valve velocity > 4.0 m/s, manifests with symptoms of heart failure, syncope, and angina. Occasionally, severe AS results in cardiogenic shock. Medical therapy in patients with severe AS is challenging due to the balance necessary between adequate preload and afterload in the setting of a severe obstruction to left ventricular outflow. Patients treated with medicines alone without subsequent aortic valve replacement (AVR) have a very poor prognosis. In the Placement of Aortic Transcatheter Valves (PARTNER) trial, the 1-year survival of medically treated patients with severe AS was only 50%.[1] Interestingly, at 5 years all except one patient died on medical management including aortic valvuloplasty without aortic valve replacement.[2]

For over two decades, before availability of transcatheter aortic valve replacement (TAVR), balloon aortic valvuloplasty (BAV) was the only percutaneous therapy for severe AS. BAV was developed in the 1980s and initially suggested as an alternative to surgical aortic valve replacement (SAVR), but was quickly recognized as inadequate therapy due to inadequate increase in aortic valve area and almost certain restenosis within a few months.[3] BAV is performed by obtaining percutaneous femoral artery access and passing a wire retrograde across the aortic valve and into the left ventricle. A balloon advanced over the wire across the aortic valve is then inflated inside the aortic valve with the aim of disrupting calcific deposits within the valve and reducing the severity of AS. BAV can also be performed antegrade via femoral venous access and transseptal puncture across the interatrial septum in patients with insufficient iliofemoral arterial anatomy for the conventional retrograde approach. In most patients treated with BAV, the mean aortic valve gradient by transthoracic echocardiogram decreases by 50% and the aortic valve area significantly increases by 0.2 to 0.5 cm^2.[4] BAV can generally be performed with moderate rates of major complications. Procedural mortality ranges from 1% to 5% and is typically a result of aortic regurgitation while 30-day mortality ranges from 6% to 10% and is a consequence of heart failure among other comorbid conditions. Vascular complications occur in 1% to 2% of cases in modern practice. Despite favorable hemodynamic results in the early postprocedure period, many patients suffer from recurrent severe AS after BAV. Between 24% and 76% of patients have been found to have restenosis of the aortic valve within 6 months after BAV, and some reports have shown restenosis as early as 2 hours after BAV.[5] Long-term outcomes after BAV without subsequent AVR are poor and similar to those of patients with severe AS treated medically. The probability of freedom from death or AVR at 1, 2, and 3 years after BAV is 40%, 19%, and 6%, respectively in a historical series.[6]

In the modern era of TAVR, BAV has been performed with increasing frequency as bridging therapy before TAVR. Between 1998 and 2010, the use of BAV increased by 158% corresponding to the advent of TAVR during that period.[7] However, even in the modern era the long-term outcomes after isolated BAV remain poor with high rates of recurrent AS and death in patients who are not treated with subsequent valve replacement. The survival of patients undergoing BAV alone remains significantly worse compared with patients who undergo BAV as a bridge to eventual TAVR. BAV may be considered as a bridging therapy in patients with severe AS admitted to the intensive care unit with heart failure, respiratory failure, or cardiogenic shock refractory to medical therapy. BAV is most useful in patients with a temporary contraindication to AVR (sepsis, multisystem organ failure, ventilator-dependent respiratory failure, coagulopathy, etc.) or in patients in whom the contribution of AS to their symptoms is uncertain. In these cases, BAV may offer a window to achieve cardiopulmonary stability or symptom improvement that may allow for bridging to subsequent AVR. BAV without plans for subsequent AVR is not a definitive therapy for severe AS and should be considered palliative.[4,8,9]

TRANSCATHETER AORTIC VALVE REPLACEMENT

In the past decade, TAVR has revolutionized the care of AS patients because it has become an established alternative to SAVR in patients with severe AS who are at more than low surgical risk (**Figure 39.1**).[10] "High risk" for SAVR is commonly defined as a Society of Thoracic Surgeons predicted risk of operative mortality (STS PROM risk score) of 8% to 15%, unsuitable anatomy for open surgery such as porcelain aorta or prior chest radiation, or significant frailty.[11] Most patients considered for TAVR are

elderly with the mean age of participants in TAVR clinical trials being over 80 years of age.[1,12,13] Patients considered for TAVR often have multiple comorbidities that may have important implications on prognosis. For this reason, patient selection is the most important aspect of a successful TAVR program. Careful clinical and geriatric risk assessment including frailty by a comprehensive heart valve team is the standard of care before TAVR in order to select patients with an anticipated benefit in terms of symptoms and longevity. The heart valve team approach to selecting patients for TAVR carries a class I indication in the most recent American College of Cardiology (ACC)/American Heart Association (AHA) guidelines.[11] Clinical risk stratification is typically performed using risk scores designed for cardiac surgery populations (STS PROM risk score or Euroscore), but it is important to recognize that these risk scores do not assess certain factors unique to TAVR, such as aortic annulus sizing, iliofemoral vascular anatomy, and coronary ostia height, among others. Risk prediction tools specific for TAVR have been proposed but have not yet been widely adopted.[14,15] In general, TAVR should not be performed in patients with a life expectancy of <12 months due to a competing noncardiac condition. Attention to risk factors

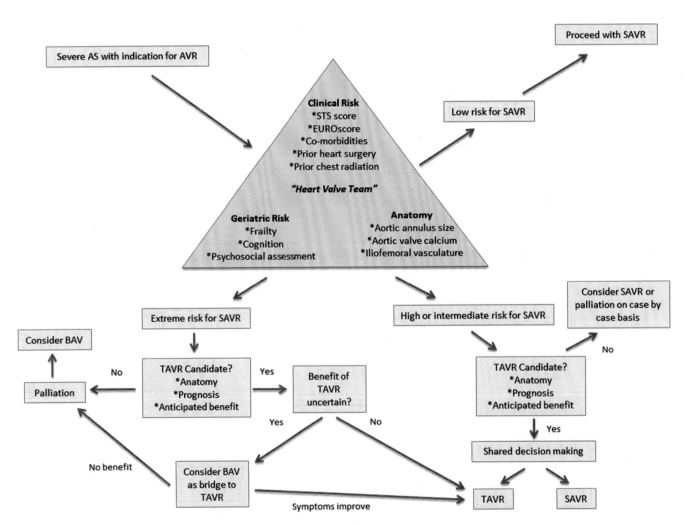

FIGURE 39.1 Decision algorithm for the interventional management of severe aortic stenosis. AS, aortic stenosis; AVR, aortic valve replacement; BAV, balloon aortic valvuloplasty; SAVR, surgical aortic valve replacement; STS, Society of Thoracic Surgeons; TAVR, transcatheter aortic valve replacement.

such as frailty, cognitive performance, and functional status is important to select patients with the greatest anticipated benefit from TAVR. Although TAVR has conventionally been applied to patients with degenerative calcific AS of a tricuspid aortic valve, it has been used effectively in carefully selected cases of severe bicuspid AS, aortic regurgitation, and within failed prior SAVR bioprosthesis as a so-called valve-in-valve TAVR.

In the United States, there are two TAVR systems commercially approved by the Food and Drug Administration (FDA) and a number of other devices currently available in clinical trials. The Edwards Sapien 3 valve[1] (Edwards Lifesciences, Irvine, CA) and the Medtronic Evolut R[16] (Medtronic, Minneapolis, MN) are the predominant TAVR platforms used in contemporary practice. Both are FDA approved for use in patients with extreme risk or high risk for SAVR. The Edwards S3 and Sapien XT valves have recently gained FDA approval in intermediate risk patients as well. However, prior generations of these valves (the Edwards SAPIEN XT valve and the Medtronic CoreValve, respectively) have only limited applications in modern practice. During TAVR, a bioprosthetic stent-mounted valve is deployed through a transcatheter system within the native aortic valve annulus (**Figure 39.2**). Unlike SAVR in which the native aortic valve is excised and replaced, during TAVR the leaflets of the native aortic valve remain in situ and are pushed aside during valve deployment. Edwards S3 valves are "balloon expandable" valves (BEV), which are bovine tissue valves deployed by inflation of a balloon mounted within the valve. The Medtronic system is a porcine tissue valve that is a "self-expandable" valve (SEV) that does not require balloon

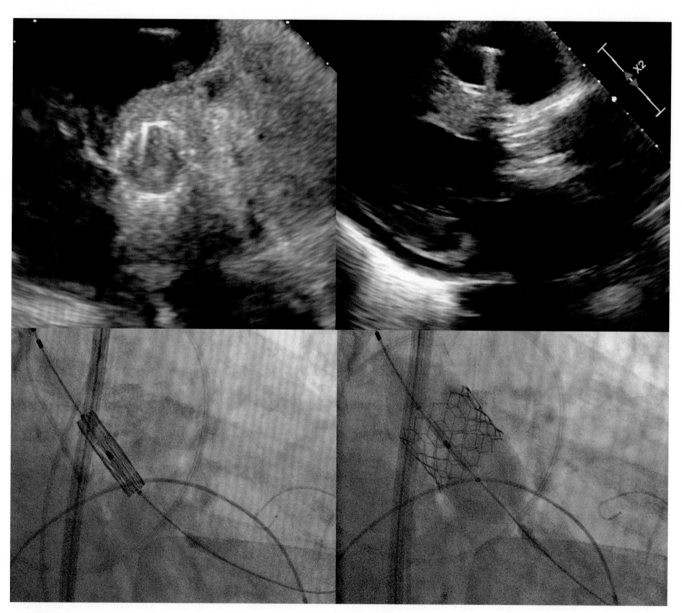

FIGURE 39.2 Echocardiography and fluoroscopy of the transcatheter aortic valve. Caval-aortic implantation of an Edwards transcatheter aortic valve for severe aortic stenosis. Top left—short-axis view of the Edwards valve by echo. Top right—long-axis view of the Edwards valve by echo. Bottom left—fluoroscopy of the Edwards valve before deployment. Bottom right—fluoroscopy of the Edwards valve during deployment with the balloon fully expanded.

inflation. BEV and SEV have distinct advantages and disadvantages, but most TAVR centers have experience with both systems. BEV may be better suited for patients at risk for paravalvular leak (eccentric aortic valve annulus, heavy annular calcification, high left ventricular outflow tract to aorta angulation), whereas SEV may be better in patients at risk for coronary occlusion during TAVR due to low clearance of the coronary ostia.[10] Only one randomized controlled trial has directly compared outcomes of the Edwards SAPIEN XT valve and the Medtronic CoreValve.[17] In 241 patients randomized 1:1 to the Edwards SAPIEN XT and the Medtronic CoreValve, the Edwards SAPIEN XT valve group had a higher rate of successful device implantation, lower rate of aortic regurgitation, and lower rate of permanent pacemaker implantation. Despite these differences, mortality at 30 days was similar between the two groups.

Most TAVR procedures (almost 90%) are performed these days by percutaneous femoral artery access ("transfemoral TAVR"), which does not require routine surgical cut-down to expose or repair the femoral access site. However, in the minority of patients in whom the iliofemoral vessels are inadequate to accommodate a percutaneous TAVR (minimal lumen area < 6 mm^2), TAVR can be successfully performed using surgical access via the ascending aorta ("transaortic TAVR") or the left ventricular apex ("transapical TAVR"). Carotid artery and axillary/subclavian artery access for TAVR with a surgical arterial exposure and repair have also been used with success. Rarely, TAVR can be performed by accessing the descending aorta via the adjacent inferior vena cava ("caval-aortic TAVR") with percutaneous femoral vein access in patients in whom surgical access carries excessive risk and the iliofemoral arterial anatomy is inadequate to accommodate a transfemoral system. Surgical access for TAVR is associated with increased risk of adverse events, longer hospital stays, and increased short- and long-term mortality due to the more invasive nature of this procedure. Since the early days of TAVR, the proportion of cases performed by a transfemoral approach has increased substantially as the delivery sheaths have decreased from 24 French (8 mm external diameter) to 14 French (<5 mm diameter) over time.

It is critical to understand the complications of TAVR that may manifest intraprocedurally or during the index hospital stay. Intraprocedural complications such as aortic annular rupture, left ventricular perforation, valve embolization, bleeding, and vascular injury can be life threatening and require immediate attention by the procedural team including the interventional cardiologist and cardiac surgeon. However, a number of complications may develop in the immediate postprocedure period. Coronary ostia occlusion may not be immediately detected and can present as an acute myocardial infarction with chest pain, ischemic ECG changes, a major rise in cardiac biomarkers, and electrical or hemodynamic instability. Coronary occlusion is typically the consequence of the native aortic valve leaflet occluding the coronary ostia because it is pushed against the aortic annulus and aortic sinuses during deployment of the TAVR valve. However, myocardial infarction after TAVR due to underlying coronary artery disease (CAD) or coronary occlusion is exceedingly rare with rates $< 0.5\%$.

Stroke is a feared complication after TAVR that occurs in 2% to 4% of cases. Most post-TAVR strokes occur within 5 days of TAVR and are related to manipulation of the native aortic valve, aortic arch, or aortic annulus. The risk of stroke after TAVR is similar between BEV and SEV and between femoral and nonfemoral access types.[18] Additionally, the rate of stroke after TAVR is similar to the rate of stroke in the SAVR arm of the PARTNER A trial and the SAVR arm of the CoreValve High Risk Study.[12,13] Embolic protection filter devices are currently under investigation as a way to mitigate the risk of stroke after TAVR, but these devices are not yet widely adopted for clinical use.

Paravalvular leak (PVL) after TAVR is a complication associated with increased long-term mortality. In a secondary analysis of the PARTNER trial, patients with moderate/severe PVL after TAVR had a 35% mortality rate at 12 months compared with 22% mortality in patients with mild PVL and 16% mortality in patients with trace or no PVL (log-rank $P < 0.0001$).[19] In that study, moderate/severe PVL was an independent risk factor for all-cause 1-year mortality in a multivariate risk adjusted model. Risk factors for PVL include anatomic considerations that contribute to poor apposition of the TAVR valve with the aortic valve annulus (annulus geometry and calcification, left ventricular outflow tract–aorta angle), prosthesis undersizing, and poor valve position either too high or too low in the annulus. Although even moderate severity PVL is associated with increased mortality, the rate of significant PVL is now much less frequent with newer generation valves and increased operator experience (<5% with both the Edwards S3 valve and the Medtronic Evolut R).[20,21]

Conduction system disease is a common complication after TAVR due to the close proximity of the aortic valve annulus to the AV node and His bundle. Patients with high-grade AV block after TAVR often require critical care monitoring with a temporary pacemaker. New left bundle branch block is common after TAVR and is of uncertain clinical significance.[22] Conduction system disease requiring a new permanent pacemaker implantation within 30 days after TAVR occurs in 3% to 4% of patients treated with BEV and nearly 20% of patients treated with SEV in early trials.[1,12,16] However, pacemaker implantation rates are lower in next generation SEVs currently being tested in clinical trials.

Survival after TAVR is superior to survival among medically treated patients with severe AS and comparable to survival among SAVR in high-risk surgical patients. In large registries from the United States and Europe, mortality at 30 days after TAVR is 5% to 12% and 1-year survival is 76% to 85%.[10] TAVR valves appear to be durable without significant valve deterioration at follow-up intervals up to 5 years. Longer-term follow-up data are not widely available because of the relative youth of the procedure, although there is no evidence to date that TAVR valves are any less durable than SAVR bioprosthetic valves. This issue will merit careful scrutiny in the coming years as TAVR is tested in younger and lower-risk populations.

A recently recognized concern is the risk of leaflet thrombosis early after TAVR. During an ongoing clinical trial, a patient who suffered a post-TAVR stroke was noted to have reduced leaflet mobility of the TAVR valve by computed tomography (CT), which prompted concern that subclinical leaflet thrombosis may be a risk factor for stroke after TAVR. In a subsequent retrospective analysis, reduced leaflet motion by CT was detected in up to 40% of patients after TAVR, although the clinical significance of this finding remains uncertain.[23] Interestingly, patients treated with therapeutic anticoagulation had return of normal leaflet motion suggesting that early anticoagulation after TAVR may reduce the risk of leaflet thrombosis. The role of anticoagulation in the post-TAVR setting is the topic of ongoing investigation in multiple clinical trials and registries.

BALLOON MITRAL VALVULOPLASTY

Severe mitral stenosis (MS) is characterized by mitral valve area < 1.5 cm^2, pressure half-time of ≥ 150 ms in diastole, a transmitral mean pressure gradient of > 5 to 10 mm Hg, and pulmonary hypertension by echocardiography.[11] The most common cause of hemodynamically significant MS is rheumatic heart disease. Calcific MS is increasingly recognized to be an import lesion in the United States.[24] In any event, MS is a far less common valvular lesion in the developed world compared with degenerative calcific AS. In the developing world, however, severe MS remains a prevalent cause of cardiovascular morbidity and mortality with over 15 million people affected with rheumatic heart disease annually.[25] Severe MS can be a challenging lesion to treat in the intensive care unit due to associated low cardiac output, pulmonary hypertension, pulmonary edema, and cardiogenic shock in severe cases. Additionally, patients with MS are often poorly tolerant of the increased chronotropy due to either endogenous catecholamine surge or pharmacologic therapy with chronotropic–inotropic medications. These patients often require correction of the valvular lesion to achieve cardiopulmonary stability.

Unlike BAV, percutaneous balloon mitral valvuloplasty (BMV), which was first introduced by Inoue in the 1980s, is effective and durable therapy for MS. BMV offers excellent long-term durability with survival free of cardiac death, repeat BMV, mitral valve surgery, or functional impairment of 69% at 7 years and 30% at 20 years.[26,27] Moreover, redo BMV can be performed with excellent safety and durability in patients with prior BMV who have restenosis of the mitral valve.[28,29] BMV can be safely performed with procedural mortality $< 0.5\%$ and severe mitral regurgitation in $< 5\%$ of cases.[25] In randomized controlled trials, BMV has shown comparable rates of success and restenosis when compared with surgical commissurotomy.[30] Therefore, in the 2014 ACC/AHA guidelines on the management of valvular heart disease, BMV has a class I indication in patients with symptomatic severe MS and favorable valve morphology and a class IIa indication even in asymptomatic patients with very severe MS and favorable valve morphology for BMV.[11] These guidelines highlight the importance of patient selection by echocardiographic assessment of the mitral valve morphology. This assessment is typically performed using the Wilkins score, also termed the "splittability" score.[31] The Wilkins score incorporates echocardiographic assessment of four parameters (mitral valve leaflet mobility, leaflet thickness, leaflet calcification, and subvalvular chordal thickening), each graded on a scale of 1 to 4, creating an overall score ranging from 4 to 16. Patients with a Wilkins score ≤ 9 are most suitable for BMV, whereas those with a Wilkins score > 9 should be considered for mitral valve surgery. Contraindications for BMV include inadequate valve morphology for BMV, left atrial thrombus, severe mitral regurgitation (MR), or concomitant valvular disease or CAD that would favor open surgery over percutaneous therapy (severe tricuspid valve disease, severe aortic valve disease, or CAD necessitating bypass surgery).

During BMV, a 14 French venous sheath and a 5 French arterial sheath are placed in the femoral vessels. The procedure is performed via transseptal puncture across the interatrial septum, and the dumbbell-shaped Inoue balloon is advanced anterograde through the left atrium and across the mitral valve. The balloon is inflated from the distal (left ventricular) edge to the proximal (left atrial) edge with a designed waist in the middle portion with the aim of reducing the severity of MS by disrupting the mitral valve commissures.[30] A successful procedure is one in which the mitral valve area post-BMV is >1.5 cm^2 and the degree of MR is not more than mild.[32] Procedural complications of the BMV include cardiac perforation (up to 2%) and transient ischemic attack or stroke (2% to 3%).

PERCUTANEOUS MITRAL VALVE REPAIR

Mitral valve regurgitation is one of the most common valvular lesions encountered in the cardiac intensive care unit. The severity of MR is characterized by several echocardiographic parameters: it is considered severe in the presence of a central MR jet $> 40\%$ of the left atrium, a holosystolic eccentric MR jet, a regurgitant volume of ≥ 60 mL, a regurgitant fraction $\geq 50\%$, a vena contracta ≥ 0.7 cm, and/or an effective regurgitant orifice of > 0.40 cm^2.[11] Degenerative MR (DMR), or "primary MR," is a lesion caused by valvular pathology (redundant and myxomatous leaflet tissue, endocarditis, rheumatic heart disease, and others) resulting in severe valvular regurgitation. In these patients, MR is often the primary cardiac pathology and symptoms of heart failure can be treated with successful valve repair or replacement. Additionally, observational data suggest improved survival with surgical repair compared with medical therapy in patients with severe symptomatic DMR. Contrary to DMR, functional MR (FMR) (also termed "secondary MR") is caused by failure of mitral valve leaflet coaptation due to annular dilatation or apical tethering of the subvalvular apparatus due to left ventricular enlargement. In these patients, MR is considered secondary to underlying myocardial dysfunction and treatments to improve cardiac symptoms require attention to both the MR and the underlying myocardial dysfunction. In FMR patients, surgery has not been shown to improve survival but has been used to palliate symptoms of heart failure in those who remain symptomatic despite optimal medical therapy. The role of mitral valve surgery in patients with FMR is controversial because it is not clear that the benefits of mitral valve surgery truly outweigh the risks.

Figure 39.3 depicts the decision algorithm for the interventional management of severe MR.

A number of percutaneous devices for mitral valve repair have been or are currently under investigation, but the most widely adopted device is the MitraClip system (Abbott, Abbott Park, IL).[33] The MitraClip is a percutaneous approach that mimics the surgical Alfieri stitch first described in 1991. In the Alfieri stich procedure, a suture is placed between the medial scallops of the anterior and posterior mitral valve leaflets (A2 and P2 leaflets) creating a double-orifice mitral valve, which reduces the degree of MR. In the MitraClip procedure, a 24-French sheath is placed in the right femoral vein and the MitraClip device (cobalt–chromium metal alloy clip covered in polypropylene fabric) is advanced transseptally across the interatrial septum into the left atrium. Using transesophageal echocardiogram (TEE) guidance, the opened clip is positioned in the left ventricle and retracted to capture the mitral valve leaflets within the arms of the clip, and the clip is then closed (**Figure 39.4**). The degree of MR and MS are assessed by TEE, and if the result is satisfactory the clip is released and left in place (**Figure 39.5**). The operator may reposition and regrasp the mitral valve leaflets up until the clip is released from the delivery system, but after the clip is released from the delivery system it cannot be repositioned. In about 40% of cases, two clips are needed to achieve a satisfactory result.[34]

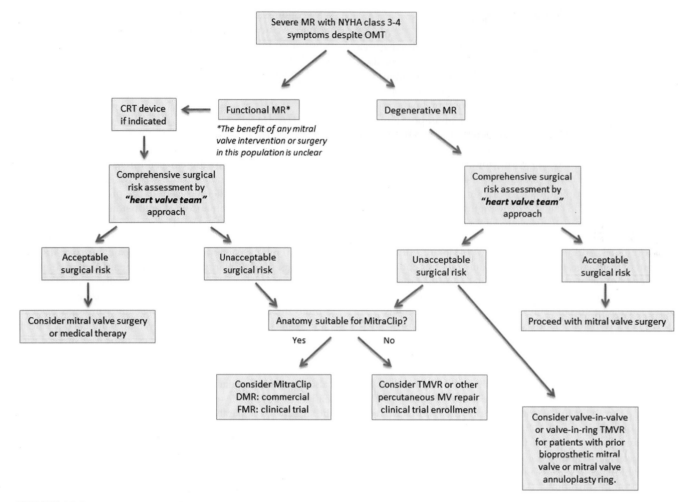

FIGURE 39.3 Decision algorithm for the interventional management of severe mitral regurgitation. CRT, cardiac resynchronization therapy; FMR, functional mitral regurgitation; MR, mitral regurgitation; NYHA, New York Heart Association; OMT, optimal medical therapy; TMVR, transcatheter mitral valve replacement.

The MitraClip is currently FDA approved in patients with severe symptomatic DMR who are deemed to have prohibitive risk to undergo mitral valve surgery. In the Endovascular Valve End-to-End Repair Study (EVEREST II), the MitraClip was compared to mitral valve surgery in 279 patients with a primary endpoint of death, mitral valve surgery, or 3+ or 4+ MR. All patients in that study were candidates for open heart surgery (inoperable patients were excluded) and most had DMR as opposed to FMR. The rate of the primary endpoint was 55% versus 73% ($P = 0.007$) at 12 months and 44% versus 64% ($P = 0.01$) in the MitraClip and surgery groups, respectively.[33,35] The difference in the primary endpoint was driven mainly by increased rates of mitral valve surgery in the MitraClip group, but mortality was comparable between arms and the rates of major adverse events were significantly lower in the MitraClip group at 12 months (15% vs 48%, $P < 0.001$). Importantly, the presence of the MitraClip did not preclude future mitral valve surgery. The clip itself can be safely explanted during subsequent mitral valve surgery, and surgical mitral valve repair and replacement are options after MitraClip. Outcomes up to 4 years from the EVEREST II trial demonstrate equal survival in the MitraClip and surgery arms and equal rates of 3+ to 4+ MR in both arms.[36] Additionally, in

the EVEREST II trial, successful MitraClip without significant residual MR was associated with improvements in quality of life and reductions in heart failure hospitalizations at 1-year follow-up in DMR patients.[37] Based on these data, the 2014 ACC/AHA guidelines give a class IIB recommendation that MitraClip may be considered in patients with severe symptomatic DMR who are not surgical candidates and have anatomy favorable for the MitraClip procedure.[11]

While the EVEREST II trial demonstrated the safety and efficacy of MitraClip in predominantly DMR patients with acceptable surgical risk, subsequent studies of the MitraClip in high-risk or inoperable patients including those with critical illness requiring inotrope therapy have demonstrated excellent procedural success rates, immediate hemodynamic improvements, and improvements in functional status.[25,38–43] Currently, the MitraClip is being compared to medical therapy in high-risk surgical patients with severe FMR and heart failure in both the Clinical Outcomes Assessment of the MitraClip Percutaneous Therapy for Extremely High Surgical-Risk Patients (COAPT) trial and the Randomized Study of the MitraClip Device of Heart Failure Patients with Clinically Significant Functional Mitral Regurgitation (RESHAPE-HF). As mentioned above, the role of mitral

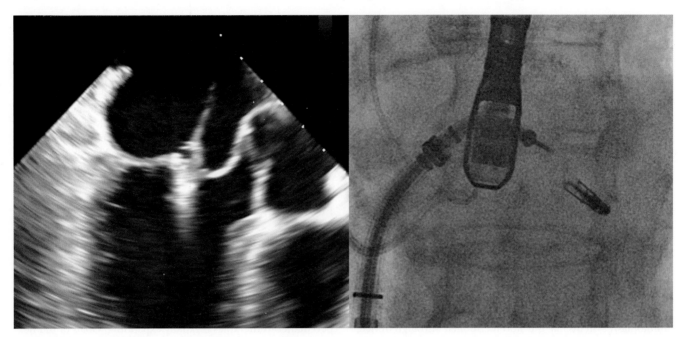

FIGURE 39.4 Echocardiography and fluoroscopy of the "MitraClip" percutaneous mitral valve repair device. Percutaneous mitral valve repair with the MitraClip device in the setting of heart failure due to severe mitral regurgitation from prolapse and flail of the posterior mitral valve leaflet. Left—Intraoperative transesophageal echo demonstrating the MitraClip device grasping the anterior and posterior leaflets of the mitral valve before deployment. Right—Fluoroscopy of the MitraClip device after deployment.

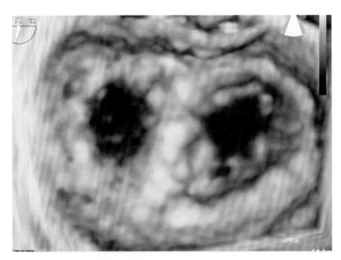

FIGURE 39.5 Three-dimensional echo of the mitral valve after percutaneous mitral valve repair with the MitraClip device. Intraoperative three-dimensional transesophageal echo of the mitral valve demonstrates the double orifice mitral valve resulting from successful percutaneous mitral valve repair with the MitraClip device.

valve surgery is unclear in patients with severe FMR because there is no randomized controlled evidence of durable benefit from mitral valve surgery in these patients, and the ACC/AHA guidelines give only a class IIB recommendation that mitral valve surgery may be considered in this high-risk group.[11] The COAPT and RESHAPE-HF trials will offer important understanding of the potential benefit of mitral valve repair in high-risk surgical patients with heart failure and severe FMR.

Several other experimental percutaneous approaches to mitral valve repair are in development. Many of these other devices employ repair mechanisms distinct from the MitraClip system. For example, the Carillon device (Cardiac Dimensions, Kirkland, WA) uses an anchor mechanism placed in the coronary sinus to create an indirect percutaneous mitral valve annuloplasty while the Mitralign percutaneous annuloplasty system uses a retrograde approach across the aortic valve into the left ventricle to deliver an anchoring system directly into the mitral valve annulus from within the left ventricle. These and other devices are currently being tested in clinical trials but have not been widely adopted in practice and remain beyond the scope of this chapter.[25,34,44]

TRANSCATHETER MITRAL VALVE REPLACEMENT

With the widespread adoption of TAVR over the past decade and its success in treating patients who were previously not candidates for AVR, there has been considerable interest in developing a transcatheter mitral valve replacement (TMVR) system. However, TMVR is far more technically challenging than TAVR for several reasons including higher-risk patient groups, larger and asymmetric valve annulus, complex subvalvular apparatus, and lack of annular calcium in many patients with severe MR that poses challenges for device anchoring. There are several TMVR devices currently in development, but these are only available in select centers on an experimental basis. Most devices were not attempted in humans until 2014 and the worldwide experience with these devices is very small to date.[25] While MitraClip and other transcatheter mitral valve repair devices can be successfully performed via a percutaneous approach, TMVR devices to date require a surgical approach with a transatrial or transapical exposure to the mitral valve. In highly selected cases of bioprosthetic mitral valve stenosis, there have been reports of placement of a TAVR device in the mitral position in a so-called valve-in-valve TMVR.[45] These valve-in-valve TMVRs have been performed with a percutaneous transseptal approach as well.[46]

TRANSCATHETER TRICUSPID VALVE INTERVENTION

Severe tricuspid regurgitation (TR) poses multiple therapeutic challenges. Most cases of severe TR are secondary to either primary right ventricular dysfunction or end-stage left-sided heart failure. Severe TR is a well-established independent risk factor for increased mortality, but the optimal treatment of severe TR remains a clinical conundrum. These patients are often quite ill and have manifestations of right-sided heart failure with peripheral edema, ascites, and congestive hepatopathy. Isolated surgical tricuspid valve repair or replacement is seldom performed due to very poor durability and outcomes in this population.[47]

There are several devices in development for transcatheter tricuspid valve repair, but none of these is available outside of early clinical trials. A variety of mechanisms has been tested including annuloplasty systems like the aforementioned Mitralign device, direct anchor-based annuloplasty systems, and transvalvular spacing devices that anchor in the right ventricular apex. However, in-human experience with each of these devices is very small and no device appears to be close to widespread clinical use.[25,48]

Transcatheter tricuspid valve replacement has also been attempted, but most in-human experience with transcatheter tricuspid valve replacement involves valve-in-valve or valve-in-ring placement of a TAVR device or pulmonic valve device within a prior failed tricuspid bioprosthesis or tricuspid annuloplasty. Such valve-in-valve and valve-in-ring procedures are rare and only described in small case reports and series.[49–51] Transcatheter tricuspid valve replacement of a native tricuspid valve poses challenges given the ability of the tricuspid valve annulus to severely dilate under conditions of right ventricular failure. No such device is currently close to clinical use. Some centers have used "heterotropic" placement of a transcatheter valve (typically a TAVR device) in the superior and inferior vena cava to alleviate symptoms of severe TR as a palliative measure, but outcomes of this approach are limited to small observational series.[52,53]

TRANSCATHETER PULMONIC VALVE REPLACEMENT

Pulmonary valve disease is exceedingly rare in adult cardiology. Adult survivors of childhood congenital heart disease will occasionally present with pulmonic valve disease in adulthood. Those who have undergone a prior Ross procedure (replacement of the aortic valve with the patient's own pulmonary valve "autograft" and placement of a new pulmonary allograft valve) may present with a failing pulmonary bioprosthesis. Patients with repaired tetralogy of Fallot may present with stenosis or regurgitation of the reconstructed right ventricular outflow conduit. Infective endocarditis and rheumatic disease rarely affect the pulmonary valve. Other rare causes of pulmonary valve disease in adulthood include obstructive lesions due to cardiac masses or vegetation.[11]

In patients with a transpulmonary gradient > 50 mm Hg, balloon pulmonary valvuloplasty is indicated with serial balloon dilation of the pulmonic valve.[25] The maximum balloon to valve annulus ratio recommended is 1.4:1 to avoid subsequent pulmonic regurgitation.

Unlike BAV, this procedure has durable efficacy with low rates of restenosis on long-term follow-up.[25,54] However, in patients with stenotic pulmonary bioprostheses or prior conduits, pulmonic valve replacement is often required rather than balloon valvuloplasty because balloon valvuloplasty does not have durable efficacy in this setting as it does in native pulmonary valve stenosis. Cases of severe pulmonary regurgitation with right ventricular enlargement or dysfunction may also warrant pulmonary valve replacement.[25] Transcatheter pulmonary valve replacement can be performed safely and effectively with the balloon-expandable Melody pulmonary valve system or with an Edwards Sapien TAVR system.

FUTURE DIRECTION

Severe valvular heart disease is commonly encountered in the critical care setting, and the management of these patients often involves an interventional or surgical approach to achieve satisfactory long-term results. For over three decades, the only percutaneous option to treat valvular heart disease among inoperable patients was balloon valvuloplasty, but in modern practice the number of percutaneous therapies is rapidly expanding. Goals of the next generation of percutaneous devices include developing smaller profiles to expand treatment to more patients, and to reduce vascular and bleeding complications. Adjunctive therapies like embolic filter protection devices to mitigate the risk of stroke are also under ongoing clinical trial investigation. In the TAVR arena, novel devices are in development with anchoring mechanisms for patients with primary aortic regurgitation and little to no aortic annular calcium. Additionally, the adoption of TAVR in low- and intermediate-risk populations remains an area of active investigation and future promise. In the field of percutaneous mitral valve repair, the coming years will demonstrate whether this technology can improve outcomes among patients with congestive heart failure due to severe FMR. Moreover, the relatively young fields of tricuspid valve intervention and percutaneous mitral valve replacement promise substantial growth and maturation over the coming decade with several experimental devices in development in both these arenas.

REFERENCES

1. Leon MB, Smith CR, Mack M, et al. Transcatheter aortic-valve implantation for aortic stenosis in patients who cannot undergo surgery. *N Engl J Med.* 2010;363(17):1597-1607.

2. Kapadia SR, Leon MB, Makkar RR, et al. 5-year outcomes of transcatheter aortic valve replacement compared with standard treatment for patients with inoperable aortic stenosis (PARTNER 1): a randomised controlled trial. *Lancet.* 2015;385(9986):2485-2491.

3. Cribier A, Savin T, Saoudi N, Rocha P, Berland J, Letac B. Percutaneous transluminal valvuloplasty of acquired aortic stenosis in elderly patients: an alternative to valve replacement? *Lancet.* 1986;1(8472):63-67.

4. Ben-Dor I, Pichard AD, Satler LF, et al. Complications and outcome of balloon aortic valvuloplasty in high-risk or inoperable patients. *JACC Cardiovasc Interv.* 2010;3(11):1150-1156.

5. Wang A, Harrison JK, Bashore TM. Balloon aortic valvuloplasty. *Prog Cardiovasc Dis.* 1997;40(1):27-36.

6. Lieberman EB, Bashore TM, Hermiller JB, et al. Balloon aortic valvuloplasty in adults: failure of procedure to improve long-term survival. *J Am Coll Cardiol.* 1995;26(6):1522-1528.

7. Badheka AO, Patel NJ, Singh V, et al. Percutaneous aortic balloon valvotomy in the United States: a 13-year perspective. *Am J Med.* 2014;127(8):744-753.e3.

8. Eltchaninoff H, Durand E, Borz B, et al. Balloon aortic valvuloplasty in the era of transcatheter aortic valve replacement: acute and long-term outcomes. *Am Heart J.* 2014;167(2):235-240.

9. Kapadia S, Stewart WJ, Anderson WN, et al. Outcomes of inoperable symptomatic aortic stenosis patients not undergoing aortic valve replacement: insight into the impact of balloon aortic valvuloplasty from the PARTNER trial (Placement of AoRtic TraNscathetER Valve trial). *JACC Cardiovasc Interv.* 2015;8(2):324-333.

10. Agarwal S, Tuzcu EM, Krishnaswamy A, et al. Transcatheter aortic valve replacement: current perspectives and future implications. *Heart.* 2015;101(3):169-177.

11. Nishimura RA, Otto CM, Bonow RO, et al. 2014 AHA/ACC guideline for the management of patients with valvular heart disease: a report of the American College of Cardiology/American Heart Association Task Force on Practice Guidelines. *J Thorac Cardiovasc Surg.* 2014;148(1):e1-e132.

12. Smith CR, Leon MB, Mack MJ, et al. Transcatheter versus surgical aortic-valve replacement in high-risk patients. *N Engl J Med.* 2011;364(23):2187-2198.

13. Adams DH, Popma JJ, Reardon MJ. Transcatheter aortic-valve replacement with a self-expanding prosthesis. *N Engl J Med.* 2014;371(10):967-968.

14. Iung B, Laouénan C, Himbert D, et al. Predictive factors of early mortality after transcatheter aortic valve implantation: individual risk assessment using a simple score. *Heart.* 2014;100(13):1016-1023.

15. Capodanno D, Barbanti M, Tamburino C, et al. A simple risk tool (the OBSERVANT score) for prediction of 30-day mortality after transcatheter aortic valve replacement. *Am J Cardiol.* 2014;113(11):1851-1858.

16. Adams DH, Popma JJ, Reardon MJ, et al. Transcatheter aortic-valve replacement with a self-expanding prosthesis. *N Engl J Med.* 2014;370(19):1790-1798.

17. Abdel-Wahab M, Mehilli J, Frerker C, et al. Comparison of balloon-expandable vs self-expandable valves in patients undergoing transcatheter aortic valve replacement: the CHOICE randomized clinical trial. *JAMA.* 2014;311(15):1503-1514.

18. Athappan G, Gajulapalli RD, Sengodan P, et al. Influence of transcatheter aortic valve replacement strategy and valve design on stroke after transcatheter aortic valve replacement: a meta-analysis and systematic review of literature. *J Am Coll Cardiol.* 2014;63(20):2101-2110.

19. Kodali S, Pibarot P, Douglas PS, et al. Paravalvular regurgitation after transcatheter aortic valve replacement with the Edwards sapien valve in the PARTNER trial: characterizing patients and impact on outcomes. *Eur Heart J.* 2015;36(7):449-456.

20. Herrmann HC, Thourani VH, Kodali SK, et al. One-year clinical outcomes with SAPIEN 3 transcatheter aortic valve replacement in high-risk and inoperable patients with severe aortic stenosis. *Circulation.* 2016;134(2):130-140.

21. Manoharan G, Walton AS, Brecker SJ, et al. Treatment of symptomatic severe aortic stenosis with a novel resheathable supra-annular self-expanding transcatheter aortic valve system. *JACC Cardiovasc Interv.* 2015;8(10):1359-1367.

22. Urena M, Webb JG, Cheema A, et al. Impact of new-onset persistent left bundle branch block on late clinical outcomes in patients undergoing transcatheter aortic valve implantation with a balloon-expandable valve. *JACC Cardiovasc Interv.* 2014;7(2):128-136.

23. Makkar RR, Fontana G, Sondergaard L. Possible subclinical leaflet thrombosis in bioprosthetic aortic valves. *N Engl J Med.* 2016;374(16):1591-1592.

24. Sud K, Agarwal S, Parashar A, et al. Degenerative mitral stenosis: unmet need for percutaneous interventions. *Circulation.* 2016;133(16):1594-1604.

25. Figulla HR, Webb JG, Lauten A, Feldman T, et al. The transcatheter valve technology pipeline for treatment of adult valvular heart disease. *Eur Heart J.* 2016;37(28):2226-2239.

26. Hernandez R, Bañuelos C, Alfonso F, et al. Long-term clinical and echocardiographic follow-up after percutaneous mitral valvuloplasty with the Inoue balloon. *Circulation.* 1999;99(12):1580-1586.

27. Bouleti C, Iung B, Laouénan C, et al. Late results of percutaneous mitral commissurotomy up to 20 years: development and validation of a risk score predicting late functional results from a series of 912 patients. *Circulation.* 2012;125(17):2119-2127.

28. Bouleti C, Iung B, Himbert D, et al. Long-term efficacy of percutaneous mitral commissurotomy for restenosis after previous mitral commissurotomy. *Heart.* 2013;99(18):1336-1341.

29. Tuzcu EM, Kapadia SR. Long-term efficacy of percutaneous mitral commissurotomy for recurrent mitral stenosis. *Heart.* 2013;99(18):1307-1308.

30. Nobuyoshi M, Arita T, Shirai S, et al. Percutaneous balloon mitral valvuloplasty: a review. *Circulation.* 2009;119(8):e211-e219.

31. Wilkins GT, Weyman AE, Abascal VM, Block PC, Palacios IF. Percutaneous balloon dilatation of the mitral valve: an analysis of echocardiographic variables related to outcome and the mechanism of dilatation. *Br Heart J.* 1988;60(4):299-308.

32. Tuzcu EM, Block PC, Griffin BP, Newell JB, Palacios IF. Immediate and long-term outcome of percutaneous mitral valvotomy in patients 65 years and older. *Circulation.* 1992;85(3):963-971.

33. Feldman T, Foster E, Glower DD, et al. Percutaneous repair or surgery for mitral regurgitation. *N Engl J Med.* 2011;364(15):1395-1406.

34. Feldman T, Young A. Percutaneous approaches to valve repair for mitral regurgitation. *J Am Coll Cardiol.* 2014;63(20):2057-2068.

35. Feldman T, Kar S, Elmariah S, et al. Randomized comparison of percutaneous repair and surgery for mitral regurgitation: 5-year results of EVEREST II. *J Am Coll Cardiol.* 2015;66(25):2844-2854.

36. Mauri L, Foster E, Glower DD, et al. 4-year results of a randomized controlled trial of percutaneous repair versus surgery for mitral regurgitation. *J Am Coll Cardiol.* 2013;62(4):317-328.

37. Lim DS, Reynolds MR, Feldman T, et al. Improved functional status and quality of life in prohibitive surgical risk patients with degenerative mitral regurgitation after transcatheter mitral valve repair. *J Am Coll Cardiol.* 2014;64(2):182-192.

38. Maisano F, Franzen O, Baldus S, et al. Percutaneous mitral valve interventions in the real world: early and 1-year results from the ACCESS-EU, a prospective, multicenter, nonrandomized post-approval study of the MitraClip therapy in Europe. *J Am Coll Cardiol.* 2013;62(12):1052-1061.

39. Reichenspurner H, Schillinger W, Baldus S, et al. Clinical outcomes through 12 months in patients with degenerative mitral regurgitation treated with the MitraClip® device in the ACCESS-EUrope Phase I trial. *Eur J Cardiothorac Surg.* 2013;44(4):e280-e288.

40. Schillinger W, Hünlich M, Baldus S, et al. Acute outcomes after MitraClip therapy in highly aged patients: results from the German TRAnscatheter Mitral valve Interventions (TRAMI) Registry. *EuroIntervention.* 2013;9(1):84-90.

41. Franzen O, Baldus S, Rudolph V, et al. Acute outcomes of MitraClip therapy for mitral regurgitation in high-surgical-risk patients: emphasis on adverse valve morphology and severe left ventricular dysfunction. *Eur Heart J.* 2010;31(11):1373-1381.

42. Franzen O, van der Heyden J, Baldus S, et al. MitraClip® therapy in patients with end-stage systolic heart failure. *Eur J Heart Fail.* 2011;13(5):569-576.

43. Pleger ST, Chorianopoulos E, Krumsdorf U, Katus HA, Bekeredjian R. Percutaneous edge-to-edge repair of mitral regurgitation as a bail-out strategy in critically ill patients. *J Invasive Cardiol.* 2013;25(2):69-72.

44. Herrmann HC, Maisano F. Transcatheter therapy of mitral regurgitation. *Circulation.* 2014;130(19):1712-1722.

45. Cheung A, Webb JG, Barbanti M, et al. 5-year experience with transcatheter transapical mitral valve-in-valve implantation for bioprosthetic valve dysfunction. *J Am Coll Cardiol.* 2013;61(17):1759-1766.

46. Bouleti C, Fassa AA, Himbert D, et al. Transfemoral implantation of transcatheter heart valves after deterioration of mitral bioprosthesis or previous ring annuloplasty. *JACC Cardiovasc Interv.* 2015;8(1 Pt A):83-91.

47. Filsoufi F, Anyanwu AC, Salzberg SP, et al. Long-term outcomes of tricuspid valve replacement in the current era. *Ann Thorac Surg.* 2005;80(3):845-850.

48. Campelo-Parada F, Perlman G, Philippon F, et al. First-in-man experience of a novel transcatheter repair system for treating severe tricuspid regurgitation. *J Am Coll Cardiol.* 2015;66(22):2475-2483.

49. Van Garsse LA, Ter Bekke RM, van Ommen VG. Percutaneous transcatheter valve-in-valve implantation in stenosed tricuspid valve bioprosthesis. *Circulation.* 2011;123(5):e219-e221.

50. Weich H, Janson J, van Wyk J, et al. Transjugular tricuspid valve-in-valve replacement. *Circulation.* 2011;124(5):e157-e160.

51. Roberts P, Spina R, Vallely M, et al. Percutaneous tricuspid valve replacement for a stenosed bioprosthesis. *Circ Cardiovasc Interv.* 2010;3(4):e14-e15.

52. Lauten A, Ferrari M, Hekmat K, et al. Heterotopic transcatheter tricuspid valve implantation: first-in-man application of a novel approach to tricuspid regurgitation. *Eur Heart J.* 2011;32(10):1207-1213.

53. Laule M, Stangl V, Sanad W, et al. Percutaneous transfemoral management of severe secondary tricuspid regurgitation with Edwards Sapien XT bioprosthesis: first-in-man experience. *J Am Coll Cardiol.* 2013;61(18):1929-1931.

54. Radtke W, Keane JF, Fellows KE, Lang P, Lock JE. Percutaneous balloon valvotomy of congenital pulmonary stenosis using oversized balloons. *J Am Coll Cardiol.* 1986;8(4):909-915.

Patient and Family Information: PERCUTANEOUS THERAPY FOR VALVULAR HEART DISEASE

INTRODUCTION

The heart is a highly complex organ involving multiple systems that work together, such as the coronary arteries that supply blood flow to the heart muscle, the electrical system that coordinates each heartbeat, and the heart muscle that pumps the blood through the body. The valves of the heart are like doors between the chambers of the heart. There are four heart valves (tricuspid, pulmonic, mitral, and aortic) with two primary roles: (1) to allow blood to pass from one chamber to the next at the right time during the heartbeat; and (2) to prevent blood from flowing backward within the heart and lungs. Valvular heart disease occurs when either of these two roles of the heart valve is compromised. A valve that does not allow blood to flow forward is called "stenotic" or narrowed, whereas a valve that allows excessive amounts of blood to flow backward is called "regurgitant" or leaky. Valves with severe stenosis or regurgitation (or both) cause heart failure due to weakening of the heart muscle and fluid buildup within the heart and lungs.

SIGNS, SYMPTOMS, AND EVALUATION

Valvular heart disease can present differently in different patients. Some patients remain asymptomatic despite severe valvular heart disease, while other patients may have symptoms of chest pain, shortness of breath, passing out, or even shock. The severity of symptoms depends on how long the valvular heart disease has been present and how well the body is able to compensate. Your doctor may find a heart murmur, engorged neck veins, fluid in the lungs, or swelling in the abdomen or legs. However, it is important to realize that some patients will have very few physical signs and symptoms of valvular heart disease and, on the contrary, not all patients with a heart murmur have severe valvular heart disease. An echocardiogram, which is an ultrasound study of the heart, is needed to study the heart valves in detail. The echocardiogram provides information on the severity of valve stenosis and regurgitation as well as the overall heart size and muscle function. In many patients, an invasive echocardiogram in which the ultrasound probe is passed into the esophagus (transesophageal echocardiogram or TEE) is needed to adequately study the heart valves. Since the ultrasound probe can be placed in closer proximity to your heart with this method, the images obtained will better elucidate the functionality of your heart valves as if having a closer look.

MEDICAL TREATMENT

Some patients with valvular heart disease can be successfully treated with medications alone. The usual goal of medical treatment is to reduce fluid buildup with diuretics ("water pills"). However, medicines cannot reverse or cure valvular heart disease in most cases. Treatment of high blood pressure and other underlying heart conditions such as CAD and arrhythmias can also help the heart valve function and to reduce symptoms because the various systems of the heart all work in concert with each other. In patients with severe valvular heart disease who have symptoms despite medications, a procedure to correct the valve problem may be needed.

HEART SURGERY

A cardiac surgeon can repair or replace a diseased heart valve in patients who can safely undergo the operation without excessive risk. In the hands of an experienced cardiac surgeon, valve repair and replacement can be performed safely and with outstanding long-term improvements in symptoms. When valve replacement is performed, either a tissue valve or a mechanical valve may be selected on the basis of a discussion between the patient and surgeon after weighing the pros and cons in each case. In some forms of valvular heart disease, heart surgery is a lifesaving procedure. However, in other patients, heart surgery carries a very high risk of complications such as major bleeding, stroke, heart attack, or death. Risk factors for heart surgery complications include weak heart function, advanced age, prior heart or chest surgery, prior chest radiation, obesity, and severe disease of other organs such as the lungs, kidney, or liver. For patients in whom heart surgery carries an unacceptable risk of a major complication, the only option may be a less invasive procedure.

PERCUTANEOUS INTERVENTION

In select patients, a cardiologist and cardiac surgeon can perform a percutaneous valve procedure. Percutaneous means that the procedure can be performed through the blood vessels by a small puncture made through the skin, so open heart surgery is not needed. Not everyone is a candidate for this type of procedure due to certain factors related to each patient's anatomy and the valve involved. Your doctor may perform testing including echocardiogram, CT scan, MRI, or heart catheterization to determine whether a percutaneous intervention will be possible. In most centers, a heart valve team including imaging cardiologists, interventional cardiologists, cardiac surgeons, nurses, and coordinators will review each case to determine whether a percutaneous heart valve procedure is possible. Currently, percutaneous interventions are commonly used for AVR and mitral valve repair. In select centers, other valve procedures such as pulmonic valve replacement, mitral valve replacement, tricuspid valve repair, and tricuspid valve replacement may be possible. Additionally, balloon valvuloplasty, which is a procedure in which a stenotic valve is opened with a balloon but the valve is not repaired or replaced, is widely available in many centers and has been used for over three decades. Percutaneous valve procedures usually have a lower risk of major complications compared with heart surgery, and may be a better option for patients who cannot undergo heart surgery due to the risk of the procedure.

WHAT TO EXPECT

Percutaneous valve procedures are typically performed in an operating room or a cardiac catheterization suite. Some percutaneous valve procedures require general anesthesia while others can be performed safely with mild sedation. A TEE may be used during the procedure to help the physician performing the procedure visualize the valve in real time. Most, but not all, percutaneous valve procedures are performed by puncture of the artery and/or vein in the groin area. The doctor will place a sheath, which is a tube through which equipment can be passed, in the groin vessels using a needle and a thin wire as a guide. The sheath can range anywhere from 5 mm in diameter to almost 9 mm in diameter. Multiple sheaths may be used for one procedure. Some valve procedures require the placement of a temporary pacemaker during and/or immediately after the procedure. These procedures usually take 1 to 2 hours. Most patients who do require general anesthesia can have the endotracheal breathing tube removed at the end of the procedure. The puncture site in the leg is repaired with sutures and several hours of bedrest are often needed immediately following the procedure to prevent bleeding complications at the puncture site. A 3- to 5-day hospital stay is common after a percutaneous procedure and varies depending on each patient's unique needs. After a percutaneous aortic valve replacement, some patients require placement of a permanent pacemaker. A few patients, especially elderly adults, may require a short stay in rehabilitation after a valve procedure, but most patients are discharged home directly. Serious procedural complications include heart attack, stroke, death, or need for an emergency surgery. Each of these complications arise in typically < 5% of cases. More common complications include bleeding or injury to a blood vessel that may require a surgical repair afterward.

Joanna Chikwe

Henry Tannous

40

Contemporary Surgical Approach to Valvular Disease

AORTIC VALVE SURGERY

PATHOPHYSIOLOGY OF AORTIC STENOSIS

Morphology

Calcium is deposited in the collagen framework of abnormal leaflets due to the shear stresses occurring with each cardiac contraction. Eventually, the aortic valve becomes a lumpy, rigid structure with a tiny orifice, with calcification extending down the membranous septum and over the ventricular surface of the anterior mitral valve leaflet. Approximately 1% to 2% of people have a congenitally bicuspid aortic valve (right and left cusp fusion is present in more than 80% of patients with bicuspid valves).[1] Shear stresses in bicuspid valves are greater and they tend to calcify decades earlier than trileaflet valves. Rheumatic disease causes fibrous leaflet thickening, rolled leaflet edges, and fusion of commissures, and eventually also results in accelerated calcific changes.

Structural and Functional Changes

The average decrease in the stenotic aortic valve is 0.1 cm^2/y. This occurs faster in degenerative and bicuspid stenosis than in rheumatic stenosis.[1] Major hemodynamic compromise does not occur until the valve is reduced to less than half the normal aortic valve area of 3 to 4 cm^2; beyond this, left ventricular (LV) outlet obstruction rapidly increases.[2] Turbulent flow in the ascending aorta may cause poststenotic dilatation. The left ventricle hypertrophies in response to outlet obstruction. The number of myocytes is fixed: hypertrophy is an increase in myofibrils, causing existing myocytes to become thicker. Concentric hypertrophy occurs in response to pressure overload seen in aortic stenosis (AS); and eccentric hypertrophy occurs in response to volume overload, for example, aortic insufficiency (AI). Concentric hypertrophy maintains ventricular volume. There is also an increase in interstitial collagen, but not much fibrosis. Initially hypertrophy (increase in LV mass from 150 g to up to 300 g) allows generation of the high interventricular pressures required to maintain LV ejection fraction and cardiac output through the stenotic lesion, despite gradients > 100 mm Hg: this is compensated AS. Eventually, hypertrophy cannot compensate for increased wall stress, and the left ventricle thins, dilates, and ejection fraction falls: this is low-gradient low-ejection fraction (also known as low-gradient low-flow) AS.

Systolic Function

In compensated AS, ejection fraction is preserved. Decompensated AS (low gradient, low flow) occurs when systolic function declines as a result of chronic afterload mismatch. The transvalvular gradient falls because cardiac output decreases, even though the valve stenosis is unchanged or worse.[2,3]

Diastolic Function

Diastole has an energy-dependent and a passive component. The passive component depends on normal compliance: this is often reduced in AS. The time required for the energy-dependent phase is greater because of impaired myocardial relaxation and decreased chamber compliance. LV end diastolic pressure is increased, eventually reducing diastolic coronary flow. Adequate LV filling is very dependent on the "atrial kick" supplied by synchronized atrial contraction and controlled heart rate.

Patients may exhibit symptoms of diastolic failure with paroxysmal nocturnal dyspnea, orthopnea, and pulmonary edema even with normal ejection fraction, and decompensate if they go into atrial fibrillation. Diastolic dysfunction may take months to years to improve after surgery and may not improve if patients are left with a significant gradient across the prosthetic valve.[2,3]

Coronary Blood Flow

In AS, the myocardial oxygen supply–demand mismatch causes angina even in patients with normal coronary arteries. This is due to increased muscle mass, which results in increased myocardial oxygen demand. This eventually outpaces compensatory increase in blood flow resulting in lower coronary blood flow per 100 g of myocardium. The increased LV end diastolic pressure reduces coronary perfusion during diastole. Increased systolic time reduces diastolic filling time. Additionally coronary vasodilatory reserve results in decreased coronary flow in exercise.

Clinical Findings in Aortic Stenosis

Patients may be asymptomatic. Most present with any of the triad of angina, exertional syncope, and dyspnea. There is a 5% incidence of sudden death. Symptom onset is closely related to survival. Clinical findings include a slow, rising, low-amplitude pulse, occasionally with a thrill at the carotids; a sustained apex beat; a soft first heart sound, sometimes preceded by fourth

433

heart sound; a single heart sound if valve is calcified; an ejection systolic murmur radiating from the aortic area to the right carotid; and a soft early diastolic murmur due to AI while leaflets become immobile.

PATHOPHYSIOLOGY OF AORTIC INSUFFICIENCY

Morphology

Pathology of any of the components of the aortic root can prevent leaflet coaptation leading to AI. In developing countries, rheumatic disease causes leaflet thickening and shortening. The main cause of AI in developed countries is annular dilatation, for example, annuloaortic ectasia caused by cystic medial dilatation associated with connective tissue disorders such as Marfan disease, or type A aortic dissection. AI may also be caused by endocarditis resulting in leaflet destruction, and calcification resulting in leaflet mobility.

Structural and Functional Changes

Acute Aortic Insufficiency

Acute AI is most commonly caused by endocarditis, aortic dissection, and trauma. Acute severe AI is usually a surgical emergency. This is because there is no time for any of the adaptive changes that characterize chronic AI to develop and the sudden volume overload results in pulmonary edema while the filling pressure increases in a noncompliant ventricle. Reduced coronary blood flow, low cardiac output, and hypoxia due to acute pulmonary results in end-organ ischemia.[2]

Chronic Aortic Insufficiency

Chronic AI is better tolerated than acute partly because of the following adaptive and maladaptive changes. AI leads to both volume overload, because of the regurgitant fraction, and pressure overload, because of the increased volume of blood ejected. Volume overload causes eccentric hypertrophy and LV dilatation. Pressure overload results in concentric hypertrophy: the same increase in myofibrils and interstitial collagen described in AS occurs in AI. Ventricular enlargement produces a larger total stroke volume (up to 10 L/min), all of which enters the aorta during systole: this is compensated AI and the resultant increase in pulse pressure causes systemic hypertension and a large increase in LV afterload. LV compliance decreases and diastolic function is compromised as hypertrophy progresses. Eventually LV end diastolic pressures and left atrial pressures begin to increase: pulmonary hypertension and congestive cardiac failure is a feature of decompensated AI as well as acute AI. Finally, as myocytes are stretched beyond their limit of effective contraction, LV systolic function decreases, and the rate of increased LV end systolic diameter accelerates to about 7 mm/y. Coronary perfusion may be reduced for the same reasons as in AS.

Clinical Findings in Aortic Regurgitation

Acute AI is characterized by cardiovascular collapse and the symptoms of pulmonary edema. Chronic AI is usually asymptomatic until LV function is significantly impaired. Symptoms eventually include angina (because of myocardial oxygen supply–demand mismatch caused by the combination of increased oxygen consumption due to ventricular hypertrophy and contractility, and decreased coronary reserve caused by the fall in diastolic pressure gradient between the aorta and left ventricle), effort dyspnea, and the symptoms of congestive cardiac failure. Fatigue may predominate.

Clinical signs include a large-amplitude collapsing or "water-hammer" pulse with a rapid upstroke; Quincke sign (capillary pulsation visible in the nail bed); Corrigan sign (visible pulsation in the neck); de Musset sign (head nodding as a result of arterial pulsation); Duroziez sign ("pistol-shot" femorals); a sustained, laterally displaced apex beat; a single second heart sound, with third heart sound; an early diastolic murmur maximal at lower left sternal edge radiating to the apex and axilla; an ejection systolic murmur may be present as well as a late diastolic murmur (Austin Flint) from fluttering of the anterior mitral leaflet as it is hit by the regurgitant jet.[2,3]

Indications for Aortic Valve Surgery

Severe AS may be defined as an aortic valve area < 1 cm^2. If the mean transvalvular gradient is over 40 mm Hg, then stenosis is severe, but severe AS may be present at lower gradients if the patient has poor LV function (see the above description of low-gradient low-flow AS).

The presence of symptoms or LV systolic dysfunction are both class I indications for aortic valve replacement in both AS and AI (**Figures 40.1 and 40.2**).

Indications for Aortic Valve Surgery

Class I indications for aortic valve replacement in AS[1]:

- Symptomatic severe AS (aortic valve area < 1.0 cm^2 or mean gradient > 40 mm Hg);
- Patients with moderate AS undergoing other cardiac surgery;
- Asymptomatic patients with severe AS and LV systolic dysfunction.

Class IIb indications for aortic valve replacement in AS:

- Asymptomatic AS and abnormal response to exercise (eg, hypotension, symptoms), or aortic valve area < 0.6 cm^2/mean gradient > 60 mm Hg if low surgical risk, or calcification/coronary disease implying rapid progression risk.

Class I indications for aortic valve replacement in AI:

- Acute severe AI, symptomatic severe AI;
- Severe AI undergoing coronary artery bypass grafting or other valve surgery;
- Severe asymptomatic AI and EF $<50\%$

Class IIa indications for aortic valve replacement in AI:

- Severe AI and LV end systolic diameter > 50 mm or LV end diastolic diameter > 65 mm

Class IIb indications for aortic valve replacement in AI:

- Severe AI with normal ejection fraction and LV end systolic diameter > 50 mm or LV end diastolic diameter > 65 mm and progressive dilatation or declining exercise tolerance;
- Indications for aortic valve replacement in endocarditis;
- Endocarditis and severe AI or AS resulting in heart failure, heart block, annular abscess, destructive penetrating lesion (class I); recurrent emboli and vegetation despite appropriate antibiotics, fungal or other virulent organism (class IIa), or large, mobile vegetation > 10 mm (class IIb).

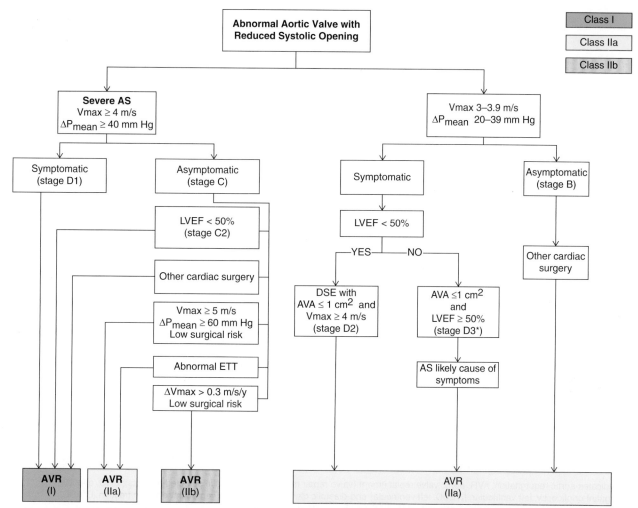

Arrow show the decision pathways that result in a recommendation for AVR. Periodic monitoring is indicated for all patients in whom AVR is not yet indicated, including those with asymptomatic AS (stage D or C) and those with low-gradients AS (stage D2 or D3) who do not meet the criteria for intervention.

*AVR should be considered with stage D3 As only if valve obstruction is the most likely cause of symptoms, stroke volume index <35 mL/m^2, indexed AVA is ≤0.6cm^2/m^2, and data are recorded when the patient is normotensive (systolic BP 140 mm Hg).

As indicates aortic stenosis; AVA; aortic valve area; AVR, aortic valve replacement by either surgical or transcatheter approach; BP, blood pressure; DSE, doubtamine stress echocardiography; ETT, exercise tredmill test; LVEF, left ventricular ejection fraction ΔP_{mean}, mean pressure gradient; and V_{max}, maximum velocity.

FIGURE 40.1 Indications for aortic valve replacement in aortic stenosis. AS, aortic stenosis; DP$_{mean}$, the mean pressure gradient across the valve; DV$_{max}$, change in maximum velocity across the valve on echocardiography. (From Nishimura RA, Otto CM, Bonow RO, et al. 2014 AHA/ACC Guideline for the management of patients with valvular heart disease: a report of the American College of Cardiology/American Heart Association Task Force on Practice Guidelines. *J Am Coll Cardiol.* 2014;63:2438-2488.)

Symptomatic Aortic Stenosis

The onset of symptoms in patients with AS is a poor prognostic sign. There is a 5% incidence of sudden death per year. Symptoms are most likely because it is as if the aortic valve area is <1 cm^2 or the transvalvular mean gradient is >40 mm Hg, and symptom onset in these patients mandates prompt aortic valve replacement in all except very high-risk cases.[2,3]

Low-Gradient Low-Ejection Fraction (Low-Flow) Aortic Stenosis

There are three main subgroups of symptomatic AS patients with transvalvular gradients of <40 mm Hg. Dobutamine infusion during echo or cardiac catheterization can help stratify patients. If cardiac output and transvalvular gradient increase in response to dobutamine, it suggests there is a true flow-limiting lesion in the setting of reversible ventricular dysfunction: surgery would be beneficial although at higher risk than in patients with normal LV function. In the irreversibly damaged left ventricle, there is little or no increase in transvalvular flow in response to inotropes, and lack of contractile reserve: these patients present with high postoperative mortality and worse survival. Finally, in patients with severe cardiomyopathy due to nonvalvular cause, with only moderate or mild AS, the aortic valve area increases during dobutamine stress testing. These patients derive minimal benefit from surgery.[2]

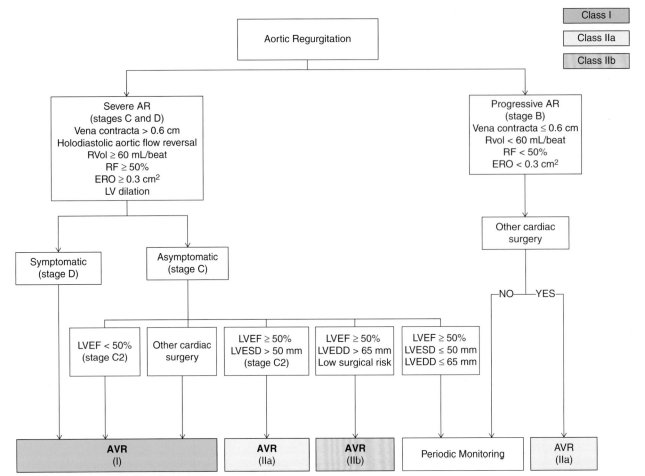

FIGURE 40.2 Indications for aortic valve replacement for aortic regurgitation. (From Nishimura RA, Otto CM, Bonow RO, et al. 2014 AHA/ACC Guideline for the management of patients with valvular heart disease: a report of the American College of Cardiology/American Heart Association Task Force on Practice Guidelines. *J Am Coll Cardiol.* 2014;63:2438-2488.)

Asymptomatic Aortic Stenosis

Most asymptomatic patients with severe AS have near-normal life expectancy without aortic valve replacement. Their 1% to 2% incidence of sudden death is less than the mortality of aortic valve replacement (which is approximately 2% overall in the United States), making it crucial to select only those patients at high risk of sudden death without surgery. Two techniques are employed: echocardiography and exercise testing. Asymptomatic patients with a peak transvalvular gradient > 64 mm Hg have an 80% chance of becoming symptomatic within 2 years (hence surgery in these patients has an ACC/AHA IIb indication if surgery is likely to be low risk). Exercise testing is safe in asymptomatic patients, and can identify the presence of exercise-induced hemodynamic compromise, which is an ACC/AHA IIb indication for aortic valve replacement. The natural history of AS in asymptomatic patients with a positive exercise test is probably very similar to that of patients with exertional symptoms.

Aortic Insufficiency

Acute severe AI is a surgical emergency because of the potentially immediately life-threatening sequelae of pulmonary edema and coronary ischemia described earlier. In infective endocarditis with lesser degrees of AI, the indications for early operation are annular abscess formation, new heart block, or evidence of heart failure. In patients who develop chronic severe AI, it may be 10 years before symptoms become severe because of the adaptive changes described earlier. The prognosis during this period is good: severe chronic AI with preserved ejection fraction has an 80% 5-year survival. Surgery should take place before permanent LV dysfunction ensues: so surgery is often indicated in asymptomatic patients. Progressive LV enlargement or decreasing ejection fraction usually precedes the onset of symptoms and decompensation. Aortic valve replacement should therefore be carried out before the LV ejection fraction falls below 50%, the LV end systolic diameter increases to >55 mm, or the LV end diastolic diameter increases to >70 mm.

Special Considerations

Elderly and High-Risk Patients

The life expectancy of octogenarians without significant comorbidity can be more than 10 years. Aortic valve replacement in selected octogenarians has <3% operative mortality and results in improved quality and length of life in patients with symptomatic AS. These patients, and younger patients adjudicated high risk, are increasingly seen as candidates for transcatheter aortic valve replacement, which in the United States is approved for use in patients with a Society of Thoracic Surgeons predicted operative mortality score of >3% (intermediate and high risk), with severe trileaflet, calcific AS.

Patient Prosthesis Mismatch

The postoperative gradient across a prosthetic aortic valve depends on the valve size and cardiac output: it is higher in small valves, large patients, anemia, fluid overload, tachycardia, and hyperdynamic left ventricles (which is why β-blockers are sometimes used to address high postoperative transvalvular gradients). Postoperative gradients 20 to 30 mm Hg are very common particularly with bioprosthetic valves, and common practice is to try to minimize a postoperative gradient by implanting the largest prosthesis that will fit in the patient's aortic annulus (AA), and not implanting a prosthesis "too small" for the patient's size. How small is "too small" is quantified by Patient Prosthesis Mismatch (PPM), defined as Indexed Effective Orifice Area (IEOA) < 0.85 cm^2/m^2.[4–8] There are, however, no strong data to show difference in survival or symptoms according to whether patients have PPM because the data are dominated by observational studies that are prone to selection bias, primarily because PPM tends to occur in patients with other risk factors for worse outcomes (females, obese, older patients).

There are several options to avoid a high transvalvular gradient after aortic valve replacement in a patient at risk for this because of a small aortic root. The theoretical long-term benefits of minimizing the residual transaortic gradient must be weighed against the incremental operative risks posed to the patient: occlusion of either coronary ostia or annular rupture due to placing an oversized prosthesis is associated with very high morbidity and mortality. Aortic root enlargement is associated with an incremental 2% to 3% risk of operative mortality in observational series, and national mortality for aortic root replacement is 7% to 10%, compared with 2% for aortic valve replacement.[9,10]

Planning before surgery may identify the potential problem in advance, allowing other modalities to be considered. For example, an annular diameter < 20 mm on preoperative echo is likely to take only a 19-mm valve. If the patient is very active or large, has diastolic dysfunction, or low-gradient low-ejection fraction AS, a 19-mm aortic valve is unlikely to be suitable. Options include transcatheter aortic valve replacement, which allows a prosthesis with a larger effective orifice area to be placed. Sutureless valves also appear to have better characteristics in this regard. Alternatively, mechanical valves have superior hemodynamics for given size, which requires a careful discussion before surgery with the patient given the need for lifelong anticoagulation and incremental risk of stroke and major bleeding events. Surgical approaches in increasing order of complexity and operative risks include stentless valves, aortic root enlargement, and aortic root replacement.

Valve Sparing Procedures

There are a large number of procedures described for patients with morphologically normal aortic valves, but with aortic regurgitation caused by pathology affecting the sinotubular junction (STJ) or the aortic annulus (AA). In patients with severe AI, a normal STJ, and normal AA, a Dacron tube graft approximately 10% smaller than the diameter of the AA is scalloped into tailored flaps that are used to recreate the sinuses of Valsalva. It is necessary to reimplant the coronary arteries. Alternatively, tailored flaps are omitted and

the valve is simply resuspended within the Dacron tube, restoring valvular competency. In patients with a normal AA but dilated STJ, which occurs in patients with chronic hypertension, poststenotic dilatation and type A dissection, a simple interposition style graft can be placed, with or without a band of PTFE (Polytetrafluoroethylene) for additional support at the level of the STJ. It is not necessary to reimplant the coronaries. In patients where both AA and STJ are enlarged due to annuloaortic ectasia that can be caused by connective tissue disorders such as Marfan syndrome, AI can be treated by valve-sparing root remodeling. A number of modifications to procedures originally separately described by Magdi Yacoub and Tirone David exist. The main principles of valve-sparing surgery in Marfan disease involve implanting a Dacron graft at the annulus. The sinus aorta is attached to the inside of the Dacron graft, with reimplantation of the coronary ostia.

Surgical Approaches

Transcatheter aortic valve replacement is described in Chapter 39, and is increasingly the procedure of choice for intermediate and high-risk patients.[11] Surgical aortic valve replacement is most commonly performed via a sternotomy or an upper hemisternotomy, which allows the incision to be 6 to 7 cm in length. Occasionally anatomy is amenable to a minithoracotomy approach, which allows a 6-to-7-cm incision via an intercostal space. The aim of smaller incisions is to limit the impact of surgery on postoperative respiratory function, pain control, bleeding and transfusion requirement, and to improve cosmesis. Cannulation for cardiopulmonary bypass is usually performed via the ascending aorta and right atrium; however femoral cannulation may be used to facilitate smaller incisions. Retrograde flow from femoral arterial cannulation is associated with higher rates of stroke in elderly patients and those with atheromatous vasculature.

Results of Aortic Valve Surgery

Early Mortality

In an analysis of 141,905 isolated valve procedures in a U.S. national database, unadjusted mortality was 1.4% for patients adjudicated "low risk" with a Society of Thoracic Surgeons predicted operative mortality score (STS-PROM) score of <4%; 5.24% in patients adjudicated intermediate risk (STS PROMO score 4% to 8%) and 11.2% in patients adjudicated high risk with an STS PROM score > 8%.[12] The biggest risk factors for operative mortality are emergency presentation, advanced age, multiple valve surgery, coronary artery disease, aortic root pathology, and endocarditis. Results have improved over recent decades despite sicker patient profiles. Most early deaths are related to cardiogenic shock, stroke, and hemorrhage. The higher mortality observed in patients undergoing bioprosthetic compared with mechanical aortic valve replacement is related to their higher preoperative comorbidity, including greater age.

Late Mortality

Overall survival (including hospital deaths) after aortic valve replacement is approximately 75% at 5 years, 60% at 10 years, and 40% at 15 years, depending on the patient's age and comorbid conditions. Type of prosthesis (mechanical versus bioprosthetic valve) has not been shown to have an impact on survival. Although patients with bioprosthetic valves have significantly worse unadjusted survival curves than patients with mechanical valves, as with early mortality, this reflects the greater age and comorbidity of this group at baseline. Survival can be described in terms of hazard phases:

the early, rapidly declining hazard phase (short-term survival) is dominated by perioperative mortality. It gives way to a phase about 6 months after operation (intermediate-term survival) where the death rate remains steady at approximately 2% per annum. This begins to rise steadily after 5 years (late-term survival). Other risk factors for late mortality include advanced age at operation (30-day mortality 1% in patients aged 40 to 50 years compared with >3% in patients aged > 80 years). Additional risk factors for operative mortality include worse New York Heart Association (NYHA) class, LV enlargement, atrial fibrillation, the number of previous aortic valve replacements, coexisting coronary artery disease, aneurysm, or LV structural abnormality.

Complications of Aortic Valve Replacement

The complications of cardiac surgery in general include re-exploration for bleeding or tamponade (2%), perioperative myocardial infarction (1%), deep sternal wound infection (1%), prolonged mechanical ventilation (2%), and organ dysfunction (5%). Complications particularly associated with aortic valve replacement are as follows:

COMPLETE HEART BLOCK

Permanent pacemakers are inserted for permanent complete heart block in about 5% of aortic valve replacement patients. Complete heart block results from trauma to the bundle of His after extensive debridement of calcium from the junction of the right and noncoronary cusp. Heart block characteristically worsens over postoperative days 1 to 3, and sometimes settles as edema improves.[13, 14]

STROKE

The overall risk of stroke is about 2% for isolated aortic valve replacement, increasing to 3% in combined aortic valve replacement with concomitant coronary bypass surgery.[15] Stroke following aortic valve replacement shares many of the same risk factors as in other cardiac surgery, including prior stroke, carotid artery disease, aortic atheroma or calcification, endocarditis, and atrial fibrillation. Removal of all calcific debris from the operative field and thorough de-airing help prevent perioperative stroke.

PROSTHETIC ENDOCARDITIS

Mechanical valves are at slightly higher risk of endocarditis up to 3 months after surgery, the risks even out by 5 years. Homografts were once assumed to carry a lower risk of early endocarditis, but this has not been supported by data. The cumulative risk of prosthetic valve endocarditis is about 1% at 1 year and 3% at 5 years post aortic valve replacement. Early endocarditis (within 3 months of surgery) is usually hospital acquired: organisms are commonly staphylococci and gram-negative bacilli. Late prosthetic endocarditis usually results from a transient streptococcal bacteremia. The mortality is up to 60%.

THROMBOEMBOLISM

The rate of valve thromboembolism is roughly 1% to 2% per year: the rate in adequately anticoagulated mechanical valves is slightly higher than that in bioprosthetic valves, which is one of the strong rationales for bioprosthetic valves.[16–20] Valve thrombosis is a rare emergency: cardiovascular collapse, venous congestion, and systemic embolization are usually acute, but may be insidious in onset. The management is intravenous heparin. If the thrombus

is greater than 5 mm, thrombolysis or reoperative bioprosthetic aortic valve replacement is indicated.

PARAPROSTHETIC LEAK

Major paraprosthetic regurgitation occurs in 5% to 10% of transcatheter aortic valve replacements. It is uncommon with surgical aortic valve replacement, and is caused most commonly by prosthetic endocarditis (late), and less commonly by technical errors in insertion (early). Patients present with hemolytic anemia, and if severe, congestive heart failure. The treatment is surgery. If the area of dehiscence is small and there is no evidence of sepsis, one or two interrupted sutures may suffice. Occasionally, paravalvular regurgitation is amenable to percutaneous closure with an Amplatzer-type device. Where this is not possible, redo aortic valve replacement is indicated.[21]

PROSTHESIS FAILURE

Failure of mechanical valves is almost exclusive to strut failure of a particular Bjork-Shiley tilting disc valve, withdrawn in 1986. Bioprosthetic aortic valve failure is age dependent: rates of failure are <10% at 10 years in the over 70s age group, but closer to 30% in the 40-to-50-year age group. Degenerative failure in cryopreserved homograft aortic valve replacement is between 5% and 10% at 10 years.

REOPERATION FOR ANY REASON

The risk of reoperation is highest in the first 6 months following aortic valve replacement due to prosthetic endocarditis and paravalvular leak. It falls to about 1% a year where it remains for mechanical valves.[13,14] The risk also falls initially in bioprosthetic valves, but begins to rise rapidly after 10 to 12 years due to structural degeneration.[15]

FAILURE TO IMPROVE SYMPTOMS AND LEFT VENTRICULAR FUNCTION

90% of patients are NYHA class I or II, 5 to 10 years following aortic valve replacement, depending on their other comorbidities, and baseline LV function. Completely normal LV mass is rarely achieved, but where the LV end diastolic pressure was low preoperatively, and the transvalvular gradient is minimal, LV mass eventually returns to near-normal values.

MITRAL VALVE SURGERY

PATHOPHYSIOLOGY OF MITRAL REGURGITATION

Morphology

The mitral valve consists of the mitral valve annulus, leaflets, chordae tendineae, papillary muscles, and the left ventricle wall. Disease involving any of these structures may result in reduced leaflet coaptation leading to mitral regurgitation, described using a functional classification, description of etiology, and segmental valve nomenclature. Leaflet dysfunction is commonly described using Carpentier's classification of leaflet motion as either type I, which is normal leaflet motion; type II, which is excessive leaflet motion or prolapse; type III, which is restricted leaflet motion; and further subdivided into type IIIa, which is restricted leaflet opening; and type IIIb, which is restricted leaflet closure.

The functional classification can be supplemented with a description of the lesion causing the functional problem. Common lesions are chordal elongation or rupture, leaflet perforation, annular dilatation, and papillary muscle displacement or rupture. Finally, the etiology underlying the lesion is described: common etiologies of mitral regurgitation include degenerative disease (which covers a range of overlapping pathology resulting in mitral valve prolapse including myxomatous disease, fibroelastic deficiency, and Barlow disease), ischemic disease (which can result in acute and chronic changes causing regurgitation), rheumatic disease, endocarditis, and dilated cardiomyopathy.

Etiology

Degenerative mitral valve disease is one of the commonest causes of mitral regurgitation in developed countries with an incidence of 1% to 2%. Typically degenerative disease causes prolapse (type II mitral regurgitation) due to chordal elongation or rupture, most commonly of the P2 segment. Histology shows myxomatous degeneration. Degenerative mitral valve disease encompasses a spectrum from single segment prolapse in small valves (fibroelastic deficiency) to multisegment prolapse in giant valves (Barlow).

Ischemic mitral regurgitation is usually due to chronic LV dysfunction and posterior displacement of papillary muscle (type IIIb) with normal leaflets. Acute papillary muscle rupture is a rare cause of acute type II mitral regurgitation after myocardial infarction. Dilated cardiomyopathy causes type I MR due to annular dilatation.

Endocarditis causes type I mitral regurgitation due to leaflet perforation and destruction, which may be extensive and involve the mitral annulus. Rheumatic disease results in type IIIa MR with restricted leaflet opening due to calcification and commissural fusion.

Less common causes of mitral regurgitation include abnormal systolic anterior motion, which results in mitral valve regurgitation and elevated LV outflow tract gradients, congenital causes such as cleft mitral valve, and connective tissue disease such as Marfan disease.

Structural and Functional Changes in Mitral Regurgitation

Chronic Mitral Regurgitation

The pathophysiologic changes associated with mitral regurgitation commonly progress through one or more of three stages: acute mitral regurgitation, chronic compensated mitral regurgitation, and chronic decompensated mitral regurgitation. Acute mitral regurgitation results in LV volume overload at end diastole, that is, increased preload and decreased afterload due to the regurgitant pathway into the left atrium. The combination of increased preload and reduced afterload means that a larger volume of blood is ejected from the left ventricle.

Because a large volume of ejected blood enters the left atrium rather than the aorta, forward stroke volume, and hence cardiac output decreases. The increased blood volume in the left atrium raises the pressure from a normal left atrial pressure of 10 mm Hg to up to 25 mm Hg. The increased preload leads to eccentric hypertrophy and LV dilatation, increasing total stroke volume and forward stroke volume to near normal levels. Left atrial enlargement accommodates volume overload at lower filling pressures (15 mm Hg), but predisposes to atrial fibrillation and mural thrombi.

Chronic decompensated mitral regurgitation exists when systolic dysfunction prevents effective ventricular contraction; stroke volume and cardiac output are reduced as blood flows into the low-resistance regurgitant pathway, and left atrial and pulmonary

pressures rise as a result. Untreated decompensated mitral regurgitation rapidly progresses to pulmonary edema and congestive cardiac failure. Symptoms, LV dysfunction, left atrial dilatation, atrial fibrillation, and pulmonary hypertension, are all associated with decreased long-term survival in the setting of chronic MR.

Clinical Findings in Mitral Regurgitation

The interval from diagnosis of mitral regurgitation to the onset of symptoms varies by etiology (it may be months in fibroelastic deficiency to many years in rheumatic or Barlow disease). LV ejection fraction remains normal despite even severe LV dysfunction because 50% of stroke volume ejects into low-pressure left atrium. While most deaths are related to heart failure, the incidence of sudden death suggests ventricular arrhythmias are an important feature of the disease process. Signs include atrial fibrillation, prominent sustained apex beat, systolic thrill, right parasternal heave reflecting right ventricular hypertrophy due to pulmonary artery hypertension, quiet first heart sound, third heart sound audible, and loud pansystolic murmur loudest at apex radiating to axilla.

Acute Mitral Regurgitation

Acute severe mitral regurgitation may be caused by chordal rupture, ischemic heart disease, or infective endocarditis, and it is an indication for urgent surgery. A sudden volume overload is imposed on the left ventricle, increasing preload and resulting in a small increase in total stroke volume. Without the compensatory left atrial and LV dilatation seen in chronic severe mitral regurgitation, however, forward stroke volume is reduced, and congestive heart failure or even cardiogenic shock may result. The patient with acute severe mitral regurgitation is always symptomatic.

PATHOPHYSIOLOGY OF MITRAL STENOSIS

Morphology

The commonest cause of mitral stenosis is rheumatic fever: the disease process causes leaflet thickening and calcification and commissural and chordal fusion. Isolated mitral stenosis occurs in 40% of all patients presenting with rheumatic heart disease, and 60% of patients with mitral stenosis give a history of rheumatic fever. The ratio of female to male patients with this pathology is 2:1. Congenital malformation of the mitral valve occurs rarely.[2,3]

Structural and Functional Changes

The cross-sectional area of the normal mitral valve is 4.0 to 5.0 cm^2. Narrowing of this area to <2.5 cm^2 means that a pressure gradient must be generated across the mitral valve in diastole in order to expel blood from the left atrium into the left ventricle. This results in elevation of left atrial and pulmonary venous pressures. Left atrial enlargement, atrial fibrillation, and thrombus formation result from chronic left atrial pressure overload. Pulmonary hypertension results from passive transmission of elevated left atrial pressures, pulmonary vasoconstriction, and irreversible pulmonary vasculature remodeling. Pulmonary edema occurs when pulmonary venous pressure is greater than plasma oncotic pressure. At rest, mitral stenosis is usually asymptomatic, but any increase in transmitral flow rates (eg, due to hyperdynamic circulation) or reduction in the diastolic filling period, such as tachycardia or atrial fibrillation, will result in an increase in the pressure gradient, causing dyspnea. Severe mitral stenosis may have a low gradient in patients with a low cardiac output.

Clinical Findings in Mitral Stenosis

The first symptoms of dyspnea in patients with mitral stenosis are usually precipitated by physical exertion including exercise, sex, emotional stress, infection, pregnancy, or rapid atrial fibrillation because of the increase in the pressure gradient across the mitral valve described earlier. Recurrent chest infections are characteristic. In advanced cases, hemoptysis may be caused by chest infections, pulmonary infarction, acute pulmonary edema, and rupture of small pulmonary vessels. Systemic embolism is frequent, particularly in atrial fibrillation.

Signs on clinical examination include a decreased amplitude pulse, atrial fibrillation, "tapping" apex beat, left parasternal heave due to right ventricular hypertrophy, thrill due to palpable opening snap, loud first heart sound, an opening snap loudest at lower left sternal edge, and a presystolic murmur, with a delayed mid-diastolic murmur.[2]

Indications for Mitral Valve Surgery

Chronic Mitral Regurgitation

The prognosis of chronic mitral regurgitation depends on both the etiology and severity of the lesion. In patients with severe symptomatic chronic mitral regurgitation of any etiology, the prognosis is poor. The average mortality rate is approximately 2% to 5% per year, and may be as high as 70% at 8 years. Patients with chronic mild to moderate mitral regurgitation are unlikely to require surgery, and therapy is aimed at treating the symptoms and preventing complications. American Heart Association (AHA) guidelines recommend that these patients are followed up on a yearly basis, with transthoracic echo if there are clinical grounds for suspecting a deterioration in LV or mitral valve function.[2,3]

In chronic ischemic mitral regurgitation, the valve itself is usually anatomically normal and the regurgitation is secondary to papillary muscle and LV dysfunction following infarction. The prognosis is poorer than in mitral regurgitation caused by nonischemic pathology. Coronary artery bypass may improve LV function and reduce mitral regurgitation. If LV dysfunction is very severe (LV end systolic diameter > 55 mm or LV ejection fraction < 30%), and repair/chordal preservation is unlikely, surgery does not extend life expectancy and is unlikely to provide symptomatic benefit.

Class I indications for mitral valve surgery therefore include chronic severe mitral regurgitation and NYHA class II to IV symptoms or mild to moderate LV dysfunction.[2,3] Additionally, class I indications include asymptomatic chronic severe mitral regurgitation with normal LV function if the likelihood of repair is more than 90%, or in the presence of new atrial fibrillation, pulmonary artery systolic pressures greater than 50 mm Hg at rest (or 60 mm Hg on exercise); or in the setting of NYHA III to IV symptoms with severe LV dysfunction if there is a primary leaflet dysfunction (ie, not secondary or functional mitral regurgitation) and repair is likely. Class IIb indications for surgery include chronic severe mitral regurgitation due to severe LV dysfunction despite optimal medical therapy that may include biventricular pacing where appropriate (**Figures 40.3 and 40.4**).[2,3]

Acute Mitral Regurgitation

Acute severe mitral regurgitation is a class I indication for urgent surgery. There is no scope for compensatory changes: cardiac output falls, left atrial pressures increase, and pulmonary edema and cardiogenic shock ensue.

Mitral Stenosis

It may be as long as 20 to 40 years between the occurrence of rheumatic fever and the onset of symptomatic mitral stenosis. Once symptoms develop, it may take up to 10 years before these become disabling. In the minimally symptomatic patient, 10-year survival is 80%, which drops to 10% to 15% once symptoms become limiting. Once there is severe pulmonary hypertension, mean survival drops to <3 years. The mortality of untreated mitral stenosis is due to heart failure in 60% to 70%, systemic embolism in 20% to 30%, pulmonary embolism in 10%, and infection in 1% to 5% of patients. Patients with a mitral valve area of <1.5 cm^2 and NYHA functional class III to IV symptoms should be referred for surgery if balloon valvotomy is not possible. There is good evidence that patients with NYHA functional class I to II symptoms and a mitral valve area <1.0 cm^2, and severe pulmonary artery hypertension (systolic pulmonary artery pressure > 60 to 80 mm Hg) benefit from surgery.[2]

Surgical Approaches

Mitral valve repair and replacement is most commonly performed via a sternotomy, and right (and very occasionally left) thoracotomy approach is very feasible. As in aortic valve surgery, the aim of smaller incisions is to limit the impact of surgery on postoperative respiratory function, pain control, bleeding and transfusion requirement, and to improve cosmesis. Cannulation for cardiopulmonary bypass is usually performed via the ascending aorta and Bicavally (Superior and Inferior Vena Cava); however, femoral cannulation may be used to facilitate smaller incisions. Retrograde flow from femoral arterial cannulation is associated with higher rates of stroke in elderly patients and those with atheromatous vasculature.

Mitral Valve Repair

Planning Mitral Valve Repair

In degenerative valve disease, mitral valve repair is associated with better early and late survival, and freedom from complications of prosthetic valve including stroke, recurrence of mitral regurgitation, and reoperation compared with mitral valve replacement. Therefore, mitral valve repair is preferable to replacement in patients with degenerative valve disease, particularly in young patients and asymptomatic patients where the sequelae of valve replacement are more serious.[2,3]

Mitral valve repair is not as reproducible as mitral valve replacement because it requires additional technical expertise primarily because mitral valve morphology is highly variable, and repair complexity depends on valve morphology. Consequently, in order to maximize the likelihood of a competent and durable mitral repair, it is important to match surgeon expertise to repair complexity. Lesions associated with a more straightforward repair include type II mitral regurgitation from isolated P2 prolapse from degenerative disease, and type IIIb P3 from ischemic disease.

Lesions associated with more complex repair include multi-segment or bileaflet prolapse, in Barlow disease, type IIIa lesion from rheumatic disease, lesions related to infective endocarditis, such as leaflet perforation and annular abscess, cleft mitral valve, primary abnormal systolic anterior leaflet motion, and previous failed mitral repair. Patients with these lesions should be seen by a surgeon with specific expertise in mitral valve repair.

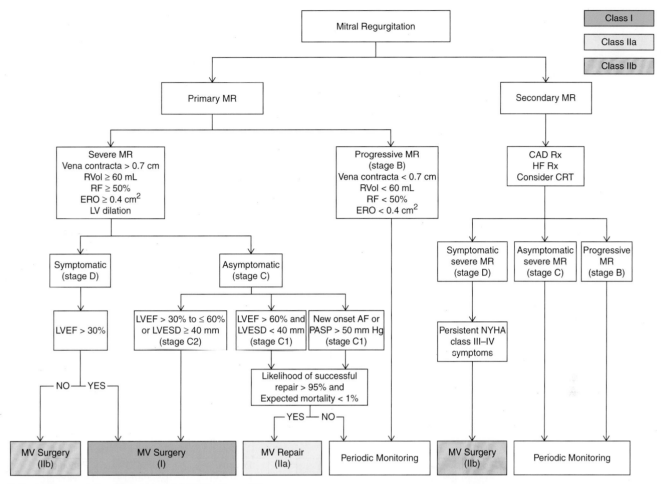

FIGURE 40.3 Indications for mitral valve repair or replacement for mitral regurgitation. (From Nishimura RA, Otto CM, Bonow RO, et al. 2014 AHA/ACC Guideline for the management of patients with valvular heart disease: a report of the American College of Cardiology/American Heart Association Task Force on Practice Guidelines. *J Am Coll Cardiol.* 2014;63:2438-2488.)

Special Considerations

Concomitant Tricuspid Annuloplasty

Functional tricuspid regurgitation commonly occurs secondary to mitral valve lesions causing pulmonary hypertension and right ventricular dilatation. When right ventricular dilatation develops, the tricuspid annulus dilates because it is not supported by a fibrous skeleton. This is most pronounced in the posterior and anterior part of the annulus because the septal annulus is relatively fixed. Leaflet coaptation is reduced leading to tricuspid regurgitation. Observational data suggest that in patients with more than 2+ tricuspid regurgitation, annular dilatation, or pulmonary artery hypertension, functional tricuspid regurgitation may not resolve with correction of the left-sided lesion, and should be repaired to avoid late severe tricuspid regurgitation, which develops in a minority of patients and is associated with high morbidity and operative mortality. Tricuspid repair can be easily accomplished using tricuspid ring annuloplasty without significant incremental morbidity.[22]

Concomitant Atrial Ablation and Left Atrial Appendage Closure

Atrial fibrillation may be addressed at the time of mitral valve surgery with concomitant ablation using a variety of energy sources: cryoablation is used most commonly. Full-thickness lesions are created around the pulmonary veins, and may include more complete left and right atrial lesions sets. The freedom from atrial fibrillation at 1 year using this technique is 60% to 70%. Cut-and-sew maze procedures, where the lesions are created by resecting and resuturing the left and right atrium, offer much greater freedom from atrial fibrillation but at the expense of increased morbidity, particularly related to bleeding risk, and are not widely performed. In patients with atrial fibrillation, it is possible to ligate the left atrial appendage either from inside the left atrium, which affords a more complete and durable closure if performed as a double layer rather than a single purse-string, or from outside using sutures or clips, which is faster but may

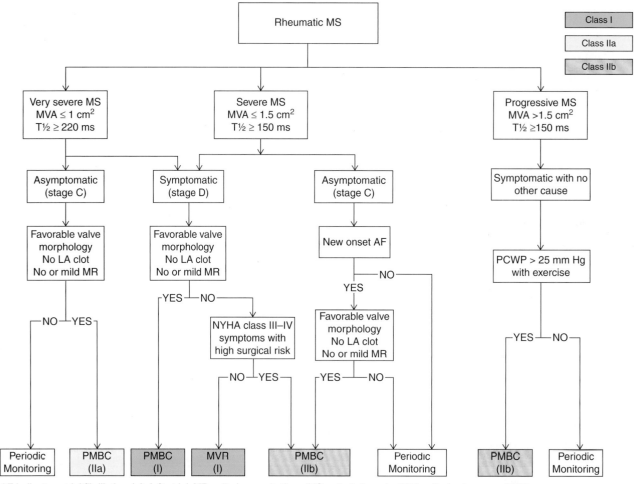

AF indicates atrial fibrillation; LA, left atrial; MR, mitral regurgitations; MS, mitral stenosis; MVA, mitral valve area; MVR, mitral valve surgery (repair or replacement); NYHA, New York Heart Association; PCWP, pulmonary capillary wedge pressure; PMBC, percutaneous mitral balloon commissurotomy; and T½, pressure half-time.

FIGURE 40.4 Indications for intervention for mitral stenosis. (From Nishimura RA, Otto CM, Bonow RO, et al. 2014 AHA/ACC Guideline for the management of patients with valvular heart disease: a report of the American College of Cardiology/American Heart Association Task Force on Practice Guidelines. *J Am Coll Cardiol.* 2014;63:2438-2488.)

not occlude the base of the appendage as reliably as a hand-sewn closure. The rationale is to reduce the risk of thromboembolic stroke, but there are little data to support the efficacy of any of the techniques, with some data showing increased stroke risk if there is residual blood flow after attempted surgical closure.

Mitral Valvotomy

Open mitral valvotomy is a historic procedure that used to be performed for mitral stenosis (usually rheumatic), before the wide availability of percutaneous balloon mitral valvotomy. It was one of the first cardiac surgical procedures performed, and the basic principles of the operation remained unchanged for three decades until the advent of cardiopulmonary bypass enabled the surgeon to work on the mitral valve under direct vision, in a still, bloodless field. Percutaneous balloon mitral valvotomy is performed using a transvenous approach with a transseptal puncture. The initial results of percutaneous versus surgical valvotomy are comparable, and both interventions have low rates of restenosis providing good functional outcomes up

to 3 years. At 3 years, however, valve areas in the balloon mitral valvuloplasty group are greater than in the surgical ones. Additionally, procedural mortality is less than that associated with mitral valve replacement. In view of this, as well as the lower cost and morbidity of the percutaneous approach, percutaneous approach is recommended in patients without any contraindications. Contraindications to percutaneous balloon valvotomy include > 2+ mitral regurgitation, left atrial thrombus, Wilkins score ≥ 8 (range 4 to 16), or Cormier group 3, severely decreased leaflet mobility, prominent leaflet or subvalvar thickening, calcification especially commissures, and severe concomitant coronary artery disease or AS requiring surgery.

Results of Mitral Valve Surgery

Early Mortality

The mortality of isolated mitral valve repair, with or without tricuspid repair, for degenerative disease in patients without pulmonary hypertension is <1%. Higher operative mortality (2% to 5%) is seen in patients with pulmonary hypertension, LV dysfunction, advanced age, ischemic mitral regurgitation, active endocarditis, and mitral replacement.

Late Mortality

Successful repair for degenerative mitral regurgitation restores life expectancy to that of an age-matched normal population. Ischemic mitral regurgitation is associated with much poorer survival: one-third of patients are dead within 5 years despite successful repair. LV end diastolic dimension greater than 65 mm is associated with worse survival with <50% of patients alive at 5 years. Rheumatic patients are usually younger, and have good long-term survival with around 80% to 90% still alive 10 years after surgery.[13]

Complications

The complications of cardiac surgery in general include reexploration for bleeding or tamponade (2%), perioperative myocardial infarction (1%), deep sternal wound infection (1%), prolonged mechanical ventilation (2%), and organ dysfunction (5%). Complications particularly associated with mitral valve surgery are as follows:

FAILURE OF REPAIR

A patient leaving the operating room with greater than 1+ mitral regurgitation is described as having residual mitral regurgitation, whereas recurrent mitral regurgitation refers to patients who initially had no mitral regurgitation after surgery, but developed mitral regurgitation later. Residual mitral regurgitation is usually due to a technical issue, such as incorrect choice of ring, failure to close cleft, inadequate treatment of prolapse, or advanced disease due to an etiology not amenable to repair (rheumatic mitral disease). Recurrent mitral regurgitation may occur early, and is also usually related to a technical problem, such as dehiscence of leaflet suture line, failure of chordal reconstruction, or very occasionally endocarditis. Late recurrent mitral regurgitation is usually due to progression of underlying disease. The late failure rate for degenerative disease is around 1% to 2% per year, and much lower than the failure rate for rheumatic and ischemic repair, reflecting the more progressive nature of the latter two etiologies.

COMPLETE HEART BLOCK

Permanent pacemakers are inserted for permanent complete heart block in about 1% to 2% of mitral valve replacement patients. Complete heart block results from trauma to the bundle of His. Heart block characteristically worsens over postoperative days 1 to 3, and sometimes settles as edema improves.

STROKE

The overall risk of stroke is about 1% for isolated mitral valve replacement, increasing to 3% in mitral valve replacement combined with concomitant aortic valve replacement or coronary bypass surgery. Stroke following mitral valve replacement shares many of the same risk factors as in other cardiac surgery, including prior stroke, carotid artery disease, aortic atheroma or calcification, endocarditis, and atrial fibrillation. Removal of all calcific debris from the operative field, and thorough de-airing help prevent perioperative stroke.

PROSTHETIC ENDOCARDITIS

Mechanical valves are at slightly higher risk of endocarditis up to 3 months after surgery, the risks even out by 5 years. Homografts were once assumed to carry a lower risk of early endocarditis, but this has not been supported by data. The cumulative risk of prosthetic valve endocarditis is about 1% at 1 year and 3% at 5 years post mitral valve replacement. Early endocarditis (within 3 months of surgery) is usually hospital acquired: organisms are commonly staphylococci and gram-negative bacilli. Late prosthetic endocarditis usually results from a transient streptococcal bacteremia. The mortality is up to 60%.

THROMBOEMBOLISM

The rate of valve thromboembolism is higher than in aortic prostheses because flow velocity across the valve is slower. It is roughly 2% per year, with adequate anticoagulation of mechanical valves, and 1% per year with bioprosthetic valves, and may present as stroke or systemic embolization.[16] The mainstay of management is intravenous heparin. Valve thrombosis is rare, and presents with acute onset of extreme dyspnea and orthopnea, but may be insidious. Fluoroscopy or echo is used to visualize if one or both leaflets are not moving. Acute thrombosis can be treated with thrombolytic therapy, but usually this is a chronic process with acute exacerbation that requires replacement (normally with a bioprosthesis to avoid a repeat episode). The thrombus is usually very organized and may be superimposed on pannus. Surgical thrombectomy may be tempting but is often ineffective because it is impossible to clear pannus and thrombus easily from ventricular aspect of prosthesis.

PARAPROSTHETIC LEAK

Paraprosthetic leak is uncommon after mitral valve replacement: immediate or early paraprosthetic leaks may be due to needle holes (tiny, and disappear after protamine), incomplete decalcification of annulus, annular tear, or suture positioning. Late new paraprosthetic leaks are more likely due to endocarditis. Narrow, high-velocity jets are high risk for hemolytic anemia that may be disabling (requiring multiple transfusions). Broader jets may be hemodynamically significant especially if mitral regurgitation was not present preoperatively. The decision to treat depends on balancing disadvantages of fixing the paravalvular leak (eg, reclamping diseased aorta, additional ischemic time in sick heart, severe mitral annular calcification making any improvement unlikely, high-risk resternotomy) against the disadvantages of leaving it. Prosthetic valve endocarditis is a strong indication for surgery in this context. In the absence of endocarditis, paravalvular regurgitation may be amenable to percutaneous closure with an Amplatzer-type device. Where this is not possible, redo mitral valve replacement may be indicated.

PROSTHESIS FAILURE

In the mitral position, the lifetime risk of reoperation for bioprosthetic failure is around 45% for a 50-year-old, and this falls by just over 10% for every additional 5 years of age at the time of implantation. At 20 years after surgery, around 10% to 15% of patients with mechanical valves will have required reoperative valve replacement for infective endocarditis, pannus, or valve thrombosis.[22]

REOPERATION FOR ANY REASON

The risk of reoperation is highest in the first 6 months following mitral valve replacement due to prosthetic endocarditis and paravalvular leak. It falls to about 1% a year where it remains for mechanical valves. The risk also falls initially in bioprosthetic valves, but begins to rise rapidly after 10 to 12 years due to structural degeneration.[22]

FAILURE TO IMPROVE SYMPTOMS AND LV FUNCTION

90% of patients are NYHA class I or II, 5 to 10 years following mitral valve replacement, depending on their other comorbidities and baseline LV function. Completely normal LV mass is rarely achieved, but where the LV end diastolic pressure was low preoperatively, and the transvalvular gradient is minimal, LV mass eventually returns to near normal values.

Atrial Fibrillation

Around 10% to 20% of patients undergoing mitral surgery have a history of preoperative atrial fibrillation and the incidence of postoperative atrial fibrillation is around 40%. Atrial fibrillation is associated with thromboembolic complications including stroke, heart failure, and decreased survival; so aggressive treatment of patients with a history of preoperative atrial fibrillation with intraoperative ablation is recommended. These patients are routinely anticoagulated for 3 months after surgery, may be at increased risk for thrombus formation in the early postoperative period, and are often pacemaker dependent for several days after surgery.

TRCIUSPID VALVE SURGERY

PATHOPHYSIOLOGY

Morphology

Functional tricuspid regurgitation commonly occurs secondary to left-sided valve lesions causing pulmonary hypertension and right ventricular dilatation. When right ventricular dilatation develops, the tricuspid annulus dilates because it is not supported by a fibrous skeleton. This is most pronounced in the posterior and anterior part of the annulus, since the septal annulus is relatively fixed. Leaflet coaptation is reduced leading to tricuspid regurgitation. Observational data suggest that in patients with more than 2+ tricuspid regurgitation, annular dilatation, or pulmonary artery hypertension, functional tricuspid regurgitation may not resolve with correction of the left-sided lesion, and should be repaired to avoid late severe tricuspid regurgitation, which develops in a few patients and is associated with high morbidity and operative mortality.

Acute tricuspid valve endocarditis is usually associated with sepsis from long-term indwelling venous catheters or intravenous drug use. Common causative organisms are *Pseudomonas aeruginosa* and *Staphylococcus aureus*. Rheumatic tricuspid valve may result in annular dilatation and functional tricuspid regurgitation secondary to severe mitral stenosis. The tricuspid leaflets are often characterized by mild restriction and leaflet thickening.

Transvenous pacing wires can lead to leaflet perforation, or more commonly scarring, causing tricuspid regurgitation. Traumatic tricuspid valve rupture is a rare sequela of severe nonpenetrating chest injury. Carcinoid valve disease results in severe leaflet thickening and immobility, causing regurgitation and stenosis.

Clinical Findings

The symptoms and natural history are determined by the dominant left-sided heart lesion. Tricuspid stenosis causes increased systemic venous pressure, resulting in hepatomegaly, ascites, and peripheral edema. A mid-diastolic murmur may be present. In tricuspid regurgitation, the progression is slower than mitral regurgitation, and many patients are symptom free for decades. The predominant clinical features are those of raised venous pressure. A pansystolic murmur may be present. Patients usually have moderate to severe right ventricular failure by the time they present for surgery, as well as severe pulmonary hypertension, and moderate to severe liver dysfunction, which is why isolated tricuspid valve surgery has such high mortality (approximately 10% to 15%) with low cardiac output, respiratory failure, and sepsis being the major problems postoperatively.

Indications for Tricuspid Valve Surgery

Class I indications for tricuspid repair include severe tricuspid regurgitation in patients having mitral valve surgery. Tricuspid repair for mild tricuspid regurgitation and pulmonary artery hypertension or tricuspid annular dilatation are class IIb indications for tricuspid repair in patients having mitral valve surgery. Severe symptomatic primary tricuspid regurgitation is a class IIa indication for isolated tricuspid valve surgery.[2,3,23]

Surgical Approach

The tricuspid valve is easily approached via either a sternotomy or a right thoracotomy. The most common procedure is tricuspid annuloplasty, which may be performed using a rigid or flexible ring, or a running stitch around the annulus known as a De Vega suture annuloplasty that is less durable. The tricuspid annulus tissue offers little support and sutures need to be placed and tied carefully to avoid tears, correcting tricuspid regurgitation by reducing the posterior and anterior annulus that are most prone to dilatation. The atrioventricular node is avoided, leaving the area at the apex of the triangle of Koch free of sutures. Tricuspid valve replacement is usually performed for failed repairs, and in operations for endocarditis or carcinoid tricuspid pathologies. A bioprosthetic replacement is usually preferred over a mechanical valve replacement, which will preclude future placement of transvalvular catheters or wires. The valve and subvalvular apparatus is excised, and the valve is inserted using horizontal everting mattress sutures with pledgets on the atrial side.

SURGERY FOR INFECTIVE ENDOCARDITIS

DIAGNOSIS

The Duke diagnostic criteria are 95% specific, with a 92% negative predictive value.

Duke criteria for infective endocarditis establish a definite diagnosis with two major or one major and three minor or five minor criteria. Possible endocarditis is defined by the presence of one major and one minor, or three minor criteria. The major Duke criteria include positive blood cultures (*Streptococcus viridans*, *Streptococcus bovis*, HACEK, *Staphylococcus aureus*, enterococci with no other primary focus from two separate cultures or persistent positive cultures more than 12 hours apart or all of three or majority of four separate cultures positive drawn over the space of >1 hour), and echo evidence including an oscillating intracardiac mass in the absence of alternative explanation, abscess or new regurgitant lesion, or new partial dehiscence of prosthetic valve. The minor Duke criteria include predisposition, fever > 38°C, emboli, or blood culture and echo signs that do not fulfill the definition of major Duke criteria.[2,3,24–30]

INDICATIONS FOR SURGERY

Surgery is indicated for structural valve lesions with evidence of hemodynamic compromise or abscess formation. The optimal time to operate after embolic stroke is 7 to 14 days if possible, but it is often necessary to operate sooner because of the patient's hemodynamic state. An accurate assessment of neurologic function is necessary before proceeding with surgery.

Acute endocarditis with stenosis or regurgitation and congestive heart failure is a class I indication for urgent surgery. Other class I indications for surgical intervention include fungal endocarditis; endocarditis complicated by heart block, annular or aortic abscess, or fistulae between right or left atrium or ventricle and sinus of Valsalva, or mitral leaflet perforation in aortic valve endocarditis; prosthetic valve endocarditis and dehiscence; or worsening valve function, heart failure, or abscess. Native valve endocarditis and recurrent emboli and persistent vegetations despite appropriate antibiotics, and the presence of prosthetic valve endocarditis and bacteremia despite appropriate antibiotics are class IIa indications for surgery. Finally, the presence of mobile vegetations > 10 mm in size are class IIb indications for surgery.[2,3]

Choosing the right time to operate can be difficult: the surgeon must define "appropriate antibiotics," and balance the need to optimize major comorbidity, often including acute embolic stroke, with the fact that these patients are liable to deteriorate irreversibly. In most cases, early surgical intervention is preferable to late: in case of preoperative embolic stroke, delay surgery for 5 to 10 days if possible; if the patient has evidence of a hemorrhagic stroke, then several weeks are usually needed to minimize the risk of additional intracerebral bleeding while on cardiopulmonary bypass or postoperatively.

SURGICAL APPROACHES

The goals of surgery are to remove infected tissue and drain abscesses, reverse hemodynamic abnormalities, and to restore cardiac and vascular architecture. Transesophageal echocardiography is critical in planning surgery that may involve drainage of abscesses, debridement of necrotic tissue, closure of acquired defects, such as ventricular septal defect, annular abscess, fistulae, and aneurysms, in addition to valve repair and replacement. The most common approach is median sternotomy, which allows assessment and treatment of all valves in the event of more extensive involvement than identified preoperatively.

Aortic valve endocarditis is not usually amenable to valve repair, and is treated with complete excision and debridement of all infected tissue, with valve replacement if extensive annular involvement is not there. Extensive destruction of the annulus and sinuses requires treatment with aortic root replacement. There is no good evidence that homograft valve replacement versus bioprosthetic or mechanical valve root replacement reduces the risk of recurrent infective endocarditis. Aortic valve abscesses are most common posterior to the membranous part of the interventricular septum, and under the left coronary ostia.

Mitral and tricuspid calve endocarditis can often be treated effectively with surgical repair after resection and debridement of all infected tissues. Mitral valve abscesses are most common in the P2 portion of the annulus. For small abscesses, evacuation and debridement is relatively straightforward, but in extensive root abscesses involving the atrioventricular and ventriculoarterial junction, debridement may cause dehiscence and abscesses around the mitral valve should also be debrided with great regard for atrioventricular discontinuity. In prosthetic valve endocarditis, extra care must be taken to debride all prosthetic material. Small vegetations can be debrided and perforations in the mitral valve may be repaired with autologous pericardium.

COMBINED VALVULAR PROCEDURES

PATHOPHYSIOLOGY OF COMBINED VALVE DISEASE

Rheumatic valve disease, infective endocarditis, and connective tissue disease are the most common causes of disease requiring surgical intervention on two or more valves. The pathophysiology is dictated by the dominant lesion. Aortic and mitral regurgitation impose a large volume overload on the left ventricle, which undergoes marked hypertrophy and eventual dilatation. Aortic and mitral stenosis result in a small, hypertrophied, noncompliant left ventricle, usually with well-preserved LV function. In patients with mitral stenosis and aortic regurgitation, the mitral stenosis is usually dominant. Mitral stenosis restricts LV, blunting the effect of AI on LV volume. Even in severe AI, hyperdynamic circulation and dilated left ventricle are absent. In AS and mitral regurgitation, the AS worsens the degree of mitral regurgitation. The mitral regurgitation causes difficulty in assessing the severity of the AS because of reduced forward flow. Patients can decompensate rapidly. In mitral stenosis or regurgitation and tricuspid regurgitation, pulmonary hypertension is usually present.

INDICATIONS FOR SURGERY IN MODERATE VALVE DISEASE

Although the nondominant lesion may be mild at the time of operation, these lesions are progressive. Rheumatic AS that was mild at the time of operation on concomitant rheumatic mitral lesion progresses to moderate to severe in one-third of patients within 5 years. The progression of AI is much slower and better tolerated, although distorting the aortic annulus by mitral annuloplasty ring or replacement may cause 2+ AI to become severe. Regurgitant combined lesions tend to progress faster, and the prognosis in combined stenotic lesions is worse than in isolated stenotic lesions. The temptation to operate on multiple valves to avoid later surgery needs to be balanced against increased perioperative mortality and long-term morbidity of valve replacement. It is sometimes reasonable to inspect the valve in question at the time of surgery to make a final decision.

PROSTHETIC VALVES

TYPES OF VALVE PROSTHESIS

Valve prostheses are either mechanical or bioprosthetic ("tissue").[31] Tissue valves are mounted on a metal frame (stented), or supported by pig aorta and cloth (stentless). Stented valves are the most commonly used bioprosthesis, and are usually either porcine aortic valves or bovine pericardium. Homografts are human cadaveric aortic roots, complete with aortic valves in situ. A pulmonary autograft is the patient's own excised pulmonary valve used in the Ross procedure.

Mechanical Valves

Over 50 models of mechanical valves exist underlying the fact that no single design meets all the criteria of the perfect prosthesis. Bileaflet valves provide the best hemodynamic profile and lowest thromboembolic risk, and so are the most widely used today. Commonly inserted models include CarboMedics (radiopaque titanium ring with carbon discs) and St Jude Medical (pyrolytic carbon, radiolucent). Tilting disc (or monoleaflet) valves have been largely superseded by bileaflet valves with better hemodynamic profile. Tilting disc valves include Metronic-Hall A770 carbon-coated disc in sewing ring and Bjork-Shiley carbon-coated disc with titanium struts. Ball-in-cage valves were the first prostheses with long-term durability, but are no longer manufactured. They are associated with higher thromboembolic rates and are bulky prostheses with Starr-Edwards the best known model.

Bioprosthetic Valves

There is a similar variety of choices of tissue valves. Discovery of glutaraldehyde fixation in the 1960s by Alain Carpentier, followed by antimineralization led to second- and third-generation tissue valves with improved durability. There are two main types: stented and stentless.[30] Stented valves are the most commonly implanted, as they are technically easier to implant. Porcine stented valves are made of pig aortic valves, usually with the porcine noncoronary cusp (which is smaller in the pig) replaced with a coronary cusp to make the valve symmetrical. Examples include Carpentier-Edwards 2625, Hancock (Medtronic), and the Hancock II with an anticalcification agent added to the fixative. Bovine stented valves are made of bovine pericardium (equine occasionally used), such as the Perimount (CE 2700/CE Magna). Stentless valves are porcine valves supported by porcine aorta. The lack of a stent means the valves have a better hemodynamic profile, but are technically trickier to implant. The most commonly used include the Freestyle, which may be implanted in the subcoronary position as a valve replacement, as an inclusion root cylinder, or as a full aortic root replacement, and hence "Freestyle."

Homografts

Homografts are aortic roots removed from cadaveric human hearts and implanted as root replacements: the graft does not express major histocompatibility complex antigen as viable endothelial cells disappear within hours of implantation and so allograft rejection does not occur. Valves are removed from disease-free cadaveric hearts, unsuitable for transplantation, of donors aged 6 months to 55 years, up to 12 hours after death. The donor heart is procured using aseptic technique, preserved in cold Ringer lactate solution, and packaged in sterile plastic bag that is buried in slush. Homograft preparation takes place in a clean not aseptic environment. The homograft block consists of all tissue between the base of the left ventricle containing the anterior leaflet of the mitral valve and the aortic annulus, to the innominate artery. The coronary ostia are preserved with a small rim of coronary artery. The annulus is sized and

the length of aorta recorded. There are three main techniques for preservation, which aim to prevent bacterial colonization and preserve fibroblasts and endothelial cells. Cryopreservation has largely superseded antibiotic preservation. Homovital preservation is a recent development. After harvest, the homograft block is stored in a culture medium that contains a low concentration of broad-spectrum antibiotics and stored at 4°C for 24 hours. The culture medium is changed and the tissue stored for a further 24 hours at 4°C. It can either be used at this time as a homovital graft or frozen in 10% fetal calf serum and 10% dimethylsulfoxide (DMSO) with controlled rate freezing (fall of 1°C/min to a target temperature of −40°C) to achieve cryopreservation.

Where root replacement is indicated, homografts are more pliable than Dacron composite valve replacements, may be more resistant to infection (although there are little data to support this), and so are favored in surgery for aortic valve endocarditis requiring root replacement where tissue is very friable and reinfection a significant risk. However, homografts are not as durable as mechanical valves, and may not be as durable as porcine or bovine valve replacement. Homograft aortic root replacement is a technically demanding operation and the results are very dependent on the surgeon, given the additional technical complexity of positioning the homograft in the correct anatomic position, dissecting out the coronary ostia and reimplanting them, and additional suture lines, all of which carry an increased risk of postoperative bleeding and prolong the time for which the patient is on bypass. The national mortality for aortic root replacement is approximately 7%,[9] compared with approximately 1% to 2% for subcoronary aortic valve replacement. There is a theoretical risk of transmitted infections; tuberculosis was transmitted in several cases before preservation and procurement protocols changed. Homografts depend on donor organ supply, which is falling. Homograft tissue is variable in quality, depending on the age of the donor, as well as the skill of the harvester: both the homograft aorta and the valve leaflets may be perforated or buttonholed, and the tissue can be very friable.

Pulmonary Autograft

Using the patient's own pulmonary valve to replace the aortic valve is known as the Ross procedure, after Donald Ross, the British surgeon who pioneered its use. The pulmonary valve is replaced with a pulmonary homograft, which has a life expectancy of 15 to 20 years. The patient's own pulmonary valve in the aortic position has better life expectancy than an aortic bioprosthesis, is resistant to infection, does not warrant formal anticoagulation, and most importantly "grows" with the patient.

Indications for the Ross procedure are controversial because of the additional mortality and morbidity associated with the operation and variable data on the freedom from need for re-operation. The use of the Ross procedure is least controversial in very young patients who will not be well served by implanting small prosthetic valves. Use of the Ross procedure in older patients with a predicted life expectancy of greater than 30 years, and in whom an active lifestyle requires good hemodynamic function and contraindicates warfarin, is thought by some clinicians to be reasonable if the surgeon can offer operative mortality of <2%, that is, comparable to isolated aortic valve replacement.

Contraindications to the Ross procedure include Marfan and other connective tissue disorders. Rheumatic valve disease is a viewed by some as a contraindication.

The drawbacks are primarily related to the technical difficulty of both procedure and reoperation, and many more surgeons have been discouraged by the steep learning curve and abandoned the operation than have managed to successfully adopt it as part of their repertoire. Mortality in one metaanalysis ranged from 1% to 7%. Reoperation for autograft dilatation is reduced by modifications where Teflon felt is used to buttress the proximal suture line.

CHOICE OF VALVE PROSTHESIS

There are no strong data showing major long-term survival difference between mechanical versus tissue valve in either aortic or mitral position.[15,22,23–36] In a patient aged over 65 years, a bioprosthetic valve will likely last the patient's lifetime, does not require long-term anticoagulation, and carries an approximate 1% annual risk of thromboembolic stroke; but valve failure becomes an increasing risk from 10 to 15 years depending on position and patient age. Mechanical valves last decades but approximately 15% will need explanting by 15 years because of endocarditis, pannus, or thrombosis; they require lifelong anticoagulation and have 3% to 4% annual risk of stroke or hemorrhage.

Bioprosthetic Valve Deterioration

Freedom from structural valve deterioration at 12 years in older patients is over 90% with third-generation tissue valves such as the Carpentier-Edwards pericardial valves in the aortic position.[22,37] Tissue valves last longer in the elderly because the hemodynamic demands on the valve are less: the chances of bioprosthetic aortic valve failure at 12 years is approximately 40% in patients aged 18 to 39 years, at least 30% in patients aged 40 to 49 years, and at least 10% in patients aged over 70 years. Lifetime risk of reoperation is similar for each age group. Tissue valves last less well in the mitral position compared with the aortic position, and redo mitral valve replacement is associated with higher risk of mortality than redo aortic valve replacement. Calcification of bioprostheses occurs in areas of greatest stress: the commissural regions of porcine valves or the zone of flexion in porcine and pericardial valves, and leads eventually to prosthesis failure. This may happen earlier in patients with renal failure, but the disadvantages of managing anticoagulation in these patients and their shorter life expectancy means bioprostheses remain a reasonable choice in these patients.

Hemodynamic Profile

In smaller sizes (eg, #19, #21), bioprostheses cause more flow obstruction than same-size mechanical valves. Stented bioprostheses are more obstructive than stentless, which are more obstructive than mechanical.

Thromboembolic and Hemorrhagic Events

Without anticoagulation, life-threatening thrombosis and thromboembolic events are inevitable. Even in an optimally anticoagulated patient (INR 2.5 to 3), the incidence of major thromboembolic events including stroke and hemorrhage is still 2% to 4% per year (and this number is higher in multiple valves and older patients).[21,38–43] Bleeding problems (pericardial effusion, late tamponade) are more common postoperatively, and valve thrombosis is a later risk in patients not therapeutically anticoagulated.

CHOICE OF VALVE PROSTHESIS IN SPECIAL GROUPS

Younger Patients

National analyses show a trend toward implanting more tissue valves in younger patients. This may reflect the lack of evidence for a long-term survival difference between mechanical and biologic valves[23,24]; greater awareness of the lifetime risk of stroke and bleeding rate and the inconvenience of lifelong anticoagulation; better durability of tissue valves; the fall in the mortality of reoperative surgery; and the increasing feasibility of transcatheter valve-in-valve replacement.[44–55]

Pregnancy

Pregnant women have increased risk of mechanical valve-related thromboembolism: anticoagulation is vital.[43–45] Warfarin, a teratogen, is contraindicated in the first trimester, and low molecular weight heparin or unfractionated heparin should be administered instead, from initial attempts to conceive up until the beginning of the second trimester or delivery. Consequently, bioprosthetic valves may be a reasonable choice for women of childbearing age, even though they will eventually need reoperative valve surgery.

Endocarditis

There are no data to suggest that choice of valve replacement affects recurrence of endocarditis. Homografts have not been shown to give increased resistance to endocarditis, and they are less durable than porcine valves: their main advantage is that they are more forgiving to implant in very friable tissue.

Atrial Fibrillation

Atrial fibrillation is no longer an indication to implant a mechanical valve: concomitant ablation means 60% of patients will be in sinus rhythm at 1 year, obviating the need for anticoagulation altogether if a bioprosthesis is implanted.

PERIOPERATIVE CARE

Preoperative Management

All patients undergoing cardiac surgery should undergo a careful history and physical examination to first confirm the indication for surgery, identify possibly contraindications to surgery, and conditions that may increase surgical risk. An accurate description of severity, duration, and nature of symptoms; a cardiovascular history including prior cardiovascular interventions, risk factors, and medications; and a comprehensive cardiovascular examination are mandatory. Assessment of respiratory, renal, and neurologic dysfunctions is indicated based on clinical history, examination, and risk factors. A recent change in symptoms or clinical examination may be an important finding that may change the timing or type of surgery.

All patients should have a recent echocardiogram clearly identifying the severity of the lesion as well as left and right ventricular function, the presence of pulmonary hypertension, and other valvular lesions. Cardiac catheterization should be performed in most patients; in young patients with no risk factors for coronary disease, a CT coronary angiogram may be sufficient to show anatomy. In patients with bicuspid valve disease, a CT scan is useful to evaluate the ascending aorta for aneurysm. Older patients, those with a history of mediastinal radiation, evidence of aortic calcification on imaging, any pulmonary history, and those patients undergoing reoperative cardiac surgery should undergo a CT scan of the chest without contrast. Lung function testing should be performed in patients with pulmonary disease or smoking history.

Antiplatelet agents and anticoagulation should be stopped several days before surgery, with appropriate bridging therapy if indicated. It is common practice to stop angiotensin converting enzyme inhibitors for 24 hours preoperatively to reduce the risk of postoperative vasoplegia. A complete blood count, coagulation profile, blood chemistry, liver function tests, and blood cross match are part of the standard panel of tests. All patients should have a 12-lead ECG and a chest X-ray. The patients must not eat or drink for 8 hours before induction of anesthesia. In diabetic patients, an insulin sliding scale may be needed.

Postoperative Management

Most patients follow the expected postoperative course, but particular vigilance is required to prevent and recognize potentially life-threatening complications including hemorrhage, cardiac tamponade, respiratory and renal failure, stroke, and arrhythmias and conduction block, which can arise unexpectedly particularly during the first 48 to 72 hours after surgery. Urinary, respiratory, and sternal wound infections are more common after postoperative day 4.

Patients arrive on the intensive care unit ventilated with a central venous line, radial arterial line, Foley catheter, and sometimes a pulmonary artery catheter in place. A chest X-ray, 12-lead ECG, complete blood count, coagulation profile, blood chemistry, liver function tests, and arterial blood gas are performed on arrival. The chest X-ray is checked to review the position of the endotracheal tube, the pulmonary artery catheter, and the presence of hemothorax or pneumothoraxes. The ventilator settings are adjusted accordingly. Inotropic support may increase but more commonly decreases during the first 6 hours, and is weaned according to hemodynamic parameters such as cardiac index and mixed venous and blood pressure. Temporary epicardial pacing may be required and it is important to understand how the pacing wires and box work, particularly in an emergency. Most patients wean from the ventilator and are extubated within 6 hours. A spontaneous diuresis of at least 1 mL/kg/h is expected. Mediastinal drainage should decrease steadily and should not be greater than 150 mL/h. Insulin requirements often increase. Prophylactic antibiotics are continued. Aspirin is given 81 mg orally or via the nasogastric tube. Preoperative antianginals are discontinued.

On postoperative day 1, the large chest drains are removed after 3 hours of consecutive zero drainage and a post drain removal chest X-ray is taken and checked for pneumothoraxes. The central line and arterial line are removed. The patient is transferred to the stepdown unit, and helped to mobilize. Routine oral medication is commenced (usually aspirin 81 mg qd, furosemide 40 mg qd, preoperative statin, paracetamol 1 g qid, lactulose 10 mL bid, senna two tablets, and low-molecular-weight heparin such as enoxaparin 40 mg qd s/c). Patients who require formal anticoagulation are started on warfarin. Patients should be sitting out of bed, and start eating and drinking.

Over the next 2 to 5 days, the Foley and any remaining central venous, arterial lines, and chest tubes are removed. The patient should complete a satisfactory stairs assessment with a physiotherapist. All blood results and imaging should be returning to normal values. Adequate pain control should be possible with regular Tylenol and occasional oral opiate analgesia. Pacing wires are removed if there is no conduction block or coagulopathy on postoperative day 4 to 6. Most valve patients should have a routine postoperative transthoracic echocardiogram. The patient should have passed stool before being discharged home.

REFERENCES

1. Verma S, Siu S. Aortic dilatation in patients with bicuspid aortic valve. *N Engl J Med.* 2014;370:1920-1929.
2. Nishimura RA, Otto CM, Bonow RO, et al. 2014 AHA/ACC Guideline for the management of patients with valvular heart disease: a report of the American College of Cardiology/American Heart Association Task Force on Practice Guidelines. *J Am Coll Cardiol.* 2014;63:2438-2488.
3. Vahanian A, Alfieri O, Andreotti F, et al. Guidelines on the management of valvular heart disease (version 2012). The Joint Task Force on the Management of Valvular Heart Disease of the European Society of Cardiology (ESC) and the European Association for Cardio-Thoracic Surgery (EACTS). *Eur Heart J.* 2012;33(19):2451-2496.
4. Pibarot P, Dumesnil JG. Prosthetic heart valves: selection of the optimal prosthesis and long-term management. *Circulation.* 2009;119:1034-1048.
5. Mohty D, Dumesnil JG, Echahidi N, et al. Moderate patient-prosthesis mismatch can impact on mortality after aortic valve replacement: influence of age, obesity and left ventricular dysfunction. *J Am Coll Cardiol.* 2009;63:39-47.
6. Pepper J, Cheng D, Stanbridge R, et al. Stentless versus stented bioprosthetic aortic valves: a consensus statement of the International Society of Minimally Invasive Cardiothoracic Surgery (ISMICS) 2008. *Innovations (Phila).* 2009;4:49-60.
7. Blackstone EH, Cosgrove DM, Jamieson WR, et al. Prosthesis size and long-term survival after aortic valve replacement. *J Thorac Cardiovasc Surg.* 2003;126:783-796.
8. Mohty D, Boulogne C, Magne J, et al. Prevalence and long-term outcome of aortic prosthesis-patient mismatch in patients with paradoxical low-flow severe aortic stenosis. *Circulation.* 2014,130.S25-S31.
9. Stamou SC, Williams ML, Gunn TM, et al. Aortic root surgery in the United States: a report from the Society of Thoracic Surgeons database. *J Thorac Cardiovasc Surg.* 2015;149:116-122.
10. Dhareshwar J, Sundt TM, Dearani JA, et al. Aortic root enlargement: what are the operative risks? *J Thorac Cardiovasc Surg.* 2007;134:916-924.
11. Reinohl J, Kaier K, Reinecke H, et al. Effect of availability of transcatheter aortic valve replacement on clinical practice. *N Eng J Med.* 2015;373:2438-2447.
12. Thourani VH, Suri RM, Gunter RL, et al. Contemporary real-world outcomes of surgical aortic valve replacement in 141,905 low-risk, intermediate-risk and high-risk patients. *Ann Thorac Surg.* 2015;99:55-61.
13. Carpentier A. Lasker clinical research award. The surprising rise of nonthrombogenic valve surgery. *Nat Med.* 2007;13:1165-1168.
14. Tannous H, Chiang Y, Cavallaro P, et al. Permanent pacemaker requirement after concomitant surgical ablation for atrial fibrillation. *Eur J Cardiothorac Surg.* 2014;46:1041.
15. Chiang YP, Chikwe J, Moskowitz A, et al. Survival and long-term outcomes following bioprosthetic versus mechanical aortic valve replacement in patients aged 50 to 69 years. *JAMA.* 2014;312:1323-1329.
16. Cannegieter SC, Rosendaal FR, Briet E. Thromboembolic and bleeding complications in patients with mechanical heart valve prostheses. *Circulation.* 1994;89:635-651.
17. Torella M, Torella D, Chiodini P, et al. LOWERing the INtensity of oral anticoaGulant Therapy in patients with bileaflet mechanical

aortic valve replacement: results from the "LOWERING-IT" Trial. *Am Heart J.* 2010;160:171-178.

18. Karthikeyan G, Senguttuvan NB, Joseph J, et al. Urgent surgery compared with fibrinolytic therapy for the treatment of left-sided prosthetic heart valve thrombosis: a systematic review and meta-analysis of observational studies. *Eur Heart J.* 2013;34:1557-1566.

19. Keuleers S, Herijgers P, Herrgods MC, et al. Comparison of thrombolysis versus surgery as first line therapy for prosthetic heart valve thrombosis. *Am J Cardiol.* 2011;107:275-279.

20. Karthikeyan G, Math RS, Matthew N, et al. Accelerated infusion of streptokinase for the treatment of left-sided prosthetic valve thrombosis: a randomized controlled trial. *Circulation.* 2009;120:1108-1114.

21. Ruiz CE, Jelnim V, Kronzon I, et al. Clinical outcomes in patients undergoing percutaneous closure of periprosthetic paravalvular leaks. *J Am Col Cardiol.* 2011;58:2210-2217.

22. Chikwe J, Chiang YP, Egorova NN, et al. Survival and outcomes following bioprosthetic vs. mechanical mitral valve replacement in patients aged 50 to 69 years. *JAMA.* 2015;313:1435-1442.

23. Chikwe J, Itagaki S, Anyanwu A, et al. Impact of concomitant tricuspid annuloplasty on tricuspid regurgitation, right ventricular function and pulmonary artery hypertension after repair of mitral valve prolapse. *J Am Coll Cardiol.* 2015;65:1931-1938.

24. Lopez J, Revilla A, Vilacosta I, et al. Definition, clinical profile, microbiological spectrum, and prognostic factors of early-onset prosthetic valve endocarditis. *Eur Heart J.* 2007;28:760-765.

25. Amat-Santos IJ, Messika-Zeitoun D, Eltchanimoff H, et al. Infective endocarditis following transcatheter aortic valve implantation: results from a large multicenter registry. *Circulation.* 2015;131:1566-1574.

26. Sohail MR, Martin KR, Wilson WR, et al. Medical versus surgical management of *Staphylococcus aureus* prosthetic valve endocarditis. *Am J Med.* 2006;119:147-154.

27. Wang A, Pappas P, Anstrom KJ, et al. The use and effect of surgical therapy for prosthetic valve endocarditis: a propensity analysis of a multicenter, international cohort. *Am Heart J.* 2005;150:1086-1091.

28. Kang DH, Kim YJ, Kim SH, et al. Early surgery versus conventional treatment for infective endocarditis. *N Engl J Med.* 2012;366:2466-2473.

29. Lalani T, Chu VH, Park LP, et al. In-hospital and 1-year mortality in patients undergoing early surgery for prosthetic valve endocarditis. *JAMA Intern Med.* 2013;173:1495-1504.

30. Habib G, Lancellotti P, Antunes MJ, et al. 2015 ESC guidelines for the management of infective endocarditis. *Eur Heart J.* 2015;36:3075-3123.

31. Chaikof EL. The development of prosthetic heart valves—lessons in form and function. *N Engl J Med.* 2007;367:1368-1371.

32. McClure RS, McGurk S, Cevasco M, et al. Late outcomes comparison of nonelderly patients with stented bioprosthetic and mechanical valves in the aortic position: a propensity-matched analysis [published online ahead of print January 15, 2014]. *J Thorac Cardiovasc Surg.* 2014;148(5):1931-1939. doi:10.1016/j.jtcvs.2013.12.042.

33. Hammermeister K, Sethi GK, Henderson WG, Grover FL, Oprian C, Rahimtoola SH. Outcomes 15 years after valve replacement with a mechanical versus a bioprosthetic valve: final report of the Veterans Affairs randomized trial. *J Am Coll Cardiol.* 2000;36(4):1152-1158.

34. Oxenham H, Bloomfield P, Wheatley DJ, et al. Twenty year comparison of a Bjork-Shiley mechanical heart valve with porcine bioprostheses. *Heart.* 2003;89(7):715-721.

35. Stassano P, Di Tommaso L, Monaco M, et al. Aortic valve replacement: a prospective randomized evaluation of mechanical versus biological valves in patients ages 55 to 70 years. *J Am Coll Cardiol.* 2009;54(2):1862-1868.

36. Van Geldorp MW, Jamieson WR, Kappetien AP, et al. Patient outcome after aortic valve replacement with a mechanical or biological prosthesis: weighing lifetime anticoagulant-related event risk against reoperation risk. *J Thorac Cardiovasc Surg.* 2009;4:881-886.

37. Koertke H, Zittermann A, Wagner O, et al. Efficacy and safety of very low dose self-management of oral anticoagulation in patients with mechanical heart valve replacement. *Ann Thorac Surg.* 2010;90:1487-1494.

38. Grunkemeier GL, Li HH, Nafetl DC, et al. Long-term performance of heart valve prostheses. *Curr Probl Cardiol.* 2000;25:73-154.

39. Makkar RR, Fontana G, Jilihawi H, et al. Possible subclinical leaflet thrombosis in bioprosthetic aortic valves. *N Engl J Med.* 2015;373:2015-2024.

40. Eikelboom JW, Connolly SJ, Brueckmann M, et al. Dabigatran versus warfarin in patients with mechanical heart valves. *N Engl J Med.* 2013;369:1206-1214.

41. Siontis GC, Juni P, Pilgrim T, et al. Predictors of permanent pacemaker implantation in patients with severe aortic stenosis undergoing TAVR: a meta-analysis. *J Am Coll Cardiol.* 2014;64:129-140.

42. Bach DS, Patel HJ, Kolias TJ, Deeb GM. Randomized comparison of exercise hemodynamics of Freestyle, Magna Ease and Trifecta bioprostheses after aortic valve replacement for severe aortic stenosis [published online ahead of print January 27, 2016]. *Eur J Cardiothorac Surg.* 2016;50(2):361-367. doi:10.1093/ejcts/ezv493.

43. Cohen G, Zagorski B, Christakis GT, et al. Are stentless valves hemodynamically superior to stented valves? Long-term follow-up of a randomized trial comparing Carpentier-Edwards pericardial valve with the Toronto Stentless Porcine Valve. *J Thorac Cardiovasc Surg.* 2010;139:848-859.

44. Brown JM, O'Brien SM, Wu C, Sikora JA, Griffith BP, Gammie JS. Isolated aortic valve replacement in North America comprising 108,687 patients in 10 years: changes in risks, valve types, and outcomes in the Society of Thoracic Surgeons National Database. *J Thorac Cardiovasc Surg.* 2009;137(1):82-90.

45. Schnittman S, Chikwe J, Toyoda N, et al. Survival and late outcomes following bioprosthetic versus mechanical aortic valve replacement in patients aged 18 to 49 years. *J Thorac Cardiovasc Surg.* In press.

46. Ruel M, Kulik A, Lam BK, et al. Long-term outcomes of valve replacement with modern prostheses in young adults. *Eur J Cardiothorac Surg.* 2005;27(3):425-433.

47. Johnston JA, Cluxton RJ, Heaton PC, et al. Predictors of warfarin use among Ohio Medicaid patients with new onset nonvalvular atrial fibrillation. *Arch Intern Med.* 2003;163:1705-1710.

48. Dvir D, Webb J, Bleiziffer S, et al. Transcatheter aortic valve replacement for degenerative bioprosthetic surgical valves: results from the global valve-in-valve registry. *Circulation.* 2012;126(19):2335-2344.

49. Regitz-Zagrosek V, Lundqvist CB, Borghi C, et al. ESC guidelines on the management of cardiovascular diseases during pregnancy: the Task Force on the Management of Cardiovascular Diseases during Pregnancy of the European Society of Cardiology (ESC). *Eur Heart J.* 2011;32:3147-3197.

50. Zuhlke L, Engel ME, Karthikeyan G, et al. Characteristics, complications, and gaps in evidence based interventions in rheumatic heart disease: the Global Rheumatic Heart Disease Registry (the REMEDY study). *Eur Heart J.* 2015;36:1115-1122.

51. Oterhals K, Fridlund B, Nordrehaug JE, et al. Adapting to living with a mechanical aortic valve: a phenomenographic study. *J Adv Nurs.* 2013;69:2088-2098.

52. Conradi L, Silaschi M, Seiffert M, et al. Transcatheter valve-in-valve therapy using 6 different devices in 4 anatomic positions: clinical outcomes and technical considerations. *J Thorac Cardiovasc Surg.* 2015;150:1557-1565.

53. Breglio A, Anyanwu A, Itagaki S, et al. Does prior coronary bypass surgery present a unique risk for reoperative valve surgery? *Ann Thorac Surg.* 2013;95:1603-1608.

54. LaPar DJ, Yang Z, Stukenborg GJ, et al. Outcomes of reoperative aortic valve replacement after previous sternotomy. *J Thorac Cardiovasc Surg.* 2010;139:263-272.

55. Ruparelia N, Predergast BD. TAVI in 2015: who, where and how. *Heart.* 2015;101:1422-1431.

Patient and Family Information for: CONTEMPORARY SURGICAL APPROACH TO VALVULAR DISEASE

WHAT THE PATIENT AND FAMILY NEED TO KNOW

The heart works by pumping blood though four one-way valves, and over time these valves may become too tight (stenosis) or leaky (regurgitation). This most commonly affects two valves on the left side of the heart—the aortic and mitral valves—and sometimes affects the first valve on the right side of the heart—the tricuspid valve. In all cases, this means that the heart has to work harder to accomplish its job of pumping 5 to 8 L of blood per minute around the body. If this happens slowly, then the heart can compensate by stretching and developing thicker muscle. But eventually the heart muscle reaches its limit, and heart failure can result. Before that, the effects of the extra work and compensation can be felt as chest pain, breathlessness, or dizziness with exercise. In advanced cases, fluids fill up in the lungs and patients may experience difficulty breathing even when lying down, and may have lower leg swelling.

Sometimes a murmur can be heard using a stethoscope, but usually the most accurate way to assess the problem is an echocardiogram, which is a type of ultrasound that measures the function and size of the chambers of the heart, and assesses the heart valves.

Mitral and tricuspid regurgitation can be repaired, which allows patients to keep their own valve tissue, with the advantage of not needing anticoagulation and less risk of needing repeat surgery in the future. Most stenotic valves cannot be repaired and need to be replaced: the options for replacement are either mechanical valves or tissue valve (biologic). Mechanical valves are very durable, but need the recipient to take a blood thinner such as Coumadin for life. The risk of stroke and major bleeding is higher than with biologic valves, which do not need blood thinners. The disadvantage with tissue valves is that some patients will need repeat surgery as the valves eventually wear out over 10 to 15 years. For most people, a tissue valve is a good option.

Transcatheter aortic valve replacement is increasingly an option for treating aortic stenosis (AS), and for some people can replace a worn-out tissue valve. For most people, valve repair or replacement surgery is low risk, and the risk of major complications such as stroke is lower than the risk of dying or having a stroke if no treatment is carried out. Surgery usually takes 3 to 4 hours and is performed on the heart-lung machine, under a general anesthetic through a 2-to-5-inch incision usually in the front of the chest. Most patients are able to walk few days after surgery, and go home after 5 days.

Aeshita Dwivedi
Karen Kan
Sujata B. Chakravarti
Dan G. Halpern

41

The Care of the Adult Patient With Congenital Heart Disease in the Cardiac Care Unit

INTRODUCTION

Congenital heart disease (CHD) is the most common congenital lesion, estimated at 0.8% of newborns.[1-4] The medical and surgical revolution in the care of children with CHD over the recent decades has led to survival rates above 90% of children reaching adulthood. There are now more adults than children with CHD, with more than 1 million cases in the United States. Adults account for approximately 66% of the overall CHD population, and 60% of those with severe CHD.[5] A recent outcome study showed that survival of patients with adult congenital heart disease (ACHD) is increased when care is rendered in a center that has expertise in ACHD care.[6]

Care for the patient with ACHD in the cardiac care unit (CCU) is often challenging and requires meticulous investigation into the patient's past medical and surgical histories to understand complex pathophysiology. The patient and, commonly, the parents are an important source of information. One should enquire about the type of congenital defects and surgeries the patient underwent as well as the baseline vital signs, functional capacity, and known residual lesions.

The physical examination may reveal and corroborate information. For example:

1. Left lateral thoracotomy scar may be a hint of a previous Blalock–Taussig (BT) shunt (communication between the subclavian and the pulmonary artery [PA] for lesions that obstruct pulmonary blood flow) or coarctation of the aorta (CoA) repair.
2. Blood pressure differences between the upper and lower extremities may suggest significant obstructive CoA.
3. Patients having Eisenmenger syndrome (ES) are cyanotic, have clubbing, an accentuated P2 component on cardiac auscultation, yet do not exhibit an impressive murmur of the original unrepaired shunt (eg, large ventricular septal defect [VSD]) because ventricular pressures have reached equilibrium.
4. Continuous murmur over the left upper chest with a wide pulse pressure may suggest a hemodynamically significant patent ductus arteriosus (PDA), aortic regurgitation (AR), or, in the relevant clinical setting, a sinus of Valsalva rupture.
5. Congenital pulmonary stenosis has a mid-systolic click on auscultation that decreases in intensity during inspiration (the only right-sided lesion that does not accentuate during inspiration).

To simplify the understanding of complex lesions and hemodynamics, the congenital clinical scenario could be deconstructed to basic components such as shunts and obstructive and regurgitant lesions. These are further incorporated to the common adult pathologies (eg, arrhythmia, heart failure [HF], ischemia, sepsis, hypovolemia, and pulmonary hypertension). A drawing of the heart with lesions may be useful.

Any evaluation of a change in the clinical status of a patient with ACHD warrants reevaluation of the anatomy using multimodality imaging (eg, transthoracic and transesophageal echocardiography [TTE, TEE], cardiac magnetic resonance imaging [MRI]) as well as a new hemodynamic assessment by a right-sided hemodynamic catheterization). Opacification of conduits, pathways, vascular structures, and baffles is often needed to further delineate the anatomy. In the setting of pulmonary hypertension, a vascular reactivity test with nitric oxide and oxygen may be useful to determine reversibility.

It is important to underscore the importance that ACHD cardiologists are to be an integral part of the care team with congenital cases in the CCU. The ACHD team is a large collaboration between adult and pediatric clinical cardiologists, congenital imagers, and those in interventional cardiology, electrophysiology, intensive care, anesthesia, obstetrics, and genetics. Weekly complex case conferences with team members are encouraged.

The following sections detail specific congenital lesions followed by several fundamental topics.

SPECIFIC LESIONS

Shunt Lesions

In normal physiology, the pulmonary blood flow (Qp) and systemic blood flow (Qs) run in parallel and maintain an equivalent ratio of blood through both the circulations at any given time (Qp:Qs = 1:1). Any abnormal connection that allows oxygenated and deoxygenated blood to mix is called a shunt. Shunt calculations of Qp:Qs > 1 signify net left-to-right shunting, whereas Qp:Qs < 1 signifies net right-to-left shunting. Shunt lesions are further divided into pre-tricuspid lesion, such as atrial septal defects (ASDs) and partial anomalous pulmonary venous connection, and post-tricuspid lesions such as VSDs and PDAs. Pre-tricuspid lesions cause right-sided heart enlargement and post-tricuspid lesions cause left-sided heart enlargement. A Qp:Qs > 1.5 commonly denotes a significant shunt. The spectrum can vary from small ASDs or VSDs to near absence of delineation between the right and left heart, causing a single-ventricular mixing physiology. Commonly, shunt lesions with chamber enlargement are an indication for closure of the communication, unless there is evidence of irreversible pulmonary hypertension, which is the unfortunate sequela of chronic volume overload with or without pressure overload through the lung vasculature.[7]

CCU care of shunt lesions warrants delineation of the anatomy, shunt calculation (Qp/Qs, most accurate by cardiac magnetic resonance [MR] and cardiac catheterization), and assessment of the pulmonary pressures (by echocardiography and cardiac catheterization). The degree of shunting is influenced by the size of the shunt, compliance of the ventricles, and the downstream pulmonary vascular resistance (PVR) and systemic vascular resistance (SVR). Altering each of these components would change the degree of shunting.

We discuss the most common congenital shunt lesions including ASD, VSD, and PDA.

Atrial Septal Defect

ASDs are among the most common CHDs encountered in adulthood (**Figure 41.1**).[8] ASDs typically cause left-to-right shunting and right-sided heart structure enlargement. The direction of the shunting occurs because of greater compliance of the right ventricle and thus lower right atrial pressure. The timing of the interatrial shunt is typically in late systole, early diastole, and during atrial systole. In situations where the right ventricular (RV) compliance is decreased and right atrial pressure is increased, ASDs may shunt right-to-left and cause cyanosis. Qp:Qs > 1.5 and an ASD larger than 1 cm are associated with a significant shunt. The clinical concern with ASDs is the development of RV enlargement and dysfunction due to volume overload, arrhythmias, paradoxic emboli, and the development of pulmonary hypertension. Although rare, the pulmonary vascular disease may

progress to a fixed state that would cause the shunt to reverse and cause cyanosis, which is referred to as ES.

Clinically, the age and degree of symptoms vary according to the size of the shunt, direction of the shunt, and presence of other associated congenital malformations. The most common type of ASD is the secundum type, which is a deficiency of the septum primum, the major membrane forming the septum. The deficiency is located in the center of the interatrial septum. Other types include primum ASD, which is an inferior defect that is part of the endocardial cushions (junction between the atria and ventricles) and is associated with a cleft anterior mitral valve; sinus venosus defect is a deficiency in the tissue at the junction between the right atrium and the superior vena cava (SVC) or inferior vena cava (IVC) and is associated with anomalous pulmonary venous connections; and unroofed coronary sinus is a defect that opens between the coronary sinus (left-sided atrioventricular [AV] groove) into the left atrium and is associated with a persistent left SVC and could present with cyanosis.

Patients with ASDs commonly present by the fifth decade with exercise intolerance and/or arrhythmia. On physical examination, RV enlargement may cause an RV heave and on auscultation a wide and fixed splitting of S2 is characteristic of ASDs. Pulmonary hypertension will have a loud P2. Owing to the increased flow across the tricuspid valve (TV), a diastolic rumble that accentuates with inspiration may be heard. In primum ASD, which is associated with cleft mitral valve, murmur of mitral regurgitation can be appreciated. If a patient has ES, cyanosis and clubbing may also be present. Electrocardiogram (ECG) in secundum ASD shows right axis deviation, whereas in primum ASD it is left axis deviation; and the P waves in sinus venosus ASD are typically negative in the inferior leads. Otherwise, ECGs have rSr′ or rsR′ pattern due to RV hypertrophy, and the Crochetage pattern is a sensitive and specific sign of ASD described as a notch on the R wave in the inferior leads.

Echocardiogram is essential for diagnosis of an ASD and is helpful in identifying associated lesions. A TTE is also useful to evaluate the size and function of the right ventricle as well as direction of the shunt. Using Doppler echocardiography, pulmonary artery systolic pressure (PASP) and the ratio of Qp:Qs can also be estimated (however, these are not always accurate and are subject to errors). TTE is often adequate for diagnosis of secundum and primum ASDs. However, it is less sensitive for diagnosis of sinus venosus ASDs. Presence of right heart dilatation in the absence of an alternative etiology should always raise suspicion for an undiagnosed ASD on a TTE. TEE is typically needed for confirming diagnosis of sinus venosus ASD and unroofed coronary sinus. A TEE can identify anomalous pulmonary venous connection associated with sinus venosus ASD. A TEE is also helpful to evaluate the size of the ASD as well as to guide treatment options. Cardiac MRI is very useful for evaluating the degree of shunting (Qp:Qs), delineating the anatomy including identifying the pulmonary veins. In patients who cannot undergo a cardiac MRI, computed tomography (CT) may be considered. Lastly, once ASD repair is being considered, a cardiac catheterization is necessary to evaluate PA pressures as well as PVR and vascular reactivity because these factors impact the management of the ASD.

Indications for closure of ASDs are RV enlargement regardless of symptoms, paradoxic embolism, or orthodeoxiaplatypnea (dyspnea and cyanosis when sitting upright or standing). Secundum ASDs may be closed percutaneously with an ASD closure device,

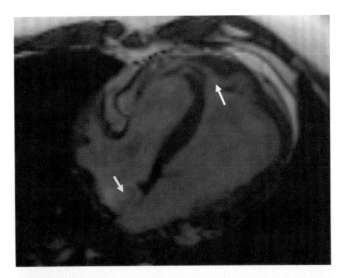

FIGURE 41.1 Shunts by CMR. Combination of a secundum atrial septal defect (*yellow arrow*) and an apical muscular ventricular septal defect (*white arrow*). The patient also has a relatively hypoplastic right ventricle compared to the left. CMR, cardiac magnetic resonance.

unless they are larger than 35 mm or have inadequate margins (<5 mm) and then surgical closure is warranted. Primum ASDs, sinus venosus defects, and unroofed coronary sinus ASDs require surgical closure using a patch repair. Contraindications for ASD closure are evidence of irreversible pulmonary hypertension (ie, ES, PVR greater than two-thirds of SVR, or commonly PVR above 5 to 7 Woods units)

Patients with small, asymptomatic ASDs (typically <10 mm) with normal RV function and absence of pulmonary hypertension should be monitored.

Ventricular Septal Defect

VSDs are the most common CHD in children (**Figures 41.1** and **41.2**). VSDs are associated with left-sided heart enlargement and dysfunction and are more prone to cause pulmonary hypertension.[9]

The most common type is the membranous VSD, which is located next to the septal leaflet of the TV. Occasionally, it is associated within an aneurysm of the TV-associated tissue and at times is occluded by the septal leaflet of the TV. Infundibular VSDs (also known as conal, supracristal, subpulmonary, subarterial, or doubly committed juxta-arterial) are common in the Asian population. These are typically located beneath the semilunar valves and are often associated with AR due to prolapse of the right coronary cusp of the aortic valve into the defect. Inlet VSD is a deficiency in the endocardial cushion (junction between the atria and ventricles) and is seen commonly in patients with trisomy 21. When associated with a primum ASD and a common AV valve, these constitute an atrioventricular canal defect (AVCD). Muscular VSDs (also called trabecular) are VSDs surrounded by muscle tissue and not infrequently are multiple. The types of VSDs that may close spontaneously in childhood (40% to 60% of VSDs) are the membranous and muscular types.

Clinically, the majority of patients in adulthood will not require any interventions, because isolated small VSDs remain asymptomatic. Moderate-sized VSDs already present with left-sided HF in childhood, and large VSDs present with HF in infancy or pulmonary hypertension in childhood. Interestingly, on physical examination the small VSDs present with a loud holosystolic murmur (large pressure gradient), whereas the large ones

are minimally heard because there is equilibrium in pressure between the ventricles. As noted before, patients with ES would have cyanosis, clubbing, and signs of right-sided HF and an accentuated P2 on auscultation. Most patients with VSDs initially have relatively normal ECGs. Subsequently, as the left ventricle develops volume overload, signs of interventricular conduction delay and left ventricular (LV) enlargement may be noted. With the presence of Eisenmenger complex, signs of RV hypertrophy, right axis deviation may also be noted.

TTE is useful in visualizing the defect and assessing LV/RV size and function as well as pulmonary pressures. Cardiac MRI would provide supplemental visualization of the defect as well as more accurate shunt calculations. Cardiac catheterization is used to delineate anatomy and assess for pulmonary pressures as well as pulmonary vascular reactivity in the setting of pulmonary hypertension. A restrictive VSD is regarded as a small shunt with Qp/Qs < 1.4 and high-pressure gradients across the VSD. Qp/Qs > 1.5 denotes significant (moderate and above) shunt. LV enlargement with a Qp/Qs ≥ 2 as well as symptoms or history of endocarditis without the presence of irreversible pulmonary hypertension are class I indications for VSD closure. Most VSDs require surgical patch repair; and if other concomitant lesions (such as aortic insufficiency) exist, they should be addressed as well. Percutaneous repair may be considered for patients with an isolated uncomplicated muscular VSD and for membranous VSD bases on the anatomy. Asymptomatic patients with small VSDs can be followed up with serial imaging and follow-up. No endocarditis prophylaxis is warranted in patients with unrepaired VSDs.

Patients with ES are managed medically, which is discussed in a separate section.

Patent Ductus Arteriosus

PDA is a persistent communication between the aortic isthmus (junction between the aortic arch and descending aorta) and the main PA that causes a left-to-right shunt that may result in left-sided volume overload and pulmonary hypertension.[10] Usually, the ductus arteriosus, which is essential to the fetal circulation for blood flow from the heart to the lower part of the body, closes within 72 hours of birth. There is a female preponderance for PDA with a 2:1 ratio compared to male, and it is associated with congenital Rubella and birth at high altitudes as well as other congenital defects (ie, ASDs, VSDs, CoA). PDAs are primarily a clinical concern because of LV volume overload and dysfunction and a risk for endarteritis or endocarditis (commonly the pulmonary valve). The latter is estimated roughly as up to 1%/year.

The PDA shunt occurs continuously throughout the cardiac cycle in systole and diastole and sounds like "machinery" on auscultation. The direction of the shunt is from the aorta into the PA (left-to-right), and in the setting of a significant shunt, akin to AR, may cause a wide pulse pressure, low diastolic coronary filling pressures, and ischemia. With time, owing to the increased flow across the pulmonary bed, the PVR may rise, eventually leading to shunt reversal, right-to-left shunt, and Eisenmenger physiology. Because the shunt is connected between the PA and the aortic isthmus, the cyanosis only appears in the lower part of the body in the setting of ES, referred to as "differential cyanosis" (**Figure 41.3**).

The clinical presentation depends mainly on the size of the shunt and the presence of any concomitant lesions. Patients with small PDAs may remain asymptomatic and be incidentally diagnosed because of the presence of a murmur, whereas those

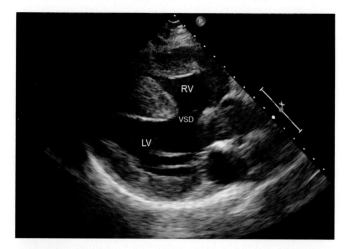

FIGURE 41.2 Large muscular VSD with Eisenmenger syndrome; transthoracic parasternal long-axis view echocardiography. The RV is severely hypertrophied. LV, left ventricle; RV, right ventricle; VSD, ventricular septal defect.

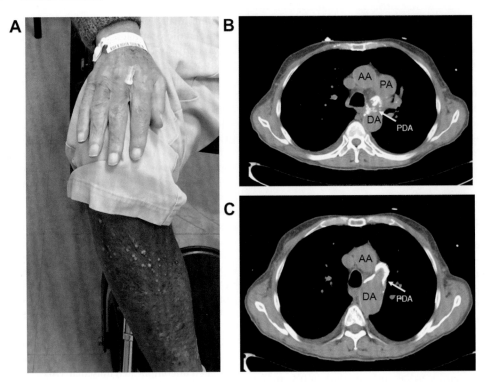

FIGURE 41.3 PDA complicated by Eisenmenger syndrome. A, "differential cyanosis," upper limbs proximal to the PDA are oxygenated and lower limbs beyond the PDA are deoxygenated, as pulmonary flow is shunting right-to-left through the PDA toward the lower body. B and C, two consecutive axial images of non–contrast-enhanced CT scan demonstrating a calcified large PDA *(arrow)* communicating between the DA and the PA. AA, ascending aorta; CT, computed tomography; DA, descending aorta; PA, pulmonary artery; PDA, patent ductus arteriosus.

with moderate-to-large PDAs typically present in early childhood and infancy, respectively, with signs of LV volume overload. Echocardiography is commonly the initial modality to make the diagnosis, and cardiac MR or CT angiography is supplemental for further delineation of the anatomy, Qp/Qs, and pulmonary pressure measurement in preparation for a catheter-based closure procedure.

Generally, any PDA that could be "heard" on auscultation during physical examination is designated for closure. According to guidelines, any PDA with LV volume overload regardless of symptoms without irreversible pulmonary hypertension should be closed. Also, patients with a history of endocarditis should have their PDA closed. PDAs are occluded with coils or closure devices such as the Amplatzer ductal occluder.

BICUSPID AORTIC VALVE, COARCTATION, AND AORTOPATHIES

Bicuspid aortic valve (BAV) is a common congenital condition with an estimated incidence of 1% to 2% of the general population. The most common cusp fusion is between the right and left. Over time, BAVs can be either stenotic or regurgitant and may require aortic valve replacement in adulthood. BAV is associated with an aortopathy and increased frequency of ascending aortic aneurysms. Aortic root replacement is recommended when the aortic diameter exceeds 5.0 to 5.5 cm or if there is a rapid enlargement of the root (>5 mm/year).[11]

Frequently associated with BAV, CoA comprises a segmental narrowing of the aorta at the ligamentum arteriosum site adjacent to the left subclavian artery (**Figure 41.4**). Patients with significant

CoA develop collateral vessels that mitigate the severity of the obstructive narrowing. More than half of patients with CoA have BAV, and about 10% of those with BAV, would be found to have CoA. Another association of CoA is Shone complex, which refers to multiple left heart obstructive lesions that include CoA, BAV, subaortic stenosis, parachute mitral valve, and supra-mitral valve ring.

Patients with CoA commonly present with hypertension, exertional headaches, and leg claudication. CoA is an important diagnosis in the evaluation of systemic hypertension in the young. On physical examination, a significant CoA may cause an abnormally lower blood pressure measured in the lower limbs. However, a significant collateral network may mask these differences and a radial–femoral delay pulse check examination may be completely normal. In addition, carotid pulses may be hyperdynamic and a murmur or bruit may be present in the left interscapular area. Chest X-ray may show the "number 3" sign and rib notching. Patients with CoA are at risk for congestive HF, aortic rupture and dissection, endocarditis and endarteritis, intracerebral hemorrhage from associated brain aneurysms (5%), and myocardial infarction. Management of these patients includes consideration of percutaneous or surgical repair and medical therapy for hypertension. Blood pressure control in the setting of CoA may be challenging because excessive reduction of pressures beyond the coarctation may cause lower body hypotension, gut ischemia, and renal failure. By guidelines, intervention is recommended for patients who have a peak-to-peak gradient across the aortic narrowing as measured on cardiac catheterization greater than or equal to 20 mm Hg. Echocardiography measurements of the maximum instantaneous gradient across the area of coarctation commonly overestimate the peak-to-peak gradient measured in

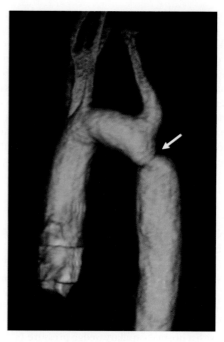

FIGURE 41.4 Coarctation of the aorta by MR angiography. Three-dimensional reconstruction of the aorta demonstrating (*arrow*) a discrete coarctation of the aorta distal to the left subclavian artery and the area of the aortic isthmus. MR, magnetic resonance.

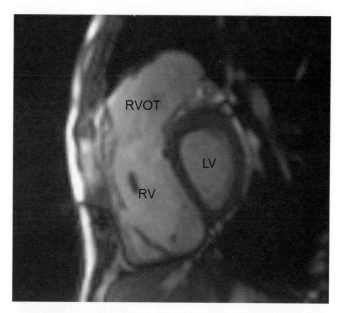

FIGURE 41.5 Repaired tetralogy of Fallot by CMR. Short-axis image demonstrating a severely dilated RV and an RVOT as well as free pulmonary regurgitation. There are no pulmonary valve leaflets identified. The septum is flat, suggesting RV volume overload compressing the LV. CMR, cardiac magnetic resonance; LV, left ventricle; RV, right ventricle; RVOT, right ventricular outflow tract.

the catheterization laboratory. The mean gradient derived by TTE across the area of coarctation has been found to be more closely related to the peak-to-peak gradient. Cardiac MRI is very useful for delineation of the anatomy, collateral identification, and flow measurements in preparation for stent implantation, which is the preferred method of intervention in the adult patient. It should be noted that patients with CoA have accelerated atherosclerosis and ischemic heart disease, and these should be suspected in the relevant scenario.

TETRALOGY OF FALLOT

Tetralogy of Fallot (TOF) represents a spectrum of disease that is classically defined by four components: (1) subpulmonary infundibular/right ventricular outflow tract (RVOT) stenosis, (2) VSD (commonly membranous), (3) overriding aorta, and (4) RV hypertrophy. Frequently, these patients have small, stenotic pulmonary valves along with PA hypoplasia and stenosis, coronary anomalies, right aortic arch, as well as ASDs.

The embryonic pathophysiology is related to one single abnormal process—the anterior and cephalad deviation of the conal septum leading to right-sided obstruction with an aortic valve overriding the two ventricles. In the neonatal period, this disease causes lack of adequate pulmonary blood flow and cyanosis; and thus the initial treatment may include a shunt between the arterial and the pulmonary circulations (eg, BT shunt between the subclavian artery and the PA) followed by definite repair that includes surgical closure of the VSD and the relief of the RVOT obstruction, commonly using the transannular patch repair.

In the era of modern cardiac surgery, nearly all patients with TOF in the United States will have had reparative surgery early in life. Because the RVOT was resected and there is no functioning pulmonary valve, the major complication related to the TOF repair is chronic pulmonary regurgitation (PR) (**Figure 41.5**). Long-standing PR further begets RV dilatation and dysfunction, tricuspid regurgitation (TR), LV dysfunction related to RV/LV interactions (up to 30%) and tachyarrhythmias (intra-atrial reentrant tachycardia [IART], atrial fibrillation [AF], and VT). Other long-term complications include residual RVOT obstruction, residual VSD from a dehiscing patch, and patch-related TR. By clinical practice guidelines, pulmonary valve replacement (PVR) is warranted for severe PR in symptomatic patients with decreased exercise tolerance or clinical HF. In addition, it is generally agreed that PVR is also reasonable in asymptomatic patients with severe PR who exhibit moderate-to-severe RV enlargement (greater than indexed end-diastolic volume 150 cc/m^2, greater than indexed end-systolic volume of 80 cc/m^2) or dysfunction (right ventricular ejection fraction [RVEF] <47%), left ventricular dysfunction (left ventricular ejection fraction [LVEF] <55%), concomitant moderate and above TR, QRS >160 ms, severe AR, RVOT obstruction/aneurysm, or significant atrial or ventricular arrhythmias related to the right ventricle.[12] New native RVOT transcatheter pulmonary valves are in the investigational phase.

Overall survival in repaired TOF is excellent, yet there is an increased risk of sudden cardiac death (SCD) later in life. Arrhythmias are related to surgical scar lines and dysfunctional right ventricle. SCD is estimated at 2% per decade in patients with repaired TOF, and overall arrhythmia frequency increases in the fifth decade. A QRS > 180 ms on ECG is a sensitive predictor of SCD in addition to morphologic findings such as RV hypertrophy and ventricular dysfunction. There is a direct relationship between the degree of RV enlargement/dysfunction and the degree of arrhythmias. Lastly, aortic root dilatation is also prevalent in patients with repaired TOF that could be explained in part by the basic overriding aorta receiving an increased cardiac output and evidence of an intrinsic aortopathy.

Arrhythmia and HF related to RV and LV dysfunction are anticipated to be the diagnoses for admission to the CCU.

EBSTEIN ANOMALY OF THE TRICUSPID VALVE

Ebstein anomaly (EA) is a rare diagnosis and entails malformation of the TV in which there is failure of delamination (separation) of the septal and posterior tricuspid leaflets from the myocardium, causing the "functional" tricuspid annulus to be apically displaced[13] (**Figure 41.6**). The portion proximal to the annulus is dilated and the right ventricle proximal to the "functional" tricuspid annulus is similar in morphology to the atrium and thus is "atrialized." Because the posterior and septal TV leaflets are malformed, the anterior leaflet is often large and redundant; and, on physical examination, a systolic "snap" can be heard. This deformity leads to varying degrees of TR and rarely stenosis. EA is also associated with atrial communications (eg, patent foramen ovale [PFO], ASD), multiple accessory conduction pathways (ie, Wolf–Parkinson–White [WPW]), LV non-compaction, pulmonary valve abnormalities, PDA, and CoA. Clinical presentation varies and depends largely on the degree of malformation of the tricuspid leaflets, RV size and function, presence of associated cardiac lesions, and accessory pathways. For example, a first presentation to the CCU of a patient with EA may be collapse or SCD due to rapidly conducting AF in the setting of WPW. Others may present with exercise-induced cyanosis due to right-to-left shunting through an ASD or, more commonly, exercise intolerance due to RV dysfunction and severe TR. ECG shows "Himalayan" P waves, and the patient may have preexcitation with short PR interval and a very wide right bundle branch block. Echocardiographic diagnosis is based on apical displacement of the septal leaflet of

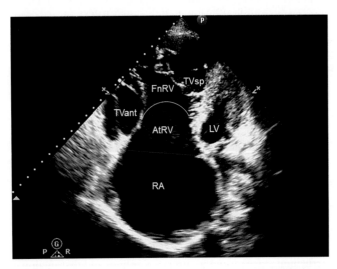

FIGURE 41.6 Transthoracic apical four-chamber view of Ebstein anomaly of the tricuspid valve demonstrating severe right ventricular dilatation, which is divided into a proximal atrialized portion (AtRV) and a distal function portion (FnRV) by the apicalized tricuspid annulus (curved yellow line). The apically displaced TVsp is diminutive in size and the TVant is large, redundant, and is connected to the anatomic tricuspid annulus (red line). The LV is small and compressed by the dilated right ventricle. Not seen in this figure, but the patient had severe tricuspid regurgitation. LV, left ventricle; AtRV, atrial right ventricle; FnRV, functional right ventricle; RA, right atrium; TVant, anterior leaflet of the tricuspid valve; TVsp, septal leaflet of the tricuspid valve.

the TV by more than 0.8 cm/m^2 from the true tricuspid annulus. TV repair of EA is surgically challenging and is warranted for decreased exercise tolerance, cyanosis, paradoxic embolism, and progressive RV enlargement and dysfunction. In the Cone procedure, the large anterior TV leaflet is manipulated to create a functional valve. If surgical repair is deemed impossible, a TV replacement is performed. In cases where the RV is considered too dysfunctional, a Glenn shunt (connection between the SVC and PA) may be performed to partially unload the right ventricle, that is, blood from the upper part of the body would directly flow to the lungs bypassing the right ventricle. Lastly, accessory pathways should be ablated (see discussion in arrhythmia in adult congenital heart disease section).

PULMONARY ARTERIAL HYPERTENSION, CYANOSIS, AND EISENMENGER SYNDROME

Pulmonary arterial hypertension (PAH) occurs in approximately 5% to 10% of ACHD. ES (**Figures 41.2** and **41.3**), which is the most extreme form of congenital PAH, is seen in about 1%.[14] The definition of PAH includes a mean PA pressure greater than or equal to 25 mm Hg with a normal capillary wedge pressure (<15 mm Hg). Congenital PAH is included in World Health Organization (WHO) group I category. ES typically occurs in patients with congenital defects that result in substantial unrestricted left-to-right shunting, most commonly VSD and AVCDs. Over time, the shunt causes detrimental hemodynamic effects with large increases in PVR (generally greater than 10 Wood units) that subsequently causes reversal or bidirectional flow across the existing shunt. Cyanosis and hemodynamic derangements depend on the degree of flow reversal across the shunt.

ES affects multiple organ systems because of the chronic cyanosis. The effects include secondary erythrocytosis with increased viscosity, iron deficiency anemia, thrombocytopenia, coagulopathy,[15] cerebral abscesses, microemboli, strokes, and renal dysfunction. Interestingly, the coronary arteries are ectatic with less atherosclerosis and calcifications.[16]

There are several unique management considerations for these patients including limitation of strenuous isometric exercise, dehydration, and chronic high altitude and warm environments. Active hydration is encouraged but may be challenging in the setting of chronic HF. Phlebotomy is offered for symptomatic patients with hyperviscosity symptoms such as severe headaches (commonly with hemoglobin >20 g%, hematocrit > 65%). Iron deficiency anemia is common and associated with increased frequency of strokes, yet careful correction is required because it increases the blood count further. Pregnancy is completely contraindicated because of the up to 50% maternal and fetal mortality, and termination of pregnancy should be counseled when possible.

Randomized controlled trials, the most notable being the BREATHE-5 (**B**osentan **R**andomized Trial of **E**ndothelin **A**ntagonist **THE**rapy-5), have demonstrated that patients with ES derive a clinical benefit from pulmonary vasodilator therapies (including prostanoids, endothelin receptor antagonists, and phosphodiesterase inhibitors). Although these patients are at an elevated risk of PA thromboembolism, the role of anticoagulation is not entirely clear because they are prone to bleeding such as hemoptysis. Oxygen supplementation has limited support but could be offered. Lastly, for those with advanced disease, heart–lung transplantation can be offered for selected patients on a case-by-case basis.

CCU care depends on the inciting pathology, yet general care of the patient with ES includes intravenous (IV) filters, oxygen support as needed, maintenance of SVR (use of vasopressors as needed) and reduction of PVR (nitric oxide inhalation, IV prostacyclin therapy), and correction of arrhythmia and iron deficiency anemia. Decision making in regard to diuresis depends on the degree of HF in the setting of limiting hypovolemia and hyperviscosity.

TRANSPOSITION OF THE GREAT ARTERIES AND SYSTEMIC RIGHT VENTRICLE

In d-transposition of the great arteries (d-TGA), the aorta originates from the right ventricle and the PA from the left ventricle.[17] The aorta is usually situated anteriorly and to the right of the PA. The immediate palliation at birth is the creation of an ASD with a balloon because the two parallel circulations are not compatible with life. The original surgical correction for d-TGA was the atrial switch operation (ie, Mustard or Senning procedures) in which the systemic venous circulation was baffled to the LV and the pulmonary venous circulation to the RV (**Figure 41.7**). Long-term complications include baffle obstruction (commonly at the SVC junction), baffle leak with paradoxic emboli, systemic RV dysfunction, TR, and tachyarrhythmia (mostly atrial that may degenerate to ventricular). CCU evaluation of the d-TGA post atrial switch should include imaging of the baffles for obstruction/leakage, correction of arrhythmia, and HF support. Baffle leaks and obstructions could be treated with stenting.

For the past 25 years, the arterial switch operation (ASO) or Jatene procedure has been the standard surgical approach to treatment of d-TGA. This procedure restores normal anatomy, yet has its own set of complications including coronary obstruction, aortic dilatation, and supra-pulmonary stenosis. A d-TGA post ASO should always raise suspicion of ischemia. Of note, the patient may have damaged cardiac innervation and not have classic complaint of angina.

In congenitally corrected transposition of the great arteries (cc-TGA or levo transposition of the great arteries [L-TGA]), the ventricles are inverted, and the morphologic right ventricle is situated on the left side and is connected to the aorta (so-called "double discordance"—AV and ventriculoarterial). The aorta is anterior and to the left of the PA. Long-term complications include TR (in 90%, the TV is abnormal), heart block (1% to 2%/year), outflow tract obstructions, and systemic RV dysfunction. Common surgeries for cc-TGA are TV repair, and at present children undergo double-switch operation with a simultaneous arterial switch and atrial switch for complete anatomic repair.

To reiterate, both d-TGA post atrial switch and cc-TGA share the same pathology of a systemic right ventricle (**Figure 41.7**). The systemic right ventricle, acting as the main pumping chamber to the aorta, is subjected to both increased pressure and volume load and thus develops HF. Interestingly, the TR seen in cc-TGA is primarily related to an abnormal TV and thus has the benefit of being corrected/replaced before worsening the systemic RV function (per guideline before RVEF of 40%); whereas in d-TGA post atrial switch, the TR seen is functional and related to systemic RV dilatation and dysfunction. Also, because the right coronary artery is still the main coronary providing blood to the chamber, ischemia may develop because of supply–demand mismatch. Potentially advanced HF therapies may be offered in the setting of intractable systemic HF (see Heart Failure in adult congenital heart disease section).

SINGLE VENTRICLE AND FONTAN PALLIATION

Single ventricle anatomy is one of the more challenging and complex ACHD pathologies (**Figure 41.8**). The term encompasses several different conditions including tricuspid atresia, mitral atresia, double-inlet left ventricle, and hypoplastic right or left ventricle. In caring for the patient with ACHD having single ventricle anatomy, it is important to note that most of these patients have had several staged procedures early in life culminating in the Fontan operation.[18] Broadly, the Fontan operation is a palliative procedure in which systemic venous return is routed directly to the pulmonary arterial circulation. The systemic venous circulation flows passively into the lungs, now propelled by the negative intrathoracic pressure, skeletal muscles, and gravity of the blood from the upper part of the body. The hemodynamic consequence of the Fontan circulation is chronically elevated systemic venous pressures that eventually cause chronic liver congestion, ascites, leg varices, and promote lymphatic congestion that may cause protein-losing enteropathy

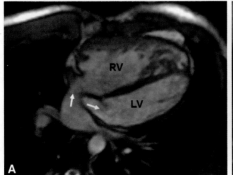
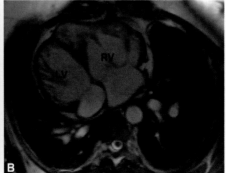

FIGURE 41.7 Transposition of the great arteries (TGA) with systemic right ventricles by CMR. A, d-TGA post atrial switch operation; white arrow denotes the pulmonary venous baffle and the yellow arrow denotes the systemic venous baffle. B, Dextrocardia with congenitally corrected TGA (cc-TGA or levo-TGA [L-TGA]). CMR, cardiac magnetic resonance; LV, left ventricle; RV, right ventricle.

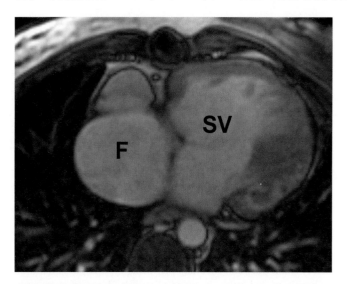

FIGURE 41.8 Fontan circulation by CMR. Baseline anatomy is double-inlet left ventricle with an atriopulmonary Fontan circulation. CMR, cardiac magnetic resonance; F, Fontan; SV, single ventricle.

(PLE)[19] and plastic bronchitis. Current Fontan surgery includes a total cavopulmonary connection that consists of an extracardiac conduit or lateral tunnel baffle (within the right atrium) connecting to the PA from the IVC and a Glenn shunt connecting the SVC to the PA from above. An older version of the Fontan palliation consisted of atriopulmonary connection (right atrium connected to the PA) that resulted in an extremely large right atrium that promoted arrhythmia and clot formation.

The patients should be followed up closely by an ACHD specialist, particularly as several characteristic long-term issues arise including atrial arrhythmias, right atrial thrombus often necessitating systemic anticoagulation, single ventricular dysfunction, systemic AV valve regurgitation, cyanosis (due to veno-veno collaterals, pulmonary arteriovenous malformations, residual shunts, open fenestration, lung disease), hepatic congestion with deterioration of liver function from fibrosis to frank cirrhosis,[20-22] PLE, and plastic bronchitis. Although the 10-year survival after a Fontan is estimated to be 90%, many of these patients do require reoperation in adulthood and the long-term survival is protracted with SCD, thromboembolism, and HF being the most common causes of death.

CCU care for the patient with a Fontan circulation requires a thorough understanding of the limitation of having a passive pulmonary circulation. Any increase in left atrial pressure (eg, LV dysfunction, AV valve regurgitation, LV outflow tract obstruction) or increase in PVR (eg, pulmonary baffle obstruction, pulmonary hypertension, pneumonia, pneumothorax, and obstructive sleep apnea) may hinder the passive flow and decrease the cardiac output. Arrhythmia is commonly supraventricular and not tolerated well, and therefore cardioversion is commonly the initial step in the treatment. A common caveat is that in such patients, a heart rate of 120 beats/min is commonly atrial flutter (IART). Furthermore, volume management is challenging because HF, cirrhosis, lymphatic obstruction, and chronic hypoalbuminemia contribute to chronic anasarca. End-stage patients require increasing dosages of diuretics and repeated paracentesis. Patients with atriopulmonary Fontan, which is the older version of the connection, may be offered a "Fontan conversion" in which the

connection would be changed to an extracardiac version with plication of the right atrium and placement of a pacing system. The conversion reduces the frequency of arrhythmia and increases the efficiency of the circuit.

GENERAL TOPICS OF DIAGNOSIS AND MANAGEMENT IN ADULT CONGENITAL HEART DISEASE

ARRHYTHMIA IN ADULT CONGENITAL HEART DISEASE

Cardiac arrhythmias are a leading cause of morbidity and mortality in the ACHD population. The burden of arrhythmias increases with age, number of cardiac surgeries, and the complexity of the congenital lesion.[23,24]

Atrial Arrhythmias

The most common atrial arrhythmia in the ACHD population is IART. It may originate within the natural conduction channels (ie, the cavotricuspid isthmus) or iatrogenic conduction channels (suture lines or patches). IART commonly occurs in patients who have undergone surgical atrial manipulation (eg, atrial switch operations or Fontan procedure). Electrocardiographically, it will appear similar to atrial flutter, yet usually slower in rate (250 to 400 ms) and frequently conduct 2:1 to 1:1. Like in AF, these patients are at risk of thromboembolic complications. Hemodynamically unstable patients should be cardioverted emergently. Antiarrhythmic drugs may be considered for rate or rhythm control but have low efficacy. Therefore, these are typically treated with catheter ablation. The success of ablation procedures ranges from 55% to 90% depending on the anatomy of the burden of fibrosis in the atrium. These arrhythmias may recur post ablation; and in select patients, surgical (intraoperative) ablation may be indicated.

AF is also a commonly encountered arrhythmia in ACHD and its frequency increases with age. Because AF arises from the left atrium, lesions affecting the left-sided structures are associated with AF; for example, mitral valve deformities and single ventricle or aortic stenosis. It should be noted that often times AF may occur in association with sinus node dysfunction with a slow ventricular response. Treatment strategies include class III antiarrhythmics and may warrant catheter or surgical pulmonary vein isolation. Anticoagulation should be prescribed in accordance with the AF guidelines to prevent thromboembolic complications.

Accessory pathways predispose patients with ACHD to tachyarrhythmias, and some may be life-threatening. WPW syndrome is commonly associated with EA (found in about 20% of patients), and congenitally corrected TGA with an Ebstenoid malformation of the left-sided TV. The location of the multiple accessory pathways is usually in the vicinity of the tricuspid annulus. The treatment typically includes catheter ablation of the pathway; however, it is often challenging because of the altered anatomy and the presence of multiple pathways.

Ventricular Tachycardias and Sudden Cardiac Death

The overall incidence of SCD in patients with ACHD is about 1% per decade but may be higher in more complex lesions and typically increases with age. The highest risk lesions include repaired TOF, EA, and congenital aortic stenosis. As in patients with HF, systemic ventricle dysfunction is the major risk factor for SCD. Any hemodynamic compromise or stress on the ventricles can increase the risk of malignant arrhythmias. In TOF, the risk of SCD is approximately 2% until adolescence, but acutely rises to 6% to 10% per decade in adulthood. RV enlargement and longer duration of the QRS width have also been correlated with SCD. Holter monitor and in select patients electrophysiologic (EP) study may be performed for risk stratification. Evidence of non-sustained ventricular tachycardia (VT) on Holter or inducible VT on EP study has been shown to predict risk of SCD in patients with TOF. In patients with congenital aortic stenosis or CoA, the risk of SCD directly correlates with the severity of the gradient across these lesions. VTs should be managed similarly to the general population, whereby hemodynamically unstable patients warrant emergent defibrillation. Implantable cardioverter defibrillators (ICDs) are indicated for prevention of SCD. The indication for ICD implantation in patients with ACHD is largely similar to the general adult population. ICD implantation can often be challenging and have higher risk because of the distorted anatomy and prior surgeries. At times, epicardial ICDs may be implanted if venous access cannot be obtained. In select patients, subcutaneous ICDs are implanted. Patients with monomorphic VT can also be considered for VT ablations. Cardiac resynchronization therapy (CRT) is a primarily effective therapy for restoring electromechanical synchrony in the morphologic left ventricle. Owing to the altered anatomy, CRT is less effective in patients with ACHD with systemic right ventricles or single ventricles.[25]

Bradyarrhythmias

Sinus node dysfunction is common as a result of direct injury after a surgery. Rarely is the sinus node congenitally absent. Sinus node dysfunction is commonly seen after atrial switch operations (ie, Mustard and Senning) for d-TGA or after a Fontan operation. The bradycardia may predispose patients to higher incidence of atrial tachyarrhythmias. Because the AV node is embryologically a part of the AV canal, congenital anomalies including AV canal defects can lead to AV block. cc-TGA is also a common congenital cause of complete heart block as the AV node has an aberrant location. Similar to sinus node dysfunction, AV block can also occur post surgically (eg, post VSD or TOF repair). Treatment inevitably includes a pacemaker implantation. However, it should be noted that transvenous pacemaker implantation in the patient with ACHD is often challenging and requires thoughtful planning based on the anatomy, presence of intracardiac shunts, and patency of the venous system. Transvenous pacemakers are contraindicated in patients with atrial or ventricular shunts because of the risk of thromboembolism. In such cases, epicardial lead placement may be considered; however, this requires surgical access and is technically a more arduous procedure.

HEART FAILURE IN ADULT CONGENITAL HEART DISEASE

HF portends worse prognosis and increased mortality in patients with ACHD and is a major mode of death.[26,27] Of note, patients with ACHD may present with atypical symptoms compared to the general population; hence, a high index of suspicion must be maintained for the diagnosis. More commonly, patients with ACHD develop heart failure with reduced ejection fraction (HFrEF), which can be due to pressure or volume overload, valvular dysfunction, alteration in the myocardial architecture (eg, non-compaction), ischemia, or arrhythmias.[28] However, heart failure with preserved ejection fraction (HFpEF) is probably under-recognized and has been implicated in patients with

obstructive physiology (eg, Shone complex) or restrictive physiology. Presenting symptoms vary according to the affected ventricle. Involvement of the systemic ventricle regardless of morphology typically leads to symptoms of pulmonary congestion including shortness of breath, orthopnea, paroxysmal nocturnal dyspnea, wheezing, and reduced exercise tolerance. If the sub-pulmonic ventricle is involved, the symptoms are typically that of "right-sided HF," which include fatigue, weight gain, increased abdominal girth, and bloating. A combination of the symptoms will occur in patients with biventricular failure. Patients with shunts may present with worsening cyanosis and, frequently, the first presentation is new onset of arrhythmia.

During the diagnostic investigation, laboratory testing, imaging, and, frequently, a new hemodynamic study (ie, right heart catheterization) is performed. Imaging is important to assess ventricular and valve function as well as conduit/baffle/pathway patency and functionality. Commonly, an echocardiogram is initially performed and cardiac MRI or CT (for pacemaker-dependent patients) is added for supplementation of data. Cardiopulmonary exercise test is helpful to determine the exercise capacity and the peak oxygen consumption (VO_2). Lower VO_2 values predict higher mortality and can help guide the need for advanced HF therapies, commonly peak VO_2 less than 14 cc/kg/min.[29]

When patients with ACHD have IV access, air filters should be placed on IV tubing to prevent paradoxic embolization of air and thrombus, because many patients will have residual shunts. In addition, establishment of arterial and central venous access can be difficult because the vascular anatomy may be altered and the patients frequently have occlusion of multiple arteries and central veins due to prior procedures. In patients with Glenn shunts (ie, communication between the SVC and PA), namely, most patients with Fontan circulation, the tracing in a central line represents the pulmonary pressures and not the right atrium.

B-type natriuretic peptide (BNP) and N-terminal pro-BNP (NT-proBNP) are helpful for management and prognostication. BNP levels correlate with the functional class and degree of shunt severity. However, in asymptomatic patients, there is no significant correlation between the degree of hypoxia and BNP levels. High BNP levels typically reflect elevated cardiac filling pressure, worsening valvular function, and chamber enlargement. In TOF patients, studies have found a correlation between BNP levels and the degree of RV dilatation as well as the severity of PR. In addition, the BNP levels decrease after pulmonary valve replacement. Rather than the absolute BNP value, the trend in BNP may be more helpful in evaluation of patients with HF. In addition, presence of anemia, liver/renal dysfunction, and hyponatremia portend a worse prognosis.

Limited data exists regarding the medical and surgical management of HF in patients with ACHD. However, understanding the underlying pathophysiology is key to tailoring the management in this patient population. For example, vasodilator therapy for HFrEF of the LV in a patient with right-to-left shunt will cause increase in shunt flow and should be used cautiously.

Medical management of HFrEF of the morphologic left ventricle is similar to the general management of HF, which includes diuretics, β-blockers, angiotensin-converting enzyme inhibitors/angiotensin receptor blockers, and mineralocorticoid receptor antagonists. For HFrEF of a systemic RV (eg, cc-TGA, d-TGA post atrial switch) data are extremely limited. Symptomatic patients with signs of congestion may be treated similar to LV failure with diuretics, β-blockers, and neurohormonal blockade. However, in asymptomatic patients, the utility of β-blockers and neurohormonal blockade is not known and cannot be routinely recommended. In addition, in patients with d-TGA post atrial switch, venodilators that reduce preload may impair ventricular filling and cardiac output, and β-blockers should be used cautiously because sinus node dysfunction is common. Morphologic right ventricle in the subpulmonary position (normal anatomy) is commonly managed with diuretics, possibly digoxin, and in the setting of pulmonary hypertension with pulmonary vasodilators (ie, phosphodiesterase inhibitors, endothelin antagonists, or prostacyclins). Single ventricle post Fontan operation patients with HFrEF are commonly treated with diuretics and standard HF therapy as well as advanced PH therapies when applicable, yet data are scarce. In regard to HFpEF management, no medications have been found to improve survival in this group of patients with HF. For symptomatic relief of volume overload, diuretics should be used.

In critically sick patients with acute HF, extracorporeal membrane oxygenation and ventricular assist devices (VADs), right or left sided, may be considered. A VAD also has a role in bridge to transplant in patients with advanced HF. A thorough evaluation of the vascular anatomy and patency should be conducted before deployment of these therapies.

Ultimately, patients with irreversible and medically refractory HF should undergo evaluation for heart transplant. A very detailed workup is performed to evaluate candidacy for heart transplant. Irreversible pulmonary hypertension should be ruled out before transplant to ensure favorable outcomes, or the patient should be considered for a heart–lung transplant.

Lastly, cardiopulmonary rehabilitation is recommended because limited data have demonstrated improved quality of life measures and safety.

PREGNANCY IN ADULT CONGENITAL HEART DISEASE

Medical care for these patients begins in the preconception period with careful planning that takes into account anticipated hemodynamic shifts and possible complications throughout pregnancy and labor orchestrated by a multidisciplinary team.[30] Although a detailed discussion of management strategies for specific congenital disorders is beyond the scope of this chapter, it is important to note that the normal hemodynamic changes in pregnancy may unmask previously undiagnosed CHD or exacerbate residual lesions. Several disease conditions have been designated as contraindicated to undergo pregnancy (according to the modified WHO classification), including PAH, severe systemic dysfunction (LVEF < 30%, NYHA class III to IV), severe mitral stenosis, severe symptomatic aortic stenosis, Marfan syndrome with dilated aorta >4.5 cm, BAV with aortic dilatation >5 cm, and severe CoA. As a general rule, with the increased blood volume and decreased SVR, regurgitant lesions tend to be tolerated (eg, PR in TOF, TR in EA), moderate and above stenotic lesions may become symptomatic and hemodynamically significant (eg, aortic stenosis), aortic dimensions enlarge (patients with connective tissue disease are most susceptible), systemic ventricular dysfunction may worsen, and the frequency of arrhythmia may increase. Fetal ultrasound is recommended at 18 weeks of gestation owing to the increased likelihood of CHD in the offspring of a patient with ACHD (from 0.8% in the general population to 3% to 6%) as well as genetic evaluation.

INFECTIVE ENDOCARDITIS IN ADULT CONGENITAL HEART DISEASE

Patients with ACHD have inherently the highest risk of contracting infective endocarditis (IE) among the different cardiovascular populations owing to the abundant use of prosthetic material and the presence of shunts within their hearts.[31] In the CCU setting, any patient with ACHD who presents with clinical sepsis should immediately raise suspicion of IE, especially if the patient has had a recent dental procedure. Vegetations tend to develop on prosthetic material or in areas of turbulent flow that damage the endothelium (eg, septal leaflet of the TV from a membranous VSD jet or the pulmonary valve from a PDA jet). Treatment considerations are the same as those for the general population. Right-sided lesions such as pulmonary or TV endocarditis are usually well tolerated and the risk of systemic embolization depends on the presence of a concomitant shunt. Long-term follow-up of prosthetic conduits or graft endocarditis may be performed by serial positron emission tomography-fluorodeoxyglucose studies and inflammatory markers.

Primary prevention according to guidelines[32] currently recommends antibiotic prophylaxis for IE before dental procedures for ACHD with history of IE; prosthetic valves; uncorrected/palliated cyanotic CHD (including with shunts/conduits); completely repaired CHD (surgically or with a device) for the first 6 months and repaired CHD with residual defects at the site or adjacent to the site of a prosthetic patch/device that inhibits endothelization. In addition, the ACHD guidelines recommend IE prophylaxis before vaginal delivery in patients with prosthetic valves.[1]

COMORBID CONDITIONS

Noncardiac comorbidities are common in patients with ACHD. Renal dysfunction is present in up to 50% of young patients with ACHD, with up to 10% having moderate-to-severe dysfunction with a glomerular filtration rate <60 mL/min.[33] Similarly, restrictive lung disease is prevalent and results from prior sternotomies and thoracotomies, diaphragm dysfunction, parenchymal lung disease from perioperative insults, and cardiomegaly. These patients may also develop plastic bronchitis.[34] Patients with ACHD having chronic elevation in central venous pressure, such as patients with Fontan physiology or RV dysfunction, may have hepatic dysfunction and cirrhosis that may lead to abnormalities in coagulation, as well as to portal hypertension and esophageal varices.[20] Fontan patients are also at risk for the development of PLE.[19] In patients with cyanosis, hematologic abnormalities are common and include iron deficiency despite erythrocytosis, thrombocytopenia, platelet dysfunction, and factor deficiencies.[15] Longitudinal studies of the neurocognitive development of patients with CHD have also revealed that neurodevelopmental and behavioral abnormalities are common in this population, as are abnormalities on brain MRI.[35] Presence of noncardiac abnormalities may significantly impact overall outcomes in patients with ACHD.

CONCLUSION

The majority of patients with CHD are reaching adulthood and require a new knowledge base and management considerations by the treating cardiologist. ACHD specialists are a valuable resource for the care of these fascinating and complicated patients.

ACKNOWLEDGMENTS

The authors wish to acknowledge Dr. Frank Cecchin for his valuable suggestions.

REFERENCES

1. Warnes CA, Williams RG, Bashore TM, et al. ACC/AHA 2008 guidelines for the management of adults with congenital heart disease: executive summary: a report of the American College of Cardiology/American Heart Association Task Force on Practice guidelines (writing committee to develop guidelines for the management of adults with congenital heart disease). *Circulation.* 2008;118(23):2395-2451.

2. Baumgartner H, Bonhoeffer P, De Groot NM, et al. ESC Guidelines for the management of grown-up congenital heart disease (new version 2010). *Eur Heart J.* 2010;31(23):2915-2957.

3. Bhatt AB, Foster E, Kuehl K, et al. Congenital heart disease in the older adult: a scientific statement from the American Heart Association. *Circulation.* 2015;131(21):1884-1931.

4. Webb G, Mulder BJ, Aboulhosn J, et al. The care of adults with congenital heart disease across the globe: current assessment and future perspective: a position statement from the International Society for Adult Congenital Heart Disease (ISACHD). *Int J Cardiol.* 2015;195:326-333.

5. Marelli AJ, Ionescu-Ittu R, Mackie AS, Guo L, Dendukuri N, Kaouache M. Lifetime prevalence of congenital heart disease in the general population from 2000 to 2010. *Circulation.* 2014;130(9):749-756.

6. Mylotte D, Pilote L, Ionescu-Ittu R, et al. Specialized adult congenital heart disease care: The impact of policy on mortality. *Circulation.* 2014;129(18):1804-1812.

7. Sommer RJ, Hijazi ZM, Rhodes JF Jr. Pathophysiology of congenital heart disease in the adult: Part I: Shunt lesions. *Circulation.* 2008;117(8):1090-1099.

8. Geva T, Martins JD, Wald RM. Atrial septal defects. *Lancet.* 2014;383(9932):1921-1932.

9. Minette MS, Sahn DJ. Ventricular septal defects. *Circulation.* 2006;114(20):2190-2197.

10. Schneider DJ, Moore JW. Patent ductus arteriosus. *Circulation.* 2006;114(17):1873-1882.

11. Verma S, Siu SC. Aortic dilatation in patients with bicuspid aortic valve. *N Engl J Med.* 2014;370(20):1920-1929.

12. Geva T. Indications for pulmonary valve replacement in repaired tetralogy of fallot: the quest continues. *Circulation.* 2013;128(17):1855-1857.

13. Attenhofer Jost CH, Connolly HM, Dearani JA, Edwards WD, Danielson GK. Ebstein's anomaly. *Circulation.* 2007;115(2):277-285.

14. Opotowsky AR. Clinical evaluation and management of pulmonary hypertension in the adult with congenital heart disease. *Circulation.* 2015;131(2):200-210.

15. Komp DM, Sparrow AW. Polycythemia in cyanotic heart disease—a study of altered coagulation. *J Pediatr.* 1970;76(2):231-236.

16. Halpern DG, Steigner ML, Prabhu SP, Valente AM, Sanders SP. Cardiac calcifications in adults with congenital heart defects. *Congenit Heart Dis.* 2015;10(5):396-402.

17. Warnes CA. Transposition of the great arteries. *Circulation.* 2006;114(24):2699-2709.

18. Elder RW, Wu FM. Clinical approaches to the patient with a failing fontan procedure. *Curr Cardiol Rep.* 2016;18(5):44.

19. Feldt RH, Driscoll DJ, Offord KP, et al. Protein-losing enteropathy after the Fontan operation. *J Thorac Cardiovasc Surg.* 1996;112(3):672-680.

20. Kiesewetter CH, Sheron N, Vettukattill JJ, et al. Hepatic changes in the failing Fontan circulation. *Heart.* 2007;93(5):579-584.

21. Wu FM, Kogon B, Earing MG, et al. Liver health in adults with Fontan circulation: a multicenter cross-sectional study. *J Thorac Cardiovasc Surg.* 2016;153(3):656-664.

22. Wu FM, Jonas MM, Opotowsky AR, et al. Portal and centrilobular hepatic fibrosis in Fontan circulation and clinical outcomes. *J Heart Lung Transplant.* 2015;34(7):883-891.

23. Khairy P, Van Hare GF, Balaji S, et al. PACES/HRS expert consensus statement on the recognition and management of arrhythmias in adult congenital heart disease: developed in partnership between the Pediatric and Congenital Electrophysiology Society (PACES) and the Heart Rhythm Society (HRS). Endorsed by the governing bodies of PACES, HRS, the American College of Cardiology (ACC), the American Heart Association (AHA), the European Heart Rhythm Association (EHRA), the Canadian Heart Rhythm Society (CHRS), and the International Society for Adult Congenital Heart Disease (ISACHD). *Can J Cardiol.* 2014;30(10):e1-e63.

24. Walsh EP, Cecchin F. Arrhythmias in adult patients with congenital heart disease. *Circulation.* 2007;115(4):534-545.

25. Cecchin F, Frangini PA, Brown DW, et al. Cardiac resynchronization therapy (and multisite pacing) in pediatrics and congenital heart disease: five years experience in a single institution. *J Cardiovasc Electrophysiol.* 2009;20(1):58-65.

26. Stout KK, Broberg CS, Book WM, et al. Chronic heart failure in congenital heart disease: a scientific statement from the American Heart Association. *Circulation.* 2016;133(8):770-801.

27. Budts W, Roos-Hesselink J, Rädle-Hurst T, et al. Treatment of heart failure in adult congenital heart disease: a position paper of the Working Group of Grown-Up Congenital Heart Disease and the Heart Failure Association of the European Society of Cardiology. *Eur Heart J.* 2016;37(18):1419-1427.

28. Kantor PF, Redington AN. Pathophysiology and management of heart failure in repaired congenital heart disease. *Heart Fail Clin.* 2010;6(4):497-506, ix.

29. Ross HJ, Law Y, Book WM, et al. Transplantation and mechanical circulatory support in congenital heart disease: a scientific statement from the American Heart Association. *Circulation.* 2016;133(8):802-820.

30. European Society of Gynecology (ESG), Association for European Paediatric Cardiology (AEPC), German Society for Gender Medicine (DGesGM), et al. ESC Guidelines on the management of cardiovascular diseases during pregnancy: the Task Force on the Management of Cardiovascular Diseases during Pregnancy of the European Society of Cardiology (ESC). *Eur Heart J.* 2011;32(24):3147-3197.

31. Mulder BJ. Endocarditis in congenital heart disease: who is at highest risk? *Circulation.* 2013;128(13):1396-1397.

32. Wilson W, Taubert KA, Gewitz M, et al. Prevention of infective endocarditis: guidelines from the American Heart Association: a guideline from the American Heart Association Rheumatic Fever, Endocarditis, and Kawasaki Disease Committee, Council on Cardiovascular Disease in the Young, and the Council on Clinical Cardiology, Council on Cardiovascular Surgery and Anesthesia, and the Quality of Care and Outcomes Research Interdisciplinary Working Group. *Circulation.* 2007;116(15):1736-1754.

33. Dimopoulos K, Diller GP, Koltsida E, et al. Prevalence, predictors, and prognostic value of renal dysfunction in adults with congenital heart disease. *Circulation.* 2008;117(18):2320-2328.

34. Alonso-Gonzalez R, Borgia F, Diller GP, et al. Abnormal lung function in adults with congenital heart disease: prevalence, relation to cardiac anatomy, and association with survival. *Circulation.* 2013;127(8):882-890.

35. Bellinger DC, Wypij D, Rivkin MJ, et al. Adolescents with d-transposition of the great arteries corrected with the arterial switch procedure: neuropsychological assessment and structural brain imaging. *Circulation.* 2011;124(12):1361-1369.

V

INTENSIVE CRITICAL CARE

Janet M. Shapiro
Vishal P. Patel

42

Mechanical Ventilation in the Cardiac Care Unit

MECHANICAL VENTILATION

Mechanical ventilation is a life support method by which a device supports the partial or total transport of oxygen and carbon dioxide between the environment and the pulmonary capillary bed. Mechanical ventilation itself is not a treatment modality, but rather a supportive measure. The physiologic and clinical objectives are to restore homeostasis and support respiration as the underlying pathology is being treated (**Table 42.1**).

The causes of respiratory failure may be divided into hypoxemic and hypercapneic (**Table 42.2**). The majority of patients being admitted to a cardiac care unit with respiratory failure falls into the category of hypoxemic respiratory failure due to cardiogenic pulmonary edema. Cardiogenic pulmonary edema causes decreased lung compliance, ventilation-perfusion mismatching, and diffusion impairment. Hypoxemia of mild-to-moderate severity can often be managed by the administration of oxygen through delivery systems ranging from nasal cannula to facemasks. However, it can be increasingly difficult to maintain adequate oxygenation and oxygen delivery with more severe hypoxemia, and these patients may require positive-pressure ventilation (PPV).

Physiologic derangements and clinical findings will determine the need for mechanical ventilation, which should be considered early in the course and not be delayed until the need becomes emergent. Patients suffering from cardiogenic shock will have an increased respiratory workload and reduced cardiac output

delivered to the muscles of respiration. They are often described as "tiring out" or developing respiratory muscle fatigue and may show physical examination findings such as nasal flaring, use of accessory muscles of respiration (sternocleidomastoids or intercostals), paradoxic or asynchronous movements of the rib cage and abdomen, and an increased pulsus paradoxus. If the mechanical workload progressively increases, the breathing demand at some point will exceed the respiratory pump capabilities. The patient

TABLE 42.1	Objectives of Mechanical Ventilation

- Improve pulmonary gas exchange by supporting alveolar ventilation and arterial oxygenation
  - Improve hypoxemia
  - Improve acute respiratory acidosis
- Decrease the metabolic cost of breathing by unloading the muscles of respiration
  - Ease respiratory distress and respiratory muscle fatigue
- Reduce systemic or myocardial oxygen consumption
- Prevent or improve atelectasis
- Reduce the risk of ventilator-associated lung injury

TABLE 42.2	Causes of Respiratory Failure

Hypercapnic respiratory failure
- Increased respiratory workload due to
  - Airway resistance (asthma, airway obstruction)
  - Elastic workload (pulmonary fibrosis, pneumonia, congestive heart failure)
  - Severe metabolic acidosis
  - Carbon dioxide production
  - Copious secretions in the airways
- Diminished central respiratory drive due to
  - Sedative or analgesic medications
  - Central nervous system injury
- Diminished respiratory muscle function due to
  - Mechanical disadvantage from
    - Chest wall deformities
    - Dynamic hyperinflation (COPD)
  - Respiratory muscle weakness from
    - Electrolyte abnormalities
    - Myopathies or neuropathies
    - Deconditioning

Hypoxemic respiratory failure
- Ventilation-perfusion mismatching
- Right-to-left shunt
- Alveolar hypoventilation
- Diffusion impairment
- Reduced inspired oxygen concentration

COPD, chronic obstructive pulmonary disease.

will be unable to sustain adequate levels of ventilation to effectively eliminate carbon dioxide, and progressive hypercapnia will ensue. A substantial proportion of patients who require mechanical ventilation have relatively normal arterial blood gases, but show the other signs of respiratory failure mentioned. Therefore, the decision to place a patient on mechanical ventilation should not be determined by abnormalities of the arterial blood gas.

Increased respiratory work may markedly raise the oxygen cost of breathing, so that the respiratory muscles disproportionally consume oxygen at the expense of aerobic metabolism of other vital organs such as the heart, brain, and kidneys. Under these circumstances, mechanical ventilation decreases the work of breathing, decreases the oxygen cost of breathing, and redistributes oxygen delivery to the respiratory system and thereby improving oxygen delivery to other bodily organs.

If the underlying pathology is readily reversible and the clinician believes there is time, a trial of oxygen or noninvasive support can be initiated. However, those patients who are post cardiac arrest, are undergoing therapeutic hypothermia, experiencing ongoing cardiac ischemia, demonstrating cardiac or airway instability, exhibiting altered mental status, or having copious secretions are not candidates for noninvasive ventilation (NIV) and they require endotracheal intubation with PPV.

Working closely with the respiratory therapist is essential in decision making and implementation of respiratory support for critically ill patients.

HIGH-FLOW NASAL CANNULA

High-flow nasal cannula (HFNC) is emerging as a new mode of oxygen support for patients with acute hypoxemic respiratory failure with mild-to-moderate work of breathing.[1] Traditional nasal cannulas or masks can deliver flows up to 15 L/min. HFNC is a new form of oxygen support in which oxygen is delivered at very high flow (**Figure 42.1**). Humidified air is delivered at flows up to 60 L/min. In states of high patient workload, room air is entrained and there is dilution of the administered oxygen. With HFNC, the flow rate matches the patient's inspiratory flow and so there is less dilution of the administered oxygen. With HFNC, there is a small amount of positive pressure generated and an increase in lung volume. Compared with conventional oxygen therapy, patients demonstrate a decrease in respiratory rate and greater synchrony. HFNC may be better tolerated than conventional oxygen or NIV.

Thus, HNFC may be effective in patients in the CCU with hypoxemia who are able to sustain the work of breathing.

NONINVASIVE VENTILATION

NIV refers to a method of delivering ventilatory assistance through the use of a mask interface rather than through an invasive interface, such as an endotracheal tube (ETT) or tracheostomy. NIV may provide respiratory support to selected patients while avoiding complications of invasive mechanical ventilation.[2] Cardiogenic pulmonary edema and chronic obstructive pulmonary disease (COPD) exacerbation are two acute disorders for which NIV has proved beneficial.[2]

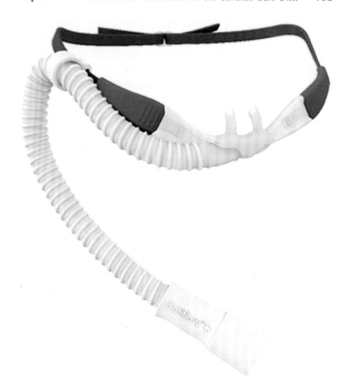

FIGURE 42.1 High-flow nasal cannula.

NIV reduces respiratory muscle work and facilitates a slower and deeper pattern of breathing, thus improving minute ventilation and alveolar ventilation. NIV has been shown to improve gas exchange, normalize arterial carbon dioxide, increase arterial oxygen, increase pH, increase tidal volume, and decrease respiratory muscle work in acute and chronic respiratory failure. Its use can also stabilize certain metabolic parameters such as heart rate, respiratory rate, and blood pressure.

The modes that are most commonly used in the critical care setting are PPV modes of continuous positive airway pressure (CPAP) and bilevel positive airway pressure (BPAP).

In acute cardiogenic pulmonary edema, both CPAP and BPAP have been shown to reduce the work of breathing and intubation rates.[3,4] CPAP has been shown to improve oxygenation, reduce respiratory rate, and reduce the rate of intubation compared to standard oxygen therapy. BPAP similarly has demonstrated lower intubation and complication rates compared to standard oxygen therapy. Although a trial comparing standard oxygen therapy with NIV (CPAP or BPAP) found no significant difference in 7- or 30-day mortality between either of the two groups, the NIV group did achieve more rapid improvement in respiratory distress and metabolic disturbances than did oxygen therapy alone.[5]

For patients with acute cardiogenic pulmonary edema who are hemodynamically stable and meet criteria for NIV, we recommend BPAP as the initial ventilatory mode.

PATIENT SELECTION

Successful application of NIV may obviate the need for endotracheal intubation in select patients. A trial of NIV is therefore worthwhile in most patients who do not require emergent intubation, assuming

TABLE 42.3	**Potential Indicators of Success with Noninvasive Ventilation**

- Younger patient
- Lower severity of illness (APACHE score)
- Ability to cooperate, coordinate breathing with ventilator, less air leaking
- Moderate degree of hypercapnia ($Paco_2 > 45$ mm Hg, <92 mm Hg)
- Moderate degree of acidemia (pH > 7.1, <7.35)
- Improved gas exchange, heart rate, and respiratory rate within 2 h

APACHE, *A*cute *P*hysiologic *A*ssessment and *C*hronic *H*ealth *E*valuation.

that they have no contraindications. Potential indicators of success with NIV use are listed in **Table 42.3**. The clinician must exclude patients in whom the use of NIV would be unsafe. Patients who are at risk of imminent respiratory or cardiac arrest or who have already sustained arrest should be promptly intubated. Patients with unstable conditions such as shock, myocardial ischemia, or life-threatening cardiac arrhythmias should not be managed with NIV. Patients who are comatose, agitated, or uncooperative also cannot undergo NIV. Patients being considered for NIV should be able to manage their secretions, and those with copious amounts should be considered for intubation. Facial surgery, trauma, or deformities that may prevent adequate fitting of the mask interface, and patients with gastric distension and vomiting are relative contraindications.

INITIATION AND SETTINGS

Once the patient has been selected to receive a trial of NIV, it should be initiated as soon as possible. Any delay may result in further deterioration of the patient's condition and increase the likelihood of failure. The oronasal mask should be selected for most patients (**Figure 42.2**). This mask is secured to the patient's face by the use of adjustable Velcro straps. Parameters that need to be set with the BPAP mode of ventilation include inspiratory positive airway pressure (IPAP), expiratory positive airway pressure (EPAP), fraction of inspired oxygen (Fio_2), and a backup respiratory rate.

IPAP is used synonymously with the term *pressure support* and EPAP is regarded as *positive end-expiratory pressure (PEEP)*. Therefore, an IPAP of 15 cm water and an EPAP of 5 cm water are equivalent to a pressure support of 10 cm water and a PEEP of 5 cm water. The initial target IPAP and EPAP should be selected on the basis of bedside observation and determined primarily by patient tolerance. A minimum IPAP of 10 cm water and EPAP of 5 cm water is usually appropriate, because giving the patient higher initial pressures may result in intolerance and early failure. The tidal volume delivered with this mode depends on the difference between IPAP and EPAP. For example, the tidal volume will be greater using an IPAP of 15 cm water and an EPAP of 5 cm water (difference of 10 cm water), than an IPAP of 10 cm water and EPAP 5 cm water (difference of 5 cm water). The goal tidal volume to be delivered in most patients is usually 6 to 8 mL/kg predicted body weight.

The BPAP machine is a pressure-limited device that supports a spontaneous mode of ventilation. That is, the breath will be

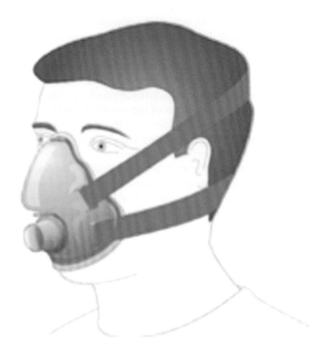

FIGURE 42.2 Oronasal noninvasive ventilation mask.

delivered only if there is a recognized patient effort. If the physician wishes to add a mandatory minimum machine-directed breath, he can set a backup rate of 10 to 12 breaths/min. However, these forced breaths are commonly not synchronized with the patient's effort.

A practical approach is to set the initial Fio_2 to 100%. Arterial blood gas analysis should then be performed after 1 to 2 hours of initiation of BPAP, and the Fio_2 can be titrated down if the Pao_2 is at an acceptable level. It is then reasonable to further titrate down the Fio_2 in small decrements based on the patient's oxygen saturation on pulse oximetry (usually to a goal greater than or equal to 90%). **Table 42.4** shows a protocol to guide the initiation of NIV. Adjustment of IPAP and EPAP may be necessary to achieve optimal tidal volumes and tolerance of NIV.

MONITORING AND TROUBLESHOOTING

Patients who are started on NIV for acute respiratory failure should be monitored in the same way as patients who are mechanically ventilated through an ETT. Patients should be observed closely for the first 2 hours after initiation to troubleshoot, provide reassurance, and monitor for deterioration. If there is no stabilization or improvement over this time, NIV should be considered a failure and the patient should be promptly intubated. If the patient is clearly failing immediately after initiation, the clinician should not wait but should proceed to intubation. Clinical signs of failure include worsening gas exchange, worsening encephalopathy or agitation, inability to clear secretions, inability to tolerate any of the mask interfaces, persistent signs and symptoms of respiratory fatigue, and hemodynamic instability. Reductions in respiratory rate and accessory muscle use, coupled with improvement in thoracoabdominal synchrony and gas exchange, suggest a favorable response and good prognosis if seen within 2 hours.

TABLE 42.4	**Protocol for Initiation of NIV**

1. Appropriately monitored location, with monitoring of pulse oximetry and vital signs

2. Patient in bed or chair at >30° angle

3. Connect all tubing, turn on ventilator, and select and fit mask interface

4. Start with low pressure with backup rate; 8 to 12 cm water IPAP; 3 to 5 cm water EPAP; back up rate of 12 breaths/min

5. Gradually increase IPAP (by 2 cm increments up to 10 to 20 cm water) as tolerated to achieve alleviation of dyspnea, decreased respiratory rate, increased tidal volume, and good patient–ventilator synchrony

6. Provide F_{IO_2} supplementation as needed to keep oxygen saturation >90%

7. Check for air leaks and readjust straps if needed

8. Monitor initial blood gas (1 to 2 h after initiation) and then as needed

9. Encouragement, reassurance, and frequent checks and adjustments as needed

EPAP, expiratory positive airway pressure; IPAP, inspiratory positive airway pressure; NIV, noninvasive ventilation.

Many patients do not tolerate BPAP, and this is usually due to patient–ventilator asynchrony (when the phases of inspiration and expiration do not match that of the patient). Waveform displays of breath-by-breath delivered flow, volume, and pressure are available on most intensive care unit (ICU) ventilators (**Figure 42.3**). If the alarms for these parameters are triggered (ie, low tidal volume or pressures), this is most likely due to a mask leak. Patients can often be satisfactorily ventilated despite such leakage because most pressure-limited ventilators are able to compensate for leaks by sustaining airflow to maintain mask pressure. If the leak is large enough to interfere with ventilatory support, readjusting the position of the mask on the face with tightening of the Velcro straps may help. Also, the mask size itself may have to be changed to ensure a proper fit. Air leaks may also be present if ventilator tubing becomes disconnected from the ventilator or facemask, or if nebulization ports remain open to the atmosphere.

Some of the other problems that may be encountered with NIV are nasal congestion or dryness, nasal bridge redness or ulceration produced by excessive mask tension, irritation of the eyes causing conjunctivitis, and gastric insufflation leading to distension. Major complications such as aspiration, hypotension, and pneumothorax are seldom seen, and these events can be prevented by carefully selecting patients for NIV.

Patients With Do Not Intubate Order

NIV is frequently used in patients who have a directive for no intubation but have a potentially reversible cause of respiratory failure such as cardiogenic pulmonary edema. These patients may be good candidates for NIV because their short-term prognosis may be significantly improved. In contrast, NIV is also initiated in patients with advanced-stage diseases who have poor prognosis.

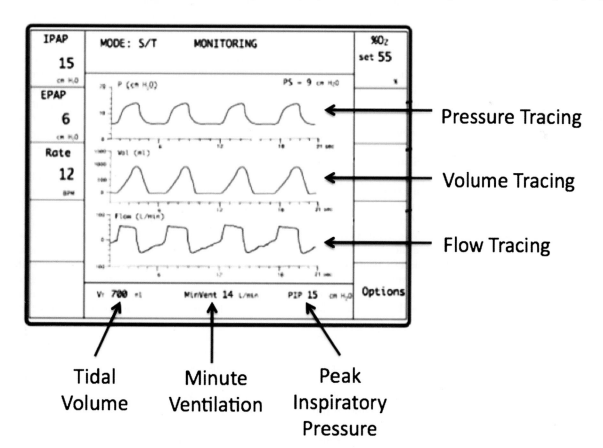

FIGURE 42.3 Waveform display in NIV. EPAP, expiratory positive airway pressure; IPAP, inspiratory positive airway pressure; NIV, noninvasive ventilation; PIP, peak inspiratory pressure. (Philips Respironics BiPAP Vision, Respironics Inc., Murrysville, PA.)

It is a life support measure and its use should be guided by the goals of care, because it may still offer benefits in alleviating respiratory distress or suffering. More information regarding this topic can be found in the chapter on *End-of-Life Care in the CCU.*

INVASIVE MECHANICAL VENTILATION

Invasive mechanical ventilation is usually initiated in the CCU for patients with acute respiratory failure, cardiogenic shock, and cardiac arrest. If a patient with pulmonary edema has a contraindication to or fails NIV, he/she should be promptly intubated.

UNDERSTANDING THE MECHANICAL VENTILATOR

The mechanical ventilator gives the patient each breath based on the settings selected by the clinician.[6] Understanding a few basic terms is helpful. The term *cycling or control* refers to the way the ventilator determines that the inspired breath is complete and signals to stop inspiration. This can be sensed either by volume (inspiration stops once the target volume is delivered), pressure (inspiration stops once the target pressure is reached), flow (when flow decreases to a given level, inspiration is terminated), or time (inspiration stops after a preset time interval). The term *limit* refers to a factor that limits the rate at which gas flows into the lungs and causes inspiration to end before cycling is complete. A limit can be pressure, volume, or flow. *Triggering* is the signal that opens the inspiratory valve, allowing air to flow into the patient. To initiate a breath, the ventilator must recognize that a set value has been reached. The trigger can be set to time, volume, pressure, or flow.

Breath types can be classified in several different ways. If the patient determines the beginning, duration, and end of a breath, the breath is termed *spontaneous*. If the ventilator controls for any of these aspects, the breath is considered to be either *assisted* or *mandatory (controlled)*.

Tidal volume (V_T) is the amount of air delivered with each breath. The normal V_T in a 70-kg person is roughly 500 mL. *Minute ventilation* (MV_E) is the product of tidal volume and the respiratory rate, and is the amount of air inhaled or exhaled in 1 minute. The normal MV_E is 5 to 8 L/min. *Fraction of inspired oxygen* (FiO_2) is the percentage of oxygen in the inspired air, and can range from 21% (room air) to 100%. *PEEP* is the pressure set on the ventilator to prevent expiratory alveolar collapse.

The selection of ventilator mode for a critically ill patient is generally based on the experience of the clinician and institutional preference. PPV can be either volume controlled or pressure controlled.[6] In *volume control (volume preset* or *volume cycled)* ventilation, the machine delivers a preset volume determined by the physician and, within limits, delivers that volume irrespective of the pressure generated within the system. The amount of pressure necessary to deliver this volume can fluctuate based on the resistance and compliance of the patient and ventilator circuit. If the tidal volume is set at 500 mL, the ventilator will continue to deliver gas until it reaches this goal. Upon completion of the inspired volume, the ventilator will open a valve allowing the patient to passively exhale.

In *pressure control (pressure preset* or *pressure cycled)* ventilation, the ventilator applies a predefined pressure target set by the physician. The ventilator will flow gas into the patient until this set pressure is reached. Upon reaching the preset pressure, the ventilator allows for passive exhalation. The resulting tidal volume will vary according to airway resistance and lung compliance.

The mode is also classified on the basis of how the breath is initiated—whether by the ventilator, the patient, or both. In *controlled mechanical ventilation (CMV)*, the MV_E is determined entirely by the set respiratory rate and the set control (volume or pressure control). The patient does not initiate additional MV_E above that set by the ventilator (ie, there is no ventilator triggering by the patient). For example, in volume-controlled CMV, if the set respiratory rate is 12 breaths/min and the preset tidal volume is 500 mL, the patient will be guaranteed an MV_E of 6 L/min (no lower and no higher). Patients are unable to alter their MV_E if the clinical situation changes such as hypoxemia or worsening acidosis, and acid–base maintenance is solely the responsibility of the physician. If placed on this mode, patients who are awake or spontaneously triggering may generate asynchronous respiratory efforts that may contribute to increased work of breathing, patient discomfort, and worsening gas exchange.

During assist-control (AC) *AC ventilation*, the physician determines the minimum MV_E by setting the respiratory rate and control (volume or pressure control). The patient can increase his own MV_E by triggering additional breaths (by flow or pressure) above the set respiratory rate. Each time the patient triggers, the ventilator will generate a fully supported breath according to the volume or pressure preset. For example, in volume-controlled AC, if the respiratory rate is set to 12 breaths/min and the tidal volume to 500 mL, the minimum MV_E will be 6 L/min. If the patient triggers an additional 8 breaths/min, the MV_E then becomes 10 L/min. This mode is the most commonly used mode of ventilation in ICUs and is best suited for those who are awake or still have spontaneous respiratory efforts, and can even be used in those who do not generate any respiratory efforts.

Pressure-regulated volume control (PRVC) is a dual-control mode available on many ventilators. Its basic features are similar to those of AC ventilation, with the main difference being that the ventilator is able to auto-regulate the inspiratory time and flow to deliver the preset tidal volume at the lowest possible plateau airway pressure.

Pressure support ventilation (PSV) differs from the other modes of mechanical ventilation discussed in that it is a flow-cycled mode and is intended to support spontaneous respiratory efforts. The ventilator delivers inspiratory pressure until the inspiratory flow decreases to a predetermined percentage of its peak value (usually 25%). In this mode, the physician sets the pressure support level, PEEP, and FiO_2. The patient must trigger each breath because there is no set respiratory rate. Work of breathing is inversely proportional to pressure support level and inspiratory flow rate. Tidal volumes are therefore determined by a combination of PSV settings, the patient's effort, and underlying pulmonary mechanics. An adequate MV_E cannot be guaranteed and it cannot be used in patients who are heavily sedated, paralyzed, or who cannot generate spontaneous efforts.

CPAP is a mode of support that is also applied to spontaneously breathing patients. During the respiratory cycle, a constant pressure is applied to the airway throughout inspiration *and* expiration. The ventilator does not cycle during CPAP, and all breaths must be initiated by the patient. CPAP is commonly combined with PSV or may be used alone in patients weaning from mechanical ventilation.

Additional modes of ventilation (such as airway pressure release ventilation) are used mainly for patients with acute respiratory distress syndrome (ARDS) and are beyond the scope of this discussion.

ENDOTRACHEAL INTUBATION

Endotracheal intubation should only be performed by an experienced clinician or anesthesiologist. Patients are often intubated using an induction agent (ie, propofol, etomidate) and in some instances undergo rapid sequence intubation with the addition of neuromuscular blocking agents. A specific neuromuscular blocking agent, succinylcholine, may cause a sudden release of potassium into the bloodstream and should be avoided in patients with renal failure or hyperkalemia because it may lead to sudden cardiac arrest. Induction agents have a common problem of causing peripheral vasodilation. This effect may become even more pronounced if there is significant dehydration, hypovolemia, or underlying acidosis. Critically ill patients in a state of compensated shock maintain their circulation by vasoconstriction and tachycardia. The use of a vasodilating induction agent can blunt this response and reduce systemic blood pressure by reducing peripheral vascular resistance.

When positive pressure is applied to the airway, there is an increase in intrathoracic pressure and a decrease in venous return to the heart causing reductions in ventricular filling pressures, stroke volume, and cardiac output. The effects of initiating PPV on blood pressure and cardiac output can usually be treated with the administration of saline boluses. Intravenous fluid preparations should always be prepared for the intubation process in anticipation of such adverse effects. If the effects of vasodilation caused by induction agents cannot be reversed with saline infusion, the temporary use of vasoconstrictor agents (ie, phenylephrine, norepinephrine) may be required. Complications of intubation include local trauma and aspiration of gastric contents.

Once the ETT is advanced through the vocal cords, the tube is secured and the cuff is inflated. Placement is clinically confirmed by the symmetric rise and fall of the chest wall, the presence of bilateral breath sounds, and end-tidal carbon dioxide measurement during manual ventilation. If placement is adequate and oxygen saturation is sufficient, the patient can then be attached to the mechanical ventilator. ETT cuff inflation pressure should not exceed 30 cm water to avoid complications such as tracheal rupture, pressure necrosis, or tracheo-innominate artery erosion and fistula. A chest radiograph should be obtained to ensure ideal location of the tip of the ETT, which should be between 3 and 5 cm above the carina.

PHYSIOLOGIC AND PATHOPHYSIOLOGIC CONSEQUENCES OF POSITIVE-PRESSURE VENTILATION

PPV can produce complex interactions in the patient's cardiopulmonary state.[7] PPV results in an increased mean intrathoracic pressure; the clinical effect on cardiac output is variable and depends on the patient's intravascular volume status/ventricular filling pressures, underlying left ventricular compliance, and ejection fraction.

Increases in intrathoracic pressure can decrease venous return to the right heart. The amount of venous return is determined by the pressure gradient from the extrathoracic veins to the right atrium. The intrathoracic and right atrial pressures increase during PPV, which reduces the gradient for venous return. This effect may be overexaggerated by increases in PEEP or in those with intravascular volume depletion. Right ventricular output can also be reduced by increased alveolar inflation and compression of the pulmonary vascular bed, resulting in increased pulmonary artery pressures and pulmonary vascular resistance. In addition, left ventricular output may be compromised from shifting of the interventricular septum toward the left ventricle leading to impaired diastolic filling.

In contrast to these adverse effects, PPV can be beneficial in patients with left ventricular failure and pulmonary edema.[7] Transmyocardial pressures can be reduced by increases in intrathoracic pressure, resulting in a decreased left ventricular afterload and overall improved left ventricular performance. This effect is most likely to be seen when filling pressures are high and ventricular performance is poor.

Measurements of pressure, airflow, and volume can reveal basic physiologic properties of the respiratory system (**Figure 42.4**). *Peak inspiratory pressure (PIP)* is the maximal airway pressure recorded in the patient–ventilator circuit. It represents the total pressure needed to overcome resistance related to the ventilator tubing, ETT, and patient airways in addition to the elastic recoil of the lungs and chest wall.

The end-inspiratory pressure is measured by applying an inspiratory pause at the end of passive inflation; this will result in an immediate drop in airway opening pressure to a lower initial value, followed by a gradual decrement until a *plateau airway pressure* is reached. Because plateau pressure is measured when there is no airflow, it reflects the static compliance of the respiratory system. Increases in plateau pressures can be seen in patients with decreased lung compliance (ie, ARDS, congestive heart failure, multilobar pneumonia, severe atelectasis) or decreased chest wall compliance (ie, morbid obesity, kyphoscoliosis, abdominal distension, tension pneumothorax) (**Table 42.5**).

Normally, a transpulmonary pressure of 35 cm water would inflate the lungs to near-total lung capacity. In patients with acute lung injury (ALI) or pulmonary edema, total lung capacity may be reduced because of alveolar collapse. Therefore, V_T delivered with each assisted breath may result in heterogeneous ventilation and over-distension of the more compliant regions of the lungs, and subsequent increased plateau/alveolar pressures. This may cause *volutrauma* to the alveoli as a result of the shear mechanical forces applied to the alveoli because they are repeatedly opened and closed. This damage is termed *ventilator-associated lung injury* and is often indistinguishable from other causes of ALI clinically and radiographically. Primary interventions to reduce this injury include preventing alveolar over-distension through the use of smaller V_T (6 mL/kg of predicted body weight) and keeping plateau pressures to a goal of less than 30 cm water.[8]

Pneumothorax, subcutaneous emphysema, pneumomediastinum, and other forms of extra-alveolar air are generally referred to as *barotrauma*. Barotrauma is usually the result of disruption of the pulmonary parenchyma and alveolar rupture from elevated airway pressures or volumes.

Extrinsic PEEP is generally added to prevent alveolar collapse, and increasing levels may be required depending on the clinical situation. In the setting of respiratory failure from ARDS or congestive heart failure, decreased lung compliance may lead to significant alveolar collapse and refractory hypoxemia due to increased shunt fraction. In these settings, extrinsic PEEP

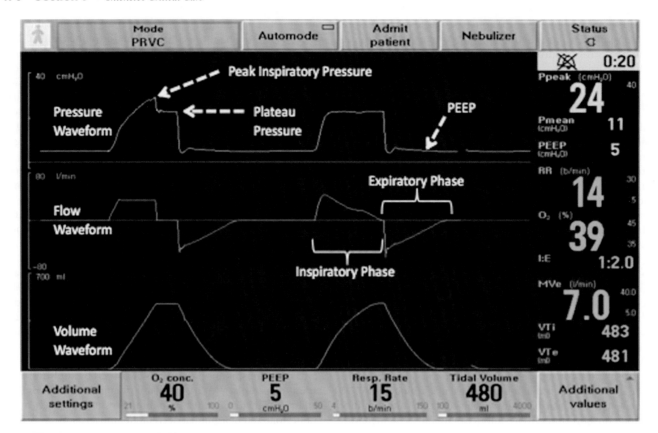

FIGURE 42.4 Waveform and pressure analysis on the invasive mechanical ventilator. PEEP, positive end-expiratory pressure; PRVC, pressure-regulated volume control. (SERVO-i, Maquet, Tastatt, Germany.)

has been used to prevent alveolar collapse, recruit alveoli, and improve oxygenation.

Intrinsic PEEP (PEEP$_i$, auto-PEEP, or *breath stacking)* is present when alveolar pressure exceeds atmospheric pressure at the end of expiration in the absence of a set ventilator PEEP level. When inspiration is initiated before expiratory flow from the preceding breath has ceased, air trapping will occur. Auto-PEEP can develop for numerous reasons including high minute volume (due to high V_T, respiratory rate, or high trigger sensitivity), prolonged inspiratory times (leading to obligatory decrease in expiratory time), and expiratory flow resistance or limitations (due to small-bore ETT or obstructive airways disease). Consequentially, it may potentiate the aforementioned hemodynamic effects of PPV by further increasing intrathoracic pressure. Auto-PEEP will also increase the risk of pulmonary barotrauma and the work of breathing by making it more difficult for the patient to trigger a ventilator-assisted breath. Treatment for auto-PEEP involves adjusting ventilator settings (decreasing inspiratory time, increasing inspiratory flow rate, decreased V_T, decreasing respiratory rate, decreasing trigger sensitivity), maintaining adequate anxiolysis and analgesia to reduce ventilatory demand, and reducing expiratory flow resistance (suctioning, bronchodilators).

Although supplemental oxygen is necessary and valuable in many clinical situations, inappropriate or excessive therapy can be detrimental. The effects of normobaric hyperoxia on the respiratory system have been extensively studied, showing effects ranging from mild tracheobronchitis to diffuse alveolar damage or ARDS. Hyperoxia appears to produce cellular injury

through increased production of reactive oxygen species, which can ultimately result in cell death.[9] In general, attempts are made to decrease the F_{IO_2} to less than 60% to a goal Pa_{O_2} of 60 to 65 mm Hg or Sp_{O_2} greater than or equal to 90% as soon as patients are able to tolerate it. Optimal selection of PEEP may also help decrease oxygen requirements.

SETTINGS FOR MECHANICAL VENTILATION IN THE CCU

This section covers the basic initial settings for the volume-controlled AC mode. The settings that need to be considered with this mode include the V_T, respiratory rate, extrinsic PEEP, and F_{IO_2}.

In principle, the ventilatory management of patients with cardiogenic shock and pulmonary edema is similar to that of patients with noncardiogenic pulmonary edema (ARDS). In addition, patients in the CCU, especially those following cardiac arrest, may suffer ARDS due to aspiration at the time of the cardiac arrest. Many of the recommendations regarding ventilatory strategies for these groups of patients are based on avoiding the pulmonary complications of alveolar over-distension. These strategies are called *lung protective strategies.* Owing to the overwhelming evidence that inflating the lungs to near-total lung capacity or above can damage normal lung units in patients with ARDS and worsen mortality, the current recommendations for ARDS are to set the tidal volume to 6 mL/kg of predicted body weight.[8] It is reasonable to use V_T of 6 to 8 mL/kg predicted body weight in patients ventilated for reasons other than ARDS. Predicted

TABLE 42.5	Causes of Respiratory Distress in the Patient on Mechanical Ventilation

Ventilator issues
- Inadequate minute ventilation (tidal volume or respiratory rate), F_{IO_2}, inspiratory flow rate, PEEP, or trigger sensitivity
- Ventilator circuit leak
- Ventilator malfunction

Increased peak inspiratory pressures with unchanged plateau pressures
- Endotracheal tube problems
  Examples: patient biting, increased resistance in tubes by heat and moisture exchange, obstruction by secretions, blood, or foreign object
- Bronchospasm (asthma or COPD)
- Obstruction of lower airways (secretions, blood, or foreign object)
- Aspiration of oropharyngeal or gastric contents

Increased peak inspiratory pressures with increased plateau pressures
- Pneumonia
- Atelectasis
- ARDS and pulmonary edema
- Migration of ETT into a mainstem bronchus
- Pneumothorax
- Abdominal distension

Extrapulmonary issues
- Delirium, anxiety, or pain
- Acute neurologic event
- Sepsis

ARDS, acute respiratory distress syndrome; COPD, chronic obstructive pulmonary disease; ETT, endotracheal tube; PEEP, positive end-expiratory pressure.

body weight is based on height and gender, and so the height should be measured in all ventilated patients to set the proper tidal volume.

PEEP can potentially improve oxygenation by recruiting collapsed and flooded alveoli for gas exchange, diminishing intrapulmonary shunting of blood, improving ventilation-perfusion mismatching, and also redistributing intra-alveolar edema.

Initial Settings

Tidal volume V_T: 6 to 8 mL/kg predicted body weight.
Respiratory rate: at least 12/min. Higher rates may be required, for example, in patients with severe underlying acidosis or patients being ventilated for ARDS.
F_{IO_2}: set to 100% after intubation. The lowest possible F_{IO_2} necessary to meet oxygenation goals should be used. Arterial blood gas analysis should then be performed after 1 hour to ensure adequate oxygenation. F_{IO_2} should then be rapidly titrated down (by 10% to 20% every 30 minutes) to a goal Pao_2 of 60 to 65 mm Hg or Spo_2 greater than or equal to 90% to avoid complications of high inspired oxygen concentration.
PEEP: A typical initial PEEP of 5 cm of water is often applied to prevent atelectasis. Higher levels of PEEP may be required to recruit alveoli and improve gas exchange; however, attention must

be paid to airway pressures to avoid complications of alveolar over-distension. PEEP above 20 cm water should rarely be used.

MONITORING PATIENTS ON INVASIVE MECHANICAL VENTILATION

Patient–ventilator asynchrony is commonly manifested as respiratory distress with "bucking" or "fighting" the ventilator. This happens when the phases of the breath delivered by the ventilator do not match that of the patient. Clinical signs include anxiety, agitation, tachypnea, tachycardia, use of accessory muscles of respiration, and uncoordinated thoracic wall and abdominal movements. Asynchrony can lead to dyspnea and increased work of breathing. Bedside observation and examination of ventilator waveforms can help detect the presence and identify the cause of asynchronous ventilation.

Asynchrony or respiratory distress may signify a life-threatening complication, and so rapid assessment is required. In addition to clinical examination, the clinician must monitor ventilator parameters such as tidal volume, respiratory rate, peak inspiratory pressure, plateau airway pressure, and auto-PEEP values. It should be noted that patient–ventilator asynchrony need not be present for possible pulmonary complications associated with mechanical ventilation to arise. In addition, extrapulmonary processes such as fever, pain, delirium, and anxiety may also increase respiratory drive and lead to patient–ventilator asynchrony. **Figure 42.5** offers an algorithmic approach to the mechanically ventilated patient in respiratory distress.

Chest radiographs should be followed to ensure proper positioning of the ETT (optimal 3 to 5 cm above the carina), because cephalad or caudad migration is very common.

Arterial blood gas analysis is usually performed at the initiation of mechanical ventilation and then periodically based on the disease process and ventilator changes. Acid–base disturbances may require adjustments of minute ventilation, because they can lead to significant and potentially life-threatening cellular dysfunction or hemodynamic consequences. F_{IO_2} will be adjusted to assure adequate oxygenation and avoid potential oxygen toxicity.

SEDATION IN THE MECHANICALLY VENTILATED PATIENT

The majority of mechanically ventilated patients will require sedation and/or analgesia to facilitate ventilator synchrony, and alleviate pain and discomfort from critical care procedures and treatments.[10] A number of different agents can be used alone or in combination to achieve consistent sedation, anxiolysis, and analgesia. Common medication classes include benzodiazepines, opioid analgesics, and neuroleptic agents. A neuroleptic agent may be used if medication for delirium is indicated. Each class differs in the amount of anxiolysis, analgesia, amnesia, and hypnosis provided. Elimination half-life, volume of distribution, and drug clearance may be significantly altered in critically ill patients. No single agent is sufficiently superior to other agents to recommend its standard use in all patients. Selection must therefore be individualized according to the patient's distress, physiologic parameters, expected duration of therapy, and potential interactions with other medications. Careful attention should also be paid to the possible development of adverse reactions. Brief descriptions regarding drug classes, effects, and pharmacokinetics are presented in **Table 42.6**.

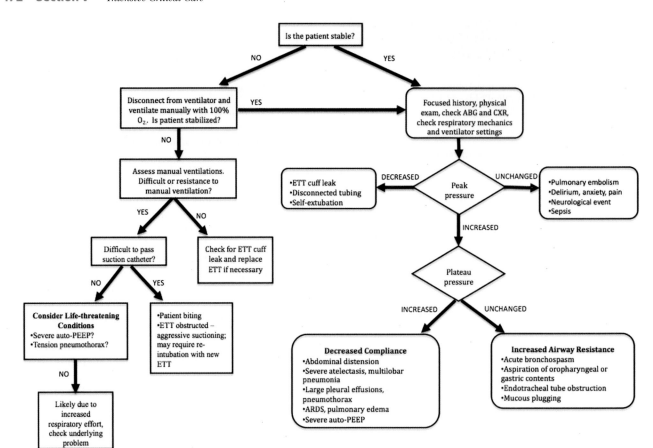

FIGURE 42.5 Approach to the mechanically ventilated patient in respiratory distress. ABG, arterial blood gas; ARDS, acute respiratory distress syndrome; CXR, chest X-ray; ETT, endotracheal tube; PEEP, positive end-expiratory pressure.

TABLE 42.6	Characteristics of Sedative Medications Commonly Used in the ICU Setting		
DRUG	**ONSET**	**DURATION**	**EFFECTS**
Opioids			Potent sedative/analgesic effects, without causing anxiolysis, hypnosis, or amnesia
• Morphine	5–10 min	4 h	
• Fentanyl	<0.5 min	30–60 min	
Benzodiazepines			Sedative anxiolytic, hypnotic, and amnesic effects without analgesic effects
• Lorazepam	5–20 min	6–8 h	
• Midazolam	1–5 min	30 min	
• Diazepam	1 min	20–60 min	
Neuroleptic			Potent sedative anxiolytic with minimal hypnotic and amnesic effects; no analgesia provided
• Haloperidol	30–60 min	0.5–6 h	
Anesthetic–sedative			Potent sedative hypnotic, with minimal amnesic effects; anxiolysis seen at low doses; no analgesia provided
• Propofol	<1 min	3–10 min	
Central α₂ agonist			Sedative sympatholytic with moderate anxiolysis and analgesia; no hypnosis or amnesia; no significant effect on respiratory drive
• Dexmedetomidine	5–10 min	1–2 h	

ICU, intensive care unit.

A goal depth of sedation should be determined before initiating sedative–analgesic regimens and the goal should be individualized on the basis of the clinical situation.[10] Patients expected to have a shorter duration of mechanical ventilation may require lighter sedation or no sedation at all. On the other hand, patients being mechanically ventilated for severe hypoxemia or ARDS may require deeper sedation. The goal depth of sedation should be frequently assessed and titrated using validated and reliable scales for mechanically ventilated patients (eg, Richmond Agitation-Sedation Scale).

TABLE 42.7	Criteria for a Successful Ventilator Weaning Trial

- Pressure support ≤ 8 cm water (ideally <5 cm water)
- PEEP ≤ 5 cm water
- Spo$_2$ > 92% while breathing ≤ 50% Fio$_2$
- Respiratory rate < 35 breaths/min
- Heart rate < 140 beats/min
- Systolic blood pressure <180 mm Hg but >90 mm Hg
- No diaphoresis or signs of respiratory fatigue
- Tolerated for at least 30 min to 2 h

PEEP, positive end-expiratory pressure.

VENTILATOR-ASSOCIATED COMPLICATIONS

Critically ill patients requiring mechanical ventilation are at risk for clinically important upper gastrointestinal hemorrhage due to stress ulceration.[11] Histamine-2 receptor antagonists and proton pump inhibitors reduce the frequency of overt upper gastrointestinal hemorrhage in patients in the ICU when compared to no prophylaxis.

A ventilator-associated pneumonia (VAP) may complicate the course of patients requiring mechanical ventilation. The Centers for Disease Control has introduced the surveillance definition of a ventilator-associated event as worsening oxygenation for 2 days following a period of stability. On the basis of current definitions, a VAP requires sustained worsening oxygenation, along with fever, leukocytosis, need for antibiotics, purulent endotracheal secretions, and growth of a pathogenic organism. The most common cause of VAP is aerodigestive tract colonization, followed by aspiration of contaminated secretions into the lower airways. Proper specimens should be collected before beginning empiric antibiotic coverage. Steps to reduce the risk and prevent development of VAP should be employed routinely in mechanically ventilated patients.[12] These include semi-recumbent positioning, oral care, and compliance with strict hand washing and other infection control protocols.

WEANING AND EXTUBATION

Weaning refers to the process of liberating the patient from the mechanical ventilator. The use of weaning protocols, generally involving respiratory therapists and nurses, has been shown to reduce the duration of mechanical ventilation.[13] Readiness testing refers to the use of objective clinical criteria to determine whether a patient is ready to begin weaning. The reason for the patient's respiratory failure should have been identified and the patient should have shown a favorable response to the treatment. Chest radiograph should demonstrate improvement in pulmonary edema. Oxygenation should be satisfactory: Spo$_2$ greater than or equal to 90% while receiving less than or equal to 50% Fio$_2$ and PEEP less than or equal to 5 cm water. Patients should be hemodynamically stable with minimal or no need for vasopressor support, and without myocardial ischemia or unstable cardiac arrhythmias. Sedative drugs should be discontinued, and the patient should be awake and alert, or easily arousable, and be able to manage secretions. In addition, significant fluid, electrolyte, and metabolic disorders should be corrected before weaning attempts.

A once-daily spontaneous breathing trial should be initiated when the patient meets readiness criteria. A weaning trial can be performed using a T-piece or PSV.

A T-piece trial involves removing the ventilator with the ETT in situ connected to oxygen and monitoring spontaneous respirations. In a PSV trial, a pressure support level of approximately 5 cm water is added to the CPAP mode. We prefer using the PSV approach over the T-piece because PSV provides reassurance of ventilator alarm features and backup ventilatory assistance in case of apnea, extreme tachypnea, or inadequate minute ventilation. In addition, PSV overcomes the increased work of breathing from resistance of the ETT that may be seen with T-piece trials. A successful weaning trial meets the criteria outlined in **Table 42.7**. If the patient meets all of the weaning criteria, the patient may be extubated. If the patient fails to meet all of the criteria, ventilatory support should be resumed and another weaning trial should be attempted the following day. In the case of cardiogenic pulmonary edema, the administration of diuretics before extubation may be beneficial even if the patient is not in overt heart failure, because the cardiovascular effects of PPV discussed earlier will be reversed once positive pressure is removed.

For extubation, the patient should be placed in the upright position and the oropharynx and trachea via the ETT should be suctioned to remove secretions. The ETT cuff is then deflated and the ETT is removed. Immediately after removal, any secretions that are coughed up and present in the oropharynx should be promptly suctioned and supplemental oxygen should be provided. Physical examination including auscultation of the lungs to confirm bilateral air entry and the upper airway to exclude the presence of inspiratory stridor (which would suggest laryngeal edema) should be performed.

Respiratory distress following extubation may be due to airway disease, recurrent pulmonary edema, secretions, or laryngeal edema. In many cases, early and aggressive management with suctioning, bronchodilator therapy, diuresis, or NIV can prevent re-intubation. If laryngeal edema is present, the administration of intravenous glucocorticoids and inhaled racemic epinephrine may lessen the need for re-intubation. In patients with respiratory distress following extubation, NIV may prevent re-intubation if applied early.[14] If the patient fails a trial of NIV or meets any of the contraindications to the use of NIV discussed earlier in this chapter, he/she should be promptly re-intubated followed by a thorough evaluation and treatment of the cause of the post-extubation respiratory failure.

CONCLUSION

Mechanical ventilation provides life-saving support in the CCU. Clinicians must closely attend to the goals, ventilator settings, and patient–ventilator monitoring to utilize mechanical ventilation to the greatest benefit and prevent complications. Understanding and utilizing sedation goals and daily weaning assessments will assure that patients are promptly liberated from mechanical ventilation.

REFERENCES

1. Roca O, Hernandez G, Diaz-Lobato S, et al. Current evidence for the effectiveness of heated and humidified high flow nasal cannula supportive therapy in adult patients with respiratory failure. *Critical Care*. 2016;20:109. doi: 10.1186/s 13054-01601263-z.

2. Liesching T, Kwok H, Hill NS. Acute applications of noninvasive positive pressure ventilation. *Chest.* 2003;124:699–713.

3. Bersten AD, Holt AW, Vedig AE, Skowronski GA, Baggoley CJ. Treatment of severe cardiogenic pulmonary edema with continuous positive airway pressure delivered by face mask. *N Engl J Med.* 1991;325:1825–1830.

4. Nava S, Carbone G, Dibatista N, et al. Noninvasive ventilation in cardiogenic pulmonary edema. *Am J Respir Crit Care Med.* 2003;168:1432–1437.

5. Alasdair G, Goodacre S, Newby D, et al. Noninvasive ventilation in acute cardiogenic pulmonary edema. *N Engl J Med.* 2008;359:142–151.

6. Oeckler RA, Hubmayr RD, Irwin RS. Mechanical ventilation part I: invasive. In: *Irwin and Rippe's Intensive Care Medicine.* 7th ed. Philadelphia, PA: Lippincott Williams and Wilkins; 2012:624–641, 643–659.

7. Pinksy MR. Cardiovascular issues in respiratory care. *Chest.* 2005;128:592S–597S.

8. The Acute Respiratory Distress Syndrome Network. Ventilation with lower tidal volumes as compared with traditional tidal volumes for acute lung injury and the acute respiratory distress syndrome. *N Engl J Med.* 2000;342:1301–1308.

9. Jackson RM. Pulmonary oxygen toxicity. *Chest.* 1985;88:900–905.

10. Barr J, Fraser GL, Puntillo K, et al. Clinical practice guidelines for the management of pain, agitation, and delirium in adult patients in the intensive care unit. *Crit Care Med.* 2013;41:263–306. doi: 10.1097/CCM.0b013e3182783b72.

11. Dellinger RP, Levy MM, Rhodes A, et al. Surviving sepsis campaign: international guidelines for management of severe sepsis and septic shock: 2012. *Crit Care Med.* 2013;41:580–637.

12. American Thoracic Society, Infectious Diseases Society of America. Guidelines for the management of adults with hospital-acquired, ventilator-associated, and healthcare-associated pneumonia. *Am J Respir Crit Care Med.* 2005;171:388–416.

13. Blackwood B, Alderdice F, Burns K. Use of weaning protocols for reducing duration of mechanical ventilation in critically ill adult patients: Cochrane systematic review and meta-analysis. *BMJ.* 2011;342:c7237. doi:10.1136/bmj.c7237.

14. Cabrini L, Landoni G, Oriani A. Noninvasive ventilation and survival in acute care settings: a comprehensive systematic review andmetaanalysis of randomized controlled trials. *Crit Care Med.* 2015;43:880–888.

Patient and Family Information For: MECHANICAL VENTILATION

A mechanical ventilator is a machine that helps patients breathe when they are not able to breathe enough on their own. It is commonly referred to as a *breathing machine or respirator.* Most patients who require help breathing with mechanical ventilators are cared for in the ICU or cardiac care unit. Many people think of mechanical ventilators as a way to treat breathing-related issues. However, patients are placed on ventilators to support their breathing function while giving time for treatments to improve their condition. Being on a respirator means the patient is critically ill—it is life support.

There is always a team taking care of the patient, including the physician, nurse and respiratory therapist.

WHY MECHANICAL VENTILATORS ARE USED

Mechanical ventilators help support the patient by pushing breaths with oxygen into the lungs, as well as removing carbon dioxide from the lungs. There are some patients who are in an ICU in whom breathing is difficult—they may feel short of breath and tired from the work that their breathing requires. This is called *respiratory failure* and is often due to the cardiac disease where poor pumping leads to fluid buildup in the lungs. Some patients also have pneumonia, COPD, or asthma, or too much mucus present in the windpipe or airways; and these conditions make it even more difficult to breathe. Mechanical ventilators can help ease the work of breathing for these people and prevent their condition from getting worse. If a patient does not get help early enough, the condition can worsen very quickly and ultimately cause the heart and lungs to stop.

Other patients may not be breathing at all because they are in a coma, have brain damage or injury, very weak muscles, or because they suffered a cardiac arrest. In this case, a ventilator must be used to breathe for the patient.

HOW MECHANICAL VENTILATORS WORK

There are two basic types of ventilators that are available. The first is called a *noninvasive ventilator* or *BiPAP machine*. This device pushes air into the lungs through tubing that is connected to the patient by way of a mask, which covers the nose and mouth. It can help improve oxygen levels in the blood and lessen the amount of work that the muscles need to do to in order for the patient to breathe. Patients can sometimes still speak to their family and friends while on this machine, and some may also be able to eat provided it is safe to do so. This type of ventilator is commonly used in the cardiac care unit for patients suffering from shortness of breath due to heart failure.

Patients on BiPAP have to be monitored very closely. Even with the help of this device, some patients will continue to have a great deal of trouble breathing. If the patient has not improved within a few hours of this device being started, then this machine is not successful and the patient will need a second type of machine, called the *invasive mechanical ventilator*. Also, not all patients are good candidates for BiPAP and we may decide that it is more harmful than beneficial to use it.

The invasive mechanical ventilator is connected to the patient through a tube (called an ETT) that is placed in the mouth or nose and down into the windpipe. The process of placing the tube into the patient's windpipe is called *intubation*. The device blows air into the lungs and it can help a person by doing all of the breathing for them or just assisting their breaths. The difference between BiPAP and the invasive ventilator is that with the invasive ventilator the doctors have more control over a person's breathing and are able to completely rest the muscles used for breathing.

HOW PATIENTS FEEL WHILE ON INVASIVE MECHANICAL VENTILATORS

The ventilators themselves do not cause pain, but most people who require invasive ventilators do not like the feeling of having a tube in their mouth or nose. They cannot talk because the tube passes through the voice box into the windpipe. They also cannot eat when the tube is in place, and so they need a temporary feeding tube from the mouth to the stomach until the breathing tube is removed. Some people will feel some discomfort as air from the machine is being pushed into the lungs and they will try to breathe out while the machine is trying to push air in. This is called *fighting* against the ventilator and makes it more difficult for the ventilator to help. In addition, people undergo many diagnostic tests and therapies that can cause physical discomfort or pain. For these reasons, patients are often given medications such as sedatives or painkillers to make them feel more comfortable.

HOW PATIENTS ARE MONITORED

Anyone on a ventilator will be hooked up to a monitor that measures heart rate, breathing rate, blood pressure, and oxygen levels at regular intervals. Other tests that may be done routinely include chest X-rays and blood tests that will measure the amount of acid, oxygen, and carbon dioxide in the blood. The doctors, nurses, and respiratory therapists use this information to gauge how well the patient is doing and to see if any adjustments need to be made to the ventilator.

RISKS OF MECHANICAL VENTILATION

Some risks of mechanical ventilation do exist. However, if the doctors feel that the patient needs to be on a ventilator, the benefits of placing the patient on one are always greater than these potential risks.

When a person is first placed on a respirator, he/she may experience a drop in blood pressure. This can usually be reversed with the use of intravenous fluids, but some patients may temporarily require medications to keep their blood pressure normal.

Sometimes, a part of the lung that is weak can become too inflated with air and start to leak. This leaked air collects in an empty space between the lungs and the chest wall. Because there is a limited amount of space in the chest, the leaked air starts to take up more space and the lung begins to collapse. This is called a *pneumothorax*. This air needs to be removed as soon as possible because it can result in life-threatening complications. It is drained by a *chest tube*, which is likely to remain until the patient no longer requires the ventilator.

The pressure from the ventilator to put air into the lungs can also damage the lungs. Doctors try to keep this risk to a minimum using the lowest amount of pressure that is needed. In addition, very high levels of oxygen may be harmful to the lungs. Unfortunately, patients who already have damaged lungs may need very high levels of oxygen until the lungs start to heal, which makes it difficult to reduce this risk.

As mentioned, many patients on mechanical ventilation will need some level of sedation. Different patients will react to each medication differently. At times, sedation medications can build up and the patient may remain in a deep sleep for hours or days, even after the medication is stopped. The doctors and nurses try to adjust the medications so that the right amount is being delivered at all times.

The breathing tube can allow germs and bacteria from the mouth to get into the lungs more easily. This can cause an infection such as pneumonia, which can be a serious problem and could mean that the patient has to stay on the machine longer. People who are very sick can be more prone to infection than others. All members of the medical staff take maximum precautions to prevent this from happening; however, if an infection occurs, it can be treated with antibiotics.

HOW LONG ARE MECHANICAL VENTILATORS USED?

Ventilators can be lifesaving, but they do not fix the primary disease or injury. Ventilators help support a patient until other treatments become effective. The medical team will always try to help patients get off the ventilator at the earliest possible time, but will not do so until there has been an improvement or a reversal of the problem at hand.

Weaning refers to the process of getting the patient off the ventilator. Depending on the patient, this process may take a few hours up to a few days or longer. Specific criteria are used to decide whether a patient is ready to come off of the respirator including blood oxygen levels, chest X-ray results, and physical examination. Some patients will never improve enough to be taken off the ventilator completely and may require long-term ventilator support.

Not all patients improve just because they are on a ventilator, and patients can die even though they are on a respirator. It is hard to predict or know for sure whether a person will recover with treatment. Sometimes, doctors feel very sure the ventilator will help and the patient will recover. Other times, the doctors only have a rough idea of the chances a person will survive. For patients who are very sick and at the end of life, mechanical ventilation sometimes only postpones death.

Matthew Durst
Hooman Poor

43

Pulmonary Embolism and Deep Vein Thrombosis

Pulmonary embolism (PE) and deep vein thrombosis (DVT) are two categories of a broader disease known as venous thromboembolism (VTE). VTE can have a wide range of clinical presentations ranging from an asymptomatic incidental finding to hemodynamic collapse and death. The incidence of VTE is estimated at approximately 200,000 new cases per year in the United States, with a slightly higher predominance of DVT compared to PE.[1]

Not only is VTE a fairly common disease but it is also a significant cause of mortality. Previous autopsy studies have demonstrated PE as a direct cause of, contributing to, or accompanying death in approximately 15% of hospitalized patients over the past 40 years.[1] In the International Cooperative Pulmonary Embolism Registry (ICOPER) study published in 1999, the 3-month mortality rate of all patients diagnosed with PE before autopsy was 15.3% and it increased to 58.3% in patients who presented with hemodynamic instability.[2]

PATHOGENESIS

While the exact cause of VTE is unknown, it has been associated with a number of factors and is likely dependent on the interplay between them. Three of these factors, venous stasis, endothelial injury, and a hypercoagulable state, oftentimes referred to as Virchow triad, are all associated with the development of VTE.[1] The likelihood of developing VTE is significantly increased when multiple risk factors are present simultaneously.

Pulmonary emboli typically originate from thrombi present in the deep veins. The proximal veins of the lower extremities, specifically the iliac and femoral venous system, are believed to be the source of most diagnosed pulmonary emboli. Right heart, pelvic vein, renal vein, and upper extremity thrombi are also potential sources of pulmonary emboli. Patients with PE are also found to have clots in the right heart, otherwise known as emboli in transit, and are at high risk of mortality.[1]

PHYSIOLOGY OF THE RIGHT VENTRICLE AND THE PULMONARY VASCULATURE

The pulmonary circulation can be modeled similarly to electrical circuits using Ohm's law, which states that voltage difference (V) equals the current of electrons (I) multiplied by the resistance (R). The pressure difference between the pulmonary artery (P_{PA}) and the left atrium (P_{LA}) in the pulmonary circulation is analogous to the voltage difference in the electrical circuit. The cardiac output (CO), which is the flow of blood through the pulmonary artery (PA), is analogous to the current in the electrical circuit. And, the pulmonary vascular resistance (PVR) is analogous to the resistance in the electrical circuit (**Figure 43.1**).

The normal pulmonary circulation is a low-pressure and low-resistance circuit due to differences in blood vessel structure compared to the systemic circulation. The structure and function of the right ventricle (RV) are different compared to that of the left ventricle (LV), because the RV does not have to generate nearly as much pressure to produce the same CO as the LV. The RV is crescentic and relies more heavily on longitudinal shortening for force generation, whereas the LV is concentrically shaped and relies more on circumferential constriction. Overall, the RV is a thinner walled, more compliant, and more energy-efficient chamber than the LV. However, the operating characteristics of the RV are heavily dependent upon the low-pressure nature of the pulmonary circulation, leaving the RV very susceptible and poorly equipped to handle acute increases in RV afterload.[3]

PATHOPHYSIOLOGY OF INCREASED PULMONARY VASCULAR RESISTANCE

Emboli cause an increase in PVR through two mechanisms. The primary mechanism for the increase in PVR is mechanical obstruction of the vasculature. The relationship between clot burden and PVR is hyperbolic. At low levels of mechanical obstruction, blood is able to be diverted to regions of distensible vasculature, which minimizes the increase in PVR. However, with more significant clot burden, this compensatory mechanism is overwhelmed as the remaining vessels become over-distended, leading to rapid rises in PVR for small increases in obstruction. The second mechanism for increased PVR is the release of humoral factors, leading to vasoconstriction of the pulmonary vasculature.[4] The major humoral factors that have been associated with changes in PVR following PE are thromboxane-A_2, which is an end product of arachidonic acid metabolism, and serotonin.[5] Thromboxane-A_2 is both a systemic and pulmonary

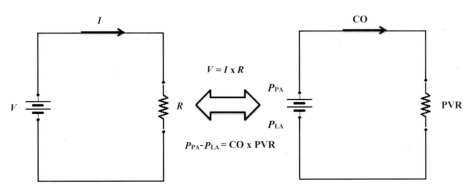

Ohm's law: $V = I \times R$

Physiologic correlate for pulmonary circulation:

$$P_{PA} - P_{LA} = CO \times PVR \qquad P_{PA} = (CO \times PVR) + P_{LA}$$

FIGURE 43.1 Circuit diagram of the pulmonary circulation. CO, cardiac output; I, current; PLA, left atrial pressure; PPA, mean pulmonary artery pressure; PVR, pulmonary vascular resistance; R, resistance; V, voltage.

vasoconstrictor that is released by platelets with the purpose of causing vasoconstriction to achieve homeostasis. Platelets are also the likely source of serotonin release because serotonin plays an important role in platelet aggregation and is a very potent pulmonary vasoconstrictor despite causing systemic vasodilation. Because pulmonary emboli are composed primarily of fibrin and small amounts of platelets, it is unlikely that the embolus itself is the source of thromboxane-A_2 and serotonin release. Instead it is probable that fresh platelets that have amassed around the embolus are activated and release these vasoactive substances which then lead to significant pulmonary vasoconstriction. The roles that these two substances play in pulmonary vasoconstriction are supported by multiple animal studies looking at receptor antagonists that demonstrate significant attenuation to abolishment of the rise in PVR with blockade of the receptors.[5] The initial symptomatic relief resulting from treatment with heparin that is observed within hours likely stems from blockade of platelet activation and prevention of further release of humoral vasoconstrictors, not clot resolution, because not enough time has elapsed for significant fibrinolysis to have occurred.

EFFECTS ON HEMODYNAMICS

PE increases PVR both through mechanical obstruction as well as through substrate-mediated pulmonary vasoconstriction. In non–hemodynamically significant PE, obstructing emboli and local vasoconstriction divert blood flow to unaffected regions of the vasculature, causing them to dilate and thus minimizing the overall increase in PVR. If enough of the vasculature is obstructed or constricted, PVR rises significantly and the RV afterload increases. To maintain CO, the RV must generate higher pressures. Although the RV is able to generate higher pressures to some degree, as discussed earlier, the RV in a healthy individual without prior cardiopulmonary disease is ill-equipped to deal with significant increases in afterload.

The maximal mean PA pressure that can be generated by a normal RV is approximately 40 mm Hg.[6] Increases in RV afterload beyond this point result in decreases in RV CO. The decreased RV CO leads to a drop in LV preload and subsequent LV CO. Increases in RV afterload lead to increased RV wall stress, which results in increased RV ischemia that can decrease RV CO. In addition, because of the compliance of the RV, increases in RV afterload result in RV dilation, which further exacerbates RV wall stress. As the RV dilates, the leaflets of the tricuspid valve are pulled apart, leading to poor coaptation and worsening tricuspid regurgitation, which leads to decreased RV output. Because the heart is encased in the pericardium, the free wall of the dilating RV cannot expand outward, and, instead, RV dilation leads to a leftward shift of the intraventricular septum, causing a decrease in the size of the LV cavity and a further decrement in LV preload. Notably, because of the drop in LV CO, there is a decrease in right coronary artery (RCA) perfusion, leading to further RV ischemia. These events continue to cascade in a downward spiral leading to further deterioration in RV function and resultant declines in CO, ultimately progressing to cardiogenic shock (**Figure 43.2**).[7,8] This vicious cycle can be exacerbated by additional factors. Excessive fluid loading will cause worsening RV dilation. Although sometimes unavoidable, intubation is especially dangerous because the sedatives used for induction can cause peripheral vasodilation, leading to decreased RCA perfusion pressure and RV ischemia. Furthermore, positive intrathoracic pressure from mechanical ventilation can lead to increased RV afterload because of the compression of pulmonary vessels.

For patients with underlying chronic cardiopulmonary disease resulting in pulmonary hypertension, the RV has been chronically exposed to increased afterload, and thus has had time to adapt by undergoing hypertrophy, allowing it to generate pressures significantly higher than that which a normal RV can generate.[9] Nevertheless, patients with underlying cardiopulmonary disease are at increased risk for hemodynamic decompensation in the setting of a significant PE because of their baseline compromised state.

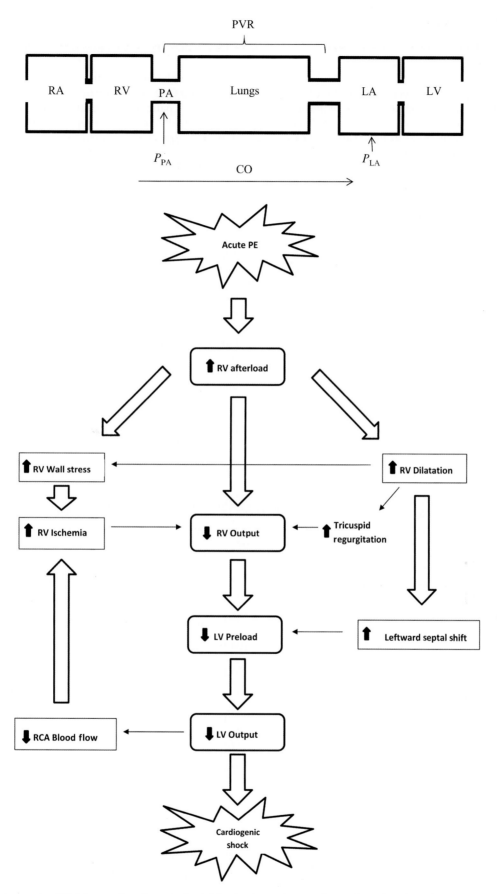

FIGURE 43.2 Vicious cycle of RV failure and cardiogenic shock following hemodynamically significant PE. CO, cardiac output, LA, left atrium; LV, left ventricle; PA, pulmonary artery; PE, pulmonary embolism; P_{LA}, left atrial pressure; P_{PA}, mean pulmonary artery pressure; PVR, pulmonary vascular resistance; RCA, right coronary artery; RV, right ventricle.

EFFECTS OF PULMONARY EMBOLISM ON GAS EXCHANGE

One of the major physiologic effects of PE is the creation of dead-space ventilation, which is defined as areas of the lung that receive ventilation but no perfusion. An increase in dead-space ventilation would normally result in hypercapnia because of a reduced ability to eliminate carbon dioxide from the blood stream; however, hypercapnia is not a common finding in PE because patients compensate by hyperventilating other areas of the lung that are participating in gas exchange. Typically, if the clot burden is severe enough to cause hypercapnia, the hemodynamic effects often prove fatal.[10]

Hypoxemia is a common finding in PE and is due to a combination of multiple factors. One factor is the development of an intrapulmonary shunt, defined as blood traversing areas of the lung that receive no ventilation. This lack of ventilation may occur because of effects from the embolism, which includes atelectasis, pulmonary infarction, and bronchoconstriction. Shunt physiology is also present in a small subset of patients who develop intracardiac shunting, typically through a patent foramen ovale that has opened because of increased right atrial pressure from RV failure. Low mixed venous saturations from decreased CO may contribute to hypoxemia because the venous blood starts at a lower oxygen saturation before traversing abnormal lungs. Hypoxemia is typically accompanied by an increased gradient between the alveolar oxygen concentration (PaO_2) and the arterial oxygen concentration (PaO_2). An increased gradient may even be present in patients with a normal PaO_2 because of the effects of hyperventilation on arterial CO_2 partial pressure.[10]

DIAGNOSIS OF DEEP VEIN THROMBOSIS

DVT, although not fatal by itself, has the potential to fragment and cause a fatal PE. On the other hand, inappropriate anticoagulation of patients exposes them to unnecessary risks, such as a potentially life-threatening hemorrhage. Therefore, it is important to make a proper diagnosis in patients suspected to have a DVT. The gold standard for diagnosis of DVT is venography, which involves the injection of iodinated contrast dye into a dorsal foot vein to outline the entire venous system of the lower extremity. Venography has been demonstrated to have a risk of approximately 1.2% for the development of symptomatic DVT or PE during 3 months of follow-up after a normal venogram. Venography is no longer commonly used to establish or rule out the diagnosis of DVT because of its invasive nature, associated risks, high cost, lack of availability at many centers, and the fact that it is contraindicated in some patients, such as those with renal dysfunction or severe allergies to the contrast material.[11]

Current practice typically uses combinations of clinical probability assessments, D-dimer assays (high sensitivity and moderate sensitivity), and imaging such as venous ultrasonography (US), computed tomography (CT) venography, or magnetic resonance imaging (MRI). The decision on the combination of tests used is dependent upon the pretest probability of the presence of DVT, the suspected location (lower vs upper extremity), and suspected first episode versus recurrence.[11]

Multiple clinical probability assessments for DVT exist. One of the more commonly used tools, known as the Wells score (**Table 43.1**), was developed by Wells et al.[12] and classifies the

TABLE 43.1	Wells Scores			
DVT			**PE**	
Active cancer (treatment within 6 mo or palliative)	+1		Clinically suspected DVT	+3.0
Calf swelling ≥ 3 cm compared to asymptomatic calf (measured 10 cm below tibial tuberosity)	+1		Alternative diagnosis is less likely than PE	+3.0
Swollen unilateral superficial veins (nonvaricose, in symptomatic leg)	+1		Tachycardia (heart rate > 100)	+1.5
Unilateral pitting edema (in symptomatic leg)	+1		Immobilization (≥ 3 d) or surgery in previous 4 wk	+1.5
Previous documented DVT	+1		History of DVT or PE	+1.5
Swelling of the entire leg	+1		Hemoptysis	+1.0
Localized tenderness along the deep venous system	+1		Malignancy (treatment within 6 mo or palliative)	+1.0
Paralysis, paresis, or recent cast immobilization of lower extremities	+1			
Recently bedridden ≥ 3 d, or major surgery requiring regional or general anesthetic in the past 12 wk	+1			
Alternative diagnosis at least as likely	−2			
High probability	>2		High probability	>6.0
Moderate probability	1–2		Moderate probability	2.0–6.0
Low probability	<1		Low probability	<2.0

DVT, deep vein thrombosis; PE, pulmonary embolism.

pretest probability of patients who are suspected of having DVT into three categories: low, moderate, or high probability. The scoring system consists of multiple questions with one point assigned for each question that is answered in the affirmative followed by a subtraction of two points if there is an alternative diagnosis to DVT that is at least equally as likely as the diagnosis of DVT. A score of less than 1 is considered low probability, 1 to 2 is considered moderate probability, and 3 or more is considered high probability of having a DVT. In the initial study of 593 patients, 3% in the low-probability group, 17% of the moderate-probability group, and 75% of the high-probability group were ultimately diagnosed with DVT.[12] A modified version of the Wells score, which incorporates the presence of prior DVT and divides patients into either low- or high-probability groups, can also be used.[13]

The D-dimer, a degradation product of cross-linked fibrin, has a high sensitivity for the presence of VTE; however, it has a poor specificity because of numerous conditions other than VTE that can cause an elevation in D-dimer levels. This makes the D-dimer assay a useful test in low-risk patients as a test to rule out the presence of DVT. Unfortunately, the test is much less useful in acutely ill or hospitalized patients because of the high occurrence of false-positive results.[11] Multiple versions of the test exist, each with its own sensitivity and specificity.[14]

Owing to its noninvasive nature, low cost, and lack of radiation or contrast dye, US is the most commonly used modality to diagnose DVT. The two types of US studies include proximal compression US and whole-leg US. In both cases, the US probe is used to assess for the presence of a clot within the vein by compression, a positive study defined as the inability to fully compress any segment of the vein under gentle pressure with the probe. The proximal study assesses the femoral and popliteal veins, but not the calf veins. Whole-leg US assesses the proximal veins as well as the calf veins.

For patients in whom US cannot be obtained, such as those who are in a cast, or in whom US is nondiagnostic, CT venography or MRI may be used to further evaluate for DVT. CT venography requires the injection of iodinated contrast, typically into an arm vein, with CT imaging timed for opacification of the deep veins. CT venography can be combined with computed tomography pulmonary angiography (CTPA) to evaluate for both PE and DVT. MRI may be used in a variety of ways to establish the diagnosis of DVT. Magnetic resonance venography can be done without contrast; however, the use of contrast agents such as gadolinium improves visualization of the vasculature. MRI can also be used to directly image thrombi using techniques to take advantage of the composition of clots. MRI is less frequently used because of higher costs and lack of availability for this purpose at most centers.[11]

DIAGNOSIS OF PULMONARY EMBOLISM

Combinations of clinical probability calculators, D-dimer assays, and imaging modalities such as pulmonary angiography, CT angiogram, lung scintigraphy (ventilation-perfusion [VQ] scan), and echocardiography are used to make the diagnosis of PE.[15]

Similar to how venography was the gold standard for the diagnosis of DVT, pulmonary angiography was previously the gold standard for the diagnosis of PE. It is done by performing a right heart catheterization and injecting contrast dye into the pulmonary arteries. The vasculature is then examined

for filling defects or amputation of a branch of the PA. One benefit of pulmonary angiography over CT angiography is the ability to simultaneously obtain invasive hemodynamic measurements. With the improvement in CT imaging, pulmonary angiography has fallen out of favor because of its invasive nature and cost.[15]

Multiple clinical prediction rules are available to determine the pretest probability of PE. The most frequently used scoring system was again developed by Wells et al.[12], which classifies patients into three groups: low likelihood, moderate likelihood, and high likelihood with rates of diagnosed PE of approximately 10%, 30%, and 65%, respectively (**Table 43.1**). A simplified version of the Wells score separates patients into two groups.[15]

CTPA is currently the diagnostic imaging modality choice for evaluation of patients with suspected PE. CTPA involves the injection of iodinated contrast, typically into an arm vein, with imaging timed for opacification of the pulmonary arterial circulation. This allows for adequate visualization of the pulmonary vasculature at least down to the level of the segmental pulmonary arteries, providing a sensitivity and specificity of 96% and 95%, respectively.[15] CTPA also allows for evaluation of the lung parenchyma that may reveal diagnoses other than PE that may be the cause of the respiratory problems.

VQ scans are another imaging modality that can be useful for the diagnosis of PE, particularly in patients who cannot undergo CTPA because of contrast allergies, renal insufficiency, or any other reason. The test involves the injection of technetium (Tc)-99m–labeled macroaggregated albumin particles that ultimately get lodged in the pulmonary capillaries and are viewable by scintigraphy, allowing for evaluation of pulmonary perfusion. The perfusion studies are then matched with ventilation studies, which require the inhalation of radio-labeled gas or microparticles that can be imaged to evaluate ventilation of the lungs. The matched scans are then examined, looking for areas of the lung with poor perfusion but preserved ventilation, which would signify a PE. VQ scans have the benefit of requiring significantly less radiation exposure when compared to CTPA. VQ scans are frequently classified into one of the following categories, considered diagnostic in most patients: normal or near normal, low probability, intermediate probability (nondiagnostic), and high probability.[15]

Echocardiography may also be helpful in making the diagnosis of PE and is a useful tool for prognostication. Signs such as RV dilatation and signs of RV pressure overload are highly suggestive of PE. McConnell sign, defined as a decreased contractility of the RV free wall compared to the apex, can sometimes be seen in patients with PE. Mobile right heart thrombi seen on echocardiography essentially confirm the diagnosis of PE; however, they are a rare finding. Because the overall negative predictive value of echocardiography is low, it is a poor test to rule out PE.[15]

RISK STRATIFICATION FOR PATIENTS WITH PULMONARY EMBOLISM

To determine the optimal management of patients with PE, it is crucial to assess their risk of short-term decompensation. Patients with a higher risk of decompensation are likely to benefit more from aggressive therapies compared to patients with a lower risk profile.

The Pulmonary Embolism Severity Index (PESI) score is a tool that was developed to help risk stratify patients diagnosed with PE. The model utilizes 11 criteria to stratify patients into 5 classes of risk (PESI classes I to V), the lowest group having a 30-day mortality of 0% to 1.6% and the highest class having a 30-day mortality rate between 10% and 24.5%.[16] The PESI score is particularly useful for identifying low-risk patients (PESI I and II) who can be safely treated as outpatients.[17]

For patients in higher PESI classes, it is important to further stratify based on risk of short-term morbidity and mortality. On the basis of the Management Strategies and Determinants of Outcome in Acute Pulmonary Embolism Trial (MAPPET), hemodynamic status on presentation, specifically systolic blood pressure (SBP) <90 mm Hg, not clot burden, is the major determinant of short-term mortality. The trial included patients with PE and overt signs of impending right heart failure, noting in-hospital mortality rates of 8.1%, 25%, and 65% in patients with RV dysfunction but SBP > 90 mm Hg, cardiogenic shock, and those requiring cardiopulmonary resuscitation at presentation, respectively.[18] On the basis of this elevated risk of death, the American Heart Association defines massive PE as acute PE with sustained hypotension (SBP < 90 mm Hg for at least 15 minutes or requiring inotropes in the absence of another cause of hypotension), pulselessness, or persistent profound bradycardia (heart rate < 40 beats/min with signs or symptoms of shock) (**Figure 43.3**).[19] Owing to the high risk of early mortality in these patients, immediate intervention to restore pulmonary perfusion is required.

Normotensive patients with RV dysfunction and/or myocardial injury are at a slightly increased risk of deteriorating into a massive PE compared to those who are low risk, and are thus classified as "submassive" PE.[19] Tests that can be used to determine whether a patient has RV dysfunction or myocardial injury include echocardiography, CT scans, electrocardiography, brain natriuretic peptide (BNP), N-terminal (NT)-proBNP, troponin I, and troponin T. Evidence of RV dysfunction on echocardiography includes RV free wall hypokinesis, RV dilatation, increased ratio of RV to LV diameter, and elevations in calculated RV systolic pressures. CT scans can also be used to evaluate for RV dilatation and increased ratio of RV to LV diameter. Electrocardiographic findings of sinus tachycardia, new-onset atrial arrhythmias, new right bundle branch block, Qr pattern in V1, an S1Q3T3 pattern, negative T waves in V1 to V4, and ST segment shift over V1 to V4 have been associated with higher short-term risk. BNP and NT-proBNP, which are released in states of RV pressure overload that lead to increased myocardial stretch, can also be useful tests because patients with normal BNP and NT-proBNP

PE CLASSIFICATIONS

Massive PE = Acute PE + one of the following:

1. Sustained Hypotension
   - SBP < 90 mmHg for at least 15 minutes or requiring inotropic support
   - Not due to another cause such as arrhythmia, hypovolemia, sepsis, or LV dysfunction
2. Pulselessness
3. Persistent Profound Bradycardia
   - Heart rate < 40 bpm with signs or symptoms of shock

Submassive PE = Acute PE without systemic hypotension (SBP ≥ 90 mmHg) + one of the following:

1. RV Dysfunction: defined as the presence of at least one of the following
   - RV dilation (echocardiography or CT)
   - Elevated BNP or NT-proBNP
   - EKG changes (new or incomplete RBBB, anteroseptal ST elevation or depression, or anteroseptal T-wave inversion)
2. Myocardial necrosis: defined as an elevation in troponin I or troponin T

FIGURE 43.3 PE classification from the scientific statement from the AHA. AHA, American Heart Association; PE, pulmonary embolism.

levels have a high negative predictive value for increased risk of poor outcome. Finally, troponin levels also have a good negative predictive value because patients without troponin elevations are at low risk for early adverse outcomes.[15,19] **Table 43.2** represents a risk stratification schematic.

TREATMENT OF DEEP VEIN THROMBOSIS

Because DVT itself is not a fatal condition, the decision whether to treat a DVT and the choice of treatment involves weighing the risks of the progression to PE and recurrence versus the risks of treatment. Factors involved in determining whether to treat include location of the thrombus, the presence or absence of a known provoking factor, any underlying hypercoagulable state,

TABLE 43.2	PE Risk Stratification for Early Mortality Risk			
EARLY MORTALITY RISK	**SHOCK OR HYPOTENSION**	**PESI CLASS III–V**	**RV DYSFUNCTION ON IMAGING**	**+ CARDIAC BIOMARKERS**
High risk	+	N/A	+	N/A
Intermediate-high	–	+	+	+
Intermediate-low	–	+	Either one or neither +	
Low risk	–	–	Assessment unnecessary, both—if done	

PE, pulmonary embolism; PESI, Pulmonary Embolism Severity Index; RV, right ventricle.
Adapted from ESC Committee for Practice Guidelines (CPG), Endorsed by the European Respiratory Society (ERS), European Heart Journal. 2014; 35(43):3033-3073.

prior history of VTE, bleeding risk, and patient preference. Potential treatment options include monitoring, anticoagulation (**Table 43.3**) used to prevent further clots and promote passive reduction of thrombus size, thrombolysis which actively promotes clot breakdown, catheter-directed thrombolysis (CDT), inferior vena cava (IVC) filter placement, and thrombectomy.[20]

In the case of patients with a first occurrence of DVT, the location of the thrombus will play a significant role in the treatment decision. For patients with clots distal to the popliteal vein (isolated distal DVT) without severe symptoms or risk factors for extension such as positive D-dimer without an alternative reason, extensive thrombosis (>5 cm in length, involving multiple veins, or >7 mm in maximal diameter), close to proximal veins, no reversible provoking factor, active cancer, prior VTE, or inpatient status, monitoring with repeat US in 2 weeks is preferred to treatment with anticoagulation. If repeat US is unable to be performed or any risk factors are present, anticoagulation is preferred in patients with low-moderate bleeding risk. In patients with high bleeding risk, serial monitoring is preferred. If extension is seen on the repeat US, then anticoagulation should be initiated. For patients with proximal leg DVT, anticoagulation is recommended if tolerated and preferred over CDT. The use of an IVC filter in addition to anticoagulation is not recommended; however, an IVC filter should be used in patients who cannot tolerate anticoagulation due to bleeding, have a contraindication to anticoagulation, or have developed VTE despite being anticoagulated. For patients with proximal upper extremity DVT (axillary or more proximal veins), typically occurring in the setting of central venous catheter usage, treatment with anticoagulation is preferable to CDT and the catheter should be removed if still present. For patients with

a recurrent episode of VTE while not on anticoagulation, initiation of anticoagulation is the preferred method of treatment.[20]

The initial choice of anticoagulation is based on multiple factors such as presence of active malignancy, presence of renal dysfunction, planned procedures, prior treatment failures, need for monitoring, and cost. For patients with active malignancy, low-molecular-weight heparin (LMWH) is the preferred agent. For patients without active malignancy, novel oral anticoagulants (NOACs) such as dabigatran, rivaroxaban, apixaban, and edoxaban are preferred to vitamin K antagonists (VKAs) such as warfarin, and VKAs are preferred to LMWH. For patients who have recurrent VTE despite anticoagulation, LMWH is recommended. If the recurrence occurs while the patient is compliant with LMWH treatment, the dose of the LMWH can be increased. In both cases of treatment failure, the presence of an underlying malignancy should be considered.[20]

The duration of anticoagulation is dependent upon whether the DVT was provoked by a known reversible factor, whether it is an initial clot or a recurrence, presence of active malignancy, presence of known hypercoagulable state, and bleeding risk. For patients with a first occurrence with a known reversible risk factor such as surgery, pregnancy, leg injury, or a flight >8 hours, 3 months of therapy is the recommended duration. For patients who are low-moderate bleeding risk with unprovoked DVT, recurrent DVT while off anticoagulation, or who have an active malignancy, indefinite treatment with anticoagulation is preferred to 3 months of treatment. In patients with similar high bleeding risk, 3 months of treatment is recommended over indefinite treatment. Patient preferences should also be taken into account when deciding on treatment duration.[20]

TABLE 43.3	Available Anticoagulants			
ANTICOAGULANT	**DOSE**	**ROUTE**	**RENAL ADJUSTMENT**	**REVERSAL AGENT**
Apixaban	10 mg twice daily for 7 d, then 5 mg twice daily	Oral	Yes	No
Argatroban	2 µg/kg/min Titrate to aPTT goal	IV	No	No
Bivalrudin	0.15–0.2 mg/kg/h Titrate to aPTT goal	IV	No	No
Dabigatran	150 mg twice daily	Oral	Yes	Idraucizumab
Edoxaban	60 mg daily 30 mg daily if ≤ 60 kg	Oral	Yes	No
Fondaparinux	Weight based <50 kg = 5 mg daily 50–100 kg = 7.5 mg daily >100 kg = 10 mg daily	SubQ	Yes	No
LMWH	1 mg/kg every 12 h	SubQ	Yes	Protamine for partial neutralization
Rivaroxaban	15 mg twice daily for 21 d, then 20 mg daily	Oral	Yes	No
Unfractionated heparin	80 U/kg bolus, then 18 U/kg/h Titrate to aPTT goal	IV	No	Protamine
Warfarin	Individualized dosing Titrate to goal INR	Oral	No	Vitamin K

aPTT, activated partial thromboplastin time; INR, international normalized ratio; IV, intravenous; LMWH, low-molecular-weight heparin; SubQ, subcutaneous.

TREATMENT OF PULMONARY EMBOLISM

Unlike in patients with DVT alone, patients with PE may present with hemodynamic instability and respiratory abnormalities such as hypoxemia. The initial step in management should be to provide adequate support to maintain organ perfusion and gas exchange. As discussed earlier, the etiology of hypotension and shock from PE is RV failure secondary to an increase in RV afterload. Aggressive volume expansion should be avoided because it may further exacerbate RV dilation and wall stress. Vasopressors such as norepinephrine should be used to maintain arterial pressure and inotropes such as dobutamine should be used to support RV

contractility. The role of inhaled pulmonary vasodilators such as epoprostenol and nitric oxide is unclear, but may improve hemodynamics given the presence of pulmonary vasoconstriction from humoral factors. Hypoxemia should be treated with supplemental oxygen and mechanical ventilation should be initiated if required; however, if intubation and mechanical ventilation is required, special care should be taken because inducing agents and the use of positive-pressure ventilation can cause further hemodynamic compromise in these very unstable patients.

The mainstay of therapy for PE is anticoagulation, which prevents the formation of new thrombi and allows the patient's endogenous fibrinolytic system to resolve the clots that are present. Because

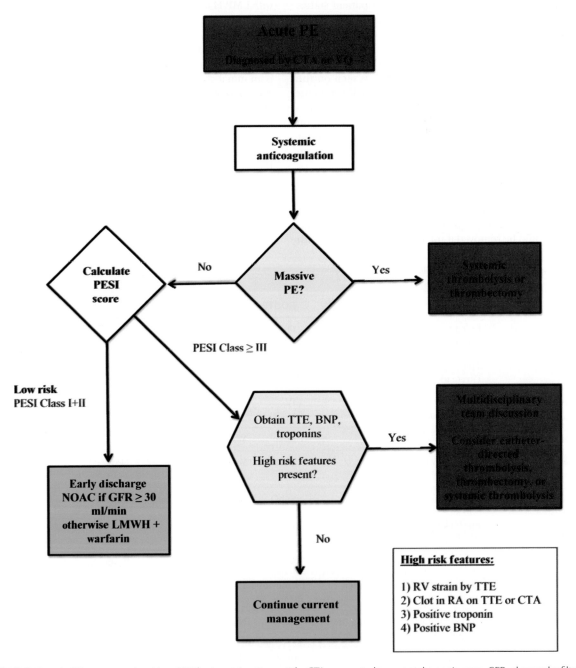

FIGURE 43.4 Sample PE treatment algorithm. BNP, brain natriuretic peptide; CTA, computed tomography angiogram; GFR, glomerular filtration rate; LMWH, low-molecular-weight heparin; NOAC, novel oral anticoagulant; PE, pulmonary embolism; PESI, Pulmonary Embolism Severity Index; RA, right atrium; RV, right ventricle; TTE, transthoracic echocardiogram; VQ, ventilation-perfusion.

PE is a potentially life-threatening condition, empiric anticoagulation should be started in patients with intermediate-high clinical probability of PE during the diagnostic workup. In patients with a low probability of PE, anticoagulation can be withheld until a diagnosis of PE is confirmed. Recommended initial anticoagulation choices include subcutaneous LMWH, unfractionated heparin with monitoring of the activated partial thromboplastin time, or subcutaneous fondaparinux. In cases where heparin products cannot be used, such as with heparin-induced thrombocytopenia, non–heparin-based anticoagulation should be used. Once the diagnosis of PE is confirmed, it is crucial to risk stratify patients to help decide the most appropriate treatment and level of monitoring. A sample algorithm is provided in **Figure 43.4**.

For patients who are low risk (PESI I and II), no further workup for risk stratification is necessary, and these patients can be considered for early discharge home with anticoagulation. As with DVT, the NOACs and VKAs are preferred to LMWH except for in-patients with active malignancy or recurrence while taking another form of anticoagulation. For patients at intermediate to high risk (PESI classes III to V), cardiac imaging and biomarkers should be obtained to evaluate for signs of RV dysfunction and/or myocardial necrosis.

For patients with massive PE, aggressive therapies to restore pulmonary perfusion should be undertaken given the high mortality risk. If there are no absolute contraindications, systemic thrombolysis is recommended (**Table 43.4**). Surgical embolectomy may also be considered in centers with experience with the procedure. Surgical embolectomy is also a good option in cases of clot in transit (right atrial or RV thrombus), which have a high risk of embolizing into the pulmonary vasculature.

While the mortality rate for submassive PE is higher than that for low-risk PE, the role of thrombolysis in this population is controversial. Thrombolysis has been shown to reduce the rate of hemodynamic decompensation in patients with submassive PE; however, this benefit has not translated into a reduction in mortality, likely because of the increase in adverse events, particularly intracranial hemorrhage, which occurs in about 2% of patients receiving systemic thrombolysis. To reduce the bleeding risks of thrombolysis, lower doses can be administered. Ultrasound-assisted, catheter-directed, low-dose thrombolysis has been investigated as a potential treatment. The rationale of this therapy is to administer the thrombolytic directly at the clot while using high-frequency US to increase thrombus permeability to thrombolytic agents, allowing for use of even lower doses of thrombolytics and theoretically decreasing the risk of bleeding.[21]

Given the lack of clear consensus guidelines for the treatment of massive and submassive PEs, the use of multidisciplinary teams, often comprising physicians from cardiology, pulmonology, critical care, interventional radiology, cardiothoracic surgery, and emergency medicine, can help determine the best treatment strategy and provide a multidisciplinary recommendation along with rapid mobilization of resources.

TABLE 43.4	**Contraindications to Systemic Thrombolysis**

1. Prior intracranial hemorrhage
2. Structural intracranial cerebrovascular disease
3. Malignant intracranial neoplasm
4. Ischemic stroke within 3 mo
5. Suspected aortic dissection
6. Active bleeding or bleeding diathesis
7. Recent surgery encroaching on the spinal canal or the brain
8. Recent facial or closed-head trauma with evidence of bony fracture or brain injury

Adapted from 2014 AHA Statement.[19]

REFERENCES

1. Kroegel C, Reissig A. Principle mechanisms underlying venous thromboembolism: epidemiology, risk factors, pathophysiology and pathogenesis. *Respiration.* 2003;70(1):7-30.
2. Goldhaber SZ, Visani L, De Rosa M. Acute pulmonary embolism: clinical outcomes in the International Cooperative Pulmonary Embolism Registry (ICOPER). *Lancet.* 1999;353(9162):1386-1389.
3. Sheehan F, Redington A. The right ventricle: anatomy, physiology and clinical imaging. *Heart.* 2008;94(11):1510-1515.
4. Halmagyi DF, Starzecki B, Horner GJ. Humoral transmission of cardiorespiratory changes in experimental lung embolism. *Circ Res.* 1964;14:546-554.
5. Smulders YM. Pathophysiology and treatment of haemodynamic instability in acute pulmonary embolism: the pivotal role of pulmonary vasoconstriction. *Cardiovasc Res.* 2000;48(1):23-33.
6. McIntyre KM, Sasahara AA. The hemodynamic response to pulmonary embolism in patients without prior cardiopulmonary disease. *Am J Cardiol.* 1971;28(3):288-294.
7. Matthews JC, McLaughlin V. Acute right ventricular failure in the setting of acute pulmonary embolism or chronic pulmonary hypertension: a detailed review of the pathophysiology, diagnosis, and management. *Curr Cardiol Rev.* 2008;4(1):49-59.
8. Poor HD, Ventetuolo CE. Pulmonary hypertension in the intensive care unit. *Prog Cardiovasc Dis.* 2012;55(2):187-198.
9. McIntyre KM, Sasahara AA. Determinants of right ventricular function and hemodynamics after pulmonary embolism. *Chest.* 1974;65(5):534-543.
10. Elliott CG. Pulmonary physiology during pulmonary embolism. *Chest.* 1992;101(4 suppl):163s-171s.
11. Bates SM, Jaeschke R, Stevens SM, et al. Diagnosis of DVT: antithrombotic therapy and prevention of thrombosis, 9th ed: American College of Chest Physicians evidence-based clinical practice guidelines. *Chest.* 2012;141(2 suppl):e351S-e418S.
12. Wells PS, Anderson DR, Bormanis J, et al. Value of assessment of pretest probability of deep-vein thrombosis in clinical management. *Lancet.* 1997;350(9094):1795-1798.
13. Wells PS, Anderson DR, Rodger M, et al. Evaluation of D-dimer in the diagnosis of suspected deep-vein thrombosis. *N Engl J Med.* 2003;349(13):1227-1235.
14. Di Nisio M, Squizzato A, Rutjes AW, Büller HR, Zwinderman AH, Bossuyt PM. Diagnostic accuracy of D-dimer test for exclusion of venous thromboembolism: a systematic review. *J Thromb Haemost.* 2007;5(2):296-304.
15. Konstantinides SV, Torbicki A, Agnelli G, et al. 2014 ESC guidelines on the diagnosis and management of acute pulmonary embolism. *Eur Heart J.* 2014;35(43):3033-3069, 3069a-3069k.
16. Aujesky D, Obrosky DS, Stone RA, et al. Derivation and validation of a prognostic model for pulmonary embolism. *Am J Respir Crit Care Med.* 2005;172(8):1041-1046.
17. Aujesky D, Roy PM, Vershuren F, et al. Outpatient versus inpatient treatment for patients with acute pulmonary embolism: an international, open-label, randomised, non-inferiority trial. *Lancet.* 2011;378(9785):41-48.

18. Kasper W, Konstantinides S, Geibel A, et al. Management strategies and determinants of outcome in acute major pulmonary embolism: results of a multicenter registry. *J Am Coll Cardiol.* 1997;30(5):1165-1171.

19. Jaff MR, McMurtry MS, Archer SL, et al. Management of massive and submassive pulmonary embolism, iliofemoral deep vein thrombosis, and chronic thromboembolic pulmonary hypertension: a scientific statement from the American Heart Association. *Circulation.* 2011;123(16):1788-1830.

20. Kearon C, Akl EA, Ornelas J, et al. Antithrombotic therapy for VTE disease: chest guideline and expert panel report. *Chest.* 2016;149(2):315-352.

21. Kucher N, Boekstegers P, Müller OJ, et al. Randomized, controlled trial of ultrasound-assisted catheter-directed thrombolysis for acute intermediate-risk pulmonary embolism. *Circulation.* 2014;129(4):479-486.

Patient and Family Information for: PULMONARY EMBOLISM AND DEEP VEIN THROMBOSIS

Deep Vein Thrombosis (DVT) and Pulmonary Embolism (PE) are blood clots that occur in the blood vessels of the limbs, primarily the legs, and the lungs, respectively. They are part of a spectrum of disease known as Venous Thromboembolism (VTE). Typically, the body maintains a balance where blood remains fluid while inside the blood vessels, but clots whenever it exits the blood vessels. This mechanism is how the body stops bleeding after a cut occurs. DVTs occur when the blood clots inappropriately inside the body and can occur if the blood flow through those veins is sluggish, as can occur during prolonged surgery or very long periods of immobility such as a long plane flight. In other cases, patients may have a "hypercoagulable state," a condition where the blood is intrinsically more likely to form clots. Occasionally, pieces of these clots from the blood vessels of the limbs may break off and travel to the lungs and get lodged in the blood vessels of the lung, a process known as pulmonary embolism. The blood clots cause symptoms by blocking the blood flow in the blood vessels they reside.

The symptoms of blood clots are variable and depend on the location. For DVTs, the most common symptoms are swelling, pain, and redness near the location of the blood clot. Some patients may have no symptoms at all. Blood clots in the lung (PE) may cause shortness of breath, chest pain, a rapid pulse, and coughing up blood. Occasionally, some people with PE do not have any symptoms at all and the blood clots are found incidentally.

Of the two, PE is the more dangerous, life-threatening form of blood clot. In severe cases of PE, the blood clots can impair the ability of the flowing blood to take up oxygen and can also prevent blood from circulating through the lungs, possibly leading to death. DVTs themselves do not cause these problems, but pieces can break off and result in PE.

If your doctor suspects that you have a PE or DVT, there are numerous tests that may be ordered to find the clot. These tests include imaging tests such as CT scans, VQ scans, and ultrasound of the limbs. A blood test, known as the D-dimer, which is often abnormally elevated in people with blood clots, can be helpful to rule out the presence of PE or DVT.

The treatment depends upon the severity of the clots. Simple blood clots are treated with blood thinners, otherwise known as anticoagulants, to prevent growth of current clots and also to prevent the formation of new blood clots. All patients with VTE are treated for at least 3 months, and treatment may be longer depending on the cause of the blood clot. In some patients who are unable to take blood thinners, such as people with recent bleeding or some recent surgeries, a device called an IVC filter may be placed in one of the veins in the abdomen to try to prevent blood clots that form in the lower limbs from reaching the lungs.

In very severe cases where patients have very low blood pressure, medications called thrombolytics may be given to try to dissolve the blood clots. In some cases, this may be determined to be unsafe and the person with the clot may have to undergo surgical removal of the blood clots.

Louis Brusco
Diana Anca

44

Sedation and Analgesia in the Cardiac Care Unit

INTRODUCTION

Patients in a cardiac care unit (CCU) experience pain, anxiety, stress and, at times, delirium, and altered mental status. Sedation and analgesia of these patients is not only a humane way to treat their discomfort but it also is an integral part of their therapy to allow them to tolerate the various other therapies, treatments, and instrumentations that they are subjected to in the critical care setting. It also is integral in reducing the metabolic response and oxygen demands of the critically ill cardiac patient.

Sedatives and analgesic medications carry with them hemodynamic, respiratory, neurologic, and other side effects, so that proper sedation is a balance between adequacy of sedation and minimizing these other effects. In addition, development of delirium in the cardiac care setting is a complication that dramatically impacts on the survival and quality of life of patients after they have recovered from their illness. Recently, the implication of the very choice of agent in the development of delirium has led to a reevaluation of the impact of all sedative/analgesic regimens in the context of their propensity to cause or help delirium.

The desired level of sedation in the cardiac care setting can vary widely between the awake, alert, conversant, oriented and comfortable patient, and the patient who is in a drug-induced coma and therapeutically paralyzed. The precise level of sedation and the agents used are determined by the indications for sedation, whether they are anxiety, insomnia, agitation, coordination with a mechanical ventilator, prevention of removal of tubes or lines, protection against myocardial ischemia, or the need for amnesia during paralysis. Agents are chosen depending on the relative amounts of the different components of analgesia, anxiolysis, amnesia, sleep, and muscle relaxation that are needed.

Although use of pharmacologic agents is the main way to achieve these goals, it cannot be stressed enough that other measures that reduce the need for amounts or even the very need for sedation are tremendously beneficial to patients, their comfort, and the avoidance of confusion and delirium. Such measures include frequent reorientation, assurance, and communication from the nursing staff; proper environmental controls such as lighting, temperature, and noise control; assessment and management of sensations such as hunger, thirst, and need to void; providing a variety of stimuli, such as visitors and media; and maintenance of a diurnal variation, with, if possible, a window facing the outside.

EVALUATION OF LEVEL OF SEDATION

One goal of management of critically ill cardiac patients is maintaining an optimal level of pain control and sedation. Unfortunately, pain and anxiety are subjective and somewhat difficult to consistently measure from caregiver to caregiver. Over 50% of patients who were interviewed after their intensive care unit (ICU) stays rated their pain as moderate to severe, during rest as well as during procedures.[1-3] Thus, the assessment of pain and anxiety must be discussed first before moving on to the pharmacology of the agents.

Although patients in a CCU are being monitored with highly sophisticated equipment, technological methods of measuring pain and anxiety such as those using electroenphalography (EEG), cerebral function analyzing monitors, lower esophageal contractility, combinations of physiologic variables or serum concentrations of medications, among others, have all proved to be no more reliable and a lot more complicated and expensive as simple, clinically based scoring systems. Properly designed scoring systems can be used not only to assess and record pain and anxiety but also to allow bedside nurses to titrate therapy in a more tightly defined window on their own, meeting regulatory requirements without needing repeated orders from a practitioner who is licensed to prescribe the medications.

The most basic of clinical methods of pain assessment is simply asking the patient to rate the pain on a scale of 0 to 10, with 0 being no pain at all and 10 being the worst pain imaginable. Although simple and widely used, and despite those instructions being given, the very fact that not infrequently some patients will answer "11" shows that when pain is being experienced acutely, the overall severity of the pain seems much greater than some historical control. One step up from a simple number scale is the use of a "Visual Analog Scale" (VAS)—which is simply a line that has the scale marked off in measured intervals. This scale is highly reliable and valid from patient to patient and caregiver to caregiver.[4] It can be further modified to have pictures of happy and unhappy patients or faces on the scale in varying degrees instead of numbers. Unfortunately, it is limited because it ignores qualitative aspects of pain, and many critically ill cardiac patients are not strong enough or awake enough to use such a system.

Measuring sedation and level of consciousness is similarly difficult, and requires the use of assessment of a practitioner observing the patient. The most basic method is to perform a mental status and neurologic examination and report the results. This is not practical on a repeated basis and does not allow the easy determination of changes that would allow titration of medications from time to time. The Glasgow Coma Scale (GCS) is widely used for the assessment of level of consciousness, but it was designed and validated for patients with neurologic deficits, and is not designed for assessment of sedation.

Sedation scales are subjective tools that, in general, measure the patient's responsiveness to verbal, auditory, and or physical stimuli. The ideal scale would determine the degree of sedation and agitation, be applicable in a wide variety of patient situations, have a well-defined sedation goal, include behavioral descriptors, be easy to measure and score with minimal training, and be reproducible, reliable, and valid across caregivers. Proper use of such a scale can reduce the duration of mechanical ventilation and also reduce length of stay in both the CCU and the hospital.[5] However, even though this has been known for over 10 years, the clinical use of scoring systems still remains low.[6] It is therefore imperative that every patient care area or unit that sedates critically ill patients chooses a sedation scale that best fits its patients, trains the caregivers in its use, and develops procedures to use that information in the sedation of the patients in the cardiac care area.

One of the most widespread of the currently used sedation scales is the Ramsay Sedation Scale (RSS), introduced in 1974 and modified slightly since then. The modified scale is shown in **Table 44.1**. As it was designed primarily for use during research into sedative agents, it was at the same time both groundbreaking but less than ideal for clinical use. Since its debut, many others have been developed for different reasons. Some of the more commonly referenced or clinically used ones include the Sedation Agitation Scale (SAS, **Table 44.2**),[7] the Motor Activity Assessment Scale,[8] the Vancouver Interactive and Calmness Scale (VICS),[9] the Richmond Agitation–Sedation Scale (RASS, **Table 44.3**),[10] the Adaptation to Intensive Care Environment (ATICE) instrument,[11] and the Minnesota Sedation Assessment Tool (MSAT).[12]

A thorough review and comparison of these scales can be found here.[13] The decision to use one scale or the other is many times a local, multidisciplinary decision. What is important is that

TABLE 44.1	Modified Ramsay Sedation Scale
SCORE	**DEFINITION**
1	Anxious and agitated or restless or both
2	Cooperative, oriented, and tranquil
3	Responds to commands only
4	Brisk response to a light glabellar tap or loud auditory stimulus
5	Sluggish response to a light glabellar tap or loud auditory stimulus
6	No response to a light glabellar tap or loud auditory stimulus

Performed using a series of steps: observation of behavior (score 1 or 2), followed (if necessary) by assessment of response to voice (score 3), followed (if necessary) by assessment of response to loud auditory stimulus or light glabellar tap (score 4 to 6).

TABLE 44.2	Sedation–Agitation Scale	
SCORE	**TERM**	**DESCRIPTOR**
7	Dangerous agitation	Pulling at ET tube, trying to remove catheters, climbing over bedrail, striking at staff, thrashing side to side
6	Very agitated	Requiring Restraint and frequent verbal reminding of limits, biting ETT.
5	Agitated	Anxious or physically agitated, calms to verbal instructions.
4	Calm and cooperative	Calm, easily arousable, follows command.
3	Sedated	Difficult to arouse but awakens to verbal stimuli or gentle shaking, follows simple commands but drifts off again.
2	Very sedated	Arouses to physical stimuli but does not communicate or follow commands, may move spontaneously.
1	Unarousable	Minimal or no response to noxious stimuli, does not communicate or follow command.

Guidelines for SAS assessment

1	Agitated patients are scored by their most severe degree of agitation as described.
2	If patient is awake or awakens easily to voice ("awaken" means responds with voice or head shaking to a question or follows commands), that is a SAS 4 (same as calm and appropriate—might even be napping).
3	If more stimuli such as shaking are required but patient eventually does awaken, that is a SAS 3.
4	If patient arouses to stronger physical stimuli (may be noxious) but never awakens to the point of responding yes/no or following commands, that is a SAS 2.
5	Little or no response to noxious physical stimuli represents a SAS 1.

ET, endotracheal; SAS, Sedation–Agitation Scale.

a scale is indeed used and that it is performed in a standard and consistent manner.

ANALGESIC AND SEDATIVE AGENTS

Critically ill cardiac patients are often treated with continuous infusions of potent medications. Some, such as sedative-hypnotics, have sedation as a primary action; whereas others, such as opioids, have a sedative action that is a secondary effect to the primary analgesic effect. Patients require sedatives because of pain, anxiety, delirium, and the desire to keep them from remembering an uncomfortable time in their lives. Especially when patients are on

TABLE 44.3	Richmond Agitation–Sedation Scale	
SCORE	**TERM**	**DESCRIPTION**
+4	Combative	Overtly combative or violent, immediate danger to staff
+3	Very agitated	Pulls on or removes tube(s) or catheter(s) or exhibits aggressive behavior toward staff
+2	Agitated	Frequent nonpurposeful movement or patient–ventilator dys-synchrony
+1	Restless	Anxious or apprehensive, but movements not aggressive or vigorous
0	Alert and calm	
−1	Drowsy	Not fully alert, but has sustained (>10 s) awakening, with eye contact, to voice
−2	Light sedation	Briefly (<10 s) awakens with eye contact to voice
−3	Moderate sedation	Any movement (but no eye contact) to voice
−4	Deep sedation	No response to voice, but any movement to physical stimulation
−5	Unarousable	No response to voice or physical stimulation

Performed using a series of steps: observation of behaviors (score +4 to 0), followed (if necessary) by assessment of response to voice (score −1 to −3), followed (if necessary) by assessment of response to physical stimulation such as shaking shoulder and then rubbing sternum if no response to shaking shoulder (score −4 to −5).

mechanical ventilation, it is most often much easier to administer such medications via continuous infusion. Use of such agents via continuous infusion, however, is associated with prolonged mechanical ventilation and a longer stay in the CCU, whereas daily interruption of sedative treatment has been shown to reduce the duration of mechanical ventilation and CCU duration.[14] Thus, it is no longer considered acceptable to sedate patients to a deep, deep state but rather to move to a lighter plane of sedation. This is much more difficult and requires both the use of sedation scales as mentioned, sedation protocols, and the selection of agents that are somewhat easier to titrate and have somewhat shorter durations of action than in use previously. It has also been shown that a shift toward more of an analgesic-based sedation instead of a sedative-hypnotic–based regimen is beneficial.[15,16] We therefore now review the most commonly used agents in the CCU for sedation.

Some definitions are needed to help in the classification and description of the various agents. "Analgesic agents" have as their primary mode of action the reduction of patients' pain. They usually will have as a side effect the sedation of patients, but the sedative effect and the analgesic effect may have different potencies and durations of action. Analgesics can be broadly divided into "opioids," meaning morphine-like in action, and "nonopioids" which are medications such as nonsteroidal anti-inflammatory agents and acetaminophen.

"Sedative-hypnotics" are medications that have as their primary effect the reversible depression of the central nervous system, inducing sleep, allaying anxiety, and causing amnesia.

Other drugs used in sedation are such drugs as "psychotropic medications," such as haloperidol or risperidone; they are antipsychotic medications that interfere with neurotransmitters in the brain that affect the way the cerebral neurons interact with each other.

OPIOIDS

Opioids are the mainstay of analgesic therapy in the CCU patient. Opioid analgesics, such as morphine, have as their mechanism of action the means of acting selectively on neurons that transmit and modulate nociception, leaving other sensory modalities and motor functions intact. Opioid receptors are found in the brain, spinal cord, and peripheral tissues. When bound to receptors, opioids produce analgesia, drowsiness, changes in mood, and mental clouding. An important feature of opioid analgesia is that it is not associated with loss of consciousness except at extremely high doses.

All opioids depress respiratory drive in a dose-dependent manner, and this depression is increased when opioids are given in conjunction with sedative-hypnotic medications. In general, opioids have minimal hemodynamic effects when given to patients who are not volume depleted, but can cause hypotension in patients who are volume depleted because of veno-dilatation. The primary problems with long-term administration of opioids are tachyphylaxis and dependence and withdrawal symptoms with discontinuation of long-term continuous infusion. A dosing summary is contained in **Table 44.4**.

Morphine

Morphine is the prototypical opioid. It was discovered in 1804 and is the most abundant alkaloid found in opium. It has been sold commercially for almost 200 years and remains a mainstay in

TABLE 44.4	Analgesics Used in the Cardiac Care Unit		
DRUG	**ELIMINATION HALF-LIFE**	**PEAK EFFECT (IV) (min)**	**STARTING DOSE**
Morphine	2–4 h	10–30	1–4 mg bolus 1–5 mg/h infusion
Hydromorphone	2–4 h	10–20	0.2–1 mg bolus 0.5–2 mg/h infusion
Fentanyl	2–5 h	2–3	25–100 µg bolus 25–200 µg/h infusion
Remifentanil	4 min	1.5	6–9 µg/kg/h infusion
Methadone	12–24 h	30–60	5–50 mg every 6–12 h based on previous opioid dose

IV, intravenous.

the sedation of critically ill cardiac patients. This is primarily due to cost and familiarity factors, because other opioids lack some of the problems associated with morphine. The dose required to produce analgesia, as with most opioids, varies and is dependent on such factors as tolerance, tachyphylaxis, and metabolic and excretory ability. Although morphine is metabolized in the liver, 6% to 20% of the metabolites are morphine-6-glucoronide, a metabolite that is excreted by the kidneys;[17,18] and while the data is variable, it is anywhere from half as potent to 20 to 40 times more potent than morphine itself[18,19] and can accumulate in renal failure. For this reason, hydromorphone is the long-acting opioid that is preferred in renal failure. When given via bolus injection, morphine causes histamine release, but this is not a factor when used via infusion in patients in the CCU. However, when given by bolus, it was one of the classical treatments for cardiogenic pulmonary edema, because the vasodilation and preload reduction it causes, along with the analgesia and anxiolysis, made patients in cardiogenic pulmonary edema much more comfortable.

It is the most hydrophilic of the opioids and therefore has the slowest onset of action. A bolus dose of morphine will take effect in 5 to 10 minutes with peak analgesic effect in 90 minutes and lasting for 2 to 3 hours—after continuous infusion, it does not exhibit prolongations in half-life (known as "context-sensitive half-life") such as happens with fentanyl and, to a lesser extent, with sufentanil and alfentanil.[20]

Usual doses to start morphine via infusion are 0.5 to 2 mg/h. Bolus doses of morphine can be given at 2 to 4 mg every 1 to 2 hours as a start, but doses can increase as tolerance develops. It is not unusual to see patients require morphine infusions of 15 mg/h or more.

Hydromorphone

Hydromorphone, the most common name for the drug actually called either dihydromorphone or dimorphone, is a semi-synthetic derivative of morphine. It was synthesized and researched in the 1920s. It is slightly more lipophilic than morphine and thus exhibits superior fat solubility and speed of onset than morphine.[21] It is thought to be three to four times stronger than morphine but with a lower risk of chronic dependency. It lacks the renally excreted active metabolites of morphine. It also has a slightly longer duration of action than morphine—roughly 3 to 4 hours. Its duration of action makes it slightly more cumbersome to adjust via continuous infusion, but, because it does not exhibit the context-sensitive half-life prolongation of fentanyl, it is sometimes preferable to fentanyl via infusion for long durations of sedation.

Most clinicians will start with hydromorphone at 0.1 to 0.2 mg/h and titrate as needed. Bolus doses of 0.5 mg given every 2 to 4 hours can be a starting point for intermittent intravenous (IV) dosing.

Fentanyl

Fentanyl is a fully synthetic opioid that was first developed in 1960 and has served as the parent molecule to the synthetic opioids that have been developed since then—sufentanil, alfentanil, and remifentanil. It is far more potent than morphine—roughly 40 times more potent on an mg/mg basis. As with other opioids, it works by binding to opioid receptors in the brain, spinal cord, and periphery, but its highly lipophilic chemistry causes it to cross the blood–brain barrier very easily, giving it an extremely short onset of action. It does not cause histamine release, and,

similar to other opioids, is neither an arterial vasodilator nor a negative inotrope.[22] It can, however, cause veno-dilatation and hypotension in a patient who is volume depleted. It is a potent blocker of endogenous catecholamines, which can be beneficial (in preventing a patient from becoming hypertensive and/or tachycardic with procedures) and detrimental (causing hypotension in patients whose hemodynamics are dependent on an elevated level of endogenous catecholamines).

Fentanyl is primarily metabolized in the liver to inactive metabolites, but its cessation of action is primarily through redistribution from the brain to the peripheral tissues rather than metabolism of active drug. Therefore, while a single or a few bolus doses have a shorter duration of action than morphine, on the order of 60 to 90 minutes, when given by infusion, even after 2 hours, the time to decrease by 50% concentration goes from 30 minutes for a bolus dose to 120 minutes with the infusion, and the time to decrease by 80% goes from 60 minutes with a bolus to over 600 minutes with the infusion.[20] This "context-sensitive half-life" is due to slow release from the fatty compartments that fentanyl has such an affinity for, and causes a greatly prolonged effect for fentanyl when given by infusion—to an effective half-life much longer than morphine after a few hours of infusion.

Fentanyl also has a particular problem in many patients of having rapidly escalating dosing requirements.[23] It is not uncommon for patients to start out on one dose and 24 to 48 hours later be requiring four to five times as much as they were just a day or two earlier. This tolerance seems greater for many patients than with the longer acting opioids and, combined with the context-sensitive half-life prolongation, makes fentanyl a less than ideal medication to use for critically ill cardiac patients for any longer than 24 to 48 hours.

Fentanyl dosing usually starts at 50 to 100 µg for a bolus dose or 50 to 100 µg/h via infusion with titration—it is not uncommon to rapidly (over 24 to 72 hours) require 500 to 750 µg/h via infusion.

Sufentanil

Sufentanil is similar to fentanyl in every way except that it is more potent—roughly 10 times more potent than fentanyl and almost 400 times more potent than morphine. It does not exhibit quite the same context-sensitive half-life prolongation as fentanyl. It was synthesized in 1974. It is perhaps the most potent sympatholytic opioid in clinical practice. Its use in critically ill cardiac patients has been minimal because, until recently, it was under patent protection and was much more expensive than fentanyl when used for sedation in the CCU.

Remifentanil

Remifentanil is a potent ultrashort-acting synthetic opioid.[24] It is unique in that it has a rapid onset of action, and it has an ester linkage that undergoes rapid hydrolysis by nonspecific tissue and plasma esterases, which means that it has an organ-independent metabolism and does not accumulate in either renal or hepatic failure. Its context-sensitive half-life remains at a flat 4 minutes even after prolonged infusions.[25] It is fairly potent—roughly twice as potent as fentanyl and 100 times as potent as morphine. It is very hemodynamically stable but, unlike fentanyl, it does cause histamine release when given as a bolus; and many times an antihistamine such as diphenhydramine is given as an adjunct when it is used for sedation. It is a potent respiratory depressant, and practitioners familiar with its use commonly see patients who are awake but will not breathe until it is fully worn off, which happens minutes later.

Remifentanil seems to have all the makings of an ideal sedative agent for critically ill cardiac patients. Although studies have been promising, review of a meta-analysis of studies in critically ill patients[26] shows that while remifentanil use is associated with a reduction in time to tracheal extubation, there was no reduction in mortality, duration of mechanical ventilation, length of ICU stay, or risk of agitation. The other reason it is not currently a viable analgesic for CCU use is that it is still on patent and extremely expensive—recent change in marketing arrangements for the drug have caused the price to double in the United States. Until the price significantly decreases, remifentanil remains a theoretical but not a practical answer to analgesic needs in the CCU.

Methadone

Almost polar opposite in pharmacology to remifenanil is methadone, among the longest acting of the opioids.[27] It is a synthetic opioid that is structurally unlike morphine but still acts on opioid receptors and produces many of the same effects. It was developed in 1937 and has been used commonly because of its long duration of action and low cost. High doses of methadone can block the euphoric effects of other opioids such as heroin and morphine, and it has become a mainstay in the treatment of patients addicted to opioid narcotics. Although that is its most common use, it does have other uses as well, and one of those is in the long-term critically ill patients. Methadone has an excellent oral bioavailability (80% to 90%), an elimination half-life of 12 to 24 hours, and is equipotent with morphine. It can be given via oral tablets or suspension, or intravenously.

Patients who are on long-term opioid infusions may suffer withdrawal symptoms on cessation—others, although not experiencing true withdrawal symptoms, simply need the medication slowly tapered off to allow the patient to gradually reach a state of no sedation. Frequently, this will take place when the patient is ready to leave a CCU but is prevented from leaving by the presence of a sedative infusion. Using methadone to transition a patient from a continuous IV infusion of opioid sometimes can be an ideal way to bridge this gap. Commonly, the patient will be given methadone at a dose of 0.5 to 0.75 mg/d of the equivalent amount of morphine the patient is on. The availability of methadone in an oral suspension makes it even easier to give to patients receiving tube feeds. It has been studied in pediatric patients, but the pharmacology is applicable to adult patients as well.[28]

One consideration in patients receiving methadone that does not exist with the other opioids is that methadone is associated with prolongation of the QTc interval in high doses, and has been implicated in progressing on to torsade de pointes. The mean daily dose in one study was over 350 mg/d, a very high dose; and in usual use it is easy to limit doses to below that, but especially in cardiac patients who may be more predisposed to arrhythmias and QT prolongation, this must be considered.[29]

SEDATIVE HYPNOTICS

In addition to opioids for analgesia, patients in cardiac care settings require sedation for anxiety, restlessness, agitation, and to decrease chances of remembering bad experiences in the CCU. Anxiety is best treated after pain is controlled with analgesics and reversible conditions such as hypoxia, infections, renal or hepatic failure, and metabolic abnormalities are corrected. Most sedative-hypnotics work by binding to the inhibitory gamma-aminobutyric acid (GABA) receptor, which counterbalances the action of excitatory neurotransmitters. By themselves, they have minimal respiratory depressant effect unless patients are made unresponsive to outside stimuli, but with even minimal doses of opioids the respiratory depression is significantly augmented. The clinical effects are very, very similar—so are the differences in pharmacokinetics, cost, and side effects of administration. A dosing summary is contained in **Table 44.5**.

Lorazepam

Lorazepam is a moderately slow-onset intermediate-acting benzodiazepine that is available to be given either via IV bolus or infusion or via the oral route. Its initial onset is in 5 to 10 minutes, but a wide therapeutic dosing range means that some patients will be fairly well sedated with a small initial dose and others will require multiple, higher doses.[30] For example, patients who are withdrawing from alcohol will sometimes require very high doses, whereas elderly patients will sometimes become heavily sedated with minute doses. Elderly patients may sometimes also "disinhibit" and become very agitated with all benzodiazepines, so they should be used with caution in the elderly.[31]

Lorazepam is metabolized in the liver to inactive metabolites; it has an elimination half-life of 10 to 20 hours, and an effective duration of action of 3 to 6 hours. It is glucuronidated in the liver, and because the glucuronidation system is less affected in liver dysfunction than in the oxidative system, lorazepam may not be as affected by hepatic dysfunction as are other medications, but it should still be used with caution in patients with liver dysfunction.

TABLE 44.5	Sedatives Used in the Cardiac Care Unit		
DRUG	**ELIMINATION HALF-LIFE (h)**	**PEAK EFFECT (IV) (min)**	**STARTING DOSE**
Midazaolam	3–5	1–2	1–2 mg bolus 0.5–10 mg/h infusion
Lorazepam	10–20	2–20	1–2 mg bolus 0.5–10 mg/h infusion
Propofol	20–30	1–2	20–70 mg bolus (sedation) 100–200 mg bolus (intubation) 25–100 µg/kg/min infusion
Halperidol	10–24	3–20	2–10 mg bolus 2–10 mg/h infusion
Dexmedetomidine	2	5–15	0.2–1.5 µg/kg/h

IV, intravenous.

It is not unusual for a patient to receive 24 hours of a moderate dose of lorazepam and take 5 to 7 days to wake up.

Like all members of this class of drugs, lorazepam will cause hypotension via arterial dilatation, and will cause a more pronounced hypotension via veno-dilatation in patients who are volume depleted. Lorazepam is diluted in propylene glycol, and with long-term high-volume infusions propylene glycol toxicity, causing acute tubular necrosis, lactic acidosis, and a hyperosmolar state, can occur.[32]

Initial bolus doses of lorazepam are typically from 0.5 to 2 mg, and infusion rates usually start at 0.5 to 1 mg/h and can go as high as 20 to 25 mg/h, with rates of over 100 mg/h not unheard of for patients in severe alcohol withdrawal.

Midazolam

Midazolam is a rapid-onset, short-acting benzodiazepine. It has the characteristic of causing anterograde amnesia (amnesia after administration) perhaps better than any other sedative. When given in small doses, it is not unusual to have patients arousable and talking and later have no recollection of those events. It has a short onset of perhaps 1 to 2 minutes; and while the half-life is 1 to 4 hours, its duration of action after a single bolus dose is less than 15 minutes. It is water soluble in the bottle and becomes highly lipophilic at body pH. Its short duration of action is due to rapid equilibration and redistribution among the various bodily compartments. Owing to its lipophilic nature, it has a prolonged context-sensitive half-life due to a high volume of distribution in fatty compartments and also due to accumulation of an active metabolite, alpha1-hydroxymidazolam.[33] The half-life more than doubles, but, more importantly, because the short duration of action after bolus dose is due to redistribution, the effective duration of action after infusions of greater than 24 hours approaches that of lorazepam.

Midazolam is the drug of choice for short-term sedation in the non-intubated patient, especially for procedures. It has minimal respiratory depressant effects when given alone, but it highly potentiates the respiratory suppression of opioids. Dosing information is found in **Table 44.5**.

Propofol

Propofol is a rather unique drug that is not a benzodiazepine and has no other drugs in its class, as an alkylphenol. It is highly lipophilic and totally insoluble in water and is thus prepared in a 10% lipid emulsion at a concentration of 10 mg/mL. Similar to the benzodiazepines, it works on the GABA receptor, and it has excellent sedative and hypnotic properties, adequate amnestic properties, and has no analgesic properties. By itself, it has minimal respiratory depressant properties at lower doses but will suppress respiration at doses used for induction of general anesthesia, 1.5 to 2 mg/kg. Rapid equilibration across the blood–brain barrier is the reason for its extremely rapid onset of action.[34] Unlike benzodiazepines, in addition to vasodilatation it also is a myocardial depressant and thus can cause hypotension after large bolus dosing in hemodynamically unstable patients.

Propofol shows a short duration of action after less than 24 hours of infusion, and infusions of longer than 24 hours show only a slight prolongation of effect; after 24 hours, patients wake up much faster than they do with midazolam or lorazepam. It is metabolized in the liver, but there is extrahepatic metabolism as well,[35] so there is little or no prolongation of effect in renal or hepatic failure.[36]

Because of its formulation, a number of considerations must be mentioned. Because it is an emulsion in lipid, with high volumes of administration fat overload is a concern, especially in patients also receiving lipid formulations as part of total parenteral nutrition. Nutritional lipids should be adjusted downward to compensate for the lipid administered with the propofol, and patients should be followed up for hypertriglyceridemia and, with longer infusions, for pancreatitis.[37] The lipid nature of the propofol emulsion makes it an excellent medium to grow bacteria, and to reduce the chances of bacterial overgrowth propofol in the United States has additives to act as bacteriostatic agents. Depending on the formulation, propofol will have either ethylenediaminetetraacetic acid, sodium metabisulfite, or alcohol. Patients who are sulfite allergic could have an adverse reaction to the propofol solution.[38]

Propofol has also been implicated in a sometimes fatal syndrome termed "propofol infusion syndrome" (PRIS).[39] Because propofol has properties similar to barbiturates such as sodium pentothal and pentobarbital in lowering cerebral metabolic rate for oxygen and decreasing intracranial pressure, it became popular to use it at fairly high doses for prolonged periods of time in patients with head injury and elevated intracranial pressure from cerebral edema. In 2001, the first series of cases of patients receiving propofol at doses over 5 mg/kg/h who developed progressive myocardial failure with dysrhythmias, metabolic acidosis, hyperkalemia, and evidence of muscle cell destruction.[40] Other studies have confirmed a dose-dependent connection, but there also have been some patients with some of the features of PRIS who received it at lower doses for only a few hours. Therefore, anyone receiving propofol infusion must be observed for the signs of PRIS, and most institutions have installed a cap of 5 mg/kg/h on dosage of propofol for durations over 24 hours.

Dexmedetomidine

Dexmedetomidine is another unique medication with a novel mechanism of action. It binds to the α_2 receptors in the brain as an agonist, and the location of the receptors determines the action of the medication. Dexmedetomidine binds to α_2 receptors in the locus ceruleus of the brain stem, giving it its sedative and anxiolytic effects, and in the dorsal horn of the spinal cord, releasing substance P and producing its analgesic effects.[41] It causes less hypotension than another medication that is also an α_2 receptor agonist, clonidine, and much more sedation and analgesia. The hallmark of dexmedetomidine therapy is mild sedation and induction of sleep, anxiolysis, analgesia with minimal respiratory depression, and reduction of stress response to surgery and other stimuli. The type of sleep is also important, because it comes closer than any other sedative to causing a sleep that mimics normal rapid eye movement sleep. Patients sedated with dexmedetomidine appear tranquil and comfortable, yet being readily arousable and interactive and oriented when stimulated, only to fall right back to that tranquil, sleeping state when the stimulus is discontinued.[42]

The dosing of dexmedetomidine is also different from the other sedatives mentioned earlier. Bolus doses are poorly tolerated, do not have a good clinical effect, and are rarely used. A loading infusion may be used at the start of the therapy, with a dose of 1 μg/kg of actual body weight given as an infusion over 10 minutes (which translates into 6 μg/kg/h rate of infusion for 10 minutes). Alternatively, an infusion may just be started at the desired rate. Although in the United States, the approved dose range is from 0.2 to 0.7 µg/kg/h for up to 24 hours, doses higher than that for longer periods of time have been safely used.[43] Distribution half-life is 6 minutes, and elimination half-life is 2 hours, but effective duration of action is different—after a loading infusion, onset of sleep sensation starts during the loading and is at its peak 10 to 20 minutes after the load is complete. After cessation of therapy, there is a gradual return to baseline mental status—but because the sleep is so mild and so natural, plus other medications are usually being given, it is very difficult to indeed tell when the effect of the drug has lessened significantly.

The adverse effects of dexmedetomidine include paradoxical hypertension, especially during the bolus dose, followed by hypotension and bradycardia from the sympathetic inhibition. These can be beneficial, but they also may require the adjustment of other medications, such as beta-blockers or calcium channel blocker medications.

The biggest drawback to using dexmedetomidine is a practical one. The other sedatives used via infusion in a cardiac care setting can be given via bolus, and, when given via bolus or at high enough rates of infusion, reliably produce a patient who is essentially unresponsive to painful stimuli. This level of sedation is difficult, if not impossible, to attain with dexmedetomidine alone. Thus, other medications often need to be used for sudden breakthroughs of agitation and pain, and the need for those additional medications many times discourages caregivers from gaining extensive experience with dexmedetomidine.

Because of the more natural sleep pattern that is produced by dexmedetomidine, there has been hope that it will reduce the amount of delirium seen in critically ill patients. Delirium has become an important topic of discussion in critical care, as can be seen in the next section.

DELIRIUM

Over the past 10 years delirium in all types of critically ill patients has become an important area of concern. As medical knowledge and technology over time have improved survival of severely ill patients, many times their mental state after such recovery was less than optimal. Patients would recover from their multisystem organ dysfunction, only to be left with a delirious mental status that required long-term sedation, rehabilitation, or institutionalization in a skilled nursing facility. Elderly patients in particular seemed more susceptible to the onset of delirium, and it has been diagnosed in up to 60% to 80% of patients requiring mechanical ventilation.[44] Having delirium in a CCU is associated with a higher re-intubation rate, a higher mortality, and a longer length of stay. It also has a high rate of progression to permanent cognitive impairment. Thus, it is no longer a condition that can be expected to clear once the patient leaves the CCU.

Delirium is a disturbance of consciousness with inattention accompanied by a change in cognition or perceptual disturbance that develops acutely over a short period of time, from a few hours to a few days.[45] It can be further broken down into hyperactive and hypoactive forms.[46] The hyperactive form, commonly mislabeled "ICU psychosis" in the past, is characterized by agitation, restlessness, attempting to remove catheters and tubes, and emotional lability. It has a better long-term prognosis. The hypoactive form is characterized by withdrawal, lethargy, flat affect, apathy, and decreased responsiveness. It is sometimes erroneously termed ICU or critical care "encephalopathy." Making the diagnosis of either type with precision is sometimes difficult, and can be done with one of two validated tools that can be found here.[44,47]

For the purposes of this chapter, it is important to recognize a number of aspects of delirium in critically ill cardiac patients. First is to diagnose it, and to rule out other organic causes of the condition. Second is to realize that sedative regimens that are used in the CCU have been implicated in the development of delirium. Sedatives and analgesics work by altering neurotransmitter levels and the exposure to benzodiazepines and/or opioids are involved in 98% of patients with delirium.[48] Some agents within a class have at times been shown to be more causative of delirium than others. Morphine,[49] fentanyl,[50] midazolam,[50] and lorazepam[51] have all been implicated in the development of delirium, with lorazepam probably being the most consistently implicated one. Conversely, the newer, more expensive agents, dexmedetomidine[52] and remifentanil,[53] may have lower incidences of delirium. It has not yet been established, however, if the costs involved in using remifentanil or dexmedetomidine, among the other disadvantages, are worth the reduction in delirium.

Lastly, it is important to know what can be used to treat the hyperactive type of delirium and what else can be done to prevent delirium in the first place. As far as treatment of the delirium goes, in the past it was thought that patients needed to be "unscrambled" and so potent antipsychotic medications, such as haloperidol or risperidone, were used. Indeed, the very initiation of using a delirium assessment tool can increase the use of haloperidol dramatically.[54] Haloperidol is the only parenteral medication available to use in the patient with delirium, because benzodiazepines do not seem to be helpful.[55] Use of an atypical antipsychotic, quetiapine, seems to be the best studied and shows promise in treating patients with delirium in combination with haloperidol.[56] We are still in an early phase of this research, and much more work needs to be done.[57] Finally, it is important not to underestimate the importance of nonpharmacologic therapy. Such things as cognitive stimulation, reorientation prompts, a sleep protocol, visual and hearing aids, reminders to prevent volume depletion, and walking/exercise all reduced the incidence of delirium, and, while labor intensive, are absolutely essential in reducing and treating delirium in the CCU.[58]

SEDATION AND ANALGESIA IN DIAGNOSTIC AND THERAPEUTIC PROCEDURES IN THE CARDIAC CARE UNIT

Increasingly, diagnostic and therapeutic procedures are performed in the CCU at the bedside, both because of lack of timely access to the operating room (OR) and cost savings.

Both pain medications, sedatives and hypnotics, are used alone or in combination to facilitate the performing of bedside procedures. Concerns related to the patient physiology and to transport to the OR have made performing bedside procedures a more viable and safer option.

Care in the CCU setting is similar to the one in the OR from the point of view of both equipment and personnel. The monitors are nearly identical to the ones in the OR, and the ventilators have the same capabilities and more regarding mechanical ventilation of patients, despite the lack of inhalational agents. CCU nurses are also similar to the ones in the OR with regard to many skills and capabilities.[59]

There are multiple diagnostic and therapeutic procedures done at the bedside in the CCUs for many different indications. Even though the concept and goal of sedation and analgesia is the same for all of them, there are small but important differences between each procedure. Some of these procedures are more or less specific to the CCU and the field of cardiology; others are common in other critical care settings and involve other subspecialties as well.

The following are common cardiovascular procedures in the CCU requiring sedation and/or analgesia.

TRANSESOPHAGEAL ECHOCARDIOGRAPHY

Transesophageal echocardiography (TEE) is an invaluable, semi-invasive, diagnostic modality that is increasingly used both in the CCU setting as well as in the OR for structural and functional study of the heart. Owing to its proximity to posterior cardiac structures, the TEE probe offers superior visualization of these posteriorly located structures; and because use of higher frequency probes is possible with this anatomical proximity, it offers better spatial resolution compared to transthoracic echocardiography (TTE). The indications are broad, including assessment of structure and function of native or prosthetic valves, infective endocarditis, cardiac sources of emboli, acute aortic syndrome, tumors, and congenital heart diseases.[60] When performed in the OR, patients are almost always under general anesthesia, but in the CCU setting, the patients are usually consciously sedated.

Patients undergoing TEE examination in the CCU tend to be more frail, with other comorbidities (cardiovascular, cerebrovascular, heart failure, and coronary or valvular heart disease) and usually have more acute clinical scenarios, making them at least intermediate risk for anesthesia most of the times.

TEE is generally regarded as a safe procedure. It involves the placement of the ultrasound probe via the oropharynx into the esophagus and down into the stomach, which might cause nausea, shortness of breath, agitation, and pain due to pharyngoesophageal intubation, symptoms that might be alleviated by use of local anesthetics and sedation.

There is significant variation with regard to sedation for TEE. Some centers use benzodiazepines alone, specifically midazolam, whereas others use a combination of opiates, either as a bolus or infusion, in addition to midazolam.

Several studies have explored the use of different combinations of sedatives, alone or combined, and the use of local anesthetics to the oropharynx.[62,63]

The medications used, either alone or in combination, were propofol, midazolam, alfentanil, remifentanyl, and dexmedetomidine.[63–65]

Although TEE is regarded as a safe procedure and the complications are rare, they exist and mostly involve the gastrointestinal (GI), cardiovascular, and respiratory systems. These complications are mostly related to probe insertion, medications used for sedation, and operator experience.[61,66]

Given the potentially serious complications, especially in the particularly frail CCU patient population, careful pre-procedural evaluation and monitoring during the procedure should take place. These include careful assessment of medical history, particularly assessing history of esophageal and gastric pathology or history of bleeding disorders. Performing a thorough physical examination with particular emphasis on the examination of the airway, cervical spine mobility, and dentition is important. Fasting 6 to 8 hours before the procedure should be ascertained,

and monitoring of vital signs at baseline and throughout the procedure should take place.

Supplemental oxygen should be administered and emergency airway equipment should be available.

Dentures should be removed when present, and bite guards should be placed on patients with full dentition.

After local anesthetic spraying of the oropharynx and/or sedation, the TEE probe is lubricated and then inserted, avoiding any resistance. Supplemental doses of the medications can be administered during the procedure to assure the patient's comfort and optimal examination.

Obese patients pose a particular challenge both from the standpoint of safe sedation and analgesia and optimal examination. They have a higher incidence of coronary artery disease, hypertension, and sleep apnea; hence there is a higher potential for complications such as hypoxemia, especially in class III obesity.[67]

DIRECT CURRENT CARDIOVERSION

External electric cardioversion is used to treat abnormal heart rhythms to restore the normal sinus rhythm. Most non-emergent cardioversions in the CCU are performed to treat atrial fibrillation or atrial flutter. It is also performed on an emergent basis to correct dangerous rhythms when they are associated with hypotension, chest pain, confusion, or shortness of breath. The procedure can be quite painful and requires sedation. Performing the procedure involves coordinating several teams: cardiology/electrophysiology, anesthesiology, and, when a prior TEE is required, the echocardiography team. This coordination can be sometimes difficult, because it could be needed at short notice. The ideal medication for sedation for cardioversion would have rapid onset and offset, cardiovascular stability, and no respiratory depression. Propofol has been the most widely used drug followed by etomidate and often a short-acting opiate.[68,70] The goal of sedation for cardioversion is a short period of deep sedation or general anesthesia using agents with a rapid recovery. Considering the potential risk of hypotension and respiratory depression associated with the procedure, the presence of an anesthesiologist to assure airway control is required. Supplemental oxygen and proper monitoring with blood pressure (invasive or noninvasive), pulse oximetry, electrocardiogram (ECG), and capnography are required.[69]

Because of the strong jolt associated with the electric shock and the resultant skeletal muscle contraction, lip and tongue laceration can occur despite sedation; it is therefore important to insert a soft bite block between the teeth right before induction of the sedation/anesthesia.

PERICARDIOCENTESIS

Pericardial effusion is accumulation of fluid around the heart, which in time can lead to pericardial tamponade and can be life threatening if not evacuated in a timely manner.

Pericardiocentesis is the aspiration of the fluid from the pericardial space and it can be lifesaving. Cardiac ultrasound is the gold standard for detection and assessment of the pericardial effusion.

Typically, the drainage of the pericardial fluid is performed by pericardiocentesis in the catheterization laboratory under fluoroscopic or echocardiographic guidance, or by establishing a pericardial window in the OR. When there are acute signs of pericardial tamponade, the pericardiocentesis can be performed at the bedside under echocardiographic guidance.[71]

The procedure involves scanning with the ultrasound for the place where the effusion is the largest, sterile skin preparation, sterile drape cover, and requires local anesthetic injection and IV sedation, especially for anxious patients. If the decision is made for use of sedation, utmost care must be taken to use drugs with the least amount of hemodynamic impairment, because these patients are already in a very frail hemodynamic state. Drugs such as midazolam and short-acting opiates are a good choice. If a deeper level of sedation is needed for a short period of time, etomidate and etamine are other good options.

INTRA-AORTIC BALLOON PUMP

Intra-aortic balloon pump (IABP) is a device that improves cardiac function by balancing the myocardial oxygen demand and supply. It inflates during diastole, increasing the coronary perfusion pressure and then deflates during systole leading to decreased afterload and left ventricular work. It is usually placed in the catheterization laboratory under fluoroscopy guidance but occasionally it is necessary to place the IABP in the CCU setting in unstable patients in cardiogenic shock, acute myocardial infarction, acute severe mitral regurgitation, or ischemic ventricular septal defect. IABP is placed percutaneously via the femoral artery using a Seldinger technique and rarely via the subclavian, axillary, or iliac artery. Considering the large lumen of the device, and the need for the patient to be still during insertion, local anesthetic and mild sedation might be necessary, with careful monitoring of the cardiovascular and respiratory status, especially because some patients might already be in pulmonary edema.

TEMPORARY TRANSVENOUS PACEMAKER

Emergent insertion of a temporary transvenous pacemaker is the treatment of choice for patients with different conduction abnormalities, such as Mobitz II, symptomatic bradycardia, complete heart block, and ischemic or nonischemic new-onset bifascicular block. It is usually used as a bridge to more permanent solutions for underlying conduction abnormality, such as treating the reversible underlying cause or insertion of a permanent pacemaker.[72]

Temporary transvenous pacing involves two components: obtaining central venous access and intracardiac placement of the pacing wire. The preferred route is the internal jugular vein, followed by the subclavian and femoral veins. The central venous access is obtained under ultrasound guidance and requires local anesthetic infiltration of the skin and sometimes mild sedation, especially because the procedure can be slightly prolonged by the need for proper positioning of the intracardiac wire, which is achieved by following the ECG waves.

MISCELLANEOUS PROCEDURES IN THE CARDIAC CARE UNIT

1. Upper GI endoscopy is sometimes performed at the bedside in patients in the CCU, to assess upper GI tract pathologies, such as bleeding or esophageal pathologies. The sedation and analgesia are similar to the ones for performing a TEE, because the procedure is quite similar and involves the same steps.
2. Placement of invasive monitoring or access lines, such as arterial and central venous lines, is a common procedure in patients in the CCU. Arterial line insertion involves placement of a catheter inside an artery (radial, brachial, femoral, or dorsalis

pedis) for the purpose of continuous blood pressure monitoring on patients who are on inotropes or pressor infusions, or require multiple arterial blood sample drawings. The vast majority of times, the procedure only requires injection of a local anesthetic at the site, but on occasion, on very anxious or agitated patients, addition of other medication is required. Small, divided doses of benzodiazepines, opiates, or a combination of both are warranted in these settings with close monitoring of the patient's hemodynamic and respiratory status.

Because of necessity of patient positioning in a Trendelenburg position for central venous line placement with the head turned to the side and the need to cover the face with sterile drapes, and the slightly longer time for insertion, the central line placement poses more challenges than arterial placement; hence more frequent requirements for sedatives and analgesics in addition to the local anesthetic infiltration.

CONCLUSION

Patients in a cardiac care setting often need sedative or analgesic medications to help them through their course of CCU stay and while undergoing different therapeutic or diagnostic modalities. These medications have benefits but also side effects that need to be considered before administering the medications. The choice of medications may have long-lasting implications for patients in their recovery phase. Using a method of treating these patients that is balanced between personal professional experience and judgment and an evidence-based approach is the best way of properly choosing the optimal regimen.

REFERENCES

1. Carroll KC, Atkins PJ, Herold GR, et al. Pain assessment and management in critically ill postoperative and trauma patients: a multisite study. *Am J Crit Care*. 1999;8:105-117.
2. Puntillo KA. Pain experiences of intensive care unit patients. *Heart Lung*. 1990;19:526-533.
3. Stanik-Hutt JA, Soeken KL, Belcher AE, Fontaine DK, Gift AG. Pain experiences of traumatically injured patients in a critical care setting. *Am J Crit Care*. 2001;10:252-259.
4. Chapman CR, Casey KL, Dubner R, Foley KM, Gracely RH, Reading AE. Pain measurement: an overview. *Pain*. 1985;22:1-31.
5. Brook AD, Ahrens TS, Schaiff R, et al. Effect of a nursing implemented sedation protocol on the duration of mechanical ventilation. *Crit Care Med*. 1999;27:2609-2615.
6. Payen JF, Bosson JL, Chanques G, Mantz J, Labarere J; DOLOREA Investigators. Pain assessment is associated with decreased duration of mechanical ventilation in the intensive care unit: a post hoc analysis of the DOLOREA Study. *Anesthesiology*. 2009;111:1308-1316.
7. Riker RR, Picard JT, Fraser GL. Prospective evaluation of the Sedation-Agitation Scale for adult critically ill patients. *Crit Care Med*. 1999;27:1325-1329.
8. Devlin JW, Boleski G, Mylnarek M, et al. Motor Activity Assessment Scale: a valid and reliable sedation scale for use with mechanically ventilated patients in an adult surgical intensive care unit. *Crit Care Med*. 1999;27:1271-1275.
9. de Lemos J, Tweeddale M, Chittock D. Measuring quality of sedation in adult mechanically ventilated critically ill patients: the Vancouver Interaction and Calmness Scale. *J Clin Epid*. 2000;53:908-919.

10. Sessler CN, Gosnell MS, Grap MJ, et al. The Richmond Agitation-Sedation Scale—validity and reliability in adult intensive care unit patients. *Am J Respir Crit Care Med.* 2002;166:1338-1344.

11. De Jonghe B, Cook D, Griffith L, et al. Adaptation to the Intensive Care Environment (ATICE): development and validation of a new sedation assessment instrument. *Crit Care Med.* 2003;31:2344-2354.

12. Weinert C, McFarland L. The state of intubated ICU patients: development of a two-dimensional sedation rating scale for critically ill adults. *Chest.* 2004;126:1883-1890.

13. Sessler CN. Sedation scales in the ICU. *Chest.* 2004;126:1727-1730.

14. Kress JP, Pohlman AS, O'Connor MF, Hall JB. Daily interruption of sedative infusions in critically ill patients undergoing mechanical ventilation. *N Engl J Med.* 2000;342:1471-1477.

15. Karabinis A, Mandragos K, Stergiopoulos S, et al. Safety and efficacy of analgesia-based sedation with remifentanil versus standard hypnotic-based regimens in intensive care unit patients with brain injuries: a randomized, controlled trial. *Crit Care.* 2004;8:R268-R280.

16. Park G, Lane M, Rogers S, Bassett P. A comparison of hypnotic and analgesic based sedation in a general intensive care unit. *Br J Anasth.* 2007;98:76-82.

17. Hasselström J, Säwe J. Morphine pharmacokinetics and metabolism in humans. Enterohepatic cycling and relative contribution of metabolites to active opioid concentrations. *Clin Pharmacokinet.* 1993;24:344-354.

18. Van Dorp ELA, Romberg R, Sarton E, Bovill JG, Dahan A. Morphine-6-glucuronide: morphine's successor for postoperative pain relief? *Anesth Analg.* 2006;102:1789-1797.

19. Frances B, Gout R, Monsarrat B, Cros J, Zajac JM. Further evidence that morphine-6β-glucuronide is a more potent opioid agonist than morphine. *J Pharm Exp Ther.* 1992;262:25-31.

20. Shafer SL, Varvrel JR. Pharmacokinetics, pharmacodynamics and rational opioid selection. *Anesthesiology.* 1991;74:53-63.

21. Murray A, Hagen NA. Hydromorphone. *J Pain Symptom Manage.* 2005;29:S57-S66.

22. Stanley TH, Webster LR. Anesthetic requirements and cardiovascular effects of fentanyl-oxygen and fentanyl-diazepam-oxygen anesthesia in man. *Anesth Analg.* 1978;57:411-416.

23. Arnold JH, Truog RD, Scavone JM, Fenton T. Changes in the pharmacodynamic response to fentanyl in neonates during continuous infusion. *J Pediatr.* 1991;119:639-643.

24. Glass PS, Hardman D, Kamiyama Y, et al. Preliminary phramcokinietic and pharmacodynamics of an Ultra-Short-Acting Opioid:Remifentanil (GI87084B). *Anesth Analg.* 1993;77:1031-1040.

25. Hughes MA, Glass PSA, Jacobs JR. Context-sensitive half-time in multicompartment pharmacokinetic models for intravenous anesthetic drugs. *Anesthesiology.* 1992;76:334-341.

26. Tan JA, Ho KM. Use of remifantanil as a sedative in critically ill adults patients: a meta-analysis. *Anesthesia.* 2009;64:1342-1352.

27. Sim SK. Methadone. *Can Med Assoc J.* 1973;109:615-619.

28. Siddappa R, Fletcher J, Heard AM, et al. Methadone dosage for prevention of opioid withdrawal in children. *Paediatr Anaesth.* 2003;13:805-810.

29. Krantz MJ, Kutinsky IB, Robertson AD, et al. Dose-related effects of methadone on QT prolongation in a series of patients with Torsade de Pointes. *Pharmacotherapy.* 2003;23:802-815.

30. Wagner BK, O'Hara DA. Pharmacokinetics and pharmacodynamics of sedatives and analgesics in the treatment of agitated critically ill patients. *Clin Pharmacokinet.* 1997;33:426-453.

31. Greenblatt DJ, Sellers EM, Shader RI. Drug disposition in the elderly. *N Engl J Med.* 1982;306:1081-1088.

32. Horinek EL, Kiser TH, Fish DN, MacLaren R. Propylene glycol accumulation in critically ill patients receiving continuous intravenous lorazepam infusions. *Ann Phramcother.* 2009;43:1964.

33. Malacrida R, Fritz ME, Suter PM, Crevoisier C. Pharmacokinetics of midazolam administered by continuous intravenous infusion to intensive care patients. *Crit Care Med.* 1992;20:1123-1126.

34. Barr J, Egan TD, Sandoval NF, et al. Propofol dosing regimens for ICU sedation based upon an intergrated pharmacokinetic-pharmacodynamic model. *Anesthesiology.* 2001;95:324-333.

35. Veroli P, O'Kelly B, Bertrand F, Trouvin JH, Farinotti R, Ecoffey C. Extrahepatic metabolism of propofol in man during the anhepatic phase of orthotopic liver transplantation. *Br J Anaesth.* 1992;68:183-186.

36. Nathan N, Debord J, Narcisse F, et al. Pharmacokinetics of propofol and its conjugates after continuous infusion in normal and in renal failure patients: a preliminary study. *Acta Anaesthesiol Belg.* 1993;44:77-85.

37. Possidente CJ, Rogers FB, Osler TM, Smith TA. Elevated pancreatic enzymes after extended propofol therapy. *Pharmacotherapy.* 1998;18:653-655.

38. Langevin PB. Propofol containing sulfite-potential for injury. *Chest.* 1999;116:1140-1141.

39. Wong JM. Propofol infusion syndrome. *Am J Ther.* 2010;17:487-491.

40. Cremer OL, Moons KG, Bouman EA, Kruijswijk JE, de Smet AM, Kalkman CJ. Long-term propofol infusion and cardiac failure in adult head injured patients. *Lancet.* 2001;357:117-118.

41. Kamibayashi T, Maze M. Clinical uses of alpha2-adrenergic agonists. *Anesthesiology.* 2000;93:1345-1349.

42. Coursin DB, Coursin DB, Maccioli GA. Dexmedetomidine. *Curr Opin Crit Care.* 2001;7:221-226.

43. Tan JA, Ho KM. Use of dexmedetomidine as a sedative and analgesic agent in critically ill adult patients: a meta-analysis. *Intensive Care Med.* 2010;36:926-939.

44. Pun BT, Ely EW. The importance of diagnosing and managing ICU delirium. *Chest.* 2007;132:624-636.

45. American Psychiatric Association. *Diagnostic and Statistical Manual of Mental Disorders.* 4th ed, text revision. Washington, DC: American Psychiatric Association; 2000.

46. Meagher DJ, MacLullich AM, Laurila JV. Defining delirium for the International Classification of Diseases, 11th Revision. *J Psychosom Res.* 2008;65:207-214.

47. Ely EW, Margolin R, Francis J, et al. Evaluation of delirium in critically ill patients: validation of the Confusion Assessment Method for the Intensive Care Unit (CAM-ICU). *Crit Care Med.* 2001;29:1370-1379.

48. Ely EW, Gautam S, Margolin R, et al. The impact of delirium in the intensive care unit on hospital length of stay. *Intensive Care Med.* 2001;27:1892-1900.

49. Dubois MJ, Bergeron N, Dumont M, Dial S, Skrobik Y. Delirium in an intensive care unit: a study of risk factors. *Intensive Care Med.* 2001;27:1297-1304.

50. Granberg Axèll AI, Malmros CW, Bergbom IL, Lundberg DB. Intensive care unit syndrome/delirium is associated with anemia, drug therapy and duration of ventilation treatment. *Act Anaesth Scand.* 2002;46:726-731.

51. Parndaripande P, Shintani A, Peterson J, et al. Lorazepam is an independent risk factor for transitioning to delirium in intensive care unit patients. *Anesthesiology.* 2006;104:21-26.

52. Riker RR, Shehabi Y, Bolesch PM. Dexmedetomidinevs midazolam for sedation of critically ill patients: a randomized trial. *JAMA.* 2009;301:489-499.

53. Radtke FM, Franck M, Lorenz M, et al. Remifentanil reduces the incidence of post-operative delirium. *J Int Med Res.* 2010;38:1225-1232.

54. van den Boogaard M, Pickkers P, van der Hoeven H, Roodbol G, van Achterberg T, Schoonhoven L. Implementation of a delirium assessment tool in the ICU can influence haloperidol use. *Crit Care.* 2009;13:R131.

55. Lonergan E, Luxenberg J, AreosaSastra A. Benzodiazepines for delirium. *Cochrane Database Syst Rev.* 2009;(4):CD006379.

56. Devlin JW, Roberts RJ, Fong JJ, et al. Efficacy and safety of quetiapine in critically ill patients with delirium: a prospective, multicenter, randomized, double-blind, placebo-controlled pilot study. *Crit Care Med.* 2010;38:419-427.

57. Girard TD, Panharipande PP, Carson SS, et al. Feasibility, efficacy, and safety of antipsychotics for intensive care unit delirium: the MIND randomized, placebo-controlled trial. *Crit Care Med.* 2010;38:428-437.

58. Lundström M, Edlund A, Karlsson S, Brännström B, Bucht G, Gustafson Y. A multifactorial intervention program reduces the duration of delirium, length of hospitalization, and mortality in delirious patients. *J Am Geriatr Soc.* 2005;53:622-628.

59. Dennis BM, Gunter O. Surgical procedures in the intensive care unit: a critical review. *OA Crit Care.* 2013;1(1):6.

60. Hutterman E. Transesoephageal echocardiography in critical care. *Minerva Anes.* 2006;72(11):891-913.

61. Daniel W, Erbel R, Kasper W, et al. Safety of transesoephageal echocardiography. A multicenter survey of 10419 examinations. *Circulation.* 1991;83:817-821.

62. Sutaria N, Northridge D, Denvir M. A survey of sedation and monitoring practices during transesoephageal echocardiography in the UK: are recommended guidelines being followed? *Heart.* 2000;84(suppl II):ii19.

63. Schelling V, Mattle D, Stahli C, et al. Sedation during transesoepahgeal echocardiography. *Cardiovascular Med.* 2015;18(7-8):215-219.

64. Renna M, Chung R, Li W, et al. Remifentanil plus low dose of midazolam for outpatient sedation in transesophageal echocardiography. *Int J Cardiol.* 2009;136:325-329.

65. Toman H, Erkilinic A, Kocak T, et al. Sedation for transesophageal echocardiography: comparison of propofol, midazolam and midazolam-alfentanil combination. *Med Glas (Zenica).* 2016;13(1):18-24.

66. Mathur SK, Singh P. Transesoephageal echocardiography related complications. *Indian J Anes.* 2009;53(5):567-574.

67. Garimella S, Longaker RA, Stoddard MF. Safety of transesophageal echocardiography in patients who are obese. *L Am Soc Echocardiogr.* 2002;15(11):1396-1400.

68. Harrison SJ. Cardioversion and the use of sedation. *Heart.* 2004;90(12):1374-1376.

69. James S, Broome IJ. Anaesthesia for cardioversion. *Anaesthesia.* 2003;58:291-292.

70. Lewis SR, Nicholson A, Reed SS, Kenth JJ, Alderson P, Smith AF. Anaesthetic drugs for cardioversion. *Cochrane Database Syst Rev.* 2015;(3):CD010824.

71. JungHO. Pericardial effusion and pericardiocentesis: role of echocardiography. *Korean Circ J.* 2012;42(11)725-734.

72. Gammage MD. Temporary cardiac pacing. *Heart.* 2000;83(6):715-720.

Patient and Family Information for: SEDATION AND ANALGESIA IN THE CARDIAC CARE UNIT

WHY PATIENTS NEED SLEEP OR PAIN MEDICATIONS IN THE CARDIAC CARE UNIT

Patients who are in a CCU can experience pain, anxiety, stress and, at times, an altered mental status. Quite simply, a CCU is a stressful and uncomfortable place to be in for any length of time. Many patients need some form of medication to help them cope with these conditions. Often, it is the most severely ill patients who require the most sedation.

Patients in a CCU will, at the very least, have attached to them a number of wires connecting them to the monitor, in addition to some sort of IV catheter. Patients who are more seriously and acutely ill may have IV catheters in their neck or chest, or larger tubes in their groin supporting their hearts. The most seriously ill patients will have a tube in their mouth, an endotracheal tube, to connect their lungs to an artificial respirator. Usually, the more support or monitoring an apparatus provides to the patient, the more uncomfortable it tends to be. The endotracheal tube, being hard plastic in contact with the main airway, is quite possibly the most irritating. Although some patients can tolerate an endotracheal tube without sedation, most patients need some sedation to tolerate the tube.

Treatments given to patients also tend to be, at best, uncomfortable, and, at worst, painful. Critically ill patients in a CCU do not tend to cough or breathe deeply enough and need help getting phlegm up from their lungs. Sometimes this is done by clapping on their backs, which can be uncomfortable. Sometimes, however, that maneuver is not enough, and a small tube needs to be placed into the patient's nose or mouth and into their lungs to get the phlegm out before the patient develops pneumonia.

Increasingly, diagnostic and therapeutic procedures are performed in the CCU at the bedside, both because of lack of timely access to the OR and acuity of patients' condition. These procedures are often uncomfortable and sometimes painful, and patients need appropriate means to decrease their pain and suffering while undergoing a procedure.

In addition to being able to tolerate devices in the CCU, there is also the need for patients to get some sleep. It is very, very difficult to sleep in a CCU, because things are happening at all hours of the day and night, and it is difficult to make it dark enough for people to fall asleep. In addition, the monitors make noises, often with each heartbeat, and the attached cables and tubes frequently pull and wake patients up as they turn. The beds in a CCU are optimized for both durability and to keep from damaging the skin, but may not be the most comfortable for sleeping.

For these and other reasons, many times it is necessary to give patients either pain medications or sleep-inducing medications as part of their treatment in a CCU.

GOALS OF SEDATION AND PAIN MANAGEMENT IN THE CARDIAC CARE UNIT

Very often, family members do not have the same goals in mind as their caregivers when it comes to the treatment of pain or of the sedation of a loved one in the CCU. Some families think it is bad for the patient to be sedated, and want them to be more awake and interactive, going so far as to overstimulating the patient during visits. They get the mistaken impression that if the patient is not awake, he/she is in either an unintended or an induced coma which they perceive as a bad thing. They repeatedly ask for the sedation to be turned down. Other families are concerned that the patient is feeling too much discomfort or will remember too much of these traumatic events and want them more deeply sedated.

It is important to realize that sedation of patients in the CCU has become an important area of research and concern over the past 15 years. It was always known that patients needed sedation and pain medication in a CCU for them to not pull out their tubes or hurt themselves. It was also felt that sedating patients fairly heavily was a good thing, to reduce the stress of being in the CCU, and, simply, to just be humane to the patient. Although there were always concerns that too much sedation was a bad thing, it was not until the year 2000 that research was published showing clearly that it was important not to over-sedate patients. That one study, and others following it, showed that waking patients up every day—even for a short period of time—and then reevaluating the need and dose of sedation leads to less time on the respirator, less time in the CCU, and an improved survival rate. But it is not an easy thing to do—there is a risk of patients getting too awake and hurting themselves, and so it must be done in the right patients at the right time and speed. It also has become clear through recent research that the type and amount of sedation can have a strong influence on the patients' mental state, long after they have recovered from their physical ailments and have left the CCU.

Usually, some type of rating scale that makes it very easy to tell if the patient is at the desired level of sedation or not is used. The scales are generally of two types. In the more basic scale, a patient is asked to rate the pain either on a number scale or by pointing at a line or chart, sometimes with happy or sad faces on it, sometimes with just a line or ruler on it. These are used primarily to rate the patient's pain, and will be used before and after every dose of pain medication to try to put a number rating to the pain a patient is feeling. In this way, the doctors caring for the patients can adjust the amount of medication by seeing what dose produces what response.

The other type of scale is one where the nurse evaluates a patient, and many times will do something like talk to a patient or touch a patient, to see the reaction, then gives the patient a number scale rating to determine their level of sedation. The physicians taking care of the patient, or the CCU nurse, will sedate the patient according to those ratings. Many sedation scales have been developed over the years.

It is important to have discussions with the physicians and nurses taking care of a family member about the precise goals of sedation. To be able to fully understand the sedation of a family member, ask to see the sedation scale in use in that particular CCU, discuss the desired level of sedation, and ask whether they perform a daily wake-up test. A family could also offer to help in the daily wake-up test, but that takes a skilled staff of the CCU and a family member who can avoid getting too emotional at the bedside, as the wake up may not be pleasant sometimes to watch. Once a family member understands the goals of sedation, then the member can try to help the staff in the CCU keep the patient at the desired level of sedation.

NONSEDATIVE METHODS OF KEEPING PATIENTS COMFORTABLE

Using medications is not the only method we have to keep patients comfortable in the CCU. There are a number of other methods that are tried and true. The most important among these is to continually reorient the patient to the time, place, and, if necessary, names. The CCU is a very confusing place, and lack of sleep plays havoc with the patient's ability to keep track of time. It is not unusual for patients in a CCU to become confused and not know where they are, or what day it is, or to overestimate the amount of time that has passed since they have seen a family member. This is much more common with older patients, but younger patients can also be affected. Families tend to get very depressed and upset at such actions. Some even can get angry at their family member. It is important to remember that this happens all the time, and is not at all unusual. It also does not signify any permanent damage. This is probably where family members can be the most help to the staff in the CCU and to the patient. It may have to be done more than once on a visit. Another good thing for family members to do is to try to get patients to remember things from outside the CCU—bringing up events, people, foods, clothing, and so on. Bringing pictures to the CCU, especially with the patient in them with other people, is a very good way to aid in this process. Repeatedly reorienting patients, telling them the day, reminding them what day or what hour they last saw one or another family member can help the staff in the CCU use less sedating medications and ultimately help get the patient out of CCU faster and in better mental shape.

SEDATIVE AND PAIN MEDICATIONS IN THE CARDIAC CARE UNIT

It is helpful for the family to understand the different types of medications that are used in the CCU to promote sleep and treat pain. This is because some of them may have different meanings to the lay person, incorrect meanings that may have a negative connotation. For patients in the CCU, most of the time they get either strong pain relievers such as morphine, strong sleep medications such as Ativan (lorazepam), or tranquilizers such as haloperidol. It is important for the family member to understand why each of those is used.

PAIN MEDICATIONS

Patients in the CCU have pain—if they are on the respirator, just the breathing tube alone causes a fair amount of discomfort and pain. Lying in bed for long periods of time is also uncomfortable. They may have surgical incisions, and many of the procedures that are done are painful. To treat those pains, most often patients are given medications such as morphine—others might receive Dilaudid (hydromorphone), fentanyl, or even methadone. This class of drugs is commonly called "opiates" or "narcotics." They are given via the IV line, either continuously all the time or intermittently. They differ primarily in how long they last, and some of the minor side effects. For example, morphine and hydromorphone may have more of a mind-altering quality to their effect than methadone or fentanyl. Fentanyl is the shortest acting, at about 45 minutes to an hour; then morphine which lasts 2 to 3 hours; hydromorphone, which lasts 3 to 4 hours, and, finally, methadone which can last 8 to 12 hours. Patients who are less ill may be able to receive pain medications by mouth—these generally last longer, from 6 to 24 hours each dose.

Pain medications such as these have a number of effects. First, they are used to reduce the amount of pain a patient feels. It is important to realize that these medications do not work like when something is taken for a headache—1 minute, there is pain; soon afterwards, the pain is totally gone. Most often, the patient will still feel the sensation that was painful, but it will not be as intense, they may not care that they feel it, they will be more comfortable; they may even say that the sensation is still there but it does not hurt. Second, these medications will have somewhat of a sleep-inducing effect, but this effect is shorter than the pain-relieving effect and if small enough doses are given may be minimal, if present at all. The most common side effects that are concerning about these medications is that they interfere with the patient's desire to breathe—so, if they go to sleep, they may not breathe, which is why they are monitored after they receive the medications. The other major side effect these medications have is that they can cause nausea and vomiting. So when these medications are given, physicians and nurses have to balance the desirable effects with the undesirable side effects.

When to give these medications is usually decided in a number of ways. If the patient is awake, it might only be given when they ask for them and at no other times. Sometimes, a patient might be connected to a patient-controlled analgesia (PCA) pump where the patient gets small amounts of pain medication through the IV line whenever they push the button. The safety mechanism with both of these is that if the patient is too sleepy to either ask for the medication or push the button—they will not get too much and they will not make themselves too sleepy. This is why a nurse might be heard saying that the patients have to ask for the medication themselves, that they cannot give it just because family members want the patients to get more medication because they are grimacing or making a look on their face that looks like pain—it might be dangerous to give patients the pain medication in that state. For sicker patients, the nurse might be instructed by the physicians to use a pain scale such as described earlier to administer medications. Lastly, patients, especially those on mechanical ventilators, may be on a continuous amount of the medications so that they are getting a small amount every minute to provide constant comfort, and the rate at which they give the pain medication is determined by the scales mentioned earlier.

SEDATIVE (SLEEP) MEDICATIONS

In addition to medications to treat pain, to treat patients' anxiety and help them sleep, patients may also get sedative medications such as midazolam (Versed) or lorazepam (Ativan), which are more modern versions of a similar drug many people know about called diazepam (Valium). These medications have a wide range of effects that depend on dose, ranging from treating anxiety and making a patient feel calm, to inducing a comfortable sleep, to rendering a patient unconscious. Even low doses can cause amnesia, and the patient may not remember things that happen while under the influence of these medications. Although this may many times be a beneficial effect, because the CCU can be a scary place, it also can make it more difficult for the family to reorient the patient the way discussed earlier. Also, elderly patients can sometimes get wild and agitated with these medications and lose control of inhibitions—a side effect called "dis-inhibition." When combined with the pain medications described earlier, they can enhance the pain medications' ability to depress breathing, so they have to be used with caution when used together. Also, the combination of the deep sleep of the sedatives and the nausea and vomiting from the pain medications can be dangerous because patients can then have stomach contents go into the lungs and cause pneumonia. This is not at all to say that they cannot be used together, just that these are concerns that need to be watched for. Both lorazepam and midazolam can be given either intermittently or continuously via the IV line. They differ only in that midazolam, when given once or twice, is very short acting, on the order of 15 to 30 minutes, whereas lorazepam can last for 2 to 4 hours. When given continuously, depending on what dose is required and how long the infusion is running for, can take a few hours to a few days to wear off.

Another medication that can be used continuously, usually in patients on mechanical ventilation, is called propofol. Propofol is easy to remember because it is a milky white liquid, sometimes nicknamed "milk of anesthesia." It is a powerful sleep-inducing agent, and is usually not used to just treat anxiety, but, rather to go further and either makes patients very, very sleepy or even unconscious. Its ability to cause amnesia is not quite as great as for lorazepam or midazolam, so patients need to be more asleep with this medication if the goal is to keep them from remembering things. It is very, very short acting, which is why it usually is used only continuously. Similar to lorazepam or midazolam, it can cause blood pressure to drop; and when given with the narcotic pain relievers, it can cause a patient to stop breathing.

Still a different type of medication used in these settings is a relatively new drug called dexmedetomidine (Precedex). This drug causes a very natural and restful sleep, and does not work like other drugs to depress the patient's drive to breathe. The sleep it causes is totally different from other medications—the patient will appear to be asleep, not responsive to verbal stimulation, yet, with gentle touch, will wake up and be totally coherent and appropriate, only to drift back to sleep when the stimulus is removed. It also has very nice pain-relieving qualities, and treats pain in a manner different from that of narcotics, so the combination of the two is a very effective way to treat pain. It does not have any amnesia effects, so it is not useful to make patients not remember their time in the CCU. It has a ceiling effect, so that it never will produce the deep sleep or near coma condition as midazolam, lorazepam, or propofol will produce, and it cannot be given intermittently, only continuously, and takes a while both to work and stop working, about 20 to 30 minutes on either end. It is most useful in combination with the other medications. Its main advantage is that it recently has been shown to cause less delirium in the CCU, as is discussed here.

DELIRIUM

When a patient is in the CCU and is subject to all the stresses of being there, the constant stimulation, the lights, the noise, the lack of natural sleep, and the administration of the medications, can all sometimes result in the patient developing a state of altered consciousness, called "delirium." Delirium is an acute state of confusion. It is characterized by some combination of drowsiness, disorientation, hallucination, a sudden inability to focus attention, sleeplessness, and severe agitation and irritability. When it develops, it carries with it a longer time in the CCU and the hospital and a higher rate of complications such as infections and death. It is much more common in older patients, and one out of four elderly patients admitted to the hospital will suffer some form of delirium. Preventive measures include the daily wake up and lessening the use of sedatives mentioned, and the reorientation and helping the patient focus also help tremendously. Use of dexmedetomidine for sedation, with its more natural sleep tendencies, has been shown in some studies to decrease the incidence of delirium. Once it starts, it may require the use of tranquilizers that act on the chemicals in the brain that are out of balance and help straighten them out again. A number of tranquilizers can be used. If it is decided that the patient needs to get the medication fast, a medication called haloperidol (Haldol) can be given either via IV or into the muscle. If they are given orally, in addition to haloperidol, another common one is risperidone, and there are others as well. Tranquilizers such as these will cause a dazed and stunned look, and the patient will frequently be awake, answer questions in a rather flat toned voice, show little emotion, and have a very slow reaction to any stimuli. This is just a phase the patient will go through on the way to recovery, but it can last a while, sometimes days or weeks, until the patient is back to the usual state of mind.

ADDICTION

A very common reaction of families to hearing that their relative is getting these medications, some of them whose names they associate with drug abuse, is "Will they become addicted?" Strong pain killers such as morphine cause two types of dependence, commonly termed "addiction." Patients may get chemically or physically dependent, where their bodies cannot tolerate a sudden withdrawal of the drug and it needs to be reduced slowly over time; otherwise the patient can get withdrawal symptoms. This is easily treated with slowly tapering off the medication over time, and the risk for it goes up depending on the dose and the duration of medications the patient received in the CCU, which is another reason to give as little as possible. However, people mistake this for psychological dependency, in which the patient mentally craves for the drug and needs it from a mental standpoint. Only a minute fraction of patients receiving morphine-like drugs in the CCU ever become psychologically dependent on the medications, and the risk is considered small for the benefit most patients get from these important medications. The sedative drugs such as lorazepam are much less likely but still can cause a physical dependence.

ANESTHESIA AND PAIN CONTROL FOR BEDSIDE PROCEDURES IN THE CARDIAC CARE UNIT

Patients in the CCU oftentimes require certain procedures, either for diagnostic purposes or for therapeutic purposes.

Examples of different procedures done in the CCU include the following.

TRANSESOPHAGEAL ECHOCARDIOGRAPHY

TEE is a special form of echocardiogram, performed by esophageal placement of a probe with a transducer at its tip. It is very similar to the probe used by gastroenterologists to perform upper endoscopies. It is performed in patients who either await heart surgery to give the cardiac surgeon and anesthesiologist more information about the heart structures, confirm the success of the surgical repair or if additional repair is needed, or in patients who are treated in the CCU to assess and monitor medical treatment. It gives a very good image of the heart because the esophagus or swallowing tube is very close to the heart. An approximately 6- to 8-hour fasting is required before undergoing the procedure.

For the patient to tolerate this procedure, a combination of local anesthetic to the back of the throat and IV sedation are frequently used.

The local anesthetic is usually lidocaine spray or a solution to be gurgled to numb the oropharynx, and the tolerance of the procedure is enhanced by administering IV sedatives and analgesics. The combination of local anesthetics and IV sedatives and analgesics blocks the stress response, the laryngeal reflex to the TEE probe insertion, and the pain, and is very useful especially for very anxious patients or patients who are unable to cooperate.

The medications used are usually a combination of pain relievers such as morphine and fentanyl, and sleeping medications such as midazolam or lorazepam. On occasion, a stronger sleeping medication might be used, such as propofol. The amount of medications used differs depending on the patient's weight, age, and how strong the heart is. Patients with weaker hearts might require less medication and it might take longer to achieve the desired effect. The same pattern is true for older patients.

Heavier patients might require more medication, although this pattern does not always stay true; however, the patients require more careful monitoring of their breathing, because they are prone to obstruct the air passage secondary to obstruction by the back of the tongue and might require additional maneuvers or equipment (such oral airways to lift the tongue and clear the throat to allow free air movement) to ensure safety.

CARDIOVERSIONS

If the heart has an irregular, abnormal rhythm or is beating too fast, a cardioversion might be necessary. The most commonly treated arrhythmias are atrial fibrillation and flutter.

Cardioversion is a procedure that includes applying an external electrical shock to the chest wall to restore the normal heart rhythm. The procedure involves placement of patches on the chest and back, in addition to the existing monitors already in place. Because the procedure can be painful, it requires deep sedation or general anesthesia. The shock lasts only a fraction of a second and it might need to be repeated. The whole procedure might last 20 to 30 minutes.

The sedatives will be administered via the IV catheter already in place, and the shock will be delivered through the patches on the patient's chest, once the patient is rendered unconscious. Sometimes more than one shock needs to be delivered to convert to the normal rhythm. Once the procedure is completed, the medication is stopped and the patient will wake up shortly. There are few potential complications that can occur with the cardioversion and they are related to the sedation used for the patient to tolerate the procedure, new arrhythmias, stroke, lip or tongue lacerations, or skin burns.

The deep sedation used to allow the delivery of the shock can result in aspiration of the stomach content into the lungs, which could lead to pneumonia. Also, the sedation can cause obstruction of breathing, especially in heavier patients or in those who have sleep apnea, so careful, divided administration of medication for sedation and careful monitoring of breathing has to take place.

The shock is timed with the heart beat so it does not produce dangerous rhythms after cardioversion, but sometimes the heart is slow to go into the normal rhythm and a temporary pacemaker might be necessary to bridge this period.

Stroke can happen as a result of a preexisting, or a newly formed clot which can travel to the brain. The use of blood thinners before the cardioversion greatly reduces the risk of stroke.

An oxygen mask will be placed on the patient's face and a soft block will be placed between the teeth to avoid lip or tongue injury.

INSERTION OF CATHETERS AND DEVICES

Oftentimes the patients in the CCU require insertion of catheters for continuous monitoring of the blood pressure and access to frequent blood draws, such as arterial lines, which consists of placement of a small catheter into an artery, either at the wrist (most commonly), groin or foot (rarely).

Central venous catheters are inserted for both monitoring of pressures inside the heart and as the means of administering potent medications or blood if needed. They are typically placed in the veins in the neck (most frequently) or groin (rarely).

On occasion, a critically ill patient might require placement of a device called IABP to help with heart function and oxygen delivery to the heart. It is placed via one of the arteries in the groin and advanced all the way in the chest to the aorta, which is the main artery carrying blood out of the heart. It requires the patient to keep the leg straight afterwards, often being accomplished by placing a brace on the leg.

When patients have rhythm problems, the placement of a temporary transvenous pacemaker is required. It involves the placement of a catheter into one of the veins in the neck or in the groin and then advancing a wire into the heart.

The insertion of the central venous catheters or the IABP necessitates the patient to be still, on his/her back, in a "head down "position, sterile preparation of skin, and placement of sterile drapes which sometimes cover the patient's face, and can lead to significant anxiety.

The insertion of these catheters is facilitated by injecting the skin with local anesthetic, such as lidocaine, and most of the times is sufficient to assure the patient's comfort, especially for the small catheters (arterial lines, central venous catheters), but the larger catheters, such as IABP or temporary transvenous pacemakers, require the administration of sedatives, such as midazolam, and analgesics, such as fentanyl.

PLACEMENT OF A BREATHING TUBE

Critically ill patients might need to be intubated, which involves deep sedation with drugs such as propofol or etomidate and placement of a breathing tube in the wind pipe, to adequately oxygenate them. After the intubation, to tolerate the breathing tube and the mechanical ventilation they will need continuous sedation with drugs such as midazolam, lorazepam, propofol, or etomidate. Sometimes pain medication such as opiates can also be added.

A careful balance has to be achieved by the CCU team between administering drugs for sedation and pain and maintaining stable blood pressure and breathing, and hence the need for multiple monitors.

CONCLUSION

It is important to understand the choice of medications and why each is used. The doctors and nurses must balance the need to treat pain and the need to reduce stress and anxiety with the very real side effects all of these medications can cause. By discussing with the doctors and nurses exactly what medications the patient is receiving, and what the goals of therapy are, helps understand better the treatment plan and also be more helpful to both the staff and to the patient, because the best calming effect usually is a calm family member being at the bedside working with the CCU staff to keep a patient oriented, calm, and tranquil. It will also allow the family member to endure the stay of the relative in the CCU with less stress to the member as well.

Karim El Hachem
James Jones
Ira Meisels

Renal Failure in the Cardiac Care Unit

INTRODUCTION

Acute kidney injury (AKI), previously called acute renal failure, is a common problem in the cardiac care unit (CCU) and is characterized by an abrupt decline (over hours to weeks) in the glomerular filtration rate (GFR), leading to accumulation of nitrogenous waste products. AKI can result in uremia, oliguria, or anuria, and volume imbalance as well as electrolyte and acid base abnormalities. AKI is independently associated with an increased length of stay, increased morbidity, and short- and long-term mortality and imposes a heavy economic burden on the health care system.

There is substantial interaction between the heart and the kidneys that is now referred to as cardiorenal syndrome (CRS). In patients admitted to the CCU, AKI frequently complicates acute coronary syndromes, revascularization procedures, coronary artery bypass graft (CABG) surgery, decompensated heart failure, cardiogenic shock, and cardiac arrest. In critically ill patients, more often than not, AKI is multifactorial resulting from several insults occurring at once.

Early recognition, adequate hemodynamic support, and withdrawal of nephrotoxic agents are of paramount importance to help reduce the risks and the costs associated with AKI. AKI is associated with worsening outcomes, particularly if occurring in critical illness and if severe enough to require renal replacement therapy (RRT). Hence, preventive measures should be part of appropriate management.

DEFINITIONS

AKI is diagnosed by an increase in serum creatinine (SCr) and blood urea nitrogen (BUN) on routine laboratory examination and/or by a decrease in urinary volume over a certain period of time. With the development of the RIFLE[1] classification and subsequently the acute kidney injury network (AKIN) criteria[2] (**Table 45.1**), the definition of AKI became more objective. Both criteria were very useful for quantitating renal function and for research purposes but less so for clinical practice.

More recently, building off the previous criteria, the Kidney Disease: Improving Global Outcomes (KDIGO) clinical practice guidelines[3] simplified the definition of AKI (**Table 45.1**); KDIGO defines AKI as any of the following:

1. An increase in SCr by at least 0.3 mg/dL within 48 hours; or
2. An increase in SCr to ≥1.5 times baseline, which is known or presumed to have occurred within the prior 7 days; or
3. A decline in urine volume to <0.5 mL/kg/h for 6 hours.

A new terminology, CRS[4], has been proposed to define the spectrum of disorders secondary to the hemodynamic interdependence between the heart and the kidneys. It includes those disorders of the heart and kidneys where acute or chronic dysfunction in one organ induces acute or chronic dysfunction of the other. Five subtypes have been defined:

Type 1 acute CRS: Acute worsening of cardiac function leading to renal dysfunction;

Type 2 chronic CRS: Chronic cardiac dysfunction (ie, chronic heart failure) leading to renal dysfunction;

Type 3 acute renocardiac syndrome: Acute worsening of renal function (due, eg, to renal ischemia or glomerulonephritis) causing cardiac dysfunction (eg, heart failure);

Type 4 chronic renocardiac syndrome: Primary chronic abnormalities in renal function leading to cardiac disease (eg, coronary disease, heart failure, or arrhythmia);

Type 5 secondary CRS: Acute or chronic systemic conditions (eg, sepsis or diabetes mellitus) causing simultaneous dysfunction of the heart and kidney.

EPIDEMIOLOGY

Prior to the RIFLE criteria,[1] more than 30 different definitions of AKI were reported in the literature. Consequently, epidemiologic studies used various clinical and physiologic endpoints, yielding a discrepant incidence of AKI in different clinical settings ranging from 1% to 31% in hospitalized patients (with an average incidence of 5% to 7%)[5] and 35% to 40% in the critically ill.[6] The diagnosis of AKI independently increases the risk of mortality by 5.5- to 6.5-fold as compared to a similarly ill patient without AKI. The incidence of AKI requiring RRT was 5% in a large, multicenter study[7] with a 90-day mortality in the range of 50% to 60%.

TABLE 45.1		Summary of the RIFLE Classification, the AKIN Criteria, and the KDIGO Classification and Staging for AKI							
RIFLE[1]				AKIN[2]			KDIGO[3]		
RIFLE Criteria	SCr Increase	GFR Decrease	Urine Output	AKI Stage	SCr Increase	Urine Output	AKI Stage	Serum Creatinine	Urine Output
Risk	1.5 × ULN	>25% decrease	<0.5 mL/kg/h for 6 h	Stage 1	1.5–2 × baseline	<0.5 mL/kg/h for 6 h	Stage1	SCr 1.5–1.9 times baseline OR > 0.3 mg/dL	<0.5 mL/kg/h for 6–12 h
Injury	2 × ULN	>50% decrease	<0.5 mL/kg/h for 12 h	Stage 2	2–3 × baseline	<0.5 mL/kg/h for 12 h	Stage 2	2.0–2.9 baseline	<0.5 mL/kg/h for >12 h
Failure	3 × ULN (or rise by 0.5 mg/dL if baseline SCr > 4 mg/dL)	>75% decrease	<0.3 mL/kg/h for 24 h OR anuria for 12 h	Stage 3	>3 × baseline (also if on RRT)	<0.3 mL/kg/h for 24 h OR anuria for 12 h	Stage 3	3.0 × baseline OR increase in SCr to >4 mg/dL OR initiation of renal replacement therapy	<0.3 mL/kg/h for >24 h OR Anuria for >12 h
Loss	Persistent acute kidney disease > 4 wk								
ESRD	End-stage renal disease (requiring dialysis > 3 mo)								

ESRD, end-stage renal disease; RRT, renal replacement therapy; SCr, serum creatinine; ULN, upper limit of normal.

RISK FACTORS

In a large tertiary center CCU, characteristics such as older age, African-American race, diabetes, hypertension, previous coronary disease, and heart failure were incrementally more common across increasing renal dysfunction patient strata.[7] Decompensated heart failure, cardiogenic shock, use of iodinated contrast media, aggressive diuresis, and use of nephrotoxic medications are common precipitants of AKI. Patients with underlying chronic kidney disease are also at higher risk of developing AKI, referred to as acute on chronic kidney injury.

RENAL NEUROHORMONAL REGULATION AND RESPONSE TO RENAL HYPOPERFUSION

The kidney plays a central role in maintenance of fluid balance and excretion of waste products. Renal hypoperfusion is initially compensated for by various systemic mechanisms in an attempt to restore tissue perfusion. Hypovolemia, of any cause, reduces release of atrial natriuretic peptide, increases production of antidiuretic hormone, and increases sympathetic (and decreases parasympathetic) activity through the baroreceptor reflex. In the

kidney, the combination of hypotension and sympathetic activation leads to reduced perfusion pressure in the afferent arteriole and a decrease in the GFR. A decrease in tubular sodium chloride (due to slower transit and increased proximal reabsorption) is sensed by the macula densa in the distal convoluted tubule, and this causes the juxtaglomerular apparatus to release renin. Renin activates angiotensin, which is converted peripherally to angiotensin II. Apart from being a potent vasoconstrictor, angiotensin II also acts on the adrenal cortex to produce aldosterone, which increases salt and water reabsorption in the kidney. In addition to these mechanisms, the kidney possesses the ability to autoregulate, that is, to maintain its perfusion pressure despite changes in the mean blood pressure over a wide range of 80 to 180 mm Hg. As a consequence of this compensatory mechanism, the renal tubules remain intact despite renal hypoperfusion. When normal renal perfusion is restored, urine flow returns to normal.

A concept important to understanding the pathophysiology of AKI in the CCU is effective circulating volume (ECV). ECV is the arterial blood volume effectively perfusing tissue. ECV is a dynamic quantity and not a measurable distinct compartment, which normally varies directly with extracellular fluid (ECF). The ECV may not vary directly with the ECF volume in certain diseases, such as congestive heart failure (CHF) or hepatic cirrhosis;

therefore, in these clinical settings, renal hypoperfusion may occur despite apparent volume excess.

In contrast to prerenal AKI, if the hypovolemia is severe or sustained, the renal tubules can become necrotic and lose their ability to conserve salt and water. Tubular obstruction by necrotic cells at the pars recta (where the proximal tubule narrows into the descending loop of Henle) leads to a rise in the intraluminal pressure, decreasing the glomerular tubular gradient. This reduction in GFR may persist even after restoration of normal hemodynamics. Furthermore, injury to the tubular basement membrane can result in back leak of tubular fluid into the interstitial tissue. In this situation, urine flow may not be restored despite restoration of normal renal perfusion.

ETIOLOGIES OF ACUTE KIDNEY INJURY

Based on this pathophysiology of renal adaptation to injury, AKI is classically divided into three large pathophysiologic categories of prerenal, renal, and postrenal AKI (**Table 45.2**).

Prerenal azotemia results from ineffective renal perfusion and is the most common cause of AKI in patients presenting to the emergency room. Renal or intrinsic AKI in the CCU most commonly results from ischemic or toxic acute tubular necrosis (ATN). The prerenal and intrinsic renal categories are not mutually exclusive but rather represent a continuum of renal injury where persistence of the ischemic insult may deteriorate into ATN.

TABLE 45.2	**Common Etiologies of AKI**

Prerenal AKI

1. Hypovolemia, eg, renal (overly aggressive diuresis) or extrarenal fluid loss (bleeding, diarrhea, vomiting, sequestration)
2. Decreased renal perfusion: decreased forward flow secondary to low cardiac output, renal vasoconstriction, systemic vasodilatation, hepatorenal syndrome, impairment of renal autoregulation (NSAIDs, ACEIs, ARBs)

Renal AKI

1. Acute tubular necrosis
   a. Ischemic
   b. Toxic, eg, use of radiocontrast media, aminoglycosides, amphotericin B, calcineurin inhibitors, mannitol, hemolysis, rhabdomyolysis
   c. Infection, with or without sepsis
2. Glomerular diseases or vasculitis
   a. Glomerulonephritis, eg, as a complication of bacterial endocarditis, lupus nephritis
   b. Thrombotic microangiopathies, eg, malignant hypertension, scleroderma crisis
3. Interstitial nephritis commonly related to antibiotic use
4. Renovascular obstruction, eg, atheroembolic disease, arterial dissection

Postrenal AKI

Urinary retention owing to use of anticholinergic agents, obstruction, and compression by hematoma or mass

ACEIs, angiotensin converting enzyme inhibitors; AKI, acute kidney injury; ARBs, angiotensin receptor blockers; NSAIDS, nonsteroidal anti-inflammatory drugs.

A prerenal state also sensitizes the kidney to nephrotoxic insults, thus accounting for the increase in the incidence of AKI owing to nephrotoxic agents in hypovolemic states. Postrenal AKI due to obstruction in the urinary collecting system is an uncommon cause of AKI in the CCU but should always be ruled out promptly because of its reversibility. Nephrotoxicity can result from various drugs, such as aminoglycosides, amphotericin, calcineurin inhibitors, foscarnet, ifosfamide, cisplatin, and crystal-forming drugs. Additionally, conditions such as multiple myeloma and rhabdomyolysis can cause nephrotoxicity resulting in AKI. The pathophysiologic mechanism for renal injury differs among the agents and conditions.

CLINICAL EVAULATION

Either a rise in BUN and SCr or a drop in the urine output should alert the clinician to the presence of AKI. One of the earliest signs of AKI may be oliguria that is usually defined as decline in urine output to <0.5 mL/kg/h. However, a patient who is fluid overloaded or with a high catabolic rate may require a urine flow rate considerably higher than this minimum standard. A number of etiologies of AKI present with nonoliguric rises in the BUN and creatinine; therefore, absence of oliguria does not preclude an evaluation of renal injury.

The history should be focused on identification of risk factors of AKI, determination of baseline renal function to ascertain the presence of CKD if possible, careful assessment of symptoms and precipitants of volume depletion (careful review of the intake and output), careful review of vital signs to identify episodes of hypotension, and a thorough review of all home medications as well as all recently administered in-hospital medications to identify potential nephrotoxins. The history is essential in determining the etiology of AKI because it may help the clinician to prevent further exposure to ongoing nephrotoxic insults.

Another important historic feature is the temporal correlation between the possible nephrotoxic insult and the clinical course of AKI. The SCr rises rapidly (within 24 to 48 hours) in patients with AKI following renal ischemia and radiocontrast exposure. Peak SCr concentrations are usually seen after 3 to 5 days with contrast nephropathy and return to baseline after 5 to 7 days. In contrast, SCr concentrations usually peak later (7 to 10 days) in ATN and sometimes even later in atheroembolic disease. The rise in SCr seen with many tubular epithelial cell toxins (eg, aminoglycosides) or in the setting of drug-induced acute interstitial nephritis usually happens 7 to 10 days after onset of therapy, although the latent period may be as short as 1 day after some antibiotics or as long as several months with nonsteroidal antiinflammatory drugs (NSAIDs).

Information from the physical examination is invaluable and must be integrated with the historic and laboratory data. The patient's volume status must be carefully assessed by examination of skin turgor, edema, jugular venous distension, orthostatic hypotension, and pulmonary vascular congestion. In addition, certain findings on physical examination can be diagnostic, for example, the presence of a distended bladder in a patient with urinary retention, a skin rash in suspected drug-induced interstitial nephritis, papilledema in malignant hypertension, or retinal cholesterol plaques in a patient with atheroembolic disease.

DIAGNOSTIC EVALUATION

Even with a careful history and examination, the determination of the etiology of AKI may be challenging. **Figure 45.1** is a clinical pathway that simplifies the diagnostic approach to AKI.

Microscopic examination of the urine and urinary indices can be informative. Certain findings on urinalysis can point toward specific diagnoses as shown in **Table 45.3**. In prerenal or postrenal AKI, the urinalysis should be devoid of cells and protein. The absence of casts is usual in postrenal kidney injury but hyaline casts can be present in the setting of prerenal AKI.

Various urinary indices are commonly used to differentiate prerenal AKI from renal AKI. Urinary sodium concentration varies with the rate of water reabsorption. A patient who is in a prerenal state (both sodium and water avid) could have a decreased amount of sodium content in the urine but at a relatively high urine concentration (more than 20 to 40 mEq/L) due to a low urine volume in the setting of concurrent water avidity. Fractional excretion of sodium (FeNa) is a more reliable index since it does not vary with urine volume. FeNa measures the

percentage of filtered sodium that is excreted in the urine. FeNa is calculated as follows:

$$FeNa = [(\text{urine sodium}/\text{plasma sodium})/(\text{urine creatinine}/ \\ \text{plasma creatinine})] \times 100.$$

A FeNa < 1% is indicative of a prerenal etiology. It is important to recognize that the FeNa value of 1% that distinguishes prerenal disease from acute tubular necrosis applies only in patients with a markedly reduced GFR. It is also important to remember that diuretics inhibit tubular sodium reabsorption so that in the CCU, patients receiving diuretics can have a FeNa > 1% despite intravascular volume depletion. A fractional excretion of urea nitrogen (FeUrea) and fractional excretion of uric acid (FeUric acid) may be more helpful in this setting. Similarly, the FeNa can be >1% despite volume depletion in patients with underlying CKD secondary to impaired tubular function at baseline. Also, prerenal states are not the only causes of low FeNa; it can also be low in acute glomerulonephritis, early obstructive nephropathy, liver failure, contrast nephropathy, pigment-induced nephropathy, and normal renal function.

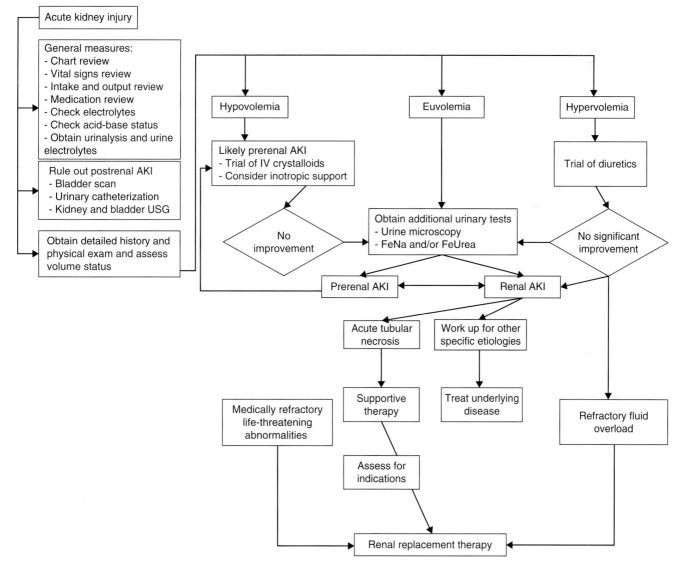

FIGURE 45.1 AKI pathway. AKI, acute kidney injury; FeNa, fractional excretion of sodium; FeUrea, fractional excretion of urea USG: Ultrasonogram.

TABLE 45.3	Urinalysis in Acute Kidney Injury
FINDING	**SUGGESTED DIAGNOSIS**
Muddy brown granular casts or epithelial cell casts	Acute tubular necrosis
RBC casts, dysmorphic RBCs	Acute glomerulonephritis
WBC casts, eosinophils	Acute interstitial nephritis
Large blood on dipstick with no RBCs	Hemoglobinuria or myoglobinuria
Specific crystals	Crystalline nephropathies, eg, Indinavir, Trimethoprim-sulfamethoxazole, or acyclovir associated, urate nephropathy

RBC, red blood cell; WBC, white blood cell.

TABLE 45.4	Diagnostic Indices to Differentiate Prerenal and Renal Acute Kidney Injury	
DIAGNOSTIC INDEX	**PRERENAL AKI**	**RENAL AKI**
Serum BUN to creatinine ratio	>20	<10–15
Urine Na (mEq/L)	<10	>20
Urine/serum creatinine ratio	>50	<20
Urine osmolality	>500	Variable
Urine specific gravity	>1.020	~1.010
FeNa (%)	<1	>1
FeUrea (%)	<35	>50
FeUric acid (%)	<12	>20

AKI, acute kidney injury; BUN, blood urea nitrogen; FeNa, fractional excretion of sodium; FeUrea, fractional excretion of urea; FeUric acid, fractional excretion of uric acid; Na, sodium.

Some of the other diagnostic indices in this regard are listed in **Table 45.4**.

Because the most commonly used marker of AKI, that is, SCr only rises 24 to 48 hours after the inciting injury, there is active research toward identifying newer serum and urine biomarkers for the early diagnosis of AKI. Some of the most promising markers are serum and urine neutrophil gelatinase-associated lipocalin (NGAL),[8,9] interleukin 18 (IL-18),[10] kidney injury molecule-1 (KIM-1),[11] and cystatin C.[12] Further research is needed before these markers replace SCr as a marker of AKI in the clinical setting.[13]

Although glomerular diseases are an uncommon cause of AKI in the CCU, the finding of red blood cell casts or dysmorphic casts should prompt further evaluation. Estimation of urinary protein excretion is an important adjunct to further classify these patients. The use of random, spot urine protein/urine creatinine ratio as an estimate of 24-hour protein excretion has simplified this task by eliminating the need for cumbersome and often inaccurate 24-hour urine collections. A random urine protein/creatinine ratio >1 g protein/g of creatinine is usually seen in the presence of glomerular diseases. This ratio should be used only when kidney function is in steady state because the result may not be accurate

in the setting of AKI. A number of serologic tests for secondary etiologies could help narrow the differential diagnosis; however, a definite diagnosis would require a kidney biopsy.

All patients with AKI should have periodic monitoring of serum electrolytes (sodium, potassium, magnesium, calcium, and phosphorus) and acid-base status because these are frequently abnormal and can become life threatening, for example, severe hyperkalemia or severe metabolic acidosis.

Even though postrenal AKI is relatively uncommon in the CCU, a renal ultrasound should be obtained in all cases of unexplained AKI. A false negative study may be due to concomitant volume depletion or extrinsic compression, for example, secondary to a retroperitoneal hematoma. In the latter scenario, a noncontrast CT scan of the abdomen may be diagnostic.

DRUG DOSING

AKI affects renal drug elimination and other pharmacokinetic processes involved in drug disposition (eg, absorption, drug distribution, and metabolism). Drug dosing errors are common in patients with renal impairment and can cause adverse effects and poor outcomes. Dosages of drugs cleared renally should be adjusted according to estimated creatinine clearance. The most commonly used formulas are listed in **Table 45.5**. We recommend using the Cockcroft–Gault formula where creatinine clearance is estimated as a function of age, sex, and body weight. However, all those formulas were studied in patients with CKD with stable creatinine clearances and not in patients with AKI who have a day-to-day variation in the GFR. The actual GFR is much lower than the estimated GFR (often <10 mL/min in oliguric patients) for patients who are developing AKI and higher than the estimated GFR in patients who are in the recovery phase of AKI.

Loading doses of medications should not be decreased in patients with AKI or CKD. Recommended methods for maintenance of dosing adjustments are dose reductions, lengthening the dosing interval, or both. Physicians should be familiar with commonly used medications that require dose adjustments;

TABLE 45.5	Common Formulas Used to Estimate Glomerular Filtration Rate or Creatinine Clearance
NAME	**FORMULA**
MDRD formula, estimates GFR	$\text{eGFR (mL/min/1.73 m}^2) = 175 \times [\text{serum creatinine (µmol/L)} \times 0.0113]^{-1.154} \times \text{age (years)}^{-0.203}]$ ($\times$ 0.742 if female)
Cockcroft–Gault, estimates creatinine clearance (C_{Cr})	$C_{Cr} = [(140 - \text{age}) \times \text{weight (kg)} / (72 \times \text{Cr})] (\times 0.85 \text{ if female})$
CKD-EPI, estimates GFR	$\text{eGFR} = 141 \times \min (\text{SCr}/\kappa, 1)^{\alpha} \times \max(\text{SCr}/\kappa, 1)^{-1.209} \times 0.993^{\text{age}} \times 1.018 \text{ [if female]} \times 1.159 \text{ [if black]}$

κ is 0.7 for females and 0.9 for males, α is –0.329 for females and –0.411 for males, min indicates the minimum of SCr/κ or 1, and max indicates the maximum of SCr/κ or 1.

CKD-EPI, chronic kidney disease epidemiology collaboration; eGFR, estimated glomerular filtration rate; MDRD, modification of diet in renal disease; SCr, serum creatinine.

however, it is impossible to be aware of all the subtle adjustments that are often needed. Before prescribing any new medication, dosing in AKI/CKD should be verified using any reliable print or electronic resource. Careful monitoring of drug levels, when available, can ensure therapeutic efficacy while minimizing toxicity.

In patients who are on RRT especially those on intermittent hemodialysis (IHD), the drug dosing for those drugs that are significantly dialyzed should be scheduled to be given post dialysis. Some of the common drugs used in the CCU that are likely to be significantly dialyzed include aspirin, dabigatran, atenolol, lisinopril, and antimicrobials like cefepime.

PREVENTION OF ACUTE KIDNEY INJURY

Because very few specific treatments are available for renal AKI, the key is prevention. This is especially true for patients who are at higher risk for developing AKI, for example, patients with advanced age, preexisting renal impairment, diabetes, hypertension, CHF, sepsis, or hypovolemia.

In addition to patients with prerenal azotemia, specific groups of patients may benefit from fluid administration to prevent AKI (ie, patients with early sepsis, rhabdomyolysis, and those receiving drugs such as amphotericin B and contrast media, or drugs associated with crystal deposition such as acyclovir and sulfonamides). Overaggressive fluid resuscitation should be avoided to prevent complications of fluid overload.

Maintenance of a mean arterial blood pressure > 65 mm Hg with optimization of volume status and use of vasoactive agents is critical to maintain optimal renal perfusion. In the setting of decompensated heart failure, the judicious use of inotropes can be necessary to prevent and treat AKI. Low-dose dopamine does increase renal plasma flow; however, clinical studies do not support the use of "renal dose" dopamine to prevent AKI or reduce the requirement of RRT.[14,15] The use of dopamine (or of fenoldopam,[16] a short-acting dopamine receptor-1 agonist) for this purpose is not recommended at present.

When using potentially nephrotoxic antimicrobials, attention to drug levels, adjusted dosing, and dose interval may minimize the risk of drug-induced nephrotoxicity. Furthermore, daily assessment of continued need for broad-spectrum antibiotics based on culture results is essential. Early identification of drug-induced AKI and discontinuation of the offending agent can prevent further renal injury.

ACUTE KIDNEY INJURY—SPECIAL SITUATIONS

CONTRAST-INDUCED NEPHROPATHY

Contrast-induced nephropathy (CIN) or contrast-induced acute kidney injury is generally defined as an increase in serum creatinine concentration of >0.5 mg/dL or 25% above baseline within 48 hours after contrast administration. Risk factors for CIN include advanced age, preexisting CKD, dehydration, hypotension, intra-aortic balloon pump, concomitant administration of nephrotoxic drugs, sepsis, diabetes mellitus, and CHF requiring active diuretic use. Various scoring systems are available to quantify this risk.[17] In patients with established AKI, avoiding the use of contrast media if possible until AKI has resolved should be considered.

Certain measures such as the following may be useful in minimizing the risk of CIN:

1. The use of low osmolar or isoosmolar contrast media and use of lowest possible volume (eg, avoiding left ventriculogram in patients at risk);
2. Optimization of volume status: Discontinuation of diuretics and use of isotonic saline starting 6 to 8 hours before contrast administration to ensure adequate hydration is a commonly used strategy.
3. Discontinuation of angiotensin converting enzyme inhibitors (ACEI)/angiotensin receptor blockers (ARBs) prior to contrast administration can sometimes be done but this strategy is not routinely recommended because data have shown conflicting results.
4. Isotonic sodium bicarbonate has been shown to be superior to isotonic saline in some studies but the evidence is equivocal.[18]
5. Another agent sometimes used is oral *N*-acetylcysteine (NAC). Evidence for the preventive efficacy of NAC is equivocal and cannot be routinely recommended at this time.[19]
6. Recent data suggest a beneficial effect of statin administration although the quality of this data is weak.
7. All other potential nephrotoxins should be discontinued when possible.
8. Periprocedural hemodialysis has no role in the prevention of CIN.[20]

ACUTE KIDNEY INJURY POST CARDIAC SURGERY

AKI complicates up to 30% of cardiac surgery. The risk factors most commonly associated with AKI in this setting include female sex, left ventricular dysfunction, diabetes, peripheral vascular disease, chronic obstructive pulmonary disease, emergent surgery, use of intra-aortic balloon pump, prolonged cardiopulmonary bypass time, and, most importantly, preoperative elevations in SCr.[21] The avoidance of cardiopulmonary bypass has been shown to be associated with lower incidence of postoperative AKI[22] and should be considered whenever possible. Recently, nesiritide,[23] a recombinant human BNP and fenoldopam, a renal vasculature dilator, have shown mixed results in preventing postcardiac surgery AKI.

TREATMENT OF ACUTE KIDNEY INJURY

The treatment of AKI depends on its etiology. In postrenal AKI, rapid relief of obstruction will reverse the AKI. Prerenal AKI owing to hypovolemia should be managed with prompt restoration of the effective circulatory volume, usually by administration of crystalloid solutions. Hypovolemia can be caused by renal or extrarenal causes, and careful history and examination as outlined earlier is essential to determine absolute or effective hypovolemia. The adequacy of restoration of intravascular volume can be guided by periodic assessment of the central venous pressure (CVP). However, the possibility of right-sided heart failure, pulmonary arterial hypertension, or positive pressure ventilation can elevate CVP; this needs to be kept in mind while interpreting the results. The use of Swan-Ganz catheter guided therapy has fallen out of favor after the results of trials showed that use of these catheters increased anticipated adverse events and did not have any effect on overall mortality and hospitalization length.

In acute decompensated CHF, preload and afterload reduction with diuretics and vasodilators are the cornerstones of therapy. The judicious use of diuretics with close monitoring of hemodynamics and renal parameters can increase cardiac output and lower renal venous hypertension, thereby improving renal perfusion. Appropriate use of inotropes may restore normal renal perfusion especially in patients with acute systolic heart failure or advanced left ventricular systolic dysfunction. The temporary discontinuation of ACEIs or ARBs and avoidance of NSAIDs may also help increase renal perfusion.

The management of intrinsic AKI depends on the underlying etiology. The management of individual diseases, especially that of glomerular diseases, is beyond the scope of this chapter.

We focus on the special considerations in patients with ATN, which is a common cause of renal AKI in the CCU. In case of any doubt regarding whether the patient has prerenal AKI or established ATN secondary to sustained renal hypoperfusion, an adequate trial of crystalloids and/or the use of vasoactive agents may be the only differentiating feature; rapid reversibility indicates a prerenal mechanism. While fluid resuscitation is ongoing, frequent monitoring of respiratory status in patients with heart failure is essential to avoid pulmonary edema. Withdrawal of all possible nephrotoxic agents to avoid further injury to the kidney should be done concurrently. Once ischemic or nephrotoxic ATN is established, there is no specific therapy. The main goal of treatment is to treat the complications of AKI and prevent further injury.

A number of drugs have been tried to reduce the requirement for RRT and to accelerate renal recovery in ATN but none has shown a conclusive benefit. Diuretics are commonly used in oliguric AKI; however, randomized controlled trials have failed to show a reduction in the need for RRT. Hence the role of diuretics in AKI is limited to management of volume overload and/or hyperkalemia in the setting of AKI. Similarly, the use of selective renal vasodilators such as dopamine or fenoldopam is not supported by current clinical evidence and thus is not recommended.[13]

RENAL REPLACEMENT THERAPY

Conventional indications for initiation of RRT include refractory fluid overload, intractable hyperkalemia and metabolic acidosis, and uremic syndrome. Other indications include uremic pericarditis, uremic encephalopathy, uremic neuropathy, and suspected drug/toxin overdose with a dialyzable substance. Traditional triggers for treatment were based on studies in CKD patients, whereas patients with AKI who are critically ill may have a reduced tolerance of metabolic derangements.

Furthermore, the identification that iatrogenic fluid overload may play a role in perpetuating multiorgan dysfunction in critically ill patients has led to the belief that early initiation of RRT in this population may have beneficial effects on overall morbidity and mortality. However, timing of RRT initiation in critically ill patients remains unclear. Recently, a French multicenter trial showed no benefit of early versus late RRT initiation,[24] in discordance with another recent German single center trial that suggested that early initiation reduced mortality at 90 days as compared to late initiation.[25]

The available modalities for RRT include IHD, continuous renal replacement therapy (CRRT), hybrid therapies such as sustained low-efficiency dialysis and peritoneal dialysis. The choice of modality depends on institutional availability, physician preference, patient hemodynamic status, and the presence of other comorbidities. CRRT has been postulated to be more physiologic owing to its continuous nature. It is especially useful in the hemodynamically unstable patients with AKI where use of IHD could lead to further ischemic insult and delay in renal recovery. However, no randomized study has proven this theoretical benefit over conventional, intermittent dialysis.

One modality of CRRT, especially useful in the CCU, is slow continuous venovenous ultrafiltration that can allow removal of large amounts of fluid from the patient while minimizing the risk of hemodynamic instability. It can be considered as a therapeutic option in the management of a fluid overloaded patient with diuretic resistance even in the absence of AKI.

RECOVERY FROM ACUTE TUBULAR NECROSIS

Recovery from ATN is the rule rather than the exception. More than 90% of patients with ATN recover renal function sufficient to discontinue dialysis. The timing of this recovery varies among individual patients and can happen even after weeks of AKI. A post-ATN diuresis can commonly be seen in the recovery phase owing to osmotic diuresis. It is important to monitor these patients closely as they are often at the risk of developing new prerenal azotemia and electrolyte derangements if volume intake does not match urinary loss.

DEDICATION

This chapter is dedicated to the memory of Dr. James Jones who was a cherished colleague in the Division of Nephrology at Mount Sinai, St. Luke's and West. His untimely passing at the end of 2016 has left a void in our hearts and minds.

REFERENCES

1. Bellomo R, Ronco C, Kellum JA, et al. Acute renal failure—definition, outcome measures, animal models, fluid therapy and information technology needs: the Second International Consensus Conference of the Acute Dialysis Quality Initiative (ADQI) Group. *Crit Care.* 2004;8:R204-R212.

2. Mehta RL, Kellum JA, Shah SC, et al. Acute Kidney Injury Network: report of an initiative to improve outcomes in acute kidney injury. *Crit Care.* 2007;11:R31.

3. Kellum JA, Lamiere N, Aspelin P, et al. "Work group membership." KDIGO clinical practice guideline for acute kidney injury. *Kidney Int Suppl.* 2012;2:8.

4. Ronco C, Haapio M, House AA, et al. Cardiorenal syndrome. *J Am Coll Cardiol.* 2008;52(19):1527-1539.

5. Uchino S, Bellomo R, Ronco C, et al. An assessment of the RIFLE criteria for acute renal failure in hospitalized patients. *Crit Care Med.* 2006;34(7):1913-1917.

6. Bagshaw SM, George C, Bellomo R, et al. A multi-center evaluation of the RIFLE criteria for early acute kidney injury in critically ill patients. *Nephrol Dial Transplant.* 2008;23(4):1203-1210.

7. Uchino S, Kellum JA, Bellomo R, et al. Acute renal failure in critically ill patients: a multinational, multicenter study. *JAMA.* 2005;294(7):813-818.

8. Mishra J, Dent C, Tarabishi R, et al. Neutrophil gelatinase-associated lipocalin (NGAL) as a biomarker for acute renal injury after cardiac surgery. *Lancet.* 2005;365:1231-1238.

9. Haase M, Bellomo R, Devarajan P, et al. Accuracy of neutrophil gelatinase-associated lipocalin (NGAL) in diagnosis and prognosis in acute kidney injury: a systematic review and meta-analysis. *Am J Kidney Dis.* 2009;54(6):1012-1024.

10. Parikh CR, Abraham E, Ancukiewicz M, et al. Urine IL-18 is an early diagnostic marker for acute kidney injury and predicts mortality in the intensive care unit. *J Am Soc Nephrol.* 2005;16(10):3046-3052.

11. Han WK, Bailly V, Abichandani R, et al. Kidney Injury Molecule-1 (KIM-1): a novel biomarker for human renal proximal tubule injury. *Kidney Int.* 2002;62(1):237-244.

12. Bongiovanni C, Magrini L, Salerno G, et al. Serum cystatin C for the diagnosis of acute kidney injury in patients admitted in the emergency department. *Dis Markers.* 2015:416059.

13. Brochard L, Abourg F, Brenner M, et al. Prevention and management of acute renal failure in the ICU patient: an International Consensus Conference in Intensive Care Medicine. *Am J Respir Crit Care Med.* 2010;181(10):1128-1155.

14. Lauschke A, Teichgräber UK, Frei U, et al. "Low-dose" dopamine worsens renal perfusion in patients with acute renal failure. *Kidney Int.* 2006;69(9):1669-1674.

15. Friedrich JO, Adhikari N, Herridge MS, et al. Meta-analysis: low-dose dopamine increases urine output but does not prevent renal dysfunction or death. *Ann Intern Med.* 2005;142(7):510-524.

16. Landoni G, Biondi-Zoccai GG, Tumulin JA, et al. Beneficial impact of fenoldopam in critically ill patients with or at risk for acute renal failure: a meta-analysis of randomized clinical trials. *Am J Kidney Dis.* 2007;49(1):56-68.

17. McCullough PA, Adam A, Becker CR, et al. Risk prediction of contrast-induced nephropathy. *Am J Cardiol.* 2006;98(6A):27K-36K.

18. Hoste EA, De Waele JJ, Gevaert SA, et al. Sodium bicarbonate for prevention of contrast-induced acute kidney injury: a systematic review and meta-analysis. *Nephrol Dial Transplant.* 2010;25(3):747-758.

19. Subramaniam RM, Suarez-Cuervo C, Wilson RF, et al. Effectiveness of prevention strategies for contrast-induced nephropathy: a systematic review and meta-analysis. *Ann Intern Med.* 2016;164(6):406-416.

20. Cruz DN, Perazella MA, Bellomo R, et al. Extracorporeal blood purification therapies for prevention of radiocontrast-induced nephropathy. *Am J Kidney Dis.* 2006;48:361-371.

21. Suen WS, Mok CK, Chiu SW, et al. Risk factors for development of acute renal failure (ARF) requiring dialysis in patients undergoing cardiac surgery. *Angiology.* 1998;49(10):798-800.

22. Massoudy P, Wagner S, Thielmann M, et al. Coronary artery bypass surgery and acute kidney injury—impact of off-pump technique. *Nephrol Dial Transplant.* 2008;23(9):2853-2860.

23. Mentzer RM Jr, Oz MC, Sladen RN, et al; on behalf of the NAPA Investigators. Effects of perioperative nesiritide in patients with left ventricular dysfunction undergoing cardiac surgery: the NAPA trial. *J Am Coll Cardiol.* 2007;49:716-726.

24. Gaudry S, Hajage D, Schortgen F, et al. Initiation strategies for renal-replacement therapy in the intensive care unit. *N Engl J Med.* 2016;375(2):122-133.

25. Zarbock A, Kellum JA, Schmidt C, et al. Effect of early vs delayed initiation of renal replacement therapy on mortality in critically ill patients with acute kidney injury. The ELAIN Randomized Clinical Trial. *JAMA.* 2016;315(20):2190-2199.

Patient and Family Information for: RENAL FAILURE IN THE CARDIAC CARE UNIT

WHAT ARE THE KIDNEYS?

The kidneys are two bean-shaped organs located in the middle of the back, one on each side. Each measures about the size of a fist. These are vital organs and each is made up of about 1 million nephrons (filters) and tubules that process approximately 2 L of blood every 5 minutes.

WHAT ARE THE FUNCTIONS OF THE KIDNEY?

The human body consists of 60% to 70% water. This water also contains a variety of dissolved materials such as different salts (sodium chloride, potassium chloride, sodium bicarbonate, etc). All the water in the body is distributed between three spaces: the intracellular compartment (in the cells), interstitial spaces (between the cells), and intravascular (the blood). In an ideal setting, there is a perfect balance of water and salts between all these compartments. If any deregulation occurs, for instance if we get dehydrated (eg, diarrhea) or if we get fluid overloaded (eg, in patients with heart failure leading to lower extremity swelling and/or pulmonary edema), the kidneys jump into action to restore the equilibrium. Therefore, control of fluid and salt balance is an essential function of the kidneys.

Another important function of the kidneys is to excrete toxic wastes (such as urea, acid, etc) produced by the body on a daily basis. The kidney does this by filtering the blood that flows through it. In other words, the urine is actually a filtered form of blood that has all the waste material in it (urea, extra water, acid, salts, etc).

The third function of the kidney is to act as an endocrine organ. The main hormone that the kidneys produce is erythropoietin that is required by the body to produce red blood cells (that carry oxygen in the blood). In addition, the kidneys also activate other inactive products such as vitamin D (helps maintain healthy bones).

WHAT ARE THE TYPES OF KIDNEY DISEASE?

Depending on the duration of onset, kidney disease can be acute, chronic, or acute on chronic.

Acute: Such patients may have normal functioning kidneys at baseline. AKI is a potentially life-threatening condition and may require intensive care treatment. ATN is one of the most common subtypes of AKI in a critically ill patient. In ATN, the kidney tubules get damaged owing to various reasons (infections/pneumonia, low blood pressure resulting from heart failure/heart attack, etc). With time, and if the reason for damage is fixed, the tubules may start functioning again as before.

Chronic (when decrease in function takes place gradually over time): Common causes are hypertension and diabetes. Such patients may have CKD. Those who have had regular follow-up with their primary doctors may be aware of their underlying CKD. However, as kidney disease is usually painless, it is not uncommon for patients not to know of their underlying CKD until the disease is in an advanced stage.

Acute on chronic: Such patients have acute worsening of their CKD owing to critical illness, for example, pneumonia, heart attack, and heart failure.

WHAT ARE THE COMMON CAUSES OF ACUTE KIDNEY INJURY?

An injury to the kidneys is generally because of another disease process. Sometimes there may be more than one cause, and therefore it may be impossible to pinpoint the exact cause of AKI. Death is most common when AKI is caused by surgery, trauma, or severe infection in someone with heart disease, lung disease, or recent stroke. Old age, infection, loss of blood from the intestinal tract, and progression of kidney failure also increase the risk of death.

Some of the common causes of AKI are as follows:

Shock: Shock is a life-threatening condition that may accompany severe injury or illness, whereby the body suffers from insufficient blood flow to its vital organs. This can therefore result in decreased oxygen delivery to the organs (hypoxia) leading to organ failure, for example, kidney failure, heart attack (cardiac arrest), and so on. Shock may be of different type/causes: septic (owing to an infection in the body, pancreatitis, etc), hemorrhagic (owing to acute blood loss—as in a patient with bleeding from a stomach ulcer), cardiogenic (owing to heart failure from a weak heart or acute heart attack), and hypovolemic (eg, excess fluid loss from body after severe diarrhea or excessive use of diuretics).

Damage from medicine/dyes: Unfortunately, many of the medications used to treat patients may themselves cause kidney damage. People who have serious, long-term health problems are more likely than others to have such adverse effects. Some examples of such medications are as follows:

- Antibiotics used to treat life-threatening infections
- Pain medicines such as ibuprofen (and all other NSAIDs)
- Some blood pressure medicines and ACEIs (such as enalapril)
- The contrast/dyes used in imaging (CAT scan as discussed in the ensuing section)
- Some of the HIV medications, for example, tenofovir.

Urinary tract obstruction: This may happen in patients with a known history of kidney stones, benign prostate hypertrophy, or rarely in patients with cancers that invade or press on the urinary tract system.

WHAT ARE THE SIGNS AND SYMPTOMS OF KIDNEY FAILURE?

Kidney failure is almost always painless. In the setting of an intensive care unit, the following signs and symptoms may point toward a failing kidney:

Accumulation of fluid/water: Because the failing kidneys are unable to excrete water, accumulation of water in the body manifests as swelling of the feet, lower legs, face, and/or the hands. Sometimes when the kidneys fail, a lot of protein is lost in the urine, which can also cause worsening edema and labored breathing owing to accumulation of fluids in the lungs. If this is severe, the patient may require intubation (whereby the patient is sedated and a breathing tube is inserted in the windpipe) and breathing support with the help of a machine (ventilator).

Irregular heart rate: Owing to the accumulation of toxins and electrolyte imbalance (hyperkalemia or high potassium), the heart rhythm may become irregular or dangerously slow, leading to cardiac arrest.

Symptoms resulting from accumulation of toxins/waste products such as urea: Loss of appetite, nausea, vomiting, weight loss, fatigue, sleepiness, itching, twitching, and a metallic taste in the mouth. They often indicate that the person is accumulating dangerous amounts of waste products (urea) because the kidneys are not working to excrete them.

Abnormal blood tests suggesting impaired kidney function: Sometimes the patient may be totally asymptomatic but the blood tests may suggest severe kidney failure, for example, hyperkalemia (high potassium), increased blood acidity, high creatinine, and BUN levels.

HOW TO DIAGNOSE KIDNEY FAILURE?

Nephrologists are specialists in kidney diseases. When a patient has evidence of kidney failure, the intensive care team will seek the help of nephrologists to manage it. The following tests will help to determine the severity and cause of kidney failure:

Blood test: In most cases, two parameters in the blood, namely the BUN and creatinine, can give a fair assessment as to the degree of kidney failure. Urea is a byproduct of protein breakdown, and creatinine is a byproduct of normal muscle functioning. In a normal person, the level of creatinine is 0.7 to 1.2 mg/dL and that of BUN is 12 to 24 mg/dL. In addition, blood levels of some important electrolytes such as potassium are also taken into consideration while treating a patient with kidney failure.

Urine tests: Microscopic analysis of patients' urine can give some indication as to the type of kidney failure (eg, AKI owing to ATN). Other urine tests such as urine protein concentration and urine electrolytes (sodium, creatinine) can also prove helpful in making the diagnosis: for example, a high protein and blood concentration in the urine with AKI may be suggestive of lupus nephritis (owing to autoimmune disease called systemic lupus nephritis).

Imaging tests: Noninvasive procedures such as ultrasound and CAT scan help in assessing the condition of the kidneys.

Ultrasound: It is a painless, harmless (uses sound waves that bounce off structures in the body and give images), and quick way to assess the size and texture of the kidneys. Kidneys are usually normal in size in patients with AKI unless the patient also has some underlying CKD. Ultrasound is also the procedure of choice to diagnose any obstruction of the urinary tract and it is important to rule this out as the cause of kidney injury in all patients.

Computed axial tomography scan: A CAT scan uses X rays to produce pictures in crosswise slices. CAT scans can detect kidney stones, blockage, tumors, cysts, and so on. In addition to the kidneys, an abdominal CAT scan can also be used to assess other abdominal organs. Sometimes CAT scans require using contrast dye, which itself carries the risk of causing kidney injury, especially in people who already have reduced kidney function.

Kidney biopsy: Very rarely would a nephrologist decide to do a kidney biopsy in a patient with AKI. He/she may decide on doing this if conventional analysis is unable to provide sufficient clues as to the underlying cause of AKI and/or if the treatment modality would require the exact diagnosis rather than the most probable cause of AKI. In kidney biopsy, a piece of kidney tissue is taken out under guidance of ultrasound or CAT scan. This tissue is then analyzed by experts to provide the exact cause of kidney failure. Kidney biopsy unfortunately carries a high risk of bleeding (10%) and even death in <1% of patients.

HOW TO MANAGE A PATIENT WITH KIDNEY FAILURE (HEMODIALYSIS)?

The most definitive treatment of kidney failure is to fix the underlying cause. For example, if the patient is having severe heart failure, the optimization of the heart failure will most likely help in resolving acute kidney failure. However, treating the underlying disease may take time, thus necessitating the initiation of renal replacement therapy (RRT). The decision to start RRT may be taken if the patient's serum potassium levels are dangerously high and/or if the patient has mental status changes, and/or if the patient has too much fluid, and/or if the patient develops pericarditis (inflammation of the heart covering owing to high urea). RRT basically implies the use of artificial methods (dialysis) to carry out the function of the kidneys. The commonly used technique for acute kidney failure is hemodialysis.

Hemodialysis is the most common intermittent method of artificial RRT, wherein the blood is allowed to flow through a special filter that removes waste and extra fluids. The clean blood is then returned to the body. For hemodialysis, the patient needs to have a large bore catheter in one of the deep veins of the body (such as a nontunneled catheter that has to be typically changed after a few days of placement, and, a tunneled catheter that can be used for a longer period of time). It is therefore placed either in the neck or the groin. Each session of hemodialysis lasts for 3 to 4 hours and is done either daily or three times a week. However, the frequency may be adjusted based on the blood tests, degree of edema, and so on.

HOW LONG WILL THE PATIENT NEED HEMODIALYSIS?

Acute kidney failure is a potentially life-threatening condition and may require intensive care treatment. However, the kidneys usually start working again within several weeks to months after the underlying cause has been treated. Such patients may therefore require hemodialysis temporarily.

The recovery also depends on the baseline function of the kidneys, the underlying cause, and the severity of the AKI. In some cases, chronic kidney failure or end-stage kidney disease may develop, thus requiring hemodialysis lifelong.

Elissa K. Fory
Stephan A. Mayer

46

Acute Neurologic Emergencies in the Cardiac Care Unit

Some of the most feared complications from acute cardiac disease are neurologic in nature. When acute brain injury occurs, significant morbidity and mortality may follow. A team-based approach that incorporates cardiology, neurology, and critical care expertise is desirable to maximize patient outcomes and address each patient's complexities. There are four common neurologic emergencies in the cardiac care unit (CCU): delirium, hypoxic ischemic encephalopathy (HIE), acute ischemic stroke, and intracranial hemorrhage (**Table 46.1**). This chapter is tailored to patients admitted to or being admitted to a CCU, and so a broader differential diagnosis is applicable to patients in other care environments (such as the emergency department or general medical floor).

DELIRIUM

Delirium is acute brain dysfunction characterized by a change in both the level and content of consciousness. The Diagnostic and Statistical Manual of Mental Disorders (DSM-5) defines delirium as a "disturbance in attention (ie reduced ability to direct, focus, sustain, and shift attention) and awareness (reduced orientation to the environment)" that occurs over hours to days, often fluctuates (waxes and wanes), and is different from the patient's normal state of being. There may also be abnormalities of higher cognitive function or even focal neurologic deficits such as language difficulty, visuospatial changes, or changes in perception. In delirium, the symptoms are not due to an underlying or preexisting condition such as dementia. Finally, there needs to be evidence from the history, examination, or supporting data that the cause is due to a medical condition or is multifactorial. Synonyms for delirium include encephalopathy, acute brain failure, intensive care unit (ICU) psychosis, acute confusional state, and altered mental status. A diagnosis of delirium implies that there is no other underlying primary neurologic condition

accounting for the patient's syndrome, such as a stroke causing aphasia or nonconvulsive status epilepticus.

RECOGNITION OF DELIRIUM

As with any medical problem, the diagnosis of delirium starts with a history and physical examination. With delirium, key questions include the following:

- How is the patient confused? Is he or she seeing objects, having difficulty speaking, or is he or she somnolent?
- When did the change start? Has this ever occurred before? Are the patient's symptoms coming and going or are they constant?
- Does the patient have pain?
- What are the vital signs?
  - Fever suggests infection. Tachycardia may be due to fever, dehydration, or atrial fibrillation. Severe hypertension should bring hypertensive encephalopathy into the differential diagnosis.
- What is the blood glucose?
  - Hypoglycemia can cause acute confusion and should be immediately treated with oral or intravenous glucose, as appropriate. Thiamine 100 mg intravenous (IV) should precede any IV dextrose administration whenever possible. Fingerstick glucose can be falsely normal or high from many factors, including sugars on uncleaned skin; a venous glucose or chemistry should be sent to the laboratory. To avoid prolonged profound hypoglycemia that can lead to permanent coma, thiamine and IV dextrose should be given while awaiting the venous glucose result if there is *any* clinical suspicion for hypoglycemia as the cause of acute encephalopathy.
- What is the past medical history?
  - Patients with known dementia are at higher risk for delirium.
  - Patients with acute or chronic kidney or liver dysfunction are at risk for uremic or hepatic encephalopathy, respectively, as well as increased risk for medication toxicities if doses are not adjusted or organ function is changing rapidly over time.
- What is the patient's history regarding tobacco, alcohol, and substance abuse?
  - Delirium tremens should be considered in patients admitted to the hospital in the previous 12 to 72 hours.

TABLE 46.1	Common Acute Neurologic Emergencies in the CCU
Delirium	
Hypoxic ischemic (anoxic) encephalopathy	
Acute ischemic stroke	
Intracranial hemorrhage	

CCU, cardiac care unit.

TABLE 46.2	Common Medications in the CCU That Can Cause Delirium

Antibiotics: cefepime, flouroquinolones
Anticonvulsants: phenytoin, phenobarbital, levetiracetam, valproic acid
Antihistamines: diphenhydramine, dextromethorphan, famotidine
Benzodiazepines, zolpidem
Corticosteroids
Dopaminergic drugs: L-dopa, rotigotine
Digoxin
Lidocaine
Opiates

CCU, cardiac care unit.

- Cocaine and amphetamine withdrawal can result in a somnolent, stuporous state.
- Nicotine withdrawal can be prevented by prescribing a 21 mg nicotine transdermal patch for chronic smokers.
- Did the patient recently receive any medications (**Table 46.2**)?
  - Thoroughly review the patient's home medications, scheduled medications, and the medication administration record for one-time or as-needed doses.
  - If the patient received opiates and has other signs of opiate intoxication such as pinpoint pupils or hypoventilation, consider naloxone 0.4 mg IV.

BEDSIDE EXAMINATION IN DELIRIUM

Make a general assessment of the patient. Does he or she appear disheveled to suggest underlying psychiatric or dementing process? Is there nuchal rigidity? Auscultate heart and lungs to evaluate for tachypnea, rhonchi, or decreased breath sounds, irregular rhythms, or cardiac valvular abnormalities. Make note of Janeway lesions, splinter hemorrhages, hepatomegaly, abnormal bowel sounds, or jaundice.

The neurologic examination starts when you first enter the room, in how the patient is able to (or unable to) give a history. Note the level of alertness. Using terms such as "lethargic" or "stuporous" can be nebulous and easily misinterpreted, making it difficult for another practitioner to later discern if the patient has had a change in his or her examination. Instead, consider describing how long the patient can sustain attention (for a few seconds, or a minute or 2), and what intensity of stimulus was required to awaken them (voice, nonnoxious tactile stimuli, noxious stimulus, or continuous noxious stimulation). For alert patients, the mental status examination starts with orientation questions. Simple tests of attention include counting backward from 20 to 1 and naming the days of the week or months of the year in reverse order. Formal language testing can include the naming of objects, repetition, and the ability to follow verbal commands (either simple such as "show me two fingers" or more complex like "touch your left ear with your right thumb"). Do not simultaneously demonstrate the verbal command, so that the request is testing receptive language and not the patient's ability to mimic. Depending on the patient's attention and ability to participate, further mental status testing might include a formal score such as the Montreal Cognitive Assessment (MoCA, available free at mocatest.org), Confusion Assessment Method for the ICU (CAM-ICU, icudelirium.org), or Intensive Care Delirium Screening Checklist (ICDSC).

The rest of the neurologic examination is focused on finding clues to a metabolic or systemic cause for delirium and identifying focality that would suggest a primary neurologic problem as opposed to delirium. Small pinpoint but reactive pupils suggest opiate effect. Eye motion abnormalities and nystagmus can be seen with Wernicke encephalopathy or with posterior fossa pathology. Facial movements should be assessed for symmetry. The precision of the motor exam will depend on the patient's ability to participate. In a severely encephalopathic patient, strong and symmetrical withdrawal to pain in all extremities is reassuring that intracranial pathology is absent. With more cooperative patients, subtler signs of weakness such as pronator drift may be elicited. Additionally, arms should be held with elbows and wrists extended ("as if you are stopping traffic") to test for asterixis—a sign of hepatic or uremic encephalopathy. Asterixis is also called negative myoclonus and manifests as a "quick release" or fast drop from a sustained posture with a return close to the previous posture. Tremulousness can be seen with alcohol withdrawal. Tone can be tested in all patients. Deep tendon reflexes and Babinski signs should be checked. Sensory examination is almost always unreliable during a delirium evaluation and generally does not help narrow the diagnosis.

INITIAL LABORATORY AND IMAGING WORKUP FOR DELIRIUM

After evaluating the patient clinically and ensuring the fingerstick glucose is normal, the following tests should be considered:

- Chemistry, ammonia, complete blood count, therapeutic drug levels, urine toxicology:
  - Abnormalities of sodium, calcium, and glucose can cause encephalopathy and/or seizures. Profound uremia and hyperammonemia can cause metabolic encephalopathy.
- Urinalysis and urine culture; blood cultures;
- Arterial blood gas:
  - Acute respiratory acidosis or hypoxia can cause stupor. Respiratory alkalosis can suggest hyperventilation and tachypnea from sepsis. Hypoxia can be seen with pneumonia or pulmonary embolus.
- Chest X-ray should be ordered for any patient with fever, tachypnea, or hypoxia.
- Noncontrast head computed tomography (CT) should be considered for all patients and ordered emergently for any patient with a focal neurologic examination. If the patient has a new acute focal neurologic examination or an examination concerning for posterior fossa pathology, a CT angiogram (CTA) of the head and neck should be immediately and simultaneously acquired to rule out large vessel occlusion (LVO) causing stroke, which is treatable and reversible.
- Electroencephalograph (EEG) may give additional information. Triphasic waves suggest toxic or metabolic encephalopathy. Diffuse slowing of the background can be seen in either delirium or dementia. Epileptiform discharges do not diagnose seizures but may change one's post-test probability for seizures as a cause of change in mental status.

TREATMENT OF DELIRIUM

Ultimately, the treatment of delirium requires diagnosis and correction of the underlying cause. If acute pain is the cause, pain medications should be given. If agitation limits the ability to obtain initial studies, or if the patient is a threat to himself/herself or to others, then IV medications should be given with the goal of resolving the agitation (**Table 46.3**). Antipsychotics are first-line treatment for acute agitation.[1] Benzodiazepines are first line in the treatment of alcohol-withdrawal delirium, benzodiazepine-withdrawal associated delirium, or in acute hepatic failure.[2] Additionally, benzodiazepines may be considered as first-line treatment in patients with extreme or life-threatening prolongation of the QT interval. Overall, however, the total dose of benzodiazepines is associated with an increase in delirium, and so they should not be the initial treatment in a generalized patient population. Dexmedetomidine (Precedex) infusion may be used for patients who are intubated or spontaneously breathing. Dexmedetomidine has the advantages of being associated with a decreased prevalence of delirium and a decrease in ventilator days in intubated patients compared with benzodiazepines or morphine.[3] Side effects of dexmedetomidine include hypotension and bradycardia.

Nonpharmacologic treatments for delirium include frequent verbal redirection, ensuring comfort, and isolated hand restraints to prevent pulling of lines while allowing for freedom of movement. Wrist restraints and 4-point restraints may worsen agitated delirium. Treatment and prevention of delirium also include maintaining normal sleep-wake cycles: minimizing sleep interruptions at night, decreasing light stimulus to the eyes at night (including televisions and smartphones or tablets), and increasing stimulation during the day including mobilization and physical therapy. Indwelling urinary catheters, nasogastric tubes, and multiple IV lines not only serve as a source of discomfort and potential infection, but also physically restrain patients; they should be discontinued or minimized as soon as they are no longer medically necessary. Finally, protocols and automatic order sets should avoid deliriogenic medications, such as diphenhydramine for sleep.[4]

HYPOXIC ISCHEMIC ENCEPHALOPATHY

The number one cause of morbidity and mortality post cardiac arrest is continued coma and persistent encephalopathy after resuscitation. Treating patients aggressively gives the best chance

for neurologic recovery and prevents the self-fulfilling prophecy of a poor neurologic prognosis.

RECOGNITION OF HYPOXIC ISCHEMIC ENCEPHALOPATHY

Any patient who is not awake and following commands after return of spontaneous circulation (ROSC) after cardiac arrest should be considered to have HIE. The initial neurologic examination should include pupil size and reactivity, corneal reflexes, oculocephalic reflexes (barring any concern for cervical spine injury), cough reflex, gag reflex, motor response, and verbal response. The Glasgow Coma Scale (**Table 46.4**) is a simple tool that communicates the level of coma and easily tracks changes in the neurologic examination. Note any extraneous movements such as myoclonus, nystagmus, flexor or extensor posturing, or shivering.

It is extremely important to provide aggressive care to all patients on admission to the emergency department or hospital, regardless of their neurologic examination, to prevent the self-fulfilling prophecy of a poor neurologic outcome. Patients with coma shortly after ROSC, including those with some absence of cranial nerve function, can improve and even regain consciousness with aggressive medical care. Even if the patient meets criteria for brain death immediately after resuscitation or soon thereafter, aggressive critical care allows time for family discussions and for consideration of organ donation.

DIAGNOSTIC EVALUATION

Neuron-specific enolase (NSE) should be sent between 24 and 72 hours post arrest to assist with prognosis. Without hypothermia, an NSE of greater than 33 µg/L is associated with a poor prognosis. With hypothermia, patients may have a higher number (up to 80 to 100 µg/L have been reported) and still have a good outcome, although the higher the value, the less likely a good neurologic outcome.

Many centers perform noncontrast head CTs in the emergency department or directly after stabilization from cardiac arrest to rule out massive intracranial hemorrhage or acute hydrocephalus as the cause for cardiac arrest. This is a reasonable practice, but

TABLE 46.3	Drugs for the Treatment of Acute Agitated Delirium	
	INITIAL DOSE	**SELECTED SIDE EFFECTS**
Antipsychotics		
Haloperidol	1–10 mg IV/IM/po	Prolonged QT, EPS
Olanzapine	5–10 mg po/IM	Hyperglycemia
Quetiapine	25–50 mg po	
Benzodiazepines		
Lorazepam	1–4 mg po/IV/IM	
Midazolam	1–4 mg po/IV/IM	
Alpha 2 adrenergic agonists		
Dexmedetomidine	0.4 µg/kg/h IV infusion	Hypotension, bradycardia

IV, intravenous; IM, intramuscular. EPS, Extrapyramidal symptoms.

TABLE 46.4	Glasgow Coma Scale	
EYE OPENING	**BEST MOTOR RESPONSE**	**BEST VERBAL RESPONSE**
4—eyes open spontaneously	6—follows commands	5—oriented
3—eyes open to voice	5—localizes to pain	4—disoriented
2—eyes open to pain	4—withdraws from pain	3—inappropriate words
1—none	3—flexor posturing to pain	2—incomprehensible sounds
	2—extension posturing to pain	1—none
	1—none	

not one that is required if there is a known precipitant of cardiac arrest such as prolonged QT interval or a preceding period of hypoxia. Noncontrast head CTs have not been validated for use in neurologic prognostication, although the degree of changes can give the treating neurologist a flavor of the severity of the initial brain injury (**Figures 46.1–46.3**).

Magnetic resonance imaging (MRI) should not be ordered acutely after a cardiac arrest. However, noncontrasted MRI of the brain may be helpful in prognostication (**Figure 46.4**). The volume and intensity of Diffusion-Weighted Imaging (DWI) and Fluid-Attenuated Inversion Recover (FLAIR) signal changes in the cortex of the brain have prognostic value for neurologic recovery, when the MRI is performed between days 3 and 6 after the cardiac arrest. A greater amount of change prognosticates a poor neurologic outcome.[5]

Seizures and nonconvulsive status epilepticus are common in the setting of HIE, occurring in approximately 20% of patients. Continuous EEG should be considered for all patients and started as soon as possible on any patient with myoclonus or suspicion for ongoing seizure.

Finally, somatosensory evoked potentials (SSEPs), where available, are a useful prognostic tool. Traditionally, absence of the N20 cortical responses bilaterally after median nerve stimulation prognosticates a poor neurologic outcome with a 0% false negative rate. The lack of bilateral cortical SSEP responses in patients after hypothermia continues to be highly predictive

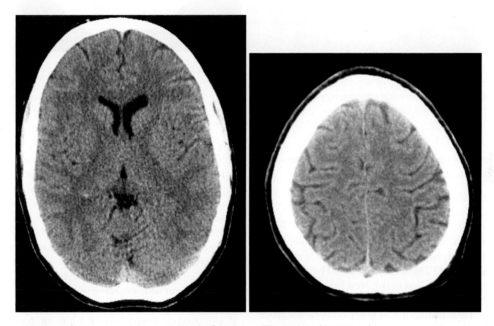

FIGURE 46.1 Two axial images from a normal noncontrast CT of the brain. CT, computed tomography.

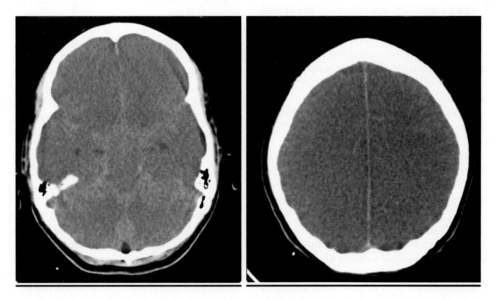

FIGURE 46.2 Noncontrasted CT scan of the head of a patient approximately 100 hours after an out-of-hospital asystolic cardiac arrest. The left panel shows pseudosubarachnoid hemorrhage and blurring of the gray-white junction throughout all the structures of the brain. The right panel shows blurring of the gray-white junction with sulcal effacement. The patient's admission noncontrast CT scan of the brain was unremarkable. At this time, the patient had flexion posturing and nonreactive pupils. The patient expired on hospital day 7 after removal of life support. CT, computed tomography.

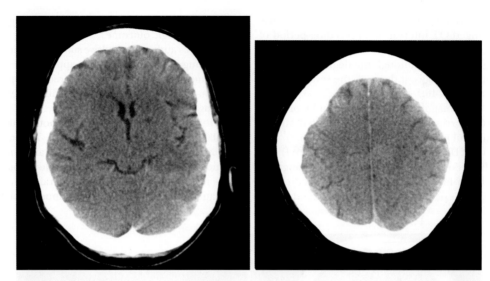

FIGURE 46.3 These two images are axial cuts of a noncontrasted head CT of a patient approximately 8 days after an out-of-hospital PEA cardiac arrest. There is loss of gray-white differentiation throughout the cerebral hemispheres, including loss of differentiation in both the basal ganglia and internal capsule (left panel), as well as the cortex. There is sulcal effacement especially at the vertex (right panel). These findings are consistent with diffuse anoxic injury. CT, computed tomography. PEA, pulseless electrical activity.

of a poor neurologic outcome. SSEPs can be performed as soon as 24 hours after cardiac arrest.[6]

TREATMENT

The only therapy shown to improve mortality and neurologic outcomes for patients with coma after cardiac arrest is targeted temperature management (TTM; hypothermia). The landmark hypothermia trials were published in the New England Journal of Medicine in 2002.[7] These studies evaluated patients after out-of-hospital ventricular fibrillation or ventricular tachycardia cardiac arrest. Hypothermia at a depth of 32°C to 34°C was started post arrest and maintained for 12 to 24 hours. The hypothermia group had a 20% absolute increase in survival and good neurologic outcome. However, in these studies, the patients in the standard therapy arm had fever to approximately 38°C. In 2013, the TTM study[8] demonstrated no differences in mortality or neurologic outcomes with the temperatures post cardiac arrest actively controlled at either 33°C or 36°C. The American Heart Association guidelines[9] now recommend using TTM for all cardiac arrest patients with coma after ROSC, at a constant temperature goal chosen between 32°C and 36°C, and maintained for at least 24 hours.

Only core temperatures should be used during hypothermia or TTM. Rectal, bladder (urinary catheter), or esophageal probes provide reliable and continuous temperature measurement. Temperature can be controlled in many ways. Simple methods include ice packs to the groin, axilla, and around the neck; rapid infusions of 4°C cold saline (useful for induction); cooling blankets; and fans. Most temperature-regulating technologies use feedback mechanisms that continuously measure the body's core temperature and automatically adjust the amount of cooling by the device to maintain a consistent body temperature. Examples include body-wrapping pads through which cold water circulates to cool the skin, central venous catheters through which cold water circulates in a closed loop and cools the surrounding venous

blood as it passes, and esophageal probes with internally circulating cold water that cools the core via surrounding soft tissues.

There are no randomized controlled trial data on blood pressure management. Hypotension can worsen cerebral perfusion and observational data suggests worse outcomes with hypotension. Significant hypertension could be associated with cerebral edema if cerebral autoregulation is impaired. Overall, hypotension should be aggressively treated to maintain systolic blood pressure ≥90 mm Hg and mean arterial pressure ≥65–80 mm Hg.[9]

Any patient with suspicion for seizure should be treated with a stable continuous infusion of benzodiazepines (such as midazolam at a starting dose of 0.05 to 0.1 mg/kg/h) or propofol, and an EEG ordered as soon as feasible. Until the EEG interpretation is obtained, the goal of treatment should be suppression of the abnormal movements, including subtler movements such as nystagmus or eye or facial twitching. Whether or not to start a nonsedating antiepileptic drug such as levetiracetam, phenytoin, or valproic acid depends on the clinical suspicion for seizure and/or nonconvulsive status epilepticus as a cause for the abnormal movements. Seizure-like activity at ictus of the cardiac arrest is not necessarily indicative of ongoing seizure activity or of primary seizure as the cause of the arrest; it can occur due to cerebral ischemia during the no-flow or low-flow period.

Prognosis in Hypoxic Ischemic Encephalopathy

Prognostication of neurologic outcome is based on a collection of physical examination findings and diagnostic tests. In the prehypothermia era, and today in patients who have not received hypothermia, the physical examination can be used to guide prognosis between 24 and 72 hours. Patients who have received hypothermia may continue to have an improving motor response for up to 7 days post arrest. The reason may be related to increase in sedation given during the hypothermia protocol, slowed metabolism of sedation during hypothermia, and actual delay in the recovery of the brain due to slowed metabolic processes during hypothermia.

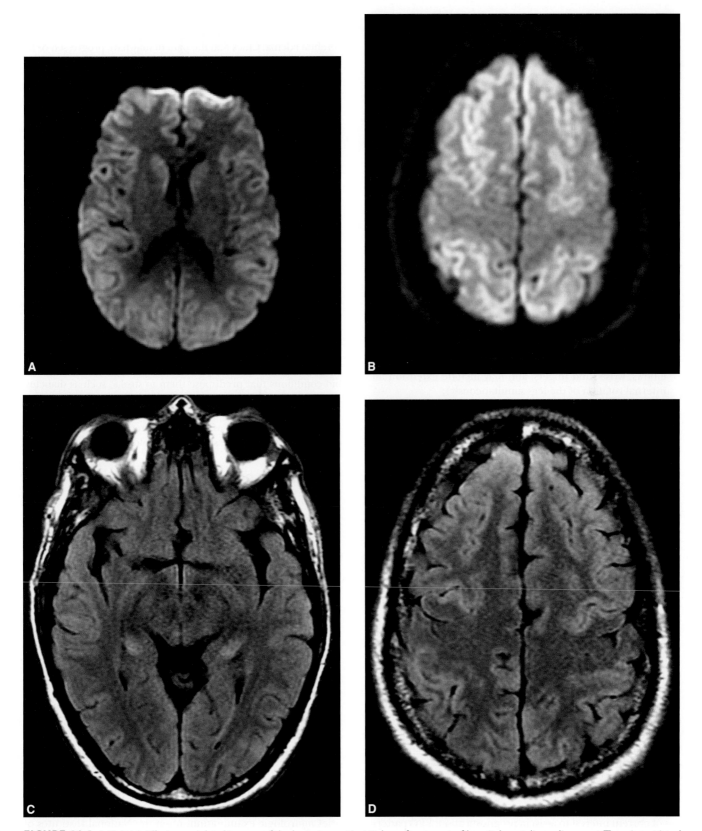

FIGURE 46.4 A, B, Axial diffusion-weighted images of the brain in a patient 5 days after an out-of-hospital asystolic cardiac arrest. There is restricted diffusion throughout the cortical ribbon. C, D, Axial FLAIR images of the brain. There is FLAIR signal hyperintensity throughout the cortical ribbon, and especially prominent in the lateral temporal lobes, occipital lobes, and frontal lobes. The total cortex score for this patient was 27, consistent with a poor neurologic prognosis.[5]

In patients who did not receive hypothermia, any one of the following findings traditionally predicts poor neurologic prognosis: lack of pupillary responses at days 1 to 3 post arrest, lack of corneal reflexes at days 1 to 3 post arrest, NSE > 33 µg/L, lack of bilateral cortical responses on SSEPs on day 1 or later, myoclonic status epilepticus, or no motor response better than extension posturing at 3 days post arrest. The lack of these findings does not ensure a good prognosis but makes the prognosis indeterminate. A poor prognosis is defined as one of severe neurologic disability, where the patient has limited understanding or consciousness and requires long-term, full nursing care.[10]

In patients who did receive hypothermia, at least 7 days should be given for the motor examination to be used in prognostication.[6] The motor response in the neurologic examination is done without sedation or paralytics and is best described in terms of the Glasgow Coma Score. The arm movements are more reliable than the leg movements, as triple flexion in the legs can mimic withdrawal. The possible arm motor responses are as follows:

- No response/no movement;
- Extensor posturing (internal rotation of the arms with extension at the elbow, pronation of the forearm, and adduction at the shoulder, and may include extension and internal rotation of the legs simultaneously);
- Flexor posturing (a stereotyped movement of flexion at the elbows, wrists, and fingers, and may include extension and internal rotation of the legs simultaneously);
- Withdrawal (purposeful pulling away from noxious stimuli in a nonstereotyped manner);
- Localizing (reaching to a noxious stimuli at or across the midline, ie to take the examiner's hand away from a sternal rub or endotracheal suctioning);
- Following commands.

A poor neurologic prognosis can be expected if the motor response is not better than extension 7 days post cardiac arrest. Take care not to attribute purposeful intent to stereotyped movements, because this may confuse both the care team and the family, and lead to additional difficulty with discussions regarding prognosis. As patients emerge from coma, movements are often small and difficult to classify. One approach is to undercall the examination so as not to build up false hope (in other words, if the movement is so small that one cannot distinguish between flexion posturing and withdrawal, call it flexion posturing initially). Serial neurologic examinations unobscured by sedation and tincture of time will clarify the true examination. The statement that any patient who has been comatose is now following commands should be taken with the utmost seriousness; following commands implies that there is a clear and reproducible motor response to a verbal command. Generally, squeezing hands should be avoided as a command to follow due to potential confusion from a grasp reflex. Useful verbal commands for examining intubated and previously comatose patients include, "Close your eyes" followed by "Open your eyes," "Stick out your tongue," "Hold up two fingers," "Hold up your thumb," or "Wiggle your toes."

Continuous EEG and noncontrast brain MRI are two modalities of current interest to assist in prognostication. EEG patterns associated with poor neurologic outcomes after cardiac arrest include spontaneous burst suppression, status epilepticus, and an EEG without change in the background to alerting maneuvers (also known as a "nonreactive" EEG background). MRI was previously discussed in this chapter.

Some patients will progress to brain death due to the severity of the initial hypoxic ischemic injury or from herniation due to cerebral edema. Clues that the patient may have progressed or be progressing to brain death include poikilothermia and diabetes insipidus (DI). Consider DI if the urine output is greater than 300 mL/h for more than 2 consecutive hours, or with high volume urine output with hypernatremia. It is important to continue aggressive critical care and maintain metabolic homeostasis as a brain-dead patient may be an organ donor candidate. Blood pressure should be supported, generally targeting a mean arterial pressure of 65 mm Hg or greater, using fluids or pressors as needed. If there is a high volume of urine output, consider desmopressin acetate IV or vasopressin infusion, titrating to a urine output of 75 to 150 mL/h. The goal is euvolemia. Hypernatremia should be corrected with half-normal saline or D5W, as appropriate. Warming blankets may be needed. Antibiotics for intercurrent infections should be continued.

ACUTE ISCHEMIC STROKE

Acute ischemic stroke can occur in patients already admitted to the CCU from a number of causes: atrial fibrillation, systolic heart failure with left ventricular thrombus, endocarditis, prosthetic cardiac valves, aortic dissection, ventricular assist devices, or postcardiac catheterization. Patients admitted to the CCU often have comorbid conditions that predispose them to stroke, such as diabetes, hypertension, hyperlipidemia, and atrial fibrillation. Other risk factors for in-hospital strokes are vascular procedures or endovascular procedures (such as cardiac catheterization), active cancer causing hypercoagulable state, or withholding of anticoagulation.

RECOGNITION OF ACUTE ISCHEMIC STROKE

With in-hospital stroke, one major barrier to timely acute treatment is recognition by the staff of an acute stroke in the patient. Time to intravenous tissue plasminogen activator (IV tPA), the medical "clot-busting" therapy for acute stroke, with in-hospital patients has been shown to be significantly longer than for those patients admitted with acute ischemic stroke through the emergency room.[11] Reasons for this delay include lack of understanding regarding the urgency of the situation, personnel and treating teams not familiar with the protocol because it is not a part of their routine practice, retrieval of tPA itself from the inpatient pharmacy, and increased transport time to CT.

First, determine that the patient clinically seems to be having a stroke. Vital signs should be checked with particular attention to blood pressure; hypertension of greater than 185/110 mm Hg should be immediately treated with a short-acting intravenous medication to a goal of < 185/110 mm Hg. A fingerstick glucose should be obtained to rule out hypoglycemia or hyperglycemia as the cause for the neurologic deficit. Hypoxia with an oxygen saturation < 94% should be treated with supplemental oxygen. Labs should be drawn and sent stat for chemistry, complete blood count (CBC), prothrombin time (PT)/international normalized ratio (INR), partial thromboplastin time (PTT). A brief neurologic examination, often the National Institutes of Health Stroke Scale (NIHSS, **Table 46.5**), is then performed to define presence and extent of deficits. Always score what the patient *actually* does, not what you *think* they can do. An NIHSS ≥ 8 has a strong predictive value for LVO, which may be amenable to endovascular therapy.

TABLE 46.5	A Summary of the National Institutes of Health Stroke Scale (NIHSS)			
ITEM	**POINTS ON NIHSS**			
1: Level of consciousness				
1A: Alertness	0—alert	1—not alert, arousable by minor stimuli	2—not alert, repeated stimulation to attend, or obtunded	3—only reflexive movements, or completely unresponsive
1B: Month and age	0—both questions correct	1—one correct	2—none correct	
1C: Simple commands: open and close eyes, make a fist and release	0—does both correctly, or mimics both correctly	1—follows one command	2—no commands	
2: Best gaze—look to both sides	0—normal	1—partial gaze palsy	2—forced deviation	
3: Visual fields	0—normal	1—partial hemianopia or extinction	2—complete hemianopia	3—blind
4: Facial palsy	0—normal	1—minor paralysis	2—partial paralysis (upper motor neuron facial weakness pattern)	3—complete paralysis (lower motor neuron facial weakness pattern) on one or both sides
5: Motor arm 5A: left 5B: right	0—no drift	1—drifts down in 10 s but does not hit bed	2—drifts down and hits bed within 10 s	3—no effort against gravity 4—no movement
6: Motor leg 6A: left 6B: right	0—no drift	1—drifts down in 5 s but does not hit bed	2—drifts down and hits bed within 5 s	3—no effort against gravity 4—no movement
7: Ataxia	0—absent	1—one limb	2—two limbs	
8: Sensory (pinprick testing)	0—normal	1—some sensory loss	2—severe or total sensory loss	
9: Language	0—normal	1—mild to moderate aphasia	2—severe aphasia	3—global aphasia or mute
10: Dysarthria	0—normal	1—mild to moderate	2—severe or mute	
11: Extinction and Inattention: sensory or visual extinction	0—normal	1—extinction or inattention in 1 modality	2—profound hemi-inattention or deficits in more than 1 modality	

In order to determine if the patient is a candidate for IV tPA, the last known normal time must be clearly defined. This may be different from the time of discovery. For example, if the patient went to sleep and woke up with a hemiplegia, then the last known normal time is the time of sleep onset. IV tPA may be given in ischemic strokes where the last known normal time is within 3 hours,[12] or within 4.5 hours with additional contraindications.[13]

INITIAL WORKUP AND TREATMENT

After establishing that there is a new neurologic deficit, checking vital signs and glucose, and drawing appropriate labs, the patient should be taken emergently for a noncontrasted CT of the brain and a CTA of the head and neck (**Figures 46.5** and **46.6**). A CTA of the head and neck should be done with any patient with a NIHSS $\geq$ 8 or cortical signs or symptoms. In the setting of an acute stroke, CTA (which uses iodinated contrast) can and should be performed without regard to the patient's creatinine, because studies have shown the risk of acute kidney injury due to contrast in this setting to be small, and in some studies, no different than patients who did not receive a CTA.[14] A neurologist or neuroradiologist should immediately review and interpret the noncontrast head CT for contraindications for IV tPA therapy, and the CTA of the head and neck for indications that intraarterial (IA) therapy is indicated (mainly LVO).

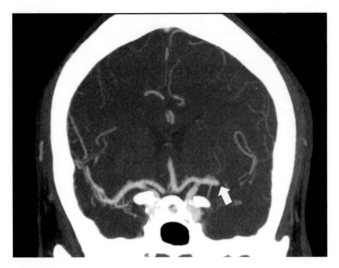

FIGURE 46.5 Coronal image of CTA of the head demonstrating an M1 segment occlusion of the left middle cerebral artery caused by thrombo-embolism. This type of lesion may be amenable to endovascular therapy. CTA, computed tomography angiogram

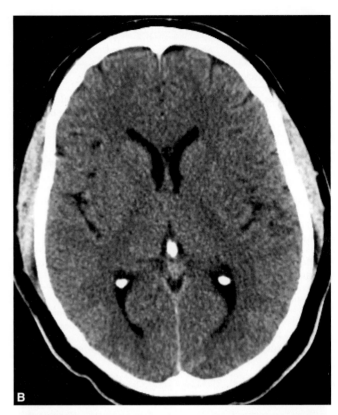

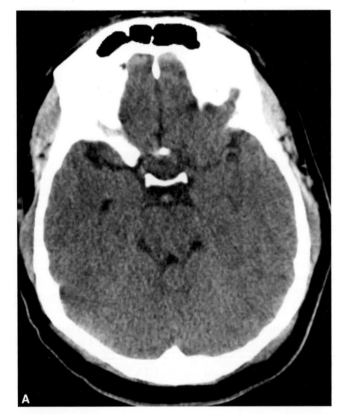

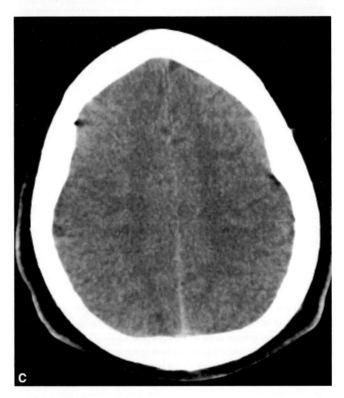

FIGURE 46.6 A-C, Initial, normal, non-contrasted head CT in a patient with an acute left internal carotid artery occlusion leading to a left middle cerebral artery syndrome (aphasia and right hemiplegia). The images were obtained 49 minutes after the onset of symptoms.

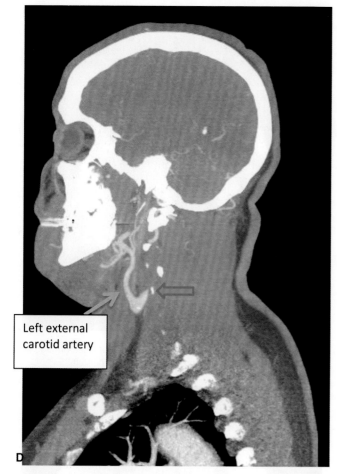

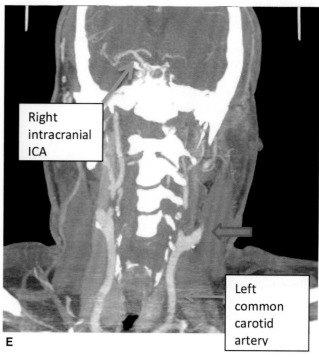

FIGURE 46.6 (*Continued*) D-E, MIPs from the CTA of the head and neck. Panel D is a sagittal MIP image at the level of the left internal carotid artery. There is no flow distally in the left internal carotid artery after this flame-shaped cutoff (large blue arrow). Panel E is a coronal MIP image showing occlusion of the cervical left internal carotid artery and the subsequent lack of opacification of the intracranial left internal carotid artery, middle cerebral artery, and anterior cerebral artery. The few vessels visualized in the left hemisphere appear to have been collateral flow from the anterior communicating artery or from meningeal collaterals. The patient was given IV tPA 153 minutes after the onset of symptoms. He underwent emergent revascularization of the left internal carotid and middle cerebral arteries. His initial NIHSS was 20; it improved to 5 by acute hospital discharge.

For patients with an acute ischemic stroke who qualify for IV tPA (**Tables 46.6** and **46.7**), it should be given as soon as possible, because there is an inverse relationship between benefit from tPA and time to administration. IV tPA is given at a dose of 0.9 mg/kg, with a maximum dose of 90 mg.[13] The first 10% is given as an IV bolus over 1 minute, and the additional 90% as an infusion over 1 hour. Blood pressure should be closely monitored and maintained at less than 185/110 mm Hg during the infusion. Neurologic checks should be performed to look for significant improvement or worsening. If the patient worsens during or after the infusion, any remaining tPA should be held and a stat noncontrast head CT obtained to rule out intracranial hemorrhage. Once tPA is given, generally no antiplatelet or anticoagulant therapy should be used for 24 hours. Blood pressures are maintained at less than 180/105 mm Hg. All patients are made nothing per oral at the time of an acute stroke, until they have a bedside swallow evaluation or a formal speech therapy evaluation.

There has been a recent revolution in acute stroke treatment, as multiple randomized controlled trials published in the last 2 years have definitively proven the benefit of IA clot extraction techniques for acute strokes caused by LVOs. Pooled analysis of the six trials

TABLE 46.6	IV tPA Inclusion Criteria

Acute ischemic stroke causing new significant neurologic deficits
Time within 3–4.5 hours of onset (last known normal time)
Blood pressure < 185/110 mm Hg

IV tPA, intravenous tissue plasminogen activator.

showed that good outcomes at 90 days increased in the intervention arm from 26% to 47% and mortality decreased from 18% to 8%.[15] Endovascular or IA therapy, combined with IV tPA when appropriate, is definitively superior to IV tPA alone for ischemic strokes due to LVO. The fastest and least invasive way to diagnose an LVO is with a CTA of the head and neck (**Figures 46.5** and **46.6**). For this reason, all patients with suspected acute stroke should get a CTA of the head and neck at the time of the initial noncontrast head CT.

For most patients with acute stroke, 162 to 325 mg of aspirin is appropriate secondary stroke prevention in the acute setting. Aspirin can be started immediately if the patient is not an IV tPA candidate; it may be given per rectum or via nasogastric tube if the patient has dysphagia. Some patients will have indications

	ADDITIONAL CONTRAINDICATIONS FOR IV TPA WITHIN 3–4.5 H OF ONSET
TABLE 46.7 **Contraindications for IV tPA**	
CONTRAINDICATIONS FOR IV TPA WITHIN 3 H OF ONSET	**ADDITIONAL CONTRAINDICATIONS FOR IV TPA WITHIN 3–4.5 H OF ONSET**
Intracranial hemorrhage on noncontrast CT[a]	Age > 80 y
CT with well-established acute or subacute infarct[a]	Anticoagulant use, regardless of INR
CT showing infarct greater than 1/3 the size of the MCA territory[a]	NIHSS ≤ 25
Active bleeding or major acute trauma[a]	History of both previous stroke and diabetes
Resolved neurologic symptoms[a]	
Rapidly improving neurologic symptoms	
Minor or nondisabling neurologic symptoms	
Suspected subarachnoid hemorrhage[a]	
Major head trauma or stroke within the last 3 mo	
Myocardial infarction in the last 3 mo	
Genitourinary or gastrointestinal hemorrhage in the last 21 d	
Major surgery in the last 14 d	
Arterial puncture at a noncompressible site or lumbar puncture in the last 7 d	
History of previous ICH	
If on oral anticoagulants, INR > 1.7	
If on heparin in the last 48 h, elevated PTT	
Receiving DOACs within 24–48 h	
Platelets < 100,000	
Blood glucose < 50 mg/dL	
Seizure at symptom onset	

[a]Absolute contraindications. CT, computed tomography; ICH, intracerebral hemorrhage; IV tPA, intravenous tissue plasminogen activator; INR, international normalized ratio; NIHSS, National Institutes of Health Strokes Scale. MCA, middle cerebral artery; DOACs, direct oral anticoagulants.

for anticoagulation for secondary stroke prevention, the most common being atrial fibrillation. When the cohort of all ischemic stroke patients is analyzed, no benefit of IV heparin is seen acutely because the risk of serious harmful effects such as intracranial hemorrhage equals the benefit of additional decrease in thromboembolic events. Instead, patients who have an indication for anticoagulation will often be bridged to warfarin with aspirin, or the initiation of new oral anticoagulants (NOACs) delayed until safe. The timing of anticoagulation initiation is an art dependent upon the size of the stroke, any hemorrhagic transformation, and the indication for anticoagulation. High dose statins should be used for all patients with low density lipoprotein (LDL) >100, unless a clear contraindications exists. Chemical deep vein thrombosis prophylaxis can be started 24 hours after tPA, or on admission if the patient did not receive tPA. Further workup and treatment of any particular stroke is beyond the scope of this chapter.

INTRACRANIAL HEMORRHAGE

Intracranial hemorrhage is classified based on the hemorrhage's location in relationship to the brain parenchyma: epidural hemorrhage is between the dura and inner table of the skull, subdural

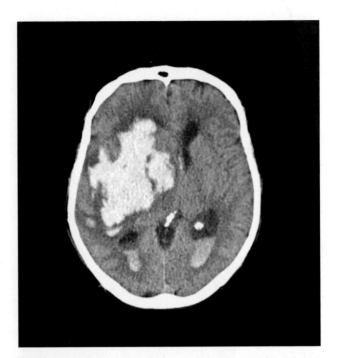

FIGURE 46.7 Large right basal ganglia intracerebral hemorrhage with intraventricular extension, hydrocephalus, and midline shift.

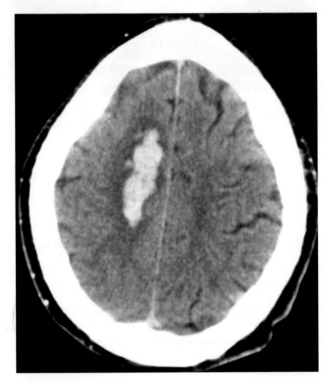

FIGURE 46.8 This axial noncontrasted head CT shows an acute right frontal intracerebral hemorrhage. CTA of the head was negative for any vascular pathology. The patient had uncontrolled hypertension and aspirin use as risk factors. He presented with acute left flaccid hemiplegia. CTA, computed tomography angiogram.

hemorrhage (SDH) is beneath the dura and above the arachnoid mater, subarachnoid hemorrhage is between the arachnoid mater and the pia mater, and intracerebral hemorrhage (ICH) is within the substance of the brain. In the absence of trauma, the common use of anticoagulants in the CCU predisposes patients to SDH or ICH.

ICH presents in a similar manner to acute ischemic stroke, with focal neurologic deficits. Headache is a common prominent symptom. If the hemorrhage is large and causing intracranial hypertension or intraventricular hemorrhage with hydrocephalus, there may also be hypertension, lethargy, nausea, or vomiting. The diagnosis of ICH is made by noncontrast head CT (**Figures 46.7** and **46.8**), where acute blood is hyperdense and seen inside the brain parenchyma. A CTA of the head and neck may still be appropriate in the initial workup, depending on the size, location, and clinical characteristics of the patient, to look for an underlying vascular malformation or the presence of a "spot sign," which can predict early hemorrhage expansion.

Initial workup and treatment for ICH parallels that of acute ischemic stroke. Always remember to first evaluate the ABCs - airway, breathing, and circulation. A common cause of intubation in patients with acute neurologic injury is obtundation and inability to adequately maintain a patent airway and ventilation. Vital signs should be monitored every 5 to 15 minutes acutely, and once the patient is stabilized every 1 hour or as per ICU protocol. Generally in ICH, targeting the systolic blood pressure (SBP) to less than 140 mm Hg is thought to be safe and may improve functional outcomes.[16] Glucose should be normalized.

As in acute ischemic stroke, when the patient is being initially assessed, laboratory studies should be sent stat for chemistry, CBC, PT, and PTT. An arterial blood gas is indicated if the patient is obtunded or was recently intubated. Hypercarbia and hypoxia can exacerbate intracranial hypertension and so should be aggressively corrected.

The size and morphology of any intracranial hemorrhage is evaluated by noncontrast CT scan of the brain. For subdural hematomas, measure the maximum width of the hematoma, as well as any midline shift. For intraparenchymal hematomas, the size of the hemorrhage can be calculated by using measurements from the CT scan, using the ABC/2 formula:

$$\text{Volume of intraparenchymal hematoma} \\ (\text{in cm}^3 \text{ or mL}) = A \times B \times C/2$$

where A = maximum hematoma width in cm; B = maximum hematoma length perpendicular to A in cm; C = height in cm (number of [0.5 cm] CT cuts the hemorrhage is seen on)/2

Hematoma volume is directly related to outcome. Look for intraventricular hemorrhage, midline shift, uncal herniation, or crowding of the basal cisterns because these can cause rapid neurologic deterioration requiring life-saving interventions such as external ventricular drains (EVDs), emergency hematoma evacuation, or hyperosmotic therapy. The ICH score (**Table 46.8**) is a useful prognostic tool that may help in medical decision making.[17]

TREATMENT OF INTRACRANIAL HEMORRHAGE

Reversal of Coagulopathies

The most common coagulopathies in the CCU are from medications. Medications that can cause or contribute to pathologic bleeding include heparin, low-molecular-weight heparins such as enoxaparin, warfarin, NOACs, aspirin, and other antiplatelet agents. Other causes of coagulopathy should also be considered, such as uremia and failure of synthetic liver function. We now review the reversal of common medication-induced coagulopathies[18] (**Table 46.9**).

Heparin is used for a wide variety of indications in the CCU, including acute myocardial infarction, stroke prevention in atrial

TABLE 46.8	The ICH Score	
		POINTS
Glasgow Coma Score: 13–15		0
5–12		1
3–4		2
ICH volume: < 30 mL		0
≥ 30 mL		1
IVH: no		0
Yes		1
Infratentorial location: no		0
Yes		1
Age: < 80 y		0
≥ 80 y		1

The ICH score predicts historic mortality in ICH.
0 = 0%, 1 = 13%, 2 = 26%, 3 = 72%, 4 = 97%, 5 = 100%.
ICH, intracerebral hemorrhage; IVH, intraventricular hemorrhage.

fibrillation, deep vein thrombosis, and left ventricular thrombus. If a patient has sudden focal neurologic deficits, any anticoagulant drip or medication should be held and a stat PT/PTT drawn. A noncontrast head CT should be obtained emergently. If an ischemic stroke without hemorrhagic transformation is discovered, no emergency reversal is necessary: whether to continue heparin would be based on a patient's specific case. If the patient has an intracranial hemorrhage and the PTT is elevated from heparin, then protamine should be given. Protamine dosing is based on the amount of heparin given and the time since the last administration of heparin. Patients are monitored for hypotension or anaphylaxis, and epinephrine should be available. Low molecular weight heparins can be reversed 60% to 75% with protamine. The factor Xa inhibitor reversal agent (andexanet alfa) being developed may play a future role in reversal of low-molecular-weight heparins.

Patients receiving warfarin and with an elevated INR should be immediately reversed, because hematoma expansion can continue for up to 72 hours in patients with vitamin K antagonist use. There are three steps to reversal of warfarin: discontinuation of warfarin, administration of vitamin K, and immediate replacement of coagulation factors with prothrombin complex concentrates (PCCs) or fresh frozen plasma (FFP). Vitamin K should be given at a dose of 10 mg IV over 10 minutes. PCCs have come into favor over FFP for immediate coagulation factor replacement. PCCs have either three factors (II, IX, and X) or four factors (II, VII, IX, and X). The United States has three brands approved by the FDA: Bebulin, Profilnine SD, and Kcentra. PCCs have the following advantages over FFP: takes no time to thaw, short preparation time, significantly lower infusion volume, rapid INR reversal, and lower risk infection. Dosing is based on both body weight and INR (**Table 46.10**). The PT/INR should be repeated 1 hour after the PCC dosing, and if it remains elevated, then PCC can be redosed. If PCC is not available, then FFP may be given at a dose of 15 mL/kg IV. Recombinant factor VIIa had previously been used and studied for the reversal of warfarin-associated coagulopathy, but it only replaces one of the factors depleted by warfarin use. With the approval of 4-factor PCC/Kcentra in the United States and high rate of thromboembolism, recombinant factor VIIa has fallen out of favor.[19]

TABLE 46.9	Anticoagulants and Their Reversal Agents	
Heparin	Protamine Maximum dose 50 mg, maximum infusion rate 5 mg/min Based on the units of heparin in the previous 2 to 3 h Time since heparin: 0 to 30 min: 1 mg protamine IV/100 units heparin 31 to 60 min: 0.75 mg protamine/100 units heparin 61 to 120 min: 0.5 mg protamine/100 units heparin >120 min: 0.4 mg protamine/100 units heparin	Immediate reversal Monitor for anaphylaxis, hypotension
Low-molecular-weight heparins	Protamine Time since enoxaparin: Less than 8 h: 1 mg protamine per 1 mg enoxaparin Greater than 8 h: 0.5 mg protamine per 1 mg enoxaparin Dalteparin: 1 mg protamine per each 100 units of dalteparin	Reverses 60%–75%
Warfarin	Vitamin K 10 mg IV PCCs OR fresh frozen plasma	May need repeated doses over hours to days
Dabigatran (Pradaxa)	Idarucizumab (Praxbind) 5 mg IV	
Factor Xa inhibitors Rivaroxaban (Xarelto) Apixaban (Eliquis)	PCC 50 IU/kg (Pending FDA Approval) Andexanet IV bolus over 15–30 min, then 2 h infusion If factor Xa inhibitor taken > 7 h ago: 400 mg bolus, 480 mg infusion If factor Xa inhibitor taken ≤ 7 h ago, or unknown: 800 mg bolus, 960 mg infusion	Andexanet is pending FDA approval.
Antiplatelet agents	DDAVP 0.3 µg/kg IV once Platelet transfusion (one apheresis unit) only if neurosurgical intervention	

IV, intravenous; FDA, US food and drug administration; PCC, prothrombin complex concentrates.

The only new oral anticoagulant agent currently with an antidote is the direct thrombin inhibitor dabigatran (Pradaxa). Idarucizumab (Praxbind) is a monoclonal antibody fragment that specifically binds dabigatran. A total of 5 mg IV is given in two doses of 2.5 mg IV no more than 15 minutes apart. Idarucizumab quickly and completely reverses the effects of dabigatran.[20] If dabigatran was taken in the preceding 2 hours, also give 50 g activated charcoal.

The oral factor Xa inhibitors currently approved by FDA in the United States and in common use are rivaroxaban (Xarelto) and apixaban (Eliquis). Andexanet alfa was developed as an antidote to the factor Xa inhibitors, and is currently pending FDA approval. With major bleeding, good or excellent clinical hemostasis is achieved in approximately 80% of patients. It

should be noted that there is an 18% rate of thrombotic events at 30 days with patients who received the drug.[21] Until andexanet alfa is available, PCCs at a dose of 50 U/kg should be strongly considered because this reverses laboratory abnormalities from rivaroxaban in nonbleeding humans.[22] If a direct factor Xa inhibitor was ingested in the preceding 2 hours, then 50 g of activated charcoal should be given.

Finally, many patients in the CCU are on antiplatelet agents. Traditionally, patients on aspirin, clopidogrel, or other antiplatelet agents were given DDAVP 0.3 µg/kg IV once (maximum dose of 20 µg) and transfused with platelets, despite lack of evidence supporting transfusion. A recent randomized trial showed that platelet transfusion in the setting of spontaneous ICH was potentially harmful, with the group receiving platelets having a statistically significant higher rate of disability than the group who did not receive platelets, and a trend toward higher mortality.[23] This study excluded patients who required neurosurgical intervention. One randomized study of patients undergoing craniectomy for hematoma evacuation after ICH showed a benefit of platelet transfusion in postoperative hemorrhage rate and volume, and in mortality, in those patients who showed aspirin-sensitivity on a platelet aggregation test.[24] Patients with thrombocytopenia and intracranial hemorrhage should be transfused platelets for a goal of greater than 70,000.

An excellent and complete review of reversal of all antithrombotic agents in the setting of intracranial hemorrhage was published in Neurocritical Care in 2016.[18]

TABLE 46.10	4-Factor Prothrombin Complex Concentrate (Kcentra) Dosing	
PRETREATMENT INR	DOSE (units/kg)	MAXIMUM DOSE (units)
2–4	25	2500
4–6	35	3500
>6	50	5000

INR, international normalized ratio.

Blood Pressure Control

Uncontrolled hypertension is a risk factor for ICH itself and for greater hematoma expansion, neurologic deterioration, dependency, and death. Current 2015 American Heart Association/American Stroke Association guidelines recommend reducing the SBP to < 140 mm Hg if the initial SBP was 150 to 220 mm Hg. This seems to be a safe target blood pressure, and may improve functional outcomes.[16] If the SBP is higher than 220 mm Hg on presentation, the goal may be adjusted. No particular agent is advantageous, although short-acting and titratable agents such as labetalol, nicardipine, or clevidipine are useful. Nitroprusside should be avoided due to a theoretical risk of increasing intracranial pressure.

Neurosurgical Intervention

Some intracranial hemorrhages may need neurosurgical intervention. Generally, symptomatic acute SDHs with mass effect or shift are evacuated. For ICH, evacuation is considered if the hematoma is large (greater than 30 mL), cortical, cerebellar, or the patient is young. New minimally invasive clot removal techniques have shown great promise, and some have even shown improvement in neurologic outcomes over medical controls. Suboccipital craniectomy is a life-saving procedure with cerebellar hemorrhages that have mass effect onto the brainstem or cause hydrocephalus. Finally, EVD placement may be needed if the patient has hydrocephalus or is somnolent, as a way to measure and treat intracranial pressure. Ultimately, an expert in neurology, stroke, or neurosurgery should be involved early in the care of patients with ICH to guide treatment, including invasive measures.

REFERENCES

1. Lonergan E, Britton AM, Luxenberg J, Wyller T. Antipsychotics for delirium. *Cochrane Database Syst Rev.* 2007;(2):CD005594.

2. Lonergan E, Luxenberg J, Areosa Sastre A. Benzodiazepines for delirium. *Cochrane Database Syst Rev.* 2009;(4):CD006379.

3. Riker RR, Shehabi Y, Bokesch PM, et al. Dexmedetomidine versus midazolam for sedation of critically ill patients. *JAMA.* 2009;301:489-499.

4. Siddiqi N, Stockdale R, Britton AM, Holmes J. Interventions for preventing delirium in hospitalized patients. *Cochrane Database Syst Rev.* 2007;(2):CD005563.

5. Hirsch KG, Mlynash M, Jansen S, et al. Prognostic value of a qualitative brain MRI scoring system after cardiac arrest. *J Neuroimaging.* 2015;25:430-437.

6. De Georgia M, Raad B. Prognosis of coma after cardiac arrest in the era of hypothermia. *Continuum.* 2012;18:515-531.

7. The Hypothermia after Cardiac Arrest Study Group. Mild therapeutic hypothermia to improve neurologic outcome after cardiac arrest. *N Engl J Med.* 2002;346:549-556.

8. Nielsen N, Wetterslev J, Cronberg T, et al. Targeted temperature management at 33°C versus 36°C after cardiac arrest. *N Engl J Med.* 2013;369:2197-2206.

9. Callaway CW, Donnino MW, Fink EL, et al. Part 8: post-cardiac arrest care. 2015 American Heart Association guidelines update for cardiopulmonary resuscitation and emergency cardiovascular care. *Circulation.* 2015;132:S465-S482.

10. Wijdicks EF, Hijdra A, Young GB, et al. Practice parameter: prediction of outcome in comatose survivors after cardiopulmonary resuscitation (an evidence-based review). *Neurology.* 2006;67:203-210.

11. Bunch ME, Nunziato EC, Labovitz DL. Barriers to the use of intravenous tissue plasminogen activator for in-hospital strokes. *J Stroke Cerebrovasc Dis.* 2012;21:808-811.

12. The National Institute of Neurological Disorders and Stroke rtPA Study Group. Tissue plasminogen activator for acute ischemic stroke. *N Engl J Med.* 1995;333:1581-1588.

13. Hacke W, Kaste M, Bluhmki E, et al. Thrombolysis with alteplase 3 to 4.5 hours after acute ischemic stroke. *N Engl J Med.* 2008;359:1317-1329.

14. Ehrlich, ME, Turner HL, Currie LJ, Wintermark M, Worrall BB, Southerland AM. Safety of computed tomographic angiography in the evaluation of patients with acute stroke. A single-center experience. *Stroke.* 2016;47:2045-2050.

15. Hussain M, Moussavi M, Korya D, et al. Systemic review and pooled analysis of recent neurointerventional randomized controlled trials: setting a new standard of care for acute ischemic stroke after 20 years. *Interv Neurol.* 2016;5:39-50.

16. Hemphill JC III, Greenberg SM, Anderson CS, et al. AHA/ASA guideline: guidelines for the management of spontaneous intracerebral hemorrhage. *Stroke.* 2015;46:2032-2060.

17. Hemphill JC III, Bonovich DC, Besmertis L, Manley GT, Johnston SC. The ICH score: a simple, reliable grading scale for intracerebral hemorrhage. *Stroke.* 2001;32:891-897.

18. Frontera JA, Lewin JJ III, Rabinstein AA, et al. Guideline for reversal of antithrombotics in intracranial hemorrhage. A statement for health care professionals from the Neurocritical Care Society and Society of Critical Care Medicine. *Neurocrit Care.* 2016;24:6-46.

19. Andrews CM, Jauch EC, Hemphill JC III, Smith WS, Weingart SD. Emergency neurological life support: intracerebral hemorrhage. *Neurocrit Care.* 2012;17:S37-S46.

20. Pollack CV, Reilly PA, Eikelboom J, et al. Idarucizumab for dabigatran reversal. *N Engl J Med.* 2015;373:511-520.

21. Connolly SJ, Milling TJ Jr, Eikelboom JW, et al. Andexanet alfa for acute major bleeding associated with factor Xa inhibitors. *N Engl J Med.* 2016;375:1131-1141.

22. Eerenberg ES, Kamphuisen PW, Sijpkens MK, Meijers JC, Buller HR, Levi M. Reversal of rivaroxaban and dabigatran by prothrombin complex concentrate: a randomized, placebo-controlled, crossover study in healthy subjects. *Circulation.* 2011;124:1573-1579.

23. Baharoglu MI, Cordonnier C, Al-Shahi Salman R, et al. Platelet transfusion versus standard care after acute stroke due to spontaneous cerebral haemorrhage associated with antiplatelet therapy (PATCH): a randomized, open-label, phase 3 trial. *Lancet.* 2016;387:2605-2613.

24. Li X, Sun Z, Zhao W, et al. Effect of acetylsalicylic acid usage and platelet transfusion on postoperative hemorrhage and activities of daily living in patients with acute intracerebral hemorrhage. *J Neurosurg.* 2013;118:94-103.

Patient and Family Information for: STROKES

WHAT IS A STROKE?

A stroke occurs when there is sudden interruption of blood flow to a specific part of the brain. When this happens, those brain cells do not get enough blood. Blood carries oxygen. All cells need oxygen to live.

TYPES OF STROKE

There are two kinds of strokes: ischemic and hemorrhagic. An *ischemic stroke* is a "nonbleeding stroke" that happens when a blood vessel leading to the brain becomes blocked. This keeps the brain cells in that area from receiving blood and oxygen. A *hemorrhagic stroke* is a "bleeding stroke" that happens when a blood vessel in or near the brain bursts. The blood is released into the brain itself or into the space between the brain and the skull. The blood then presses on and irritates the surrounding brain and keeps the cells around it from working properly.

SYMPTOMS OF A STROKE

- Sudden numbness or weakness of the face, arm, or leg, especially on one side of the body;
- Sudden confusion, trouble speaking, or trouble understanding;
- Sudden trouble seeing in one or both eyes;
- Sudden trouble walking, dizziness, loss of balance, or loss of coordination;
- Sudden severe headache with no known cause.

If you experience any of these symptoms, **CALL 911 IMMEDIATELY.** Stroke is an emergency. Do not delay. Early treatment may be able to prevent or limit permanent disability or even death.

TESTS

These tests are done to see the location of the stroke and find out its type and cause:

- **CT scan:** This is a type of X ray that takes pictures of your brain. It shows if the stroke is ischemic or hemorrhagic.
- **CTA:** This is a special CT with dye given to light up the blood vessels going to the brain. The purpose is to show a blocked blood vessel that could possibly be opened up to make the stroke better. It can also show other abnormal blood vessels such as those that cause bleeding strokes.
- **MRI:** This test uses a giant magnet instead of X rays to take pictures of the brain. The pictures have more detail than a CT scan. Because the machine is narrow and loud, some patients get nervous and may need medicine to help relax. Patients with permanent pacemakers or implanted defibrillators often cannot have MRIs. Other metal in the body may or may not be safe for MRI. You will fill out a form to see if it is safe for you to have an MRI.
- **Magnetic resonance angiography (MRA):** This takes a picture of the blood vessels with the MRI. An MRA does not usually need dye.

- **Carotid Doppler:** This test uses sound waves (ultrasound) to make pictures of the blood vessels in the front of the neck that go to the brain.
- **Transesophageal echocardiogram (TEE):** For this test, the patient is given some medicine to help relax. The patient then swallows a small tube. The tube uses sound waves to make pictures of the heart and large blood vessels around the heart. This can show if there is a blood clot in the heart, a hole in the heart, or large plaque in the blood vessel just outside the heart. These types of problems can cause a stroke.

MEDICATIONS

Most people who have a stroke need several medicines. These medicines decrease the risk of having another stroke.

- Antiplatelet medications such as aspirin, clopidogrel (Plavix), and dipyridamole with aspirin (Aggrenox) are used to prevent new ischemic strokes in many patients.
- Anticoagulants are blood thinners. These are stronger than the antiplatelet drugs and are used to prevent new ischemic strokes from specific conditions like atrial fibrillation. There are now many anticoagulants, including warfarin (Coumadin), dabigatran (Pradaxa), rivaroxaban (Xarelto), and apixaban (Eliquis). The choice of medicine is based on your body and the specific reason you need blood thinners.
- Statin medications such as simvastatin (Zocor) or atorvastatin (Lipitor) lower the cholesterol level. They can help cholesterol plaques to become smaller and smoother. This makes the plaque less likely to cause a stroke.
- Keeping a normal blood pressure with blood pressure medicines helps to prevent new strokes.

REHABILITATION

Patients usually need rehabilitation after a stroke. Rehabilitation or "rehab" involves physical therapy, occupational therapy, and/or speech therapy. There are several types of rehabilitation programs.

- **Acute rehabilitation:** This is an intensive inpatient program (in a hospital or rehab center). Every patient must be able to do at least 3 hours per day of therapy. A patient can stay here a few weeks to a few months before returning home.
- **Skilled nursing facility with rehabilitation:** In this type of program, a patient participates in therapy for 1 to 2 hours per day. The patient can stay at this facility for several months. The patient then returns home or goes to a long-term care facility.
- **Outpatient rehabilitation center:** Here, the patient comes from home for therapy. Usually it is about 1 hour of therapy, three times per week. The patient then goes back home.
- **Home rehabilitation:** This is for patients who are unable to go from their homes to an outpatient rehabilitation center. Therapy is provided in the patient's home 2 or 3 times per week.

Pavan K. Mankal
Carly E. Glick
Donald P. Kotler

47

Gastrointestinal Emergencies in the Cardiac Care Unit

INTRODUCTION

Gastrointestinal (GI) consultation for patients in the Cardiac care unit (CCU) is common in modern inpatient medicine. GI bleeding, anemia, abdominal pain, abdominal distention, nausea and vomiting, and abnormal liver function tests all occur in patients with serious cardiac diseases.

Preparation for writing this chapter began with a review of cardiology textbooks, including old texts, plus the modern GI and cardiac literature. There is not a large literature on GI emergencies in the CCU. The older literature that exists largely focuses on surgery and the cardiologist's role. Little information is given about the nature of GI complications themselves, which confounds planning.

This chapter aims to review the general principles of evaluation and management of patients with serious cardiac disease from the GI perspective, as well as the common reasons for GI consultation, using case material from our institution. The impact of anticoagulation and antiplatelet therapies on management are analyzed in detail. The safety of GI procedures in cardiac patients is also discussed.

GENERAL PRINCIPLES

Charles Friedberg captured the essence of the gastroenterologists' and cardiologists' dilemmas in approaching a GI emergency in the CCU in his discussion of surgical procedures on the cardiac patient in his textbook *Diseases of the Heart.*[1] He wrote, "In general, it may be stated that the cogency of the surgical indication is more important than the cardiac status in determining whether an operation should be performed." The first task for the gastroenterologist is to assess the acuity of the presenting problem in relation to the acuity of the cardiac disease. Three examples should suffice.

Case 1: A 78-year-old female presented with 1 day of chest pain. She was found to have a ST-elevation myocardial infarction plus congestive heart failure (CHF). Evaluation revealed multivessel coronary artery disease (CAD) plus a right ventricular thrombus and a pericardial effusion, and she underwent emergency coronary artery bypass graft (CABG). She remained in cardiogenic shock after surgery, requiring multiple pressors, and developed renal failure.

GI consultation was requested on postoperative day 10 because of a rapid rise in liver function tests, including hyperbilirubinemia, which was ascribed to shock liver. Absent bowel sounds and diffuse abdominal tenderness were noted on physical examination. Laboratory analysis revealed marked white blood cell (WBC) elevation plus persistent lactic acidosis. Noncontrast imaging studies were nondiagnostic. Because of a strong concern of bowel infarction, flexible sigmoidoscopy was performed and showed disruption of the bowel at the level of the sigmoid colon. Emergency laparotomy was performed and demonstrated infarction of the sigmoid colon and terminal ileum. The patient survived to leave the hospital 1 month later, though with very poor cardiac function.

Case 2: A 73-year-old man was transferred from another institution with hypotension and acute coronary syndrome. Cardiac catheterization revealed triple vessel disease. The patient had a history of ulcerative colitis. An intra-aortic balloon pump was placed to maintain cardiac output. The patient then developed bloody diarrhea without abdominal pain or increase in WBC count. Bowel sounds were audible. GI consultation was requested and the consultant opined that the patient had a flare of colitis rather than intestinal infarction or ischemic disease secondary to low cardiac output. Flexible sigmoidoscopy was performed while continuing ventricular assistance with the intra-aortic balloon pump, a diagnosis of active colitis was made, corticosteroids were given, the patient responded promptly, and CABG was successfully performed 5 days later. Corticosteroids were tapered relatively rapidly and replaced by other antiinflammatory therapies after surgery to facilitate healing from the thoracotomy.

Case 3: A 60-year-old male presented with an acute coronary syndrome. Cardiac catheterization showed severe stenoses and the patient underwent coronary bypass grafting. He experienced bright red rectal bleeding on the second postoperative day. The bleeding was clinically mild, without hemodynamic changes or a fall in hematocrit. The patient had a history of prostate cancer, which had been treated with radiation. A presumptive diagnosis of radiation proctitis was made, the patient was treated with stool softeners without other evaluation until the day of discharge, when flexible sigmoidoscopy was performed and documented radiation proctitis. Plans for cauterization of the rectal lesions as an outpatient were made.

In the first case, the clinical impression of an abdominal catastrophe with a 100% morality rate, if untreated, mandated the performance of an endoscopic procedure without colonic preparation as well as emergency laparotomy, despite the patient's tenuous hemodynamic state. In the second case, the patient's history and the possible deleterious effect of a serious flare of ulcerative colitis on surgical outcomes also mandated the diagnostic procedure and treatment despite clear signs of hemodynamic instability, while the need to promote postoperative healing led to a more rapid tapering of the corticosteroids than is usually done. In the third case, the blood loss appeared trivial and not immediately threatening and the patient already had undergone cardiac operation; so the GI evaluation could be safely delayed until discharge. In some cases, evaluation can even be done after discharge. In all three cases, management was aided by repeated and effective communication and collaboration between the cardiologists and gastroenterologists.

Management of GI emergencies in the CCU has evolved greatly over the past generation. In the past, noncardiac evaluations and interventions were kept to an absolute minimum. The situation changed, at least from the gastroenterologist's point of view, when a publication in the GI literature more than 20 years ago demonstrated the safety and clinical efficacy of performing endoscopy in the presence of an acute coronary syndrome.[2] A second major development has been the widespread application of anticlotting therapies in cardiac patients, both anticoagulants and antiplatelet agents. This development has brought tremendous benefits in terms of decreasing morbidity and mortality from thromboses and emboli. However, the therapies increase the risk of hemorrhage, especially in the GI tract.

The risks and benefits of anticlotting therapies follow a U-shaped curve. A greater degree of anticlotting therapy leads to a greater risk of bleeding but a lesser risk of thrombosis/embolism. Conversely, a lower degree of anticlotting therapy leads to a lesser risk of bleeding but a higher risk of thrombosis/embolism. The specific coefficients of increased or decreased risk are not entirely clear, especially with newer, short-acting agents. There are no data at all about combined antiplatelet/anticoagulant use, for example, in a patient with atrial fibrillation and an acute coronary syndrome. However, increased bleeding can be managed promptly by transfusion over the course of several hours, while thrombosis or embolism evolves over a much shorter time frame, which provides an advantage for anticlotting therapies. In addition, endoscopic or radiologic localization of a bleeding lesion may allow direct intervention for example, placing a hemostatic clip on a bleeding vessel or embolizing the bleeding vessel by interventional radiologists, which immediately reduces the risks of bleeding or rebleeding. For these reasons, gastroenterologists must learn to live with iatrogenic bleeding risks for patients in the CCU and those managing such patients must accept the attendant increased need for transfusions and invasive noncardiac therapies.

GASTROINTESTINAL BLEEDING

Gastrointestinal bleeding (GIB) potentially is a life-threatening condition affecting approximately 102 patients per 100,000 hospitalizations, with significant morbidity.[3,4] While the severity of GI hemorrhage varies greatly, anticoagulation or antiplatelet therapies complicate the situation. Around 2% of the world population is said to be on vitamin K antagonist therapy and there is increased use of direct oral anticoagulants (DOACs) inhibiting

thrombin or factor Xa in the coagulation cascade.[5] Warfarin-related major hemorrhage (irrespective of the site) is around 1% to 9% per person year, the results for newer DOACs are similar or lower than for warfarin.[6–9] On the other hand, there was an overall incidence of GI bleeding after a percutaneous coronary intervention (PCI) of 1.04% over an 8-year period, with an underlying GI malignancy being a strong predictor of such events.[10]

Although the incidence of major bleeding is low in cardiac patients, several factors are to be considered when GI bleeding is suspected: (a) the severity of bleeding; (b) antiplatelet therapy/anticoagulation type and its possible reversal; (c) potential sites and types of lesions; and (d) continuation or the timing of reintroduction of anticoagulants with careful and ongoing assessment of thrombotic risk. There are no specific guidelines on when to reverse anticoagulation effects and the optimal time for endoscopy if a lesion is suspected.

SEVERITY OF BLEEDING

Although the Glasgow-Blatchford and Rockall scoring systems, when negative, play a vital role in avoiding endoscopic intervention, the HAS-BLED scoring system attempts to estimate risk of major bleeding in patients with atrial fibrillation who are placed on anticoagulation. HAS-BLED, which includes risk factors of hypertension, abnormal renal or hepatic functional status, stroke, bleeding predilection, labile international normalized ratio (INR), age over 64 years, drugs and alcohol history, was first proposed in 2010, then introduced into guidelines. The risk stratification as low, moderate, and high risk (depending on the scores of 0, 1 to 2, and greater than 2, respectively) has been validated and found to be superior to other scoring systems (HEMORR$_2$HAGES, ATRIA, or CHA$_2$DS$_2$-VASc scores). Similarly, CRUSADE score (Can Rapid Risk Stratification of Unstable Angina Patients Suppress Adverse Outcomes with Early Implementation of the ACC/AHA Guidelines) has been used to stratify patients who undergo PCI in the setting of ST-elevation and non-ST elevation myocardial infarctions. The stratification is as follows: very low risk with score less than or equal to 20 has a 3.1% risk of major bleeding; low risk with score between 21 and 30 has a risk of 5.5%; moderate risk with score 31 to 40 has a bleeding risk of 8.5%; high risk defined as score of 41 to 50 has bleeding risk of 11.9%; and very high risk with scores above 50 has a bleeding risk of 19.5%.

While these scoring systems can help stratify some patients *prior to medical treatment*, they are, in fact, futile when a patient is in the cardiac intensive care unit with evidence of bleeding. These scoring systems do emphasize the importance of hemodynamics: blood pressure and heart rate. These two parameters can help guide medical care in patients with suspected bleeding for prompt resuscitation prior to any endoscopic intervention. Resting tachycardia, while difficult to interpret in patients with atrial fibrillation, implies mild to moderate hypovolemia, while any signs of hypotension suggest intravascular volume loss greater than 15% (if orthostatic) and 40% (if supine). Fortunately, the latter situations are infrequently seen, particularly after starting anticoagulation or antiplatelet therapy.

ANTIPLATELET THERAPY/ANTICOAGULATION

A variety of anticoagulants are used for (a) treatment of venous thromboembolism (VTE); (b) stroke prevention in patients with atrial fibrillation; and (c) prosthetic heart valves. These medications include both vitamin K antagonists (warfarin) and DOACs (rivaroxaban, apixaban, dabigatran, and edoxaban). In the setting of GI hemorrhage, the question of when to reverse anticoagulation often is difficult to answer. No specific guidelines exist for when and how to reverse the effects of anticoagulation, particularly in hemodynamically stable patients with a complicated clinical picture requiring intensive care.

In a massive bleeding emergency, vitamin K based anticoagulation can be reversed during a clinical emergency with vitamin K, fresh frozen plasma, or protein complex concentrates (clotting factors II, VII, IX, and X). Postprocedure assessment can be done with laboratory tests to confirm restoration of normal anticoagulation. However, reversing the effects of DOACs is not as straightforward. The bleeding risk profile of DOACs as compared to warfarin was assessed in various studies: Randomized Evaluation of Long Term Anticoagulation Therapy (RELY); Rivaroxaban Once-Daily, Oral, Direct Factor Xa Inhibition Compared with Vitamin K Antagonism for Prevention of Stroke and Embolism Trial in Atrial Fibrillation (ROCKET-AF), and Apixaban for Reduction in Stroke and Other Thromboembolic Events in Atrial Fibrillation (ARISTOTLE). Both dabigatran 150 mg twice daily and rivaroxaban 20 mg once daily were associated with higher incidence of massive GI bleeding compared with warfarin, while apixaban had a similar bleeding risk as warfarin. Nevertheless, in several Meta analyses of randomized controlled trials, the relative risk of massive GI bleeding was higher with DOACs compared to warfarin.[11] While the initial studies seem to convey a bleak picture, international prospective registries provide evidence of more efficacy and safety, with one study showing half the bleeding complication rate of using rivaroxaban compared to the data presented in ROCKET-AF.[12] Protein complex concentrates have been shown to attenuate the effects of the newer DOAC regimens in small studies and animal models; however, the intended correction may overshoot the "normal" target to confer a "procoagulant" environment while the additional clotting factors remain in the vasculature. Additionally, there is no laboratory support to confirm the reversal of the effects of DOACs. However, in dire life-threatening emergencies, these protein complex concentrates have been recommended as first-line agents. Nonetheless, specific drug therapies are being developed. Recently approved in the United States, idarucizumab, a monoclonal antibody therapy, binds specifically to dabigatran and rapidly neutralizes its effects in over 90% patients without any safety concerns.[13] Given the high costs, logistical issues, hospital protocols, and reimbursements, implementation is likely to lag. Additional reversal agents are in the pipeline, like andexanet alfa, for direct factor Xa inhibitors.

In the more likely scenario of nonemergent, non–life-threatening situations, DOACs fare better in reversal because they are short lived with normal restoration of coagulation profile within 12 to 24 hours after the last dose in patients without any renal compromise. Conversely, the effects of vitamin K antagonists are longer lasting and known to be effective for up to 3 days. However, the optimal timing for reversing anticoagulants' effects in nonemergent settings is not known. Given the rapid clearance of DOAC in patients with normal drug clearance, the need to use reversing agents may be unnecessary, because the drug effects dissipate within hours.

To complicate matters further, many patients have CAD requiring vascular intervention and atrial fibrillation, necessitating the use of antiplatelet along with anticoagulation therapy in an attempt to reduce their risk of both ischemic heart disease *and* stroke. Overall, the benefits from reducing adverse events with these medications is not higher than the augmented risks of bleeding, and therefore these medications are not recommended.[14] However, the concomitant use of antiplatelet therapy in patients using anticoagulation increases the risk of GI bleeding over time, which is worse with dual antiplatelet therapy and in the elderly. The risk was assessed in the APPRAISE-2 trial, and additional trials are underway to assess the risk further with other DOACs.

Nonetheless, it is important to remember that most cases of GI hemorrhage are not life-threatening. In addition, many studies mentioned earlier (ie, RELY, ROCKET-AF) have looked at outcomes to assess morbidity and mortality (including but not limited to need for reversal use, use of blood products, death after bleeding), showing a noninferior profile of DOACs when compared to older vitamin K antagonists.

LOCALIZATION: UPPER VERSUS LOWER

Whether the source of bleeding is the upper or lower GI tract is a question often faced by the critical care team. By definition, any lesion seen above the ligament of Treitz (proximal to the jejunum) is considered an upper GIB, whereas a lesion in the rest of the GI tract is considered a lower GIB. While the definitions may be clear, the attempt to localize may yield no definite source, or multiple potential sources with possible ascertainment bias. Trends in population-based evidence show that there has been a significant increase in lower sources and a decreasing trend in upper sources of GIB.[15] This is likely due to more "gut surface area" distal to the ligament of Treitz, the fact that a negative upper endoscopy will automatically characterize a bleeding episode as a lower GIB, and to the widespread use of proton pump inhibitors.[9] Although the data for DOACs are sparse, data regarding the actual source of GIBs shows 18.9% of patients have peptic ulcer disease, of which 7.2% cases required endoscopic intervention, while 9.5% of the 57.1% patients who underwent colonoscopy had lower GI findings that needed intervention endoscopically.[16] It is important to reiterate that localizing a site of bleeding may allow direct intervention, such as placement of hemostatic clips, application of a heater probe, or vascular embolization by an interventional radiologist, with abrupt cessation of bleeding and the ability to restate anticlotting therapy. In many cases, endoscopy and other studies do not reveal the source of bleeding, which is then characterized as being obscure GIB.

TIMING OF ENDOSCOPY

No evidence or guidelines exist to determine when patients on anticoagulation should/can undergo endoscopy. However, the gastroenterologists' general practice tends to be based on the clinical situation and presenting symptoms. During active bleeding, particularly when hemodynamic instability is noted (tachycardia, hypotension, bloody emesis), prompt endoscopy within 12 hours usually is performed. The use of proton pump inhibitors may reduce the yield of high-risk lesions and the need for direct intervention during endoscopy. While medical management is as important as endoscopy, urgent endoscopy (within a few hours of presentation) has not shown to improve morbidity or mortality in the general population. To complicate matters further, with anticoagulation use, iatrogenic injury to the GI tract is a valid concern; so waiting for reversal of the medication effects prior to endoscopy may be prudent.

In all cases, endoscopy should be pursued in patients who are anticoagulated as long as hemodynamic stability has been achieved, though the critical care and the gastroenterology teams must be prepared to accept a negative upper endoscopy and a negative colonoscopy during a bleeding episode (which may have resolved at this point of the work up). Although the next logical step for the bleeding work up is capsule endoscopy to assess the small bowel (the largest area of the GI tract), the procedure often is not performed in an inpatient setting. Thus, resumption of anticoagulation is often discussed prior to the completion of GI evaluation.

RESTARTING ANTICOAGULANTS/ANTIPLATELET THERAPY

Resuming anticoagulation and antiplatelet therapy after a GIB episode involves balancing the benefits of the therapy and the risks of rebleeding. Expert guidelines generally recommend that anticoagulation therapy should be resumed for stroke/systemic embolism prevention as soon as possible after a bleeding site has been treated and "stable hemostasis" has been achieved. As one strategy, warfarin could be started the day of the procedure as the effects of anticoagulation reach therapeutic values in 72 hours, while one would have to wait 48 to 72 hours before resuming shorter-acting agents. However, the situation is more complicated if the source is obscure or resolves without any intervention. Therefore, the risks of rebleeding are not often fully known in many cases. Clinical experience indicates that bleeding from peptic ulcer disease typically occurs within 72 hours of the initial bleeding episode in the absence of definitive therapy, which guides the intensity of patient follow-up.[17] The variety of difficult situations that arise, particularly in the CCU, mandates evaluating and reevaluating the risks and benefits of therapy on a daily basis or even more frequently.

Case 1: A 50-year-old man with a past medical history of atrial fibrillation, on warfarin, and chronic heart failure presented to the hospital with signs of fluid overload and melena. He underwent diuresis and upper endoscopy revealed a clean-based ulcer that needed no endoscopic intervention (ie, hemostatic clip, epinephrine injections, or electrocautery).

Case 2: A 50-year-old man with a past medical history of atrial fibrillation, on warfarin, and chronic heart failure presented to the hospital with signs of fluid overload and melena. He underwent diuresis and upper endoscopy revealed an ulcer with a visible vessel that required a hemostatic clip (which was placed adequately).

Case 3: A 50-year-old man with a past medical history of atrial fibrillation, on warfarin, and chronic heart failure presented to the hospital with signs of fluid overload and melena. He underwent diuresis and upper endoscopy revealed an ulcer with a visible vessel that required a hemostatic clip (which was placed possibly inadequately).

Although the three cases present similarly, the outcome of endoscopy can help the critical care team decide to restart anticoagulation promptly (ie, the first two cases), whereas the third case required a brief delay in restarting anticoagulation therapy. Although the use of proton pump inhibitors reduces the need for endoscopic intervention on high-risk lesions during an acute event, there is no evidence of it preventing upper GI bleeding/rebleeding when used concomitantly with anticoagulation and antiplatelet therapy.

As it is impossible to delineate all the possible scenarios of GIB episodes in patients with anticoagulation, ongoing multidisciplinary discussions in these cases is imperative. A team-based approach to help address the risks and benefits on case-by-case basis will allow stratification of patients based on their hemodynamic stability, clinical presentation, anticoagulation status and possible reversal, the benefits of endoscopy, and possibly resumption of therapy around the time of the GIB episode.

ANTICOAGULATION IN CIRRHOSIS

Cirrhotics, particularly the decompensated patients, have a higher bleeding risk profile often complicated by bleeding esophageal varices. Anticoagulation in these patients may be considered for various reasons, including portal vein thrombosis and atrial fibrillation. It is important to remember that coagulopathy from liver disease is not equivalent to medication-induced anticoagulation. While current clinical management supports use of vitamin K antagonists and low molecular weight heparin in selected compensated patients (lack of ascites, bleeding varices, encephalopathy, and hepatorenal syndrome), the use of DOACs is unclear. Those patients were excluded from the pivotal trials.

In summary, most cases of GIB in anticoagulated patients are nonlethal and do not lead to long-term adverse effects. Endoscopy should be pursued in patients who are anticoagulated or on antiplatelet therapy at a time when hemodynamic stability has been achieved, knowing that no lesion may be found or no endoscopic intervention may be pursued.

The risks and benefits should be assessed daily and the decision to resume or restart antiplatelet/anticoagulation therapy should be a team-based decision.

ANEMIA WITHOUT GASTROINTESTINAL BLEEDING

A common scenario that cardiologists are faced with in the CCU is unexplained anemia, particularly in a patient on anticoagulation or antiplatelet therapy. Clinically occult GIB is high on the list in the differential diagnosis. Although this may be the case in certain situations, having a healthy differential is prudent, especially when no overt signs of bleeding have been noted (ie, melena, hematemesis, or hematochezia). Blood in the GI tract acts like a cathartic and often presents with multiple bowel movements rather than constipation. With no clinical signs of GIB, endoscopy may not be warranted. For example, retroperitoneal bleeding or a postcatheterization hematoma in the leg may be associated with a sudden fall in hematocrit as can sepsis and disseminated intravascular coagulation.

INTESTINAL ISCHEMIA

Intestinal ischemia is an uncommon disease, particularly in cardiac patients, and may be due either to embolic or atherosclerotic disease. Intestinal ischemia encompasses acute mesenteric ischemia, nonocclusive mesenteric ischemia, and chronic mesenteric ischemia. Similar to its varied presentation from acute or chronic, the progression also embodies a large spectrum from being reversible to fatal. For example, in the acute setting of mesenteric ischemia (from embolism originating from atrial fibrillation or thrombosis from atherosclerotic disease in the superior mesenteric artery), mortality in the absence of treatment can reach up to 93% while the nonocclusive mesenteric ischemia during low-flow states can be from 50% to 90%.[18] Risk factors include history of vascular disease from smoking, diabetes, hypertension, and hyperlipidemia (similar to the risks presented in patients with CAD), as well as history of cardiomyopathies, myocardial infarctions, cardiac arrhythmias including atrial fibrillation, hypotension, recent CABG, among others.

PATHOPHYSIOLOGY

Anatomically, three major vessels supply the vasculature of the intestines: arteries from the celiac axis (supplies stomach and duodenum), superior mesenteric artery (rest of small intestine up to the splenic flexure), and inferior mesenteric artery (splenic flexure to the rectum). Although extensive collaterals help prevent ischemia in the gut, there are certain areas that are more vulnerable to injury, often labelled as watershed areas. These areas include classically the splenic flexure (Griffiths point) and the rectosigmoid region (Sudeck point).

DIAGNOSIS

Clinical presentation can vary and particularly in a cardiac patient, both acute and chronic abdominal pain should raise the possibility of "gut angina" to "gut ischemia" to "gut infarction" (similar to the workings of the heart). In textbooks, acute pain out of proportion that precedes voluminous diarrhea with or without blood noted subsequently is classic for an ischemic event. It can however present with abdominal distention (discussed later), nausea, and vomiting. Selective angiography is the most sensitive means of making a diagnosis of arterial disease and allows for the direct instillation of vasodilators.[19] Computed tomography (CT) angiography also has high sensitivity for the diagnosis of arterial disease but does not allow for therapeutic intervention. It is important to note that early diagnosis is imperative because it improves survival. If there are any signs of inflammation of the bowel wall or colitis noted on imaging, comprehensive work up to rule out infections like *Clostridium difficile* must be done.

MANAGEMENT

As with any bleeding or emergency, hemodynamic status needs to be optimized. Additionally, in intestinal ischemia, broad-spectrum antibiotics (eg, ciprofloxacin and metronidazole) need to be initiated to prevent bacterial translocation. All attempts to stop vasoactive drugs or vasoconstrictors should be made. While some data exists on use of thrombolytics on embolic events, it is not recommend given the increased risk of hemorrhage. Nonetheless, a prompt surgical consultation is necessary to remove the damaged bowel, particularly in acute mesenteric ischemia. Vasodilators like papaverine (a phosphodiesterase inhibitor) can be used particularly in nonocclusive mesenteric ischemia and chronic mesenteric ischemia. Colonoscopy can be safely done in stable patients with ischemic colitis to differentiate from other types of colitis of infectious and inflammatory origin.

ABNORMAL LIVER FUNCTION TESTS

Gastroenterologic or hepatologic consultation in the CCU may be related either to the condition that prompted CCU admission or to the same causes of liver dysfunction that might afflict anyone, such as acute or acute on chronic hepatitis, decompensated cirrhosis, cholecystitis, etc. In the latter instances, the presentation does not differ from that in the noncardiac patient and the major clinical problem is managing the disease in the face of cardiac dysfunction. In some cases, such as cholecystitis or perforation of a duodenal ulcer into the gastrohepatic ligament, the symptoms may mimic acute cardiac disease and may even cause ECG abnormalities. Drug-induced liver disease (DILI) may occur in cardiac patients, and may be caused by drugs used in the CCU. However, it is more common for GI consultation to involve circulatory failure.

CIRCULATORY FAILURE

Though the liver comprises 2.5% of body weight, it receives around 25% of cardiac output, two-thirds from the portal system and one-third from the hepatic artery. Within the liver, the pericentral areas (zone 3) are most prone to injury because of a low oxygen tension under normal circumstances. The liver is partially protected from ischemic injury because of its dual blood supply—arterial and portal venous. However, the biliary system is supplied only by the hepatic artery. Heart failure can lead to hepatic dysfunction via two mechanisms, hepatic congestion related to increased venous pressure or ischemic injury related to decreased blood flow (**Table 47.1**). Passive congestion from increased central venous pressure occurs as a result of right-sided heart failure and may be chronic or acute, the latter in the case of pulmonary embolism, especially a saddle embolus. Hepatic dysfunction from right-sided heart failure may result from constrictive pericarditis, severe pulmonary arterial hypertension, mitral stenosis, tricuspid regurgitation, cor pulmonale, or cardiomyopathy. Right ventricular dysfunction with increased hepatic venous pressure can lead to atrophy of hepatocytes and perisinusoidal edema. Chronic right-sided heart failure may lead to hepatic fibrosis, previously termed "nutmeg cirrhosis." Rheumatic heart disease was a very common cause of nutmeg cirrhosis in the past. Mortality in this condition usually was related to the severity of the heart disease, rather than the liver disease.

TABLE 47.1	**Causes of Hepatic Ischemia**

Heart failure[a]
- Right-sided heart failure
  - Right-sided myocardial infarction
  - Pulmonary embolism
  - Pulmonary hypertension
- Left-sided heart failure
  - Myocardial infarction
  - Cardiomyopathy
  - Valvular disease

Hypovolemia
  - Hemorrhage
  - Dehydration

Hypoxemia

Sepsis

Heat stroke

This is not a complete list but rather conditions that one might encounter in a CCU.
[a]In the presence or absence of cardiogenic shock.
CCU, coronary care unit.

Although the condition is termed cirrhosis, portal hypertension typically is not seen.

Right-sided heart failure in the absence of left-sided heart failure usually presents with edema, ascites, and hepatomegaly. Jaundice may be noted on physical examination. Rarely, patients can present with severe hepatomegaly and right upper quadrant pain, which is due to stretching of Glisson capsule. The liver may be pulsatile if there is tricuspid insufficiency. The liver edge typically is smooth, and hepatojugular reflux may be elicited. When present, ascites classically has elevated protein content (>2.5 g/L) and a low serum-to-ascites albumin gradient, which is different from cirrhosis secondary to alcoholic liver disease or chronic viral hepatitis. Left-sided heart failure usually does not present with these symptoms, but with symptoms of dyspnea. Mild elevations of aspartate aminotransferase (AST), alanine aminotransferase (ALT), lactate dehydrogenase (LDH), gamma-glutamyl transpeptidase, and alkaline phosphatase (ALP) typically are seen in right-sided heart failure, with elevations of up to 2 to 3 times the upper limit of normal. Bilirubin typically remains below 3 mg/dL with an elevated unconjugated fraction, but may be higher in patients with chronic, severe CHF. The rise in transaminases is greater with more acute presentations and in the presence of systemic hypotension, and may resemble acute hepatitis.

Hepatic dysfunction also may arise from low cardiac output leading to decreased perfusion and the predisposing conditions are similar to those discussed earlier. While oxygen delivery to the liver is related to both blood flow and Pao_2, hypoxemia alone rarely is sufficient to cause tissue injury. If affected by hypoxemia, the areas around the central veins are most vulnerable, because oxygen tensions are lowest under normal circumstances. Virtually any cause of hypotensive shock can result in hepatic injury, including hemorrhage, burns, heat stroke, toxic shock, sepsis, acute CHF, trauma, crush injuries, pulmonary embolism, etc. In addition to hepatic artery thrombosis and embolism, hepatic artery occlusion also may occur from sickle cell crisis, cocaine-induced arterial spasm, aortic dissection, vasculitis, hypercoagulable states, hepatic artery aneurysms, toxemia of pregnancy, embolism from tumor, endocarditis, and others (**Table 47.2**). The vulnerability of the liver to ischemic disease is greater in the presence of cirrhosis because of portosystemic shunting or portal vein thrombosis, and in CHF because of the inability of the heart to compensate for the decreased hepatic blood flow. The liver also is susceptible because of the relatively high metabolic activity of the hepatocytes. Furthermore, the liver may suffer from reperfusion injury with reactive oxygen species and lipid peroxidation as well as superoxides and hydrogen peroxide.

Hepatic injury usually is acute, but may be recognized well after the inciting event has occurred.

The diagnosis typically is made on clinical grounds. In severe episodes of hypotension, shock liver can occur in which there is a profound elevation in serum alanine aminotransferase and aspartate aminotransferase, and prolonged prothrombin time. The diagnosis of hepatic infarction can be made radiographically, with demonstration of a wedge-shaped or other defect, especially on a contrast CT study. Laboratory abnormalities in ischemic hepatitis usually peak after 1 to 3 days and normalize after 5 to 10 days. Diagnosis is typically clinical when liver tests are found to be abnormal 1 to 3 days after the episode of hypotension though the condition may mimic acute hepatitis, especially if the inciting event was missed, for example, hypotension associated with a tachyarrhythmia in an outpatient setting. There may also be concomitant elevations in

TABLE 47.2	Causes of Hepatic Infarction
Hepatic artery thrombosis
• Atherosclerosis
• Hypercoagulable states
Hepatic artery embolism
• Endocarditis
• Tumor emboli
• Therapeutic embolization
Hepatic artery aneurysm
Aortic dissection
Vasculitis involving the hepatic artery
Sickle cell disease
Vasospasm—cocaine ingestion

This is not a complete list but rather conditions that one might encounter in a CCU.
CCU, Cardiac care unit.

creatinine from acute tubular necrosis. In these episodes of severe hypotension leading to elevated liver tests, patients usually present with serum bilirubin elevations up to 20 mg/dL and AST more than 10 times the upper limit of normal. LDH typically rises and an ALT/LDH ratio of less than 1.5 can help differentiate ischemic liver damage from viral hepatitis. In addition, the transaminases tend to fall rapidly because of the acute, reversible inciting event, as opposed to viral hepatitis in which transaminase elevations are much more prolonged, lasting for a few weeks. Most cases resolve with supportive care, though hepatic decompensation may occur, especially in the presence of chronic liver disease. There is no specific therapy for ischemic injury.

The following case is an example of an acute ischemic injury to the liver.

A 36-year-old man presented to the emergency room with severe chest pain, with onset while returning from an overseas trip. CT angiogram showed no evidence of pulmonary embolism but did show aneurysmal dilatation of the ascending aorta. Transthoracic echocardiogram showed a flap in the ascending aorta plus severe aortic insufficiency. He underwent emergent aortic root replacement with reconstruction and reimplantation of coronary buttons and hemiarch replacement, with 16 minutes of circulatory arrest and a cross clamp time of 192 minutes. GI consultation was requested for marked transaminase elevations (AST, 9736 and ALT, 5731) on postoperative day 3, plus coagulopathy (INR, 3.3). Transfer to a liver transplantation center was sought but was denied due to the need for multiple pressors and other postoperative care. Continuous venovenous hemoperfusion followed by hemodialysis was started because of acute kidney injury. Doppler examination showed blood flow to both kidneys. The transaminases peaked on postoperative day 4, while the total bilirubin continued to rise until postoperative day 8. Renal recovery was noted on postoperative day 11. At discharge on postoperative day 15, both liver and kidney function tests were improving and the patient was no longer receiving hemodialysis.

DRUG-INDUCED LIVER INJURY

Medications are also a common cause of hepatic dysfunction, which may present as asymptomatic liver test elevations or even fulminant liver failure. DILI may be nonidiosyncratic or idiosyncratic. Acetaminophen is a classic nonidiosyncratic etiology of DILI because high doses of acetaminophen can lead to DILI in

TABLE 47.3	Drug-induced Liver Injury
MEDICATIONS[a]	COMMENTS
ACE inhibitors	Associated with low rate of elevated serum aminotransferases ($< 2\%$)
Alpha blockers	Associated with minimal rate of elevated serum aminotransferases (0.2%–2%)
Angiotensin II receptor antagonists	Associated with minimal rate of elevated serum aminotransferases (0.2%–2%)
Antiarrthymics	Amiodarone is associated with elevation of serum aminotransferases in 15%–50% on long-term therapy. It is recommended to have ALT and AST values checked at baseline and every 6 mo, with discontinuation of amiodarone if over twice the upper limit of normal. Using the medication intravenously may cause severe liver injury, including liver failure, with elevations in enzymes by 10–100 fold.
Hydralazine	Can cause delayed liver injury in a lupuslike syndrome or acute liver injury
Methyldopa	Chronic use is associated with mild elevation in serum aminotransferases in 5%–35% of patients. More rarely do patients present with acute liver injury.
Fibrates	Mild-to-moderate serum transaminase elevations
Niacin	Doses above 500 mg daily cause elevation >3 times ULN of transaminases. Sustained release forms may cause serious hepatotoxicity.
Statins	Associated with mild-to-moderate serum transaminase elevations. Very rarely causes acute liver failure.
Ezetimibe	Associated with transaminase elevations in 0.5%–1.5%
Aspirin	May cause elevated transaminase levels with high-dose therapy. Can have mild increase in alkaline phosphatase and bilirubin.
Clopidogrel	Associated with serum enzyme elevations in 1%–3% of patients
Prasugrel	Similar to clopidogrel
Ticlopidine	Associated with serum transaminase elevations in 4%
Dabigatran	Associated with moderate ALT elevations of >3 times ULN in 1.5%–3% in chronic use
Fondaparinux	Associated with enzyme elevation >3 times normal in 1%–3% patients
Rivaroxaban	Associated with ALT elevation of >3 times normal in 1.5%–3% patients
Apixaban	Associated with serum transaminase elevations >3 times normal in 1%–2% patients
Edoxaban	Associated with serum transaminase elevations >3 times normal in 2%–5% patients
Heparin	Associated with elevated serum transaminase 10%–60% patients
Beta-blockers	Rarely cause elevations in serum transaminase levels
Calcium channel blockers	Associated with elevated serum transaminase levels
Tolvaptan	Studies mixed: some demonstrate no hepatic damage; some show worsened outcomes in cirrhotic patients.
Sidenafil	Associated with hepatocellular and cholestatic injury
Endothelin receptor antagonists	Associated with serum transaminase elevations

[a]This is not a complete list but rather a list of medications that might be used in the CCU.
ACE, angiotensin converting enzyme; ALT, alanine aminotransferase; AST, aspartate aminotransferase; ULN, upper limit of normal.
From https://livertox.nih.gov/.

anyone. However, many medications cause idiosyncratic DILI. In fact, it is estimated that 20 new cases of DILI per 100,000 persons occur each year and that idiosyncratic DILI causes 11% of the cases of acute liver failure in the United States. DILI is classified as hepatic, cholestatic, or mixed based on the abnormalities in alanine aminotransferases and ALP. It mostly presents within 6 months of drug exposure, but can occur within days or up to a year after starting the offending agent.

There are many medications used in the CCU that may contribute to elevated liver tests (**Table 47.3**). These include, but

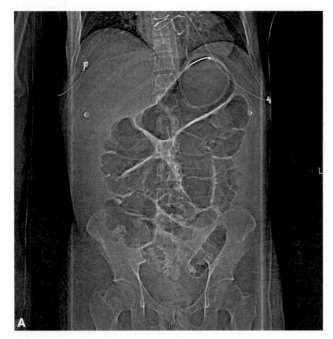 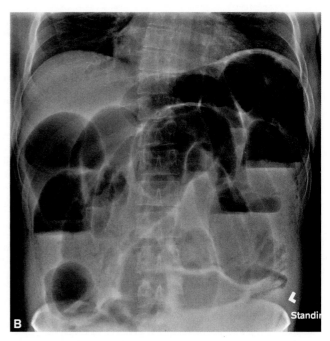

FIGURE 47.1 A, Supine abdominal film in a patient with ileus. Gaseous distention is limited to the small intestine. In this case, ileus was related to a mycotic aneurysm in a branch of the superior mesenteric artery in a patient with infective endocarditis. B, Upright plain film of the abdomen in a patient with organic obstruction, in this case volvulus associated with congenital malrotation. Note the air fluid is at different levels, which is typical for organic obstruction, as opposed to ileus.

are not limited to, aspirin, amiodarone, angiotensin converting enzyme inhibitors, angiotensin receptor blockers, statins, clopidogrel, hydralazine, and diltiazem. Liver function abnormalities during statin therapy have been widely publicized but usually are not a problem in the CCU, though they could be present on admission in a patient recently started on high dose therapy, especially simvastatin or lovastatin, and in the presence of drug–drug interactions, with agents that are CYP3A4 inhibitors. Liver function abnormalities occur less frequently than muscle injury.

Diagnosis is usually made by careful medication history and by eliminating other etiologies of abnormal liver tests with laboratory testing for viral hepatitis, autoimmune hepatitis, etc, and imaging to rule out obstruction. The ultimate diagnosis can be made by liver biopsy, but is not required. Liver tests should normalize with discontinuation of the offending agent. In some cases, the drug-induced injury is chronic. In these cases, improvement is slower, but clinical experience indicates that the transaminases will fall by at least 50% within 2 weeks of drug discontinuation.

INTESTINAL DISTENTION

Intestinal distention is a rather frequent cause of GI consultation for patients in the CCU, especially after open heart surgery. The causes may be mechanical (obstructive) or functional (nonobstructive). The major causes of mechanical obstruction are extrinsic compression, tumor, hernia, adhesion, stricture, volvulus (torsion), and intussusception, and usually are not related to the problems prompting CCU admission. In contrast, intestinal distention after cardiac surgery or myocardial infarction is more likely to be nonobstructive in nature, that is, ileus. The first task when seeing someone with intestinal distention is to differentiate obstruction from ileus. Ileus usually is reversible with treatment of

the underlying causes/exacerbating factors, whereas obstruction may require surgery, sometimes on an urgent basis. The reason for this is that ischemia/infarction occurs when intraluminal and tissue pressures are higher than mean arterial pressure, and pressures are higher in obstruction than in ileus, so that strangulation with ischemia/infarction is more likely with obstruction.

PATHOPHYSIOLOGY

The pathophysiology of ileus is incompletely understood. Historically, ileus was felt to be related to paralysis from toxins, such as in patients with peritonitis. However, experimental studies demonstrated that removal of the distended bowel and rinsing with sterile solution allowed for peristalsis to return spontaneously. Thus, ileus began to be seen as inhibited motility. Toxic megacolon is a special circumstance associated with severe, transmural inflammation, associated with ulcerative colitis or infectious colitis, such as *C. difficile*-associated colitis, which includes systemic toxicity in addition to peritoneal irritation/inflammation.

The mechanisms controlling intestinal motility include neurogenic, myogenic, and humoral factors. Intestinal motility is stimulated by cholinergic impulses and inhibited by adrenergic impulses. Ileus is related either to increased inhibition, decreased excitation, or both. Altered sympathetic/parasympathetic balance due to exaggerated sympathetic tone from retroperitoneal stimulation of thoracic sympathetic ganglia, for example, by blood products in or adjacent to the posterior peritoneum is felt to promote ileus in the small intestine (**Figure 47.1A**). The situation undoubtedly is more complicated because motility also is related to the presence of inflammatory cytokines, perhaps mediated through the activity of nitric oxide and prostaglandins.[20,21] The effects of inflammatory and other mediators are abetted by electrolyte imbalances, particularly calcium, magnesium, and phosphate, acid–base disorders,

TABLE 47.4	Causes of Ileus

Infectious/inflammatory
- Severe sepsis
- Bacterial peritonitis
- Appendicitis
- Diverticulitis
- Cholecystitis
- Pancreatitis
- Pneumonia
- Pulmonary embolism
- Intraperitoneal hemorrhage

Ischemic
- Arterial thrombosis/embolism
- Venous thrombosis
- Nonobstructive mesenteric ischemia
- Mesenteric arteritis
- Strangulation/volvulus

Retroperitoneal processes
- Pyelonephritis
- Retroperitoneal hemorrhage
- Retroperitoneal abscess
- Retroperitoneal malignancy
- Ureteropelvic lithiasis

Drug-induced
- Opiates
- Anticholinergics
- Psychiatric medications

Metabolic
- Electrolyte imbalance—Sodium, potassium, calcium, magnesium, phosphate
- Uremia
- Acidosis

Other
- Laparotomy
- Perforated viscus
- Chronic obstructive pulmonary disease
- Sickle cell disease

This is not a complete list but rather conditions that one might encounter in a CCU. CCU, Cardiac care unit.

as well as by the pharmacologic effects of opiates, calcium channel blockers, and anticholinergics. Vomiting promotes loss of potassium and hydrogen ions. Intraluminal accumulation of fluid leads to losses from the intra- and extravascular compartments, while abdominal distention may limit respiration. Gaseous distention is caused, in large part, by swallowed air, which provides a rationale for nasogastric tube decompression.

Ileus may involve the small bowel or the colon, or both sites (**Table 47.4**). The small bowel is preferentially affected by retroperitoneal processes in the thoracolumbar region, whereas the colon is preferentially affected by retroperitoneal processes in the sacral region. Of note, Ogilvie syndrome, or isolated colonic ileus, was originally related to retroperitoneal malignancies.

DIAGNOSIS

A careful history, physical examination, and review of the medical records are important to uncover historical clues suggestive of

obstructive disorders or ileus; prior abdominal surgery, prior episodes of obstruction, evidence of inguinal or abdominal hernias, prior intestinal cancer or polyps, prior radiation, inflammatory bowel diseases, gallstones, ulcers, and a history of gallstones all raise the possibility of an obstructing lesion. On the other hand, a psychiatric history, certain medications (opiates, psychiatric medications, etc), and endocrine problems such as hypothyroidism may suggest ileus. Fever, rigors, leukocytosis, or hyperlactatemia suggest infection.

It is important to remember that mesenteric ischemia can mimic ileus radiologically as well as symptomatically. Mesenteric ischemia may be arterial or venous in origin and due to atherosclerosis, embolism, or vasculitis.[22] The colon is more vulnerable than the small intestine due to a less rich collateral circulation. Increasingly severe and steady pain in the presence of abdominal distention suggests intestinal infarction, but this is a late sign; a high index of suspicion is needed to lead to a correct diagnosis before infarction occurs. Elevations in serum amylase, ALP, creatine phosphokinase, ALT, AST, and lactate dehydrogenase suggest ischemia or infarction, with enzyme leakage from damaged cells.

Radiologic studies can suggest the etiology of intestinal distention as well as its severity. Air fluid at different levels on an upright film suggests organic obstruction (**Figure 47.1B**). A jejunal diameter of > 3.5 cm is considered worrisome. The diameter of the colon to be considered worrisome is uncertain. Classically, a diameter of > 12 cm is of concern, though patients with chronic distention, such as some patients on chronic psychiatric medications, have greater diameters and are asymptomatic. On the other hand, a rapid increase in diameter is worrisome no matter what the precise diameter is. Cross-sectional studies are helpful in detecting retroperitoneal pathology such as hemorrhage or infection, which may complicate thoracic as well as abdominal surgeries.

MANAGEMENT

For the treatment of organic obstruction, the reader is referred to GI or surgical texts. For the treatment of ileus, supportive care is key, with replacement of fluids and electrolytes as necessary, and the discontinuation of agents that inhibit motility. One should consider nasogastric decompression, especially in the presence of vomiting. One may consider colonic decompression for Ogilvie syndrome if it does not respond to conservative measures with placement of a rectal tube to maintain decompression. A cecostomy should be considered for recurrence of colonic ileus or failure of colonoscopic decompression. It should be emphasized that small intestinal ileus responds to conservative measures in most cases. Endoscopy rarely is needed in patients with ileus, though it may be helpful in patients with proximal obstruction of the small bowel or distal obstruction of the large bowel. If endoscopy is performed, instilling as little air as possible is recommended so as not to exacerbate the situation and to use carbon dioxide for insufflation rather than room air, because it is resorbed much more rapidly.[23]

GASTROINTESTINAL COMPLICATIONS AFTER LEFT VENTRICULAR ASSIST DEVICE IMPLANTATION

GIB rate in patients with left ventricular assist device (LVAD) is frequent and estimated to be 18% to 44%.[24] The causes for GIB may be from use of antithrombotic agents, impaired platelet aggregation, acquired von Willebrand syndrome, and mostly commonly arteriovenous malformations (AVMs) or angiodysplasias in patients who suffer from chronic heart failure. Though the same lessons as described earlier apply to LVAD patients as well, additional precautions need to be taken with special attention to hemodynamics in this cohort. The possibility of obscure sources of GIB should be considered in these patients and a team-based approach is required to navigate these situations.

REFERENCES

1. Friedberg CK. *Diseases of the Heart.* Philadelphia, PA: Saunders; 1949: 1100.

2. Cappell MS. The safety and clinical utility of esophagogastroduodenoscopy for acute gastrointestinal bleeding after myocardial infarction: a six-year study of 42 endoscopies in 34 consecutive patients at two university teaching hospitals. *Am J Gastroenterol.* 1993;88:344-350.

3. Longstreth GF. Epidemiology of hospitalization for acute upper gastrointestinal hemorrhage: a population-based study. *Am J Gastroenterol.* 1995;90:206-210.

4. Sung JJY, Tsoi KK, Ma TK, Yung MY, Lau JY, Chiu PW. Causes of mortality in patients with peptic ulcer bleeding: a prospective cohort study of 10,428 cases. *Am J Gastroenterol.* 2010;105:84-89.

5. Radaelli F, Dentali F, Repici A, et al. Management of anticoagulation in patients with acute gastrointestinal bleeding. *Dig Liver Dis.* 2015;47:621-627.

6. Abraham NS, Singh S, Alexander GC, et al. Comparative risk of gastrointestinal bleeding with dabigatran, rivaroxaban, and warfarin: population based cohort study. *BMJ.* 2015;350:h1857.

7. Chang H-Y, Zhou M, Tang W, Alexander GC, Singh S. Risk of gastrointestinal bleeding associated with oral anticoagulants: population based retrospective cohort study. *BMJ.* 2015;350:h1585.

8. Southworth MR, Reichman ME, Unger EF. Dabigatran and post-marketing reports of bleeding. *N Engl J Med.* 2013;368:1272-1274.

9. Larsen TB, Rasmussen LH, Skjøth F, et al. Efficacy and safety of dabigatran etexilate and warfarin in 'real-world' patients with atrial fibrillation: a prospective nationwide cohort study. *J Am Coll Cardiol.* 2013;61:2264-2273.

10. Shivaraju A, et al. Temporal trends in gastrointestinal bleeding associated with percutaneous coronary intervention: analysis of the 1998–2006 Nationwide Inpatient Sample (NIS) database. *Am Heart J.* 2011;162:1062.e5-1068.e5.

11. Ruff CT, Giugliano RP, Braunwald E, et al. Comparison of the efficacy and safety of new oral anticoagulants with warfarin in patients with atrial fibrillation: a meta-analysis of randomised trials. *Lancet.* 2014;383:955-962.

12. Weitz JI, Pollack CV Jr. Practical management of bleeding in patients receiving non-vitamin K antagonist oral anticoagulants. *Thromb Haemost.* 2015;114:1113-1126.

13. Pollack CV Jr, Reilly PA, Eikelboom J, et al. Idarucizumab for dabigatran reversal. *N Engl J Med.* 2015;373:511-520.

14. Chen C-F, Chen B, Zhu J, Xu Y-Z. Antithrombotic therapy after percutaneous coronary intervention in patients requiring oral anticoagulant treatment. A meta-analysis. *Herz.* 2015;40:1070-1083.

15. Lanas A, García-Rodríguez LA, Polo-Tomás M, et al. Time trends and impact of upper and lower gastrointestinal bleeding and perforation in clinical practice. *Am J Gastroenterol.* 2009;104:1633-1641.

16. Rubin TA, Murdoch M, Nelson DB. Acute GI bleeding in the setting of supratherapeutic international normalized ratio in patients taking warfarin: endoscopic diagnosis, clinical management, and outcomes. *Gastrointest Endosc.* 2003;58:369-373.

17. Northfield TC. Factors predisposing to recurrent haemorrhage after acute gastrointestinal bleeding. *Br Med J.* 1971;1:26-28.

18. Greenwald DA, Brandt LJ, Reinus JF. Ischemic bowel disease in the elderly. *Gastroenterol Clin N Am.* 2001;30:445-473.

19. Guillaume A, Pili-Floury S, Chocron S, et al. Acute mesenteric ischemia among post-cardiac surgery patients presenting with multiple organ failure. *Shock.* 2016. doi:10.1097/SHK.0000000000000720.

20. Eskandari MK, Kalff JC, Billiar TR, Lee KK, Bauer AJ. LPS-induced muscularis macrophage nitric oxide suppresses rat jejunal circular muscle activity. *Am J Physiol.* 1999;277:G478-G486.

21. Hori M, Kita M, Torihashi S, et al. Upregulation of iNOS by COX 2 in muscularis resident macrophage of rat intestine stimulated with LPS. *Am J Physiol Gastrointest Liver Physiol.* 2001;280:G930-G938.

22. Kozuch PL, Brandt LJ. Review article: diagnosis and management of mesenteric ischaemia with an emphasis on pharmacotherapy. *Aliment Pharmacol Ther.* 2005;21:201-215.

23. Wu J, Hu B. The role of carbon dioxide insufflation in colonoscopy: a systematic review and meta-analysis. *Endoscopy.* 2012;44:128-136.

24. Harvey L, Holley CT, John R. Gastrointestinal bleed after left ventricular assist device implantation: incidence, management, and prevention. *Ann Cardiothorac Surg.* 2014;3:475-479.

Patient and Family Information for: GASTROINTESTINAL EMERGENCIES IN THE CARDIAC CARE UNIT

Being in the cardiac care unit can be an overwhelming time for both patients and their families. This can be escalated by other conditions and medical problems that present during a hospitalization. The key to understanding GI and liver diseases in a cardiac patient is to first understand that it involves interdisciplinary care and discussion among the cardiologists and gastroenterologists, with a plan individualized for each patient.

Gastro-Intestinal bleeding (GIB) can occur in any individual. This can be bleeding anywhere in the intestinal tract from the esophagus down to the rectum. Bleeding can be from the upper GI tract, which includes the esophagus, stomach, or first part of the intestines, or from the rest of the intestines, which is considered the lower GI tract. Patients may present with passing blood per rectum, black stools, or coffee-colored or bloody vomitus. If it is severe, it can cause shock with lowered blood pressure and a fast heart rate. Many different conditions can cause bleeding, ranging from an ulcer to a tear in the intestinal lining, hemorrhoids, a bleeding mass, irregular blood vessels called AVMs, to diverticulosis, which is an outpouching in the lining of the intestines. The treatment of the cause of bleed depends on the severity of the bleeding (ie, how much the blood counts drop, how much the blood pressure or heart rate changes, and how quickly blood is being lost). In some instances, it can be treated supportively with fluids, blood products, and certain medications to decrease acid secretion from the stomach. In other situations, patients may require direct visualization with endoscopy or colonoscopy, or CT studies to analyze the blood vessels. In either case, direct treatments may be used to stop the bleeding.

Some patients are at higher risk for bleeding than others. These include sick patients in an intensive care setting, and patients on blood thinners such as most patients with cardiac conditions. Although the incidence of major bleed is low in cardiac patients, it can be life threatening. The gastroenterologists and cardiologists need to assess the severity of bleeding, the potential site that the patient is bleeding from, the type of blood thinners the patient is on, and whether blood thinners can be continued or not. It is a risk and benefit conversation that will have to be individualized based on the patient. If a bleed is severe enough to cause patients to be unstable, then regardless of their cardiac status they may require an invasive procedure. The biggest discussion will be held after the bleeding is controlled about the risks and benefits of using blood thinners in somebody with a recent bleed because blood thinners increase the risk of bleeding further. Again this will be individualized for each patient with discussions among the cardiologist, gastroenterologist, and the patient.

Another problem that arises in patients in the cardiac care unit is abnormal liver function tests. This can be for a few reasons. One is mainly caused by the fact that both the heart and liver work simultaneously to help blood flow throughout the body. Many patients in the cardiac care unit have heart failure. If you can imagine, this can present in two ways. If the heart is failing to pump out blood effectively enough, then there is a lack of blood flow to all organs, including the liver. This results in less oxygen being delivered to the liver and presents as damage to the liver. On the other hand, if the heart cannot fill properly with blood, the blood will back up to all of the organs, including the liver. The liver then becomes congested with blood and can become damaged. These conditions present with elevated liver function tests and should improve with improvement of the heart failure. If heart failure is long standing and not improving, there is a chance that it can lead to liver failure and cirrhosis.

Another situation is when patients have episodes of extremely low blood pressure and decreased blood flow from the heart, which causes less oxygen to be delivered to the liver, resulting in liver damage. The treatment for this is supportive with management of the blood pressure. It will slowly resolve over time and usually does not result in liver failure.

Certain medications, both cardiac and noncardiac medications, can cause elevations in liver tests as well. Usually this is diagnosed when the liver tests get elevated after starting certain medications and after elimination of all other types of liver disease, for example, viral hepatitis. It should resolve with stopping the offending medication. The condition usually is not life threatening, but sometimes can cause chronic problems with the liver. In these instances with elevated liver tests, it is a matter of watching the laboratory values to see if they are improving and if not, patients may require a liver biopsy.

Many patients in the cardiac care unit also do not get out of bed and risk getting distension of the intestines. This differs from patients who have an actual obstruction (from a tumor, scar tissue, hernia, etc) and have a blockage in their intestines. If a patient gets distension of his or her intestines, basic radiologic workup will be done including an X-ray or a CT scan. After that, the treatment depends on whether or not the physicians believe there is an actual obstruction in the intestines. If so, the patient may require surgical intervention, because it can become life threatening. If not, the care is supportive with fluids, ensuring movement (which may be as simple as the nurse turning the patient, or walking), sometimes stopping medications that can induce distension (ie, opiate pain medications), and making sure the patient's potassium and magnesium levels are normal.

Ismini Kourouni
Gopal Narayanswami
Joseph P. Mathew

Line Access in the CCU

INTRODUCTION

Obtaining vascular access in the cardiac care unit (CCU) patient is a potentially lifesaving intervention and an important practical skill for physicians in training to acquire during their critical care rotations. Vascular access is essential for providing lifesaving medications, therapeutic interventions, and also hemodynamic monitoring. Determining the type of catheter needed, appropriate indications, contraindications, and the various considerations for the insertion, maintenance, and timely removal of arterial and venous catheters is important to prevent complications. Knowledge of vascular anatomy, familiarity with the equipment, and competency with the use of ultrasonography (US) are prerequisites for successful insertion of the catheter.

A central venous catheter (CVC) or central line (CL) is defined as a venous intravascular catheter that terminates at or close to the heart or in one of the great vessels. A CVC can be used to provide infusions of vasoactive and other medications, blood products, and also for hemodynamic monitoring. An arterial line (A-line) is an intraarterial catheter placed in a peripheral or central artery and is used for hemodynamic monitoring or for vascular access for procedures such as coronary angiography. The placement of CVCs and A-lines is routine CCU procedure, often performed at the bedside under sterile technique. Vascular access devices (VAD) that may be encountered in the CCU patient include peripheral intravenous (PIV) catheters, triple lumen catheter (TLC), introducer catheter, tunneled and nontunneled hemodialysis catheters, peripherally inserted central catheter (PICC), Swan-Ganz or pulmonary artery catheter (PAC), A-lines, and venous and arterial sheaths.

Not every CCU patient requires a CVC or A-line. The decision to place a line and the choice of site of insertion should be based on a thoughtful assessment by the operator and the CCU team of the patient's anatomy, clinical status, and coagulation profile. All lines should be placed under aseptic technique using a "bundle" or "checklist" as per institutional policy. Real-time ultrasound guidance is recommended for CVC placement in sites such as internal jugular vein (IJV) or femoral vein (FV), as well as any difficult-to-access sites. Once a VAD has been placed, there should be a daily thoughtful assessment of the need for continued use of the catheter. The best way to avoid complications of VAD is to avoid unnecessary placement and remove them as soon as they are no longer necessary.[1]

Although the authors believe that there is no substitute for bedside hands-on learning, we hope this chapter serves as a fundamental quick reference guide for physicians, nurses, physician assistants, nurse practitioners, and other health care practitioners for "frequently asked questions" about VAD encountered in the CCU.

BASIC PRINCIPLES

MATERIAL

Most catheters in the CCU, including PIVs and CVCs, are polyurethane-based catheters, which provide some rigidity to the flexible catheter and prevent kinking. The main adverse effect of these catheters is the risk of vessel perforation, namely that of the superior vena cava (SVC) from a left-sided CVC. Silicone-based catheters are more pliable and have a lower risk of vessel injury, hence are placed for long-term venous access. These catheters need a sheath introducer or an inner dilator or stylet for percutaneous insertion. Examples of silicone-based catheters encountered in the CCU include PICC and some silicone-coated sheath introducers.

SIZE

Catheter size is classified in either gauge (G) or French (F) units. In general, needles or single lumen catheters are sized by gauge and multilumen catheters are measured by French size. Whereas French size and catheter diameter are directly related (the higher the French, the larger the diameter), gauge and size are inversely related (lower gauge indicates larger diameter). The size specifications are generally indicated on the outer packet or insert.[2]

FLOW RATES

A working knowledge of the relationship between catheter size, length, and flow rates is essential in choosing the appropriate catheter for the CCU patient. The rate of flow (Q) across a catheter is directly proportional to the pressure gradient (ΔP) and inversely proportional to the resistance (R) to flow:

$$Q = \Delta P \times \frac{1}{R} \qquad \text{(Eq. 1)}$$

Resistance is directly proportional to the length of the catheter and viscosity (μ) and inversely proportional to the radius

$(r): R = 8\mu \times \text{length}/\pi r^4$. Hence the rate of flow is directly proportional to the inner radius of the catheter and the pressure gradient, and inversely proportional to the length of the catheter and the viscosity of the fluid or blood product being infused. This is based on Poiseuille's law:

$$Q = \frac{\pi r^4 \times \Delta P}{8 \mu \times \text{length}} \qquad \text{(Eq. 2)}$$

This concept is important in the resuscitation of the CCU patient, whether it is for hypovolemia or hemorrhage. Flow rates improve exponentially (r^4) with larger radius catheters, pressure bag application, and with shorter catheters. A large bore catheter that is short is optimal for volume resuscitation. **Table 48.1** lists the flow rates achieved with various devices commonly used in the CCU. So if a patient in the CCU has a major bleeding complication (eg, from femoral arterial sheath removal or gastrointestinal bleeding from antithrombotic agents), a 16-gauge antecubital peripheral IV or an introducer catheter is preferred over a long triple lumen catheter (TLC) or PICC.[3]

TABLE 48.1	Flow Rates and Catheter Size
CATHETER GAUGE AND LENGTH	**FLOW RATE (ML/MIN)**
24G × 0.75″	25
22G × 1.00″	35
20G × 1.00″	65
20G × 1.88″	55
18G × 1.16″	105
18G × 1.88″	95
16G × 1.16″	220
16G × 1.77″	205
TLC	98
16G distal lumen (brown)	52
18G medial lumen (blue)	22
18G proximal lumen (white)	24
PICC	
5F × 50 cm (single lumen)	29
5F × 50 cm (double lumen)	
18G distal lumen	9.6
20G proximal lumen	2.6
Sheath introducer	
8.5F × 10 cm	126
	333 (with pressure bag)

Source: www.BD.com, www.edwards.com, www.arrowintl.com.
PICC, peripherally inserted central catheter; TLC, triple lumen catheter.

PERIPHERAL VENOUS CATHETERS

Any patient admitted to the CCU would be considered a critically ill patient and hence needs at least one peripheral intravenous (IV) catheter. This can be potentially lifesaving when the previously stable cardiac patient becomes unstable, whether it is from a bradyarrhythmia, tachyarrhythmia, or cardiac arrest. Infusates with a pH between 5 and 9 and osmolality < 600 mOsm/L can be delivered via a peripheral catheter. Even vasopressors can be administered emergently through a properly placed peripheral catheter until central venous access is obtained. Due to increased risk of phlebitis with catheter dwell time,[4] most institutions have policies requiring change of peripheral catheters every 72 to 96 hours.[1] A recent randomized controlled study from Australia however showed no difference in adverse outcomes such as phlebitis when peripheral catheters were changed only as clinically indicated.[5]

Most institutions have one of two types of catheters: an over-the-needle cannula (ie, angiocatheter or "angiocath") or a winged catheter set (ie, butterfly) (**Figure 48.1A** and **B**). **Table 48.2** lists a step-by-step approach to placing a PIV. **Figure 48.2** illustrates the venous anatomy of the upper extremity. A proximal site is preferred if the patient is at risk for hemorrhage. In general, an 18G or 20G is preferable because it provides an adequate size for rapid infusion of medications or of contrast if the patient needs a computed tomography (CT) angiogram. Note that catheters in the antecubital fossa (eg, median cubital vein) may kink when the patient bends his or her arm, thus interfering with medication administration. If ultrasound guidance is used to cannulate the basilic or cephalic veins (**Figure 48.2**), a longer angiocatheter is preferred. Avoid sites that may appear injured or infected (ie, cellulitis). Complications include phlebitis (irritation), cellulitis, and bacteremia leading to sepsis. Hematoma, thrombus formation, and nerve injury can occur from multiple unsuccessful attempts. Infiltration of fluid around the IV site is not uncommon; however,

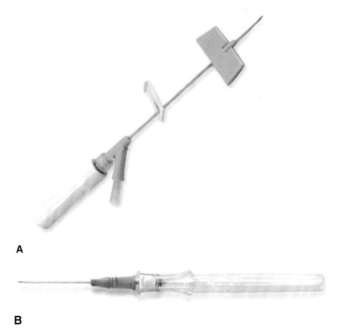

A

B

FIGURE 48.1 A, Winged peripheral IV catheter system. B, Over-the-needle angiocatheter with retractable needle.

TABLE 48.2	Peripheral IV Insertion Procedural Checklist
STEP	**DESCRIPTION**
1	Perform hand hygiene and organize equipment.
2	Explain procedure to patient.
3	Apply tourniquet on selected arm, 3 to 5 inches above the elbow.
4	Ask patient to open and close hand or hang arm to gravity.
5	Inspect arm for veins with largest diameter and fewest branch points.
6	Sterilize insertion site with chlorhexidine, alcohol, or povidone iodine.
7	Stabilize vein with nondominant hand by holding skin taut.
8	**Winged catheter system (butterfly)**
	a. Hold the system with thumb and forefinger on the finger grips.
	b. Access the vessel at a low 10 to 30 degrees angle.
	c. Visualize blood return along the catheter, then up the extension tube.
	d. Lower needle and advance the entire catheter and needle unit.
	e. Stabilize the system and pull back until the push-tab component releases from the device.
	f. Discard shielded needle into sharps container.
9	**Over-the-needle (angiocatheter)**
	a. Hold device by ribbed needle housing using dominant hand.
	b. Insert catheter using dominant hand with bevel up at 10 to 30 degrees angle in direction of vein.
	c. Observe for blood return through flashback chamber.
	d. Advance 2 to 3 mm and lower needle until flush with skin.
	e. Gently advance catheter into vein until hub rests at puncture site.
	f. Stabilize cannula and release tourniquet with nondominant hand.
	g. Use one finger to apply pressure over catheter tip to stop blood flow.
	h. Slide off needle or press safety button to retract needle.
	i. Dispose needle in sharps container.
10	Attach extension set and flush with normal saline.
11	Secure catheter with tape and transparent occlusive dressing.
12	Ensure that sterility is maintained throughout the procedure.

IV, intravenous.

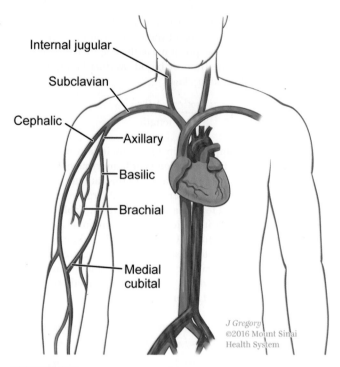

FIGURE 48.2 Venous anatomy of the neck and upper extremity.

extravasation of medications such as vasopressors and vesicants can lead to localized swelling and vascular compromise. Any early signs of minor or major complications should lead to removal of the catheter. Warm compresses and arm elevation can be used to treat phlebitis and extravasation.

CENTRAL VENOUS CATHETERS

OVERVIEW

A CVC is defined as a venous intravascular catheter that terminates at or close to the heart, in one of the great vessels. In the United States the Centers for Disease Control and Prevention (CDC) estimates that over 5 million CVCs are placed each year leading to 15 million central line days per year.[1] A CVC can be used for administration of select medications and blood products, central venous pressure (CVP) monitoring, and sampling of central venous blood. Additionally, in the CCU, an introducer catheter can allow introduction of a transvenous pacer (TVP) or a Swan-Ganz catheter. The vessels that are commonly cannulated for obtaining central venous access are the IJV, the subclavian vein (SCV) (**Figure 48.2**), and the FV. CVCs can also be used for hemodialysis, plasmapheresis, chemotherapy, and parenteral nutrition.

CVCs are available with antimicrobial impregnation (eg, chlorhexidine-silver sulfadiazine, minocycline-rifampin) and these are used when the anticipated use is over 5 days. Studies have shown a lower incidence of bacterial colonization and lower rate of central line-associated blood stream infection (CLABSI) when antimicrobial-coated CVCs are used.[6] A working knowledge of the indications and contraindications for CVC placement, as well as the principles for its insertion, maintenance, and removal is essential.

TYPES OF CENTRAL VENOUS CATHETERS

In the CCU, there are five main types of catheters that are used for central access. The most commonly used line is the TLC because it provides multiple lumens for infusion of medications and fluids (**Figure 48.3A** and **B**). Nontunneled hemodialysis catheters (**Figure 48.3C**) are often placed in the CCU for intermittent hemodialysis or continuous renal replacement therapy.

Sheath introducers (**Figure 48.3D**) are usually single lumen and can be placed in the venous or arterial system. These can be used for insertion of a temporary pacemaker (venous circulation) and are also often left in place after left heart catheterization (arterial circulation). The Swan-Ganz catheter (**Figure 48.3E**) or PAC can be placed through a sheath introducer into the pulmonary artery. See Chapter 49 for a full discussion of invasive hemodynamic monitoring including CVP and pulmonary artery

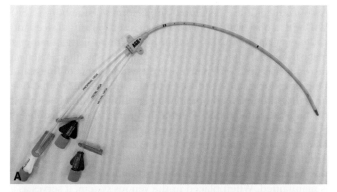

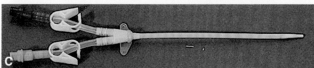

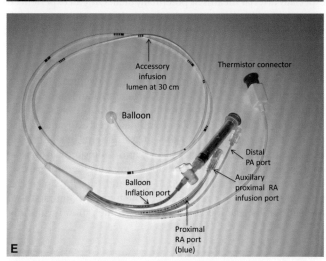

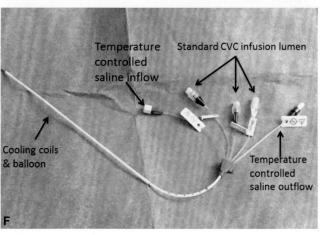

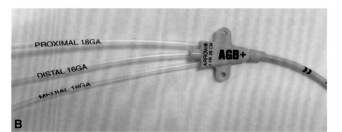

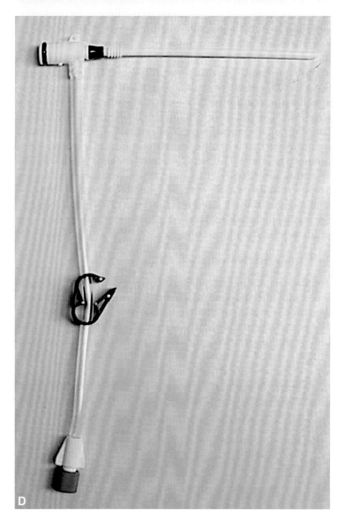

FIGURE 48.3 A, Triple lumen catheter. B, Three ports of the triple lumen catheter. C, Nontunneled hemodialysis catheter. D, Sheath introducer. E, Swan-Ganz or pulmonary artery catheter. F, Cooling catheter. CVC, central venous catheter. RA, Right atrium; PA, Pulmonary artery.

catheterization. PICC lines are often placed in the CCU patient for long-term vascular access for medications such as antibiotics. A PICC line is considered a central line as the tip ends in the SVC. Intravascular cooling catheters (**Figure 48.3F**) may be used to induce therapeutic hypothermia in the CCU patient who is post cardiac arrest. Other central catheters one may encounter in the CCU patient include long-term VADs such as tunneled hemodialysis catheters, Hickman catheters, and Ports, which are not discussed in this chapter.

Triple Lumen Catheter

The TLC has three ports: proximal (white, 18G), medial (blue, 18G), and distal (brown, 16G) in relation to the site where the line enters the patient (**Figure 48.3B**). **Table 48.3** summarizes their basic characteristics. The catheter is easily inserted at the bedside either electively or during emergencies. It is sutured at an appropriate length based on the patient's height and insertion site (see section on technique). The catheter is typically made of polyurethane and is radiopaque so the tip can be easily visualized on a chest radiograph. The tip should be in the SVC, at the junction of the SVC, and the right atrium (RA). The three lumens allow infusion of multiple, even incompatible solutions, at the same time. The distal port (brown, 16G) has the fastest flow rate and is used for resuscitation fluids and blood products, as well as for monitoring CVP because it gives the most accurate waveform. The distal port should also be used for venous blood sampling such as measurement of central venous oxygen saturation ($Scvo_2$), as it has the fastest flow rate and is closest to the pulmonary artery. The $Scvo_2$ is a surrogate for mixed venous O_2 saturation (Svo_2). TLCs with continuous measurement of $Scvo_2$ are available as well (PreSep catheter, Edwards). If hyperalimentation or total parenteral nutrition (TPN) is anticipated, the medial lumen should be dedicated solely for this purpose in order to limit risk of infection.

Nontunneled Hemodialysis Catheter

These are double lumen catheters (**Figure 48.3C**) for hemodialysis access with internal diameter of approximately 12G to accommodate high flow rates needed for hemodialysis or plasmapheresis. The catheters typically have a brown port and a blue port. The blue is the distal port from which the wire appears. Blood is drawn from the brown port into the dialyzer machine and the dialyzed blood is returned via the blue port. The ports should be reserved only for hemodialysis, except in a life-threatening emergency. Hemodialysis catheters are placed in either the IJV or CFV; the SCV is avoided due to the risk of SCV stenosis or thrombosis, especially if arteriovenous fistula (AVF) creation is anticipated for long-term access.

Sheath Introducer

An introducer is an "L-shaped" single lumen, large bore (>8F) VAD with a port, which can be used to insert various devices and catheters (**Figure 48.3D**). The short length and large diameter make it an ideal catheter for large volume resuscitation. When an introducer is used with a pressurized system, liters of fluids and blood products can be infused within minutes. Since it has one lumen, additional incompatible medications cannot be infused through the same lumen. Double and triple lumen introducers are available and have the advantage of additional ports for medication infusion, however at the expense of a lower flow rate. Additionally, in an emergency, a TLC can be potentially inserted through an introducer for additional lumen, provided sterility is maintained. When placed in the venous system, it serves as a conduit for introduction of devices and catheters, like a TVP or PAC for right heart catheterization (RHC). When placed in the arterial system, introducers are used for procedures such as left heart catheterization. Accidental removal of sheath introducers, especially arterial sheaths, is potentially fatal. Only an experienced operator should remove arterial sheaths because it carries a high risk of hemorrhage and death.

Pulmonary Artery Catheter

The PAC or Swan-Ganz catheter is a long quadruple lumen thermodilution catheter used for invasive hemodynamic monitoring (**Figure 48.3E**). It is inserted through a sheath introducer under sterile technique and the balloon inflated before advancing into the pulmonary artery. It provides measurements of right atrial, right ventricular, pulmonary artery, and pulmonary artery occlusion pressures (PAOP), and allows measurement of cardiac output and oxygenation (Svo_2). Although the PAC provides extremely useful information about the hemodynamic status of the patient, its role has diminished as studies show it does not

TABLE 48.3			Port Characteristics of the Triple Lumen Catheter		
LUMEN	**COLOR**	**GAUGE**	**LOCATION**	**RECOMMENDED USES**	
Distal	Brown	16	Catheter tip	1.	Central venous pressure monitoring
				2.	Administration of viscous, high volume of fluids, or blood products
				3.	Medication administration
				4.	Blood sampling
Medial	Blue	18	2.2 cm from distal	1.	TPN or cap for future TPN use
				2.	Medication administration (if TPN is not anticipated)
Proximal	White	18	2.2 cm from medial	1.	Medication administration
				2.	Blood administration

The colors may vary depending on the manufacturer.
TPN, total parenteral nutrition.

change clinical outcomes. Nevertheless, the PAC does provide useful information and is still utilized in CCUs and cardiothoracic ICUs, both for diagnosis and monitoring of shock states, as well as postoperative management of the cardiac surgery patient. The PAC is reviewed in detail in Chapter 49.

Intravascular Cooling Catheter

With the advent of therapeutic hypothermia after cardiac arrest, targeted temperature management of post cardiac arrest patients is often performed in the CCU. Intravascular cooling catheters can have a built-in temperature sensor that allows for precise control. It controls the temperature of saline circulating through catheter balloons via remote sensing of the patient's temperature (Zoll IVTM Catheters, Chelmsford, MA). The catheters can come with additional lumens that can be used for vascular access. The patient is cooled or warmed as venous blood passes over each balloon, exchanging heat without infusing saline into the patient. This allows for cooling to targeted temperature for the induction of hypothermia and precise temperature control during the rewarming and maintenance phase of therapeutic hypothermia.

ECMO Catheter

Extracorporeal membrane oxygenation (ECMO) is being increasingly used for prolonged mechanical cardiopulmonary support and is often delivered in the CCU or cardiothoracic ICU. Venoarterial (VA) ECMO is used for patients with cardiac failure and venovenous (VV) ECMO is used for severe acute respiratory failure. ECMO catheters are much larger (13F to 31F) and usually placed percutaneously by surgeons, typically by a modified Seldinger technique, using serial dilators to accommodate the large size. The major complications to monitor for are bleeding and limb ischemia.

Peripherally Inserted Central Catheter and Midline Catheters

PICC lines are placed for long-term venous access for intravenous medications and other therapeutics. They are usually placed in the interventional radiology (IR) suite by the IR service or at the bedside by a PICC service or an intensivist. They are inserted using ultrasound guidance into the basilic, cephalic, or brachial vein (**Figure 48.2**) through a small introducer. PICCs come with single, double, or even triple lumen and are sometimes placed in lieu of a TLC because they carry a lower risk of complications. Vasoactive agents, TPN, and caustic medications can be administered through a PICC; however, it is not an optimal line for resuscitation in a critically ill patient, especially if it is single lumen. In the CCU, they are inserted in patients with poor venous access or in patients who are being transferred to medical floor who need long-term vascular access (ie, antibiotics for endocarditis).

Midline catheters are long catheters (3 to 8 inches) that are placed in the brachial, basilic, or cephalic vein, however these are NOT considered central lines. These can remain in place for up to 30 days and often obviate the need for a central line. The infection risk with midline catheters is low and comparable to a peripheral IV.[7]

INDICATIONS FOR CENTRAL ACCESS IN THE CCU

Vascular access is crucial in the CCU patient and can often be challenging in the setting of difficult venous access, prior IV drug use, or in the context of a deteriorating patient or one in cardiac arrest. **Table 48.4** lists common indications for central access in the CCU patient. In general terms, cannulation of a central vein allows for five main scenarios:

1. Medication administration: Administration of medications contraindicated for peripheral access or when the latter is unobtainable (**Table 48.5**).
2. Hemodynamic monitoring: Measurement of parameters such as CVP and Scvo$_2$. PAC allows for measurement of cardiac output and PAOP, which can be used to guide treatment.
3. Extracorporeal therapies: Central access is needed for hemodialysis and other forms of renal replacement therapy, plasmapheresis, and ECMO.
4. Introduction of catheters: An introducer is necessary for advanced procedures performed in the CCU such as pulmonary artery catheterization and transvenous cardiac pacing.
5. Volume loading: Although fluid resuscitation is not an indication for central access, large bore introducers are very helpful in massive resuscitation with fluids or multiple blood products. Patients often are in shock and need vasoactive agents as well; hence central access is preferred.

TABLE 48.4	Indications for Central Access in the CCU
THERAPEUTIC PURPOSES	
Administration of vasoactive medications: vasopressors, inotropes	
Administration of blood products	
Aspiration for venous air embolism	
Hemodialysis	
Plasmapheresis	
INVASIVE MONITORING	
Hemodynamic monitoring	
Central venous pressure monitoring	
Central venous oxygen saturation (Scvo$_2$)	
Pulmonary artery catheterization	
Transvenous cardiac pacing	
Intra-aortic balloon pump	
Left ventricular assist device	
MEDICATION ADMINISTRATION	
Drugs with a pH < 5 and > 9	
Venous irritants regardless of pH or concentration	
Nutritional support (total parenteral nutrition)	
VASCULAR ACCESS	
Emergency venous access	
Lack of peripheral access	
Massive transfusion	

CCU, cardiac care unit.

TABLE 48.5	Medications to be Infused Through a Central Line	
DRUG	**CLASS**	**COMMENT**
Amiodarone (Cordarone)	Antiarrhythmic	Central line preferred if concentration >2 mg/mL
Calcium chloride	Electrolyte	Standard concentration (1 g/50 mL) contains three times more elemental calcium than calcium gluconate; at risk for precipitation, so CVC recommended except in case of cardiac arrest.
Dextrose in water	Nutrition/fluid	CVC preferred in high concentrations (>10%)
Dobutamine (Dobutrex)	Inotrope	Inotrope used to improve CO. Low fixed doses can be given temporarily via peripheral IV depending on institutional policy.
Dopamine (Intropin)	Adrenergic agent	Low fixed doses can be given via peripheral access depending on institutional policy.
Epinephrine (Adrenalin)	Adrenergic agent	Potent vasoconstrictor; concern for extravasation. Cardiac arrest dose (1 mg of 1:10,000) can be given peripherally.
Esmolol (Brevibloc)	Beta blocker	Short-acting beta blocker infusion; central access preferred but can be given peripherally.
Milrinone (Primacor)	Inotrope/vasodilator	Central access preferred but can be given peripherally.
Nicardipine (Cardene)	Calcium channel blocker	Venous irritant; can be infused through large peripheral IV but change site every 12 h.
Nitroglycerin	Vasodilator	Central access preferred but can be given peripherally.
Norepinephrine (Levophed)	Adrenergic agent	Potent alpha adrenergic agent, vasoconstrictor; concern for extravasation.
Phenylephrine (Neo-Synephrine)	Adrenergic agent	Works mainly on alpha adrenergic receptors. Low-dose boluses and low fixed-dose infusion can be given temporarily via peripheral access depending on institutional policy.
Potassium chloride (KCl)	Electrolyte	High concentrations (20 mEq/50 mL) infused via CVC
Sodium chloride (NaCl)	Electrolyte	Hypertonic solutions (≥ 3%) given via central line
Vasopressin (Pitressin)	Vasopressor	Vasoconstrictor; concern for extravasation

This is a limited list of medications that may be encountered in the CCU. Check your institutional policy for medications that have to be infused through a central line. Exceptions may be made during emergencies.
CCU, cardiac care unit; CO, cardiac output; CVC, central venous catheter.

PRECAUTIONS AND CONTRAINDICATIONS

Once the patient meets criteria of appropriateness for central line placement, it is the clinician's duty to assess for contraindications specific to each potential site. As CCU patients are all critically ill, contraindications are all relative. The operator must balance the risks and benefits to truly assess the need for the CVC. **Tables 48.6** and **48.7** summarize some absolute and relative contraindications, as well as site-specific relative contraindications for central line placement. Absolute contraindications at a particular site include distorted anatomy or trauma, infected skin or soft tissue, thrombosis, existing lines or devices, and vascular injury at that site. Relative contraindications include coagulopathy and bleeding disorders; however, these patients may need emergent vascular access so the benefits must be weighed against the risks. Examples include the patient with thrombotic thrombocytopenic purpura who needs plasmapheresis or the patient on aspirin, clopidogrel, and warfarin presenting with cardiogenic shock. Efforts should be made to correct major coagulopathy; however, emergent central venous access can be potentially lifesaving and should not be delayed as a result.[8]

Laboratory results and use of US may alleviate some of these contraindications. The use of ultrasound imaging is an important tool for identifying preexisting thrombus formation and anatomic variations in the IJV location, and allows for a safer and more successful line placement.[9] Additionally, operator experience is a major factor with regard to overcoming relative contraindications and limiting risk of complications. Simulation-based training has been shown to improve success rates and decrease both infectious and mechanical complications rates among trainees.[10–12]

SITE SELECTION IN THE CCU PATIENT

The operator must have an individualized approach to the CCU patient, performing a thoughtful assessment to determine the safest location of insertion, the safest method, and the appropriate periprocedural care. This will depend mostly on the experience and skill of the operator. **Figure 48.4** illustrates site-specific considerations when choosing the insertion site for central line placement. **Table 48.8** lists the anatomic landmarks to identify for each site and also the advantages, disadvantages, and complications associated with each site.

TABLE 48.6	Contraindications and Considerations for Central Line Placement

ABSOLUTE CONTRAINDICATIONS

Patient refuses

Uncooperative patient

Site specific:

- Skin or soft tissue infection

- Venous thrombosis

- Prior radiation or sclerosing agent

- Vascular injury

Superior vena cava or inferior vena cava injury or thrombosis

Expected risk outweighs any benefit

Presence of line, pacemaker, or defibrillator on the same side

Presence of fistula on the same side

RELATIVE CONTRAINDICATIONS

Moderate to severe thrombocytopenia

Uncorrected coagulopathy

Suspected stenosis of the target vein (hemodialysis patients)

Presence of arteriovenous Fistula

Multiple failed attempts (>2 attempts)

Patient cannot tolerate or has contraindication to Trendelenburg position (ie, stroke or intracranial hemorrhage with elevated intracranial pressure)

Mechanical ventilation on patient on high positive end-expiratory pressure (PEEP)

Hemothorax or pneumothorax on the contralateral side

Whole lung atelectasis or pneumonia in contralateral side

CONSIDERATIONS FOR AVOIDANCE OF CENTRAL ACCESS IN HOMONYMOUS SIDE

Anticipated need for limb alert in patient who will require long-term dialysis

Anticipated need for limb alert in patient who will require long-term implantable cardioverter defibrillator/permanent pacemaker

Lymphadenectomy in homonymous side after mastectomy or radiation therapy

TABLE 48.7	Site-specific Relative Contraindications for Central Line Placement

SUBCLAVIAN VEIN

Severe chronic obstructive pulmonary disease

Contralateral pneumothorax

Whole lung atelectasis or pneumonia in contralateral side

Mechanical ventilation with high positive end-expiratory pressure or oxygenation requirements

Morbid obesity or extreme cachexia

Major coagulopathy or bleeding risk—noncompressible site

Fracture of ipsilateral clavicle or anterior proximal ribs

Inability to lie in Trendelenburg position

Left bundle branch block—guide wire can potentially induce complete heart block

INTERNAL JUGULAR VEIN

Cervical spine immobilization

History of intravenous drug use

Inability to lie in Trendelenburg position

Whole lung atelectasis or pneumonia in contralateral side

Left bundle branch block—guide wire can potentially induce complete heart block

FEMORAL VEIN

Avoid site if possible, especially if patient is ambulatory

Ipsilateral deep vein thrombosis

Large pannus

Fungal skin infection

and attempt cannulation preferably on the same side as the lung pathology (ie, perform right IJV or subclavian CVC if the patient has pneumonia in the right lung). Causing a pneumothorax on the normal lung is potentially fatal. Always check a chest radiograph after unsuccessful attempts at IJV or subclavian CVC, prior to trying on the opposite side. Monitor for bleeding complications during and after CVC cannulation. A hematoma in the neck due to inadvertent puncture of the carotid artery can potentially lead to airway compromise by compressing the trachea. The subclavian site is noncompressible; so accidental cannulation of the subclavian artery may need intervention by a vascular surgeon. Similarly, bleeding in the FV or artery site can be very extensive before being recognized.

SITE-SPECIFIC CONSIDERATIONS

Subclavian Vein

The subclavian site is the most preferable site because it carries the lowest risk of CLABSI and thrombosis when compared to IJV

GENERAL RULES

As with any procedure, the operator should always weigh the risks and benefits of placing a central line at a particular site in order to avoid a high-risk complication. The operator should only attempt at a site where he or she is comfortable placing the CVC. With the popularity of US, many junior operators are very comfortable with US-guided CVC and may not feel as confident with SCV access. Always review the chest radiograph

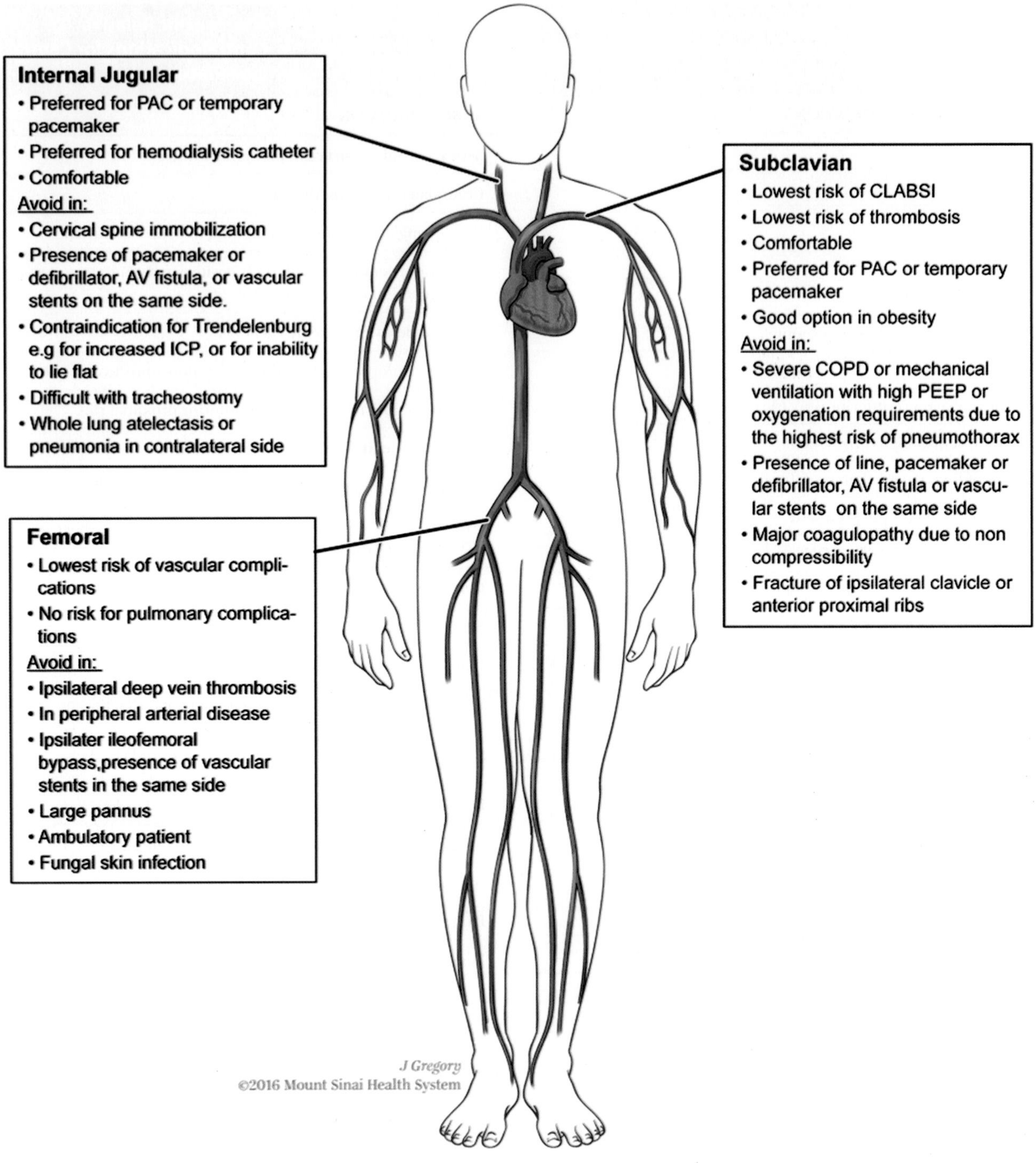

Internal Jugular
- Preferred for PAC or temporary pacemaker
- Preferred for hemodialysis catheter
- Comfortable

Avoid in:
- Cervical spine immobilization
- Presence of pacemaker or defibrillator, AV fistula, or vascular stents on the same side.
- Contraindication for Trendelenburg e.g for increased ICP, or for inability to lie flat
- Difficult with tracheostomy
- Whole lung atelectasis or pneumonia in contralateral side

Subclavian
- Lowest risk of CLABSI
- Lowest risk of thrombosis
- Comfortable
- Preferred for PAC or temporary pacemaker
- Good option in obesity

Avoid in:
- Severe COPD or mechanical ventilation with high PEEP or oxygenation requirements due to the highest risk of pneumothorax
- Presence of line, pacemaker or defibrillator, AV fistula or vascular stents on the same side
- Major coagulopathy due to non compressibility
- Fracture of ipsilateral clavicle or anterior proximal ribs

Femoral
- Lowest risk of vascular complications
- No risk for pulmonary complications

Avoid in:
- Ipsilateral deep vein thrombosis
- In peripheral arterial disease
- Ipsilater ileofemoral bypass, presence of vascular stents in the same side
- Large pannus
- Ambulatory patient
- Fungal skin infection

J Gregory
©2016 Mount Sinai Health System

FIGURE 48.4 Site-specific considerations for central line placement. AV, arteriovenous; CLABSI, central line-associated blood stream infection; COPD, chronic obstructive pulmonary disease; ICP, intracranial pressure; PAC, pulmonary artery catheterization; PEEP, positive end-expiratory pressure.

or FV catheters; however, it has a higher risk of pneumothorax.[13] Additionally, once placed, it is a comfortable site for the patient and the catheter itself is tucked under the clavicle and less likely to be manipulated with patient movement. Accessing the SCV requires placement of the cannulation needle under the clavicle and near the apex of the lung, so it is not surprising that pneumothorax is a potential complication. Avoid SCV catheterization in patients with lung hyperinflation due to severe chronic obstructive pulmonary disease (COPD) or asthma, high F_{IO_2} and positive end-expiratory pressure while on mechanical ventilation, and patients with parenchymal lung disease and limited pulmonary reserve. Also avoid subclavian access in patients with chest wall deformities, cachexia, or morbid obesity.

Internal Jugular Vein

This is a very popular site because it is easily accessed with ultrasonography.[9] The IJV is located under the sternocleidomastoid

TABLE 48.8		Site-specific Landmarks, Advantages, Disadvantages, and Complications		
SITE	**LANDMARKS**	**ADVANTAGES**	**DISADVANTAGES**	**COMPLICATIONS**
Internal jugular vein	Mandibular angle	Easy to locate, especially with US	Easily collapsible	Carotid puncture
	Heads of sternocleidomastoid (SCM)	Straight path to superior vena cava	Proximity to: • Carotid artery • Lung apex • Thoracic duct • Phrenic/vagus nerve	Infection Thrombosis
	Clavicle	Low complication rate		Pneumothorax
		Low maintenance from nursing standpoint	Higher infection rate	Arrhythmia
		Preferred site for pulmonary artery catheter (PAC)	Not preferred for short neck Difficult access during emergencies	Pleural effusion Chylothorax
		Low risk for malposition	Need chest X-ray confirmation	Brachial plexus injury
		Lower risk of pneumothorax	Dressings hard to maintain	Air embolism
Subclavian vein	Clavicle	Low infection rate	Noncompressible site if bleeding	Arterial puncture
	Suprasternal notch	Low risk for thrombosis	Avoid in coagulopathy, cachexia, high PEEP	Pneumothorax
	Manubriosternal junction	Easily maintained	Proximity to lung apex, thoracic duct	Hemothorax
	2 portions of SCM	Patient comfort	High risk for malposition (crossing to contralateral subclavian or ipsilateral internal jugular vein)	Infection Thrombosis
		Bony landmarks, even in obesity	Need chest X-ray confirmation	Arrhythmia
				Air embolism
				Chylothorax
				Pleural effusion
				Subclavian stenosis
Femoral vein	Inguinal ligament	Fast, easily accessed	Highest risk for infection	Infection
	Laterally to pubic tubercle	High success rate	Highest risk for thrombosis	Thrombosis
	VAN (from medial to lateral: *vein, artery, nerve*)	Can be used immediately	Proximity to femoral artery	Arterial puncture
		Preferred for emergencies/cardiac arrest	No central venous pressure monitoring Scvo$_2$ less reliable	Retroperitoneal hematoma
		Preferred for patient in respiratory distress or on high PEEP	Prevents mobility Dressing changes take longer	Arteriovenous fistula Pseudoaneurysm
		No risk of pneumothorax		Inferior vena cava filter dislodgement
				Air embolism

muscle (SCM) on either side of the neck. The right side of the neck is preferred because the vessels run a straight course to the RA. This side is preferred for PAC or temporary pacemaker placement, and hemodialysis catheter placement. IJV cannulation may be difficult in patients with tracheostomies because the tracheostomy holder often overlies the site. Additionally, oral and tracheal secretions from patients on mechanical ventilation often contaminate the IJV site, hence a transparent dressing is essential to secure the catheter and prevent CLABSI.

Femoral Vein

The FV site is associated with the fewest vascular and pulmonary complications; however it carries a higher infection rate and hence is discouraged by the CDC.[1] Interestingly, in a recent study comparing the three sites, there was no significant difference between the IJV and FV sites in rates of CLABSI; however, colonization rates were higher in the femoral site.[13] This site often limits the patient's ability to sit and walk, which can lead to deconditioning. Larger central catheters such as introducers and dialysis catheters are at risk for accidental displacement, which can potentially lead to massive hemorrhage. The FV is the choice of site for central venous catheterization during emergencies such as cardiac arrest (intraosseous access is another option) or in a patient who is in respiratory distress or agitated. It also has the added advantage in that placement does not have to be confirmed with a chest X-ray and so it can be used right away to administer lifesaving medications.

CATHETER-SPECIFIC CONSIDERATIONS

Introducer Catheter

An introducer for vascular access and resuscitation can be placed at any of three sites. If placing an introducer for insertion of PAC or temporary venous pacer in the CCU, right IJV access is preferred for direct access to the right heart. FV access for pulmonary artery catheterization is typically performed in the cardiac catheterization laboratory under fluoroscopic guidance.

Nontunneled Hemodialysis Catheter

A right IJV or FV catheter is preferred for central access for the initiation of hemodialysis in the CCU. The KDIGO guidelines for acute kidney injury (AKI) recommend (ungraded recommendation) in the order of preference: right IJV, followed by FV, then left IJV, and lastly, SCV with preference for the dominant side.[14] The subclavian and left IJV sites should ideally be avoided to limit risk of central venous stenosis. Although, the femoral site has been associated with increased risk of CLABSI, the CATHEDIA study demonstrated a lower catheter colonization rate in the FV site compared to IJV site in patients with body mass index (BMI) < 24.2 and a lower rate at the IJV site in patients with BMI > 28.4.[15]

CENTRAL VENOUS CATHETER PLACEMENT

Preparation and setup are key to successful CVC placement. Take time to optimize the setup by adjusting the height of the bed, procedure tray, and arrange the individual items in the order that they will be used. Always check the patient's platelet count, coagulation profile, and medication list (eg, anticoagulants, especially newer oral anticoagulants) prior to attempt.

STERILE TECHNIQUE

These catheters should be placed under the utmost sterile, operating room-like conditions. Always alert the CCU team including nursing and ancillary staff that a sterile procedure is going to be performed. Transit in and out of the room should be limited and anyone entering or leaving the room should wear a hat and a mask.

ULTRASOUND GUIDANCE

Numerous studies have shown that ultrasound guidance increases the first-attempt success rates and decreases mechanical and infectious complications.[9,11,16–18] The use of US for CVC placement is strongly advocated by various organizations such as the Agency for Health Care Research and Quality (AHRQ),[19] American Society of Anesthesiology,[20] American College of Surgeons,[21] American Society of Echocardiography, and Society of Cardiovascular Anesthesiologists.[22] Ultrasound guidance allows the operator to identify the target vessel and ensure that there is no thrombus within the vessel; it allows for real-time visualization of the needle during the cannulation. Additionally, it allows confirmation of venous placement of the guide wire before dilation and placement of the catheter. Studies have shown significant variation in the size of the central vein and its position with respect to the artery (ie, deep to the artery or directly over the artery), allowing for the possibility of arterial puncture. Landmark methods lead to failure rates as high as 36%, even in experienced hands.[9,18]

US guidance is most useful for IJV and FV cannulation. Although US guidance can be used successfully for SCV access,[16] it has a steeper learning curve and should only be performed by experienced operators due to the risk of pneumothorax. Prior to inserting a central line using US guidance, the operator should perform a preprocedural scan. The portable US machine should be set to the "vascular" preset. A high-frequency linear array (ie, vascular) transducer or probe is used for this purpose because it images superficial structures well. The operator should hold the probe like a pencil with the hypothenar eminence steady on the patient's body. This allows for a steady image during the actual procedure. The marker on the transducer should always be "operator left" to match the marker on the upper left-hand corner of the screen of the US machine. Hence, the left side of the US probe corresponds to the left side of the screen. With this setup, in order to aim the needle left, one would advance the needle to the left, and vice versa. Ultrasound gel should be used as a medium to obtain the images. The depth should be adjusted such that the vessel of interest is in the center of the screen and the gain (brightness) should be optimized to ensure the image is not too bright and not too dark. Arteries have thick walls and are pulsatile, whereas veins have thin walls and are easily collapsible when pressure is applied over the vein. Bear in mind that in profound shock states, the artery may also be collapsible; however, it will still be pulsatile. Color Doppler or pulsed Doppler can be used to further confirm arterial versus venous flow.

In the short-axis or transverse plane, the vessels will appear as round circles (**Figure 48.5A**) as the ultrasound beam intersects the vessel in a cross section at a perpendicular angle.[23] In the long-axis or longitudinal view, the ultrasound beam is parallel to the vessels and the vessels will appear as long cylinders if the beam transects the vessel in the middle along its course (**Figure 48.5B**). Ensure the vein and artery are parallel to each

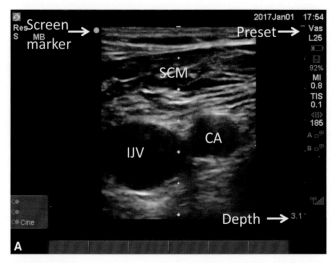
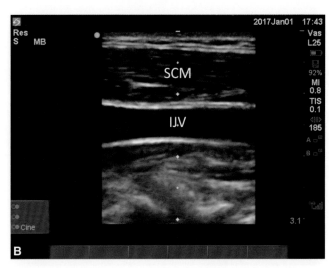

FIGURE 48.5 A, Short axis view of IJV. B, Longitudinal view of IJV. CA, carotid artery; IJV, internal jugular vein; SCM, sternocleidomastoid muscle.

other and not on top of each other. **Figure 48.6A** and **B** demonstrate examples of unsafe sites for cannulation as the carotid artery and IJV are not parallel to each other. Gentle side-to-side tilting of the transducer can often assist in optimizing the vessels such that they are parallel to each other. Image the vein up and down in the transverse view to ensure patency. Do a compression maneuver by applying gentle pressure in at least three sites to ensure there is no thrombus (**Figure 48.7**). This is a leading cause of unsuccessful CVC placement; so avoid the site and order a comprehensive study through the radiology department. **Figure 48.8A** and **B** show examples of intraluminal thrombus detected prior to IJV CVC placement. This patient actually had left IJV thrombophlebitis due to *Fusobacterium necrophorum* sepsis with septic emboli to the lungs and other organs, also known as Lemierre syndrome. **Figure 48.9A** and **B** show the CT scan of the neck to correlate with the US findings. **Table 48.9** summarizes

the steps for preprocedural ultrasound scan, which should always be done prior to US-guided line placement.

Once a safe site is identified, cannulation should be performed with the thin-walled introducer needle with the needle inserted at a steep angle (70 to 90 degrees) and directly beneath the center marker of the probe. The US probe is held steadily with the nondominant hand and the needle advanced with the dominant hand. The needle and syringe apparatus may have to be jiggled gently because it is being advanced in order to appreciate the needle on the screen. Once there is good blood flow, the angle should be decreased prior to inserting the guide wire. Alternatively, a lower angle (30 to 60 degrees) can be used with the ultrasound probe being advanced as the needle is being advanced, with gentle back-and-forth sweeping of the probe to identify and follow the tip of the introducer needle directly into the vein (**Figure 48.10**). US can also be used for confirmation that the guide wire is in the

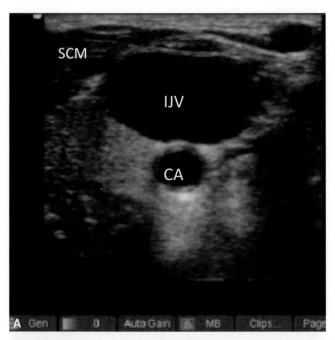
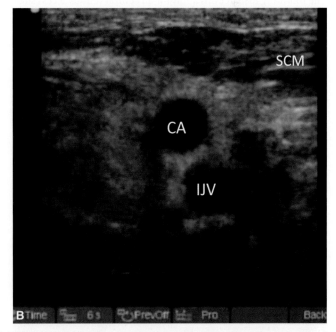

FIGURE 48.6 A, Unsafe site with carotid artery immediately beneath IJV. B, Unsafe site with carotid artery above IJV. CA, carotid artery; IJV, internal jugular vein; SCM, sternocleidomastoid muscle.

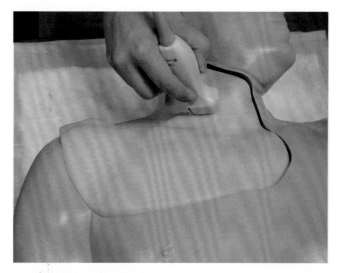

FIGURE 48.7 Image the entire length of the internal jugular vein and do a compression maneuver.

vein and not the artery. Once the guide wire is inserted, the needle should be removed and the vein imaged in both the transverse and longitudinal planes. The guide wire should be visualized in the longitudinal plane within the thin-walled vein, which will be compressible with gentle pressure (**Figure 48.11**). Be careful not to confuse this with the artery, which is immediately adjacent but will be thick walled, noncompressible, and pulsatile. A sterile probe cover should always be used in central venous catheterization. We recommend dynamic real-time use of ultrasound guidance over static US, where the skin overlying the central vein is marked due to higher success rates.[18]

LINE PLACEMENT

The following instructions apply for all central venous access sites:

Step 1: Consent

Explain the necessity and benefits of the procedure in layman terms to the patient or surrogate, as well as the risks as described earlier; convey that this is a routine and frequently performed procedure in the CCU. Assure that you will provide local anesthesia to limit pain during the procedure and that the patient will need to be under a sterile drape for an approximate period of 20 to 30 minutes. In life-threatening situations, consent may be deferred if the procedure is critical (eg, CVC placement for shock states) to treatment.

Step 2: Review Chart

It is imperative that the operator reviews the patient's laboratory data, medications, and chest radiograph to assess the safety of the procedure and for site selection. Consider platelet transfusion or reversing coagulopathy with fresh frozen plasma in the appropriate setting, if time allows.

Step 3: Prepare Equipment

Depending on the manufacturer, the central line kit will contain the basic items necessary to perform central venous catheterization (**Figure 48.12**). Many institutions have prepackaged customized procedure kits or a central line cart, which contains all the additional items necessary for CVC placement (**Figure 48.13**). Essential items to bring to the bedside include the central line kit, procedure pack or cart, ultrasound machine, ultrasound probe cover, and a bedside procedure table. **Table 48.10** contains a checklist of items necessary for central line placement.

Step 4: Time-out

Prior to performing the actual procedure, it is important to engage the CCU nurse and any procedural assistants to conduct a preprocedural verification. Perform and document a "Time-Out" as per your institution's standardized protocol. All members should agree on the following:

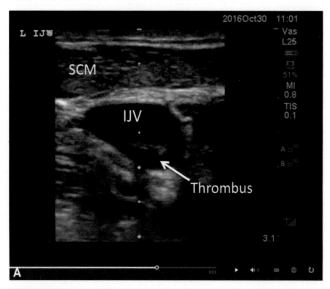

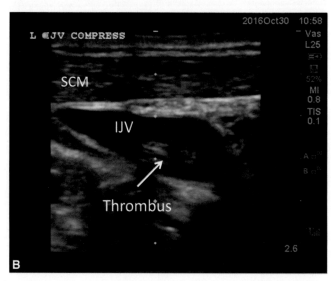

FIGURE 48.8 A, IJV intraluminal thrombus transverse view. B, IJV compression maneuver shows intraluminal thrombus with lack of compressibility. CA, carotid artery; IJV, internal jugular vein; SCM, sternocleidomastoid muscle.

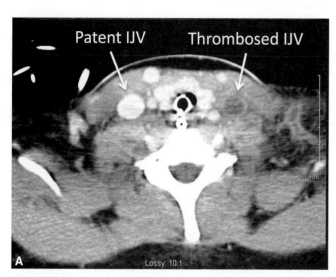

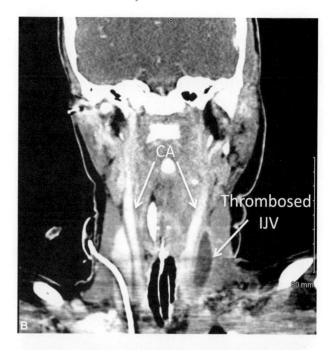

FIGURE 48.9 A, CT scan correlate of left IJV thrombosis (axial images). B, CT scan correlate of left IJV thrombosis (coronal images). CT, computed tomography; IJV, internal jugular vein.

1. Correct patient using two identifiers (name and date of birth or medical record number);
2. Correct procedure to be performed;
3. Correct site of insertion;
4. Ensure the procedural consent form is signed and dated.

Any concerns about procedural risks should be vocalized at this point. The assistant or any team member should be empowered to halt the procedure if inappropriate technique or break in sterility occurs.

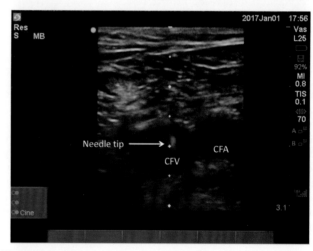

FIGURE 48.10 Echogenic needle tip visualized within common femoral vein . CFA, common femoral artery; CFV, common femoral vein.

TABLE 48.9	Steps for Line Placement: Preprocedural Ultrasound Scan
STEP	**DESCRIPTION**
1	Set ultrasound machine in "vascular" preset mode.
2	Hold vascular probe like a pencil with hand resting on patient.
3	Ensure probe marker is "operator left."
4	Identify vein and artery.
5	Optimize gain and depth, ensuring vein is in center of screen.
6	Scan up and down the vessel to ensure patency.
7	Do a compression maneuver at three sites along the vessel to ensure no thrombus.
8	Ensure vein and artery are parallel to each other.
9	Image both sides for optimal site selection.
10	Identify safest site for cannulation.

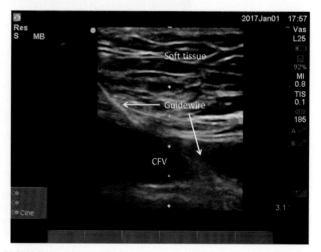

FIGURE 48.11 Echogenic guide wire visualized within common femoral vein. CFV, common femoral vein.

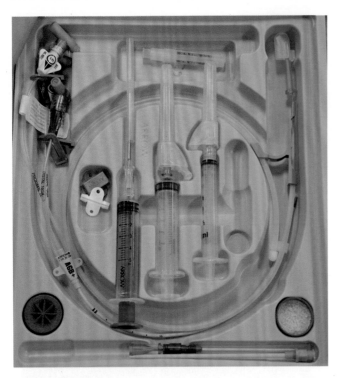

FIGURE 48.12 Central venous catheter kit.

Step 5: Patient Preparation

With an assistant's help, optimize the position of the patient and the bed before sterile barrier precautions are in place. Once the site is prepped and draped, it is difficult and inconvenient to reposition the patient and optimize the procedural settings. Ensure the patient is on a monitor. Place the patient in Trendelenburg position, with the head of the bed tilted 15 degrees posteriorly. If US is being utilized, do a prescan of the venous anatomy on both sides and identify a safe site for venous access. A disposable underpad may be placed under the proposed insertion site to prevent blood contaminating the patient's bed.

Internal Jugular Vein

Ensure the patient is in Trendelenburg position with the head slightly turned 45 degrees to the contralateral side from the intended insertion site. Anatomic landmarks for the IJV begin at the triangle formed by the heads of the SCMs and the clavicle (**Figure 48.14**). The surface projection of the IJV runs from the ear lobe to the medial clavicle, between the sternal and clavicular heads of the SCM. It increases in diameter as it descends to meet the SCV. Trendelenburg position and Valsava maneuver increase the size of the IJV. The IJV is easily collapsible and can often not be visualized due to excessive pressure by the ultrasound probe or the operator's finger. Excessive head rotation can increase the overlap of the carotid artery over the IJV, increasing risk of arterial injury. Hence, US guidance is strongly recommended for IJV cannulation. The Trendelenburg position also minimizes risk and complications of venous air embolism. Caution is advised for patients with elevated intracranial pressure, congestive heart failure, or other patients who cannot lay flat. These patients may be left in a comfortable position for most of the procedure (ie, prepping, draping) and then briefly placed in Trendelenburg position immediately before the cannulation portion.

Subclavian Vein

The SCV (**Figure 48.14**) is a continuation of the axillary vein and begins at the lateral edge of the first rib.[24] It courses anterior to the anterior scalene muscle, which separates it from the subclavian artery. It joins the IJV to form the brachiocephalic trunk. The pleural surface lies inferior and posterior to the SCV. The subclavian artery is immediately posterior to the vein. The SCV is usually not collapsible because it is tethered by fibrous connective tissue to the clavicle and first rib. This is especially helpful in the hypovolemic patient or during cardiac arrest. The thoracic duct joins the left SCV at its junction with the IJV. Right SCV cannulation is preferred in order to avoid thoracic duct injury; however, it has also been shown to have higher mechanical complications such as malpositioning.[25]

Prior to cannulation, place the patient in a 15-degree Trendelenburg position and assess the anatomic landmarks, beginning

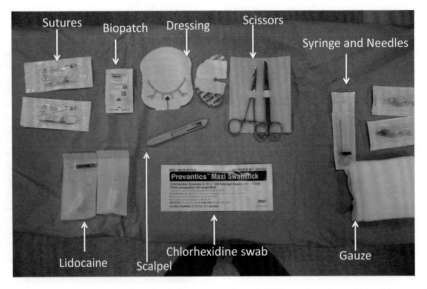

FIGURE 48.13 Additional items necessary for central line placement.

TABLE 48.10	Checklist of Items Necessary for Central Venous Catheterization

CENTRAL LINE KIT

Triple lumen catheter with Luer Lock caps

1% lidocaine 5 mL vial

25G × 1″ needle with 3 mL syringe for lidocaine administration

22G × 1.5″ "finder" needle with 5 mL syringe

18G × 2.5″ steel introducer needle with 5 mL Luer slip tip syringe

18G angiocatheter needle (in some kits)

GUIDE WIRE

Scalpel (#11)

Tissue dilator

Anchoring clips (clamp and fastener)

Needle holder

PROCEDURE CART OR PROCEDURE PACK ITEMS (IN ORDER OF USE)

2 surgical hair covers (one for assistant)

2 masks with eye shields (one for assistant)

Sterile gloves (for prepping) of appropriate size

2 chlorhexidine swabs/scrubs

Sterile gowns

Sterile gloves (for procedure) of appropriate size

Full-body fenestrated drape

3 sterile saline-filled syringes (or empty 10 mL syringe)

Medication label: 1% lidocaine

Sutures: 3.0 silk or nylon with curved or straight needle

Needle holder/driver for curved needle (if applicable)

Scissors (optional)

Gauze: 2″ × 2″ or 4″ × 4″ pads

Biopatch protective disk

Transparent, occlusive dressing

ADDITIONAL ITEMS

Portable ultrasound machine with linear array (vascular) probe

Sterile probe cover

Disposable underpad (blue Chux)

clavicle, so that the path of the needle stays parallel under the clavicle. The typical point is 2 cm lateral and 2 cm caudal to the middle third of the clavicle. Some operators place a rolled towel vertically under the spine to identify the external landmarks. Know that propping the shoulder or turning the head has been shown to decrease the size of veins. Although the traditional landmark approach is preferred by many, several articles suggest that US can increase the likelihood of success.[16,26]

Femoral Vein

For optimal exposure of the femoral region, place the patient in supine position, externally rotate and abduct the patient's leg away from midline.[27] The common FV lies medial to the common femoral artery as it runs distal to the inguinal ligament (**Figure 48.15**). The mnemonic "VAN" illustrates the contents of the femoral sheath (see **Figure 48.15**) from medial to lateral: femoral *v*ein, femoral *a*rtery, and femoral *n*erve. The femoral artery lies at the midpoint of a line connecting the pubic symphysis (PS) to the anterior superior iliac spine (ASIS). The FV lies 1 cm medial to the femoral artery. Localize the FV by palpating the artery or with US. The cannulation site must be inferior to the inguinal ligament. Reverse Trendelenburg position, with the feet tilted 15 degrees below the horizontal axis, can help engorge the FV and may aid in visualization.

Step 6: The Technique—The A to Z of Central Venous Catheterization

Dr. Seldinger developed the "Seldinger technique" in 1953.[28] More than 60 years later, the same technique is the gold standard for most vascular access procedures.[23,24] **Figure 48.16** illustrates the steps of the modified Seldinger technique where a needle is used to aspirate blood or fluid, a guide wire inserted through the needle, the tract dilated, and a catheter advanced into the vessel or desired space.

The following is a list of steps for central venous catheterization using US guidance. Don a facemask with eye shield and a surgical hat ensuring all hair is tucked away. Jewelry or watches, which may be in the field, should be temporarily removed. Assistants and all personnel in the room should also wear a hat and mask.

A. Perform hand hygiene by washing hands for 30 seconds with soap and water or using an alcohol-based hand rub, taking care to cover areas such as the wrists, finger webs, and area under fingernails.
B. Don sterile gloves in sterile fashion. Open the wrapper widely, ensuring that the sides of the wrapper do not fall back on the sterile gloves and contaminate it. Use care to touch only the inside of the glove with bare hands.
C. Prepare site using chlorhexidine-based swab or scrub with a back and forth motion for 30 seconds. Prepare a wide area and allow up to a minute for the solution to dry.
D. Deglove and perform hand hygiene once again.
E. Don sterile gown using correct technique. Put both hands into armholes and hold the gown away from the body allowing it to unfold completely. Minimize exposure of the hands outside the cuff. The assistant should pull the gown over the shoulder and tie the top portion and the inner belt of the gown, touching only the inside portion.
F. Don sterile gloves ensuring the cuffs of the gown are inside the sterile glove. Inspect the wrist to ensure that there is no exposed skin.

with the middle third of the clavicle. Follow the clavicle laterally to the "bend" where it deviates superiorly from the proximal ribs. Just medial to this point, the SCV and IJV run inferior to the clavicle. The insertion site should be somewhat removed from the

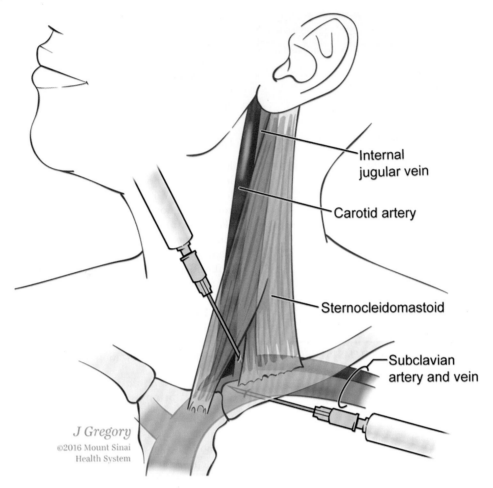

FIGURE 48.14 Internal jugular vein and subclavian vein anatomy.

G. Grasp the belt card, wait, and hand it to the assistant. Make a counterclockwise turn and retrieve the outer belt from the assistant, who holds on to the belt card. Tie the outer belt firmly.

H. Hold the sterile full-body fenestrated drape and arrange it such that the head and feet match up with that of the patient. Remove the adhesive stickers and fold it gently like a book. Place the drape on the patient ensuring the fenestrated opening is directly on the insertion site. Pat down the drape to ensure it sticks to the body before opening. With one hand keeping the drape in place, gently open the sides of the drape like a book. The assistant can help extend the full-body drape by touching only the nonsterile edges of the drape. Be careful to avoid "drape creep," whereby the drape is moved around, pulling material from the unprepped area to the sterile field.

I. The assistant should open the CVC kit and the operator should grasp the inside sterile cover and place the kit on the procedure table. Unfold the central line kit on the procedure table and position the contents at easy reach and in the order that you will use them. Take utmost care to ensure the contents do not get contaminated.

J. Prepare the TLC by placing Luer lock caps on the proximal (white) and medial (blue) ports, leaving the distal (brown) port open to allow exit of the guide wire. Flush the catheter lumens with sterile saline. If prepackaged sterile saline syringes are not available, three empty sterile syringes and a blunt needle can be used to aspirate sterile saline from a

50 mL saline bag with the assistant's help. Alternatively, sterile saline can be spurted onto the CVC kit from a prefilled 10 mL saline flush by the assistant. Prepare the guide wire by pulling back the J-shaped tip of the guide wire into the tapered hub.

K. Draw up 1% lidocaine local anesthetic using the 22G needle and syringe. Label the syringe with a lidocaine sticker. Note that the labeling is a requirement in the United States by the Joint Commission. This is done to ensure that the lidocaine is not confused with sterile saline and accidentally administered intravenously. Use a 25G needle for the initial injection over the skin.

L. If US is being utilized, drape the ultrasound probe with the sterile probe sheath. Hold the outside of the sterile cover and place sterile ultrasound gel (usually comes with the kit) inside the sheath. Have the assistant feed the nonsterile ultrasound probe into the inside of the sterile sheath, ensuring sterile gel is on the footprint of the probe. Grasp the sterile cover with the probe within and pull the sheath to cover the wire of the transducer. Do not touch the nonsterile probe or wire during this process. Place elastic bands or fasteners (comes with kit) to secure the outer cover so that it does not interfere with the procedure. Identify an area on the sterile field on which the probe can be placed when not in use. Be careful not to drag any uncovered parts of the wire into the sterile field.

M. Place gel onto the sterile probe and obtain a view where both the central vein and artery are visualized parallel to each other.

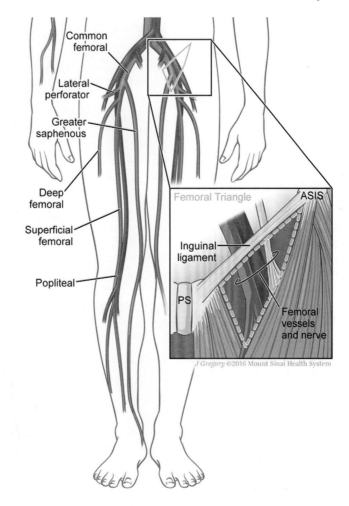

FIGURE 48.15 Venous anatomy of femoral triangle and lower extremities. ASIS, anterior superior iliac spine.

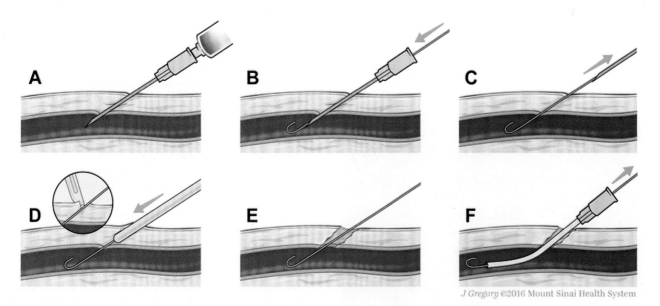

FIGURE 48.16 The Seldinger technique. A, Insert the needle into the vessel, advancing slowly until blood is aspirated. B, Stabilize the needle and insert the guide wire into the introducer needle. C, Remove the needle. D, Make a small skin incision and advance the dilator over the guide wire. E, Remove the dilator. F, Advance the catheter over the guide wire and then remove the guide wire.

The probe may need to be moved slightly up and down until the largest and safest site is identified. The assistant may need to further adjust the gain and depth to obtain an optimal view of the vein at the center of the screen.

N. Anesthetize the area over the insertion site, as well as the suture site, with 1% lidocaine. Make a wheal over the skin with the 25G needle and administer additional lidocaine in the soft tissue. Use the 22G needle if a longer needle is necessary, aspirating intermittently with the syringe to ensure a vessel is not entered. US guidance may be utilized to practice precise administration of the local anesthetic directly over the vein. Even in sedated patients, it may be wise to administer local anesthesia to ensure that they are not in pain and moving during the procedure.

O. Prior to the actual central venous catheterization, arrange your equipment on the sterile procedure table in the order that you will use them: introducer needle, guide wire, gauze, scalpel, dilator, TLC, saline flushes. Scrambling to find these items during the procedure can often result in need for multiple attempts.

P. Hold the ultrasound probe with your nondominant hand, steadying it by resting it on the patient. Obtain a transverse view and ensure the vein is at the center of the screen. Identify the distance to the vessel by looking at the distance scale on the right-hand side of the US monitor. A needle cap or the dilator can be used to apply pressure onto the skin to ensure the proposed insertion site is directly over the vein. With the dominant hand, insert the needle and slip-tip syringe (bevel up) immediately proximal to the probe at the center marker. Insert the needle using a steep angle (70 to 90 degrees) and advance the needle slowly into the vein, applying gentle negative pressure on the syringe (**Figure 48.17**). The skin may need to be made taut and a quick jab may be needed initially to pierce through the skin. The needle may need to be jiggled to identify it on the screen of the US machine. Alternatively, a lower angle (30 to 60 degrees) may be used with back and forth sweeping of the probe to follow the needle tip into the vein (**Figure 48.10**). Once the needle tip is directly over the vein, a quick jab may be needed to pierce through the vessel wall.

Q. When blood is aspirated, stop advancing and decrease the angle of the needle, ensuring good venous blood flow with

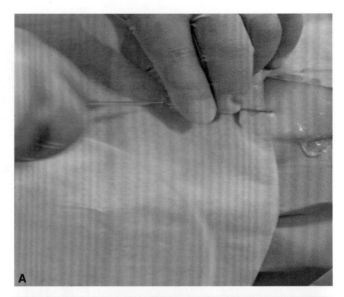

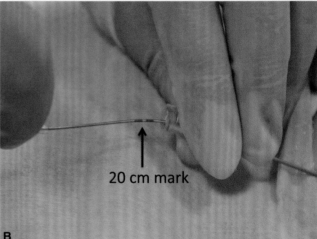

20 cm mark

FIGURE 48.18 A, Stabilization of the needle and insertion of the J-shaped guide wire. B, Advancement of the guide wire 20 to 25 cm.

negative pressure. Stabilize the needle by holding the needle with your thumb and index finger, steadying the needle by resting your hand on the body (**Figure 48.18A**). Remove the syringe from the needle making sure not to displace the needle from the vessel. Once you remove the syringe, nonpulsatile dark red blood is expected to flow gently. Pulsatile or bright red blood may indicate arterial cannulation. Remove needle and hold pressure if this occurs.

R. Insert the guide wire into the introducer needle and advance it to 20 to 25 cm (**Figure 48.18A** and **B**). Each black mark on the guide wire indicates 10 cm. Monitor for arrhythmias if IJV or SCV is being cannulated. If you meet resistance, DO NOT force the guide wire. Resistance may indicate that the introducer needle may be against the vessel wall or intersection or may have come out of the vessel altogether. If this occurs, try withdrawing the guide wire, rotating it slightly, and decreasing the angle before readvancing it. If there is resistance still, remove the guide wire and confirm again your position into the vessel with US until blood is aspirated again into the syringe.

S. Once the guide wire is in, always keep a firm grip on it, especially after dilation. Now remove the needle and confirm the

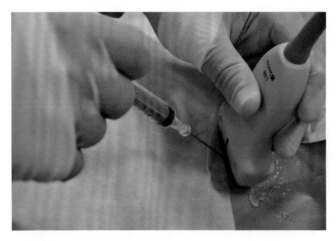

FIGURE 48.17 Needle position at center of linear array probe.

position of the guide wire with US by visualizing it in the vein in both the transverse and longitudinal views (**Figure 48.11**). In the transverse view, back-and-forth sweeping of the probe may be needed to visualize the guide wire entering the vein. In the longitudinal view, do not confuse the vein (compressible) and artery (pulsates when compressed).

T. Keeping the skin taut, make a small 1 to 2 mm nick with the number 11 blade at the insertion site with the scalpel (**Figure 48.19**). With the skin taut, advance the dilator over the wire in a twisting motion and dilate the skin and subcutaneous tissue only (**Figure 48.20**). Once the tract is dilated, remove the dilator and use gauze to control any bleeding that occurs after dilation. Keep hold of the guide wire at all times, particularly after dilation, to avoid inadvertent insertion into the vessel.

U. Thread the guide wire through the distal tip of the catheter until it comes out through the distal (brown) port of the TLC (**Figure 48.21A** and **B**). While holding the guide wire static with your nondominant hand, advance the catheter over the wire with your dominant hand to the desired depth (**Figure 48.21C**). Remove the guide wire and immediately cap the distal brown port. Confirm blood return from all ports and ensure all lumens flush without resistance. **Table 48.11** contains suggested depths to insert subclavian and IJV catheters. Depending on the height and gender of the patient, SCV and IJV CVCs can be advanced to the suggested depth. For IJV and SCV, the catheter tip should be in the SVC above its junction with the RA, with the distal tip parallel to the vessel wall. Femoral lines can generally be advanced all the way and secured.

V. Clean the site with alcohol or chlorhexidine and allow it to dry. Place the blue and white catheter anchoring clips over the catheter (SCV and IJV), and a Biopatch on the catheter at the insertion site (**Figure 48.22A**).

W. Suture the line in place. Clean and apply a sterile, transparent, occlusive dressing (**Figure 48.22B**).

X. Uncover the patient, discard all the sharps in the sharps container and order a portable chest radiograph to confirm position.

Y. Write a procedure note.

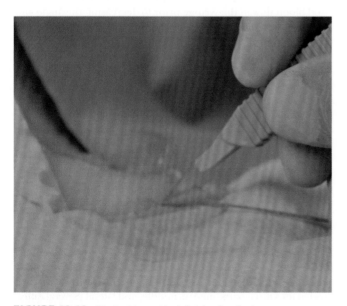

FIGURE 48.19 Skin incision with dull side of scalpel.

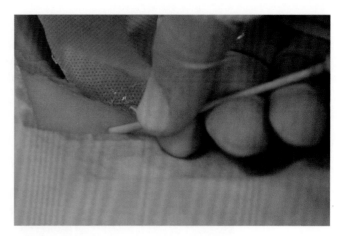

FIGURE 48.20 Dilation of the skin and soft tissue.

Figure 48.23 delineates a step-by-step algorithm of central venous catheterization using the steps already described. Additional landmark approaches and site-specific techniques are described in later sections.

SITE-SPECIFIC LANDMARKS AND ULTRASOUND-GUIDED APPROACHES

Internal Jugular Vein

Anatomic landmarks for the central approach to IJV catheterization begin at the apex of the triangle formed by the sternal (medial) head and clavicular (lateral) head of the SCM and the clavicle (**Figure 48.14**). A confluence between the IJV and the brachiocephalic vein facilitates cannulation at this location. The head should be rotated 45 degrees contralaterally, avoiding excessive rotation. With landmark approaches, a 21G or 22G "finder needle" attached to a 5 mL syringe is often used to locate the vein and estimate the distance and angle to the vein. The finder needle may be either removed or left in place for reference when the introducer needle is inserted.

Ultrasound-guided approach: This approach is the standard of care and preferred method to minimize mechanical and thrombotic complications. Do a preprocedural scan of the left and right IJV to select the best site. Place the ultrasound probe parallel and cephalad to the clavicle, at the apex of the triangle, with the probe marker "operator left." Visualize the IJV and carotid artery in the transverse view. The carotid artery will be thick walled and pulsatile while the IJV will be thin walled and easily compressible (**Figure 48.5**). Identify a safe site for cannulation where the IJV is away from the carotid artery and not overlying it (**Figure 48.6**). Position the transducer and optimize the depth such that the vein is centered on the screen. Stay in the mid-neck and avoid the lower neck region above the clavicle, because there is a risk of puncturing the apex of the lung, even with US guidance. Use a high angle (70 to 90 degrees) and advance the needle into the IJV, maintaining negative pressure until the vein is punctured. Decrease the angle of the needle prior to feeding the guide wire.

Alternatively, a lower angle may be used but the operator must follow the tip of the needle into the vein using sweeping back-and-forth motions with the transducer to identify the needle

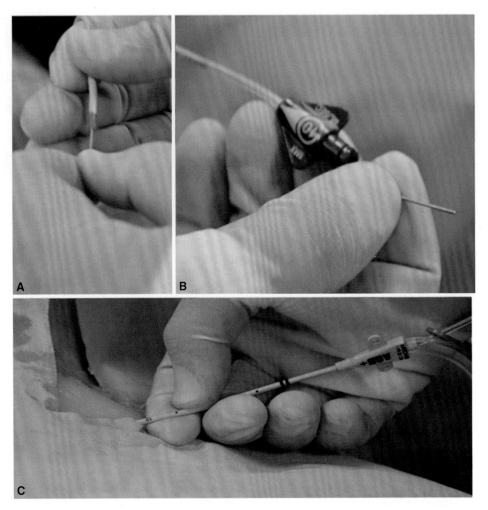

FIGURE 48.21 Advancement of the catheter over the guide wire. A, Insert the guide wire into the tip of the catheter. B, Thread the guide wire until it comes out through the distal port of the catheter and grasp the guide wire. C, Advance the catheter over the guide wire and then remove the guide wire.

tip as it is advanced into the IJV (**Figure 48.10**). Once the needle is inserted through the skin, slide or tilt the probe toward the needle tip until it is visualized on the screen. Be careful not to be confused by imaging the "shaft" of the needle, which will look similar to the tip. As the needle is advanced toward the vein, tilt the probe in the direction of the needle's trajectory to ensure you can see the needle tip at all times. Periodically

TABLE 48.11		Depth of Central Venous Catheter Insertion
SITE	**SUGGESTED DEPTH**	**FORMULA-BASED (HEIGHT IN CM)**[a]
Right SCV	15–17 cm	(Height/10) – 2 cm
Right IJV	16–18 cm	Height/10
Left SCV	18–20 cm	(Height/10) + 2 cm
Left IJV	18–20 cm	(Height/10) + 4 cm

[a]There are no well-controlled studies of height-based formulas supporting their routine use.

IJV, internal jugular vein; SCV, superior vena cava.

reposition the tip to confirm that it is directly above the vein. Make a small jab as the needle tip punctures the IJV and confirm good blood flow in the syringe prior to decreasing the angle and inserting the guide wire. Always confirm that the guide wire is in the vein prior to proceeding with the Seldinger technique (**Figure 48.24A** and **B**).

Landmark approach: The central approach is the most commonly used landmark approach. Place the index finger of the nondominant hand on the carotid artery pulse. Insert needle at apex of the triangle. The insertion point is just lateral to the carotid artery pulse. Use a 45 to 60 degrees angle and aim toward the ispsilateral nipple. The depth of the IJV using this technique is 3 to 5 cm. Sometimes the vessel will have been completely traversed by the needle with no blood return due to vessel collapse by hypovolemia or from pressure on the skin. Withdraw the needle to the subcutaneous plane and redirect the needle slightly medially.

Subclavian Vein

Landmark approach: The infraclavicular approach is most commonly used because it is quick and easy to perform, and obviates the need to set up the US machine. As part of setup, the clavicle should be divided into three parts: medial, middle, and lateral. Several different techniques and insertion sites are described in the literature:

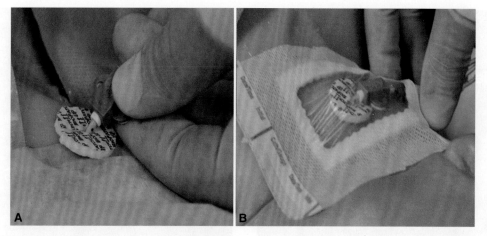

FIGURE 48.22 Securement of central venous catheter with anchoring clips, sutures, and transparent dressing.

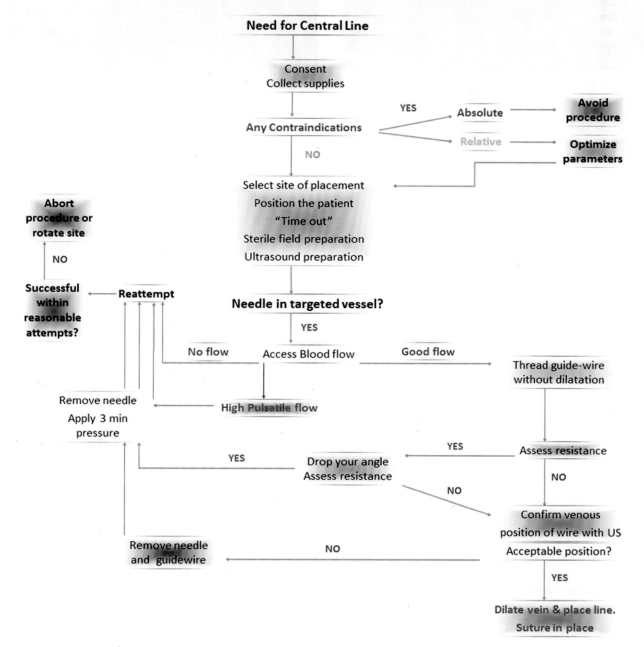

FIGURE 48.23 Central venous catheterization algorithm using Seldinger technique.

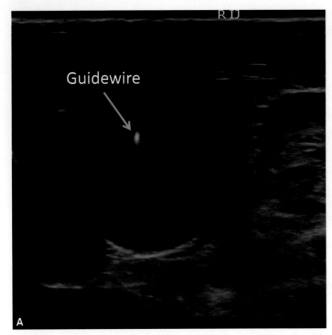
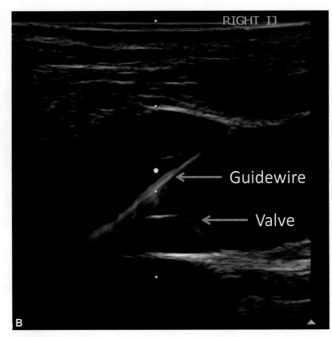

FIGURE 48.24 A, Guide wire in IJV. B, Longitudinal view of guide wire in internal jugular vein.

- Insert the needle 2 cm caudal to the mid-clavicle.
- 2 cm lateral and caudal to the bend of the clavicle.
- 1 cm caudal to the junction of the medial and middle third of the clavicle.
- Inferior to the clavicle at the deltopectoral groove.

The needle should be inserted with the bevel facing the heart at a 10-degree angle toward the sternal notch. Matching up the numbers of the syringe with the bevel will allow you to know where the bevel is facing at all times. Starting 2 cm lateral to the bend of the clavicle and approximately 2 cm caudal (usually midclavicular), insert the catheterization needle through the skin and toward the sternal notch. Keep a low (<20 degrees) angle at all times. Once the needle is under the skin, keep the needle and syringe parallel and beneath the clavicle (**Figure 48.14**). Advance the needle toward the sternal notch until venous blood is aspirated.[24] Keep the middle finger of the nondominant hand on the sternal notch and use it as a landmark. Use the thumb of the nondominant hand to depress the soft tissue adjacent to the needle, so as to get beneath the clavicle and keep the needle flat at all times. Once blood is aspirated, advance the guide wire and follow the steps of the Seldinger technique (**Figure 48.16**).

Ultrasound-guided approach: Technically speaking, we are referring to US-guided axillary vein cannulation as the insertion point is lateral to the first rib. The brachial and basilic veins combine to form the axillary vein and the SCV is the anastomosis of the axillary and cephalic veins (**Figure 48.2**). Although US-guided SCV catheterization is safe, it requires expertise with vascular ultrasound. Using the linear array probe with the orientation marker left, scan along the inferior margin of the mid-clavicular region in a sagittal plane and slide the transducer laterally toward the axillary region. In the transverse or short-axis view, identify the axillary vein where it is most superficial and separate from the axillary artery. Stay within 4 cm of the mid-clavicle to avoid brachial plexus injury. Do a compression maneuver and

use color Doppler to identify the vein from the artery. Identify the pleural line beneath the vessels. Now holding the base of the probe steady with the nondominant hand, turn the probe counterclockwise with the dominant hand and obtain a longitudinal view. Perform a compression maneuver and ensure the vessel is the vein and not the artery. While holding the probe steady with the nondominant hand resting on the body, insert the needle at the midpoint of the transducer at 45 to 70 degrees and follow the needle as it punctures the midpoint of the vein (**Figure 48.25**). Consider decreasing the angle to facilitate advancing the guide wire and the remaining steps.

Femoral Vein

Landmark approach: This is a useful approach during emergencies such as cardiac arrest. Externally rotate and abduct the patient's leg away from the midline. The FV lies caudal to the inguinal ligament and medial to the femoral artery in the femoral triangle (**Figure 48.15**). Palpate the femoral artery and insert the introducer needle 1 cm medial to this point at a 45 degree angle.[27] Advance the needle until there is a flash of venous blood. After stabilizing the needle, detach the syringe and advance the guide wire. Follow the remainder of the steps of the Seldinger technique. If the femoral artery is inadvertently punctured, hold compression for 5 to 10 minutes.

Ultrasound-guided approach: Using a linear array probe with the marker "operator left," identify the common FV and artery (**Figure 48.26**). As described previously, do a preprocedure scan to rule out deep vein thrombosis (**Table 48.9**). Identify the safest site for cannulation and holding the probe steady, insert the needle at a 45 to 70 degree angle into the vein. Once there is venous blood return, decrease the angle, ensuring there is still good blood flow. Holding the needle steady, detach the syringe and advance the guide wire. Use US to confirm that the guide wire is in the vein and not the artery. Follow the remaining steps for central venous cannulation.

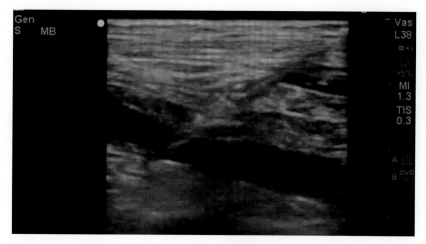

FIGURE 48.25 Ultrasound-guided cannulation using longitudinal approach.

CENTRAL LINE VERIFICATION OF POSITION

The operator must ensure the catheter is placed in the central vein and not the artery. Arterial cannulation can lead to stroke, hemorrhage, and thrombosis. Ultrasound guidance can help with ensuring venous cannulation in IJV and FV CVC placement. The tip of the CVC must lie in the SVC or IVC and never in the RA. The catheter tip may potentially perforate the thin wall of the RA, resulting in hemorrhage and cardiac tamponade. A chest radiograph must be performed immediately after IJV and SCV CVC to confirm position and rule out complications.

For an ultrasound-guided placement of central line, confirmation of position is a multistep process. Initially, dark venous blood can be aspirated in the syringe. The operator must ensure that there is no pulsatile flow or bright red blood from the introducer needle, which may indicate cannulation of the artery. After insertion of the guide wire, the position can again be confirmed by visualizing the guide wire in the vein in the transverse and longitudinal views. This step precedes dilation of the vessel with the rigid dilator and ensures that the operator will not proceed if there is false cannulation of the carotid or femoral artery. In debatable situations, blood gas analysis is useful in differentiating arterial versus venous gas pattern. Additionally, the catheter can be connected to a pressure transducer to confirm venous waveform and pressure. With the introduction of US, this is not done routinely anymore. US is emerging as a tool to rule out

malposition and pneumothorax but this is not the standard of care at this time.[29] Postprocedural chest radiography is necessary at the end of every internal jugular or subclavian venous cannulation to confirm the position of the distal tip of the catheter and the absence of immediate complications like pneumothorax.

CORRECT POSITION

For any internal jugular or subclavian central line, the catheter tip is in correct position when it lies in the lower SVC or the cavoatrial junction. On a chest radiograph, this is at the level of the first anterior intercostal space above the carina (**Figure 48.27**). Placing an IJV or SCV catheter tip too deep can result in arrhythmias or even cardiac tamponade. A catheter can be repositioned by withdrawing it and resuturing, however it can never be advanced due to the risk of infection.

ROUTINE CATHETER CARE

Patency problems are common and include sluggish flow, no flashback of blood, or complete blockage. Possible causes for that would be clotted blood in the catheter or drug precipitation from infusate (eg, parenteral nutrition) or malpositioning of the catheter from initial placement. A rescue method to restore patency is by the use of a thrombolytic agent like alteplase (Cathflo

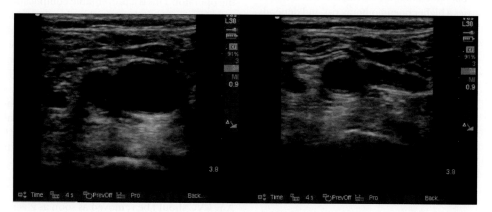

FIGURE 48.26 Common femoral vein with compression maneuver.

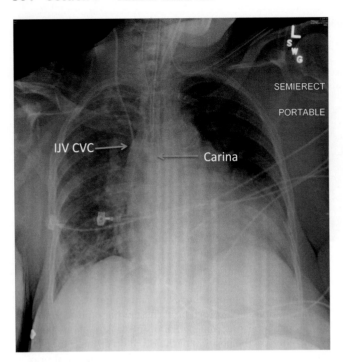

FIGURE 48.27 Central line position on chest radiograph. CVC, central venous catheter; IJV, internal jugular vein.

or t-PA). See **Figure 48.28** for an algorithm to trouble shoot a nonfunctioning CVC.

COMPLICATIONS

Central line placement is an invasive procedure and it is not uncommon to have complications. General complications of placement of central lines are site specific and are summarized in **Table 48.12**.[30,31] The choice of site should be based on patient factors and operator's experience. In general, complication rates increase with increased number of attempts.[9,32] Simulation-based training has been shown to reduce the number of mechanical and infectious complications.[10,11,33]

Infection

Observing standard infection control measures such as hand hygiene and using aseptic technique when placing CVC is paramount to preventing CLABSI.[1] The subclavian site carries the lowest risk of infection, however carries a higher pneumothorax risk and depends on operator experience.[13] The femoral site is associated with the highest risk of infectious complications. A central line bundle is essential for any CCU and includes hand hygiene, chlorhexidine skin antisepsis, and maximum barrier precautions during insertion, avoidance of the femoral site, a daily review of necessity of the CVC and removal when no longer necessary.[34] Interventions such as a daily goals sheet and simulation-based training on sterile techniques have been shown to decrease CLABSI.[35] Any central line that is placed emergently or in a nonsterile fashion should be promptly removed. Routine catheter tip cultures, CVC changes, and guide wire exchanges are not recommended.

Pneumothorax

This is by far the most common complication of the subclavian site. There is no consensus as to whether all patients need chest tubes if a pneumothorax occurs. Stable patients with small pneumothoraces may be closely observed. Patients with large pneumothoraces or those who are on mechanical ventilation require chest tube placement to manage this complication and avoid tension pneumothorax, which is life threatening.

Arterial Puncture

Arterial puncture and even cannulation is not uncommon. If recognized early (ie, with introducer needle), 5 to 10 minutes of solid pressure on the site will resolve most bleeding issues without consequence. This is different, though, if the artery has been dilated or cannulated with a TLC or introducer sheath. If this occurs, leave the line in place and consult vascular surgery immediately.

Hematoma

Femoral artery puncture can lead to hematoma. Retroperitoneal hemorrhage is a feared complication and blood can flow freely into the retroperitoneum. The FV becomes the external iliac vein superior to the inguinal ligament and retroperitoneal hemorrhage can occur if the posterior wall is punctured multiple times above the inguinal ligament. This often occurs when the landmark approach is used during cardiac arrest or other emergencies. Occasionally, the FV is cannulated after the needle has traversed the femoral artery; so the bleeding will occur when the catheter is removed. Similarly, a hematoma from carotid artery puncture can compress the trachea and hence compromise the airway. US-guidance decreases the risk of all these mechanical complications.[11]

Air Embolism

This is a rarer occurrence but can be catastrophic. This can occur during CVC placement or during its removal.[36] The patient will quickly decompensate and become short of breath, altered, and hypotensive or have a cardiac arrest. If this is suspected, place the patient in the left lateral decubitus or Trendelenburg position so as to trap the air in the right ventricle. Provide supportive care such as high-flow oxygen or mechanical ventilation, intravenous fluids, and vasopressors. The most useful technique to prevent air embolism is placing the patient in Trendelenburg when performing IJV or SCV catheterization or removal. Always cover the hub of the introducer needle or CVC once it is in the vein.

Guide Wire Embolization

Loss of a guide wire is possibly the most disturbing complication for the operator. This is a preventable complication and many institutions have policies of confirming that the guide wire was removed after the procedure. Always maintain control of the guide wire throughout the procedure and be all the more vigilant after the dilation of the vessel. If the operator does lose the guide wire, check to see if it is still in the lumen of the catheter. If so, then clamp the catheter and guide wire with a Kelly clamp or similar instrument and remove the entire apparatus, along with the guide wire. If the guide wire has embolized distally, consult vascular surgery or IR to help with retrieval. **Figure 48.29A** and **B** depict US images of guide wire embolization through the venous circulation into the RA.

CENTRAL ACCESS REMOVAL

Any CVC should be removed as soon as it is no longer necessary. Central line removal is distinct from insertion, with its own set of potential complications. Some complications of CVC removal

PATENCY ALGORITHM

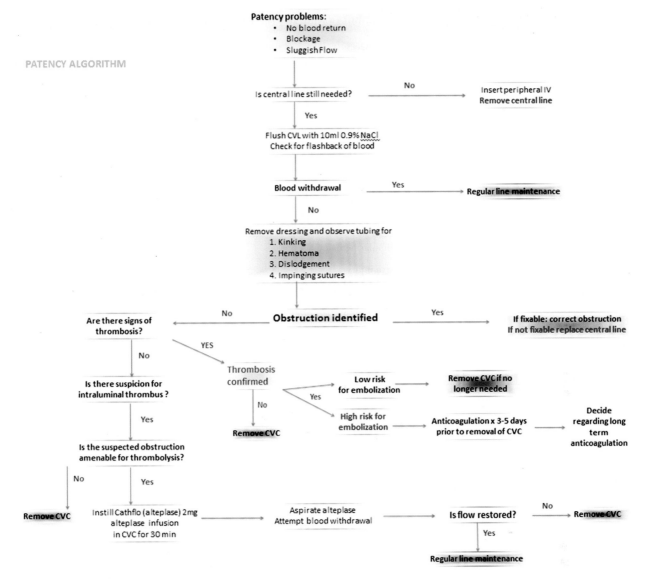

FIGURE 48.28 Central line occlusion trouble shooting algorithm.

include bleeding, air embolism, catheter fracture, and dislodgement of thrombus from the catheter tip. **Table 48.13** is a checklist of essential steps to follow during CVC removal. A working knowledge of potential complications and simulation-based training is essential for the CCU personnel removing lines. CVC removal should only be performed by professionals who have received adequate training and been assessed as competent in performing the procedure.[37]

ARTERIAL LINE PLACEMENT

Arterial catheterization is indicated when continuous beat-to-beat blood pressure monitoring is needed. This applies for patients with circulatory shock, hypertensive emergencies, aortic syndromes, acute stroke, and multiorgan failure states. Arterial access is also required for diagnostic and therapeutic interventions like coronary angiography, aortic balloon pump, or left ventricular assisted devices, and ECMO. Indications for intraarterial line placement are summarized in **Table 48.14**. See Chapter 49 for a discussion on arterial blood pressure monitoring and its uses.

Like CVCs, intraarterial lines are interventions that require patient consent, cooperation, and sterile conditions as discussed earlier. A-lines are generally placed using the Seldinger technique (**Figure 48.16**). A-lines have a lower rate of infection, but the risk of infectious and thrombotic complications does exist; so they should be discontinued as soon as they are no longer indicated. No drugs should be injected via an A-line; the direct contact of a medication with the tissues can result in cell death, severe gangrene, and limb ischemia. **Table 48.15** contains a list of contraindications for A-line placement.[32,38]

Surgical and anatomic considerations are the influencing factors when choosing the site for arterial cannulation. The radial artery is the most common site for cannulation because it is thought to have a low rate of associated complications. This low rate of complications occurs as a result of extensive collateral circulation involving the ulnar artery and palmar arches with flow to the distal limb. The anatomic landmarks and advantages/disadvantages for each site are summarized in **Table 48.16**.[39] The most common complication is arterial thrombosis. Thrombotic risk factors include larger catheter size, hypotension, smaller arterial

TABLE 48.12	Complications of Central Venous Catheterization	
MECHANICAL COMPLICATIONS	**COMPLICATIONS**	**PREVENTATIVE MANAGEMENT**
Internal Jugular CVC		
Immediate complications	Carotid puncture	Do not dilate; apply pressure.
	Pneumothorax	Insert chest tube if necessary.
	Bleeding	If severe, consider evacuation.
		Correct coagulopathy prior.
	Malposition	Correct position.
	Venous air embolism	Flush all ports with saline.
	Dysrhythmias	Retract guide wire.
	Submandibular hematoma	Watch for tracheal compression.
	Vagus nerve injury	
	Guide wire migration	Consult vascular surgery
	Thoracic duct injury (left side)	Keep NPO; requires TPN until healing; consult surgery.
Subclavian CVC		
Immediate complications	Subclavian arterial puncture	Do not dilate; apply pressure.
	Pneumothorax	Insert chest tube if necessary.
	Hematoma/hemothorax	If severe, consider surgical evacuation. Correct coagulopathy prior. Keep NPO; requires TPN until healing; consult surgery.
	Thoracic duct injury (left side)	
	Vagus nerve injury	
	Cardiac tamponade	Pericardiocentesis
	Malposition	Retract line; if needed, change.
	Venous air embolism	Flush all ports with saline.
	Dysrthymias	Retract guidewire.
	Guide wire migration	Consult vascular surgery.
Femoral CVC		
Immediate complications	Femoral artery puncture	Do not dilate; apply pressure.
	Femoral nerve puncture	Ultrasound use
	Retroperitoneal bleeding from external iliac artery puncture	Correct coagulopathy first. If severe, consider evacuation
	Venous air embolism	Flush all ports with saline.
	Guide wire migration	Might require vascular intervention.
	Punctured bladder	Urology consult
	Bowel perforation	If patient has femoral hernia

TABLE 48.12	Complications of Central Venous Catheterization (*continued*)	
MECHANICAL COMPLICATIONS	**COMPLICATIONS**	**PREVENTATIVE MANAGEMENT**
For all types of access	Bleeding	Apply pressure.
	Deep vein thrombosis (DVT)	DVT prophylaxis
	Thrombophlebitis	Prompt removal
	Infection	Early removal, antibiotics
	Extravasation	Manage as per vesicant
	Thrombosis	Consider thrombolytics.
	Nerve injury	

CVC, central venous catheter; TPN, total parenteral nutrition.

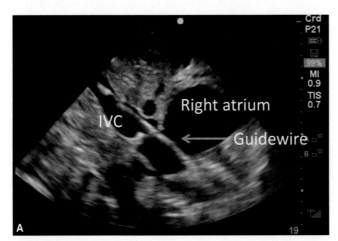
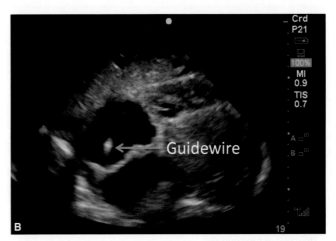

FIGURE 48.29 A, Guide wire embolization to inferior vena cava (IVC). B, Guide wire embolization to IVC/right atrium.

TABLE 48.13	Checklist for Central Line Removal

CENTRAL LINE REMOVAL CHECKLIST

Place the patient in Trendelenburg position with the CVC exit site below the level of the heart.

Ensure that all CVC lumens are capped and/or clamped.

Cover the CVC exit site with gauze and apply gentle pressure while removing the catheter in a slow, constant motion.

Have the patient perform the Valsalva maneuver as the last portion of the CVC is removed.

Place pressure on the site for at least 5 min.

Apply a sterile occlusive dressing, such as gauze filled with petroleum jelly, and cover with a transparent film dressing.

Leave dressing in place for at least 24 h and change every 24 h until the exit site has healed.

Instruct the patient to remain lying flat for 30 min after removal of the catheter.

CVC, central venous catheter.

dimension, multiple arterial sticks, duration of cannulation, and administration of vasoactive agents. The cannulation site further potentiates thrombotic propensity.[40,41]

GENERAL RULES

Multiple failed attempts might lead to arterial vasoconstriction; therefore choice of radial artery requires a level of operator's comfort that he or she will be able to place the line in with relatively low number of attempts. Prior to the procedure, the modified Allen test should be performed to assess for good collateral circulation from the ulnar artery. The modified Allen test is performed by asking the patient to make a fist. While the hand is clenched, the ulnar and radial arteries are occluded with digital pressure to obstruct blood flow to the hand. When the hand is unclenched, the pressure over the ulnar artery is released. In the presence of good circulation, the palm flushes in 5 to 10 seconds.[42] **Table 48.17** contains a list of basic items needed for arterial catheterization.

TECHNIQUE

If you are able to get arterial blood gas from radial artery, then you probably have already mastered the direct cannulation

TABLE 48.14	Indications for Intra-arterial Lines in the CCU

INVASIVE MONITORING OR AGGRESSIVE HEMODYNAMIC RESUSCITATION INTERVENTIONS

Hemodynamic monitoring:
- Continuous blood pressure
- Shock on vasoactive agents
- Hypertensive emergency
- Open heart surgery
- Hemorrhagic stroke
- Aortic syndromes
- Cerebrovascular accident after thrombolysis
- Blood pressure monitoring in obese patients, amputees, burn victims

Cardiac output monitors (ie, Flotrac)

Intra-aortic balloon pump

Left ventricular assist device

ARTERIAL BLOOD GAS ACCESS

Need for frequent arterial blood gases
Acute respiratory distress syndrome or in severe metabolic derangements

TABLE 48.15	Contraindications for Intra-arterial Lines in the CCU

Thrombocytopenia

Infection at insertion site

Traumatic injury at insertion site

Arteriovenous fistula

Peripheral arterial insufficiency of intended limb

Prior surgeries or radiation

Raynaud syndrome

Thromboangiitis obliterans (Buerger disease)

Synthetic vascular graft

CCU, cardiac care unit.

technique. Following are the basic steps of arterial catheterization. It is assumed that the operator will adhere to standard hospital policy of obtaining informed consent, performing a "time-out," and maintaining maximum barrier precautions throughout the procedure.

Catheter Over Needle Technique (Radial Artery Catheterization)

A. Palpate the radial artery and perform the modified Allen test. If you cannot feel it, aim as distally as possible, either rotate position or use US guidance to visualize the artery.

B. Once you identify the artery, position the patient with the wrist dorsiflexed using a rolled towel under the wrist and tape to maintain that position.

C. Adjust height of bed to ensure comfort during procedure.

D. Perform hand hygiene using an alcohol-based rub.

E. Don sterile gloves and prepare site using chlorhexidine swabs.

F. Don hat, mask, and sterile gown.

G. Identify the point of maximal pulsation of the radial artery and inject local lidocaine subcutaneously.

H. Hold the angiocatheter-covered needle with dominant hand while stabilizing the artery with the nondominant hand.

I. Puncture the skin at an angle of 30 to 45 degrees just distal to where the artery is palpated. Once flashback of blood is seen, advance the needle 2 mm after flash to ensure catheter placement inside the lumen. Flatten the needle slightly and advance the catheter until flashback of blood is seen in the hub of the needle. Note that some catheters have a built-in guide wire that is advanced into the artery once there is flashback and then the catheter is advanced over the wire.

J. Withdraw the needle/wire from the catheter. There should be pulsatile flow of bright red blood coming out of the catheter. Press on the catheter proximal to the hub to control the bleeding.

K. Have an assistant hand you the transducer connecting tubing and connect it to the catheter hub. Be careful not to displace the catheter or pull it out mistakenly. Check for arterial waveform on the monitor.

L. Suture the catheter in place using a securing device and/or placing a suture around the proximal hub.

M. Clear the site and place a transparent dressing.

Catheter Over Guide Wire: Seldinger Technique (Femoral Arterial Catheterization)

A. Palpate the femoral artery in the femoral triangle, staying caudal to the inguinal ligament.

B. Perform hand hygiene; don hat, mask, and sterile drape.

C. Prepare, drape, and anesthetize the skin and soft tissue over the femoral artery.

D. Puncture the skin at an angle of 40 to 60 degrees with the introducer needle/syringe, distal to where the arterial pulse is palpated (note that a long introducer needle should be used).

E. Advance the needle until the artery is punctured and bright red blood is aspirated.

F. Decrease angle slightly ensuring good blood flow.

G. Stabilize needle and remove syringe from needle, confirming free pulsatile flow of bright red blood.

H. Pass the guide wire through the needle and withdraw the needle (**Figure 48.16**).

I. Advance the cannula over the guide wire while maintaining control of the guide wire at all times. Advance the guide wire into the lumen of the artery with rotational movements. Note a thin dilator is usually available in a vessel catheterization kit if needed.

J. Remove the guide wire and expect brisk high-pressure bright red blood flow from the catheter.

K. Attach the transducer connecting tubing to the catheter and look for a good A-line waveform on the monitor.

L. Secure the cannula with sutures and cover with a transparent dressing.

TABLE 48.16		Site-specific Characteristics of Arterial Line Placement		
SITE	**LANDMARKS**	**ADVANTAGES**	**DISADVANTAGES**	**COMPLICATIONS**
Radial	Distal end of radius between tendons of brachioradialis and flexor carpi radialis	Easy to locate	Easily collapsible	Thrombosis risk
		Ease of placement	Prone to vasoconstriction if multiple attempts	Limb ischemia
		Most common site of cannulation	Difficult in profound shock	
		Presence of collateral flow (ulnar artery and palmar arch)	High thrombosis risk	
		Easily maintained		
			Frequent accidental removal	
Femoral artery	Below the inguinal ligament	Easy cannulation especially with ultrasound guidance	Highest infection rate	Retroperitoneal hemorrhage
	Palpated midway between the pubic symphysis and anterior iliac crest	Lower thrombosis risk	Compressible for bleeding control	
		Easily maintained	Avoid in peripheral arterial disease	
		Comfortable		
		Largest accessible arterial access		
Axillary artery	Palpated in the intramuscular groove between the coracobrachial and triceps muscles	Lower infection and thrombosis risk	Ultrasound guidance often needed	Brachial plexus compressive injury from hematoma
	Deep to pectoralis minor muscle	Maintains pulsation in profound shock due to proximity to aorta	High failure rate	Paresthesia
		Second largest after femoral artery	Proximity to pleural space, brachial plexus	Cannulation of left axillary is preferred compared to the right.
		Preferred in obese if radial access difficult	Right axillary line in continuity with right carotid⬚ risk for cerebral thromboembolism	
Brachial artery	Medial side of antecubital fossa	Easily accessed but lacks the anatomic benefit of collateral circulation	Highest likelihood for thrombosis and loss of radial pulsations	DO NOT USE
	Lateral border of brachial muscle			Any cannulation may lead to upper limb ischemia
				Median nerve injury

ULTRASOUND GUIDANCE

Ultrasound use is often helpful in arterial catheterization of the critically ill CCU patient. The insertion of the catheter by blind palpation can sometimes require multiple attempts and thus can cause patient discomfort and arterial vasospasm. This is particularly true in the CCU patient with profound shock. Ultrasound guidance is particularly helpful with axillary artery catheterization.

The use of ultrasound guidance has been shown to increase first-pass success rate and reduce the number of attempts.[43,44]

Prior to the procedure, clean the ultrasound transducer with an antiseptic wipe. Perform a preprocedural scan with a high-frequency linear array transducer to identify the optimal site for cannulation. Ensure the transducer marker is "operator left" and the screen marker is also on the upper left hand corner.

TABLE 48.17	Items Necessary for Arterial Line Placement
Arterial line kit	
Arterial catheter	
1% lidocaine 5 mL vial	
25G × 1″ needle for lidocaine administration	
22G × 1.5″ with 5 mL syringe for lidocaine administration	
20G steel introducer needle with 5 mL Luer slip syringe	
20G angiocatheter needle (in some kits)	
J-shaped guide wire	
Scalpel (#11)	
Thin dilator (not always used)	
Straight or curved needle with sutures	
Gauze: 2″ × 2″ or 4″ × 4″ pads	
Fenestrated drape	
Additional supplies	
Surgical caps	
Masks with eye shield	
Chlorhexidine swabs/scrubs	
Sterile gown	
Sterile gloves	
Biopatch protective disk	
Transparent, occlusive dressing	
A-line transducer setup with tubing connected to saline bag (supplied by registered nurse [RN])	
Disposable underpad (blue Chux)	
Additional items	
Portable ultrasound machine with linear array (vascular) probe	
Sterile probe cover	

Identify the artery that will be cannulated and adjust the gain and depth to optimize the image such that the vessel of interest appears in the center of the screen. Arteries will appear round, thick walled, and are pulsatile with compression. Scan up and down in the transverse view to ensure there is no tortuosity or calcification. Locate a section with the largest diameter. The radial artery will be located adjacent to the styloid process of the radial bone (**Figure 48.30A**). The femoral artery is the pulsatile vessel located in the femoral triangle (**Figures 48.15** and **48.26**). For axillary artery cannulation, have the patient place his or her arm under his or her head and scan the axillary region until the vessels are identified. **Table 48.16** lists general anatomic landmarks and considerations for each potential site.

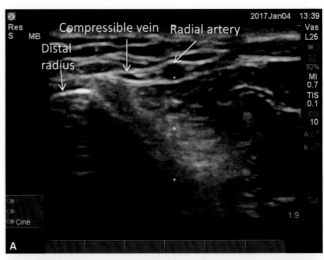

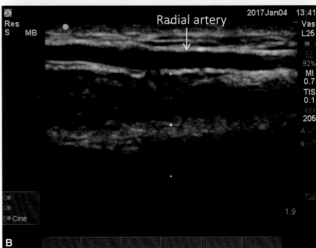

FIGURE 48.30 A, Radial artery in transverse view. B, Radial artery in longitudinal view.

Transverse Approach

Arterial catheterization can be performed in either the transverse view or longitudinal view (**Figure 48.30A** and **B**).[40] It is assumed that the operator will maintain sterility throughout the procedure and will always use a sterile sheath to cover the ultrasound transducer. Sterile gel should be applied inside the sheath without contaminating the field or the operator's sterile gloves. After locating the artery, optimize the image and center the artery in the transverse view. Anesthetize the skin and insert the angiocatheter-covered needle at the midpoint of the transducer at a 45 to 60 degree angle. Slide or angle the probe up and down until the needle tip is visualized. Make sure you are imaging the tip and not the shaft of the needle. As the needle is advanced toward the artery, follow the tip of the needle by sliding the transducer back and forth. Adjust the position of the needle until it is directly over the artery and then puncture through the vessel wall into the lumen. Follow steps for either the catheter over needle/wire technique or the Seldinger technique described previously.

Longitudinal Approach

For the longitudinal view approach, first obtain a transverse view with the vessel in the center of the screen. Hold the base

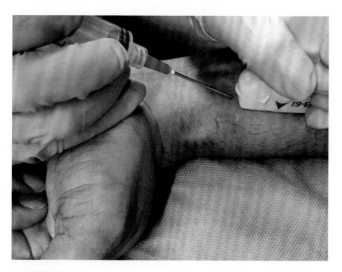

FIGURE 48.31 Transducer hold for longitudinal approach for cannulation.

of the transducer steady, turn the transducer counterclockwise with the dominant hand, and obtain a longitudinal view (**Figure 48.30B**). Notice the thick-walled vessel that is pulsatile and noncompressible. While holding the transducer steady with the nondominant hand resting on the body, insert the needle at the midpoint of the transducer at a 30 to 45 degrees angle (**Figure 48.31**) and follow the needle as it punctures the midpoint of the artery. Follow steps for catheter over needle or Seldinger techniques described earlier. The longitudinal approach can be useful for radial artery cannulation, whereas the transverse approach is preferable for femoral artery and axillary artery catheterization.

CONCLUSION

Line access is essential and allows for hemodynamic monitoring and administration of lifesaving medications in the CCU patient. A working knowledge of the types of catheters, indications, contraindications, and considerations for site selection is imperative. Knowledge of vascular anatomy, familiarity with the equipment, and competency in the procedure are prerequisites for successful insertion of the catheter. A daily assessment and early removal of the line as soon as it is no longer necessary reduces the risk of complications. Limiting the number of attempts at insertion drastically reduces both infectious and mechanical complications. Ultrasound guidance and simulation-based training are helpful in achieving competence and reducing complications.

REFERENCES

1. O' Grady NP, Alexander M, Burns LA, et al; Healthcare Infection Control Practices Advisory Committee. Guidelines for the prevention of intravascular catheter related infections. *Am J Infect Control.* 2011;39(4 suppl 1):S1-S34.

2. Sterile, single-use intravascular catheters. Part 5: over-needle peripheral catheters. *International Standard ISO* 10555-5. 1996:1-3.

3. Barcelona SL, Vilich F, Cote CJ. A comparison of flow rates and warming capabilities of the Level 1 and rapid infusion system with various-size intravascular catheters. *Anesth Analg.* 2003;97:358-363.

4. Malach T, Jerassy Z, Rudensky Z, et al. Prospective surveillance of phlebitis associated with peripheral intravenous catheters. *Am J Infect Control.* 2016;34:308-312.

5. Rickard CM, Webster J, Wallis MC, et al. Routine versus clinically indicated replacement of peripheral intravenous catheters: a randomized controlled equivalence trial. *Lancet.* 2012;380:1066-1074.

6. Casey AL, Mermel LA, Nightingale P, Elliott TS. Antimicrobial central venous catheters in adults: a systematic review and meta-analysis. *Lancet Infect Dis.* 2008;8(12):763.

7. Maki DG, Kluger DM, Crnich CJ. The risk of bloodstream infection in adults with different intravascular devices: a systematic review of 200 published prospective studies. *Mayo Clinic Proc.* 2006;81(9):1159-1171.

8. Goldhaber SZ. Counterpoint: should coagulopathy be repaired prior to central venous line insertion? No. *Chest.* 2012;141(5):1142-1144.

9. Karakitsos D, Labropoulos N, De Groot E, et al. Real-time ultrasound-guided catheterisation of the internal jugular vein: a prospective comparison with the landmark technique in critical care patients. *Crit Care.* 2006;10:R162.

10. Khouli H, Jahnes K, Shapiro J, et al. Performance of medical residents in sterile techniques during central vein catheterization: randomized trial of efficacy of simulation-based training. *Chest.* 2011;139(1):80-87.

11. Sekiguchi H, Tokita JE, Minami T, Eisen LA, Mayo PH, Narasimhan M. A prerotational, simulation-based workshop improves the safety of central venous catheter insertion: results of a successful internal medicine house staff training program. *Chest.* 2011;140(3):652-658.

12. Mathew JP, Desai A, Yedowitz-Freeman, et al. Perceptions of medical residents regarding central venous catheter placement before and after simulation-based training. *Crit Care Med.* 2015;43:226.

13. Parienti JJ, Mongardon N, Megarbane B, et al. Intravascular complications of central venous catheterization by insertion site. *N Engl J Med.* 2015;373:1220-1229.

14. Palevsky PM, Liu KD, Brophy PD, et al. KDOQI US Commentary on the 2012 KDIGO Clinical Practice Guideline for acute kidney injury. *Am J Kidney Dis.* 2013;61(5):686-688.

15. Parienti JJ, Thirion M, Mégarbane B, et al. Femoral versus jugular venous catheterization and risk of nosocomial events in adults requiring acute renal replacement therapy: a randomized controlled trial. *JAMA.* 2008;299:2413-2422.

16. Fragou M, Gravvanis A, Dimitriou V, et al. Real time ultrasound guided subclavian vein cannulation versus the landmark method in critical care patients: a prospective randomized study. *Crit Care Med.* 2011;39(7):1607-1612.

17. Feller-Kopman D. Ultrasound-guided internal jugular access: a proposed standardized approach and implications for training and practice. *Chest.* 2007;132:302-309.

18. Milling TJ Jr, Rose J, Briggs WM, et al. Randomized, controlled clinical trial of point-of-care limited ultrasonography assistance of central venous cannulation: the third Sonography Outcomes Assessment Program (SOAP-3) trial. *Crit Care Med.* 2005;33:1764-1769.

19. Shekelle PG, Wachter RM, Pronovost PJ, et al. Making health care safer II: an updated critical analysis of the evidence for patient safety practices, Chapters 18. Use of Real-Time Ultrasound for central ine insertion brief update. *Evid Rep/Technol Assess.* 2013;211:1-945.

20. American Society of Anesthesiologists Task Force on Central Venous Access, Rupp SM, Apfelbaum JL, Blitt C, et al. Practice guidelines for central venous access: a report by the American Society of Anesthesiologists Task Force on Central Venous Access. *Anesthesiology.* 2012;116:539-573.

21. Pittirut M, Hamilton H, Biffi R, MacFie J, Pertkiewicz M. ESPEN guidelines on parenteral nutrition: central venous catheters (access, care, diagnosis and therapy of complications). *Clin Nutr.* 2009;28(4):365-377.

22. Troianos CA, Hartman GS, Glas KE, et al. Guidelines for performing ultrasound guided vascular cannulation: recommendations of the American Society of Echocardiography and the Society of Cardiovascular Anesthesiologists. *J Am Soc Echocardiogr.* 2011;24:1291-1318.

23. Ortega R, Song M, Hanset CJ, Barash P. Ultrasound-guided internal jugular cannulation. *N Engl J Med.* 2010;362:e57.

24. Braner DA, Lai S, Eman S, Tegtmeyer S. Central venous catheterizatin—subclavian vein. *N Engl J Med.* 2007;357:e26.

25. Yerdel MA, Karayalcin K, Aras N, Bozatli L, Yildirim E, Anadol E. Mechanical complications of subclavian vein catheterization—a prospective study. *Int Surg.* 1991;76:18-22.

26. Shiloh A, Eisen L, Yee M, Karakitsos D. Ultrasound-guided subclavian and axillary vein cannulation via an infraclavicular approach: in the tradition of Robert Aubaniac. *Crit Care Med.* 2012;40(10):2922-2923.

27. Tsui JY, Collins AB, White DW, Lai J, Tabas JA. Placement of a femoral venous catheter. *N Engl J Med.* 2008;358:e30.

28. Seldinger SI. Catheter replacement of the needle in percutaneous arteriography; a new technique. *Acta Radiol.* 1953;39:368-376.

29. Maury E, Guglielminotti J, Alzieu M, Guidet B, Offenstadt G. Ultrasonic examination: an alternative to chest radiography after central venous catheter insertion? *Am J Respir Crit Care Med.* 2001;164:403-405.

30. McGee D, Gould M. Preventing complications of central venous catheterization. *N Engl J Med.* 2003;348:1123-1133.

31. Merrer J, De Jonghe B, Golliot F, et al; French Catheter Study Group in Intensive Care. Complications of femoral and subclavian venous catheterization in critically ill patients: a randomized controlled trial. *JAMA.* 2001;286(6):700-707.

32. Eisen LA, Narasimhan M, Berger JS, Mayo PH, Rosen MJ, Schneider RF. Mechanical complications of central venous catheters. *J Intensive Care Med.* 2006;21:40-46.

33. Barsuk JH, Cohen ER, Feinglass J, McGaghie WC, Wayne DB. Use of simulation-based education to reduce catheter-related bloodstream infections. *Arch Intern Med.* 2009;169(15):1420-1423.

34. Pronovost P, Needham D, Berenholtz S, et al. An intervention to decrease catheter-related bloodstream infections in the ICU. *N Engl J Med.* 2006;355(26):2725-2732.

35. Desai A, Spiegler P, Kutzin J, et al. Impact of a daily goals sheet and simulation-based training on CLABSI incidence: a five-year analysis. *Crit Care Med.* 2015;43:204.

36. Kim DK, Gottesman MH, Forero A, et al. The CVC removal distress syndrome: an unappreciated complication of central venous catheter removal. *Am Surg.* 1998;64(4):344-347.

37. Ingram P, Sinclair L, Edwards T. The safe removal of central venous catheters. *Nurs Stand.* 2006;20(49):42-46.

38. Nuttall G, Burckhardt J, Hadley A, et al. Surgical and patient risk factors for severe arterial line complications in adults. *Anesthesiology.* 2016;124:590-597.

39. Cousins TR, O'Donnell JM. Arterial cannulation: a critical review. *AANA J.* 2004;72:267-271.

40. Ailon J, Mourad O, Chien V, Saun T, Dev S. Ultrasound-guided insertion of a radial arterial catheter. *N Engl J Med.* 2014; 371:e21.

41. Scheer B, Perel A, Pfeiffer UJ. Clinical review: complications and risk factors of peripheral arterial catheters used for haemodynamic monitoring in anaesthesia and intensive care medicine. *Crit Care.* 2002;6:199-204.

42. WHO Guidelines on Drawing Blood: Best Practices in Phlebotomy. *Annex I, Modified Allen Test.* Geneva Switzerland: World Health Organization; 2010. Available at https://www.ncbi.nlm.nih.gov/books/NBK138652/.

43. Levin PD, Sheinin O, Gozal Y. Use of ultrasound guidance in the insertion of radial artery catheters. *Crit Care Med.* 2003;31(2): 481-484.

44. Shiloh AL, Savel RH, Paulin LM, Eisen LA. Ultrasound-guided catheterization of the radial artery: a systematic review and meta-analysis of randomized controlled trials. *Chest.* 2011;139(3):524-529.

Patient and Family Information for: LINE ACCESS IN THE CCU

During a patient's stay in the coronary care unit (CCU), various lines may be placed in the veins or arteries for close monitoring and for administering potent medications. Below are some of the lines that may be placed.

CENTRAL LINE

WHAT IS A CENTRAL LINE?

A central line, also known as a central venous catheter (CVC), is a long, thin, flexible tube that is inserted in one of the large veins in the neck, upper chest, or groin region and leads to the heart. It allows delivery of fluids and necessary medications and can stay in place much longer than a regular intravenous (IV) catheter. It can also be used to measure the pressures within the heart.

WHAT ARE THE TYPES OF CENTRAL LINES?

The most common central line is called a triple lumen catheter (TLC) because it has three ports, which all end in different openings within the catheter. It is inserted in a large vein in the neck, upper chest, or groin, with its tip residing near the heart. Dialysis catheters typically have two ports (dual lumen) and can be used on a short-term basis in order to perform dialysis while in the CCU.

A peripherally inserted central catheter (PICC line) is a really long catheter that is inserted into a vein in the upper arm and is threaded until it reaches the larger vein near the heart.

Long-term-use tunneled catheters, also known as perm-a-cath, is inserted usually in a large vein in the neck. This catheter can be used for long-term dialysis, if needed.

WHY YOU NEED A CENTRAL LINE?

Your doctor or nurse will explain the reason you need a central line.

Below are some common reasons why a patient in the CCU might require a central line.

- If the small veins in the arms are not easily found or it is difficult to place a regular IV line
- If the blood pressure is low and strong medications are needed to raise the blood pressure (These medications are too strong to be given through a regular IV.)
- If the intravenous medications that have to be given can potentially burn the smaller vessels or muscles
- If blood or other blood products need to be rapidly given
- If intravenous nutrition is needed for a number of days
- If you need to undergo dialysis or plasmapheresis, where the blood is purified

WHERE IS THE PROCEDURE PERFORMED?

The procedure is typically done at the bedside in the CCU. A PICC line or perm-a-cath may be performed in the interventional radiology (IR) department or in the operating room (OR).

WHAT IS THE CARE BEFORE AND AFTER THE PROCEDURE?

Before the procedure is done, your lab work will be checked to assess your risk of bleeding, especially if you are taking any blood-thinning medications. If your platelets are low or international normalization ratio (INR) is high, a transfusion of platelets, plasma, or vitamin K may be necessary before the procedure.

An ultrasound machine is often used to guide the procedure. The blood vessels are visualized with ultrasonography in order to decide where the central line will be placed and also to prevent placement of the catheter elsewhere.

The procedure is sterile. Your body and face will be covered with a sterile drape to minimize any risks for infection during the insertion. You will be able to talk with your doctors during the procedure. You may be placed in the Trendelenburg position, where the head is lowered and the legs are raised. This position ensures safety of the central line placement.

If the central line is placed in the neck or upper chest, a chest x-ray is performed afterward to confirm the position of the central line near the heart and also in order to make sure there is no pneumothorax, which is collapse of the lung on the affected side.

IS THE PROCEDURE PAINFUL?

You will be awake and able to interact with the doctors performing the procedure. You will be given a numbing medication at the insertion area. After the initial injection of a local anesthetic, the procedure is pain free but you may experience pressure or discomfort. Your cooperation is of critical important during that time.

HOW LONG DOES IT TAKE?

No more than 30 to 45 minutes, accounting for the time of the procedure and preparation.

ARE THERE ANY POSSIBLE COMPLICATIONS?

All procedures carry some risk. This is a common procedure in CCUs and ICUs. A trained physician, physician assistant, or nurse practitioner usually places the line under sterile technique.

POSSIBLE COMPLICATIONS:

- Infection of the catheter
- Bleeding at the site or internally
- Puncture of the artery which is running next to the vein
- Pneumothorax or collapsed lung
- Heartbeat changes (arrhythmias)
- Blood clot in the vein where the line is placed
- Air bubbles entering the blood circulation

HOW TO CARE FOR THE CENTRAL LINE:

The catheter extends outside your body, allowing the nurses and doctors to access it to provide you medications, antibiotics, and fluids. The dressing will be getting changed at every nursing shift.

To avoid any infection, clotting, or other complications, meticulous care of the central line is important.

WHEN IS THE LINE REMOVED?

As soon as the central line is no longer needed, it should be removed. Gentle pressure should be applied on the area for 3 to 5 minutes.

The doctor will discuss with you if the line needs to be changed with a new one.

More Information:

1. American Thoracic Society (ATS): www.thoracic.org
2. Centers for Disease Control & Prevention: www.cdc.gov/

ARTERIAL LINE PLACEMENT

WHAT IS AN ARTERIAL LINE?

An arterial line is thin, flexible tube or catheter that is carefully inserted in the artery located in the wrist or groin. This catheter is connected through tubing to the monitor in the CCU, which will allow for beat-to-beat measurement of your blood pressure.

WHY YOU NEED AN ARTERIAL LINE?

Your doctor or nurse will explain the reason you need an arterial line.

Common Reasons for the Procedure:

- Low blood pressure (hypotension or shock) that requires medications in order to increase it
- High blood pressure (hypertension) requiring accurate measurements in order to control it with medications
- Lung problems or being on a ventilator, where the oxygen and carbon dioxide levels in the blood need to be checked frequently
- Severe respiratory or kidney problems that may require frequent checking of the acidity of the blood

WHERE IS THE PROCEDURE PERFORMED?

The procedure is typically performed at the bedside in the CCU.

WHAT IS THE CARE BEFORE AND AFTER THE PROCEDURE?

Before the procedure is performed, your lab work is checked to assess your risk of bleeding. If your platelets are low or INR is high, you might need transfusion of platelets, plasma, or vitamin K in order to lower the risk of bleeding.

The radial artery is located in the wrist and femoral artery is located in the groin region. These arteries may be palpated to locate them or an ultrasound machine may be used to guide the procedure.

The procedure itself is sterile and hence your body will be covered with a sterile drape to minimize any risks for infection during the insertion.

You will be able to move and sit up with the catheter in place. Care must be taken to prevent kinking and accidental removal of the catheter, which can lead to profuse bleeding.

IS IT PAINFUL?

You will be given a local anesthetic or numbing medication at the site of insertion. After the initial injection of the local anesthetic, the procedure is pain free but you might experience pressure or discomfort. Your cooperation is of critical importance during this time.

HOW LONG DOES IT TAKE?

No more than 20 to 30 minutes.

ARE THERE ANY POSSIBLE COMPLICATIONS?

A trained physician, physician assistant, or nurse practitioner usually places the line under sterile technique and under safe and controlled settings. All procedures have a risk of potential complications.

POSSIBLE COMPLICATIONS:

- Pain at the insertion site
- Bleeding at the site or internally
- Infection of the catheter
- Clotting of the catheter and possible low blood flow to the arm or leg

WHAT IS THE CARE FOR THE ARTERIAL LINE?

To avoid any infection, clotting, or other complications, meticulous care of the arterial line is important. Your CCU nurses and doctors will closely monitor the catheter and site.

WHEN IS THE LINE REMOVED?

As soon as the line is no longer needed, it gets removed. Gentle pressure will need to be applied on the area for 3 to 5 minutes. The site will be monitored for any further bleeding or swelling.

Gopal Narayanswami
Gabriela Bambrick-Santoyo
Joseph P. Mathew

49

Invasive Hemodynamic Assessment in the CCU

INTRODUCTION

Invasive hemodynamic monitoring is very often required in the care of a critically ill patient in the cardiac care unit (CCU) and is vital to the monitoring of the CCU patient, as well as dictating therapy. Various strategies of goal-directed fluid resuscitation utilizing dynamic measures of fluid responsiveness are available, which allow for monitoring and help direct therapy. A conservative fluid management strategy with judicious use of fluids along with monitoring of indices of tissue oxygenation is optimal in the CCU patient. Proper measurement and interpretation of the data is the key in ensuring adequate tissue perfusion and oxygen delivery, which is the goal.

PATHOPHYSIOLOGY OF HEMODYNAMICS IN A CRITICALLY ILL PATIENT IN THE CCU

It is important to understand oxygen delivery before we go into the various measures available for hemodynamic monitoring. Oxygenated blood is delivered to the tissues via the aorta, and deoxygenated blood returns to the right heart from where it enters the lungs to get reoxygenated. Tissue extraction of oxygen occurs during this transit. The normal arterial oxygen saturation (Sao_2) is 96% to 99%. The normal mixed venous saturation ($S\bar{v}o_2$) in the pulmonary artery (PA) is 65% to 75%, which denotes tissue oxygen extraction to be roughly 25% to 35%.

Determinants of cardiac output (CO) are preload, afterload, and inotropic contractility. Many monitoring systems work to incorporate these measures to determine the adequacy of CO. A hemodynamically stable patient for the most part does not require invasive hemodynamic monitoring, whereas in the hemodynamically unstable patient, invasive monitoring is frequently warranted. Such patients invariably have an arterial line and a central venous catheter (CVC), which by themselves can provide useful hemodynamic parameters. When this is not sufficient, additional invasive devices such as PA catheters (PACs) and CO monitors are utilized.

Hemodynamic data can help classify the cause of shock. The measured data can be used to calculate variables such as CO, systemic vascular resistance (SVR), and pulmonary vascular resistance

(PVR). The following equations are important to understand because they determine tissue perfusion and oxygenation:

$$CO = HR \times SV \qquad \text{(Eq. 1)}$$

$$DO_2 = CO \times Cao_2 \qquad \text{(Eq. 2)}$$

$$Cao_2 = 1.348 \times Hemoglobin \times Sao_2 + 0.003 \times Pao_2 \qquad \text{(Eq. 3)}$$

where CO is cardiac output, HR is heart rate, SV is stroke volume, DO_2 is oxygen delivery, Cao_2 is oxygen content, Sao_2 is oxygen saturation, and Pao_2 is the partial pressure of oxygen.

HEART LUNG INTERACTIONS

Both spontaneous and mechanical ventilation induce cyclical changes in intrapleural or intrathoracic pressure and lung volume. Intermittent positive pressure ventilation induces cyclic changes in the loading conditions of the left and right ventricles. This can independently affect the key determinants of cardiovascular performance, which are preload or atrial filling, afterload, heart rate, and myocardial contractility.

Spontaneous inspiration produces a negative pleural pressure, and this reduction in intrathoracic pressure is transmitted to the right atrium (RA). In contrast, intermittent positive pressure ventilation (tidal volume > 8 mL/kg ideal body weight) produces inspiratory increases in intrathoracic pressure and RA pressure decreasing venous return and right ventricular (RV) preload, and also increases RV afterload. This leads to a decrease in RV stroke volume, which is manifested as a decrease in left ventricular (LV) stroke volume, which is at its minimum during the expiratory period due to a phase lag of 2 to 3 beats (ie, pulmonary transit time). These cyclic changes are greater when patients are volume depleted and are on the steep rather than the flat portion of the Frank–Starling curve. This can lead to changes in pulse pressure (PP) variation, stroke volume variation, and inferior vena cava (IVC) size variation, indicating a patient who may be fluid responsive.[1] The biventricular dependence is confounded if the patient on a ventilator is also making spontaneous efforts or has an atrial arrhythmia. It is important to consider this while interpreting data.

ARTERIAL BLOOD PRESSURE

DEFINITION

Arterial blood pressure (ABP) is the pressure exerted by the circulating volume of blood upon the wall of the arteries. It is measured both at its peak (systolic blood pressure, SBP) and at its trough (diastolic blood pressure, DBP). The blood pressure in the aorta during systole is a clinical indicator of afterload (ie, the forces the left ventricle must overcome to eject blood).

The normal ranges in ABP are systolic 90 to 140 mm Hg and diastolic 60 to 90 mm Hg. PP is the difference between systolic and diastolic pressure. If BP is measured in the brachial artery, the average PP is approximately 40 mm Hg. Above 60 mm Hg, the risk of coronary events and all-cause mortality increases. The main determinant of PP is large artery compliance. The less compliant arteries are, the higher the PP, which is why PP increases with age, as elastin fibers of the arterial walls are weakened by years of stress.

ABP and PP can be affected by various factors as illustrated in **Tables 49.1** and **49.2**.

Mean Arterial Pressure

Mean arterial pressure (MAP) is often used as a surrogate indicator of blood flow and a better indicator of tissue perfusion than SBP because it accounts for the fact that two-thirds of the cardiac cycle is spent in diastole. A MAP of 65 mm Hg or greater is needed to maintain adequate tissue perfusion.

Systemic MAP is defined as the mean perfusion pressure throughout the cardiac cycle and it can be calculated as follows:

$$MAP - SVR \times CO \qquad \text{(Eq. 4)}$$

A more practical estimate can be obtained by the following equation:

$$MAP = \frac{2}{3} DBP + \frac{1}{3} SBP \qquad \text{(Eq. 5)}$$

TABLE 49.1	Factors Affecting Arterial Blood Pressure
SYSTOLIC BLOOD PRESSURE	**DIASTOLIC BLOOD PRESSURE**
Stroke volume	Arterial wall distensibility
Left ventricular ejection velocity	Systemic arterial resistance
End diastolic volume	Blood viscosity
Arterial wall distensibility	Length of the cardiac cycle
Systemic arterial resistance	
Blood viscosity	

TABLE 49.2	Factors Affecting Pulse Pressure
INCREASED PULSE PRESSURE	**DECREASED PULSE PRESSURE**
Fever, exercise	Cardiac tamponade
Bradycardia	Hypovolemia
Aortic regurgitation	Shock
Anemia	Massive pulmonary embolism
Hyperthyroidism	Tension pneumothorax
	Aortic stenosis

Intra-arterial Blood Pressure Monitoring

Intra-ABP is the direct measurement of arterial pressure and it involves inserting a catheter in a suitable artery. The catheter must be connected to a sterile, fluid-filled system, which is in turn connected to an electronic patient monitor.

CLINICAL UTILITY

ABP monitoring offers several advantages over noninvasive blood pressure (NIBP) monitoring. It allows continuous beat-to-beat pressure measurement and allows accurate blood pressure readings at very low pressures. It allows close monitoring of patients on vasopressors, inotropes, or vasodilators. It enables ABP measurement in patients in whom NIBP monitoring is difficult and allows for frequent arterial sampling. The waveforms can also provide useful information about the patient's cardiovascular status.

MEASUREMENT

Most of the ABP measuring systems consist of a column of fluid directly connecting the arterial catheter to a pressure transducer. The pressure waveform of the arterial pulse is transmitted via the column of fluid to a pressure transducer where it is converted into an electrical signal. This electrical signal is then processed, amplified, and converted into a visual display by a microprocessor.

WAVEFORM

The arterial pressure wave is a complex wave generated by a series of pressure changes that occur during valve closure, systole, diastole, and by reflection waves caused by the impedance of blood flow as it traverses distally. The waveform seen in the transducer is the summation of all these waves resulting in a single waveform. Each component can be assigned to a specific point of the cardiac cycle and has hemodynamic significance. This can be appreciated by looking at the waveform in **Figure 49.1**. The systolic upstroke represents the pressure generated at the beginning of systole. The dicrotic notch represents the closure of the aortic valve and the subsequent downstroke represents

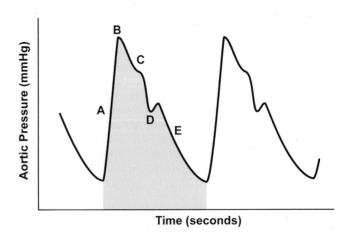

FIGURE 49.1 Arterial waveform. *A*, Systolic uptake. *B*, Peak systolic pressure. *C*, Systolic decline. *D*, Dicrotic notch. *E*, Diastolic runoff.

the rapid decline during diastole. Due to the differences in the characteristics of the vascular tree, ejection velocities, and the length of the fluid column, arterial waveforms differ depending on the site of catheter insertion. The further the catheter is from the aorta, the higher the SBP, the further the dicrotic notch, and the wider the PP. The MAP, however, will remain constant and hence is relied on as the main hemodynamic parameter to assess perfusion.

ACCURACY OF MEASUREMENTS

It is important that accuracy of the ABP measurements is maintained by reducing the length of tubing used and ensuring that there are no bubbles or clots in the system. The accuracy and interpretation of invasive pressure measurements depend on a number of physical principles of the systems used.

Damping

Anything that reduces energy in an oscillating system will reduce the amplitude of the oscillations. This is termed damping and measurements will be adversely affected if there is excessive (overdamping) or insufficient (underdamping) damping,

Factors that will cause overdamping include three-way stopcocks, bubbles, clots, long tubing, and kinks in the catheter or tubing. These may be a major source of error, causing an underreading of SBP and DBP, although the MAP is relatively unaffected.

Transducer position can be checked (ie, zeroed) by turning the stopcock off to the patient and open to air, at the level of the heart. The monitor must be adjusted to display zero. Incorrect readings may be obtained if the transducer is not releveled with changes in position of the bed or patient.

Abnormal Arterial Line Waveforms

Under certain circumstances, it is possible to correlate the shape of an arterial waveform with a specific pathology. A steep systolic upstroke can be seen in hypertension or atherosclerosis due to noncompliance of the vessels. In aortic regurgitation, the PP is widened and a second peak, bisferient pulse can also be seen (**Figure 49.2**). Aortic stenosis can cause delaying of the upstroke slope and a low systolic peak due to limited outflow (**Figure 49.3**).

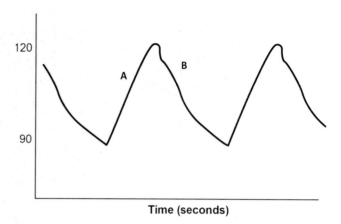

FIGURE 49.3 Arterial waveform in aortic stenosis. *A*, Slurred gradual systolic upstroke. *B*, Absent dicrotic notch.

CENTRAL VENOUS PRESSURE

DEFINITION

Central venous pressure (CVP) is the pressure measured in the lower third of the superior vena cava (SVC) and is considered a direct measurement of the pressure in the RA (ie, mean RA pressure). It is commonly used as an estimate of RV filling pressures or preload.

Some authors suggest the following equation to help health care providers:

$$CVP = \text{Mean RA pressure} = \text{Right ventricular end diastolic pressure (RVEDP)} = \text{Preload.}$$

The CVP value is determined both by the pressure of venous blood in the vena cava and the function of the right heart. The principal factors affecting CVP are shown in **Figure 49.4**. Venous return is in turn influenced by intravascular volume, compliance characteristics of the venous system (venous tone), PVR, and intrathoracic pressure. The changes in CVP are directly proportional to volume changes and inversely proportional to venous compliance.

MEASUREMENT

CVP is acquired by inserting a CVC into any of several large veins. It is threaded so that the tip of the catheter rests in the lower third of the SVC. The pressure monitoring assembly is attached to the distal port of a multilumen CVC. The CVP can be measured manually (using a manometer) or electronically (using a transducer). Normal CVP is 2 to 6 mm Hg. The CVP must be set at zero at the level of the RA with the patient lying supine (the "phlebostatic axis"—usually 4th intercostal space in the midaxillary line). In the thorax, extravascular pressures should be close to zero at the end of expiration; hence, CVP is measured at end expiration and at end diastole.

CLINICAL UTILITY

Traditionally, CVP has been utilized to assess volume responsiveness, with a low CVP thought to predict fluid responsiveness whereas a patient with a high CVP is thought to be fluid

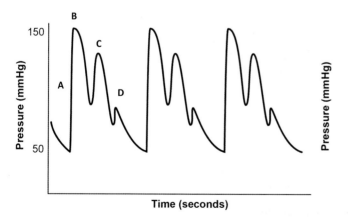

FIGURE 49.2 Arterial waveform in aortic regurgitation. *A*, Widened pulse pressure. *B* and *C*, Bisferiens pulse, peak *C* is a reflected wave. *D*, Dicrotic notch.

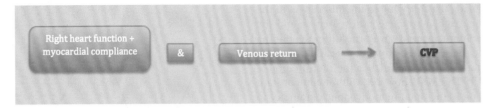

FIGURE 49.4 Factors affecting CVP. CVP, central venous pressure.

replete. These concepts have been challenged based on meta analysis that have questioned the use of static measures of fluid responsiveness.[2]

CVP is elevated in conditions such as RV failure, tricuspid stenosis, or regurgitation, pericardial disorders, and mechanically ventilated patients on high positive end-expiratory pressure (PEEP) settings and does not reflect fluid status. For the last decade, the utility of CVP measurement to determine volume responsiveness has been questioned. Because of this debate, its use should be in association with information relating to other hemodynamic variables.

WAVEFORM

In sinus rhythm, the CVP waveform reflects changes in right atrial pressure during the cardiac cycle and contains five components:

- Two major positive deflections: *a* and *v* waves
- Two negative deflections: *x* and *y* descents
- A third positive wave: the *c* wave, which is not consistently observed

Figure 49.5 shows this anatomy of a CVP waveform in correlation with the cardiac cycle with the help of a simultaneous ECG tracing. The first peak is the *a* wave, which immediately follows the *P* wave of the ECG. This *a* wave (atrial) represents the pressure increase due to atrial systolic contraction. The *a* wave is followed by the *x* descent, which is the drop in atrial pressure during ventricular systole caused by atrial relaxation and the downward movement of the atrioventricular junction during early ventricular systole. The trough of the *x* descent is followed by the *v* wave, which represents the increase in pressure generated by the passive filling of the atria during ventricular systole. The *v* wave corresponds to the end of the *T* wave in the ECG. The *y* descent results from the drop in atrial pressure as the blood enters the ventricle during diastole. The *c* wave represents closure of the atrioventricular valves and is seen as a small positive wave early on in the interrupts the *x* descent. The waveform components and their timing in the cardiac cycle are listed in **Table 49.3**. Understanding the CVP waveform can help the clinician to interpret the various abnormalities that can be seen in certain clinical conditions. The waveform abnormalities and the conditions associated with them are listed in **Table 49.4**.

CURRENT CONCEPTS

CVP AND ITS USEFULNESS IN GUIDING FLUID THERAPY

CVP is a static measure of right atrial pressures. Traditionally, clinicians have used the concept that a low CVP will be a measure of fluid responsiveness and a high CVP will predict someone who

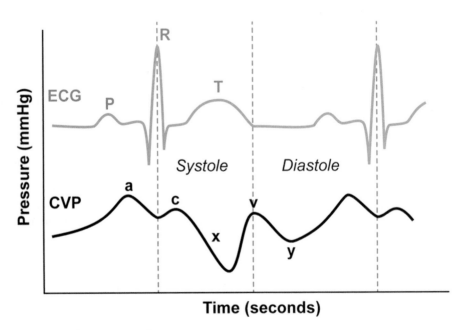

FIGURE 49.5 Anatomy of CVP waveform. CVP, central venous pressure.

TABLE 49.3	Components of the Central Venous Pressure Waveform	
WAVEFORM COMPONENT	**PHASE OF CARDIAC CYCLE**	**MECHANICAL EVENT**
a wave	End diastole	Atrial contraction
c wave	Early systole	Tricuspid bulging (inferior vena cava)
v wave	Late systole	Systolic atrial filling
x descent	Mid systole	Atrial relaxation
y descent	Early diastole	Early ventricular filling

TABLE 49.4	Abnormal Central Venous Pressure Waveforms
WAVEFORM ABNORMALITY	**CLINICAL CORRELATION**
Dominant *a* wave	Pulmonary hypertension Tricuspid stenosis Pulmonary stenosis
Canon *a* wave	Complete heart block Ventricular tachycardia with atrioventricular dissociation
Dominant *v* wave	Tricuspid regurgitation
Exaggerated *x* descent	Pericardial tamponade Constrictive pericarditis
Slow *y* descent	Tricuspid stenosis Atrial myxoma
Absent *y* descent	Tamponade
Prominent *x* and *y* descent	Constrictive pericarditis

will not respond to a fluid challenge. This concept was promoted by the Surviving Sepsis Campaign (SSC) guidelines based on the Early Goal Directed Therapy trial by Rivers, which showed that using a target CVP goal of 8 to 12 mm Hg (12–15 mm Hg in mechanically ventilated patients) for fluid resuscitation, along with other early interventions, led to decreased mortality in patients with severe sepsis and septic shock.[3,4] However, this relationship between CVP and intravascular volume as well as its usefulness to predict fluid responsiveness has been questioned.[5] In 2008, Marik et al[2]. conducted a systematic review of the literature on this topic that included 24 studies and 805 patients. The studies analyzed demonstrated that patients with low CVPs may not be fluid responsive and patients with high CVPs may be fluid responsive. They found that there is a very poor correlation between CVP and blood volume as well as the inability of CVP or ΔCVP to predict the hemodynamic response to a fluid challenge. They concluded that CVP should not be used to make clinical decisions regarding fluid management.[2,6]

Overall, the methods for assessing fluid responsiveness have evolved over time from static parameters to dynamic measures based on either a passive leg raise (PLR) or a real fluid challenge, both of which have a higher degree of accuracy in predicting fluid responsiveness.[7] However, these dynamic measures have not been fully incorporated into clinical practice. Although static measures of fluid responsiveness such as the CVP have fallen out of favor, extremes of CVP values still have clinical utility. Septic shock is associated with low CVP, high CO, and low SVR. In contrast, cardiogenic shock is associated with high CVP, low CO, and high SVR. A low CVP is useful because it suggests a low volume state whereas a high CVP is less useful because the patient may have fluid overload or have normal volume status with heart failure. A very high CVP in the absence of right-sided heart disease represents a patient who will likely not be fluid responsive. Although the CVP measurement has been heavily criticized in the literature, when measured correctly it is one of the few tools that is devoid of subjective interpretation by the end user. Additionally, it is a value that is easily obtained in the CCU patient and can be interpreted by various members of the health care team. A CVP should never be interpreted in isolation and should be used in context with one's physical examination, echocardiogram (ECG), and other dynamic measures of fluid responsiveness, which are described later in this chapter. For example, it should not be assumed that a patient is adequately fluid resuscitated if the CVP is normal. Similarly, a patient with right heart dysfunction with elevated CVP may be fluid responsive despite an elevated CVP. In summary, the CVP provides insight into the patient's hemodynamic status and is a useful adjunct when used in combination with other predictors of fluid responsiveness.

CENTRAL VENOUS OXYGEN SATURATION AND OXYGEN DELIVERY

The central venous oxygen saturation ($Scvo_2$) is obtained from a from a central line, preferably from an internal jugular or subclavian vein catheter, and serves as a surrogate of mixed venous oxygen saturation ($S\bar{v}o_2$). It is estimated that the $Scvo_2$ is 3% to 5% higher than $S\bar{v}o_2$. The femoral $Scvo_2$ is less reliable. $Scvo_2$, along with the CVP, can help guide further fluid management.

A low $Scvo_2$ serves as an indicator of poor oxygen delivery (ie, low CO, low hemoglobin or low Sao_2) or increased consumption by tissues (eg, fever, hyperthyroidism). A high $Scvo_2$ indicates poor extraction by tissues (eg, sepsis, hypothyroidism, cyanide poisoning) or arteriovenous shunting. The SSC sepsis guidelines recommend a target $Scvo_2$ of $>70\%$[4] as a target for resuscitation for patients with severe sepsis and septic shock; however, these protocoled recommendations have since been challenged.[8–10]

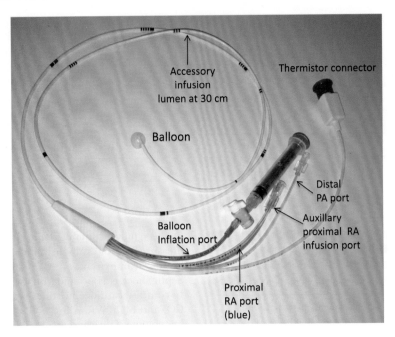

FIGURE 49.6 Standard pulmonary artery catheter.

THE PULMONARY ARTERY CATHETER

In 1970, Swan and his colleagues[11] described PAC with a balloon proximal to the tip, which could be directed to the branches of the PA. It permits measurement of intracardiac filling pressures. The catheter is inserted into the RA, RV, and when in position with the balloon inflated in the PA, a "wedge" pressure is obtained. This wedge pressure provides an indirect measure of LV filling pressure, which can guide the clinician in the management of fluid therapy in patients with shock and respiratory failure. CO measurements obtained by the thermodilution method and the derived SVR measurement can help distinguish mixed shock states and assist in titrating vasopressors and inotropic medications. The PAC can assist in the management of patients with acute myocardial infarctions, valvular dysfunction, intracardiac shunts, pericardial tamponade, and pulmonary hypertension. Additionally, it can help with the diagnosis and management of mechanical complications of myocardial infarction, such as ventricular septal rupture, papillary muscle rupture, and RV infarction. Contraindications to PAC include severe coagulopathy or thrombocytopenia, RV thrombus, tricuspid or pulmonic valve prosthesis, and right-sided endocarditis. In patients with left bundle branch block, passage of the catheter can induce complete heart block.

DESCRIPTION

A PAC or Swan-Ganz catheter is a flexible, balloon-tipped, flow-directed catheter that is guided through the right side of the heart and into a branch of the PA. Under sterile conditions, the catheter is generally inserted through the subclavian, internal jugular, or femoral, vein. The right internal jugular vein and left subclavian vein are ideal because the curvature of the PAC facilitates passage through the heart. The procedure, also known as right heart catheterization, may be performed with or without the use of fluoroscopy.[12]

The typical PAC is 110 cm long and has four lumens: the distal, proximal, thermistor, and inflation lumen. The distal lumen port is located at the tip of the catheter. This port allows monitoring of systolic, diastolic, and mean pressures in the PA and allows visualization of the waveform to guide proper placement. It can also be used for drawing mixed $S\bar{v}o_2$ samples. The proximal port, located approximately 30 cm from the tip of the catheter, is used to monitor RA pressure, CVP, and to inject the solution used to assess intermittent CO by thermodilution. Additionally, there may be an accessory RA proximal port with its lumen at 30 cm from the catheter tip, which may be used for infusion of medications. **Figure 49.6** shows a standard PAC with the balloon inflated.

Thermodilution involves injection of a known amount of solution with a known temperature rapidly into the RA lumen of the catheter. Usually cold fluid is injected into the proximal lumen and the temperature of the blood is measured downstream in the PA by a thermistor. This information is plotted on a time–temperature curve that represents the time it takes for the blood to change from a warmer baseline temperature to a cooler temperature after the injection and then back to the baseline temperature as the blood circulates. The rate of blood flow is inversely proportional to the change in temperature over time. When CO is low, it takes longer for the blood temperature to return to baseline; when CO is high, the cooling fluid is carried faster through the heart, and the temperature returns to baseline faster.

The inflation lumen connects to a balloon that is located less than 1 cm from the catheter tip, which is inflated with 1.5 mL air to advance into the PA. The waveform is constantly observed on the monitor during advancement until a wedged position is obtained. It is important that on deflation of the balloon, a PA waveform is obtained so as to avoid over wedging. It is used to obtain PAWP, which is also called pulmonary artery occlusion pressure (PAOP) or pulmonary capillary wedge pressure (PCWP).

Once lodged in the PA, the inflated balloon serves as a continuous conduit from the catheter tip through the pulmonary vein, left atrium (LA), and open mitral valve into the left ventricle. This allows

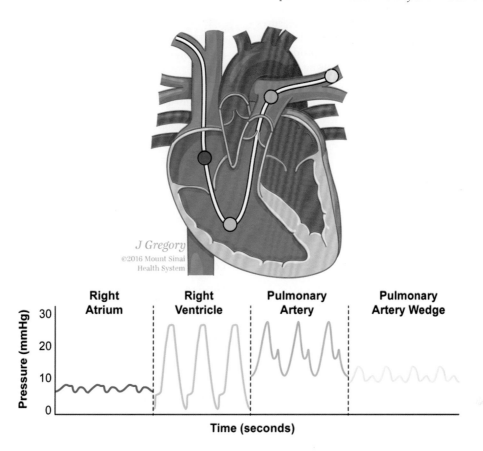

FIGURE 49.7 Waveforms during right heart catheterization.

the distal lumen to indirectly measure LV pressure. The balloon should be deflated once PAOP measures are obtained. The pulmonary artery diastolic pressures (PADP) can also serve as a surrogate to PAOP. Newer catheters come with continuous cardiac output (CCO) and continuous Sv̄o₂ monitoring. In order to measure CO continuously, thermal energy emitted by the filament located on the catheter is used to calculate CO using thermodilution principles.

INSERTION

Prior to PAC insertion, the system must be zeroed to ambient air pressure. The reference point for this is the midpoint of the LA, estimated at the fourth intercostal space in the midaxillary line with the patient lying in supine position. With the transducer at this height, the membrane is exposed to atmospheric pressure and the monitor is then adjusted to zero. The PAC should be checked for cracks and kinks. The balloon should be checked and all lumens flushed to remove air bubbles.

The catheter is inserted through an introducer catheter sheath and advanced using continuous pressure monitoring from the distal lumen (**Figure 49.7**). It is recommended to insert the catheter 15 cm so that the tip is outside of the sheath. The balloon is then inflated before advancing into the PA. **Figure 49.7** shows the various waveforms obtained during right heart catheterization. If an RV waveform is still present approximately 20 cm after the initial RV pattern appears, the catheter may be coiling in the RV. The catheter is withdrawn slowly and advanced again until the

PA tracing is obtained and even further until a wedge tracing is obtained. Sometimes fluoroscopy is necessary in difficult cases. Measure CO by connecting the thermistor to a computer and perform thermodilution. The assistant should note down the systolic, diastolic, and mean pressures in the right heart, including the PAOP at end expiration.

An ideal positioning of the PAC is one which shows the PA tracing with the balloon deflated and a pulmonary occlusion tracing with the balloon inflated. It is important to deflate the balloon after acquiring readings and values. A chest X-ray is obtained to ensure proper placement preferably in West Zone 3, where the pulmonary capillary pressure exceeds the mean alveolar pressure.[13] This zone is located in the most dependent portion of the lung, where vascular pressures are the highest. If the PAOP is greater than the PA diastolic pressure or if there is marked respiratory variation, this may be a clue that the catheter has not migrated into Zone 3. The tip of the catheter should therefore be ideally positioned below the level of the LA. In a patient on a ventilator, high PEEP can alter the baseline intrathoracic pressure. However if it is located in the right zone as mentioned earlier, the effects of PEEP on PAOP are usually small, and often do not affect clinical management.

The PAOP waveform is similar to the CVP waveform obtained from the proximal port, which reflects RA pressures. However, it is important to recognize that the PAOP waveform is shifted to the right by 80 to 120 ms in relation to the ECG because of the time delay in the waveform travelling through the pulmonary circuit.

As a review, let us contrast PAOP versus CVP. PAOP measures left atrial pressure, and approximates left ventricular end diastolic pressure (LVEDP) when the mitral valve functions properly.

Some authors simplify this concept by the following formula:

$$PAOP = Mean\ LA\ pressure = LVEDP,$$

while

$$CVP = Mean\ RA\ pressure = RVEDP = Preload.$$

MEASUREMENTS

Direct measurements that can be obtained from an accurately placed PAC are the following:

    Central venous pressure
    Right atrial pressure (RAP)
    Right ventricular pressure (RVP)
    Pulmonary arterial pressure (PAP)
    Pulmonary artery occlusion pressure
    Cardiac output
    Mixed venous oxyhemoglobin saturation ($S\bar{v}o_2$)

The PAC can also indirectly measure the following:

    Systemic vascular resistance
    Pulmonary vascular resistance
    Cardiac index (CI)
    Stroke volume index (SVI)
    Left ventricular stroke work index (LVSDI)
    Right ventricular stroke work index (RVSI)
    Oxygen delivery (DO_2)
    Oxygen consumption (VO_2)

INTERPRETATION

Right ventricle: During catheter insertion using the distal tip, the peak RV systolic pressure and the RVEDP are measured from the RV pressure waveform. Normal RV systolic pressure varies from 15 to 30 mm Hg and normal RVEDP varies from 1 to 7 mm Hg. Elevations in RV pressure are associated with diseases that elevate the PAP, pulmonic valve disorders, and diseases that primarily affect the RV.

Pulmonary artery: Normal PA systolic pressures range from 15 to 25 mm Hg, whereas PA diastolic pressures range from 8 to 12 mm Hg. The mean PAP (mPAP) is typically 16 mm Hg (10 to 22 mm Hg). Pulmonary hypertension is defined as mPAP ≥ 25 mm Hg. The PA tracing is similar in appearance to the systemic arterial pressure tracing, except that the PAPs are normally much lower.

Pulmonary artery occlusion pressure: The PAOP or PCWP estimates the left atrial pressure. This is measured when the catheter tip is in the PA with the balloon inflated. Normal wedge pressures vary from 8 to 12 mm Hg, with a mean of 10 mm Hg. The PAOP usually estimates the LVEDP, which gives an idea of LV preload, assuming that there is no obstruction to flow between the LA and left ventricle and that the compliance of the left ventricle is normal. The PAOP may not reliably indicate LV preload when compliance of the left ventricle is abnormal (eg, LV hypertrophy, ischemia, or restrictive cardiomyopathy). Valvular pathology such as mitral stenosis, myxoma, or mitral regurgitation will overestimate PAOP, whereas PAOP will underestimate LVEDP

TABLE 49.5	Abnormal PAOP Values
Conditions that cause a high PAOP	
Left ventricular systolic heart failure	
Left ventricular diastolic heart failure	
Mitral and aortic valve disease	
Hypertrophic cardiomyopathy	
Hypervolemia	
Large right-to-left shunts	
Cardiac tamponade	
Constrictive and restrictive cardiomyopathies	
Conditions that cause a low PAOP	
Hypovolemia	
Pulmonary venoocclusive disease	
Obstructive shock due to pulmonary embolism	

PAOP, pulmonary artery occlusion pressure.

in aortic regurgitation. **Table 49.5** outlines the conditions that cause abnormal PAOP values.

ABNORMAL PAOP WAVEFORMS

Physiologically, the PAOP tracing has similar components to the RA with three positive and two negative deflections. The abnormal waveform seen in the PAOP tracing reflects changes on the left side of the heart. Electrocardiographic correlation is required for correct identification of these events. The PAOP waveform is delayed by >120 ms when compared with the ECG.

Large *a* waves: Increased amplitude of the *a* wave in the PAOP tracing can be seen with increased resistance to LV filling of any cause such as mitral stenosis or decreased LV compliance. Cannon *a* waves can also be seen with complete atrioventricular block due to atrial contraction against higher ventricular pressures.

Large *v* waves: The common cause of large *v* waves on a PAOP tracing is mitral regurgitation (MR). Other conditions such as ventricular septal defects can also cause large *v* waves due to increased atrial pressures. Giant *v* waves can be seen in cases of severe MR and often this may be mistaken for a PA tracing. This can be avoided by using the ECG tracing and understanding that the peak of the systolic PAP occurs within the *T* wave whereas the giant *v* wave occurs after it.

Conditions such as cardiac tamponade and constrictive pericarditis may present hemodynamic alterations prior to clinical manifestations. Whereas both conditions may produce equalization of diastolic pressures (RAP = RV diastolic pressure = PADP), waveform identification can assist in differentiating the two. In cardiac tamponade, all right-sided pressures will be elevated and there is a prominent *x* descent and a loss of the *y* descent in a PAOP or RA tracing as a result of higher diastolic values. In constrictive pericarditis, there are exaggerated *y* descents from rapid diastolic filling as a result of the rigid pericardium.

Acute ventricular septal defect (VSD) can also produce low CO when the blood volume from the left ventricle shunts over to the right ventricle. This shunting causes a "step-up" of oxygen saturation from the right ventricle to the PA. By determining saturation values in the PA, a VSD can be detected. In severe cases, a resultant elevation in the v wave during a wedge recording may also be seen. This is due to the increase in blood volume from the left ventricle, which during atrial filling, records as an elevation in the v wave.

MEASURING THE PAOP

The correct reading of a PAOP waveform in relation to an ECG strip is shown in **Figure 49.8**. As opposed to a CVP tracing, there is a delay of two to three squares of the waveform in the PAOP tracing. The "Z point" (occlusion pressure at end diastole) is measured by any one of the following methods (see **Figure 49.8**):

1. The pre c wave location
2. Mean of the highest and lowest pressure of the a wave:

$$\text{PAOP} = \frac{a + x}{2}$$

3. The Z point, a perpendicular line drawn two to three squares after the QRS complex

The abnormal waveform seen in the PAOP tracing reflects changes on the left side of the heart. The objective of placing a Swan-Ganz catheter is to obtain LVEDP, which is used to estimate LV end diastolic volume (LVEDV). The location of the end diastole period correlates to the point just before the c wave. If the c wave is not located, then the next approach would be to measure the mean of the highest and lowest pressures of the a wave. A third method is to find the Z point that correlates with the wedge pressure. This is located on the PAOP tracing by drawing a line, two to three boxes (0.08 to 0.12 seconds) after the QRS segment of the ECG tracing.

It must be remembered that respiratory efforts strongly affect the waveforms. Spontaneous ventilation tends to drop vascular pressures, whereas positive pressure ventilation raises the pressures in the inspiratory cycle. Pleural pressures become negative during inspiration in a spontaneously breathing patient and positive during the inspiratory cycle of a mechanically ventilated patient. Since expiration is the longer and more stable phase, pressures are measured at the end of expiration, when pleural pressures are close to zero.

In summary, an ideal measurement of wedge pressure involves obtaining simultaneous tracings of ECG, respiration, and the PAOP tracing, then identifying the Z point using the ECG at the end of expiration, or measuring the average of the highest and lowest pressures of that a wave. Other interpretations of the waveforms are similar to what was mentioned in the CVP tracings except that they reflect left-sided function.

CALCULATION OF CARDIAC OUTPUT

Thermodilution Method

The thermodilution method has been well validated and is performed as specified earlier. Approximately 10 mL of cold or room temperature saline is injected into the proximal lumen and the temperature difference is sensed by the distal lumen. The bedside computer monitor integrates the time–temperature curve and calculates CO using the Stewart–Hamilton equation. The area under the temperature–time curve is inversely proportional to CO. Usually three CO measurements are performed in rapid succession and averaged.[14]

Clinicians should be aware of several important sources of error such as tricuspid regurgitation and intracardiac shunts. Tricuspid regurgitation leads to an underestimation of CO. Right-to-left and left-to-right intracardiac shunts can produce falsely elevated cardiac output measurements by the thermodilution technique.

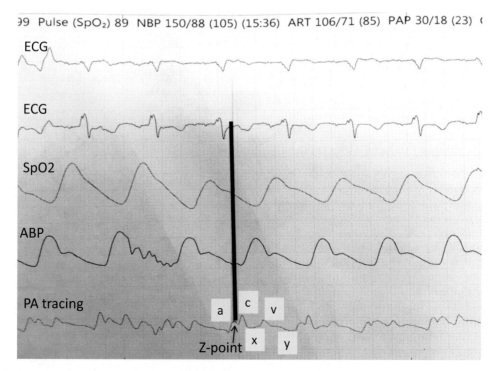

FIGURE 49.8 Pulmonary artery occlusion pressure waveform in relation to ECG. ECG, Electrocardiogram.

Variations in temperature (eg, after cardiopulmonary bypass) can also falsely affect the measurements. Accurate measurements also depend on calibration of transducers and a fluid-filled system that is devoid of air bubbles and blood clots. The CO can also be elevated physiologically. A high CO with or without heart failure can also be seen in a number of conditions such as sepsis, hyperthyroidism, anemia, Beriberi, renal disease, hepatic disease, and systemic arteriovenous malformation.

Fick Method

Fick's concept proposes that the uptake or release of a substance by an organ is the product of blood flow through that organ and the difference between arterial and venous values of that substance. Although the Fick method is considered the gold standard for CO measurement, it is not widely applied outside the cardiac catheterization laboratory, because it has many limitations including a patient who is in steady state and the requirement of simultaneous expired air and blood samples.[14]

$$CO = \frac{\dot{V}o_2}{Cao_2 - Cvo_2} \qquad (Eq.\ 6)$$

where $\dot{V}o_2$ is oxygen consumption, Cao_2 is normal arterial oxygen content, and Cvo_2 is normal venous oxygen content.

Oxygen consumption is either measured by exhaled breath analysis or estimated from a nomogram that is based on age, sex, height, and weight. The arteriovenous oxygen difference requires additional calculations:

$$Cao_2 - Cvo_2 = 1.34 \times Hgb \times (Sao_2 - S\bar{v}o_2) \times 10 \qquad (Eq.\ 7)$$

$$S\bar{v}o_2 = Sao_2 - \frac{\dot{V}O_2}{1.34 \times Hgb \times CO} \qquad (Eq.\ 8)$$

where Hgb is the hemoglobin, $S\bar{v}o_2$ is the mixed venous oxygen content and the Sao_2 is the arterial oxygen content.

DETECTION OF LEFT-TO-RIGHT SHUNTS

Arterial blood sampling from the RA, right ventricle, and PA provides helpful information when evaluating a suspected intracardiac (left to right) shunt. Detection of an oxygen saturation "step-up" in the right-sided chambers allows confirmation of the left-to-right shunt and determination of its location.

SYSTEMIC AND PULMONARY VASCULAR RESISTANCE

Once the CO has been determined, SVR and PVR can be estimated. Since the calculations of vascular resistance are based on direct measurements (ie, pressures) and indirect measurements (i.e., CO), each one can has its own intrinsic sources of error, giving rise to incorrect calculated values. Nonetheless, SVR can provide valuable information when distinguishing the classes of shock from each other and PVR is often useful when determining the prognosis of patients with pulmonary hypertension. **Table 49.6** lists the common formulas used for interpretation of Swan-Ganz values and **Table 49.7** lists the normal values. The derived values are illustrated in **Table 49.8**. Obtaining these values is very useful in creating a hemodynamic profile of the critically ill patient in the CCU. The commonly observed hemodynamic profile in the critically ill patient in various conditions is listed in **Table 49.9**.

TABLE 49.6	Formulas for Swan-Ganz Interpretation
FORMULAS	

$$DO_2\ (mL/min) = CO \times Cao_2$$

$$CO\ (mL/min) = HR \times SV$$

$$Cao_2\ (mL\ O_2/dL) = 1.34 \times Hb \times Sao_2 + 0.003 \times Po_2$$

$$Vo_2\ (mL\ O_2/min) = CO \times (Cao_2 - Cvo_2)$$

$$SVR\ (dyne \cdot s/cm^5) = \frac{MAP - CVP}{CO} \times 80$$

$$PVR\ (dyne \cdot s/cm^5) = \frac{MPAP - PAOP}{CO} \times 80$$

$$CI\ (L/min/m^2) = \frac{CO}{BSA}$$

$$SVI\ (mL/m^2/beat) = \frac{CI}{HR}$$

$$LVSWI\ (g/m^2/beat) = (MAP - PAOP) \times SVI \times 0.136$$

$$RVSWI\ (g/m^2/beat) = (MPAP - CVP) \times SVI \times 0.136$$

BSA, body surface area; Cao_2 oxygen content; CI, cardiac index; CO, cardiac output; Cvo_2 venous oxygen content; CVP, central venous pressure; DO_2, oxygen delivery; HR, heart rate; LVSWI, left ventricular stroke work index; MAP, mean arterial pressure; MPAP, mean pulmonary artery pressure; PAOP, pulmonary artery occlusion pressure; PVR, pulmonary vascular resistance; RVSWI, right ventricular stroke work index; SV, stroke volume; SVI, stroke volume index; SVR, systemic vascular resistance; Vo_2, oxygen consumption

TABLE 49.7	Normal Values
CO: 4–8 L/min	
CI: 2.5–4 L/min	
CVP: 2–6 mm Hg	
PAWP: 8–12 mm Hg	
PAP: 25/10 mm Hg	
$S\bar{v}o_2$: 0.65–0.70	

CI, cardiac index; CO, cardiac output; CVP, central venous pressure; PAP, pulmonary arterial pressure; PAWP, pulmonary artery wedge pressure.

TABLE 49.8	Derived Values
USE OF FORMULA: CO = (MAP − CVP)/SVR	
SV: 50–100 mL/beat	
SVI: 25–45 mL/beat/m²	
SVR: 900–1300 dyne · s/cm⁵	
SVRI: 1900–2400 dyne · s/cm⁵	
PVR: 40–150 dyne · s/cm⁵	
PVRI: 120–200 dyne · s/cm⁵	

PVR, pulmonary vascular resistance; PVRI, pulmonary vascular resistance index; SV, stroke volume; SVI, stroke volume index; SVR, systemic vascular resistance; SVRI, systemic vascular resistance index.

TABLE 49.9	Hemodynamic Profile in Common Critical Conditions				
CONDITION	CVP	PAOP	CO	PVR	SVR
Right heart failure	↑		↓	↑	
Left heart failure		↑	↓		↑
Pericardial tamponade	↑	↑	↓		↑
Hypovolemia	↓	↓	↓		↑
Cardiogenic shock	↑	↑	↓		↑
Distributive shock	↓	↓	↑		↓

CO, cardiac output; CVP, central venous pressure; PAOP, pulmonary artery occlusion pressure; PVR, pulmonary vascular resistance; SVR, systemic vascular resistance.

CONTROVERSIES ON THE MODERN USE OF THE PAC

PA catheterization is no longer routinely performed, perhaps due to a combination of overuse by inexperienced operators and lack of validity in various studies. Although it is an invasive and expensive technique, it remains a useful bedside tool in the management of select patients such as those with acute respiratory distress syndrome (ARDS) and sepsis, pulmonary hypertension, cardiogenic shock, or patients who have more than one condition.

Early studies showed that the PAC predicted hemodynamic profiles correctly in only 53% of critically ill patients; however in a subgroup analysis, PAC reduced mortality in patients with shock compared to those managed without a PAC.[15] Later studies showed that the PAC does not change clinical outcomes and that physicians had a poor understanding of how to interpret the hemodynamic data.[16] Gore et al[17] showed in a retrospective review of 3263 patients that patients managed with a PAC had a higher case fatality rate. An accompanying editorial called for a moratorium on the PAC.[18]

Additional studies in the 1990s, including the SUPPORT trial, showed that in critically ill patients, the PAC was associated with increased cost, length of stay, and mortality.[19] In patients with congestive heart failure, it was shown that management with a PAC increased anticipated adverse events and, in fact, did not affect overall mortality or hospitalization.[20] A large metaanalysis of 14 trials by Shah et al. further validated that the PAC neither decreased mortality nor hospital stay.[21] The PAC-Man study evaluated the effects of PAC-driven therapy in 65 British intensive care units (ICUs) and concluded that the PAC conferred neither benefit nor harm when used to manage critically ill patients.[22] The "nail in the coffin" was evidence from the U.S. National Institutes of Health sponsored FACTT trial, which showed that in patients with acute lung injury (ALI), PAC-guided therapy did not improve survival or organ function but was associated with more complications than CVC-guided therapy. These results, when considered with those of previous studies, suggested that the PAC should not be routinely used for the management of ALI.[23]

Overall, there has been a downward nationwide trend in the use of the PACs up to 65% between 1993 and 2004, most notably after acute myocardial infarction.[24] Nevertheless, PACs continue to be used in CCUs and cardiothoracic ICUs internationally, so one must still maintain a good understanding of its functionality.

Although they are no longer used on a routine basis, they certainly provide valuable hemodynamic information in postoperative cardiac patients and in certain CCU patients who need close hemodynamic monitoring. One of the arguments in favor of ongoing management with PAC is that prior trials included broad populations of cardiac patients in shock states and acute respiratory failure and may not have identified the exact population who may benefit from PAC monitoring. Along with its overuse in the 1990s and a lack of proper understanding of the hemodynamic data, these factors likely contributed to the fallout of the PAC.

ESOPHAGEAL DOPPLER

Esophageal Doppler monitoring involves placement of a probe in the esophagus of the patient and measuring blood flow velocity in the descending aorta. By measuring aortic blood flow (ABF), esophageal Doppler monitoring allow a reliable estimation of CO.[25] This can be done with transesophageal echocardiography or with a commercially available device that can track changes in SV and CO after a volume challenge or vasoactive agents. Probes are inserted orally to a depth of 35 to 40 cm from the incisors or nasally to 40 to 45 cm. The probe is manipulated till the distinct descending aorta waveform shape is visualized. From the aortic Doppler waveform that is obtained, valuable information such as preload and SV can be obtained.

Application of esophageal Doppler may be used intraoperatively in the recovery room or the CCU. Generally speaking, a change in ABF of 10% or higher is considered to indicate that the patient is fluid responsive. An actual fluid challenge or a PLR can be performed to see if the SV increases and this can guide further fluid management.[26] In a study of mechanically ventilated patients in normal sinus rhythm, Monnet et al[27] showed that a respiratory variation in ABF before volume expansion of at least 18% predicted fluid responsiveness with a sensitivity of 90% and a specificity of 94%. Intraoperative esophageal Doppler-guided fluid management has been shown to improve postoperative outcomes, including length of stay, after abdominal surgery and orthopedic procedures.[28,29] Precise, goal-directed fluid management in the operating room has now become standard of care and a prerequisite by many insurance companies in the United States.

PULSE PRESSURE VARIATION AND STROKE VOLUME VARIATION

The principles underlying pulse pressure variation (PPV) and stroke volume variation (SVV) are based on simple physiology that intermittent positive pressure ventilation induces cyclic changes in the loading conditions of the left and right ventricles. Mechanical insufflation increases intrathoracic pressure, decreases preload, and increases afterload of the right ventricle. The inspiratory reduction in RV ejection fraction leads to a decrease in LV filling after a phase lag of two or three heart beats because of the long pulmonary transit time. Thus, the LV preload reduction may induce a decrease in LV stroke volume, which is at its minimum during the expiratory period. Therefore, the magnitude of the respiratory changes in LV stroke volume is an indicator of biventricular preload dependence

It should be appreciated that both arrhythmias, low tidal volumes (<8 mL/kg ideal body weight [IBW]), and spontaneous breathing activity, even on mechanical ventilation, will lead to misinterpretations of the respiratory variations in PPV and SVV.[26] Hence, when measuring PPV or SVV, the patient should be passive on the ventilator, on ≥ 8 mL/kg IBW tidal volume, and in normal sinus rhythm.

$$PPV\% = \frac{PPmax - PPmin}{PPavg} \times 100$$

Figure 49.9 shows PPV measurement.

Seminal studies by Michard and others have found that a PPV of > 12%, in the appropriate patient, predicts fluid responsiveness with a sensitivity of 94% and specificity of 96%.[30,31] Based on this data, the patient in Figure 49.9 would be fluid responsive.

Goal-directed fluid management in the operating room (OR), with minimizing of PPV, has been shown to improve postoperative outcomes and decrease length of stay in high-risk surgical patients.[32]

NEWER HEMODYNAMIC MONITORING DEVICES

Various commercially available devices utilize the concepts described above in providing hemodynamic data.

FLOTRAC/VIGELEO

The FloTrac device (Edwards Lifesciences, Irvine, CA) is a CO monitor that uses pulse contour analysis to provide hemodynamic data. It requires a specialized sensor with a proprietary transducer attached to a radial or femoral arterial catheter. It analyzes the shape of the arterial pressure readings and calculates CO and other derived parameters such as SV, SVV, SVR, and CI. It updates key flow-based parameters such as CO, SV, and SVV every 20 seconds. Although the variables themselves are not always exact, when compared to the PAC, variability and trends are helpful in the management of critically ill patients. Additionally, the autocalibration feature is advantageous and make it user-friendly for all CCU staff.

PICCO TECHNOLOGY

PiCCO (Maquet, Rastatt, Germany) is a CO monitor that combines pulse contour analysis and transpulmonary thermodilution technique. The pulse contour analysis provides continuous

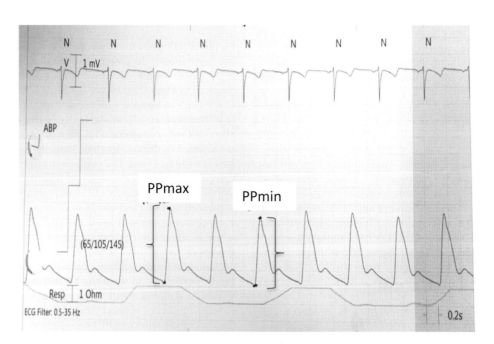

$$PPV\ \% = \frac{PPmax - PPmin}{Mean\ of\ the\ 2\ PP} \times 100$$

FIGURE 49.9 Pulse pressure variation. PPV, pulse pressure variation.

information while transpulmonary thermodilution provides static measurements. It requires a central venous line as well as the PiCCO arterial catheter, which has a thermistor on the end. For the transpulmonary thermodilution measurement, a defined bolus (eg, 10 mL cold 0.9% normal saline) is injected via a CVC. The cold bolus passes through the right heart, the lungs, and the left heart and is detected by the PiCCO catheter, commonly placed in the femoral artery. Using intermittent thermodilution and arterial pulse contour analysis, along with proprietary algorithms, various parameters such as CO, PPV, SVV, extravascular lung water, and global end diastolic volume can be obtained.

LITHIUM DILUTION CARDIAC OUTPUT (LIDCO)

LiDCO (LiDCO, London, UK) is another noninvasive method of CO measurement that utilizes thermodilution. A small dose of intravenous lithium is injected through a peripheral or central venous line, and subsequently the lithium concentration is measured by a lithium ion-sensitive electrode placed in a peripheral arterial line. A concentration–time curve is thus created, and from that curve, CO is calculated. This measurement is then used to calibrate the pulse contour analysis software. This initial calibration enables continuous subsequent CO measurement by analyzing the arterial pressure waveform. The LiDCOplus system also calculates the PPV and SVV during the respiratory cycle but uses different processing software from that used in PiCCO. This system has the advantage of not requiring a CVC but does require intermittent thermodilution.

These less-invasive hemodynamic devices have become more popular over the past decade. Data from a pooled analysis show that SVVs from these devices have a sensitivity of 82% and specificity of 86%.[31] These devices may also be useful in determining the hemodynamic response to a PLR. In this regard, an increase in CO by more than 10% in response to a PLR has been shown to accurately predict volume responsiveness in mechanically ventilated patients with spontaneous breathing activity.[33]

CONCLUSION

Invasive hemodynamic monitoring is essential to the care of the critically ill patient. Clinicians should be aware of the various modalities available and their respective advantages and pitfalls. CVP has become controversial in fluid management. Although the PAC provides extremely useful information about the hemodynamic status of the patient, its role has diminished because studies show it does not change clinical outcomes. Heart–lung interactions can be utilized to look for dynamic changes in pulse pressure and stroke volume. No measurement should be used in isolation to make clinical decisions with regard to fluid management. Proper measurement and interpretation of the data is the key to ensuring adequate oxygen delivery and tissue perfusion, which is the goal of successful hemodynamic monitoring.

REFERENCES

1. Michard F, Boussat S, Chemla D, et al. Relation between respiratory changes in arterial blood pressure and fluid responsivness in septic patients with acute circulatory failure. *Am J Respir Crit Care Med.* 2000;162:134-138.

2. Marik PE, Baram M, Vahid B. Does central venous pressure predict fluid responsiveness? A systematic review of the literature and the Tale of the Seven Mares. *Chest.* 2008;134:172-178.

3. Rivers E, Nguyen B, Havstad S, et al. Early goal-directed therapy in the treatment of severe sepsis and septic shock. *N Engl J Med.* 2001;345:1368-1377.

4. Dellinger RP, Carlet JM, Masur H, et al. Surviving Sepsis Campaign guidelines for management of severe sepsis and septic shock. *Crit Care Med.* 2004;32:858-873.

5. Osman D, Ridel C, Ray P, et al. Cardiac filling pressures are not appropriate to predict hemodynamic response to volume challenge. *Crit Care Med.* 2007;35:64-68.

6. Marik PE, Cavallazzi R. Does the central venous pressure predict fluid responsiveness? An updated meta-analysis and a plea for some common sense. *Crit Care Med.* 2013;41(7):1774-1781.

7. Marik PE, Monnet X, Teboul JL. Hemodynamic parameters to guide fluid therapy. *Ann Intensive Care.* 2011;1:1-11.

8. ProCESS Investigators, Yeal DM, Kellum JA, Huang DT, et al. A randomized trial of protocol-based care for early septic shock. *N Engl J Med.* 2014;370:1683-1693.

9. ProMISE Investigators, Mouncey PR, Osborn TM, Power GS, et al. Trial of early, goal-directed resuscitation. *N Engl J Med.* 2015;372:1301-1311.

10. ARISE Investigators, Peake SL, Delaney A, Bailey M, et al. Goal-directed resuscitation for patients with early septic shock. *N Engl J Med.* 2014;371:1496-1506.

11. Swan HJ, Ganz W, Forrester J, Marcus J, Diamond G, Chonette D. Catheterization of the heart in man with use of a flow-directed balloon-tipped catheter. *N Engl J Med.* 1970;283:447-451.

12. Kelly CR, Rabbani LE. Pulmonary-artery catheterization. *N Engl J Med.* 2013;e35(1-5).

13. John WB. *Respiratory Physiology: The Essentials.* Philadelphia, PA: Wolters Kluwer Health/Lippincott Williams & Wilkins; 2012.

14. Schroeder B. *Chapter 45: Cardiovascular Monitoring in Miller's Anesthesia.* Boston, MA: Elsevier; 2015:1345-1395.

15. Mimoz O, Rauss A, Rekik N, et al. Pulmonary artery catheterization in critically ill patients: a prospective analysis of outcome changes associated with catheter-prompted changes in therapy. *Crit Care Med.* 1994;22(4):573-579.

16. Iberti TJ, Fischer EP, Leibowitz AB, Panacek EA, Silverstein JH, Albertson TE. A multicenter study of physicians' knowledge of the pulmonary artery catheter. *JAMA.* 1990;264(22):2928-2932.

17. Gore JM, Goldberg RJ, Spodick DH, et al. A community wide assessment of the use of pulmonary artery catheters in patients with acute myocardial infarction. *Chest.* 1987;92:721-727.

18. Robin ED. Death by pulmonary artery flow-directed catheter: time for a moratorium? *Chest.* 1987;92:727-731.

19. Connors AF Jr, Speroff T, Dawson NV, et al; for the SUPPORT Investigators. The effectiveness of right heart catheterization in the initial care of critically ill patients. *JAMA.* 1996;276:889-897.

20. The ESCAPE Investigators, ESCAPE Study Coordinators. Evaluation study of congestive heart failure and pulmonary artery catheterization effectiveness: the ESCAPE trial. *JAMA.* 2005;294:1625-1633.

21. Shah MR, Hasselblad V, Stevenson LW, et al. Impact of the pulmonary artery catheter in critically ill patients: meta-analysis of randomized clinical trials. *JAMA.* 2005;294:1664-1670.

22. Harvey S, Harrison DA, Singer M, et al. Assessment of the clinical effectiveness of pulmonary artery catheters in management of patients in intensive care (PAC-Man): a randomised control trial. *Lancet.* 2005;366:472-477.

23. Wheeler AP, Bernard GR, Thompson BT, et al. Pulmonary-artery versus central venous catheter to guide treatment of acute lung injury. *N Engl J Med.* 2006;354:2213-2224.

24. Wiener RS, Welch HG. Trends in the use of the pulmonary artery catheter in the United States, 1993-2004. *JAMA*. 2007;298:423-429.

25. Valtier B, Cholley BP, Belot JP, de la Coussaye JE, Mateo J, Payen DM. Noninvasive monitoring of cardiac output in critically ill patients using transesophageal Doppler. *Am J Respir Crit Care Med*. 1998;158:77-83.

26. Monnet X, Rienzo M, Osman D, et al. Passive leg raising predicts fluid responsiveness in the critically ill. *Crit Care Med*. 2006;34:1402-1407.

27. Monnet X, Rienzo M, Osman D, et al. Esophageal Doppler monitoring predicts fluid responsiveness in critically ill ventilated patients. *Intensive Care Med*. 2005;31:1195-1201.

28. Gan TJ, Soppitt A, Maroof M, et al. Goal-directed intraoperative fluid administration reduces length of hospital stay after major surgery. *Anesthesiology*. 2002;97(4):820-826.

29. Sinclair S, James S, Singer M. Intraoperative intravascular volume optimisation and length of hospital stay after repair of proximal femoral fracture: randomised controlled trial. *BMJ*. 1997;315(7113):909-912.

30. Michard F, Boussat S, Chemla D, et al. Relation between respiratory changes in arterial pulse pressure and fluid responsiveness in septic patients with acute circulatory failure. *Am J Respir Crit Care Med*. 2000;162:134-138.

31. Marik PE, Cavallazzi R, Vasu T, Hirani A. Dynamic changes in arterial waveform derived variables and fluid responsiveness in mechanically ventilated patients. A systematic review of the literature. *Crit Care Med*. 2009;37:2642-2647.

32. Lopes MR, Oliveira MA, Pereira VO, Lemos IP, Auler JO Jr, Michard F. Goal-directed fluid management based on pulse pressure variation monitoring during high-risk surgery: a pilot randomized controlled trial. *Crit Care*. 2007;11:R100.

33. Biais M, Vidil L, Sarrabay P, Cottenceau V, Revel P, Sztark F. Changes in stroke volume induced by passive leg raising in spontaneously breathing patients: comparison between echocardiography and Vigileo/FloTrac device. *Crit Care*. 2009;13:R195.

Patient and Family Information for: INVASIVE HEMODYNAMIC ASSESSMENT IN THE CCU

WHAT IS HEMODYNAMIC MONITORING?

Invasive hemodynamic monitoring allows doctors and nurses to closely monitor the patient's clinical status. Using catheters that are placed into veins and arteries, measurements can be made of the patient's blood pressure and the pressures within the chambers of the heart. These measurements can be used to guide the clinical team to determine fluid and medical therapy.

WHAT IS THE PREPARATION?

The clinical team will explain the type of invasive hemodynamic monitoring that is being planned, including its purpose, risks, and benefits. Most procedures in the cardiac care unit (CCU) that are performed for hemodynamic monitoring are done at the bedside. Occasionally, invasive procedures will be performed in the cardiac catheterization lab. Be sure to wear your hospital gown, as parts of your body may be uncovered to facilitate the exam. You may be asked to position yourself a certain way and lay still for the procedure. Local anesthesia or numbing medication will be administered to prevent pain. Sometimes, an intravenous antianxiety medication may be given to help facilitate the procedure.

HOW LONG DOES IT TAKE?

It can take anywhere from 15 to 30 minutes to insert catheters for invasive hemodynamic monitoring. Once the catheter is in place, it may be left in place for anywhere from 1-2 days to the entire stay in the CCU. The catheter will be removed as soon as it is no longer necessary.

WHAT IS THE PROCESS?

Measurements from invasive hemodynamic monitors will be displayed on the patient monitor in the room and also at the nursing station. These measurements will help your clinical team to guide your medical management.

WHAT ARE THE RISKS AND COMPLICATIONS?

Your clinical team will weigh the risks and benefits before proceeding with catheters for invasive hemodynamic monitoring. The main risks of any catheter placement are bleeding, infection, clotting of the catheter or vessel, and damage to the blood vessel or nearby structures. There may be risks of abnormal heart rhythms when the catheter is being placed and also risk of air entering the circulation. Your clinical team will take appropriate precautions to ensure that it is a safe procedure.

WHAT ARE SOME TYPES OF INVASIVE HEMODYNAMIC MONITORING?

1. CENTRAL VENOUS PRESSURE (CVP) MONITORING

A central venous catheter (CVC) or a central line is a sterile, flexible, small hollow tube inserted into the internal jugular vein in the neck or the subclavian vein in the upper chest. The tip of catheter rests within a vein connected to the heart called the superior vena cava. When this catheter is connected to additional tubing from the patient monitor, the CVP can be measured.

Normal CVP is between 8 to 12 cmH2O. A very low CVP can indicate that you may need additional intravenous (IV) fluids, and a very high CVP can mean that you do not need any additional IV fluids. Keep in mind that CVP monitoring has come under controversy recently, and hence your clinical team will interpret the numbers in conjunction to their clinical exam and other available data to help guide your treatment.

2. ARTERIAL BLOOD PRESSURE (ABP) MONITORING

An arterial line (or A-line) is a small, sterile tube that is inserted into an artery, commonly either in the wrist (radial artery) or groin (femoral artery). When this catheter is connected to additional tubing from the patient monitor, it can obtain beat-to-beat measurements of the arterial blood pressure. These measurements are much more accurate that the regular blood pressure (BP) that is obtained from a standard BP cuff. These accurate measurements will help guide your doctors and nurses in adjusting your medications. In addition, A-lines can be used for obtaining frequent blood samples to assess the degree of acidity and levels of oxygen and carbon dioxide in the blood.

3. PULMONARY ARTERY CATHETERIZATION OR SWAN-GANZ CATHETERIZATION

A pulmonary artery catheter (PAC) is a thin tube or catheter that is placed into the right side of the heart and the artery leading to the lungs (pulmonary artery). An experienced physician, physician assistant, or nurse practitioner typically performs the procedure with local anesthesia and under sterile conditions. The catheter is generally inserted into one of three veins: the right internal jugular (RIJ) vein, located in the neck, which is the shortest, most direct path to the heart; the left subclavian vein, located under the clavicle or collar bone; or the femoral veins in the groin. During the procedure, your heartbeat and electrocardiogram will be closely monitored. A PAC measures how well the heart is functioning and monitors pressures within the heart and lungs. It is routinely used during heart surgery or when large amounts of certain heart support medications are needed. Occasionally, the catheter may damage the pulmonary artery or lung. It can also cause irregularity of the heart rhythm usually during insertion. Chest X-rays are routinely done to check for any complications.

The PAC travels through the right side of the heart and the tip rests in the pulmonary artery. Using the PAC, pressures can be obtained from the right-sided chambers of the heart and the pulmonary arteries. There is a balloon at the tip of the PAC, which can be inflated to obtain the pulmonary artery occlusion pressure (PAOP). This provides an estimate of the pressures in the left side of the heart. These measurements can help guide your clinical team to make crucial decisions about your treatment. That said, the usefulness of the PAC has also come under controversy recently, and in light of the invasive nature of the procedure, this is no longer a routine procedure done in the CCU.

Yuvrajsinh J. Parmar
Itzhak Kronzon

50

Noninvasive Hemodynamic Assessment in the CCU

Hemodynamic assessment using Doppler echocardiography in the evaluation of transvalvular gradients, valvular regurgitation, and certain clinically important variables such as pulmonary artery (PA) pressures is common among echocardiographers. In comparison, the use of echocardiography in measuring intracardiac pressures as it is done during cardiac catheterization is an underutilized tool. These measurements done by echocardiography can aid in the assessment and management of patients in the intensive care unit. This chapter focuses on the practical aspects of such an examination with the demonstration of a comprehensive hemodynamic evaluation in a patient. The information in this chapter is based on known and accepted hemodynamic and Doppler echocardiographic techniques. More data and references can be found in larger, more detailed textbooks.[1]

The simplified Bernoulli equation is the basis for the calculation of most intracardiac pressures.[2]

$$\Delta P = 4V^2$$

where ΔP = pressure gradient in mm Hg and V = velocity in m/s.

EVALUATION OF RIGHT ATRIAL PRESSURE

The evaluation of the inferior vena cava provides information regarding right atrial pressures (RAPs). With the transducer in the subxiphoid position, the inferior vena cava can be evaluated as it travels through the liver into the right atrium. During its course, the inferior vena cava becomes perpendicular to the ultrasound interrogation beam, allowing for its size and changes in its diameter during the respiratory cycle to be recorded by M-mode echocardiography. The normal diameter of the inferior vena cava in adults is 1.5 to 2.5 cm measured just proximal to its entrance into the right atrium. Normally, with inspiration, there is a decrease of 50% or more in its diameter. Failure to collapse with respiration and a dilated inferior vena cava suggests elevated RAPs.[3,4] **Table 50.1** correlates inferior vena cava characteristics (diameter and respiratory changes) and RAP. **Figure 50.1** shows a two-dimensional image and M-mode echocardiogram of a patient with a markedly elevated RAP.

EVALUATION OF RIGHT VENTRICULAR SYSTOLIC PRESSURE

Echocardiographic measurement of right ventricular systolic pressure (RVSP) is related to the velocity of flow across the tricuspid valve during systole. **Figure 50.2** shows the superimposed pressure curves of the right atrium and right ventricular and PA pressure. Under normal circumstances, there is a negligible gradient across the tricuspid valve during diastole and a negligible gradient across the pulmonic valve during systole. These gradients are so small that their measurement is beyond the sensitivity of cardiac catheterization. During systole, with the tricuspid valve closed, there is a pressure gradient between the right ventricle and the right atrium. Approximately 90% of normal adults have some degree (usually trace or mild) of tricuspid regurgitation. The velocity of the tricuspid regurgitant (TR) jet, as measured by continuous wave Doppler, is related to the pressure gradient between the right ventricle and right atrium. Using the simplified Bernoulli equation, the tricuspid regurgitation gradient can be calculated. The RVSP equals the TR gradient plus the RAP.

TABLE 50.1		IVC Size and Respiratory Variation in the Evaluation of RA Pressure[3]
IVC (CM)	Δ WITH RESPIRATION (%)	RA PRESSURE (MM HG)
≤2.1	>50	0–5
≤2.1	<50	5–10
≥2.1	>50	10–15
≥2.1	<50	15–20

IVC, inferior vena cava; RA, right atrial.

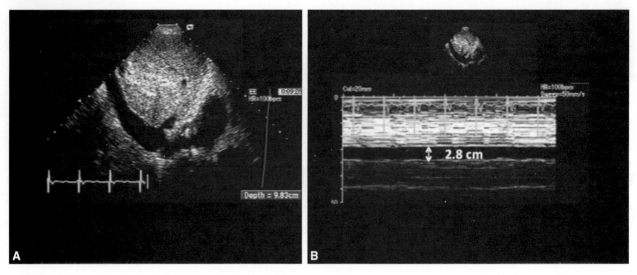

FIGURE 50.1 Assessment of right atrial pressure (RAP). A, The inferior vena cava (IVC) is markedly dilated at its entrance to the right atrium (2.8 cm). B, The M-mode recorded demonstrates lack of respiratory variations in diameter. RAP is estimated to be 15 to 20 mm Hg

$$RVSP = TR \text{ gradient} + RAP$$

Calculating RVSPs in patients who have a ventricular septal defect (VSD) with a left-to-right shunt requires measuring the gradient across the right and left ventricles. This gradient is related to the defect jet velocity between the ventricles. In the absence of aortic stenosis, the systolic pressure in the left ventricle equals the systolic blood pressure (SBP) measured by a blood pressure cuff. Thus, the RVSP equals SBP minus the systolic ventricular septal defect (SVSD) gradient.

$$RVSP = SBP - SVSD \text{ gradient}$$

The lower the SBP and the higher the RVSP, the smaller the interventricular gradient. VSDs that are associated with lower blood pressure and with high RVSP (as may be the case in VSD during acute myocardial infarction) will have a lower VSD systolic flow velocity and lower systolic VSD gradient. **Figure 50.3** shows an example of calculating RVSP in a patient after a myocardial infarction that developed a VSD with a left-to-right shunt.

FIGURE 50.2 Assessment of RV systolic pressure (see text). The diagram shows normal right-sided pressures with no significant systolic gradient across the pulmonic valve and no significant diastolic gradient across the tricuspid valve. The gradient across the tricuspid valve in systole (green arrow) is responsible for the tricuspid regurgitation velocity seen in the upper left corner. With a peak regurgitant velocity of 2.5 m/s, the gradient between the right ventricle and right atrium is 25 mm Hg. PA, pulmonary artery pressure; PVC, pulmonic valve closure; RA, right atrial pressure; RV, right ventricular; TVC, tricuspid valve closure.

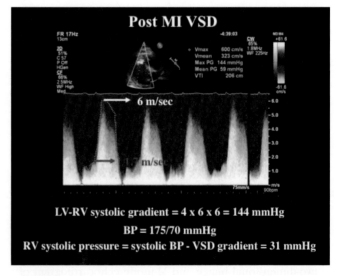

FIGURE 50.3 Assessment of right ventricular systolic pressure in a patient with a ventricular septal defect after myocardial infarction. Note that there is flow in both systole (white arrow) and diastole (red arrow). BP, blood pressure; LV, left ventricle; MI, myocardial infarction; RV, right ventricle; VSD, ventricular septal defect.

EVALUATION OF RIGHT VENTRICULAR DIASTOLIC PRESSURE

In the absence of tricuspid stenosis, there is a negligible gradient between the right atrial diastolic pressure and the right ventricular diastolic pressure (RVDP), and this gradient can therefore be ignored. As a result, it can be said that RVDP equals RAP.

$$RVDP = RAP$$

In the presence of VSDs with left-to-right shunt, the left ventricular diastolic pressure (LVDP) is usually higher than the RVDP. Therefore, there is flow between the left ventricle and right ventricle that continues throughout diastole. However, this velocity is significantly smaller when compared to the velocity of the jet across the VSD during systole (**Figure 50.3**). If the LVDP is known, then the RVDP can be calculated as the LVDP minus the diastolic ventricular septal defect (DVSD) gradient.

$$RVDP = LVDP - DVSD\ gradient$$

EVALUATION OF PULMONARY ARTERY SYSTOLIC PRESSURE

In the absence of pulmonic stenosis (PS), the pressure gradient between the right ventricle and the PA is negligible and can be ignored. It can be assumed that the pulmonary artery systolic pressure (PASP) equals the RVSP. Therefore, the PASP equals the tricuspid regurgitation (TR) gradient plus the RAP.

$$PASP = TR\ gradient + RAP$$

However, in the presence of PS, the gradient across the pulmonic valve must be accounted for. The flow velocity across the stenotic pulmonic valve can be evaluated and the PS gradient can be calculated. In these patients, the PASP equals the RVSP minus the PS gradient.

$$PASP = RVSP - PS\ gradient$$

EVALUATION OF PULMONARY ARTERY DIASTOLIC PRESSURE

The majority of patients normally have some degree (trace to mild) of pulmonic regurgitation (PR). The velocity of the PR is defined by the diastolic pressure gradient between the PA and the right ventricle. Thus, the pulmonary artery diastolic pressure (PADP) equals the pulmonary regurgitation gradient plus the RVDP.

$$PADP = PR\ gradient + RVDP$$

Because the RAP (in the absence of tricuspid stenosis) is approximately equal to the RVDP, this equation can be simplified to the PADP equaling the PR gradient plus RAP.

$$PADP = PR\ gradient + RAP$$

The ability to measure the PR velocity may be helpful in the evaluation of the PA pressure in patients who do not have tricuspid regurgitation. **Figure 50.4** shows a continuous wave Doppler tracing of pulmonic valve flow in a patient evaluated for significant pulmonary hypertension (HTN) who did not have tricuspid regurgitation. The end-diastolic velocity of the pulmonic

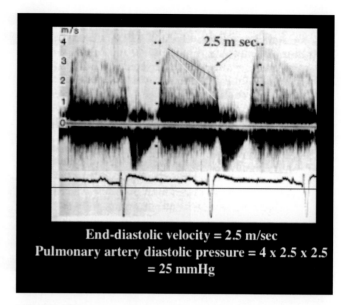

End-diastolic velocity = 2.5 m/sec
Pulmonary artery diastolic pressure = 4 x 2.5 x 2.5
= 25 mmHg

FIGURE 50.4 Assessment of pulmonary artery diastolic pressure in a patient with pulmonary hypertension. The continuous wave Doppler of the pulmonic valve shows an end-diastolic velocity of 2.5 m/s. This indicates an end-diastolic gradient of 25 mm Hg between the pulmonary artery and the right ventricle.

regurgitant flow is 2.5 m/s, which indicates an end-diastolic gradient of 25 mm Hg across the pulmonic valve. Therefore, the diastolic pulmonary artery pressure is at least 25 mm Hg, a markedly elevated value.

An estimation of PA pressures in the absence of tricuspid regurgitation or PR can be obtained with M-mode echocardiography and pulse wave Doppler. The characteristic M-mode pattern of the pulmonic valve in patients with severe pulmonary HTN (>70 mm Hg) includes absence of "a" deflection during atrial contraction (in spite of normal sinus rhythm), "flying W" appearance of the systolic opening, and lack of backward motion of the diastolic closure line (**Figure 50.5**). A more accurate estimation of mean PA pressures can be obtained by measuring the systolic acceleration time of the antegrade flow velocity measured by pulse wave Doppler just proximal to the pulmonic valve. The acceleration time is inversely proportional to the mean PA pressure.[5] The equation used for this estimation is

$$PAMP = 79 - (0.45 \times AcT)$$

where PAMP is mean PA pressure in mm Hg and AcT is acceleration time in milliseconds.

A normal acceleration time is greater than 120 ms. Values less than 90 ms are associated with a PA mean pressure of 40 mm Hg or more.

EVALUATION OF LEFT VENTRICULAR SYSTOLIC PRESSURE

In patients without aortic valve or left ventricular outflow disease, the gradient between the left ventricle and the aorta during systole is negligible. Therefore, left ventricular systolic pressure (LVSP) is equal to the SBP.

$$LVSP = SBP$$

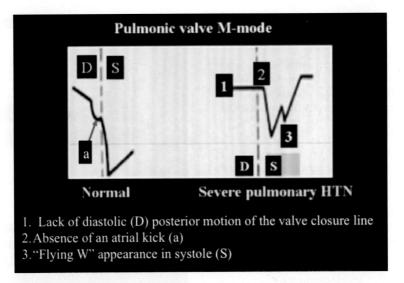

FIGURE 50.5 Comparison M-mode echocardiography of the pulmonic valve in individuals with and without severe pulmonary hypertension (HTN).

However, patients with aortic valve, subvalvular, or supravalvular stenosis have a gradient between the left ventricle and the ascending aorta. Because the systolic ascending aortic pressure equals the SBP, the LVSP equals the SBP plus the systolic pressure gradient across the aortic valve (or other subvalvular or supravalvular sites).

$$LVSP = SBP + \text{aortic stenosis gradient}$$

Gradients across the aortic valve can be measured using the Doppler examination. The maximal gradient that is recorded is the maximum instantaneous gradient (MIG), which differs from the peak-to-peak (P2P) gradient which is the gradient between peak aortic systolic pressure and peak LVSP. The P2P gradient is frequently measured and reported during cardiac catheterization. The value of the MIG is typically higher than that of the P2P gradient. In most cases of severe aortic stenosis, the P2P gradient is approximately 70% of the MIG. Both Doppler echocardiography and pressure measurement during invasive procedures are able to calculate a mean pressure gradient across the aortic valve (**Figure 50.6**). When using Doppler for the calculation of left ventricular pressure, the P2P gradient is estimated by taking 70% of the MIG and adding it to the SBP. Therefore,

$$LVSP = SBP + 70\% \text{ MIG}$$

EVALUATION OF LEFT VENTRICULAR DIASTOLIC PRESSURE

In the absence of mitral stenosis, the gradient between the left atrium and the left ventricle during diastole is small and can be ignored. Therefore, the left atrial pressure (LAP) is similar to the LVDP. The LAP can be estimated and will approximate left ventricular end-diastolic pressure (LVEDP).

$$LVEDP = LAP$$

In patients who have aortic regurgitation (AR), the regurgitant jet velocity is a function of the diastolic gradient between the aorta and the left ventricle. If the aortic diastolic pressure is known, then the LVEDP equals the diastolic blood pressure (DBP) minus the AR gradient at end diastole. In most patients, the aortic pressure equals the cuff pressure in the arm.

$$LVEDP = DBP - \text{end-diastolic AR gradient}$$

In patients with VSD with a left-to-right shunt, the LVEDP can be calculated if the RAP, which estimates RVDP (in the absence of tricuspid stenosis), is known. In these patients, the addition of the RAP and the VSD end-diastolic gradient equals the LVEDP.

$$LVEDP = RAP + \text{VSD end-diastolic gradient}$$

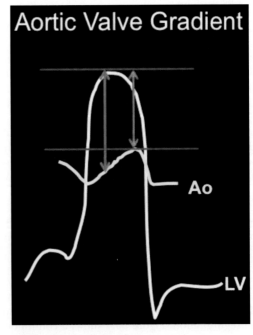

FIGURE 50.6 Left-sided pressure curves in aortic stenosis demonstrating maximum instantaneous gradient (blue arrow) and the peak-to-peak gradient (green arrow). Ao, aorta; LV, left ventricle.

Figure 50.7 demonstrates a continuous wave Doppler tracing taken from a patient with both aortic stenosis and AR. The aortic stenosis peak velocity jet is 4 m/s and AR end-diastolic velocity is also 4 m/s. The blood pressure during the examination was 150/80 mm Hg. Therefore, the LVSP equals the SBP (150 mm Hg) plus 70% of the aortic systolic gradient. Because the maximum instantaneous aortic gradient is 64 mm Hg, the P2P gradient is 70% of 64 mm Hg, which is 45 mm Hg. The LVSP is therefore 150 + 45 = 195 mm Hg. The LVDP equals the DBP (80 mm Hg) minus the aortic diastolic gradient (64 mm Hg), which equals 16 mm Hg. Therefore, this patient's left ventricular pressure is 195/16 mm Hg.

EVALUATION OF LEFT ATRIAL PRESSURE

Estimation of LAP by Doppler echocardiography can be performed in the absence of atrial fibrillation, ventricular pacing, left bundle branch block, left ventricular assist device, or mitral valve disease (mitral stenosis, moderate mitral annular calcification, more than moderate mitral regurgitation [MR], and mitral valve repair or replacement). Pulsed Doppler of the transmitral and pulmonary venous flow, along with tissue Doppler of the lateral and septal mitral annulus allows for the estimation of LAP. Under normal flow patterns, the pressure in the left atrium is 6 to 12 mm Hg. Impaired relaxation results in a flow pattern with a low E-wave and high A-wave on pulse Doppler. This corresponds with a normal or minimally elevated LAP of 13 to 19 mm Hg. In pseudonormalization of transmitral flow, the LAP is elevated ranging from 20 to 24 mm Hg. Lastly, a restrictive pattern with a high E-wave, low A-wave, and rapid transmitral deceleration time (150 ms or less), the LAP is usually at least 25 mm Hg. A simpler alternative to calculating LAP uses the ratio of the transmitral flow E-wave velocity and the tissue Doppler (E'). In general, as the LAP increases, E-wave becomes higher and the E' becomes lower. An E/E' ratio of less than 9 is associated with normal LAPs, whereas a ratio of greater than 14 is highly specific for elevated LAPs (>14 mm Hg). An equation reported by Nagueh et al[6] describes the relation between LAP and E/E'.

$$LAP = 1.24[(E/E') + 1.9]$$

A more simplified equation that may be used is

$$LAP = E/E' + 4 \text{ mm Hg}$$

PASPs can also be used to increase the accuracy of estimated LAP. **Table 50.2** provides estimations of LAP based on Doppler findings.[7] A more comprehensive analysis of diastolic dysfunction and estimation of LAP can be found by Nagueh et al.[8]

In patients with MR and without aortic stenosis, the LAP during ventricular systole (LAS) equals the SBP minus the MR gradient. In the absence of aortic stenosis, the LVSP equals the SBP.

$$LAS = SBP - MR \text{ gradient}$$

In patients with mitral stenosis, the LAP during ventricular diastole (left anterior descending [LAD]) equals the LVEDP plus the mean transmitral gradient.

$$LAD = LVEDP + \text{transmitral gradient}$$

CALCULATION OF CARDIAC OUTPUT

Cardiac output (CO) can be calculated by measuring blood flow in either the left heart (systemic blood flow [SBF]) or right heart (pulmonary blood flow [PBF]). In the absence of shunts, the PBF is equal to the SBF. SBF is best calculated by evaluating the left ventricular outflow tract (LVOT). The cross-sectional area (CSA) of the LVOT can be calculated by measuring its diameter. The product of LVOT CSA and the velocity time integral (VTI) of the LVOT is the stroke volume (SV). Multiplying the SV with the heart rate (HR) provides the CO (**Figure 50.8**).

$$SV = CSA_{LVOT} \times VTI_{LVOT}$$

$$CO = SV \times HR$$

Similarly, calculation of PBF can be done at the right ventricular outflow tract just proximal to the pulmonic valve.

CALCULATION OF SHUNT FLOW

The evaluation of shunt flow in patients with an atrial septal defect (ASD) or VSD with a left-to-right shunt can be performed by subtracting the SBF from the PBF.

$$\text{Shunt flow} = PBF - SBF$$

Alternatively, the product of the defect orifice area (DOA), the shunt VTI and HR equals the shunt flow across an ASD or VSD. **Figure 50.9** is an example of the calculation of ASD flow with a left-to-right shunt with an orifice area of 1.2 (radius of 0.6 cm), a VTI of 80 cm, and HR of 80 beats/minute. Using the equation given, the shunt flow is calculated.

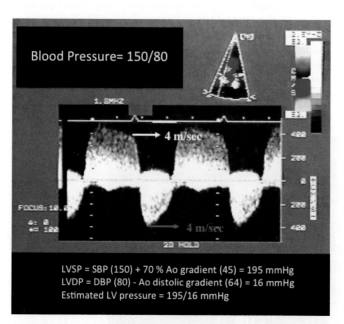

Blood Pressure= 150/80

4 m/sec

4 m/sec

LVSP = SBP (150) + 70 % Ao gradient (45) = 195 mmHg
LVDP = DBP (80) - Ao distolic gradient (64) = 16 mmHg
Estimated LV pressure = 195/16 mmHg

FIGURE 50.7 Continuous wave (CV) Doppler in the calculation of LV pressures in a patient with aortic stenosis and insufficiency (see text). Aortic stenosis peak velocity (red arrow) and aortic regurgitation end-diastolic velocity (white arrow) both measure to be 4 m/s. Ao, aorta; DBP, diastolic blood pressure; LV, left ventricular; LVDP, left ventricular diastolic pressure; LVSP, left ventricular systolic pressure; SBP, systolic blood pressure.

TABLE 50.2	Estimation of LAP Based on Doppler Findings		
DOPPLER FINDING	MILD LAP ELEVATION (13–19 MM HG)	MODERATE LAP ELEVATION (20–24 MM HG)	SEVERE LAP ELEVATION (>25 MM HG)
E/A	0.8–1	1.2–1.5	>2
Deceleration time (ms)	N/A	N/A	<150
Average (E/E′)	9–12	13–18	>20
Estimated PASP (mm Hg)	35–40	45–55	>60

The predictive accuracy is enhanced with the presence of three to four of the above findings.[7]
LAP, left atrial pressure; PASP, pulmonary artery systolic pressure.

$$\text{Shunt flow} = \text{DOA} \times \text{VTI}_{\text{shunt}} \times \text{HR}$$

ESTIMATION OF PULMONARY VASCULAR RESISTANCE

Pulmonary vascular resistance (PVR) is defined as the ratio between the pressure gradient and the blood flow across the pulmonary vascular tree, measured in Wood's units. Invasively, PVR can be calculated using the following equation:

$$\text{PVR} = (\text{PAMP} - \text{LAMP})/\text{PBF}$$

where PAMP is pulmonary artery mean pressure in mm Hg, LAMP is left atrial mean pressure in mm Hg, and PBF is the pulmonary blood flow in liters/minute. In patients with a normal PAMP (15 mm Hg), normal LAMP (5 mm Hg), and normal PBF (5 L/min), the calculated PVR is approximately 2 units.

The PVR is directly related to the PA pressure (and therefore to the maximal TR jet velocity) and inversely related to the SV in the RVOT (which can be measured noninvasively by pulsed Doppler, using the VTI at the RVOT, just proximal to the pulmonic valve). PVR can therefore be calculated by Doppler using the following equation[9]:

$$\text{PVR} = 10\left[(\text{peak TR velocity}/\text{VTI}_{\text{RVOT}}) + 0.16\right]$$

where PVR is expressed in Wood's units, TR = tricuspid regurgitation in m/s, and VTI$_{\text{RVOT}}$ = velocity time integral at the right ventricular outflow tract in centimeters (**Figure 50.10**).

CLINICAL CASE

COMPREHENSIVE HEMODYNAMIC EVALUATION

A complete echocardiographic examination can provide important information on a patient's hemodynamic profile. The information obtained may be comparable to invasive methods of hemodynamic evaluation and can guide therapy. The next few paragraphs evaluate the hemodynamic profile by means of echocardiography of a 63-year-old male with acute shortness of breath.

His vital signs during the evaluation showed a blood pressure of 100/55 mm Hg and HR 70 beats/minute. His physical examination was notable for a regular HR, an apical diastolic rumble (mitral stenosis), apical holosystolic murmur (MR), a basal systolic ejection murmur radiating to the carotids (aortic stenosis), basal diastolic murmur (AR), and presence of jugular venous distension. **Figure 50.11** shows the hemodynamic information that was

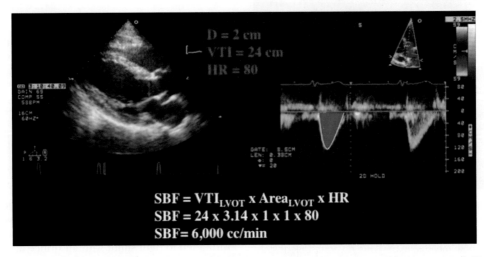

FIGURE 50.8 Calculation of systemic blood flow. The diameter (D) is measured at the LVOT in parasternal long axis view (left) and the VTI (right) is determined by pulse wave Doppler at the LVOT. HR, heart rate; LVOT, left ventricular outflow tract; SBF, systemic blood flow; VTI, velocity time integral.

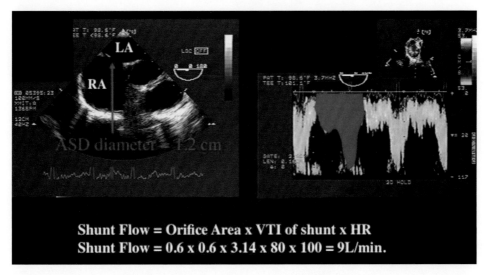

FIGURE 50.9 Calculation of ASD with left-to-right shunt flow. The red arrow marks the ASD orifice diameter (left). The VTI of the shunt flow is shown in the shaded red area (right). ASD, atrial septal defect; HR, heart rate; LA, left atrium; RA, right atrium; VTI, velocity time integral.

available at this stage. It is assumed that the aortic pressure was the same as the blood pressure measured by a blood pressure cuff.

The evaluation begins with the inferior vena cava with subxiphoid echocardiography. As can be seen in **Figure 50.12A**, the inferior vena cava measured to be 2 cm and there was less than 50% respiratory collapse. Therefore, the inferior vena cava and the RAP (and also the superior vena cava) are slightly elevated (5 to 10 mm Hg); and for the sake of simplicity, a value of 10 mm Hg will be used. At this point, the known hemodynamic profile can be seen in **Figure 50.12B**.

The right ventricular pressures can be estimated by evaluating flow across the tricuspid valve. The peak jet velocity of the tricuspid regurgitation (**Figure 50.13A**) is 3.7 m/s and, therefore,

the gradient between the right ventricle and the right atrium is 56 mm Hg. The RVSP equals the RAP (10 mm Hg) plus the tricuspid regurgitation gradient (56 mm Hg), which equals 66 mm Hg. In the absence of tricuspid stenosis, the RVDP equals the RAP. Therefore, the pressure in the right ventricle is 66/10 mm Hg (**Figure 50.13B**).

The PA pressure can now be calculated. In the absence of PS, the RVSP (66 mm Hg) practically equals pulmonary arterial systolic pressure. As demonstrated in **Figure 50.14**, this patient has PR. The pulmonary diastolic pressure can be calculated by measuring the PR velocity at end diastole. The velocity of the PR jet is 2.2 m/s, which indicates a pulmonic regurgitant gradient of 20 mm Hg. The PADP is therefore the pulmonary

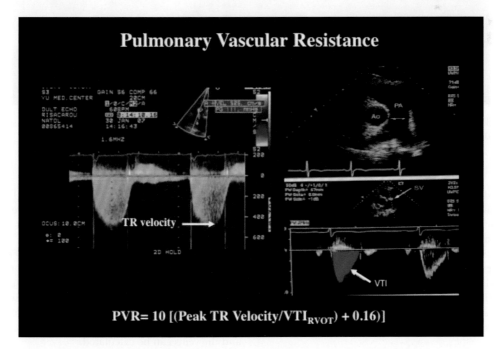

FIGURE 50.10 Noninvasive calculation of PVR in Wood's units using the peak TR velocity and VTI at the RVOT. PVR, pulmonary vascular resistance; RVOT, left ventricular outflow tract; TR, tricuspid regurgitant; VTI, velocity time integral.

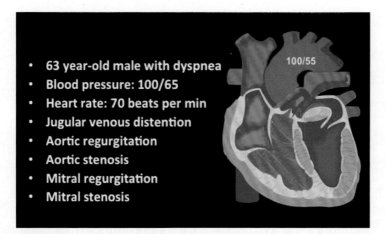

FIGURE 50.11 Initial hemodynamic profile and synopsis of history on presentation.

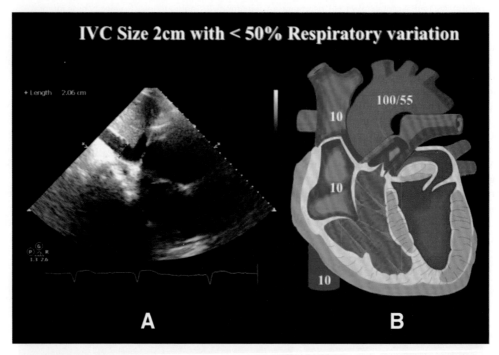

FIGURE 50.12 Calculation of right atrial pressure. A, IVC measuring 2 cm with less than 50% respiratory variation suggestive of slightly elevated right atrial pressure (5 to 10 mm Hg). B, The hemodynamic diagram shows a right atrial pressure of 10 mm Hg. IVC, inferior vena cava.

regurgitation gradient (20 mm Hg) plus RAP (10 mm Hg), which equals 30 mm Hg.

Left ventricular pressures are calculated by evaluating flow across the aortic valve. The patient has AR (**Figure 50.15**). The end-diastolic velocity of the AR jet is 3 m/s and therefore the aortic end-diastolic gradient is 36 mm Hg. Therefore, the LVEDP equals the aortic diastolic pressure (55 mm Hg) minus the AR gradient (55 mm Hg), which equals 19 mm Hg. In addition, this patient has aortic stenosis (**Figure 50.16**) with a peak instantaneous aortic flow velocity of 4 m/s, which is equivalent to a MIG

of 64 mm Hg. Because the P2P gradient is 70% of the MIG, the P2P equals 45 mm Hg. The LVSP is therefore the aortic systolic pressure (100 mm Hg) plus 70% of the MIG (45 mm Hg), which equals 145 mm Hg.

Finally, this patient has mitral stenosis (**Figure 50.17**). The mean mitral gradient was calculated to be 7 mm Hg. The LAP, therefore, equals the LVDP (19 mm Hg) plus the mitral valve mean gradient (7 mm Hg), which equals 26 mm Hg. Thus, with the use of echocardiography and without the use of invasive measures, the pressures in the cardiac chambers, the great arteries, and the veins can be calculated.

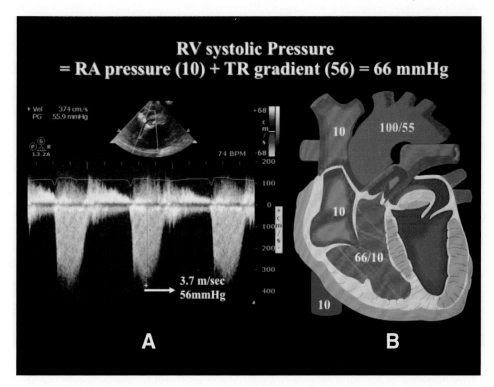

FIGURE 50.13 Calculation of right ventricular pressures. A, Tricuspid regurgitation velocity showing the gradient between the right ventricle and RA of 56 mm Hg. B, The hemodynamic diagram shows a right ventricular pressure of 66/10 mm Hg. RA, right atrium; RV, right ventricle; TR, tricuspid regurgitant.

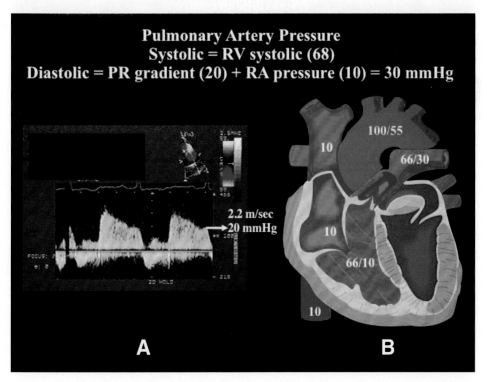

FIGURE 50.14 Calculation of pulmonary artery pressures. A, PR end-diastolic velocity of 2.2 m/s showing the gradient between the pulmonary artery and right ventricle of 20 mm Hg. B, The hemodynamic diagram shows a right pulmonary pressure of 66/30 mm Hg. RA, right atrium; RV, right ventricle; PR, pulmonic regurgitation.

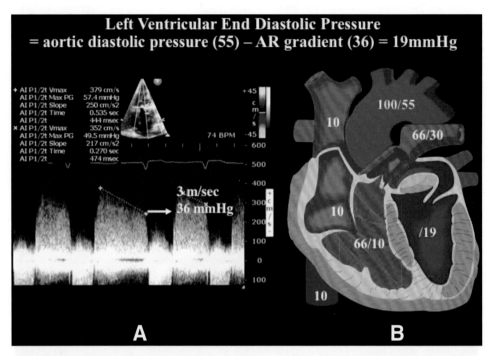

FIGURE 50.15 Calculation of left ventricular diastolic pressure. A, AR end-diastolic velocity of 3 m/s showing the gradient between the aorta and left ventricle of 36 mm Hg. B, The hemodynamic diagram shows a left ventricular diastolic pressure of 19 mm Hg. AR, aortic regurgitation.

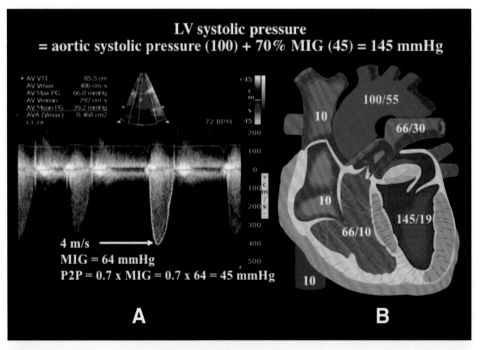

FIGURE 50.16 Calculation of LV systolic pressure. A, The peak instantaneous velocity of 4 m/s is used to calculate the MIG between the left ventricle and the aorta, which equals 64 mm Hg. Peak-to-peak (P2P) gradient, which is 70% of the MIG, equals 45 mm Hg. B, The hemodynamic diagram shows a left ventricular systolic pressure of 145 mm Hg. LV, left ventricular; MIG, maximum instantaneous gradient.

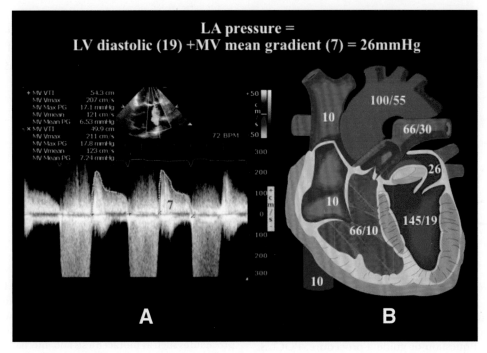

FIGURE 50.17 Calculation of LA pressure. A, Flow across the MV showing a mean mitral gradient of 7 mm Hg. B, The hemodynamic diagram shows an LA pressure of 26 mm Hg. LA, left atrial; LV, left ventricular; MV, mitral valve.

This hemodynamic evaluation provides an example of non-invasive pressure measurements in a patient with heart failure and valvular disease. Although these data are not available in all patients, some information is available in most. Invasive studies may be required when the clinical picture is not consistent with the echocardiography findings.

REFERENCES

1. Oh JK, Seward JB, Tajik JA, eds. *Chapter 4: The Echo Manual. Doppler Echocardiography and Color Flow Imaging: Comprehensive Non Invasive Hemodynamic Assessment.* 3rd ed. Philadelphia, PA: Lippincott, Williams and Wilkins; 2007:59-79.

2. Hatle L, Angelsen B. *Doppler Ultrasound in Cardiology.* 2nd ed. Philadelphia, PA: Lea & Febiger; 1985.

3. Otto C, ed. *Textbook of Clinical Echocardiography.* 5th ed. Philadelphia, PA: Elsevier–Saunders; 2013:159.

4. Rudski LG, Lai WW, Afilalo J, et al. Guidelines for the echocardiographic assessment of the right heart in adults: a report from the American Society of Echocardiography endorsed by the European Association of Echocardiography and the Canadian Society of Echocardiography. *J Am Soc Echocardiogr.* 2010;23:685-713.

5. Mahan G, Dabestani A, Gardin J, et al. Estimation of pulmonary artery pressure by pulsed Doppler echocardiography. *Circulation.* 1983;68(suppl III):III-367.

6. Nagueh SF, Middleton KJ, Kopelen HA, et al. Doppler tissue imaging: a noninvasive technique for evaluation of LV filling pressure. *J Am CollCardiol.* 1997;30:1527-1533.

7. Quinones, MA. Estimation of left ventricular filling pressures, ASE's comprehensive echocardiography, 2nd ed. *Elsevier Health Sciences.* 2016;41:185-187.

8. Nagueh SF, Smiseth OA, Appleton CP, et al. Recommendations for the evaluation of left ventricular diastolic function by echocardiography: an update from the American Society of Echocardiography and the European Association of Cardiovascular Imaging. *J Am SocEchocardiogr.* 2016;29:277.

9. Scapellato F, Temporrelli PL, Eleuteri E, et al. Accurate noninvasive assessment of pulmonary vascular resistance in patients with chronic heart failure. *Am J Cardiol.* 2001;37:1813-1819.

Ismini Kourouni
Gopal Narayanswami
Joseph P. Mathew

51

Noncardiac Point-of-Care Ultrasound in the CCU

INTRODUCTION

Goal-directed point-of-care ultrasound (POCUS) is real-time, organ-focused ultrasonography (USG) performed by a nonradiologist to answer a clinical question or guide a procedure. POCUS, also referred to as critical care ultrasonography (CCUS) or goal-directed USG, is performed and interpreted by clinicians at the point of clinical care.[1-3] Over the past decade, POCUS has become essential in the early diagnosis and treatment of critically ill patients. It allows for rapid, safe, and accurate assessment of a patient's condition and has great utility in guiding invasive bedside procedures. Safe application and interpretation of ultrasound (US) findings requires knowledge of the basic principles of USG and familiarity with the equipment and the modalities.

POCUS requires that all image acquisition, interpretation, and clinical application is performed by the clinician at the point of care, allowing for rapid integration of the results with the history and physical, laboratory, and imaging data to guide diagnosis and treatment.[4] When POCUS is performed with a focused clinical question and goal in mind, it serves as a valuable adjunct to the physical examination. We believe that POCUS is the most important contemporary innovation in critical care—an extension of the physical examination or "visual stethoscope," so to speak—and its adoption and incorporation into clinical care will certainly prove of value in the diagnosis and treatment of the patient in the cardiac care unit (CCU). We highlight the role of POCUS in making a rapid and acceptably accurate differential diagnosis of the patient in the CCU who is hypotensive, in respiratory distress, or in multiorgan failure.[5]

HISTORY

Although clinicians in these specialties such as radiology, cardiology, and obstetrics have been doing point-of-care bedside USG for the past several decades, bedside POCUS did not really advance until the 1990s, when more compact and affordable machines led to adoption by specialties such as emergency medicine (EM), anesthesiology, and pulmonary-critical care medicine. Early use of US in CCUs and intensive care units (ICUs) were driven by its success with improving the success and safety of central line placement.[6] Trauma surgeons and EM physicians started assessing patients with trauma using US, and the FAST (Focused Assessment with Sonography in Trauma) examination became fully integrated into Advanced Trauma Life Support (ATLS) guidelines.[7] US guidance is now standard of care for procedures such as thoracentesis and internal jugular vein central line placement.[8,9] Focused USG has now become part of nearly every specialty's practice in some form.[5]

THE CASE FOR POINT-OF-CARE ULTRASONOGRAPHY

Traditionally, USG and echocardiography are performed by a technician and interpreted by a radiologist or cardiologist. Patients have to be transported for these examinations and the services are often only available during daytime hours on weekdays, thus leading to delays in performance, interpretation, and communication of the results. This is very limiting to units such as the CCU where questions need to be answered at all times of day or night and on weekends. POCUS is performed at the bedside by the treating clinician, interpreted right away, and the results applied right away in conjunction with the clinical presentation and laboratory data. POCUS by no means is a replacement for a comprehensive examination and consultation by radiology or cardiology services.[4] Although POCUS is often limited to one organ system, multiple systems may have to be assessed for diagnostic purposes; but this can be done in a quick and efficient manner by the trained sonographer.[10] In addition, just like the physical examination, the sonographic examination can be repeated to reassess the patient.

The current evidence supporting the use of POCUS is overwhelming. Early studies by Lichtenstein and Axler[11] showed that focused sonography changed management in one out of every four patients in the ICU. In patients with trauma, the FAST examination has a sensitivity of 94% and specificity of 98% with a high negative predictive value for clinically significant intra-abdominal injury.[12] Multiorgan POCUS was shown to correlate accurately with the final diagnosis in patients in the emergency department (ED) with undifferentiated hypotension.[13] Lichtenstein's pioneering research showed that bedside USG could identify the correct diagnosis of acute respiratory failure, shock states, and even function as a noninvasive Swan Ganz catheter to guide fluid resuscitation.[10,14,15] Focused goal-directed echocardiography (GDE) can be helpful in the evaluation of shock states, and assessment of inferior vena cava (IVC) variability in mechanically ventilated patients has been used to accurately predict fluid responsiveness.[16,17] Work by Kory and Blaivas showed that non-radiologists could accurately detect deep vein thrombosis (DVT) at the point of care, saving time and expediting treatment.[18,19]

BASIC PRINCIPLES OF ULTRASONOGRAPHY

USs are sound waves with frequencies that exceed those perceived by the human ear (>20 kHz). Medical USG uses sound waves (2 to 10 MHz) created by a vibrating crystal within a ceramic probe (also called a transducer) that can both send and receive sound waves. Images are created on the basis of the piezoelectric principle, by which electric current causes crystals to vibrate and returning sound waves create electric current that the machine translates into real-time images. The strength or amplitude of the returning echo waves determines the brightness (ie, whiteness) of the echo pixel. Modern-day US machines generate B-mode or two-dimensional USG from an array of crystals (>128) across the footprint of the transducer.[5,20]

US waves travel through different tissue and are partly reflected at each tissue interface. They penetrate well through solid organs and fluid; however, they do not penetrate air or bone, limiting the usefulness. Hence, the ribs are often an impediment when doing echocardiography and thoracic USG. Air is completely reflected back to the transducer. If air is in the way of sound waves, it generates "A-lines" or "air lines," which are a reverberation artifact. Bone typically has a white leading edge and then a black shadow due to near-total reflection of US waves.

Bright structures are referred to as *hyperechoic*. These "white" areas represent echogenic structures that transmit and reflect US waves. "Black" areas represent areas that are *anechoic*. This occurs when US waves encounter a structure that does not reflect any waves and no waves return to the transducer (eg, fluid). Sound waves propagate through fluid and thus fluid is a great window to see other nearby structures. US waves often lose energy after their interaction with a structure and return with a low amplitude. These low-amplitude waves are translated into shades of gray or *hypoechoic* regions. Lastly, lines occur at boundaries between two markedly different tissue reflectors, delineating the two structures. Soft tissue often has white, gray, and black planes and borders, representing different speeds of propagation and reflection of US waves.[20] **Table 51.1** lists examples of structures of different echogenicity. **Figure 51.1** shows the parasternal long-axis (PLAX) view of a patient with a posterior mediastinal mass presenting with rapid atrial fibrillation demonstrating the echogenicity of different structures in the thorax.

EQUIPMENT AND IMAGE ACQUISITION

Modern US machines are portable and consist of multiple transducers or probes (**Figure 51.2**). Linear array transducers emit high-frequency US waves at a frequency of 5 to 15 MHz and provide excellent resolution of superficial structures such as vascular structures. For POCUS, this transducer is mainly used for US guidance for vascular access and to assess for DVT. Because

TABLE 51.1	Differences in Tissue Echogenicity		
GRAY SCALE	**TERMINOLOGY**	**STRUCTURE**	**EXAMPLE**
	Anechoic	Pure fluid	Pleural or pericardial effusion Ascites Bladder Veins and arteries
	Hypoechoic	Thick fluid Thrombosis Consolidation Tissue/organs	Hemothorax or hemoperitoneum DVT Pneumonia Liver, spleen, kidney, bowel Fat, lymph nodes, nerve
	Hyperechoic	Bone/calculus Strong interface	Ribs; kidney or gallstones Pleura, pericardium Diaphragm, nerve, tendon

DVT, deep vein thrombosis.

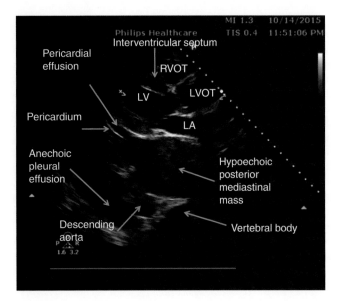

FIGURE 51.1 Differences in tissue echogenicity. LA, left atrium; LV, left ventricle; LVOT, left ventricular outflow tract; RVOT, right ventricular outflow tract.

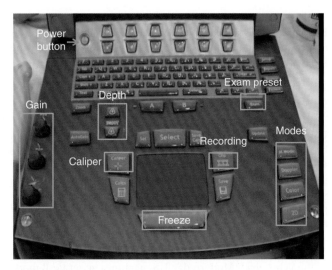

FIGURE 51.2 Portable ultrasound machine.

of its high resolution, it can be used to assess the pleura for pneumothorax. It has poor penetration and so is not used to image deeper structures. Phased array transducers are low-frequency transducers (1 to 5 MHz) and have good penetration; hence, they are used to image deeper structures. The small footprint of the transducer allows for image acquisition between the ribs, and is hence used for lung, pleural, and cardiac USG. This transducer can also be used for abdominal and pelvic imaging. The curvilinear transducer is a hybrid, multipurpose probe that images at lower frequencies ranging between 1 and 8 MHz. It has a larger footprint, which generates a beam that fans outward, resulting in a wide field of view. These probes are most often used for abdominal and pelvic applications and the FAST examination where the subcostal (SC) cardiac view can also be obtained. The microconvex probe has a small footprint that fits in between the rib interspace and can be used for thoracic imaging. **Table 51.2** summarizes the basic characteristics and uses of the different types of transducers.

Transducer orientation and manipulation is of utmost importance in obtaining good images for diagnostic purposes or procedural guidance. The transducer should be held steady, as if holding a pencil (**Figure 51.3**). All US probes have a marker that correlates with the side of the marked screen. Structures adjacent to the probe marker will appear on the same side of the image as the screen marker, helping to orient the viewer and guide probe manipulations. The operator should always be aware of the orientation of the probe marker in relation to the marker on the monitor screen. Structures closest to the footprint of the transducer will appear on the top of the screen (near field) and those furthest away will appear on the bottom (far field). Portable US machines have preset examination settings (eg, abdomen versus cardiac) for each type of examination, which sets the resolution, frame rates, and the location of the screen marker.

ULTRASOUND MANIPULATION

To obtain quality images, the gain and depth of imaging have to be optimized. *Depth* is manipulated on the console such that the structure of interest should always be in the center of the screen. The depth of interrogation is usually shown on a scale on the monitor. *Gain* adjusts the brightness of the entire image and should be adjusted such that there is maximal resolution between the different tissues that are imaged. Failure to adjust gain can lead to misinterpretation of image. Ensure that gain is uniform in both near (top half of screen) and far field (bottom half). The operator should be familiar with other features of the machine such as how to *freeze* and measure structures using the *caliper* button, how to *save* images and clips, and utilize features such as *M-mode* (motion mode) and *Doppler*. The operator must always ensure that the portable US machine is in the appropriate exam preset. For example, the frame rates acquired in abdominal preset are not optimal for cardiac imaging and the screen marker on the opposite side will reverse all the cardiac images.

IMAGE MANIPULATION

In general, the probe marker should be pointed to the operator's left side when imaging in the transverse (short-axis) plane or cephalad when imaging in the coronal or sagittal (long-axis) planes. Additional maneuvers that are used to optimize the views include *moving* the probe such that the entire transducer is moved on the body (eg, from one rib interspace to another). This maneuver helps find the optimal location and view to locate the structure of interest. *Sliding* the probe is a maneuver that slides the transducer along the course of the structure of interest (eg, blood vessel). *Compression* allows visualization of deeper structures and allows one to differentiate structures (eg, vein from artery and nerve) based on their compressibility. *Rocking* involves angling the transducer side to side and extends the plane of imaging. This is useful to center the image on the screen (eg, centering a central vein and separating it from the artery). *Rotation* is used to switch between short-axis and long-axis imaging. This is useful for

TABLE 51.2	Transducer Characteristics		
TRANSDUCER	**FREQUENCY**	**CHARACTERISTICS**	**USES**
Linear array	5–15 MHz	High frequency Excellent resolution of superficial structures Loss of depth	Vascular access DVT study Pleural lines Soft tissue and musculoskeletal imaging
Phased array	1–5 MHz	Low frequency Small footprint Deep penetration	Cardiac Lung/pleural Abdomen
Microconvex	5–8 MHz	Small footprint Good resolution	Lung Abdomen Vascular Nerve
Curvilinear	1–8 MHz	Low frequency, low resolution Multipurpose Full depth of penetration	Abdominal/pelvic imaging FAST exam Lung/cardiac

DVT, deep vein thrombosis; FAST, focused assessment with sonography in trauma.

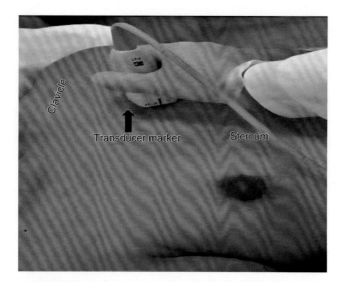

FIGURE 51.3 Transducer position for thoracic ultrasonography.

vascular access procedures and for obtaining short-axis cardiac views. *Tilting* (also called *fanning* or *sweeping*) allows the operator to scan along the course of a structure along a narrow acoustic window that is used. The transducer is held in place on the skin and angled on the long axis of the transducer face to aim the US beam in different planes (eg, obtaining multiple short-axis views of the heart).

MODES

The standard mode used for POCUS is *B-mode* or 2D USG. *M-mode* is used to display and measure the movement of structures over time. This feature is used to assess variation in the IVC diameter, diaphragmatic excursion, and to assess the pleura in the evaluation of pneumothorax. *D-mode* or *Doppler* mode evaluates the characteristics of direction and speed of blood flow (and tissue motion) through a structure. This is presented in audible, color, or spectral display.[20] Color Doppler converts measurements into an array of colors to visualize speed and direction. This is particularly useful in vascular imaging to distinguish arteries from veins. The conventional color code is such that flow toward the transducer is depicted as red and flow away from the transducer is blue ("BART": blue away, red toward). Spectral Doppler is used mainly in echocardiography and displays the movement of blood in a graph depicting flow velocities with respect to time. **Table 51.3** lists examples of the imaging modes used in POCUS.

PRACTICAL APPLICATION OF POINT-OF-CARE ULTRASONOGRAPHY IN THE CCU

The standard critical care US examination involves scanning the major regions that would answer the question about the presenting condition. The standard multiorgan POCUS examination generally includes four organ systems: thoracic (lung and pleural), cardiac, and limited abdominal and vascular imaging.

The organ of interest is often scanned first (eg, heart in shock or lungs in respiratory failure), although a standardized multiorgan approach can be used for the critically ill patient in the CCU. Although a focused examination is often all that is needed, studies have shown that a multiorgan or whole-body approach leads to a more accurate diagnosis.[13,21] The US examination should always be performed in conjunction with the patient's clinical data. It should be repeated to reassess the patient and to see if certain therapeutic interventions were effective.

The most common indication for a point-of-care examination in the CCU is for cardiopulmonary failure. POCUS is indicated in the evaluation of the patient with undifferentiated shock and can help distinguish between obstructive, cardiogenic, hypovolemic, and distributive shock states.[4,13,21,22] Another major indication would be in the setting of acute respiratory failure. A focused US examination of the heart, lungs, and deep veins can be useful in diagnosing various causes of respiratory failure.[10] Overadministration of fluids in the patient in the CCU with limited cardiopulmonary reserve can be harmful and leads to increased days of ventilator support. Assessing IVC size and variation, as well as the heart and lungs, can help guide fluid resuscitation.[17] US is very helpful in the patient whose condition suddenly deteriorates. It can be used to quickly rule out pneumothorax, massive pulmonary embolism (PE), pericardial tamponade, valvular rupture, and intra-abdominal bleeding.

FUNDAMENTALS OF THORACIC ULTRASONOGRAPHY IN THE CCU

BASIC PRINCIPLES

The utility of bedside lung ultrasound (LUS) is gaining increasing popularity as an attractive alternative to chest radiography. Easily performed by the trained intensivist, it is safe, accurate, and cost-effective. Conventionally, thoracic US is limited to the evaluation of pleural effusions; however, more recently LUS has become an attractive new tool for assessing lung status in hypoxemic critically ill patients. A frontline intensivist, Dr Daniel Lichtenstein, has been largely responsible for developing the field of critical care LUS, publishing a series of definitive reports in the 1990s that established the basis for the field.[23–26]

Traditionally, the lungs were not considered an organ amenable to USG, because US waves are not transmitted through air-filled structures. When air is displaced from the lung by a disease process, US findings change in a predictable manner. Because the lung parenchyma is normally filled with air, which is a near-total reflector, the healthy or "unhealthy" pleural line serves as the generator of reflecting signs, which can be interpreted. Lung disorders can be separated into dependent disorders and nondependent disorders, whereby fluid descends and air rises. The findings of LUS relate to the ratio of air to fluid within the lung. Most lung processes that are pertinent to the patient in the CCU (eg, pulmonary edema, pneumonia, pneumothorax, pleural effusion, and atelectasis) all extend to the lung periphery allowing the US machine's ability to distinguish air and water to produce artifacts. These artifacts are used to diagnose various disorders such as alveolar-interstitial syndrome and accurately assess lung aeration in patients with acute lung injury. LUS is therefore based on the clinical interpretation of a number of mostly dynamic artifacts.

TABLE 51.3	Modes of Ultrasonography
MODES	
B-mode	Brightness mode 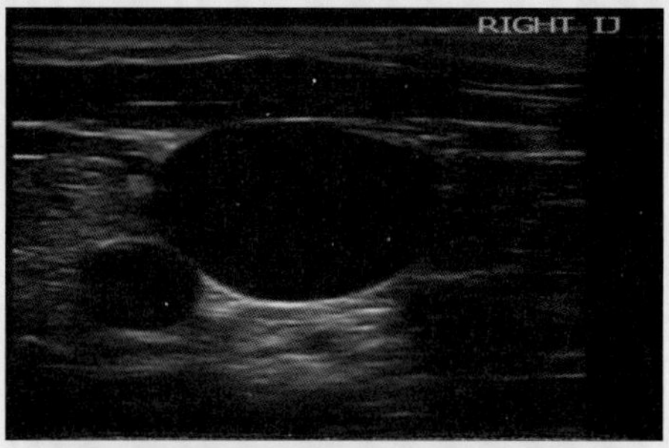
M-mode	Motion mode 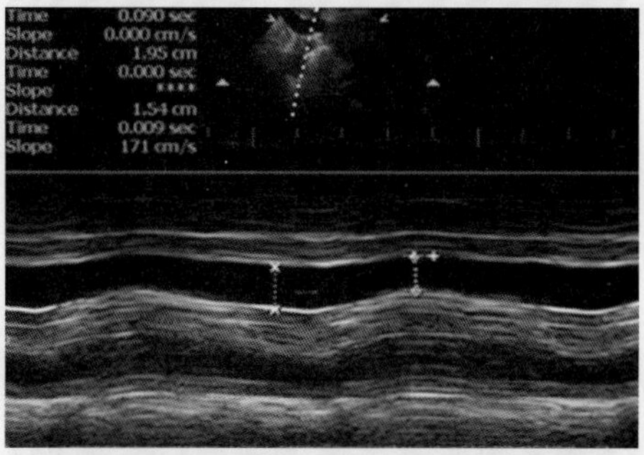
D-mode	Examines the characteristics of direction and speed of blood flow (and tissue motion) • Color Doppler • Spectral Doppler • Power Doppler • • • • 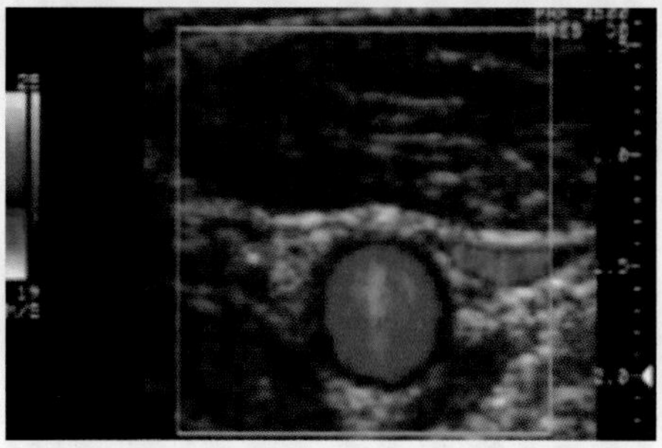

THE LUNG EXAMINATION

To examine the thorax, a micro-convex (5 to 8 MHz) transducer is preferable or, alternatively, a low-frequency (1 to 5 MHz) phased array transducer can be used because it fits in the rib interspace (**Table 51.2**).[27] A high-frequency linear array transducer (5 to 15 MHz) can be used to visualize the superficial pleural line; however, it is limited by the depth of penetration and the linear trajectory of the US beam.

The scanning of the lung occurs in the intercostal spaces. The transducer is held in a longitudinal orientation and perpendicular to the skin surface, with the marker facing cephalad (**Figure 51.3**). Initial scanning should be performed at a maximum depth (around 16 cm) and then the gain and depth must be adjusted to optimize and center the image. By moving the transducer along a series of longitudinal scan lines while imaging through adjacent intercostal spaces, the examiner can perform a complete lung examination and construct a 3D image of the thorax. The thorax can be divided into three zones: anterior, lateral, and posterior zones and then further into upper and lower zones (**Figure 51.4**).[27] Thus, a complete examination consists of 12 imaging regions, 6 in each hemithorax.

The sternum and the anterior axillary line border the *anterior lung zone*, whereas the *lateral zone* lies between the anterior and posterior axillary lines. The *posterior lung zone* lies behind the posterior axillary line. The anterior lung zone is assessed for alveolar-interstitial syndromes, lung consolidation, and pneumothorax. When examining the lateral zone, it is important to identify the hemi-diaphragm, which appears as a hyperechoic structure that separates the lungs from abdominal contents. Pleural effusions, atelectasis, and consolidation can often be seen above the hemi-diaphragm in this region. The posterior lung zone is a forgotten region where dependent pleural effusions and lung consolidation may be seen, so it is important to turn the critically ill patient to assess this area. Alternatively, Lichtenstein describes four points that can be quickly assessed as part of the BLUE (bedside lung ultrasound in emergency) protocol (**Figure 51.5**), a goal-directed LUS examination that can be performed in <3 minutes.[10]

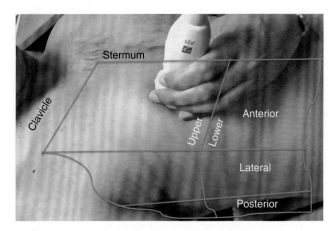

FIGURE 51.4 Lung zones for thoracic ultrasonography.

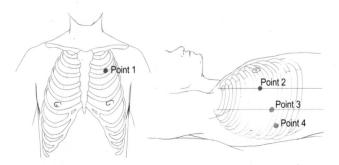

FIGURE 51.5 Bedside lung ultrasound in emergency (BLUE) protocol.

LUNG SIGNS

There are five cardinal lung signs to look for when performing thoracic USG. **Table 51.4** describes these and additional signs that are described in LUS and pleural USG. **Table 51.5** summarizes common LUS patterns seen in common disease processes that may be encountered in the CCU.

Lung Sliding

This is a subtle shimmering of the hyperechoic pleural line (**Figure 51.6**). It represents movement of visceral pleura past the parietal pleura during respiration. It must be present at multiple sites and will be present more often at the lung base. The presence of lung sliding rules out pneumothorax with 100% certainty at that particular site on the thorax.[26,27] The presence of lung sliding strongly suggests that two conditions are met: the pleural surfaces are adjacent (ie, no pneumothorax) and that the lung volume is changing. The examiner can also use a high-resolution linear array transducer because it images the pleura well. A similar analogous sign can be from *lung pulse*, which is produced when cardiac motion causes pulsations of the pleural line. Air in the pleural space (ie, pneumothorax) will cause absence of lung sliding and lung pulse. Other conditions can also cause lack of lung sliding, including apnea or hypoventilation (eg, contralateral bronchial intubation), pleurodesis, and dense lung consolidation.

A-Lines

Sonographic A-lines are visualized as hyperechoic lines perpendicular to the US beam (**Figure 51.7**). They are reverberation artifacts that arise when the US beam reflects off the pleura; therefore, these lines are below the pleural line. There is equal distance between the transducer, pleural line, and each subsequent A-line. A-lines can be thought of as "air" lines, but the air can be either in the pleural space or in the lung parenchyma. The presence of sliding lung determines that the air is in the lung parenchyma and its absence indicates that the air may be in the pleural space (ie, pneumothorax). Hence, the presence of A-lines and sliding lung means the lungs are normal at that particular site. The standard view of the upper rib, pleural line, and lower rib has the appearance of a bat flying out of the screen, and hence is called a *batwing sign* (**Figures 51.6** and **51.7**).[10,28]

B-Lines

B-lines are vertical raylike projections that start from the pleural line and continue to the bottom of the screen (**Figure 51.8**). They are also known as comet tails or lung rockets because of their sonographic similarity with comets and rockets. B-lines follow the motion of the lung sliding and efface the normal A-lines at the point of their intersection. B-lines are generated when the interlobular septa become abnormally thickened with fluid or when the alveoli become abnormally filled with fluid, blood, or purulent material. Although isolated B-lines in any given region may be a normal finding, seeing more than three lines is considered abnormal. It is not uncommon to find B-lines at the lung bases in the hospitalized patient; however, the presence of >3 B-lines in the anterior lung zones is abnormal. The focal location of B-lines may be suggestive of local infiltration (eg, focal pneumonia). A generalized B-line pattern represents an interstitial syndrome such as pulmonary edema, pneumonia, acute respiratory distress syndrome (ARDS), or interstitial lung disease.[10,23,24]

Alveolar Consolidation

When the alveoli become devoid of air and are filled with pus, fluid, or blood, the lungs develop echogenicity. Consolidated lung adjacent to the pleura will permit the transmission of US waves. In the circumstance of lung consolidation, the lung appears sonographically similar to the liver; therefore, the term "lung hepatization" has been descriptively utilized.[10,27] In addition, sonographic air bronchograms or punctate hyperechoic foci within the consolidated lung may be visualized, which indicates that air still remains in the bronchioles. The presence of mobile or dynamic air bronchograms has high specificity (94%) for the diagnosis of pneumonia, as compared to static air bronchograms, which is seen in resorptive atelectasis.[29] **Figure 51.9** shows an example of a patient with lung consolidation as a result of severe pneumonia with parapneumonic effusion.

Pleural Effusion

One of the most important uses of US in thoracic pathology is the ability to detect, quantify, and characterize pleural effusion. Pleural USG is superior to standard upright chest radiography and supine chest radiography for detecting pleural effusions.[30]

TABLE 51.4	Normal and Abnormal Signs in Lung Ultrasonography	
SIGN	**LUNG ULTRASOUND PATTERN**	**CLINICAL SIGNIFICANCE**
A-line	Horizontal reflections or reverberations of pleural line Hyperechoic and equal in distance from skin to pleural line	Present in normal lung, "air" line indicates air in lung or pleural space
B-lines	"Comet tail" or "lung rockets"—vertical hyperechoic reverberation artifacts that arise from the pleural line and extend to the bottom of the screen Move synchronously with lung sliding and efface A-lines; implies fluid-filled subpleural interlobular septa	>3 B-lines = interstitial pathology Multiple diffuse B-lines indicate interstitial syndrome Focal B-line can be seen in pneumonia, infarct, and cancer
Lung sliding	Sliding or shimmering of the pleural line that occurs with respiration Indicates intact visceral and parietal pleura	Present in normal lung Absent in pneumothorax, apnea, fibrosis, ARDS, and pleurodesis
Lung pulse	Subtle rhythmic movement of the visceral upon the parietal pleural with cardiac oscillations	Present in normal lung Rules out pneumothorax
Seashore sign	Normal M-mode image with lines above echogenic pleura and speckled pattern deep to it, indicating normal lung sliding	Normal aeration pattern No pneumothorax
Bar code or stratosphere sign	Abnormal M-mode image showing a linear pattern above and below the pleura	Signifies absence of lung sliding; can be seen with pneumothorax
Lung point	Transition point where visceral and parietal pleura separate— image changes from the intermittent presence and then absence of lung sliding	Pathognomonic sign for pneumothorax
Lung hepatization/ consolidation	Loss of aeration of lung leads to a hyperechoic appearance of lung; alveoli are filled with fluid or inflammatory cells or are atelectatic	Can be seen with atelectasis or pneumonia
Dynamic air bronchograms	Dynamic echogenic foci within consolidated lung that fluctuate with the respiratory cycle	Seen with pneumonia
Static air bronchograms	Hyperechoic foci that do not move with respiration	Seen with atelectasis
Shred sign	Border between consolidated and aerated lung	Seen with consolidation but not translobar consolidation
Curtain sign	Intermittent obscuration of underlying organs by intervening air-filled lung	Can be normal finding
Hematocrit sign	Effusion is separated into different echogenicity with a layering effect	Seen in hemothorax or highly cellular effusions (eg, malignant effusion)
Flapping lung (jellyfish sign)	Floating movement of collapsed lung within a pleural effusion	Atelectatic lung in effusion
Sinusoid sign	In a pleural effusion, M-mode appearance of the pleura moving toward and away from the parietal pleura	Can be used to distinguish pleural thickening from effusion
Plankton sign	Particulate matter in lung effusion	Complex effusion

ARDS, acute respiratory distress syndrome.

On a portable chest radiograph in the patient in the CCU, both lung consolidation and pleural effusion will appear "white." POCUS is particularly helpful in these patients, because it will help differentiate the two. Pleural fluid is typically anechoic, whereas consolidated or atelectatic lung is echogenic. It is important to also distinguish pleural effusion from pericardial effusion in such patients. In the PLAX view, pleural effusions lie posterior to the descending aorta and pericardial effusions anterior and within the pericardium. In addition, scanning the lateral or posterior lung zone (**Figure 51.4**) further helps differentiate the two effusions. The use of US also allows for the identification of a safe puncture site to perform thoracentesis, even in mechanically ventilated patients in the CCU.[8] Before thoracentesis, ensure the three cardinal features of a pleural effusion: an anechoic space; anatomic boundaries of chest wall, diaphragm and lung; and dynamic changes of the atelectatic lung and diaphragm related to respiration and cardiac motion.[28]

Pleural USG can further help characterize the pleural effusion and can even identify septations within it. Simple anechoic

TABLE 51.5	Lung Ultrasound Patterns
LUNG ULTRASOUND PATTERN	**CLINICAL SIGNIFICANCE**
A-lines with lung sliding	Normal aeration pattern
A-lines without lung sliding and +lung point	Pneumothorax
B-7 lines	Interlobular septal pathology
B-3 lines	Alveolar-interstitial syndrome
Focal absence of B-lines	Pulmonary embolus, cancer
Lung hepatization + dynamic air bronchograms	Pneumonia
Lung hepatization ± static air bronchograms	Atelectasis
Anechoic collection without septations	Simple pleural effusion
Echogenic fluid with septations	Complicated effusion

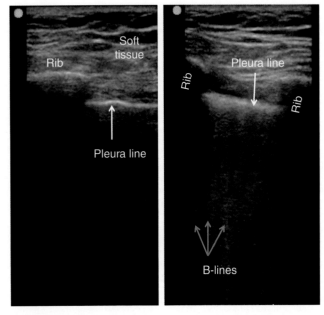

FIGURE 51.6 Normal pleural line with lung sliding imaged with linear array transducer.

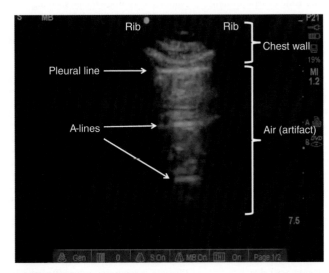

FIGURE 51.7 Standard view of A-line from anterior lung zone imaged with phased array transducer.

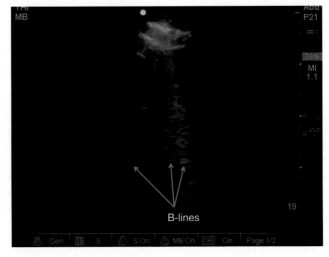

FIGURE 51.8 B-line pattern.

fluid suggests a noncomplicated pleural effusion, which may or may not be a transudate. The *flapping lung* or *jellyfish sign* is the oscillating movement of a collapsed lung in a pleural effusion (**Figure 51.10**). Strands of echogenic floating matter suggest complex fluid; this is called the *plankton sign*.[31] Septated or loculated effusions imply complicated effusions that require sampling of the fluid and usually warrant a chest tube placement or surgical drainage. **Figure 51.11A** demonstrates the multiple septations within the pleural fluid of a patient with pneumonia and empyema. This patient was a poor surgical candidate, and so was treated with a small-bore chest tube and intrapleural alteplase and deoxyribonuclease (DNase). Similarly, pleural effusions can demonstrate the *hematocrit sign*, where an echogenic or highly

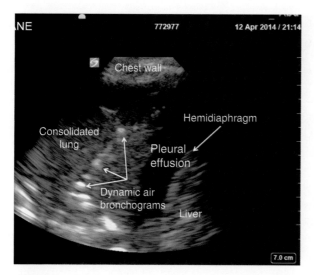

FIGURE 51.9 Lung consolidation with sonographic air bronchograms.

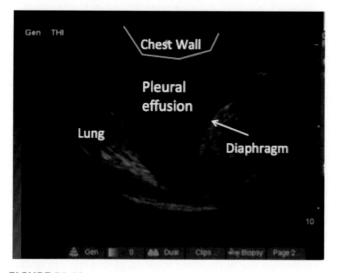

FIGURE 51.10 Moderate pleural effusion with flapping lung.

cellular effusion (ie, blood) has gravity-dependent fading of echogenicity.[31] **Figure 51.11B** is that of a patient with trauma who presented with a hemothorax.

CLINICAL SCENARIOS ENCOUNTERED IN THE CCU

Detection of Pneumothorax

Pneumothorax can occur spontaneously in the CCU and is potentially fatal. Patients on mechanical ventilation with underlying emphysema or those undergoing central line placement are at risk for pneumothorax. Lung ultrasonography carries a >95% sensitivity in the detection of pneumothorax.[32] The examination requires, on an average, 2 to 3 minutes. The transducer is placed longitudinally in the mid-clavicular line at the level of the second to third intercostal space. Sequential movement of the transducer inferior and lateral across multiple rib interspaces will allow for a comprehensive examination of the pleural space.[27] The presence of lung sliding is characteristic of normal visceral and parietal pleural layers and carries a 100% negative predictive value in the diagnosis of pneumothorax.[26] In contrast to normal lung, when air is trapped between the visceral and parietal pleural layers, lung sliding will not be detected. Nevertheless, absence of lung sliding may not always be due to the presence of pneumothorax because it has also been observed in massive atelectasis, ARDS, pleural adhesions, and severe lung fibrosis. The presence of B-lines or lung pulse also rules out pneumothorax.[24,33]

In the occasion that lung sliding is difficult to visualize, additional information is obtained with the assistance of M-mode analysis. Characteristically, M-mode analysis of normal lung tissue demonstrates the *seashore sign*, a characteristic linear wave pattern representing the motionless chest wall, and below the pleural line a granular pattern represents normal lung motion (**Figure 51.12**A). If present, it confirms the presence of lung sliding and therefore the absence of pneumothorax. When there is air in the pleural space, this morphology is replaced on M-mode imaging by parallel linear lines called the *stratosphere sign* or *bar code sign* (**Figure 51.12**B).[32] The visualization of the *lung point* may also be used in the diagnosis of pneumothorax, having a specificity of 100%. The lung point represents the transition point between normal lung sliding and to an area of absent lung sliding (**Figure 51.13**).[25] Lung point is helpful to also quantify how

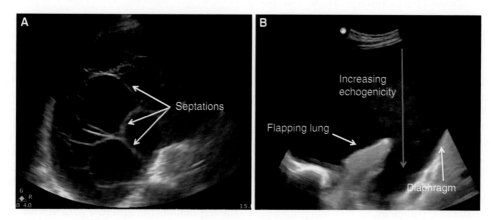

FIGURE 51.11 A, Empyema with thickened pleura and multiple septations within pleural effusion. B, Hemothorax with increasing echogenicity of fluid in the pleural space.

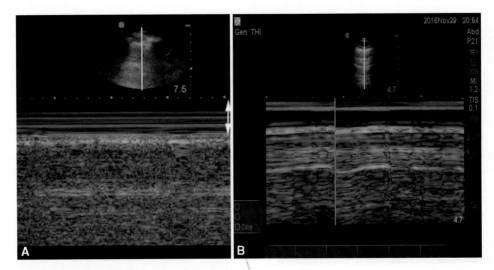

FIGURE 51.12 A, Seashore sign. B, Stratosphere or bar code sign.

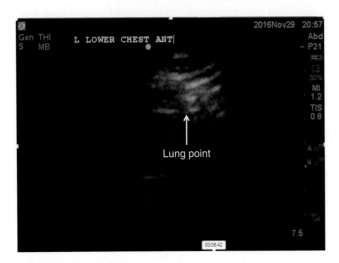

FIGURE 51.13 Lung point.

large a pneumothorax is and helps with procedural guidance for chest tube placement. One approach during central line placement would be to check for lung sliding before and after line placement to quickly rule out a pneumothorax. These concepts can be applied within seconds to the patient in the CCU who is quickly decompensating to rule out pneumothorax.

Detection of Lung Alveolar-Interstitial Syndrome

Alveolar-interstitial syndrome is a common entity in the CCU, caused by a variety of conditions, including acute pulmonary edema, ARDS, and interstitial pneumonias. B-lines 7 mm apart, called *B-7 lines*, correspond to edematous or thickened interlobular septa and extravascular lung volume (similar to Kerley B-lines on a chest radiograph). Lichtenstein also described *B-3 lines*, which are B-lines that are 3 mm apart and more confluent, indicating alveolar edema or an alveolar process such as pneumonia. The more B-lines that are present anteriorly, the lower the air to fluid and the more severe the lung pathology.

LUS is very sensitive in detecting early pulmonary vascular congestion, much more than a chest X-ray. In an acutely dyspneic patient, the detection of diffuse B-lines allows the intensivist to immediately differentiate acute pulmonary edema from chronic obstructive pulmonary disease (COPD).[23] Even while administering fluids in the CCU, the appearance of new B-lines corresponds to early pulmonary edema and correlates to elevated pulmonary artery occlusion pressures (>18 mm Hg).[14] Similarly, while administering diuretics in patients with acute pulmonary edema, one can assess for reduction in the number of B-lines and also reduction in the volume of pleural effusions.

Differentiating Between Types of Lung Alveolar-Interstitial Syndrome

Diffuse B-lines suggest an interstitial pattern, and the presence of a diffuse B-line pattern in both lungs suggests a diffuse alveolar interstitial syndrome such as pulmonary edema, pulmonary fibrosis, or ARDS. The presence of a smooth pleural line may be seen in pulmonary edema, whereas with lung fibrosis, an irregular or "lumpy bumpy" pleural line may be visualized with a high-frequency linear array transducer. In ARDS, subpleural consolidation may be visualized below the pleural line with sparing of certain areas.[28] **Table 51.6** summarizes the main characteristics that can be used to distinguish these entities.

Assessing Diaphragmatic Function

The diaphragm is hyperechoic and easily visualized by USG. Diaphragmatic function can be quickly assessed in the patient in the CCU or the patient post cardiac surgery with acute respiratory failure or inability to wean from mechanical ventilation, obviating the need for fluoroscopy. The technique involves scanning the lateral lung zone, along the anterior or mid-axillary line, and identifying the liver or spleen. M-mode imaging can be utilized to obtain a quantitative measure of diaphragmatic excursion. Normal diaphragmatic excursion for a male in quiet breathing is 1.8 and 7.5 cm during deep breathing. Sonographically detected diaphragmatic dysfunction, defined as <10 mm or paradoxical motion, can identify patients who are difficult to wean. **Figure 51.14** represents 2D and M-mode imaging of the left hemidiaphragm in a patient with amyotrophic lateral sclerosis who presented with Takotsubo cardiomyopathy and acute respiratory failure.

TABLE 51.6	Differentiating causes of the interstitial syndrome			
	ACUTE PULMONARY EDEMA	**CHRONIC HEART FAILURE**	**ARDS**	**PULMONARY FIBROSIS**
Clinical setting	Acute	Chronic	Acute	Chronic
B-lines number	++++	+/++/+++	++++	+/++/+++
B-lines distribution	Multiple, diffuse, bilateral	Multiple, diffuse, bilateral following dependent regions	Non-homogenous distribution, spared areas	More frequently posterior at lung bases
Other Lung US signs	Small bilateral pleural effusions	Bilateral pleural effusions	Subpleural consolidations, possible effusion	Irregular pleural line
Echo	Abnormal	Abnormal	Likely normal	Likely normal

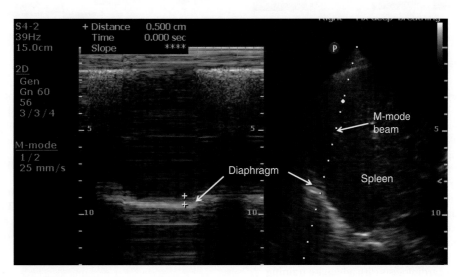

FIGURE 51.14 Decreased diaphragmatic excursion on M-mode.

Rapid Assessment of the Acutely Decompensating Patient in the CCU

Using the concepts described in this section, the CCU practitioner can rapidly assess the patient with acute respiratory failure and find the etiology of the decompensation. If there is an A-line pattern and absence of lung sliding, then pneumothorax has to be ruled out. Presence of diffuse B-lines and pleural effusions bilaterally detected on POCUS points to a pulmonary edema picture. Unilateral B-lines or a consolidation pattern can be seen with pneumonia. If lung sliding is present with a normal A-line pattern in all the lung zones, then the etiology of the respiratory decompensation has to be either due to airways disease (ie, asthma/COPD) or pulmonary vascular disease (ie, PE). Combining thoracic US with GDE can detect findings such as right ventricular (RV) strain or clot-in-transit, leading to a diagnosis of acute PE.[34]

Lichtenstein summarized these concepts in what he called the BLUE protocol, a simple, goal-directed LUS examination combined with a DVT study for acute respiratory failure. Blinded investigators scanned the four BLUE points (**Figure 51.5**) and performed compression US of the lower extremities, following a standardized algorithm (**Figure 51.15**). They were able to rapidly make an accurate diagnosis in 90% of the cases. In addition, the profiles described had very good sensitivity and excellent specificity to diagnose the conditions correlating with each profile.[10] The concepts of thoracic USG can be easily learned by house staff and other clinicians and utilized to make accurate diagnosis in patients presenting with dyspnea.[35]

FUNDAMENTALS OF ULTRASONOGRAPHY IN UNDIFFERENTIATED SHOCK: MULTIORGAN POINT-OF-CARE ULTRASONOGRAPHY

Shock is a commonly encountered condition in the CCU but is not always associated with cardiac causes. Physical examination and laboratory parameters, along with multiorgan POCUS, guide the evaluation and management. POCUS techniques involving the heart, lungs, abdomen, and vasculature are performed on

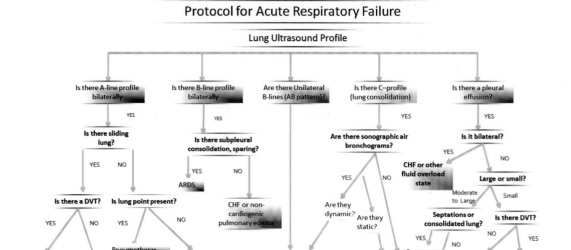

FIGURE 51.15 Lung ultrasound profiles and algorithm for the evaluation of acute respiratory failure. ARDS, acute respiratory distress syndrome; CHF, congestive heart failure; COPD, chronic obstructive pulmonary disease; CT, computed tomography; DVT, deep vein thrombosis. (Modified from Lichenstein D. Relevance of lung ultrasound in the diagnosis of acute respiratory failure: the BLUE protocol. *Chest.* 2008;134: 117-125.)

the basis of the appropriate clinical setting in an attempt to identify the cause of hypotension and optimize management. The goal-directed evaluation of a new, unexpected, or unexplained shock state in a patient in the CCU requires a structured approach that will diagnose or rule out reversible causes such as cardiac tamponade, tension pneumothorax, pulmonary embolus, ruptured aortic aneurysm, and intra-abdominal hemorrhage.

GDE allows the intensivist to assess for RV or left ventricular (LV) failure, pericardial effusion, major valvular failure, and fluid responsiveness. The statement on training in CCUS makes the recommendation that training in critical care includes training in basic critical care echocardiography.[1–3] GDE can be learned and performed well by non-cardiologists with adequate training.[36–38] Combining GDE with sonography of other organs (multiorgan or whole-body USG) adds to the diagnostic yield when evaluating the patient in shock.[4,13] One can perform a goal-directed multiorgan POCUS examination in an efficient and systematic way to discern the etiology of shock:

1. Basic critical care echocardiography to evaluate LV and RV function; rule out tamponade and valvular failure
   a. PLAX, parasternal short-axis (PSAX), apical four-chamber, and SC views
2. IVC imaging to assess volume status in the setting of hypovolemia or sepsis
3. Thoracic US to rule out pneumothorax, hemothorax
4. Limited abdominal examination
   a. Right and left flank to rule out hemoperitoneum
   b. Abdominal aorta to evaluate for dissection
   c. Kidneys and bladder to rule out hydronephrosis in the setting of sepsis or renal failure
5. Compression US of lower extremities to evaluate for DVT

A systematic approach to the patient with shock in the CCU also employs the following questions while performing POCUS[22]:

1. Is there an imminently life-threatening cause of shock?
2. Is there evidence of pump failure: LV or RV failure?

3. Is the shock state likely to be fluid responsive?
4. Is there more than one cause for the shock state?
5. Is it noncardiac in origin?
6. Is there evidence of life-threatening hemorrhage?

Figure 51.16 illustrates an algorithmic approach to the patient in the CCU who is hypotensive. Many POCUS protocols exist for the evaluation of shock. Essentially, they all incorporate multiorgan POCUS to evaluate the etiology of shock. **Table 51.7** summarizes a few of these protocols and the organs that are assessed.[39–41] Further discussions on cardiac etiologies of shock are found in other sections of this textbook.

INFERIOR VENA CAVA IMAGING: EVALUATING FLUID STATUS AND FLUID RESPONSIVENESS IN SHOCK

The IVC caliber is altered by respiration, blood volume, and right heart failure. The IVC can be used to assess intravascular volume status. Fluid responsiveness is by definition an increase in cardiac output (generally >15%) after an adequate volume challenge. Interpretation of IVC size and variability is dependent on whether a patient is spontaneously breathing or on mechanical ventilation. In the spontaneously breathing patient, IVC imaging helps estimate right atrium (RA) pressures (ie, as a "noninvasive" central venous pressure [CVP] reading). In the patient on mechanical ventilation in the CCU, respiratory variation of the IVC can predict fluid responsiveness, in the appropriate settings.

TECHNIQUE

Multiple ways have been described to image the IVC. With the patient in supine position (and knees bent if possible), the IVC can be visualized from the SC cardiac view by placing the phased array transducer in the SC space with the marker facing the patient's head. Alternatively, obtain an SC four-chamber view by positioning the probe flat just below the xiphoid, with the probe

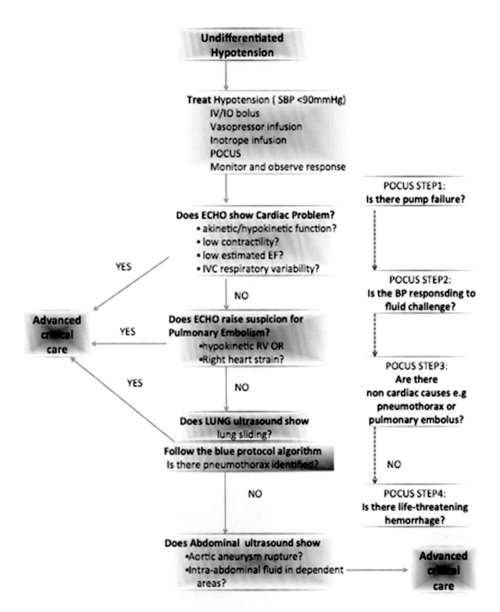

FIGURE 51.16 Approach to undifferentiated shock. BP, blood pressure; EF, ejection fraction; IO, intraosseous; IV, intravenous; IVC, inferior vena cava; POCUS, point-of-care ultrasonogaphy; RV, right ventricle; SBP, systolic blood pressure.

marker facing the patient's left side (**Figure 51.17**). Identify the RA at the top of the screen and track it while turning the probe counterclockwise and slightly perpendicular to the body such that the marker is facing the patient's head. The IVC will appear within the liver with a hepatic vein joining it and emptying into the RA. **Table 51.8** delineates basic characteristics used to identify the IVC and differentiate it from the aorta, which runs alongside the IVC. The IVC can be measured using 2D imaging or via M-mode imaging using the caliper feature. The "sniff" maneuver can be used in spontaneously breathing patients to estimate RA pressures. In patients on mechanical ventilation, the maximal and minimal diameter can be calculated to assess for respiratory variability.

SPONTANEOUSLY BREATHING PATIENT

In the spontaneously breathing patient, IVC size and the degree of collapse correlate to CVP. An IVC >2 cm in diameter, with

inspiratory collapse <50% approximates a CVP of 15 cm H_2O. When the IVC is narrow (<1.5 cm) and collapses a large amount (>50%), the CVP will be low and a hypovolemic (dehydration, hemorrhage) or distributive (sepsis, anaphylaxis) cause of shock is likely (**Table 51.9**).[42] When the IVC is dilated (>3 cm) and non-collapsing, it usually indicates volume unresponsiveness unless the patient has right heart strain. On the other hand, when the IVC is extremely small or a "virtual IVC," it likely indicates that the patient is fluid depleted (**Table 51.10**).

MECHANICALLY VENTILATED PATIENT

Studies have shown that dynamic measures of fluid responsiveness (eg, IVC variation) are more reliable than static measures (eg, CVP).[43] During mechanical ventilation of a sedated or paralyzed patient, pleural and juxtacardiac pressures increase during inspiration, causing RA pressures to rise and decreasing

TABLE 51.7	Standardized POCUS Protocols in the Evaluation of Shock		
NAME	**PROBE LANDMARKS**	**VIEWS/STRUCTURES**	**EVALUATION GOALS**
RUSH examination *Rapid Ultrasound in SHock*	PLAX/PSAX A4C/SC views SC Neck Right flank/RUQ Left flank/LUQ Suprapubic Anterior chest Chest/abdomen Femoral, popliteal veins	LV, RV, valves, pericardium IVC IJV Hepatorenal, splenorenal recess Splenorenal recess pelvis (FAST) Lung/pleura Aortic slide view Limited DVT study	**"Pump"**—LV failure, RV strain from PE, tamponade **"Tank"**—IVC and IJV collapsibility to evaluate volume status Hemoperitoneum, hemothorax, ascites Pneumothorax and pulmonary edema **"Pipes"**—ruptured aortic aneurysm, DVT/PE DVT/PE
EFAST examination *Extended Focused Assessment of Sonography in Trauma*	Anterior chest Subxiphoid Right flank/RUQ Left flank/LUQ Suprapubic	Lung/pleura SC cardiac Hepatorenal, splenorenal recess Pleural space Retrovesicular	Pneumothorax, pulmonary edema Pericardial tamponade Hemoperitoneum Splenic rupture Hemothorax Free fluid/pelvic hemorrhage
FALLS *Fluid Administration Limited by Lung Sonography*	PLAX/PSAX/A4C/SC Lung US (BLUE protocol)	Basic cardiac views Lung/pleura	Rules out tamponade and PE Rules out pneumothorax Determine A-line vs B-line profile A-line profile—gives fluids until improvement or B-line appears (points to septic or distributive shock) B-line profile—suggests cardiogenic shock

A4C, apical four chamber; BLUE, bedside lung ultrasound in emergency; DVT, deep vein thrombosis;, EFAST, Extended Focused Assessment with Sonography in Trauma; FAST, Focused Assessment with Sonography in Trauma; IVC, inferior vena cava; IJV, internal jugular vein; LUQ, left upper quadrant; LV, left ventricle; PE, pulmonary embolism; POCUS, point-of-care ultrasonography; PLAX, parasternal long axis; PSAX, parasternal short axis; RUQ; right upper quadrant; RV, right ventricle; SC, subcostal; US, ultrasound.

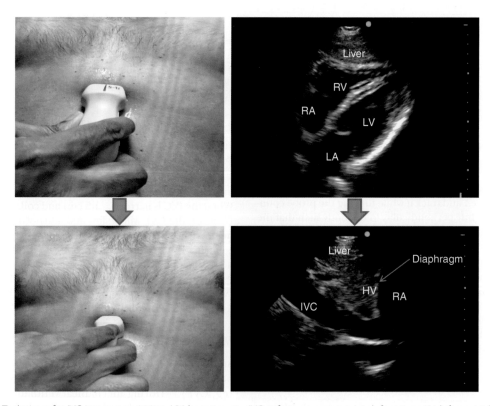

FIGURE 51.17 Technique for IVC image acquisition. HV, hepatic vein; IVC, inferior vena cava; LA, left atrium; LV, left ventricle; RA, right atrium; RV, right ventricle.

TABLE 51.8	Distinguishing IVC from Aorta	
	IVC	**AORTA**
Direction	Goes through the liver	Goes through the liver
Relation to heart	Merges with right atrium	Continues down the heart
Flow	Continuous, changes with respiration	Pulsatile
Walls	Thin-walled, may not be visible	Thick-walled, hyperechoic
Respiratory variations	May be present	No
Collateral vessels	Sub-hepatic veins merge with the IVC	Not visible from this approach

IVC, inferior vena cava.

TABLE 51.9	IVC Size, Collapsibility, and Estimation of CVP in Spontaneously Breathing Patients	
IVC DIAMETER (cm)	**INSPIRATORY COLLAPSE (%)**	**CVP (mm Hg)**
Normal: <2.1	>50	0–5 (mean 3)
IVC findings other	±	5–10 (mean 8)
High: >2.1	<50	10–20 (mean 15)

CVP, central venous pressure; IVC, inferior vena cava.

TABLE 51.10	IVC Variability and Fluid Responsiveness in Critically Ill Patients

EVALUATING FLUID STATUS VIA INFERIOR VENA CAVA SIZE AND VARIABILITY

Fluid responsiveness: clinically relevant increase in cardiac output (>15%) after a volume challenge

Spontaneously breathing patients
- Measure IVC size 2–3 cm from the right atrium using M-mode:
- Static:
  - <1 cm → likely volume depleted
  - >3 cm → sufficient volume status

Patients on mechanical ventilation (criteria)
- On mechanical ventilation
- Tidal volume >8 mL/kg ideal body weight
- Passive on ventilator support (no spontaneous breaths)
- Normal sinus rhythm

Patient is fluid responsive if:
- (Maximum diameter–minimum diameter)/minimum diameter >18% OR
- (Maximum diameter–minimum diameter)/average diameter >12%

IVC, inferior vena cava.

filling of the right heart. This causes a reduction in RV stroke volume (SV) and less filling of the left ventricle, thus reducing LV SV several cardiac cycles later. These respiratory changes are exaggerated in the hypovolemic patient and these variations in SV can be used to predict fluid responsiveness.[22] Respiratory variation of the IVC diameter has been shown to accurately predict fluid responsiveness.[17,44] **Tables 51.9** and **51.10** summarize interpretation of IVC size and variation. **Figure 51.18** shows examples of measurement of IVC diameter and respiratory variability using M-mode. **Figure 51.19** show examples of small and dilated IVCs.

FUNDAMENTALS OF ABDOMINAL ULTRASOUND IN CRITICAL ILLNESS

Abdominal USG has several applications in the evaluation of the critically ill patient in the CCU. Intraperitoneal or retroperitoneal

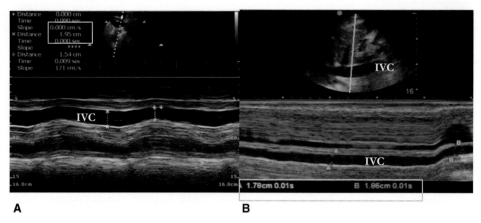

FIGURE 51.18 A, M-mode image showing respiratory variation of the IVC. B, M-mode image showing lack of respiratory variability of the IVC. IVC, inferior vena cava.

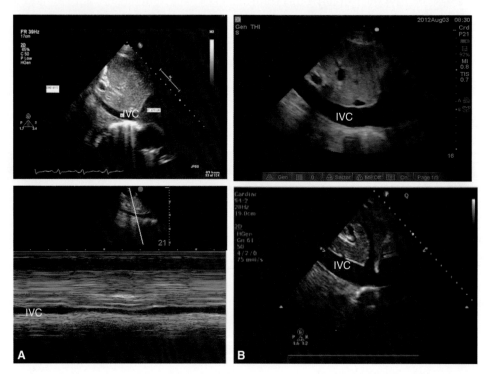

FIGURE 51.19 A, Small IVC. B, Dilated IVC. IVC, inferior vena cava.

bleeding may be the etiology of hemorrhagic shock in a patient who recently underwent a cardiac catheterization, an intra-aortic balloon pump placement, or an intravascular cooling catheter placement. Not uncommonly, patients get subjected to invasive procedures involving femoral venous or arterial sheath placement and are at risk for hemorrhage both during insertion and after removal. In addition, patients in the CCU are frequently on dual antiplatelet agents and anticoagulation, and are at high risk for intra-abdominal bleeding.

FOCUSED ASSESSMENT WITH SONOGRAPHY IN TRAUMA EXAMINATION

The FAST examination has been demonstrated to have 90% sensitivity in the detection of intra-peritoneal free fluid.[12] An approximate volume of at least 200 mL of free fluid is required for the test to have high sensitivity. In other words, a smaller volume of free blood may not be demonstrated on initial FAST examination; therefore, repeat testing may be warranted.[7]

A curvilinear transducer or, alternatively, a low-frequency phased array transducer is used for the FAST examination. The duration of the examination averages <3 minutes and is best performed in the supine position. These windows used serve to conduct the sound wave to the three most dependent areas of the peritoneal cavity in the supine patient as well as to the costophrenic angles bilaterally. The fourth view provides a view of the heart and pericardium, typically obtained from the subxiphoid region. The order of obtaining these views is not as important as systematically evaluating each quadrant for pathology.

For the right-sided evaluation, the probe is placed in the right mid-axillary line at the level of the xiphoid process in the longitudinal view (probe marker pointing cephalad and slightly posterior). This obtains a coronal view of the right hemidiaphragm, liver, and kidney. Morrison's pouch or the hepatorenal space is a site where free fluid can be detected very early (**Figure 51.20A**). Scan above the diaphragm to evaluate for a pleural fluid collection as well. For the left-sided evaluation, the probe is placed in the posterior axillary line at the level of the xiphoid process, in the longitudinal view. The left hemidiaphragm, spleen, kidney, and splenorenal space can all be identified from this view. The suprapubic region should be scanned for free fluid in the pelvis by placing the transducer in the midline of the pubic symphysis and tilting down (**Figure 51.20B**). A transverse (probe marker pointing to patient's right) and longitudinal view (probe marker facing cephalad) should be obtained to assess for free fluid in the pelvis. An SC echocardiographic view should be obtained to evaluate for pericardial fluid. The extended FAST examination also includes an examination of the anterior lung zone to rule out pneumothorax (**Table 51.7**). **Figure 51.21A** and **B** shows examples of hemoperitoneum where blood is seen as layering with increasing echogenicity, and echogenic material in the retroperitoneum (hematoma). USG does not have high sensitivity to detect retroperitoneal bleeding; hence, a computed tomography of the abdomen should be performed.

ABDOMINAL AORTIC ULTRASONOGRAPHY

Aortic sonography allows for detection of aortic syndromes such as thrombosis, dissection, or rupture. Abdominal USG serves as a rapid noninvasive test that provides important clinical information without the need for radiation or intravenous contrast. Conventionally, an abdominal aortic aneurysm (AAA) is diagnosed when the diameter of the aorta exceeds 4 cm. The risk of rupture at this level is <4% within a year, but it exponentially increases for AAA of larger diameter (>5 cm). The presence or absence of AAA can be evaluated with POCUS with high sensitivity and specificity; however, it has poor sensitivity for extraluminal blood. Nevertheless, in one ED study it was shown to improved diagnosis of ruptured AAA in the appropriate clinical setting and resulted in the correct decision to perform surgery.[45]

Sonographic visualization of the abdominal aorta is achieved through a trans-abdominal approach. The proximal aorta can be visualized with a curvilinear transducer. Ideal conditions for scanning are a thin body habitus and a non–gas-filled transverse colon. Scanning of the aorta is done between the xiphoid process and the umbilicus, because these two areas correspond to the 12th thoracic and 4th lumbar vertebral bodies where the aorta enters the abdominal cavity and bifurcates to the iliac arteries. This area below the diaphragm within a distance of 1 cm is where the aorta gives rise to its three major branches: the celiac trunk (immediately below the diaphragm) giving rise to the common hepatic artery and splenic artery (called *seagull sign*), the superior mesenteric artery, and the renal arteries. The majority (>90%) of all aortic aneurysms occur distal to the point of the renal arteries. **Figure 51.22** shows examples of the appearance of the aorta at different branch points in the abdominal aorta.

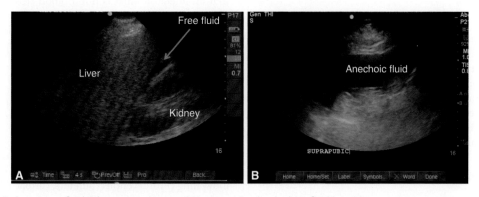

FIGURE 51.20 A, Early ascites—fluid in hepatorenal recess. B, Ascites—simple anechoic fluid in pelvis.

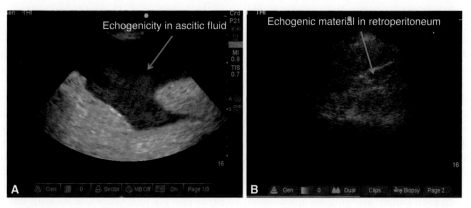

FIGURE 51.21 A, Hemoperitoneum. B, Retroperitoneal hematoma.

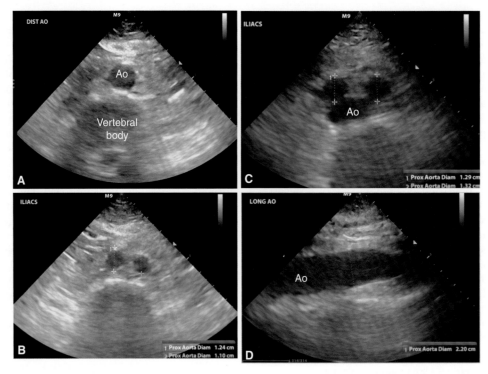

FIGURE 51.22 A, Distal aorta. B, Aorta bifurcating in iliacs. C, Aorta at the level of bifurcation to the common iliac arteries. D, Proximal aorta; longitudinal view. Ao, aorta.

ASCITES

Bedside USG is an easy way to assess for ascites in the patient with cirrhosis or right heart failure. US also facilitate paracentesis by assisting in selection of the best pocket for sampling and by avoiding nearby structures such as bowel and vasculature. US guidance has shown to lead to successful paracentesis with up to a 95% success rate in one study as compared to traditional methods (61% success rate).[46] Similarly, simulation-based training on US guidance using a paracentesis trainer has been shown to improve procedural competence of medical residents.[47]

KIDNEY AND BLADDER

In the patient with acute renal failure or abdominal pain in the CCU, bedside POCUS can serve to quickly eliminate a post-obstructive etiology. The normal kidney has a hyperechoic medulla and a relatively hypoechoic cortex. With increasing obstruction, the collecting system will become dilated and extend to the major and minor calyces and eventually thin the cortex of the kidney. Fluid is anechoic; so if the center of the kidney becomes dilated with anechoic fluid, suspect hydronephrosis. Similarly, in a post-obstructive state, one can visualize a dilated, fluid-filled (anechoic) bladder **(Figure 51.23A and B).** It is not uncommon to see a Foley balloon in a dilated anechoic bladder, indicating the catheter itself is obstructed.

Using a low-frequency phased array or curvilinear probe, obtain transverse and longitudinal views of the kidneys and bladder. The landmarks for scanning are the same as those for the FAST examination, described earlier. Fan the probe anteriorly and posteriorly through each kidney, assessing for any dilation of the collecting system. Color Doppler can be used to ensure

that an anechoic duct is not a blood vessel. Rotate the probe 90° counter clockwise and fan the probe superior to inferior to scan through the entire kidney. Place the transducer over the pubic symphysis and evaluate the bladder in the transverse and longitudinal views.[48]

DIAGNOSTIC VASCULAR ULTRASOUND

DEEP VENOUS THROMBOSIS

Critically ill patients are at higher risk for development of venous thromboembolism due to risk factors such as immobility, indwelling central venous catheters, cardiac failure, dehydration, and inflammatory states. The examination for lower extremity DVT is performed with a high-frequency linear transducer. US evaluation of venous thrombosis consists of verifying vein patency or the lack thereof. The gold standard for venous patency is the ability of a vein to collapse completely under pressure, with the lumen disappearing entirely under direct visualization with US. The diagnosis is confirmed when echogenic thrombus is observed in the vascular lumen or when the vein is not completely collapsible during compression.

To allow for better visualization of the vessels, the patient is supine, with the leg externally rotated and with the knee slightly bent. Once the common femoral vein (CFV) is identified, compressions should begin above the inguinal ligament at the proximal portion of the external iliac vein. Downward pressure should be applied to the transducer and the vein should collapse completely. The operator should then compress every 1 to 2 cm while moving distally along the CFV, the greater saphenous vein, over the lateral perforator-CFV

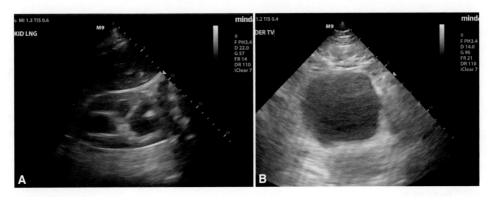

FIGURE 51.23 A, Hydronephrosis. B, Full bladder.

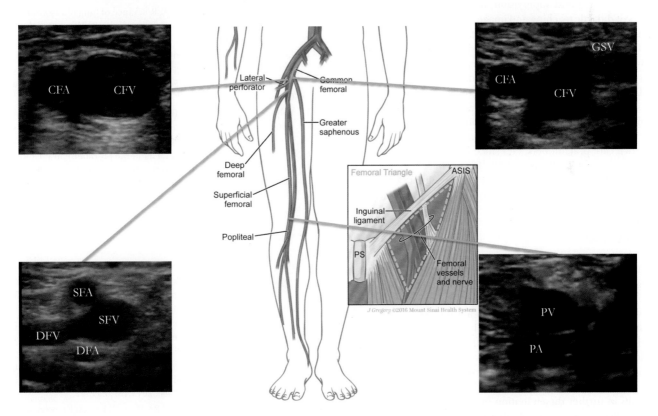

FIGURE 51.24 Compression ultrasonography to assess for DVT. ASIS, anterior superior iliac spine; CFA, common femoral artery; CFV, common femoral vein; DFA, deep femoral artery; DFV, deep femoral vein; DVT, deep vein thrombosis; GSV, great saphenous vein; SFA, superficial femoral artery; SFV, superficial femoral vein; PA, pulmonary artery; PS, pubic symphysis; PV, pulmonary vein.

junction until the CFV is seen branching into the superficial and deep branches (**Figure 51.24**). The examination then moves to the popliteal region. The knee is flexed 45 degrees and externally rotated, with the transducer placed transversely over the mid-fossa. The popliteal vein is identified overlying the artery. Even minimal pressure can compress the popliteal vein. Sequential compression at approximately 1-cm intervals should occur while moving distally to the trifurcation of the popliteal vein. Color Doppler and pulse-wave Doppler give the traditional venous US examination its name, "duplex." Studies have shown that using compression US alone, nonradiologists such as EM physicians and intensivists can accurately diagnose DVT with 95% accuracy and reducing the time to diagnosis.[18,19]

PROCEDURAL GUIDANCE FOR VASCULAR ACCESS

This is one of the highest utilization indications for POCUS in the CCU. The topic is discussed in detail with regard to both CVC placement and arterial line placement in Chapter 48 of this volume from the same authors.

LIMITATIONS OF POINT-OF-CARE ULTRASONOGRAPHY

USG has developed as an irreplaceable tool in for the critical care physician in the management of a critically ill patient. Patient factors such as obesity, body habitus, rib shadows, artifacts, the presence of edema, subcutaneous emphysema, or suboptimal patient position can be a limitation. It is also operator dependent, so adequate training and a proper certification process is required.

EDUCATION IN POINT-OF-CARE ULTRASONOGRAPHY

Studies have shown that bedside sonography can be taught to both early and advanced learners. With the popularity of POCUS, many medical schools are now adopting US education into undergraduate medication education, as early as in first year anatomy courses to fourth year electives.[49,50] Basic cardiac echocardiography, which may seem intimidating to the novice, can be easily learned with proper training and supervision. Resident physicians, after 12 hours of didactic teaching and image interpretation, were able to accurately identify LV failure, RV dilatation, pericardial effusion, and IVC dilatation.[38] Similarly, intensivists were able to successfully obtain and interpret images after 10 1-hour tutorial sessions by cardiologists.[36] Large 3-day hands-on educational courses led by Dr Paul Mayo and the American College of Chest Physicians, in which the authors have been course faculty (GN, JM), have trained thousands of physicians (eg, pulmonologists, intensivists, cardiologists, anesthesiologists, hospitalists, critical care fellows, advance care practitioners, etc) since its inception in 2007. This multiday format has been shown to be an effective way to train a large group of clinicians in POCUS with excellent performance in image acquisition, interpretation, and subject knowledge.[51]

CONCLUSIONS

POCUS has evolved into an invaluable tool in facilitating the diagnosis and treatment of acutely ill patients. With the advent of portable US machines, POCUS has revolutionized the way that patients are managed and has drastically improved the safety of procedures. Goal-directed USG readily answers clinical questions in the management of critically ill patients in the CCU with conditions such as shock, acute respiratory failure, and multiorgan failure. With proper training and supervision, POCUS is easily learned both by early and advanced learners. Challenges that remain in further dissemination of the use of POCUS include appropriate training, credentialing, and reimbursement. As medical societies make inroads into these hurdles, POCUS will continue to diffuse into medical education and daily practice.

REFERENCES

1. Mayo PH, Beaulieu Y, Doelken P, et al. American College of Chest Physicians/La Société de Réanimation de Langue Française statement on competence in critical care ultrasonography. *Chest.* 2009;135:1050-1060.

2. Expert Round Table on Ultrasound in ICU. International expert statement on training standards for critical care ultrasonography. *Intensive Care Med.* 2011;37:1077-1083.

3. Levitov A, Frankel HL, Blaivas M, et al. Guidelines for the appropriate use of bedside general and cardiac ultrasonography in the evaluation of critically ill patients—part II. *Crit Care Med.* 2016;44:1206-1227.

4. Narasimhan M, Koenig SJ, Mayo PH. A whole-body approach to point of care ultrasound. *Chest.* 2016;150:772-776.

5. Moore CL, Copel JA. Point-of-Care Ultrasonography. *N Engl J Med.* 2011;364:749-757.

6. Karakitsos D, Labropoulos N, De Groot E, et al. Real-time ultrasound-guided catheterisation of the internal jugular vein:a prospective comparison with the landmark technique in critical care patients. *Crit Care.* 2006;10:R162.

7. Scalea TM, Rodriguez A, Chiu WC, et al. Focused Assessment with Sonography for Trauma (FAST). *J Trauma.* 1999;46:466-472.

8. Mayo PH, Goltz HR, Tafreshi M, Doelken P. Safety of ultrasound-guided thoracentesis in patients receiving mechanical ventilation. *Chest.* 2004;125:1059-1062.

9. Troianos CA, Hartman GS, Glas KE, et al. Guidelines for performing ultrasound guided vascular cannulation: recommendations of the American Society of Echocardiography and the Society of Cardiovascular Anesthesiologists. *J Am Soc Echocardiogr.* 2011;24:1291-1318.

10. Lichtenstein DA, Mezière GA. Relevance of lung ultrasound in the diagnosis of acute respiratory failure*: the BLUE protocol. *Chest.* 2008;134:117-125.

11. Lichtenstein D, Axler O. Intensive use of general ultrasound in the intensive care unit. *Intensive Care Med.* 1993;19:353-355.

12. Lingawi SS, Buckley AR. Focused abdominal US in patients with trauma. *Radiology.* 2000;217:426-429.

13. Volpicelli G, Lamorte A, Tullio M, et al. Point-of-care multiorgan ultrasonography for the evaluation of undifferentiated hypotension in the emergency department. *Intensive Care Med.* 2013;39:1290-1298.

14. Lichtenstein DA, Mezière GA, Lagoueyte J-F, Biderman P, Goldstein I, Gepner A. A-lines and B-lines: lung ultrasound as a bedside tool for predicting pulmonary artery occlusion pressure in the critically ill. *Chest.* 2009;136:1014-1020.

15. Lichtenstein D, Karakitsos D. Integrating lung ultrasound in the hemodynamic evaluation of acute circulatory failure (the fluid administration limited by lung sonography protocol). *J Crit Care.* 2012;27:533.e11-e19.

16. Frankel HL, Kirkpatrick AW, Elbarbary M, et al. Guidelines for the appropriate use of bedside general and cardiac ultrasonography in the evaluation of critically ill patients—part I. *Crit Care Med.* 2015;43:2479-2502.

17. Feissel M, Michard F, Faller JP, Teboul JL. The respiratory variation in inferior vena cava diameter as a guide to fluid therapy. *Intensive Care Med.* 2004;30(9):1834-1837.

18. Kory PD, Pellecchia CM, Shiloh AL, Mayo PH, DiBello C, Koenig S. Accuracy of ultrasonography performed by critical care physicians for the diagnosis of DVT. *Chest.* 2011;139:538-542.

19. Blaivas M, Lambert MJ, Harwood RA, Wood JP, Konicki J. Lower-extremity Doppler for deep venous thrombosis—can emergency physicians be accurate and fast? *Acad Emerg Med.* 2000;7:120-126.

20. Bakhru RN, Schweickert WD. Intensive care ultrasound: I. Physics, equipment, and image quality. *Ann Am Thorac Soc.* 2013;10:540-548.

21. Laursen CB, Sloth E, Lambrechtsen J, et al. Focused sonography of the heart, lungs, and deep veins identifies missed life-threatening conditions in admitted patients with acute respiratory symptoms. *Chest.* 2013;144:1868-1875.

22. Schmidt GA, Koenig S, Mayo PH. Shock: ultrasound to guide diagnosis and therapy. *Chest.* 2012;142:1042-1048.

23. Lichtenstein D, Mezière G. A lung ultrasound sign allowing bedside distinction between pulmonary edema and COPD: the comet-tail artifact. *Intensive Care Med.* 1998;24:1331-1334.

24. Lichtenstein D, Mezière G, Biderman P, Gepner A. The comet-tail artifact: an ultrasound sign ruling out pneumothorax. *Intensive Care Med.* 1999;25:383-388.

25. Lichtenstein D, Mezière G, Biderman P, Gepner A. The "lung point": an ultrasound sign specific to pneumothorax. *Intensive Care Med.* 2000;26:1434-1440.

26. Lichtenstein DA, Menu Y. A Bedside Ultrasound sign ruling out pneumothorax in the critically ill. Lung sliding. *Chest.* 1995;108:1345-1348.

27. Volpicelli G, Elbarbary M, Blaivas M, et al. International evidence-based recommendations for point-of-care lung ultrasound. *Intensive Care Med.* 2012;38:577-591.

28. Doerschug KC, Schmidt GA. Intensive care ultrasound: III. Lung and pleural ultrasound for the intensivist. *Ann Am Thorac Soc.* 2013;10:708-712.

29. Lichtenstein D, Mezière G, Seitz J. The dynamic air bronchogram. *Chest.* 2009;135:1421-1425.

30. Kelbel C, Börner N, Schadmand S, et al. Diagnosis of pleural effusions and atelectases: sonography and radiology compared [in German]. *Rofo.* 1991;154:159-163.

31. Mayo PH, Doelken P. Pleural ultrasonography. *Clin Chest Med.* 2006;27:215-227.

32. Lichtenstein DA, Mezière G, Lascols N, et al. Ultrasound diagnosis of occult pneumothorax. *Crit Care Med.* 2005;33:1231-1238.

33. Lichtenstein DA, Lascols N, Prin S, Mezière G. The "lung pulse": an early ultrasound sign of complete atelectasis. *Intensive Care Med.* 2003;29:2187-2192.

34. Mathew JP, Kourouni I, Noronha S, Narayanswami G, Shapiro JM. A woman in her 70s with profound hypoxemia. *Chest.* 2016;150:e13-e17.

35. Filopei J, Siedenburg H, Rattner P, Fukaya E, Kory P. Impact of pocket ultrasound use by internal medicine housestaff in the diagnosis of Dyspnea. *J Hosp Med.* 2014;9:594-597.

36. Manasia AR, Nagaraj HM, Kodali RB, et al. Feasibility and potential clinical utility of goal-directed transthoracic echocardiography performed by noncardiologist intensivists using a small hand-carried device (SonoHeart) in critically ill patients. *J Cardiothorac Vasc Anesth.* 2005;19:155-159.

37. Melamed R, Sprenkle MD, Ulstad VK, Herzog CA, Leatherman JW. Assessment of left ventricular function by intensivists using hand-held echocardiography. *Chest.* 2009;135:1416-1420.

38. Vignon P, Mücke F, Bellec F, et al. Basic critical care echocardiography: Validation of a curriculum dedicated to noncardiologist residents. *Crit Care Med.* 2011;39:636-642.

39. Kirkpatrick AW, Sirois M, Laupland KB, et al. Hand-held thoracic sonography for detecting post-traumatic pneumothoraces: the Extended Focused Assessment With Sonography For Trauma (EFAST). *J Trauma.* 2004;57:288-295.

40. Lichtenstein DA. BLUE-protocol and FALLS-protocol. *Chest.* 2015;147:1659-1670.

41. Perera P, Mailhot T, Riley D, Mandavia D. The RUSH exam: Rapid Ultrasound in SHock in the evaluation of the critically Ill. *Emerg Med Clin North Am.* 2010;28:29-56.

42. Rudski LG, Lai WW, Afilalo J, et al. Guidelines for the Echocardiographic Assessment of the Right Heart in Adults: A Report from the American Society of Echocardiography. *J Am Soc Echocardiogr.* 2010;23:685-713.

43. Marik PE, Baram M, Vahid B. Does central venous pressure predict fluid responsiveness?*: A systematic review of the literature and the tale of seven mares. *Chest.* 2008;134:172-178.

44. Barbier C, Loubires Y, Schmit C, et al. Respiratory changes in inferior vena cava diameter are helpful in predicting fluid responsiveness in ventilated septic patients. *Intensive Care Med.* 2004;30(9):1740-1746.

45. Shuman WP, Hastrup W Jr, Kohler TR, et al. Suspected leaking abdominal aortic aneurysm: use of sonography in the emergency room. *Radiology.* 1988;168:117-119.

46. Nazeer SR, Dewbre H, Miller AH. Ultrasound-assisted paracentesis performed by emergency physicians vs the traditional technique: a prospective, randomized study. *Am J Emerg Med.* 2005;23:363-367.

47. Barsuk JH, Cohen ER, Vozenilek JA, O'Connor LM, McGaghie WC, Wayne DB. Simulation-based education with mastery learning improves paracentesis skills. *J Grad Med Educ.* 2012;4:23-27.

48. Boniface KS, Calabrese KY. Intensive care ultrasound: IV. Abdominal ultrasound in critical care. *Ann Am Thorac Soc.* 2013;10:713-724.

49. Bahner DP, Royall NA. Advanced ultrasound training for fourth-year medical students. *Acad Med.* 2013;88:206-213.

50. Rao S, van Holsbeeck L, Musial JL, et al. A pilot study of comprehensive ultrasound education at the Wayne State University School of Medicine. *J Ultrasound Med.* 2008;27:745-749.

51. Greenstein YY, Littauer R, Narasimhan M, Mayo PH, Koenig SJ. Effectiveness of a critical care ultrasonography course. *Chest.* 2017;151:34-40.IVC.

Janet M. Shapiro

52

End-of-Life Care in the CCU

Patients in the cardiac care unit undergo intensive and heroic treatments intended to save and prolong life. The cardiac care unit has evolved over the past several decades such that the current CCU provides care to patients with advanced age and increasing cardiac and noncardiovascular critical illness, including sepsis, acute renal injury, and acute respiratory failure.[1] Patients in the CCU are frequently managed with life support measures including mechanical ventilation, cardio-vascular support, and renal replacement therapy. Thus, the CCU clinician is faced with critically ill patients on life support measures, some of whom may be at the end of life. The major cardiology societies encourage provision of supportive and palliative care in cardiac patients at the end of life. The goal of this chapter is to provide practical information about end-of-life decision making and the process of withdrawal of life-sustaining treatments in the CCU.

Decision making about end-of-life care in the CCU is challenging for several reasons. Many patients do not have an advance directive. Even in cardiac patients with advanced interventions, including implantable electronic devices, discussions about advance directives are uncommon.[2] Clinicians face difficulty in prognostication for critically ill patients in general. In patients with heart failure, variability in the course makes identifying the end of life especially complicated. The guidelines of the Heart Failure Society of America and the American College of Cardiology/American Heart Association promote consideration of end-of-life care in patients with advanced heart failure, including decisions about inactivation of implantable defibrillators.[3,4] Aggressive and invasive treatments are often initiated for patients in the CCU in the hope of restoring life, and this initial aggressive support is construed by the family as the optimistic expectation that the patient will recover. This is especially true for patients following cardiac arrest, in whom therapeutic hypothermia is initiated. The hope from this treatment must be tempered with the reality that the majority of patients still suffer neurologic injury. The need for sedation and the post-arrest state require time for neurologic prognostication. During this time, communication with the family about uncertain prognosis and the possibility of anoxic encephalopathy is important. A multidisciplinary team approach must include the neurologist for prognostication and decision making.

GOALS OF CARE

As clinicians, our goals for patients are to save lives, return to health or an acceptable existence, alleviate suffering, and provide the dying with a peaceful death. The transition of the goal from curative treatment to comfort care is one of the most challenging aspects of critical care. It is possible to combine a palliative approach even when life-sustaining treatments are in place, so that clinicians may still focus on alleviation of symptoms and overall goals of care.

The goals of palliative care can be applied to many patients, even those receiving aggressive interventions: control of symptoms such as pain, dyspnea, and discomfort; effective communication about appropriate goals of treatment and concordance of treatment with patient preferences; and enhancing quality of life. The role of palliative care in the CCU includes providing guidance and support, so that care will be consistent with the patient's values.[5]

Effective communication is the means to achieving patient preferences in end-of-life care. The landmark SUPPORT (Study to Understand Prognoses and Preferences for Outcomes and Risks of Treatments) revealed that the wishes of dying patients were often unexplored by physicians and those patients received potentially undesired treatments at the end of life.[6] Clinicians must also recognize that their own wishes may not coincide with those of their patients, because physicians and nurses may be less likely to desire life support than patients and families. Decision making that is shared between the patient/family and the clinicians is the model process supported by American and European critical care societies.[7,8] The evolution of critical care decision making from a paternalistic model to the current standard of shared decision making is predicated on respect for patient autonomy and values. In the cardiac care unit, the majority of patients may be unable to participate in decisions owing to the severe illness, need for life support, and sedative medications. Therefore, the legally recognized appropriate surrogate often assumes the decision-making role to represent the patient's values and preferences. The family-centered approach respects the patient's values, and also acknowledges that many patients would want their family members to participate in decision making.

ETHICAL PRINCIPLES IN END-OF-LIFE DECISION MAKING

Patient *autonomy* is a foundation ethical principle for patient care. U.S. Supreme Court cases such as the Quinlan and Cruzan cases established that patients have a right to determine which medical treatments to accept or refuse, even when refusal leads to death.[9] Often, in the critical care unit, the patient is incapable of participating in the decision making. However, the patient may have left guidance in the form of an advance directive, such as a proxy, living will, or oral statements articulating his or her wishes concerning life support at the end of life. The patient may have assigned a health care proxy to make decisions if he or she becomes unable to do so. If no proxy has been assigned, the surrogate decision maker is chosen from the patient's close relatives or friends based on a priority order. In this way, the patient's values and preferences can still guide the decision-making process when decision-making capacity is lost.

The principle of *beneficence* maintains that physicians will work to provide the best course of treatment for the patient. Physicians see the goal of preserving life, but beneficence also means the support of the patient's informed decision even when refusal of therapy may lead to death. *Nonmaleficence* means not inflicting harm. This principle instructs the physician to weigh potential harms of treatments against potential benefits and not provide interventions that will not benefit the patient.

Conflict may arise when the patient, family, and clinician disagree about the appropriateness of an intervention. Nonabandonment is an important principle that obliges the physician to help the family understand the situation and support the family's decision. Physicians are not obligated to disregard their own beliefs and so, if the physician disagrees with the patient and family decision, the principle of nonabandonment requires the physician to try to transfer care to another physician who will pursue the desired plan of care. The hospital administration or ethics committee may be involved to assist in resolution of these complicated situations.

ADVANCE DIRECTIVES

As stated, patient autonomy is the strongest ethical principle driving medical decision making, so that patients have the right to make decisions for themselves; and when conscious capacity is lost, this right remains protected. Advance directives, such as the health care proxy and living will, provide for decision making based on patient values and preferences when the patient loses decision-making capacity. Respect for patient autonomy underlies the federal Patient Self-Determination Act of 1990, which requires hospital personnel to ask patients whether they have an advance directive and inform patients of their right to accept or refuse medical treatments and to create an advance directive.[10] A Do Not Resuscitate (DNR) order is one kind of advance directive that addresses interventions in the setting of a cardiopulmonary arrest. A DNR order means that if the patient suffers a cardiopulmonary arrest, the interventions of intubation, cardiopulmonary resuscitation (CPR), and advanced cardiac life support will be withheld. A DNR order is often issued for patients at the end of life, and in patients with chronic or terminal illnesses. In some patients with DNR orders, the patient may be expected to benefit from and will receive intensive care interventions, but CPR will be withheld in the event of cardiac arrest. A DNR order is often a first step in the family's decision-making process.

COMMUNICATION

Achieving appropriate decision making is based on effective communication, family comprehension of the information, and sharing of the patient's values. It should not be assumed that families grasp the severity of their relative's illness or the ramifications of life support measures. Family understanding of critical illness and intensive care treatments has been shown to be inadequate. Knowledge about CPR is especially poor, with a prevalent unrealistic expectation of survival among patients with serious medical illness and their families.[11] Accordingly, assessing family members' understanding of the patient condition is vital and will be part of the communication strategy in a family meeting.

FAMILY MEETING

Communication with the family occurs in several venues: bedside discussions, conversations with the nurse, telephone updates, as well as a formal family meeting. The contributions of the entire team are invaluable. The bedside nurse usually has important insight into the patient's condition and the family understanding of the patient's condition. A family meeting is an opportunity to present and review the situation and treatments, provide information on short-term and long-term prognoses, answer questions, explore patient and family values and wishes, and assess the family's understanding of the patient's condition. Investigators have examined family meetings and found missed opportunities in time allotted for family speech, articulating a prognosis, emphasizing the process of surrogate decision making, supporting the decision, and assuring nonabandonment. Family satisfaction with the meeting was associated with increased time for family speech; presumably this is their opportunity to make the patient and his values known.[12] Prognostication is important for family members, but the meetings often lacked discussion of prognosis for survival. Although families may doubt the accuracy of the prognosis given by physicians, that prognostic information is desired and important in the family's understanding and deliberation.[13]

Here, we can make some points about the family meeting.

- The medical team should prepare for the family meeting. The clinicians should discuss the goals of the family meeting, review the patient's condition, and achieve consensus concerning prognosis and treatments to be administered. The team should be aware of specific issues or problems related to the family situation. The bedside nurse may have great insight into the patient's condition and family situation and should be included in the meeting. It may be helpful to include team members such as the neurologist, and primary cardiologist, if applicable.
- The physician will lead the discussion in a private, quiet place. All participants should be introduced. The family should be asked their understanding of the condition and treatments. The physician should provide information about the illness, treatments including life support measures, and prognosis in a meaningful and compassionate manner, avoiding excessive

medical jargon. The clinicians should explain surrogate and shared decision making.

- The clinicians should allow time for the family to speak about the patient's values and preferences, to demonstrate their understanding of the situation, and to ask questions.
- The physician leader should judge how the family has understood the information and whether they are ready to discuss goals and end-of-life decisions. For some meetings, it is sufficient to provide the medical information and it may be better to discuss end-of-life decisions in a subsequent meeting.
- Often, the family members report that they never discussed end of life with the patient. Some ways to elucidate patient wishes include asking whether they ever had a conversation about the patient's own wishes, in the setting of another family member's illness or even related to a topic in the news; how the patient lived life, what it may mean to be dependent in all aspects of care; and what they think the patient might say about life support measures if he or she were in this meeting. The leader may ask the family what they believe is a meaningful and acceptable quality of life for the patient.
- If withdrawal of life support is discussed, the clinicians should emphasize that this does not mean withdrawal of *care* and that supportive and comfort care will be provided.
- The staff should offer support for the decision of the family, whether the decision is to withdraw or not withdraw life support. The team should assure the family that the patient will not be abandoned and all measures will be taken to prevent suffering.
- The family cannot be rushed to make a decision. The clinicians should understand that the family may not yet accept the expressed prognosis.
- The meeting may conclude with a plan to reconvene in the following days to review the situation.

It is important that clinicians do not relinquish medical decisions to the family. The physicians must give information, prognosis, and advice on how to proceed. The family provides information about the values and preferences of the patient. The transition from aggressive CCU care to comfort care is often made quickly by clinicians who have the benefit of medical knowledge of disease and prognosis, but families may need time for this adjustment and should not be rushed to make a decision. Planning a follow-up conversation within a specified time period allows the clinicians to further assess the patient's trajectory and permits the family time to grasp the information and condition. Families need ongoing contact and communication. Families need assurances that all efforts will be made to maintain comfort. Involving the palliative care service may be beneficial in optimizing the medical and nursing treatments for palliation.

Cultural values and beliefs may exert a profound influence on decision making. Domains affecting decisions include attitudes about truth telling concerning illness and prognosis, religious and spiritual beliefs, historical and political context, perception of illness, and the decision-making process in the group. The not uncommon clinician impression that the family is not accepting a dire diagnosis and prognosis may therefore at times be explained by cultural factors.[14] Recognizing the influence of cultural factors may lead to enhanced understanding and compassionate and effective communication.

Conflicts may develop between family and physicians, within families, as well as among the health care team. Given physicians' inability to be certain of the outcome, the family may be reluctant to accept a poor prognosis. The CCU team may involve other disciplines such as the patient's primary care physician, other involved subspecialties, palliative care, pastoral care, and social work. For conflicts that reveal marked differences in desires among the patient, family, and physicians, the hospital ethics committee may be involved. Ethics committee consultations may be beneficial in resolving conflicts, establishing desired care, and limiting non-beneficial life support measures. In addition, legal affairs involvement may be required in rare, complicated situations.

WITHDRAWAL OF LIFE SUPPORT

Ethical principles described previously support the decision to withdraw or withhold life-sustaining treatments. The U.S. Supreme Court cases confirmed that patients or surrogates can refuse life-sustaining therapies.[9] The decision to withdraw life support is based on patient values and preferences as articulated by the patient or his proxy or surrogate. Withdrawal of life support would be allowing the patient to die from the underlying disease. Withholding and withdrawing life support are considered equivalent, although clinicians may be more uncomfortable with the withdrawal of treatment.

Decisions to withhold or withdraw life support are common among critically ill patients, and frequently precede intensive care unit (ICU) deaths. All forms of life support may be withheld or withdrawn, including mechanical ventilation, vasopressors, antibiotics, blood product transfusions, hydration, and nutrition. Sometimes all treatments are discontinued at once, sometimes in a stepwise manner. With the exception of the withdrawal of mechanical ventilation, withdrawing these other treatments does not often lead to an evident clinical change. The decision to withdraw mechanical ventilation may be a more difficult decision for families as well as for clinicians. With the assurance that withdrawal would be the patient's wish and that medications will be provided for comfort, withdrawal of mechanical ventilation is often desired at the end of life.

At the time of withdrawal of life support, there should be written documentation of the prognosis, discussion, and decision making with the patient/surrogate, goals of care and plan, including orders to discontinue specific therapies. In particular, an order for removal of mechanical ventilation or deactivation of an implantable device should be entered.

The process of withdrawal of life support is delineated in **Table 52.1**. This process involves the actual withdrawal of life support measures as well as the palliative medications that may be required.

ORGAN DONATION

A minority of deaths in the CCU is determined by brain death criteria. Most deaths in CCU are expected and are due to progression of the cardiac and other organ failures.

Patients in the CCU may be candidates for organ donation based on brain death criteria or donation after cardiac death.[15] Institutions have policies for determination of brain death, organ donation following brain death, and organ donation after cardiac death. Patients who are admitted following cardiac arrest who suffered anoxic encephalopathy may progress to brain death. Patients should be referred to the organ procurement organization if they meet specific triggers. The actual brain death

TABLE 52.1	Withdrawal of Life Support: Process of Withdrawal of Mechanical Ventilation in the Cardiac Care Unit

Ask if family wishes to be present for extubation. Explain the process. May request chaplain presence, palliative care, and hospice services

Do Not Resuscitate Order is placed. Documentation in the medical record should reflect the discussions and decision to withdraw life support

If patient has an ICD, discuss inactivation of device

Discontinue previous orders for routine vital signs, routine laboratory tests, and radiographs

Discontinue enteral tube feedings several hours before extubation

Discontinue nonessential medications
Continue only palliative medications and necessary medications (such as anticonvulsants)

Change ventilator setting to spontaneous breathing mode (such as pressure support 5 cm H_2O) to assess palliative medication needs. Adjust palliative medications to goal of comfort and unlabored breathing. Consider opiates for dyspnea, benzodiazepines for seizures, anticholinergics for secretions, acetaminophen for fever, and antipsychotic medications for delirium.

Optimize the environment:
• Remove unnecessary equipment, provide space for family
• Discontinue monitor alarms
• Discontinue inappropriate television

Extubate patient with respiratory therapist assistance

Room air or 2–4 L of oxygen by nasal cannula if this improves comfort

ICD, implantable cardioverter defibrillator.

determination is performed by a qualified attending physician. In patients who have undergone therapeutic hypothermia following cardiac arrest, additional vigilance is recommended in initiating the brain death determination.

For patients who have a nonrecoverable neurologic injury but not brain death, the family may make the decision to withdraw life support. These patients may be candidates for organ donation following cardiac death. Institutional policies address the referral, process, and management of patients. The cardiac team will generally involve specialists including intensivists and neurologists to confirm the neurologic prognosis. Only after the decision to withdraw life support will the organ donor network approach the family concerning organ donation.

WITHDRAWAL OF MECHANICAL VENTILATION

Communication with the family about the process of withdrawing ventilation and what to expect is essential. Although it is difficult to be certain, the physician should provide an estimation of duration of survival following extubation. The family may want to be present and may desire pastoral care to be present for support. All nonbeneficial treatments, including vasoactive medications, should be discontinued, and alarms should be silenced. Palliative medications should be adjusted before extubation while the patient is on a spontaneous breathing mode. The endotracheal tube is removed and the family should remain with the patient for as long as desired.

WITHDRAWAL OF CARDIOVASCULAR IMPLANTABLE ELECTRONIC DEVICE THERAPY

Implantable defibrillation and pacing devices provide life support that can be declined or withdrawn based on patient values

and preferences.[16] The dying patient or surrogate may request inactivation, if the device effectiveness is outweighed by burdens experienced by the patient: prolonging the dying process, preventing a natural death, and suffering the loss of dignity and quality of life. The Heart Rhythm Society published a consensus statement on the management of cardiovascular implantable electronic devices in patients nearing the end of life.[16] This document sets out the ethical principles, concerns, and practical management of withdrawal of cardiovascular implantable electronic device therapy. Deactivation may prevent uncomfortable shocks in dying patients. In pacemaker-dependent patients, the device sustains life and may, like other life-sustaining treatments such as mechanical ventilation, be discontinued on the basis of the patient's right to decline therapy. If cardiac resynchronization is aiding cardiac function, then inactivation may lead to increased symptom burden. So each therapy must be addressed in light of the overall goals. The Heart Rhythm Society consensus statement offers practical advice for communication, assessing patient understanding of the device, and utilizing the overall care goals to guide management of the cardiac device. The patient's cardiologist and electrophysiologist should be involved in these discussions about deactivation.

NONINVASIVE VENTILATION

Many physicians use noninvasive ventilation for respiratory failure near the end of life.[17] Its use should be guided by the goals of care. A patient who declines mechanical ventilation may receive noninvasive ventilation with the goal of survival: in patients with heart failure, noninvasive ventilation may successfully prevent intubation and the patient may survive the episode. In patients at the end of life, noninvasive ventilation has been used for palliation of dyspnea as well as a means to give more time for family to arrive and communicate with the patient. However, if noninvasive ventilation becomes uncomfortable or burdensome, it should be removed. Noninvasive ventilation should be addressed with the patient and family as a life support measure that can be continued or discontinued based on the goals of care. Use of high-flow nasal cannula may be a good choice for patients who require O_2 support for comfort and have high ventilatory requirements.

SYMPTOM MANAGEMENT

Most critically ill patients experience pain and discomfort related to procedures and nursing care in the ICU. The possibility of pain in patients unable to report their symptoms is a great concern for families and clinicians. Dyspnea is a common symptom in critically ill patients. When withdrawal of mechanical ventilation is being discussed, a frequent concern of the family is that the patient will experience respiratory distress. The clinicians should assess the patient with input from the bedside nurse and family.

Management is individualized, based on the patient's level of consciousness, underlying disease, and reason for respiratory failure. The patient's prior use of and response to opiates is important in dosing this medication. Route of administration and dosages must be adjusted, often with the assistance of the critical care pharmacist and palliative care specialist. **Table 52.2** shows common medications used during withdrawal of life support in the critical care unit. The intravenous route of administration is often used for these patients; however, enteral, sublingual, subcutaneous, rectal, and transdermal routes can also be used for medications. **Table 52.2** shows initial doses. Patients with severe dyspnea or pain at the end of life may require much higher dosages and infusion rates. It is important to provide

these medications, even at high rates, for the goal of comfort. Goals are relief of dyspnea, resolution of tachypnea and tachycardia, and lack of indication of pain by verbal response or clinical appearance.

Opioid analgesia is a basic medication class for patients at the end of life. The desired effects are analgesia and sedation, but there is also a respiratory depressant effect on the medullary respiratory center. Opioid medications are useful in management of the symptoms and signs of respiratory distress. Morphine is often chosen for management of pain or dyspnea. In patients with renal failure, there may be accumulation of active metabolite. In these patients, hydromorphone is often used. It is important to remember that hydromorphone is 5 to 10 times as potent as morphine. These medications are given at the dosages necessary to relieve symptoms.

The concern about hastening a patient's death by administering opiate analgesia is overridden by the intention of providing comfort and relieving suffering. Studies have demonstrated that the use of palliative medications at the end of life does not hasten death.[18,19] In fact, adequate pain management may mitigate the systemic effects of severe pain. In addition to respiratory depression, attention must be directed to several effects of opioid analgesia: inhibition of peristalsis with constipation, nausea and vomiting; and myoclonus and seizures.

Benzodiazepine medications provide sedation and anxiolysis. These medications do not provide analgesia but may be useful in combination with an opioid to prevent the anxiety related to pain. Side effects also include depressed level of consciousness and respiratory depression. Delirium, in the form of either an agitated or a calm state, is a common symptom in dying patients in the ICU. Although haloperidol is the standard medication for the management of delirium, the team should implement nonpharmacologic measures such as removing restraints, reducing

TABLE 52.2	Withdrawal of Mechanical Ventilation: Initiation of Palliative Medications
PAIN OR DYSPNEA[a]	
Morphine 1–4 mg intravenous every hour as needed Continuous infusion start at 2 mg/h	If requiring continued hourly dosing, change to continuous infusion For continued symptoms, administer bolus doses of 2x hourly rate, increase infusion (range: 2–30 mg/h)
Hydromorphone 0.5–1 mg intravenous every 3 h as needed Continuous infusion 0.5–1 mg/h	If requiring continued dosing, change to standing or continuous infusion For continued symptoms, increase infusion to 3 mg/h
ANXIETY OR AGITATION	

Lorazepam
  0.5–1 mg intravenous every hour as needed
  Continuous infusion start at 2 mg/h
Haloperidol
0.5–1 mg intravenous every 4 h as needed	

TERMINAL SECRETIONS	
Scopolamine patch 1.5–3 mg every 3 d Glycopyrrolate 0.2 mg subcutaneously every 4–6 h	

[a]If patient is comfortable on stable doses of opioid, continue current dose when starting withdrawal of ventilation. If the patient is not already receiving these medications, consider starting before extubation.

activity and noise, and having family members at the bedside to calm and orient the patient.

AT THE TIME OF DEATH

Notification to the family, optimally in person, using unambiguous language that the patient died is the initial duty. A minority of deaths is determined by brain death criteria and selected patients undergoing withdrawal of life support may be candidates for organ donation following cardiac death. This process requires a specialized protocol for the withdrawal of life support and management in collaboration with the organ donor organization. The staff may assist the family by providing information about the next steps, including autopsy, funeral, and bereavement services.

The critical care unit staff can also benefit from a debriefing about the patient's course, the end-of-life care, and the death. Physicians and nurses have different perspectives on end-of-life decision making, intensity of interventions, symptom management, and the quality of death and dying.[20] The burdens experienced by ICU nursing staff may lead to burnout, moral distress, and post-traumatic stress disorder. Communication to improve collaboration and the ethical climate may improve the environment for clinicians as well as the care of dying patients.

CONCLUSION

Patients and their families should expect excellence in all treatments in the cardiac care unit, including care at the end of life. Patients deserve humanity, compassion, and respect for autonomy. End-of-life care in the cardiac care unit requires expertise on many levels: assessing prognosis, communicating information, understanding patient values and preferences for life support, and implementing a patient's end-of-life decision. The CCU team can utilize the expertise of consultants, including palliative care specialists, in optimizing end-of-life care. Clinicians' management will be rewarded by alleviating a patient's suffering, facilitating a peaceful and dignified death, and providing peace and satisfaction for the patient's family.

REFERENCES

1. Katz JN, Shah BR, Volz EM, et al. Evolution of the coronary care unit: clinical characteristics and temporal trends in healthcare delivery and outcomes. *Crit Care Med.* 2010;38:375-381.

2. Goldstein NE, Lampert R, Bradley E, et al. Management of implantable cadioverter defibrillators in end-of-life care. *Ann Intern Med.* 2004;141:835-838.

3. Heart Failure Society of America. Executive summary: HFSA 2006 Comprehensive Heart Failure Practice Guideline. *J Card Fail.* 2006;12:10-38.

4. Hunt SA, Abraham WT, Chin MH, et al. 2009 focused update incorporated into the ACC/AHA 2005 guidelines for the diagnosis and management of heart failure in adults: a report of the American College of Cardiology Foundation/American Heart Association Task Force on Practice Guidelines: developed in collaboration with the International Society for Heart and Lung Transplantation. *Circulation.* 2009;119:e391-e479.

5. Swetz KM, Mansel JK. Ethical issues and palliative care in the cardiovascular intensive care unit. *Cardiol Clin.* 2013;31:657-668.

6. The SUPPORT Principal Investigators. A controlled trial to improve care for seriously ill hospitalized patients. The study to understand prognoses and preferences for outcomes and risks of treatments (SUPPORT). *JAMA.* 1995;274:1591-1598.

7. Truong RD, Campbell ML, Curtis JR, et al. Recommendations for end-of-life care in the intensive care unit: a consensus statement by the American Academy of Critical Care Medicine. *Crit Care Med.* 2008;36:953-963.

8. Davidson JE, Powers K, Hedayat KM, et al. Clinical practice guidelines for support of the family in the patient-centered intensive care unit: American College of Critical Care Medicine Task Force 2004-2005. *Crit Care Med.* 2007;35:605-622.

9. Luce JM. End-of-life decision making in the intensive care unit. *Am J Respir Crit Care Med.* 2010;182:6-11.

10. Patient Self-Determination Act of 1990. Omnibus Budget Reconciliation Act of 1990, Pub Law No. 101-508 (1990).Accessible at: https://www.congress.gov/bill/101st-congress/house-bill/4449

11. Heyland DK, Frank C, Groll D, et al. Understanding cardiopulmonary resuscitation decision making. Perspectives of seriously ill hospitalized patients and family members. *Chest.* 2006;130:419-428.

12. Curtis JR, White DB. Practical guidance for evidence-based ICU family conferences. *Chest.* 2008;134:835-843.

13. Zier LS, Burack JH, Micco G, et al. Doubt and belief in physicians' ability to prognosticate during critical illness: the perspective of surrogate decision makers. *Crit Care Med.* 2008;36:2341-2347.

14. Ford D, Zapka J, Gebregziabher M, et al. Factors associated with illness perception among critically ill patients and surrogates. *Chest.* 2010;138:59-67.

15. Kotloff RM, Blosser S, Fulda GJ, et al. Management of the potential organ donor in the ICU: Society of Critical Care Medicine/American College of Chest Physicians/Association of Organ Procurement Organizations Consensus Statement. *Crit Care Med.* 2015;43(6):1291-1325.

16. Lampert R, Hayes DL, Annas GJ, et al. HRS expert consensus statement on the management of Cardiovascular Implantable Electronic Devices (CIEDS) in patients nearing the end of life or requesting withdrawal of therapy. *Heart Rhythm.* 2010;7:1008-1026.

17. Sinuff T, Cook DJ, Keenan SP, et al. Noninvasive ventilation for acute respiratory failure near the end of life. *Crit Care Med.* 2008;36:789-794.

18. Sykes N, Thorns A. Sedative use in the last week of life and the implications for end-of-life decision making. *Arch Intern Med.* 2003;163:341-344.

19. Chan JD, Treece PD, Engelberg RA, et al. Narcotic and benzodiazepine use afterwithdrawal of life support: association with time to death? *Chest.* 2004;126:286-293.

20. Hamric AB, Blackhall LJ. Nurse-physician perspectives on the care of dying patients in intensive care units: collaboration, moral distress and ethical climate. *Crit Care Med.* 2007;35:422-429.

Patient and Family Information for:
END-OF-LIFE CARE IN THE CCU

The doctors, nurses, and the entire CCU team treat patients with the goal of curing disease, prolonging life, and making the patient better. The team also works to relieve pain and suffering. Even with all the medical care, technology, and life support machines, patients may not get better or survive. Sometimes, the patient has an incurable illness, such as advanced heart disease, which has led to damage to all the vital organs and also led to coma. These patients are in a terminal condition and the use of life support may only postpone death. For patients and families, it is very important to communicate with the cardiac care unit team to understand the illness and outlook (prognosis) and to make decisions so that the patient's wishes and values are respected.

HOW ARE END-OF-LIFE DECISIONS MADE?

Decisions in the cardiac care unit are based on shared decision making between the physicians and the patient and family. Communication is the key to decision making for a critically ill patient. The wishes of the patient are most important. If the patient does not want life-sustaining measures, they can be stopped. This is respect for the patient's autonomy, which means control over his/her own body. The law states that the patient has a right to agree to or refuse treatments, including life support.

The decision to limit or stop life support measures is based on the wishes of the patient, as well as the patient's best interest if the exact wishes are unknown. Often, patients in a critical condition cannot communicate or participate in making decisions and trust their closest relatives to make the decisions. The patient may have prepared for this by appointing a health care proxy to make medical decisions if the patient is unable to speak. A surrogate is a close relative or friend who will make decisions if a proxy has not been appointed and the patient is unable to make decisions. If the patient has not assigned a proxy, a surrogate is chosen from the patient's close relatives or close friends based on a priority order. Some patients have filled out a proxy or living will; these documents can spell out the care or treatment that the patient wants or does not want in the case of a terminal illness or condition.

Remember that decisions about life support are made on the basis of careful, thorough discussions with doctors, patient, and family/proxy/surrogate. Patients and family members should be sure that the doctors and nurses are aware of wishes concerning the end-of-life care.

FAMILY MEETING

The CCU team will provide information to the patient and family about the patient's condition and treatment. Often, the patient is very ill and unable to understand or participate, and so the physicians will speak with the family and health care proxy. A family meeting is often convened to talk about the patient's condition, treatments, and obtain information about the patient's wishes and values. It is often very difficult to be sure of the patient's outcome (prognosis); however, the physicians should give some information about whether the patient is expected to survive and what the function might be if he/she survives. If one member of the family becomes the contact person for the CCU staff, this will help the communication process.

WHAT IS LIFE SUPPORT?

Life support measures are treatments or procedures that support or replace body functions that are failing. When patients have curable or treatable conditions, life support is temporary until the organ function improves. With advanced illness and advanced age, certain diseases lead to a continued decline in function of the organs and of the entire person. Sometimes, the body never recovers and the patient would not be able to survive without life support.

It is important to understand the benefits and burdens of life support treatments. A treatment may be beneficial if it restores functioning, improves quality of life, and relieves suffering. The same treatment could be a burden if it causes pain, prolongs the dying process, or decreases the quality of life. The decision about whether a treatment is a benefit or a burden is a personal decision based on the patient's preferences and values. If the patient is able to tell the doctors, his/her decision will be respected. If the patient is unable to express his/her wishes, the doctors will meet with the family and proxy/surrogate to learn the patient's preferences and values.

WHAT ARE LIFE SUPPORT MEASURES?

CPR (Cardiopulmonary Resuscitation) is a set of treatments given when a patient's heart and breathing stop in order to restart the heart and breathing. It involves breathing for the patient using a mask or tube placed into the patient's airway. The team will compress the chest and may apply electric shocks to get the heart beating again.

In certain conditions, CPR can be very effective, for example, if a patient has a sudden heart attack. However, in patients at the late stages of a terminal illness who are at the end of life, CPR is usually not successful. Even if the heart does start beating, often the patient remains in a coma or dies within a short period of time. Making a decision about whether the patient should go through CPR is an important decision. In patients at the end of life, when the heart stops, this would be a natural death. A DNR (Do Not Resuscitate) order means that if the heart stops, CPR will not be done and the patient would die a natural death.

Mechanical ventilation is the use of a *ventilator* to support the breathing function of the lungs. Ventilator and *respirator* both mean the same machine. A tube is inserted through the mouth into the trachea (windpipe) and this tube is connected to a ventilator that gives the breaths to the patient. Patients on a ventilator are not able to speak, sometimes are awake enough to communicate, and often require sedation so that they are not anxious or uncomfortable. Mechanical ventilation may be used for a short period, such as in heart failure or pneumonia, and can also be used for a long time in patients with neurologic disorders, who may still be satisfied with the quality of their life. However, in a dying patient, mechanical ventilation will not improve the condition or the quality of life. In a patient who is dying, being on a respirator may prolong the dying process.

Noninvasive mechanical ventilation is the use of a ventilator machine that is attached to a special face mask. The ventilator will force air through the mask so the patient will feel some pressure of air moving in. Some patients can work well with the mask and even speak; for others, it is uncomfortable. This is a kind of life support that can be used if helpful; if it becomes uncomfortable and is not beneficial, it can be stopped.

Hemodialysis is used to replace the function of failed kidneys, which will clean the blood of wastes that normally accumulate. Dialysis requires placement of a large catheter and long periods on the dialysis machine. Some patients with kidney failure can live for years while receiving dialysis treatments several times each week. For patients at the end of life, dialysis cannot be expected to restore health.

Artificial nutrition and hydration can be given by a feeding tube placed into the stomach, which replaces normal eating and drinking. Artificial feeding may be necessary in some patients undergoing a prolonged illness until their bodies recover. In patients at the end of life, artificial nutrition and hydration still cannot restore health.

WHAT HAPPENS IF THE DECISION IS MADE TO WITHDRAW LIFE SUPPORT?

The decision to withdraw life support is made after careful discussion of the prognosis and patient preferences and values. All forms of life support can be withdrawn. The doctors may suggest placing an order for no CPR—a DNR order and not administering certain medications.

The mechanical ventilator can be removed, based on patient desires and values. The physician and nurse will assure that the patient is comfortable. The family can be present during this process if they wish.

HOW WILL THE DYING PATIENT BE TREATED?

The goal of the health care team is to provide the desired and beneficial care. In a dying patient, p*ain management and comfort care* will always be provided. Pain and discomfort can be managed by medications and also by working on the environment, such as having family present. Certain medications such as morphine are used to relieve pain and can also make the patient sleepy. All medications and treatments have other effects, so the overall goal of comfort must be a priority. The physicians and nurses will monitor the patient and also rely on the family to tell the staff whether the patient is comfortable.

There are clinicians who specialize in palliative care who may be consulted to assist the team with care. Patients and families may want the services of pastoral care.

The overall goal is for the cardiac team to work with the patient and his/her family, health care proxy, and surrogate to provide care that is beneficial and desired. Comfort and respect are priorities. It is important that there is communication and understanding in the shared responsibility for decision making and care for each patient.

VI

RISK FACTORS: FROM THE ACUTE SETTING TO CHRONIC MANAGEMENT

Ashish Correa
Petra Zubin Maslov
Emad F. Aziz
Eyal Herzog

53

Hypertension in the Cardiac Care Unit

The Committee on Public Health Priorities to Reduce and Control Hypertension in the U.S. Population concluded that "the Centers for Disease Control (CDC)'s cardiovascular disease program in general, and the HTN program in particular, are dramatically under-funded relative to the preventable burden of disease."[1] The global burden of hypertension (HTN) is tremendous. HTN is a risk factor for essentially every medical condition that would warrant admission to a hospital's cardiac care unit (CCU); in fact, the CCU is where the most severe forms of the HTN burden can be seen. HTN can be defined as a sustained rise in blood pressure (BP) that increases the risk of cerebral, cardiac, and renal events. In industrialized countries, the risk of becoming hypertensive during a lifetime exceeds 90%. The clinical spectrum of HTN ranges from mild elevations in BP to hypertensive emergencies requiring immediate therapy. Patients may be asymptomatic despite marked elevation in systemic BP, yet the resultant end-organ damage is a major cause of morbidity and mortality; hence the designation of HTN as the "silent killer."

At our institute, we have created a pathway for the management of in-hospital HTN, with a particular focus on the management of HTN in the CCU (**Figure 53.1**).

HYPERTENSION: DEFINITION AND PATHOPHYSIOLOGY

The 2014 Guidelines of the Eighth Joint National Committee (JNC 8) and the 2013 European Society of Hypertension (ESH)/European Society of Cardiology (ESC) define hypertension in a non-elderly (<60-year-old) patient without diabetes and chronic kidney disease (CKD) as BP of ≥140/90 mm Hg.[2,3] JNC 8 recommends initiating treatment beyond this threshold and aiming for goals of systolic blood pressure (SBP) <140 mm Hg and diastolic blood pressure (DBP) <90 mm Hg. Although the recommendations of JNC 8 are largely based on consensus expert opinions, high-quality evidence from several randomized control trial supports their recommendation to initiate treatment for HTN in patients ≥60 years when BP is only ≥150/90 mm Hg. Additional recommendations of JNC 8, in terms of thresholds for initiating treatment and BP goals, include initiating treatment for HTN in patients <60 years

with CKD or diabetes mellitus (DM) when BP ≥140/90 mm Hg, aiming for SBP <140 mm Hg and DBP <90 mm Hg. In the diabetic population, the recommendation is based largely on the results of the ACCORD-BP (Action to Control Cardiovascular Risk in Diabetes–Blood Pressure) trial, which found that aiming for lower BP goals did not reduce the risk of nonfatal and fatal major adverse cardiovascular events.[4] The more recent SPRINT (*Systolic Blood PRessure INTervention*) trial suggests that intensive treatment to a lower BP goal may improve cardiovascular outcomes and reduce mortality in elderly patients with increased cardiovascular risk; it may be noted, however, that the trial excluded patients with diabetes and prior strokes, including a large proportion of patients with increased cardiovascular risk.[5]

HTN is a frequent reason for admission to the CCU. More commonly, however, a patient is admitted to the CCU for a condition related secondarily to HTN, with high BP being a critical target of therapy and of future risk reduction. For example, although the patient with acute coronary syndrome (ACS) or heart failure (HF) is not admitted primarily for HTN, HTN is one of the mediators of the ongoing myocardial oxygen supply–demand imbalance in ACS, and of pump failure in HF, and thus is a critical target of therapy.

BP is determined by the product of heart rate, stroke volume, and systemic vascular resistance. Heart rate is determined largely by sympathetic activity. Stroke volume depends on cardiac preload and afterload, which in turn depend on multiple variables affecting vascular tone, as well as on myocardial contractility that is determined, among other things, by sympathetic activity. It follows that BP can be reduced by reducing heart rate, stroke volume, and/or vascular resistance.

HTN can be essential or secondary. Secondary HTN is due to a discernible cause, such as renal or endocrine disease, whereas essential HTN, which is responsible for the majority of cases, is not. HTN can also be thought of as an elevation of BP due to one or more abnormalities in cardiac function, vascular function, renal function, and/or neuroendocrine function.

Cardiac: A hyperkinetic circulation due to excessive sympathoadrenal activity or increased sensitivity of the heart to baseline neurohormonal regulators increases cardiac output and causes HTN with normal systemic vascular resistance, often in younger patients.

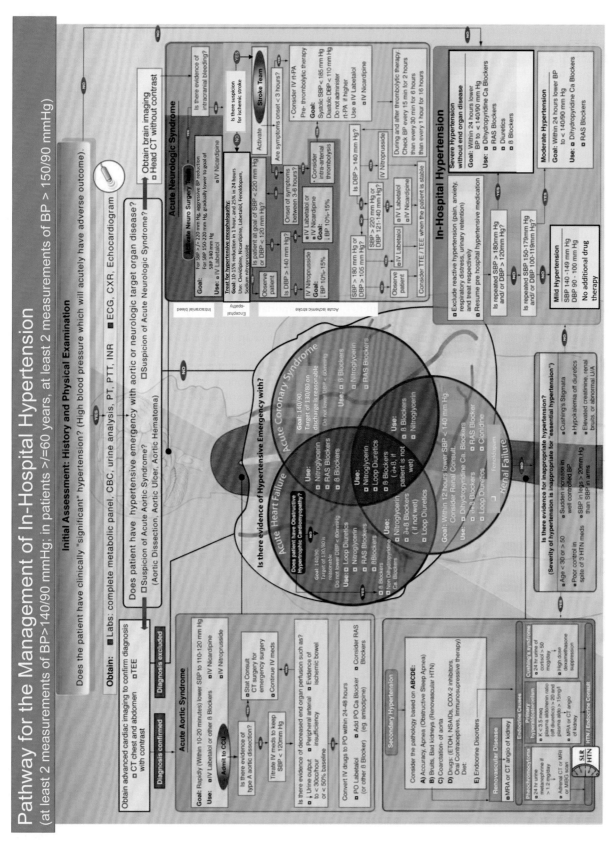

FIGURE 53.1 Pathway for the management of in-hospital hypertension. BP, Blood pressure; /=CBC, complete blood count; CCU, cardiac care unit; COX-2, Cyclooxygenase-2; CT, computed tomography; CXR, chest X-ray; DBP, diastolic blood pressure; ECG, electrocardiogram; ETOH, ethanol; HTN, hypertension; INR, international normalized ratio; MIBG, metaiodobenzylguanidine; MRA, magnetic resonance angiogram; MRI, magnetic resonance imaging; NSAIDs, non-steroidal anti-inflammatory drugs; PO, Per Os (Oral); PT, prothrombin time; PTT, partial thromboplastin time; RAS, renin–angiotensin system; SBP, systolic blood pressure; TEE, transesophageal echocardiogram; TTE, transthoracic echocardiogram.

Vascular: Elevated vascular resistance, more common in the elderly, due to abnormal blood vessel responsiveness to sympathetic outflow, endothelial damage that disrupts vasodilatory/vasoconstrictor balance, and ion channel defects will raise BP.

Renal: Renovascular disease leads to increased production of angiotensin II and aldosterone, which increase vasomotor tone and sodium/water retention leading to increased cardiac output and systemic vascular resistance.

Neuroendocrine: Neuroendocrine dysfunction as in pheochromocytoma and primary hyperaldosteronism can alter cardiac, vascular, and renal function to cause HTN via a number of mechanisms.

GENERAL PRINCIPLES ABOUT THE PHARMACOLOGIC MANAGEMENT OF HYPERTENSION

The fundamental concept of HTN treatment is that BP can be decreased by reducing heart rate, stroke volume, and/or systemic vascular resistance. These factors are interrelated, and many pharmacologic agents affect more than one of these determinants of BP. The drugs used to treat HTN are many, but when grouped into classes they are surprisingly few. It is important to remember that it is degree of BP reduction and control that is the major determinant of prevention of major adverse cardiovascular outcomes, and not class of antihypertensive drug; this fact has been accepted by major societies such as the ESH and ESC.[3] The armamentarium of drugs used to treat systemic HTN includes those that reduce intravascular volume (diuretics), downregulate sympathetic tone (β-blockers, α-blockers, and central sympatholytics), modulate vascular smooth muscle tone (calcium channel blockers [CCBs] and potassium channel openers), and inhibit the neurohormonal regulators of the circulatory system (angiotensin-converting enzyme inhibitors [ACEIs] and angiotensin receptor blockers [ARBs]). These drug classes make up the bulk of medications used to treat not only HTN but also the most common disease processes that warrant a CCU admission. β-Blockers, for example, are antihypertensives fundamentally important for reasons that go beyond their antihypertensive effects, in the treatment of HF, ACS, acute neurologic syndrome, and acute aortic syndrome. It is useful to organize drugs in classes and by mechanism of action because an understanding of how the drug class works helps one understand why it is effective for a disease process.

DIURETICS

Diuretics, which function to reduce intravascular volume and vasodilate, increase renal excretion of sodium and water. Diuretics include thiazide (thiazide-type and thiazide-like) diuretics and loop diuretics. Thiazide diuretics (thiazide-like—chlorthalidone, indapamide; thiazide-type diuretics—hydrochlorthiazide) have a long duration of action and moderate intensity of diuresis, making them more suitable for chronic HTN treatment than for short-term aggressive diuresis. After the publication of the ALLHAT (Antihypertensive and Lipid Lowering Treatment to Prevent Heart Attack) trial in 2002, thiazides became the initial antihypertensive monotherapy of choice.[6] However, recent evidence has challenged that notion; the ACCOMPLISH (*A*voiding *C*ardiovascular Events in *COM*bination Therapy in *P*atients *LI*ving with *S*ystolic *H*ypertension) trial in 2008 showed that the combination of benazepril

and amlodipine was superior to the combination of benazepril and hydrochlorthiazide in reducing cardiovascular outcomes in hypertensive patients with increased cardiovascular risk.[7] Despite this, thiazides are still among the four main classes of antihypertensive drugs recommended for initial monotherapy (in addition to ACEI, ARBs, and dihydropyridine CCBs), as recommended by the expert panel of JNC 8.[2] If a thiazide is to be used, it is always preferable to use chlorthalidone, which is more potent and longer acting than hydrochlorthiazide (despite increased risk of glucose intolerance, hyperuricemia, and hypokalemia).

Loop diuretics (eg, furosemide) have a relatively short duration of action (4 to 6 hours) and are useful more for brisk diuresis than antihypertensive efficacy, making them critical in the treatment of HF exacerbations. However, in patients with CKD and glomerular filtration rate (GFR) of less than 30 mL/min, thiazides are less effective. In such patients, loop diuretics are much more effective as antihypertensives. In patients with a low GFR, their volume status is a major determinant of BP; as such, loop diuretics play a major role in BP management by rapidly modulating volume status. Interestingly, when HTN persists even at high doses of loop diuretic, a thiazide (such as chlorthalidone, hydrochrothiazide, or metolazone) can enhance diuresis. Although ACEI forms the most important therapy for patients with CKD with proteinuria, in the absence of proteinuria or in the presence of edema, loop diuretics form an initial component of initial therapy for BP management in such patients.

Another diuretic, spironolactone, has recently gained attention after the publication of the PATHWAY-2 (*P*revention *A*nd *T*reatment of *H*ypertension *W*ith *A*lgorithm-based therap*Y*) trial.[8] Spironolactone has been shown to be the most effective add-on drug for the treatment of resistant HTN, defined as suboptimal BP control despite treatment with at least three blood-lowering drugs. This effectiveness of spironolactone in the treatment of HTN supports sodium retention as an underlying pathophysiologic cause of resistant HTN. It is important to monitor electrolytes and renal function during initiation of spironolactone.

ADRENERGIC BLOCKADE: α- AND β-BLOCKERS

β_1 Receptors found on myocardial cells, when activated, increase heart rate (chronotropy) and contractility (inotropy). α_1 Receptors found on vascular smooth muscle promote contraction and thus vasoconstriction.

β-Adrenergic antagonists or β-blockers (eg, metoprolol) have negative chronotropic and negative inotropic effects as well as effects on resistance vessels. In addition, they protect against the cardiac remodeling imposed by adrenergic stimulation and have shown long-term benefit in coronary artery disease (CAD) and HF. α-Blockers (eg, doxazosin), on the other hand, promote peripheral vasodilation, leading to a decrease in peripheral vascular resistance. Some β-blockers (labetalol, carvedilol) block α- and β-receptors, thus mediating vasodilatation (α-blockade) and decreased reflex tachycardia, along with decreased heart rate and decreased cardiac contractility. However, decades ago, the MRC (Medical Research Council) Study in the United Kingdom showed that β-blockers were less effective than other agents as antihypertensives.[9] This has been shown again by several systematic reviews and meta-analyses,[10–12] and none of the major professional societies support the use of β-blockers as initial monotherapy for HTN. Further, in the ALLHAT trial, the doxazosin arm had to be stopped early because of adverse cardiovascular outcomes.[6] α-Blockers are never used for HTN monotherapy, except to concomitantly treat an enlarged prostate.

CALCIUM CHANNEL BLOCKERS

Calcium ions are major mediators of vascular smooth muscle cell contraction as well as inotropic and chronotropic function of the heart. Calcium enters vascular smooth muscle cells, cardiomyocytes, and pacemaker cells via voltage-dependent calcium channels. CCBs, by inhibiting calcium entry into the vascular myocytes, promote myocyte relaxation, thus leading to vasodilation. In a similar way, by inhibiting calcium entry into the cardiac myocyte, they have negative chronotropic and negative dromotropic effects.

CCBs are recommended by the expert panel of JNC 8 as agents that can be used as initial monotherapy for HTN.[2] In general, dihydropyridine CCBs (eg, amlodipine, nifedipine, felodopine, isradipine) are the preferred agents; they are highly selective for arterial tissues, including the coronary arteries, where they cause vasodilation. Intravenous (IV) nicardipine has strong antihypertensive activity; intra-arterially, it decreases vasospasm in subarachnoid hemorrhage, and it is a recommended agent for HTN after acute ischemic stroke and intracerebral hemorrhage (ICH).[13] Clevidipine, a new third-generation IV dihydropyridine CCB, has a high vascular selectivity with a fast onset and offset of BP-lowering effect, thus making it easily and rapidly titratable and an especially attractive drug for acute HTN. In perioperative patients requiring HTN treatment, clevidipine compared favorably to nitroglycerin (NTG), nitroprusside, and nicardipine in terms of BP-reducing efficacy and 30-day outcomes (death, myocardial infarction [MI], stroke, renal failure).[14]

The non-dihydropyridine CCBs (diltiazem, verapamil) bind to different sites and are less selective for vascular smooth muscle; they have negative chronotropic and dromotropic effects on sinoatrial (SA) and atrioventricular (AV) nodal conducting tissue and negative inotropic effects on cardiomyocytes, making them useful heart-rate–controlling agents as in atrial fibrillation with rapid ventricular rate. Non-dihydropyridine CCBs should be used with caution in patients with impaired systolic function or conduction system disease because these agents can exacerbate HF and SA or AV node dysfunction, especially in patients already on β-blocker therapy. As such, dihydropyridine CCBs are preferred agents for HTN monotherapy. Still, diltiazem and verapamil may be useful for HTN, when used concomitantly for some other indication, such as atrial fibrillation. Further more, they are preferred second-line agents in patients with CKD, because they help in reducing proteinuria.

ANGIOTENSIN-CONVERTING ENZYME INHIBITORS AND ANGIOTENSIN RECEPTOR BLOCKERS

ACEIs prevent the ACE-mediated conversion of angiotensin I to angiotensin II, leading to decreased circulating angiotensin II and aldosterone (angiotensin II stimulates the release of aldosterone from the adrenal glands). Angiotensin II elevates BP by causing peripheral vasoconstriction and also through sodium and water reabsorption in the distal tubules. In the long term, it promotes HTN by promoting atherosclerosis; this occurs through various mechanisms such as direct effects of angiotensin II on constriction and remodeling of resistance vessels, aldosterone synthesis and

release, enhancement of sympathetic outflow from the brain, and facilitation of catecholamine release from the adrenals and peripheral sympathetic nerve terminals. In the heart, angiotensin can cause adverse tissue remodeling. It is an important trigger of several genomic and non-genomic pathways that play a role in pathogenesis of myocardial hypertrophy and fibrosis. Angiotensin II is an upregulator of intracellular genomic pathways that lead to the activation of a hypertrophic gene transcription program and the development of myocardial hypertrophy.[15] It is also one of the stimulators of fibroblasts to myofibroblast transformation, a crucial step in pathogenesis of cardiac fibrosis. Angiotensin also stimulates release of chymase from the cardiac mast cells, which additionally upregulates fibrosis by stimulating collagen production within the fibroblasts.[16]

ACEIs decrease levels of vasoconstricting angiotensin II. By reducing aldosterone production, they also promote natriuresis and reduction of intravascular volume. By decreasing bradykinin breakdown, ACEIs promote vasodilatation. They may be nephroprotective because reducing angtiotensin II levels reduces renal efferent arteriole constriction, thus reducing intraglomerular pressures and limiting glomerular damage over time. For all these reasons, these drugs are particularly useful in patients with hypertensive diabetes and HF. ARBs, by blocking angiotensin receptors, promote vasodilation and reduction in aldosterone levels, thus aiding natriuresis. However, they do not affect the levels of bradykinin.

For HTN, ACEIs are recommended as initial monotherapy by JNC 8 for the general nonblack population. For the black population, irrespective of their diabetic status, thiazides and CCBs are preferred as initial monotherapy.[2] This is based on the findings of the ALLHAT trial, which found these classes of drugs to be superior to ACEIs in the black patient population. However, for patients with CKD having proteinuria, irrespective of their race or their diabetic status, ACEIs form the first-line monotherapy. In the absence of proteinuria, ACEIs still can be used as initial monotherapy in the patient with CKD, although diuretics should be favored when there is edema. The recommendations for ARBs are similar.

NITRATES

Organic nitrates are chemically reduced to release nitric oxide (NO), an endogenous signaling molecule that causes vascular smooth muscle relaxation. Although NO can dilate both arteries and veins, venous dilation predominates at therapeutic doses. NO-induced venodilation increases venous capacitance, leading to a decrease in the return of blood to the right side of the heart, and subsequently decreased right ventricular and left ventricular (LV) end-diastolic pressure and volume. This decrease in preload reduces myocardial oxygen demand. At higher concentrations, nitrates may cause arterial vasodilation. In the coronary circulation, NTG preferentially dilates large epicardial arteries rather than smaller coronary arterioles, thus preventing coronary steal phenomenon, encountered with such agents as dipyridamole. It is unclear to what extent nitrates' effects on coronary vasodilation benefit the patient with angina because the chronic oxygen deficit in patients with CAD causes maximal dilation of coronary arteries and because atherosclerotic coronary arteries may remain noncompliant even in the face of coronary artery vasodilators. Furthermore, doses of nitrates sufficient to vasodilate epicardial arteries can induce peripheral vasodilation, hypotension, and reflex tachycardia, which harm the delicate supply-demand balance. In patients with HF, however, reflex tachycardia is rare; the venodilation and decreased end-diastolic pressure effects of nitrates make them acceptable at certain doses for decreasing pulmonary congestion in the patient with hypertensive emergency and congestive HF. Side effects related to hypotension include dizziness and syncope; nitrates are contraindicated in hypotension, and not advised in diastolic dysfunction and hypertrophic obstructive cardiomyopathy, two disease states for which adequate preload are critical to sustain cardiac output. Also, nitrates should not be taken by patients taking phosphodiesterase inhibitors (ie, sildenafil [Viagra]).

Sodium nitroprusside is a nitrate that, like NTG, liberates NO but does so nonenzymatically; as a result, nitroprusside does not target specific vessels and consequently dilates both arteries and veins. With rapid onset of action and high efficacy, nitroprusside is useful in hypertensive emergencies, but must be infused with continuous BP monitoring. Sodium nitroprusside is metabolized to products that are potentially toxic if they accumulate excessively: cyanide (acid–base disturbance, cardiac arrythmia) is converted to thiocyanate (psychosis, spasms, convulsions).

HYPERTENSION AND THE CCU

HTN is a risk factor and target of therapy (both short term and long term) for virtually every condition that warrants a CCU admission. We review the most common CCU disease states in terms of pathophysiology, diagnosis, and management in relation to HTN. **Figure 53.2** outlines the initial assessment of a patient with HTN in the hospital who may require care in the CCU. **Figure 53.3** outlines our working group's assessment of a hypertensive emergency.

HYPERTENSION AND DISEASES OF THE AORTA

Diseases of the aorta include aortic atheroma, aneurysm, arteritis, and acute aortic syndromes (aortic dissection, intramural hematoma, penetrating ulcer). These diseases tend to follow an indolent asymptomatic progressive course until they culminate in an acute life-threatening clinical presentation. The most common of these processes is aortic dissection.

Aortic dissection is characterized by an intimal tear and formation of a false lumen within the media of the artery. Repetitive hemodynamic forces produced by the blood ejected into the aorta with each cardiac cycle contribute to the weakening of the aortic intima and to medial degeneration. Sustained HTN intensifies these forces. Acute elevations in heart rate and BP can lead to catastrophic acute worsening of the disease process. The false lumen, as it extends, can obstruct the true lumen, leading to such complications as acute MI, acute renal failure, and stroke. Many patients with aortic dissection have undermining of the elastic or muscular components of the media, which is quantitatively and qualitatively more severe than expected from aging, as seen in Marfan and Ehlers–Danlos syndromes, and congenital bicuspid aortic valve.

Patients with aortic syndrome present with acute onset of severe chest pain that typically radiates through to the back. The pain is at its most severe at onset, unlike the typically crescendo pain of ACS. Although clearly not diagnostic, terms such as "tearing," "ripping," and "stabbed me in the chest and back" should alert the caregiver to the possibility of dissection. Presentations can vary, and thus aortic disease must be considered in any patient presenting with chest pain, especially because some treatments for ACS (thrombolysis and antithrombotic therapy) can worsen acute aortic syndrome.

Therapy for aortic dissection aims to halt progression; lethal complications arise not due to the tear itself but due to the extension of the tear such that occlusion or rupture occurs.

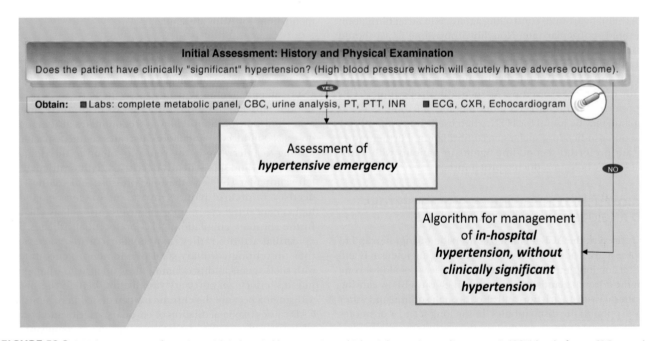

FIGURE 53.2 Initial assessment of a patient with in-hospital hypertension, which might require cardiac care unit (CCU) level of care. CBC, complete blood count; CXR, chest X-ray; ECG, electrocardiogram; INR, international normalized ratio; PT, prothrombin time; PTT, partial thromboplastin time.

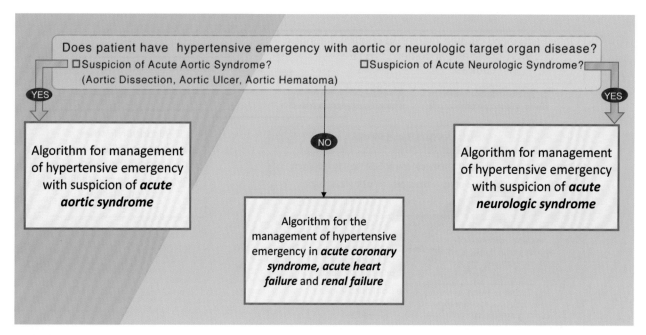

FIGURE 53.3 Assessment of hypertensive emergency.

Untreated, aortic dissection will result in death in 25% of patients in 24 hours, 50% in 1 week, and over 90% in 1 year. As the major etiologic component of the development and progression of aortic dissection, BP is the major target of treatment. Heart rate is also a major target of treatment because BP and heart rate together create a hemodynamic force that favors extension of the dissection.

Pathway Management

Figure 53.4 outlines the management of a hypertensive emergency with suspicion for an acute aortic syndrome.

The modalities available for the diagnosis of aortic dissection include computed tomography (CT), magnetic resonance imaging (MRI), transthoracic echocardiogram (TTE) or transesophageal echocardiogram (TEE), and aortography. The goals of imaging are to establish the diagnosis, determine location of the dissection (ascending, type A dissections are considered surgical emergencies), and determine extent of disease (eg, coronary or cerebral artery involvement). The choice of modality may be influenced by clinical presentation. The patient with suspected aortic dissection who also presents with physical examination findings suspicious for pericardial effusion or aortic regurgitation may benefit more from a TEE than CT, for example.

When the dissection involves the ascending aorta, the focus is surgical management. However, whether the dissection is ascending or descending, medical management to reduce BP and heart rate are critical and urgent. Labetalol, which has α_1 and β_1 and β_2 adrenergic receptor inhibitory action, is an ideal drug because it reduces BP and heart rate, and can be given intravenously for immediate onset of action and titration. We recommend lowering BP within 10 to 20 minutes to an SBP level of 110 to 120 mm Hg. Esmolol, with its short half-life and β_1 receptor selectivity, may be a good alternative for those with reactive airway disease. The CCB nicardipine is an alternative as well. Once the patient is stabilized, whether surgically for ascending

or medically for descending dissection, oral forms of the same medications (β-blocker, CCB, ACEI) are used for long-term BP control, which is crucial for secondary risk reduction.

HYPERTENSION AND ACUTE NEUROLOGIC SYNDROME

Stroke results from either ischemic or hemorrhagic causes. Ischemic stroke can be categorized by presumed mechanism of ischemia into coagulopathies (protein C deficiency, antiphospholipid antibody), small vessel-lacunar (vasculitis, embolic), large vessel-intracranial (dissection, atherosclerosis), large vessel-extracranial (Takayasu, atherosclerotic), and cardioembolic (atrial fibrillation, ventricular thrombus, infectious endocarditis). Some strokes are cryptogenic, or of undetermined cause. Hemorrhagic stroke can be categorized as intracerebral (bleeding into brain parenchyma, further classified as primary and unrelated to a brain lesion, or secondary and related to a congenital or acquired brain lesion or abnormality), subarachnoid, or intraventricular. HTN is a major risk factor for both ischemic (especially small vessel-lacunar) and hemorrhagic stroke, and thus there is little doubt that treating BP for stroke prevention (both primary and secondary prevention) is justified and very important. However, it is in the treatment of HTN for the patient in the acute phase of a stroke that there has been much controversy and ambiguity; recent data are shedding more light on this important issue.

Stroke is a major cause of morbidity and mortality; in 2014, it was the fifth leading cause of death in the United States, behind heart disease, cancer, chronic lower respiratory illnesses, and unintentional injuries.[17] Perhaps more devastating is the morbidity in survivors; stroke is the leading cause of long-term disability in adults. A total of 15% to 30% of stroke survivors are permanently disabled, and 20% require institutional care by 3 months.

Timely diagnosis of stroke, greatly dependent on history and physical examination, is critical because early implementation of treatment can improve prognosis; some treatments for ischemic

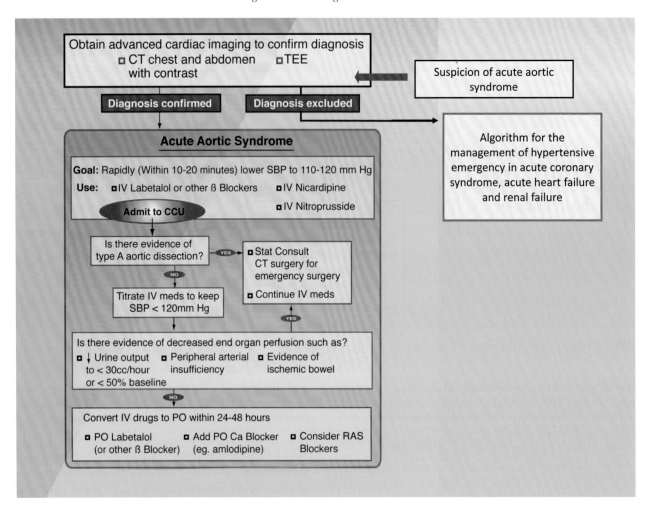

FIGURE 53.4 Management of a hypertensive emergency with suspicion of an acute aortic syndrome. CT, computed tomography; IV, intravenous; RAS, renin–angiotensin system; SBP, systolic blood pressure; TEE, transesophageal echocardiogram.

stroke, for example, are only implementable within 3 (IV recombinant tissue plasminogen activator [rtPA]) to 6 hours (intra-arterial thrombolysis) from onset of event. For this reason, the most important piece of history is time of symptom onset. Findings such as focal neurologic deficit, persistent neurologic deficit, acute onset of symptoms, and no history of head trauma favor the diagnosis of stroke; the presence of all four of these findings makes a stroke likely. Symptoms also enable the experienced clinician to determine the vascular distribution (eg, anterior or posterior) of a stroke. Once stroke is suspected, severity can be assessed with the NIH (National Institutes of Health) Stroke Scale, the diagnosis can be further pursued with imaging studies, and tests can be obtained to exclude conditions that mimic strokes (tumor, hypertensive encephalopathy, seizure, migraine variant).

The first imaging test to obtain in the acute stroke patient is a noncontrast CT scan of the brain, because this will identify most intracranial hemorrhage (ICH) and help exclude stroke mimickers such as neoplasms. Importantly, CT will not reliably diagnose ischemic stroke when early in its evolution; MRI, on the other hand, will. MRI with diffusion-weighted and perfusion-weighted imaging has a high sensitivity and specificity for ischemic lesions, even within minutes of symptom onset, and can identify brain tissue that is ischemic but not yet infarcted and therefore amenable to being rescued if successfully revascularized. CT angiogram

provides maps of cerebral blood flow, thus possibly revealing occlusion or stenosis.

An elevated BP is often detected in the first few hours after stroke. BP is usually higher for acute stroke patients with a history of HTN than in those without premorbid HTN. For ischemic strokes, the elevated BP may be a protective response of the body to maintain perfusion of partially ischemic areas. Still, for every 10 mm Hg increase above 180 mm Hg, the risk of neurologic deterioration increases by 40%, and the risk of poor outcome increases by 23% in the case of ischemic strokes. Despite this association between elevated BP and poor outcomes, the management of arterial HTN in ischemic stroke has been controversial. Investigators found a U-shaped relationship between death and admission BP; both elevated and low admission levels were associated with high rates of early and late death from stroke.[18] Elevations in mean BP during the first few days after stroke had an unfavorable effect on outcomes; death due to brain injury and brain edema correlated with high initial BP. Theoretical reasons for lowering BP include reducing brain edema, reducing risk of hemorrhagic transformation, and preventing further vascular damage. Conversely, it has been theorized that overly aggressive BP reduction may lead to neurologic worsening.[19] Furthermore, the majority of patients experience a drop in BP within the first hour of stroke without any medical treatment. Recommendations for BP control vary depending on whether it is the acute post-stroke phase or the chronic phase, and whether thrombolysis is being pursued or not; this has been discussed subsequently. In the case of hemorrhagic strokes, the issue is complex as well. Although elevated BP maintains perfusion of jeopardized brain tissues, it serves as a continued driving force for bleeding. However, rapid decrease in BP can impair perfusion and cause ischemia. Recommendations for management are discussed here.

Pathway Management

Figure 53.5 outlines the management of a hypertensive emergency with suspicion for an acute neurologic syndrome.

Our group subdivides the management of a hypertensive emergency with the suspicion of an acute neurologic syndrome into the management of three distinct clinical scenarios:

a. ICH: With respect to patients with ICH, controversy persists regarding the appropriate goal for BP management. Some studies have shown no benefit in terms of mortality and disability for aggressive BP management,[20,21] whereas others have shown reduction in hematoma size with aggressive BP control.[22] At the moment, guidelines recommend that for SBP > 220 mm Hg, rapid reduction of BP with IV agents is necessary, whereas

for SBP between 150 and 220 mm Hg, targeting an SBP of 140 mm Hg should be pursued.[23]

b. Ischemic stroke: For ischemic strokes, the management and guidelines for BP control are somewhat different. For symptoms less than 3 hours old, IV rtPA is recommended for selected patients without contraindications (eg, history of previous ICH); for symptoms 3 to 6 hours old, intra-arterial thrombolysis may be used. However, BP over 185/110 mm Hg is a contraindication to IV rtPA. In this setting, labetalol and nicardipine may be used to rapidly lower BP. During and after thrombolytic therapy, nitroprusside, labetalol, or nicardipine should be used, depending on how high the BP is, to maintain BP below 180/105 mm Hg.[24]

c. Hypertensive encephalopathy: For hypertensive encephalopathy, on the other hand, the baseline BP must be considered to avoid excessive BP lowering and prevent cerebral ischemia. Lowering the mean arterial pressure by 10% to 15% in the first hour and by 25% in the first 24 hours usually is a safe maneuver because of the pressure autoregulatory cerebral blood flow range.

Patients who were taking antihypertensive medications before their stroke or are found to have sustained HTN after their stroke will need long-term antihypertensive treatment. Historically, there

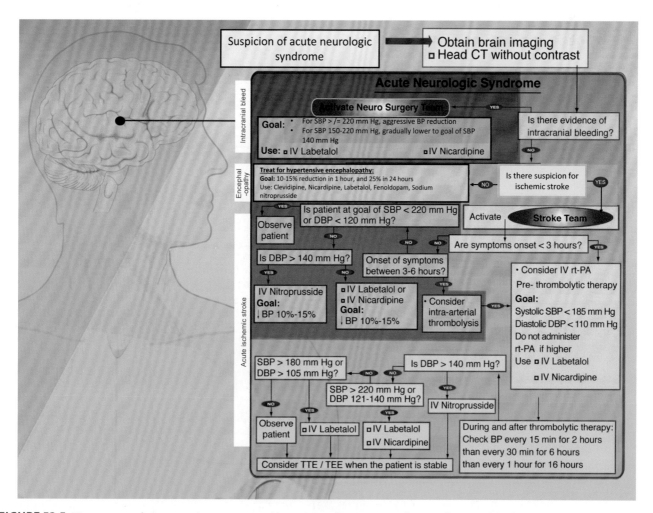

FIGURE 53.5 Management of a hypertensive emergency with suspicion of an acute neurologic syndrome. BP, blood pressure; CT, computed tomography; DBP, diastolic blood pressure; IV, intravenous; rtPA, recombinant tissue plasminogen activator; SBP, systolic blood pressure; TEE, transesophageal echocardiogram; TTE, transthoracic echocardiogram.

was a belief in the medical community that permissive HTN in the long term was protective for patients after an ischemic stroke. In fact, in patients followed up from the time of a first ischemic stroke to the time of a second stroke in the same territory, risk was increased rather than decreased with higher BP, a finding driven mainly by SBP elevations above 160 mm Hg.[25] The same facts are valid for ICH. Control of the SBP is the cornerstone of secondary prevention of recurrent ICH.[26] The timing of the reinstitution of treatment and the selection of medications will depend on the patient's neurologic status, the underlying stroke mechanism, the patient's ability to swallow medications, and the presence of concomitant disease. Presumably, most patients with mild-to-moderate stroke who are not at high risk for increased intracranial pressure may have their prestroke antihypertensive medications restarted 24 hours after their vascular event.[24]

Figure 53.6 outlines the management of a hypertensive emergency with acute HF, ACS, or renal failure.

HYPERTENSION AND ACUTE CORONARY SYNDROME

ACS refers to a spectrum of diseases that range from unstable angina and non–ST-elevation myocardial infarction (NSTEMI) to ST-elevation myocardial infarction (STEMI).

ACS is perhaps best explained in terms of the delicate balance between myocardial oxygen supply and demand. When this balance is disrupted by a disease process that affects coronary blood flow, myocardial ischemia may induce contractile dysfunction, precipitating a vicious cycle that includes tachycardia and hypotension, which may further worsen the supply–demand imbalance.

Myocardial oxygen demand is largely dependent on heart rate, myocardial wall stress (systolic pressure), and LV contractility. Myocardial oxygen supply depends on the coronary circulation. In contrast to most other vascular beds, myocardial oxygen extraction is near maximal (75% of arterial oxygen content) at rest.[27] Consequently, demand for increased myocardial oxygen consumption must be met primarily by increased oxygen delivery. A 2-fold increase in any of the determinants of oxygen consumption requires an approximately 50% increase in coronary flow.

HTN increases demand: it increases myocardial wall stress and thus requirements of coronary flow. HTN may also limit supply: it is a risk factor for vascular remodeling and atherosclerosis, the disease process that limits coronary blood flow. Even at an early age, increased vascular wall tension in people with high BP leads to thinning, fragmentation, and fracture of elastin fibers, as well as increased collagen deposition in arteries, which results in decreased compliance of these vessels. In addition to

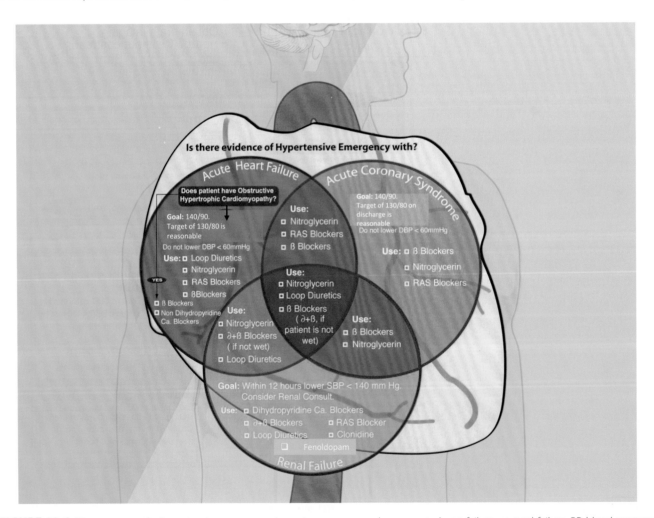

FIGURE 53.6 Management of a hypertensive emergency in acute coronary syndrome, acute heart failure, or renal failure. BP, blood pressure; DBP, diastolic blood pressure; RAA, renin–angiotensin system; SBP, systolic blood pressure.

these structural abnormalities, the HTN-mediated functional abnormality of increased arterial rigidity due to endothelial dysfunction develops over time because of aging and HTN and contributes to systolic HTN.[28]

Many of the mechanisms that initiate and maintain HTN (increased sympathetic nervous system and renin–angiotensin–aldosterone system [RAAS] activity; deficiencies in release and/or activity of vasodilators, structural and functional abnormalities in conductance and resistance arteries) are also those that mediate damage to target organs, including the coronary vessels and the myocardium.[29] This may be why antihypertensive drugs exert at least some of their beneficial effects on the vasculature by actions that are independent of BP lowering alone.

The medications used to treat ACS can be understood within the framework of the supply/demand balance. β-Blockers work to decrease BP and heart rate, two major determinants of myocardial oxygen demand. Nitrates decrease preload, and thus ventricular filling pressures and wall stress (demand). Nitrates also cause coronary vessel dilatation (supply). Morphine decreases pain and thereby heart rate, while also decreasing venous return and filling pressures (demand). Often, the patient with ACS will need a cardiac catheterization whether for diagnostic or treatment purposes. Cardiac catheterization is the gold standard for diagnosis of coronary vessel disease, and angioplasty and coronary stenting can relieve the stenosis or occlusion (supply) in a way no medication can.

Pathway Management

Detailed guidelines exist for HTN in ACS.[30] In an ACS, β-blockers are the first line of treatment based on their ability to reduce both heart rate and BP and thus myocardial oxygen demand (Figure 53.6). In the case of hypertensive emergences, an IV β-blocker may be needed. NTG has been a cornerstone of therapy for decades in ACS, and in the hypertensive patient, IV NTG is effective in the reduction of BP and symptoms. Patients need to be monitored for potential adverse effects, particularly profound hypotension, which can exacerbate ischemia. Caution should be used if there is right heart dysfunction. If β-blockers are contraindicated, a non-dihydropyridine CCB (diltiazem or verapamil) may be used, assuming there is no LV dysfunction. An ACEI or an ARB can also be considered for the management of HTN in patients with ACS, and must be added when there is LV dysfunction, anterior wall MI, diabetes, and if HTN persists. In persistent HTN even after optimization with β-blockers and ACEI/ARB, a long-acting dihydropyridine CCB (especially if there is persistent angina) or a thiazide may be used. In patients with MI and LV dysfunction, in whom HTN persists despite β-blocker and ACEI, an aldosterone antagonist may be considered. When there is symptomatic HF or CKD with GFR <30 mL/min, a loop diuretic can be used. In patients with ACS, guidelines recommend lowering BP to <140/90 mm Hg in patients who are hemodynamically stable. Targeting BP of <130/80 mm Hg at discharge is reasonable, lowering diastolic pressure <60 mm Hg should be avoided.

HYPERTENSION AND HEART FAILURE

HF can be due to a decrease in cardiac output such that end-organ perfusion is compromised (systolic dysfunction), or due to maintenance of cardiac output at the expense of increased left atrial filling pressures (diastolic dysfunction), or due to both. Both systolic and diastolic dysfunction can be understood in terms of the determinants of cardiac performance.

The determinants of cardiac performance are preload, afterload, contractility, and heart rate. As the ability of the myocardium to maintain normal forward output fails, compensatory mechanisms are activated to preserve circulatory function. Preload increases to increase stroke volume (Frank–Starling mechanism). Hemodynamic stress that cannot be compensated initiates structural changes at the cellular levels, referred to as myocardial remodeling. If the Frank–Starling and remodeling mechanisms are unable to reestablish cardiac output, neurohormonal systems are also activated. Although each of these mechanisms may contribute to maintenance of circulatory function, each may also contribute to development and progression of pump dysfunction.

HTN is intricately linked to both systolic and diastolic dysfunction by affecting each of these mechanisms. The renin–angiotensin system (RAS) that is so fundamentally linked to HTN and that recruits intravascular volume to sustain end-diastolic filling pressures may elevate preload to the point of putting a patient on the flat or descending portion of the Frank–Starling curve. HTN induces cardiac remodeling and LV hypertrophy; to decrease LV wall stress, contractile proteins are added to myocytes in parallel, thus increasing wall thickness and decreasing cavity size. Increasing thickness and decreasing cavity size relieves the increase in wall stress, but at the expense of LV remodeling and hypertrophy. Finally, the sympathetic activation that increases vascular tone also increases myocardial oxygen demand and eventually results in downregulation of β-adrenergic receptors, further impairing the ability of the system to maintain forward output.

The staples of HF treatment are diuretics, β-blockers, and ACEIs. Diuretics, specifically loop diuretics, combat the increased total body volume that is central to the pathophysiology of HF. β-Blockers and ACEIs/ARBs combat the cardiac remodeling and neurohormonal activation. Aldosterone antagonists are particularly important when there is LV dysfunction, by countering neurohormonal-mediated remodeling. The CCB amlodipine, although not first line, appears to be safe if needed for the treatment of HTN (or angina) in the patient with LV dysfunction.[31]

Pathway Management

Careful guidelines exist for the management of HTN in HF, both systolic and diastolic HF (Figure 53.6).[30,32] β-Blockers and ACEIs, which show benefit in systolic HF, should form first-line therapy. Diuretics are important for volume control and BP; although thiazides can be used, loop diuretics are key in severe HF (New York Heart Association [NYHA] Class III and IV) and in CKD when GFR is <30 mL/min. In persistent HTN in patients with LV dysfunction, aldosterone antagonists may be used. In African Americans, with LV systolic dysfunction, hydralazine and isosorbide dinitrate should be added to standard therapy. In hypertensive emergencies or in patients with severe pulmonary edema, parenteral nitrates play an important role. Although few guidelines exist for management of diastolic dysfunction, BP management—both SBP and DBP—is paramount. In addition, therapy may be directed toward management of pulmonary edema and toward rate control in atrial fibrillation. One caveat in the management of HTN in the setting of acute HF is the exclusion of hypertrophic cardiomyopathy. In patients with hypertrophic cardiomyopathy, guidelines recommend the exclusive use of a β-blocker or a non-dihydropyridine CCB (in patients with a contraindication to β-blockers) and avoidance of diuretics or NTG.

HYPERTENSION AND RENAL FAILURE

Renal failure tends not to be the primary reason for CCU admission but rather a complication or comorbidity of some other disease process requiring CCU care, such as hypertensive emergency or acute decompensated heart failure (ADHF). Nonetheless, because renal failure is associated with poor outcomes, preserving or improving the CCU patient's renal function must be a primary objective.

Severe and/or long-standing HTN induces renal microvascular damage. Mechanical stress and endothelial injury lead to increased vascular permeability, activation of the coagulation cascade and platelets, and deposition of fibrin. This fibrinoid necrosis narrows the vessel lumen, which causes renal hypoperfusion and triggers massive renin release, generating a vicious cycle of ongoing injury. RAS activation involves production of angiotensin II and release of aldosterone; this in turn leads to further vasoconstriction and sodium reabsorption, worsening HTN. Angiotensin II, acting on the efferent arteriole of the nephron, leads to pressure natriuresis, which can lead to end-organ hypoperfusion, ischemia, and dysfunction. HTN begets renal damage that begets more HTN, which if severe enough causes acute end-organ damage (hypertensive emergency).

Renal failure in the setting of acute HF is a complex issue, and an understanding of the concept of cardiorenal syndrome is essential. HF decreases renal perfusion and predisposes to renal failure. Further more, vascular congestion and increased intra-abdominal pressure in acute HF may also be implicated.[33] With worsening renal failure, there is increased fluid retention and volume overload that can worsen HF. Further more, renal failure makes diuretic dose requirements for HF higher; if HF is hemodynamically significant such that renal perfusion is compromised, inotropes or dialysis may be the only effective options. Diuretics increase solute delivery to distal segments of the nephron, resulting in epithelial cell hypertrophy and hyperplasia, which increases the solute resorptive capacity of the kidney. Reduction in renal extracellular fluid volume also leads to an increase in solute and fluid reabsorption, specifically in the proximal tubule. These mechanisms result in a state in which HF and renal failure worsen each other and make difficult the treatment of both. Although these patients may be hypotensive initially, they often eventually become hypertensive. The elevated BP may augment renal perfusion, whereas the continued venous congestion causes renal failure to persist, and the rising BP worsens HF. As such, BP management and efficient diuresis is key.

Pathway Management

For the hypertensive emergency patient in acute renal failure, the recommendation is a goal of lowering SBP to 140 mm Hg within 12 hours and considering consultation by a nephrologist (**Figure 53.6**). A recommended strategy is for a 10% to 20% reduction in mean arterial pressure during the first 1 to 2 hours, and then a further 10% to 15% reduction during the next 6 to 12 hours.

Early on, parenteral agents may be needed. Some physicians advocate the use of fenoldopam, which is unique among the parenteral BP agents because it mediates peripheral vasodilation by acting on peripheral dopamine-1 receptors, and thus, despite lowering systemic BP, by acting on these receptors in the renal vessels, it promotes renal perfusion. Thus, fenoldopam improves creatinine clearance, urine flow rates, and sodium excretion in severely hypertensive patients with both normal and impaired renal function.[34] Fenoldopam has onset of action within 5 minutes, peak action by 15 minutes, and duration of action from 30 to 60 minutes. No adverse effects have been reported.

The recommended sequence of add-on parenteral drugs is dihydropyridine CCB (nicardipine: onset 5 to 15 minutes, duration 4 to 6 hours, and increases stroke volume and reduces both cardiac and cerebral ischemia; clevidipine may also be used) and then α- + β-blocker (labetalol: liver metabolism, onset in 2 to 5 minutes, peak at 5 to 15 minutes, duration 2 to 4 hours, maintains cardiac output because of α-blocking effect). In addition, the ultimate therapy includes loop diuretics, RAS blocker, and clonidine. Loop diuretics are essential, especially in acute glomerular diseases, to reduce volume and pressure. ACEIs improve renal blood flow and reduce ischemia; they are essential in acute vascular forms of renal failure, such as scleroderma renal crisis.

Regarding long-term management, it is important to note that patients with CKD die from heart disease more than anything else. CKD is a risk factor for CAD, valvular heart disease, and other causes of heart disease. HTN control is critical to reduce the rate of development of these cardiovascular processes. If HTN is controlled, CKD progresses more slowly. Because the mechanism of HTN in the patient with CKD is RAAS activation, ACE inhibitors and ARBs are particularly valuable agents. The choice of agents often is dictated by the presence or absence of proteinuria (for which an ACEI or ARB is essential) or if edema is present (for which a diuretic is needed). In patients with proteinuric CKD, ACEI and ARB are first-line agents, irrespective of race.[2] Second-line agents include diuretics and non-dihydropyridine CCB (as they reduce proteinuria), although a diuretic is preferred in the setting of edema. In the absence of proteinuria, diuretics are preferred first-line agents, and these can be followed by dihydropyridine CCB and angiotensin blockers in patients with edema; in the absence of edema, ACEI/ARB or CCB can be used first.[7]

PLAN FOR DISCHARGE THERAPY

Once discharged from the CCU, the patient must take seriously the importance of secondary prevention, of which BP control is an important component.

Lifestyle modifications that have been associated with favorable results in hypertensive patients include weight loss, increased physical activity, smoking cessation, and a low-fat, low-sodium diet. Tightly controlled dietary modification, as in the Dietary Approaches to Stop Hypertension (DASH) study, for example, can reduce mean SBP by 3.0, 6.2, and 6.8 mm Hg in subjects on a low-, intermediate-, and high-sodium-intake diet, respectively. Weight loss, reduced sodium intake, moderation of alcohol consumption, exercise, and an overall healthy dietary pattern are entirely appropriate for patients aiming to control HTN.

Oftentimes, pharmacologic treatment is necessary to control BP, especially for patients discharged from the CCU. The most important question to ask when selecting the initial drug treatment is, which class of drug will deliver the most effective BP lowering for this patient? As mentioned, certain medications have beneficial effects for certain disease states that go beyond the medication's BP-lowering effects (β-blockers for HF). However, it must be emphasized that BP lowering is in itself a driver of benefit. In other words, regardless of the drug used, the goal should be to, lower BP. The response to different classes of drugs is similar when compared head-to-head in heterogeneous populations. However, individual responses can differ strikingly.

REFERENCES

1. Institute of Medicine (US) Committee on Public Health Priorities to Reduce and Control Hypertension. *A Population-Based Policy and Systems Change Approach to Prevent and Control Hypertension.* Washington, DC: The National Academies Press; 2010.

2. James PA, Oparil S, Carter BL, et al. Evidence-based guideline for the management of high blood pressure in adults. *JAMA.* 2013;1097(5):1-14. doi:10.1001/jama.2013.284427.

3. Mancia G, Fagard R, Narkiewicz K, et al. 2013 ESH/ESC guidelines for the management of arterial hypertension: the task force for the management of arterial hypertension of the European Society of Hypertension (ESH) and of the European Society of Cardiology (ESC). *Eur Heart J.* 2013;34(28):2159-2219. doi:10.1093/eurheartj/eht151.

4. Cushman WC, Evans GW, Byington RP, et al; ACCORD Study Group. Effects of Intensive Blood-Pressure Control in Type 2 Diabetes Mellitus. *N Engl J Med.* 2010;362(17):1575-1585. doi:10.1056/NEJMoa1001286.

5. Wright JT Jr, Williamson JD, Whelton PK, et al; SPRINT Research Group. A randomized trial of intensive versus standard blood-pressure control. *N Engl J Med.* 2015;373(22):2103-2116. doi:10.1056/NEJMoa1511939.

6. ALLHAT Officers and Coordinators for the ALLHAT Collaborative Research Group; The Antihypertensive and Lipid-Lowering Treatment to Prevent Heart Attack Trial. Major outcomes in high-risk hypertensive patients randomized to or calcium channel blocker vs diuretic. *JAMA.* 2002;288(23):2981-2997. doi:10.1001/jama.288.23.2981.

7. Jamerson K, Weber MA, Bakris GL, et al; ACCOMPLISH Trial Investigators. Benazepril plus amlodipine or hydrochlorothiazide for hypertension in high-risk patients. *N Engl J Med.* 2008;359(23):2417-2428. doi:10.1056/NEJMoa0810625.

8. Williams B, Macdonald TM, Morant S, et al; British Hypertension Society's PATHWAY Studies Group. Spironolactone versus placebo, bisoprolol, and doxazosin to determine the optimal treatment for drug-resistant hypertension (PATHWAY-2): a randomised, double-blind, crossover trial. *Lancet.* 2015;386(10008):2059-2068. doi:10.1016/S0140-6736(15)00257-3.

9. MRC Working Party. Medical Research Council trial of treatment of hypertension in older adults: principal results. *BMJ.* 1992;304(6824):405-412. doi:10.1136/bmj.304.6824.405.

10. Messerli FH, Bangalore S, Julius S. Risk/benefit assessment of beta-blockers and diuretics precludes their use for first-line therapy in hypertension. *Circulation.* 2008;117(20):2706.

11. Wiysonge CSU, Bradley HA, Mayosi BM, et al. Beta-blockers for hypertension (Review). *Cochrane Database Syst Rev.* 2012;(11). doi:10.1002/14651858.CD002003.pub2.

12. Khan N, McAlister FA. Re-examining the efficacy of beta-blockers for the treatment of hypertension: a meta-analysis. *CMAJ.* 2006;174(12):1737-1742. doi:10.1503/cmaj.060110.

13. Amenta F, Lanari A, Mignini F, Silvestrelli G, Traini E, Tomassoni D. Nicardipine use in cerebrovascular disease: a review of controlled clinical studies. *J Neurol Sci.* 2009;283(1-2):219-223. doi:10.1016/j.jns.2009.02.335.

14. Aronson S, Dyke CM, Stierer KA, et al. The ECLIPSE trials: Comparative studies of clevidipine to nitroglycerin, sodium nitroprusside, and nicardipine for acute hypertension treatment in cardiac surgery patients. *Anesth Analg.* 2008;107(4):1110-1121. doi:10.1213/ane.0b013e31818240db.

15. Wagenaar LJ, Voors AA, Buikema H, van Gilst WH. Angiotensin receptors in the cardiovascular system. *Can J Cardiol.* 2002;18(12):1331-1339.

16. Levick SP, Meléndez GC, Plante E, McLarty JL, Brower GL, Janicki JS. Cardiac mast cells: the centrepiece in adverse myocardial remodelling. *Cardiovasc Res.* 2011;89(1):12-19. doi:10.1093/cvr/cvq272.

17. National Center for Health Statistics. *Health, United States, 2015 with Special Feature on Racial and Ethnic Health Disparities.* Hyattsville, MD: National Center for Health Statistics (US); 2016:1-461.

18. Vemmos KN, Spengos K, Tsivgoulis G, et al. Factors influencing acute blood pressure values in stroke subtypes. *J Hum Hypertens.* 2004;18(4):253-259. doi:10.1038/sj.jhh.1001662.

19. Johnston KC, Mayer SA. Blood pressure reduction in ischemic stroke. *Neurology.* 2003;61:1030-1031.

20. Anderson CS, Heeley E, Huang Y, et al; INTERACT2 Investigators. Rapid blood-pressure lowering in patients with acute intracerebral hemorrhage. *N Engl J Med.* 2013;368(25):2355-2365. doi:10.1056/NEJMoa1214609.

21. Qureshi AI, Palesch YY, Barsan WG, et al. Intensive blood-pressure lowering in patients with acute cerebral hemorrhage. *N Engl J Med.* 2016;375(11):1033-1043. doi:10.1056/NEJMoa1603460.

22. Anderson CS, Huang Y, Arima H, et al. Effects of early intensive blood pressure-lowering treatment on the growth of hematoma and perihematomal edema in acute intracerebral hemorrhage: the Intensive Blood Pressure Reduction in Acute Cerebral Haemorrhage Trial (INTERACT). *Stroke.* 2010;41(2):307-312. doi:10.1161/STROKEAHA.109.561795.

23. Hemphill JC, Greenberg SM, Anderson CS, et al. Guidelines for the management of spontaneous intracerebral hemorrhage: a guideline for healthcare professionals from the American Heart Association/American Stroke Association. 2015;46:2032-2060. doi:10.1161/STR.0000000000000069.

24. Jauch EC, Saver JL, Adams HP, et al. Guidelines for the early management of patients with acute ischemic stroke: a guideline for healthcare professionals from the American Heart Association/American Stroke Association. *Stroke.* 2013;44(3):870-947. doi:10.1161/STR.0b013e318284056a.

25. Turan TN, Cotsonis G, Lynn MJ, Chaturvedi S, Chimowitz M; Warfarin-Aspirin Symptomatic Intracranial Disease (WASID) Trial Investigators. Relationship between blood pressure and stroke recurrence in patients with intracranial arterial stenosis. *Circulation.* 2007;115(23):2969-2975. doi:10.1161/CIRCULATIONAHA.106.622464.

26. Biffi A, Anderson CD, Battey TWK, et al. Association Between Blood Pressure Control and Risk of Recurrent Intracerebral Hemorrhage. *JAMA.* 2015;314(9):904-912. doi:10.1001/jama.2015.10082.

27. Feigl EO. Coronary Physiology. *Physiol Rev.* 1983;63(1):1-205.

28. Franklin SS, Gustin W IV, Wong ND, et al. Hemodynamic patterns of age-related changes in blood pressure. *Circulation.* 1997;96(1):308-315. http://circ.ahajournals.org/content/96/1/308.abstract.

29. Oparil S, Zaman MA, Calhoun DA. Pathogenesis of hypertension. *Ann Intern Med.* 2003;(139):761-776.

30. Rosendorff C, Lackland DT, Allison M, et al; on behalf of the American Heart Association, American College of Cardiology, and American Society of Hypertension. Treatment of hypertension in patients with coronary artery disease: a scientific statement from the American Heart Association, American College of Cardiology, and

American Society of Hypertension. 2015;65:1372-1407. doi:10.1161/HYP.0000000000000018.

31. Packer M, O'Connor CM, Ghali JK, et al. Effect of amlodipine on morbidity and mortality in severe chronic heart failure. Prospective Randomized Amlodipine Survival Evaluation Study Group. *N Engl J Med.* 1996;335:1107-1114.

32. Yancy CW, Jessup M, Bozkurt B, et al; American Heart Association Task Force on Practice Guidelines. 2013 ACCF/AHA guideline for the management of heart failure: a report of the American College of Cardiology Foundation/American Heart Association Task Force on Practice Guidelines. *J Am Coll Cardiol.* 2013;62(16):e147-e239. doi:10.1016/j.jacc.2013.05.019.

33. Tang WHW, Mullens W. Cardiorenal syndrome in decompensated heart failure. *Heart.* 2010;96(4):255-260. doi:10.1136/hrt.2009.166256.

34. Murphy MB, Murray C, Shorten GD. Fenoldopam: a selective peripheral dopamine-receptor agonist for the treatment of severe hypertension. *N Engl J Med.* 2002;345(21):1548-1557. doi:10.1056/NEJMra020676.

Patient and Family Information for: HYPERTENSION IN THE CARDIAC CARE UNIT

CARDIOVASCULAR SYSTEM AND HYPERTENSION

The cardiovascular system serves to propel and transport blood, which carries the elements necessary for healthy functioning of all the organs of the body. Oxygen, glucose, electrolytes, immune cells, clotting cells, and a variety of other blood components must travel to every part of the body.

The cardiovascular system is sometimes compared to a water system with a pump and water pipes. It is a closed system, in that the system is self-contained; there are no openings to the outside. All the blood that starts in the heart returns to the heart (unless, of course, there is damage to the system, as in a tear to a vessel that results in internal or external bleeding). The pipes that leave the pump are largest because they must bear the greatest volumes and pressures. The pipes let off more and more branches as they get farther from the source and therefore get smaller and thinner. The vessels that leave the heart are arteries that feed capillaries before the blood makes its way back to the heart in veins.

BP is an index of the force per unit area inside the arteries. Factors that influence BP are the rate of blood flow through the vessel and the flexibility of the blood vessel wall. The rate of blood flow ejected from the heart through the arteries and veins per minute (cardiac output) depends on the number of heart beats per minute (heart rate) and the amount of blood ejected per beat (stroke volume). The flexibility or resistance of blood vessel walls depends on many factors including age, the nervous system, and hormones. In summary, the heart pump and its cardiac output along with the blood vessels and their resistance are what determine a person's BP. This is important because it serves as the basis for understanding how such factors as age, medications, and lifestyle influence our BP.

The medical term for high BP is HTN. HTN is defined as a BP of 140/90 mm Hg or above. The first number represents the SBP; the second is the DBP. As mentioned, the heart beats to propel blood, and does so, on average, between 60 and 80 times/min. When the heart ejects blood, the pressure in the arteries goes up because the pressure generated in the heart's largest chamber is transmitted throughout the closed cardiovascular system and there is a surge in the rate of blood flow through the arteries; this yields the SBP. After the heart muscle contracts, it must relax to prepare for the next contraction and in so doing allows for blood, which returns through veins, to refill the chambers of the heart. This yields the DBP: the pressure in the arteries during the heart muscle's relaxation phase.

CCU AND HYPERTENSION

The CCU is where patients go when they are too sick to be adequately managed on a general hospital floor. The patient in the CCU needs more specialized care and to this end is managed by nurses and doctors with specialized training in critical care and cardiovascular medicine. The nurses are responsible for fewer patients than on a general floor, and thus are able to dedicate a greater level of attention to each patient. The team of doctors assigned to the CCU remains in that unit throughout the day, rather than moving throughout the hospital.

Patients can be admitted to the CCU for a variety of conditions, such as heart attack, HF, tears in the aorta (the major artery that leaves the heart), and very high BP. BP is an important component of every disease condition that warrants a CCU admission. In some cases, BP can be dangerously high; in others dangerously low. In some cases, aberration in BP (too high or too low) is the source of the problem (hypertensive emergency causing HF), whereas in others it is the result of the problem (heart attack causing dangerously low BP). Regardless, BP is something the CCU doctor must manage for every patient, and something the patient must be educated about and take seriously, both for the short term and for the long term.

DRUGS

Surely, patients and their families have heard doctors use an overwhelming number of names of drugs. Not only are there a seemingly endless number of medications but also every medication has at least two names, a generic name and a brand name (ie, metoprolol is also Lopressor and Toprol). It makes things simpler to think of drugs in terms of drug classes. This is how doctors think, and for good reason. Drugs that make up a drug class perform a similar function via a similar mechanism. β-Blockers, for example, help block activity of the β-receptor, found on the surface of many cells, including those of the heart and blood vessels. β-Blockers are very important in the treatment of HF and HTN (among other things). Furthermore, most drugs in a class have a similar-sounding generic name. β-Blockers, for example, end in "lol" (ie, metoprolol, carvedilol, atenolol). So, for example, one remembers the β-blockers as the "-lol" drugs, which are used to treat HF. ACEIs are the "-pril" drugs (ie, lisinopril, captopril, enalapril) most commonly used to treat HTN, HF, and kidney disease. A drug class that is similar to the ACEIs is the ARB family, or "-artan" drugs (ie, irbesartan, candesartan, losartan). These drugs have clinical indications similar to those of the ACE inhibitors, and have the benefit of a lesser likelihood of causing cough as an adverse effect. The CCBs can be subdivided into the dihydropyridne and non-dihydropyridines. The dihydropyridine CCBs are commonly used BP medicines, and can be remembered as the "-dipine" drugs (ie, amlodipine, nicardipine, nifedipine). The α-blocker medicines mediate their BP-reducing effects by blocking a receptor on blood vessels responsible for vessel constriction (as the vessel diameter gets smaller, the pressure within the vessel increases). These "-osin" (ie, tamsulosin, terazosin, doxazosin) medicines have a second use in relieving the symptoms of urinary frequency, hesitancy, and urgency associated with benign prostatic hyperplasia, or BPH. Thinking in terms of classes of medicines, which conveniently tend to have similar-sounding and thus easier-to-remember names, is much easier and more intuitive than remembering individual drugs.

HYPERTENSION AND ITS ROLE IN THE COMMON CCU DISEASE PROCESSES

As mentioned, patients are admitted to the CCU for a variety of conditions, most, if not all, of which have HTN as a significant consideration, either as cause, effect, or important comorbidity.

HYPERTENSION AND DISEASES OF THE AORTA

The aorta is the largest artery of the body. Because it is the first vessel that blood travels through once it leaves the heart, within it travels all of the blood that leaves the heart. All other vessels are branches of a larger vessel and therefore will only receive a fraction of the cardiac output (blood leaving the heart per minute), whereas the aorta must withstand the volume and pressure of the entire cardiac output. It is no surprise, then, that the aorta is the largest, thickest-walled blood vessel in the body. One can imagine that diseases of the aorta are potentially catastrophic; for example, a ruptured vessel in the finger will cause that vessel to spill its fraction of cardiac output, whereas a rupture of the aorta will lead to rapid loss of a huge proportion of the body's blood. Motor vehicle accidents, for example, in which the passenger is propelled forward, and then held back by a seat belt, can cause the aorta to tear, leading to immediate death.

Patients admitted to the CCU for disease of the aorta often have an acute aortic syndrome, subdivided into three conditions: aortic dissection, intramural hematoma, and aortic ulcer. An aortic dissection is a tear in the innermost lining of the aorta; an intramural hematoma is a pooling of blood in the wall of the aorta without any tear in the lining of the vessel; an aortic ulcer occurs when a plaque in the inner lining of the vessel leads to erosion of the inner part of the vessel wall and swelling of the vessel contained by the outermost lining of the wall. Patients with any of the acute aortic syndromes will usually feel sudden onset, severe, "ripping" or "tearing" pain that often feels like it goes through the chest and into the back.

Aortic dissection is a tear in the innermost lining of the aorta such that blood begins infiltrating the wall of the vessel. The problem is that this infiltrating blood pushes the inner lining into the pathway of oncoming blood, leading to obstruction to flow and an expansion of the tear. If the tear is in the first "ascending" part of the aorta, the patient needs surgery; if the tear is in the "descending" aorta, the management is medical and not surgical. Aortic dissection may be a consideration for a patient who presents with chest pain, especially patients who smoke and/or have HTN. Aortic dissection can easily be confused with heart attack; this is important because not only are the treatments different but certain treatments for heart attack, for example, clot breaking medication, can be harmful for a patient with aortic dissection.

High BP is the major risk factor for both types of aortic dissection, and BP is also the major target of medical treatment. Precipitous reductions in BP can sometimes be dangerous in other conditions such as ischemic stroke, but in the case of acute aortic dissection, the physician can and should be aggressive in lowering BP. BP reduction helps prevent extension of the tear, which could lead to stroke, cardiac tamponade, or other major complications. Every time the heart beats, a surge of blood exerts a force against the vessel wall, forcing blood into the tear and potentially causing the tear to enlarge and extend. β-Blockers, the "-lol" drugs, are often used because they lower not only BP but also the heart rate. IV β-Blockers such as labetalol are used for rapid BP and heart rate reduction to a target of under 120 mm Hg BP and under 60 beats/min heart rate, or as low as tolerated by the patient (lowering heart rate or BP too much can lead to such symptoms as dizziness). The patient is sent to the CCU to continuously monitor heart rate and BP in response to IV medication and also to monitor electrocardiogram readings in case the dissection leads to complications. Once BP is controlled, the patient can be switched to oral medications. The patient must understand the importance of compliance with medical and lifestyle recommendations to prevent future complications of aortic dissection.

HYPERTENSION AND ACUTE NEUROLOGIC SYNDROME

Patients may often be admitted to the CCU for stroke or hypertensive encephalopathy. Stroke, or cerebrovascular accident, is due to decreased oxygenated blood supply to the brain. A heart attack is death of heart muscle due to decreased blood flow to the heart, whereas stroke is death of brain cells due to impaired blood flow to the brain. If blood flow is restored before cell death occurs, brain function may recover completely; this condition is referred to as a TIA or transient ischemic attack. Stroke can be thought of as coming in two forms: stroke due to a blockage (ischemic stroke) versus bleeding (hemorrhagic stroke) of an artery supplying the brain. The end result, brain cell death, is similar for both. In addition, stroke may increase pressure in the skull and thus cause compression of surrounding healthy brain tissue because of edema or swelling in ischemic stroke and accumulation of blood in hemorrhagic stroke. In hypertensive encephalopathy, on the other hand, severe HTN causes not localized brain ischemia but rather global brain dysfunction with its associated symptoms. As a result, patients suffering from stroke often have focal neurologic deficits (weakness in a limb, slurring of speech, facial drooping), whereas patients with hypertensive encephalopathy lack focal symptoms and present instead with nausea, blurry vision, headache, and/or altered consciousness.

The first step in the assessment of a patient with suspected neurologic syndrome is a head CT scan to evaluate for bleeding in the skull. CT scans are effective for detecting blood, and although not necessarily helpful in the diagnosis of hypertensive encephalopathy or early ischemic stroke, a CT scan is the first test because an intracranial bleed, if found, might require immediate neurosurgery.

HTN is a major risk factor for acute neurologic syndrome, and a major target of therapy. For hemorrhagic stroke, BP must be lowered promptly but not to such an extent that arterial pressure becomes inadequate to sufficiently overcome intracranial pressure; cerebral perfusion pressure, or the net BP gradient responsible for blood flow to healthy brain tissue, depends on adequate arterial pressure. Generally, the BP goal is 140 mm Hg for SBP. For ischemic stroke, it has been commonly accepted in the medical community that aggressive lowering of BP may do more harm than good. On the other hand, high BP increases the risk of expansion of edema and/or conversion of an ischemic stroke into a hemorrhagic one. Many patients have spontaneous declines in BP during the first 24 hours of stroke onset. In general, the BP goals for patients with ischemic strokes are different depending on whether interventions involving "clot busters" called "thrombolytics" are undertaken to reestablish blood flow in the blocked artery. When thrombolytic therapy is undertaken, lower BP targets are aimed for during and after the procedure (around 180/105 mm Hg). When thrombolytics are not used, no treatment is required when BP is less than 220/120 mm Hg. In 2013, an expert panel reiterated these recommendations.

For hypertensive encephalopathy, the baseline BP must be taken into consideration to avoid excessive BP lowering and to prevent cerebral ischemia. Lowering the mean pressure by 10% to 15% in the first hour and by 25% over 1 day is usually safe.

HYPERTENSION AND ACUTE CORONARY SYNDROME

An ACS is a decreased blood supply to the heart (myocardial cell ischemia) that may or may not result in myocardial cell injury or death and that is due to CAD. The three forms of ACS are unstable angina, non-STEMI, and STEMI. These three entities are manifestations of the same disease process and were extensively discussed in Section A of this book.

The heart is thought of as the organ that supplies blood to the rest of the body; in fact, the heart supplies blood to the rest of the body and to itself. It does so through vessels known as coronary arteries, which come off the aorta immediately after the blood leaves the heart. There are three large coronary arteries that travel along the surface of the heart before diving deep to feed all the cells of the heart muscle. A blockage to flow in any of the coronary arteries can cut off supply enough to starve cells and lead to their death. If cells of a certain portion of the heart fail to beat adequately, the heart may not generate enough force to sustain cardiac output. A heart attack, or MI, may cause the heart to stop beating effectively (HF), or stop beating altogether (sudden cardiac death). HTN is considered a major risk factor for CAD, and thus for MI and HF.

The key concept to understand regarding coronary blood supply is that of supply and demand. The heart is unique in that it is responsible for both its supply and demand. As the heart beats harder, it supplies more blood flow, but it also demands more blood flow. HTN affects demand: higher BP forces the heart to beat harder, thus increasing the heart's demand for blood. A 70% blockage may still allow the necessary blood supply to the normotensive patient's heart, but for the hypertensive patient's more demanding heart, a 70% blockage may result in chest pain or, worse, myocardial cell damage. HTN also affects supply: higher BP leads to the development of the blockages themselves. Through mechanisms, many still to be completely understood, HTN promotes atherogenesis, or the development of plaques within the inner lining of arteries such as the coronary arteries. Not only do plaques make passageways for blood flow narrower over time but they can also rupture, releasing contents that can immediately clot and completely block blood flow. This plaque rupture is what usually causes devastating MIs.

Initial therapy of HTN in patients presenting to the CCU with an ACS should use medications that improve myocardial supply, lessen demand, or both. β-Blockers, for example, not only lower BP but they also lower the heart rate, and thus lessen the amount of energy the heart expends and the amount of blood flow it demands. Nitrates lower BP, but they also lessen the amount of blood returning to the heart, thus lessening the volume of blood the heart must pump per beat, which also lessens demand.

Nitrates and β-blockers are often first-line BP medications in patients with ACS. One exception is in the patient whose heart is so damaged that lowering the heart rate may further lessen cardiac output; in this situation, β-blockers should not be used. ACEIs and ARBs can also be used to lower BP.

Target BP is 140/90 mm Hg. DBP should not be lowered too significantly because it is the diastolic pressure that provides the force to send blood through the coronary arteries; too low a DBP may be harmful.

Upon discharge, the patient who has suffered a heart attack should be on a β-blocker and ACEI if possible. These medications lower BP and help the heart preserve or even regain function.

HYPERTENSION AND HEART FAILURE

The heart, as described, is a pump that allows for blood to be propelled throughout the cardiovascular system of blood vessels. To effectively perform this task, the heart must fill with an adequate volume of blood, pass this blood between each of its four chambers, and have sufficient muscle strength to eject blood against a significant resistance in the aorta to the entire body.

Chambers divide the heart into a right (right atrium and right ventricle) and left (left atrium and left ventricle) side. When blood returns to the heart through veins, it passes through the right atrium and ventricle before passing through the lungs to pick up oxygen and then passes to the left atrium and ventricle, where sufficient pressure is generated to propel blood to the entire body. The left ventricle is the heart's strongest and largest chamber.

HF is failure of the heart to propel blood, whether because the muscle is weak or because the heart does not fill adequately, such that either cardiac output is insufficient to meet the demands of the body's tissues or these demands are met at the expense of blood "backing up" in the direction of the lungs. In other words, HF can be due to poor forward flow or adequate forward flow but with concomitant inappropriate backward flow.

HF can be due to a multitude of abnormalities: ischemia such as in the form of a heart attack; damaged valves; drugs such as alcohol or certain chemotherapies; and, of course, HTN are among the many possible causes of HF.

HTN forces the heart to pump harder to overcome the greater resistance to forward flow, and over time the heart muscle starts to fail; it may become stiff or weak or both, resulting in forward and/or backward flow failure.

Acute HF is one of the most common reasons for admission to the CCU. A patient may have already been diagnosed with HF, and for some reason (not taking medications, not adhering to a dietary regimen, an irregular heart rhythm, a heart attack, uncontrolled BP) suffer an insult that disrupts the delicate balance and throws the patient into acutely symptomatic HF. It is also possible that a patient admitted to the CCU with HF never had any symptoms of HF. A previously adequately functioning heart may go into failure because of a heart attack, or severe damage to a heart valve, or severe HTN. A heart that is accustomed to beating against a BP of 120/80 mm Hg may fail to overcome a sudden burden of 220/120 mm Hg, or a heart that is forced to beat against a pressure of 150/100 mm Hg for years and years may do well in the beginning but with time, stretch and thicken and eventually decompensate. Regardless of the scenario, to treat HTN is to relieve the burden against which the failing heart is struggling to pump.

HTN is a common cause of HF; about 75% of patients admitted with HF have HTN. HTN is also a major target of therapy for HF. In fact, the medications that treat HF—β-blockers ("-lol" meds), ACEIs ("pril" meds), ARBs ("-artan" meds), and diuretics or water pills—also have effects on BP.

The initial urgent step is to stabilize the patient. A doctor will aim to reduce BP, ultimately to 140/90 mm Hg or lower, although not too quickly as to potentially starve certain tissues of adequate blood supply. Once the patient is stabilized, tight BP control becomes a fundamental component of long-term care. The patient with HF can easily decompensate again if he or she has a drinking binge, or salty-food binge, or skips a couple of days' doses of medicines. Managing HTN must be emphasized as crucial for preventing future decompensations and giving the heart the best chance of recovering over time.

HYPERTENSION AND RENAL FAILURE

The kidneys filter blood; they excrete much of what is not needed and retain much of what is needed. They also help maintain total body water and electrolyte (sodium, potassium, calcium, etc.) concentrations within a rather narrow healthy range. When a person becomes dehydrated, the kidneys are able to retain fluid and reduce urine output dramatically; if a person were to drink excessively, the kidneys could excrete liters and liters of free water daily. The elegant and delicate mechanism that allows such regulation involves an intricate series of blood vessels and kidney tubules and electrolyte channels; this delicate structure can be disrupted when forced to withstand the forces of high BP over many years.

Renal failure can be acute or chronic; in other words, it can develop over hours to days often with obvious symptoms, or it can develop slowly often without symptoms for several years after kidney damage first begins. HTN can cause both acute and chronic kidney damage. In fact, HTN is the second leading cause of CKD, after diabetes. Renal failure can be a reason for admission to the CCU (when due to hypertensive emergency), but more likely, it is a common complication of another disease process that warrants admission to the CCU.

Hypertensive emergency is defined as BP high enough (often DBP above 120 mm Hg) to cause end-organ damage. "End organs" most commonly affected by extremely high BP are the brain, heart, and kidneys. The high BP damages the delicate system of arteries feeding the kidney and disrupts the filtering mechanism, leading to such symptoms as decreased urine output, nausea, swelling in the legs, and generalized malaise. The goal in management of acute renal failure due to severe HTN is to limit further renal damage through BP control. The choice of optimal drug therapy is controversial. Although nitroprusside is the drug with the longest track record, it does have potential cyanide and thiocyanate toxicity, especially with prolonged infusions of high doses of nitroprusside. Fenoldopam is another useful IV agent. Other antihypertensive drugs that preserve renal blood flow are CCBs and adrenergic blocking agents.

It is worth mentioning that kidney damage is not only a consequence of HTN but also a cause of HTN. Patients with CKD, especially those on dialysis, are at very high risk for having HTN.

As mentioned, although kidney disease due to hypertensive emergency is a cause for CCU admission, more commonly a patient in the CCU for some other reason (heart attack, HF) develops renal failure concomitantly because the heart attack or HF, for example, led to decreased blood supply to the kidneys. The renal failure makes more complicated the treatment of heart disease and becomes in itself an important target of treatment. For example, diuretics, often referred to as "water pills," are critical for HF treatment. A patient in the CCU with HF is often "volume-overloaded," sometimes as much as 20 or 30 pounds heavier than usual because of water retention. The goal is to remove this water, but (1) this fluid removal can damage the kidneys, and (2) kidney damage coupled with the low output state of HF can make the fluid removal difficult. The kidney damage, at least partly brought on by the HF and/or its treatment, has made treatment of the HF more difficult. In recent years, some doctors have used the term "cardiorenal syndrome" precisely to emphasize how strongly linked are the kidney and the heart, in that function and treatment of one very often affects function and treatment of the other.

In summary, kidney damage can be a reason for CCU admission, as in the case of hypertensive emergency, but more often, kidney damage is related secondarily to, and complicates treatment of, the primary disease process that necessitated CCU admission. Good management of HTN can help preserve both kidney and cardiovascular health. When the patient with kidney damage recovers and leaves the hospital, BP control is of paramount importance.

Rodolfo J. Galindo
Mario Rodriguez Rivera
Seyed Hamed Hosseini Dehkordi
Eyal Herzog
Jeanine Albu

54

Diabetes Mellitus in the Cardiac Care Unit

INTRODUCTION

Diabetes mellitus (DM) is a complex chronic condition, with heterogeneous clinical presentation and disease progression, depending on the type of diabetes and its underlying pathophysiology. However, the defining feature of diabetes is an inappropriate elevation of blood glucose (BG), known as hyperglycemia, regardless of the underlying pathophysiologic disorder. Persistent chronic hyperglycemia leads to tissue injury resulting in micro- and macrovascular complications, such as neuropathy, retinopathy, nephropathy, and cardiovascular diseases (CVDs).

In the initial part of this chapter, we discuss the diagnostic and classification criteria of DM and general principles of care in patients with diabetes; in the latter part we focus on diabetes management in the CCU setting and discuss epidemiologic studies of patients admitted to the CCU with diabetes, outcomes in patients with hyperglycemia admitted to the CCU,

and an overview of strategies for hyperglycemia management in the CCU.

DIABETES MELLITUS: GENERAL PRINCIPLES

WHAT IS DIABETES MELLITUS? DIAGNOSIS AND CLASSIFICATION

The defining feature of DM is an inappropriate elevation of BG—hyperglycemia. This could be due to excessive glucose production, impaired glucose clearance, or both. Sustained, chronic hyperglycemia, over several years, leads to tissue injury resulting in chronic micro- and macrovascular complications such as diabetic neuropathy, retinopathy, and nephropathy and atherothrombotic vascular diseases. "Inappropriate" hyperglycemia has been defined by experts as the level which, if chronically sustained, will lead to the development of diabetic complications.

TABLE 54.1	Diagnosis of Diabetes Mellitus

CRITERIA FOR THE DIAGNOSIS OF DIABETES

1. $A_{1C} \geq 6.5\%$. The test should be performed in a laboratory using a method that is NGSP certified and standardized to the DCCT assay (http://www.ngsp.org, accessed January 2, 2017)[a]

   OR

2. FPG $\geq$ 126 mg/dL (7.0 mmol/L). Fasting is defined as no caloric intake for at least 8 h[a]

   OR

3. Two-hour plasma glucose $\geq$ 200 mg/dL (11. 1 mmol/L) during an OGTT. The test should be performed as described by the World Health Organization, using a glucose load containing the equivalent of 75 g anhydrous glucose dissolved in water[a]

   OR

4. In a patient with classic symptoms of hyperglycemia or hyperglycemic crisis, a random plasma glucose $\geq$ 200 mg/dL (11. 1 mmol/L)

CATEGORIES OF INCREASED RISK FOR DIABETES (PREDIABETES)[b]

1. FPG 100–125 mg/dL (5.6–6.9 mmol/L) [IFG]
2. Two-hour plasma glucose in the 75-g OGTT 140–199 mg/dL (7.8–11.0 mmol/L) [IGT]
3. A_{1C} 5.7%–6.4%

[a]In the absence of unequivocal hyperglycemia, criteria 1–3 should be confirmed by repeat testing.
[b]For all three tests, risk is continuous, extending below the lower limit of the range and becoming disproportionately greater at higher ends of the range.
Adapted from American Diabetes Association. Classification and diagnosis of diabetes. Sec. 2. In Standards of Medical Care in Diabetes 2017. Diabetes Care 2017;40(Suppl. 1):S11–S24.
NGSP: National Glycohemoglobin Standardization Program, DCCT: Diabetes Control and Complications Trial, FPG: Fasting plasma glucose, OGTT: Oral glucose tolerance test
IFG, impaired fasting glucose; IGT, impaired glucose tolerance.

TABLE 54.2	Classification of Diabetes Mellitus
Type 1 Diabetes	
• Due to autoimmune β-cell destruction, usually leading to absolute insulin deficiency	
Type 2 Diabetes	
• Due to a progressive loss of β-cell insulin secretion frequently on the background of insulin resistance	
Gestational Diabetes	
• Diabetes diagnosed in the second or third trimester of pregnancy that was not clearly overt diabetes prior to gestation.	
Other Specific Types	
• Monogenic diabetes syndromes • Neonatal diabetes • Maturity-onset diabetes of the young (MODY) • Diseases of the exocrine pancreas (cystic fibrosis, etc.) • Drug- or chemical-induced diabetes (treatment of HIV/AIDS, glucocorticoids, treatment after organ transplantation)	

Adapted from: American Diabetes Association. Classification and diagnosis of diabetes. Sec. 2. In Standards of Medical Care in Diabetes 2017. Diabetes Care 2017;40(Suppl. 1):S11–S24

The current criteria used to make the diagnosis of DM are listed in **Table 54.1**. According to the American Diabetes Association (ADA) 2011 criteria, either random plasma glucose, fasting plasma glucose, an oral glucose tolerance test, or a hemoglobin A_{1C} (% glycosylated hemoglobin, A_{1C}) can be used to diagnose diabetes.[1]

DM is currently classified by etiology as type 1, type 2, gestational, or other specified types (**Table 54.2**). Type 1 diabetes is characterized by an absolute or severe insulin deficiency and is immune mediated. Type 2 diabetes is a complex polygenic disease characterized by both insulin resistance and relative insulin deficiency, that is, insulin levels and secretion are inappropriate to the levels of insulin resistance and out of proportion to the glucose stimuli (dual defect).[2] Gestational DM is characterized by onset during pregnancy owing to increased insulin resistance generated by the hormonal milieu. Typically, it resolves at the end of pregnancy; however, women with gestational diabetes are at higher risk for developing type 2 diabetes later in life.[3] Other specific types of diabetes listed by etiology are a result of genetic defects in β-cell function and/or insulin action (monogenic diabetes), exocrine pancreatic disease, some endocrinopathies, drug or chemically induced (exogenous corticosteroid administration, etc.), or other rare forms (infections, immune mediated, etc.). These specific forms could manifest clinically in a manner similar to either type 1 or type 2 diabetes.

Type 1 Diabetes

Certain clinical aspects of diabetes presentation are characteristic of type 1 diabetes: diabetic ketoacidosis (DKA); signs of insulin deficiency such as weight loss and/or BG level above 250 mg/dL accompanied by non–fasting positive urine ketones; acute onset in a child or young adult; triggered by recent infection or viral illness; onset during puberty or association with other autoimmune diseases (thyroiditis, Graves disease, pernicious anemia, celiac, and Addison disease).

Type 2 Diabetes

The pathogenesis of type 2 diabetes is very different from that of type 1 diabetes. As opposed to type 1 diabetes, in type 2, insulin resistance is almost universally present, and the defect in

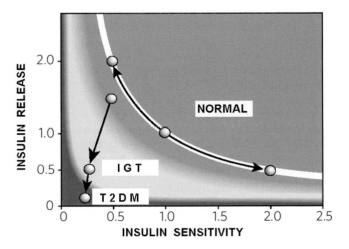

FIGURE 54.1 Relationship between insulin sensitivity and insulin release. DM, diabetes mellitus; IGT, impaired glucose tolerance.

insulin secretion is milder—just secretion is not high enough to overcome the resistance (β-cell dysfunction).

Prediabetes and Screening for Diabetes Mellitus

Type 2 diabetes is often preceded by a condition called prediabetes characterized by either abnormal fasting glucose levels (impaired fasting glucose or IFG) and/or impaired glucose tolerance (IGT, abnormal postprandial glucose), which leads to increased levels of A_{1C} (**Table 54.1**). During the prediabetes stage, there is a gradual increase in insulin resistance as a result of various causes (aging, obesity, physical inactivity, or genetics) which, when not accompanied by an increase in insulin secretion, will eventually result in elevated BG levels in the diabetic range (**Figure 54.1**). Prediabetes can be identified through the same tests used to diagnose diabetes (**Table 54.1**). It is now recommended that individuals at risk be screened for the presence of type 2 diabetes (**Table 54.3**).[1] During this screening, normal glucose tolerance, prediabetes, or full-blown diabetes can be

TABLE 54.3	**Criteria for Testing for Diabetes in Asymptomatic Adult Individuals**

1. Testing should be considered in all adults who are overweight (BMI ≥25 kg/m2 or ≥23 kg/m2 in Asian Americans) adults who have one or more of the following risk factors:

   A1C ≥ 5.7% (39 mmol/mol), IGT, or IFG on previous testing Physical inactivity

   First-degree relative with diabetes mellitus

   Members of a high-risk race/ethnicity (eg, African American, Latino, Native American, Asian American, Pacific Islander)

   Women who delivered a baby weighing >9 lb or were diagnosed with Gestational Diabetes Mellitus (GDM)

   Hypertension (140/90 mm Hg or on therapy for hypertension)

   HDL cholesterol level 250 mg/dL (2.82 mmol/L)

   Women with polycystic ovary syndrome (PCOS)

   Other clinical conditions associated with insulin resistance (eg, severe obesity, acanthosisnigricans)

   History of CVD

2. In the absence of the above mentioned criteria, testing for diabetes should begin at age 45 y

3. If results are normal, testing should be repeated at least at 3-y intervals, with consideration for more frequent testing depending on initial results and risk status

identified. The screening is very important because (a) preventive measures such as weight loss and/or increased physical activity and sometimes pharmacologic measures could prevent or delay the development of type 2 diabetes in the individuals with prediabetes and (b) early diagnosis and treatment of the clinical manifestation of type 2 diabetes could prevent chronic complications and improve chances of survival.

Metabolic Syndrome

Prediabetes and insulin resistance are integral parts of the so-called metabolic syndrome, which is defined as a clustering of risk factors that predict the development of both type 2 diabetes and CVD. More than 80% of patients with type 2 diabetes have metabolic syndrome and clustering of risk factors for CVD, which include hypertension, dyslipidemia, and associated inflammation and hypercoagulable state.[4] The clustering of these risk factors predicts the development of CVD independent of the degree of hyperglycemia. The treatment of the risk factors and the underlying pathophysiologic causes could prevent both diabetes and CVD. The most prominent underlying modifiable pathophysiologic causes are abdominal obesity and insulin resistance.[5] Inflammation and hypercoagulable states are also important factors to be addressed. The comprehensive treatment of the metabolic syndrome includes smoking cessation, assessment of diabetes risk and implementation of diabetes prevention strategies, control of blood pressure, control of glucose if type 2 diabetes is present, reduction of abdominal obesity, increase in physical activity to at least 30 minutes of activity daily (above usual), decrease in saturated fats to less than 7% of total calories, elimination of trans fat, addressing lipid levels such as low-density lipoprotein, triglycerides, and high-density lipoprotein cholesterol according to the 10-year calculated Framingham risk and eating five servings of fruits and vegetables per day.[6]

CLINICAL MANIFESTATIONS AND COMPLICATIONS OF DIABETES MELLITUS

Clinical manifestations of DM could be acute (DKA or hyperosmolar hyperglycemic state [HHS]) or chronic. The chronic complications manifest as microvascular (retinopathy, neuropathy, nephropathy) or macrovascular (cerebrovascular disease, coronary artery disease [CAD], peripheral vascular disease)

disease. Other complications are susceptibility to infections and connective tissue disorders. Positive correlations were found between glycemic control (as measured by the A_{1C} level) and prevalence and incidence of diabetic microvascular complications. Prospective randomized trials have shown that intensive control of BG significantly reduces the risk of microvascular complications in both type 1 and type 2 diabetes. The effect of tight glucose control on macrovascular complications in the absence of intensified control of other risk factors for macrovascular disease is presently controversial. It is known, however, that tight control of other CVD risk factors such as hypertension and elevated lipids does significantly reduce risk of fatal and nonfatal macrovascular events in both type 1 and type 2 diabetes patients. This reduction in risk was reported to be 20% to 50% with blood pressure control, 25% to 55% with lipid control, but only 10% to 20% with tight glucose control.[7] A comprehensive approach including tight glucose control and control of other CVD risk factors was reported to lower both micro- and macrovascular complications by 35%.[8] Unintended consequences and adverse effects of tight glucose control could be hypoglycemia, weight gain, and possible short-term worsening of proliferative retinopathy, especially and mostly when the patients require insulin, such as patients with type 1 or long-standing type 2 disease. Of particular concern is the effect of hypoglycemia on macrovascular event rates and outcomes.[7]

PHARMACOLOGIC TREATMENT OF HYPERGLYCEMIA: GENERAL PRINCIPLES IN THE OUTPATIENT SETTING

INSULIN: Patients with type 1 diabetes are always treated with insulin. In fact, one of the reasons it is very important to make the differentiation between type 1 and type 2 diabetes is to determine if there is a need for insulin at all times to avoid DKA. Patients with type 2 diabetes may also be requiring insulin for control of BG, although lack of insulin will not produce DKA except in rare cases. Insulin is used in type 2 patients when it is not possible to achieve glucose level goals with oral agents alone. Insulin treatment should be physiologic and anticipatory. That is, it should include long-acting (basal) insulin to suppress glucose production overnight and normalize fasting glucose and rapid-acting (prandial) insulin to cover meal-related glucose excursions. This physiologic concept is called the basal-bolus concept (**Figure 54.2**). Examples of different types of insulin and their peak action time and duration of action are shown in **Table 54.4**. Insulin delivered with a prefilled insulin pen, rather than from a bottle with a syringe and needle, is easier to accurately dose (**Figure 54.3A**). Similar principles, as described earlier, are used for continuous subcutaneous (SQ) insulin delivery systems utilizing an insulin pump (**Figure 54.3B**).

Oral Hypoglycemic Agents

These drugs lower glucose by several mechanisms: improve insulin resistance (sensitizers), improve insulin secretion (secretagogues), improve insulin secretion but also decrease glucagon and gastric emptying through modulation of incretin and gut hormone levels, and those which lower glucose by decreasing absorption in the gut or increase its excretion in the urine. The agents that improve insulin resistance are either biguanides (eg, metformin) or thiazolidinedione. They work through increasing insulin sensitivity in the liver, muscle, and adipose tissue. The secretagogues work directly on the β-cells (sulfonylureas, amino acid derivatives, and meglitinides). α-Glucosidase inhibitors decrease glucose absorption in the gut. Sodium-glucose co-transporter 2 inhibitors, the most recent class of oral hypoglycemic agents, reduce BG levels by increasing urinary glucose excretion. The drugs that work through modulating incretin levels (glucagon-like peptide or GLP-1 and others) are analogs of GLP-1 and dipeptidyl peptidase (DPP-4) inhibitors. DPP-4 inhibitors (eg, sitagliptin) enhance the effects of endogenous incretins by preventing their breakdown by DPP-4 as well as through other mechanisms. All these oral agents have potential side effects and have to be used with caution in hospitalized patients particularly when renal and hepatic failure are present, because they increase the risk of hypoglycemia. Combination treatments of different oral drug classes work well and are often used. Such combinations should be tried before insulin treatment is initiated. Insulin should

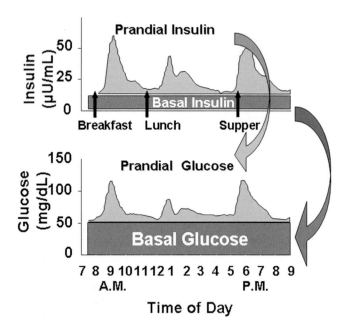

FIGURE 54.2 Physiologic insulin administration: the basal-bolus concept. The prandial insulin is 50% of the total daily dose administered before each meal to cover the prandial glucose excursions. The basal insulin is 50% of the total daily dose and controls fasting glucose by suppressing glucose production between meals and overnight. (Adapted from the Society for Hospital Medicine Glycemic Control Task Force presentation at www.hospitalmedicine.org.)

TABLE 54.4	Insulin Preparations by Subcutaneous Administration: Onset, Peak, and Duration of Action		
INSULIN, GENERIC NAME (BRAND)	**ONSET**	**PEAK**	**EFFECTIVE (h)**
Rapid-acting (prandial or correction insulin)			
Aspart (Novolog), lispro (Humalog), glulisine (Apidra)	5–15"	30–90"	<5
Short acting (prandial or correction insulin)			
Insulin regular (Novolin/Humulin)	30–60"	2–3 h	5–8
Intermediate (basal insulin q12h)			
Insulin NPH (Novolin or Humulin) (OK in pregnancy)	2–4 h	4–10 h	10–16
Long-acting (basal insulin q24h or q12h)			
Insulin glargine (Lantus) (avoid in pregnancy)	2–4 h	No peak	20–24
Insulin detemir (Levemir) (avoid in pregnancy)	3–8 h	No peak	6–23
Premixed (basal and prandial mixed)			
75% Lispro prot. susp./ 25% lispro (Humalog mix 75/25)	5–15"	DUAL	10–16
50% Lispro prot. susp./ 50% lispro (Humalog mix 50/50)	5–15"	DUAL	10–16
70% Aspart prot. susp./ 30% aspart (Novolog mix 70/30)	5–15"	DUAL	10–16
70% NPH/30% regular (Novolin or Humulin 70/30)	30–60"	DUAL	10–16

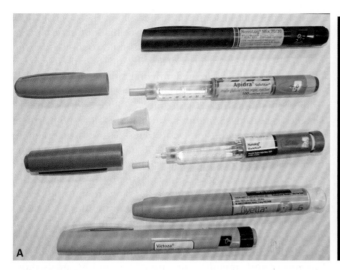
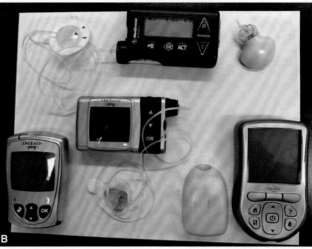

FIGURE 54.3 A, Insulin injection devices: insulin pens (short-acting, long-acting, and mixed insulins) and pens used to deliver GLP-1 analogs (Byetta and Victoza). Insulin pens are easier to use than syringes, improve patients' attitude and adherence towards the injectable treatment, and have accurate dosing mechanisms when used as prescribed. B, Insulin pumps and CGMS devices. Insulin pumps deliver insulin through a plastic catheter inserted subcutaneously; they can communicate wirelessly with a glucometer. CGMS devices measure glucose continuously through a sensor inserted subcutaneously. The hope is that in the near future, CGMS devices and insulin pumps could be combined to form an artificial pancreas. CGMS, continuous glucose monitoring system.

TABLE 54.5	Recommendations for Glycemic Control during Chronic Outpatient Management
$A_{1C} < 7.0\%$	
Preprandial capillary plasma glucose	90–130 mg/dL
Peak postprandial capillary plasma glucose[a]	180 mg/dL
Key concepts in setting glycemic goals are as follows: • A_{1C} is the primary target for glycemic control • Goals should be individualized based on	
Duration of diabetes	Known CVD or advanced microvascular complications
Age/life expectancy	Comorbid conditions
Hypoglycemia unawareness	Individual patient considerations

- Certain populations (children, pregnant women, and elderly) require special considerations
- More stringent goals ($A_{1C} < 6.5\%$) if able to achieve without significant hypoglycemia or polypharmacy for individual patients: short diabetes duration, on lifestyle or metformin only, long life expectancy, no significant CVD
- Less stringent goals ($A_{1C} < 8\%$) for patients: with history of severe hypoglycemia, advanced diabetes complications, extensive comorbid conditions, limited life expectancy, long-standing diabetes where goal is difficult to achieve despite optimal treatment
- Postprandial glucose may be targeted if A_{1C} goals are not met despite reaching preprandial goals

[a]Postprandial glucose measurements should be made 1 to 2 hours after the beginning of the meal.
CVD, cardiovascular disease.

be initiated early, however, if there is evidence of severe β-cell dysfunction, such as rapid weight loss or very high $A_{1C} > 9\%$, despite sustained efforts at diet and exercise and multiple oral agent combinations.

GLP-1 Analogs and Amylin

Amylin is a hormone that is co-secreted from the pancreas together with insulin. Amylin was shown to play a role in synchronizing the emptying of nutrients from the stomach with the secretion of insulin through acting in the brain to slow gastric emptying, lower gluconeogenesis, and decrease food intake. In type 1 diabetes, amylin levels are low, and its replacement leads to less dramatic

fluctuations of BG. GLP-1 analogs, which produce GLP 1 effects, that is, decrease in glucagon and increase in insulin and amylin secretions, have also been developed. These are drugs that need to be administered through an SQ injection, and increase GLP-1 to levels greater than those observed after administration of DPP-4 inhibitors. GLP-1 analogs promote decrease in food intake and weight loss in a large number of overweight and obese patients who take them and are frequently prescribed to obese patients with type 2 diabetes. Their development in user-friendly pens enhances their excellent results (**Figure 54.3A**). Unfortunately, some patients may not be able to tolerate them because of nausea. More severe but infrequent side effects include acute pancreatitis

TABLE 54.6	Correlation of A_{1c} With Average Glucose	
	MEAN PLASMA GLUCOSE	
$A_{1c}(\%)$	*mg/dL*	*mmol/L*
6	126	7.0
7	154	8.6
8	183	10.2
9	212	11.8
10	240	13.4
11	269	14.9
12	298	16.5

These estimates are based on ADAG data of approximately 2,700 glucose measurements over 3 months per A_{1c} measurement in 507 adults with type 1, type 2, and no diabetes. The correlation between A_{1c} and average glucose was 0.92. A calculator for converting A_{1c} results into estimated average glucose (eAG), in either mg/dL or mmol/L, is available in http://professional.diabetes.org/eAG.

and renal failure. These drugs are not indicated for use during hospitalizations.

Glycemic Targets in Outpatient Settings

It is currently recommended to aim for tight glucose control as early as possible in the course of diabetes treatment (**Table 54.5**).[1] The target A_{1c} level recommended by the ADA is less than 7% or as close to normal as is safely possible to achieve in most nonpregnant adults.[1] More stringent goals (such as 6.5%) could be sought if achieved without significant hypoglycemia or other adverse effects of treatment. This stringent goal could be recommended in patients with recent-onset diabetes, those treated with lifestyle or metformin only, those with long life expectancy, and/or no significant CVD. Less stringent goals (A_{1c} of 8% or less) are recommended for patients with a history of severe hypoglycemia, limited life expectancy, extensive complications and/or comorbid conditions, or those with long-standing diabetes in whom the goal is difficult to achieve despite appropriate education, monitoring, and appropriate use of multiple glucose-lowering agents including insulin.

The A_{1c} should be tested every 6 months if the value is at target or every 3 months when not at target or when treatment changes. Levels of A_{1c} together with the prevalence of hypoglycemia will dictate the management of glucose control. Correlation of A_{1c} with average glucose level is seen in **Table 54.6**. If A_{1c} is less than 7% and the hypoglycemia is not frequent and/or severe, then the treatment can be maintained at the current level. If A_{1c} is between 7% and 8%, this is likely due to 2-hour postprandial elevations, the following need to be reviewed: meal and activity plans, glucose monitoring techniques and frequency, compliance with medication administration and schedule, and sick day management. If A_{1c} is more than 8%, in addition to previous recommendations, goal setting, assessment of psychosocial issues, DSME (diabetes self-management education workshops) referral and medication adjustments are likely all needed (**Table 54.5**).

Hypoglycemia Management

The correct management of hypoglycemia is crucially important in all patients with diabetes who receive insulin or insulin secretagogue medications but especially in those with CVD or advanced complications. The hypoglycemia should be correctly evaluated and treated. It is defined as mild to moderate when levels of BG range from 50 to 70 mg/dL and/or patients can treat it themselves. It can be treated with oral, simple, easily absorbable carbohydrate, such as glucose tablets or gel, orange juice, or soft drinks containing 15 to 20 g of glucose. Glucose levels should be checked again in 15 minutes, and patients must be instructed to carry glucose with them at all times. Severe hypoglycemia is usually when glucose is less than 50 mg/dL, it is accompanied by altered consciousness, and patients need assistance. They need to take 20 to 30 g of simple glucose by mouth (if able), be given glucagon by intramuscular (IM) injection, or be rescued by emergency medical personnel with intravenous (IV) glucose administration. If any severe hypoglycemia episodes occur, then precipitating causes should be assessed, patients should be referred to DSME, use of glucagon IM injections should be taught to family members or care takers, and BG goals should be revised. If patients have frequent severe hypoglycemia or have hypoglycemia unawareness, then support of families and friends is absolutely needed, patients should wear identifying bracelets, and driving is not recommended.

IDENTIFYING AND TREATING COMPLICATIONS OF DIABETES

The treatment of chronic diabetes complications should be conducted according to published standards of care to ensure early diagnosis and prevent progression. These standards of care are published yearly by the ADA.[1] For microvascular disease, retinopathy, nephropathy, and neuropathy are targeted.

Retinopathy

Retinopathy is one of the ophthalmic complications of DM. It could be background or proliferative and could lead to retinal detachment, vitreous bleeding, and blindness if not treated. Early laser treatment could prevent blindness. Diabetes is also a risk factor for development of cataracts and glaucoma. Patients should have annual dilated eye examinations after 3 years from onset of type 1 diabetes and at onset of type 2 diabetes. Prevention of background or proliferative retinopathy occurrence or worsening is not only through continuing tight control of BG but also by smoking cessation and control of blood pressure and lipids.

Nephropathy

Diabetic nephropathy manifests itself as proteinuria, glomerulosclerosis, and renal failure. Nephropathy should be screened for annually with a urinary microalbumin/albumin determination. Goal is <30 mg/g creatinine, which corresponds roughly to 30 mg protein per 24 hours. In addition, glomerular filtration rate (GFR) and creatinine level need to be monitored at least annually. The prevention of nephropathy should be done through tight glucose and blood pressure control and through administration of agents that lower proteinuria, such as angiotensin-converting enzyme inhibitors and angiotensin receptor blockers. Treatment of nephropathy presenting with hematuria and nephrotic-range proteinuria include dietary protein reduction, blood pressure lowering to less than 125/75 mm Hg and revised glucose management for reduced GFR as well as a nephrology consult. If GFR < 30 mL/min, chronic kidney disease (CKD) management principles apply. Oral hypoglycemic agents' safety should be reassessed with worsening GFR.

Neuropathy

Diabetic neuropathy could be peripheral or autonomic and could lead to diabetic foot ulcer, diabetic arthropathy, and deformities with pathologic fractures, cellulitis, osteomyelitis, and amputations. The annual screening of feet for diabetes includes a complete assessment of sensation. Inspection of feet should be done at every visit; feet at high risk should be referred to podiatric care and for orthotics.

OTHER ASPECTS OF DIABETES MANAGEMENT

For all newly diagnosed diabetics, essential care should also address the following: (a) diabetes self-management education and nutrition education; (b) psychosocial screening; (c) pregnancy, contraception, and osteoporosis in women, and erectile dysfunction in men; and (d) dental care and vaccinations. A minimum amount of diabetes education (survival skills) should be taught in the hospital before discharge, and patients should be referred to an outpatient ADA-certified diabetes self-management education program. In such programs, there is an initial workshop that follows a core curriculum so core knowledge reaches all patients. Usually this is completed in about 6 hours. Self-knowledge assessment tests are given before and after the teaching sessions. Patients should attend a refresher course each year for up to 4 hours/year. Diabetes self-management nutrition education addresses diet and energy balance: weight loss issues if needed, need for carbohydrate counting in insulin-requiring patients, risk of low BG with decreased energy intake, increase in physical activity, increase in dietary fiber (14 g/1,000 kcal) and alcohol intake (maximum one drink per day for women and two drinks per day for men). Physical activity is recommended to be of both aerobic and resistance-type training and should be done in combination. Aerobic activity should be at least 150 min/week and it should be of moderate intensity, 50% to 70% of maximum heart rate (220-age). Resistance exercise should be done 3 times a week if there are no contraindications, such as the presence of proliferative diabetic retinopathy. A screening is needed to assess the literacy level that is essential for diabetes self-management education of glucose monitoring and medication adherence. Mood disorders such as depression and anxiety must be addressed because they can influence diabetes control as well as coping. Social barriers (family and economic issues) and physical barriers (blindness, amputations, etc.) are all likely to affect diabetes management and should be addressed accordingly.

DIABETES MELLITUS IN THE CARDIAC CARE UNIT

HYPERGLYCEMIA AND DIABETES IN THE CCU

Hyperglycemia is a common condition among hospitalized patients with and without diagnosed diabetes. Hyperglycemia on admission can affect up to 50% to 60% of patients admitted with acute coronary syndrome (ACS) and acute decompensated heart failure (HF), which varies based on the definition applied. More importantly, it has been reported that 14% to 50% of those presenting with ACS and hyperglycemia on admission were never diagnosed with diabetes.[9]

Hyperglycemia in patients admitted to the cardiac care unit (CCU) can be seen in three main scenarios: (1) those with previously known diagnosis of DM (of any type), (2) those with undiagnosed DM but meeting criteria for diagnosis during admission, and (3) those with stress hyperglycemia. Patients with previously diagnosed diabetes will commonly have worsening of their glycemic status—partly due to stress hyperglycemia, as explained here. Hyperglycemia in hospitalized patients with ACS has been associated with increased morbidity, mortality, and poor hospital-related outcomes, regardless of their previous status.[10]

INPATIENT HYPERGLYCEMIA AND STRESS HYPERGLYCEMIA—BRIEF DEFINITION

In the general hospitalized population, acute—or inpatient—hyperglycemia was traditionally considered as an admission or random BG ranging from >110 to >200 mg/dL in several studies.[10] Subsequently, the ADA, the AACE and the Endocrine Society defined inpatient hyperglycemia as a BG ≥ 140 mg/dL on admission or at any time during the hospitalization, or an admission HgA$_{1c}$ > 6.5%, in patients with or without diabetes.[11]

In hospitalized patients with ACS, the American Heart Association, in the scientific statement on "Hyperglycemia and Acute Coronary Syndrome" similarly defined inpatient hyperglycemia as an admission BG > 140 mg/dL during an admission, and recommended intensive glucose control in patients with BG > 180 mg/dL, regardless of their prior diabetes status. These recommendations are supported by several observational studies demonstrating that admission, mean 24-hour or mean in-hospital BG > 140 mg/dL is associated with increased mortality in the ACS population, and that lowering glucose to <140 mg/dL is associated with improved survival.[12]

Stress hyperglycemia refers to a transient elevation of BG occurring during acute illnesses, which resolves spontaneously after the acute insult dissipates. This disorder can occur in patients with or without diabetes, and has been associated with higher risk of complications and mortality compared to patients with previously diagnosed DM.[13] Trauma, infection, and surgery result in remarkable metabolic stress on the human body. Stress associated with critical illness is characterized by the activation of inflammatory cellular mediators and the hypothalamic pituitary-adrenal axis. In addition, the level of insulin is decreased, along with associated insulin resistance, at least partially from stress hormones in acutely ill patients.

In patients with ACS and "isolated" stress hyperglycemia (without previously known diabetes), the risk of mortality increases as the BG levels go above 120 to 140 mg/dL; whereas in patients with known DM and ACS, the risk of mortality starts to increase when the BG is >200 mg/dL.[14] These patients are also at increased risk of developing diabetes in the future. Greci et al. demonstrated that up to 60% of patients with stress hyperglycemia may be diagnosed with DM at 1 year[15]; therefore, screening and follow up after discharge are essential in these patients.

INCIDENCE AND PREVALENCE OF HYPERGLYCEMIA AND DIABETES IN THE CCU

According to the International Diabetes Federation, there were over 415 million people worldwide with DM in 2015 (http://www.diabetesatlas.org, accessed January 1, 2017). From 1980 to 2014 in the United States, the number of people with diabetes has increased by 4-fold, from 5.5 million to 22.0 million (https://www.cdc.gov/diabetes/statistics, accessed January 1, 2017).

There is a direct relationship between the increased prevalence of obesity and DM2 in the United States over the past two to three decades, escalating to epidemic numbers. Patients with metabolic syndrome usually have visceral obesity and insulin resistance, and are at risk for developing DM2 and CVD. Patients with DM2 and those with associated metabolic syndrome, in particular, are at high risk for CAD, cerebrovascular events, nonischemic cardiomyopathy, peripheral vascular disease, and death.[16]

The overall prevalence of hyperglycemia among hospitalized patients ranges from 32% to 42% in critically ill patients to 20% to 35% in non–critically ill patients.[11] Hospitalized patients with CVDs may have a higher burden of diabetes. In the CRUSADE study, up to 36.3% of patients with non-ST segment elevation myocardial infarction had known diabetes.[17]

In patients with ACS, hyperglycemia (with or without previously recognized diabetes) ranges from 25% to >50%, depending on the definition used by the different studies (> 110 vs 140 vs >180 mg/dL).[12] Unfortunately, the higher burden of diabetes may commonly be unrecognized by patients already presenting to the hospital with diabetes-related complications such as CVDs. In several large studies, the scenario of unrecognized diabetes has been reported in 10% to 50% of those presenting with ACS and hyperglycemia.[18]

Hyperglycemia in patients admitted for HF is also common. It has been reported that the prevalence of hyperglycemia in this population is about 42% in patients without diabetes and up to 40% to 50% in patients with diabetes.[19]

HYPERGLYCEMIA AND OUTCOMES IN HOSPITALIZED PATIENTS WITH DIFFERENT CARDIAC DISORDERS

Hyperglycemia in hospitalized patients has been associated with increased mortality and adverse outcomes. Paradoxically, patients admitted with hyperglycemia without a prior diagnosis of DM have been shown to have worse outcomes compared to those with previously diagnosed DM.[10]

Hyperglycemia and Acute Coronary Syndromes

In patients with known diabetes admitted with ACS, several studies have demonstrated that admission hyperglycemia is associated with increased risk of hospital mortality and hospital-related complications. A meta-analysis of patients with diabetes admitted with ACS reported that admission BG ≥ 180 mg/dL was associated with a 70% relative risk increase in hospital mortality, compared with normoglycemic patients on admission.[10]

Whether hyperglycemia on admission predisposes the patient to myocardial injury or is just a marker of disease severity is unclear. Hyperglycemia on admission is well accepted to be an independent predictor for poor outcomes in patients with and without diagnosed diabetes presenting with ACS. However, admission BG only represents a very specific time in the hospitalization. Persistent hyperglycemia during a hospitalization for ACS was found to be a better predictor of mortality than admission BG. Thus, some authors advocate the use of mean hospital glucose as the most accurate and practical glucometric tool in this population.[10]

In patients admitted with ACS and unrecognized DM, a meta-analysis reported that mortality increases as BG increases above 110 mg/dL, compared with normoglycemic patients.[10] Similarly, the HI-5 study showed that the 6-month mortality rate was higher in patients with BG > 144 mg/dL.[20]

Hyperglycemia and Heart Failure

With regard to patients admitted with acute HF, several studies reported an increased risk of in-hospital and overall mortality in patients with hyperglycemia.[21,22] A recent report from the "Swedish National Diabetes Registry" reported that patients with type 1 diabetes have 4-fold increased risk for HF hospitalizations, whereas poor glycemic control and albuminuria were considered strong risk factors.[22]

Hyperglycemia and Atrial Fibrillation

Atrial fibrillation (AF) is the most common chronic cardiac arrhythmia, and its prevalence is directly related to advancing age. The prevalence of DM2 is about 7% to 16% in patients with AF. A recent meta-analysis of patients with DM2 reported a 40% increased risk of AF, compared to unaffected patients. DM2 has also been found to be an independent risk factor for AF hospitalization.[23]

Hyperglycemia and Outcomes of Coronary Artery Bypass Grafting

Diabetes can affect up to 30% to 40% of patients undergoing coronary artery bypass graft (CABG) surgery. In a retrospective study at the Mayo Clinic, patients with intraoperative hyperglycemia were found to have a higher rate of mortality and complications, such as AF, sternal wound infections, prolonged mechanical ventilation, urinary tract infection, delirium, and strokes, following CABG surgery, regardless of whether they had previously recognized diabetes or not.[24] In the recent GLUCO-CABG trial, Umpierrez et al. randomized patients with inpatient hyperglycemia (BG > 140 mg/dL) to receive an intensive glycemic control; aiming BG targets between 100 and 140 mg/dL, versus a more conservative target of 141 to 180 mg/dL. The authors found similar results regarding a composite of outcomes, including mortality, wound infection, pneumonia, bacteremia, acute kidney injury, and major adverse cardiovascular events (42% vs 52%, $P = 0.08$). However, patients without known diabetes, so-called stress hyperglycemia, had a significantly lower rate of complications (34% vs 55%, $P = 0.008$).[25]

Hyperglycemia and Outcomes of Heart Transplant Surgery

Heart transplant recipients will sometimes be cared for by the CCU staff. Pre-transplant DM is a common comorbidity, presenting in up to 25% of patients undergoing heart or lung transplantation. Lang et al.[26] reported similar rates of acute rejections, graft vasculopathy, and infections in recipients with pre-transplant DM, whereas others reported higher rates of infections and posttransplant CAD/graft vasculopathy.[27]

HYPOGLYCEMIA AND OUTCOMES IN PATIENTS HOSPITALIZED WITH CARDIAC CONDITIONS

Several professional societies recommended glucose control in hospitalized patients admitted to critical settings, including those admitted with ACS. However, hypoglycemia is an inevitable consequence of glycemic management and has been associated with increased morbidity and mortality.[28]

Extensive literature has shown that hypoglycemia is a common event in the hospitalized patient. Patients with acute

CVDs are very vulnerable to the deleterious effects of hypoglycemia. Hypoglycemia is associated with increased risk of arrhythmias, ranging from bradycardia to ventricular ectopic beats and QT prolongation, mostly because of sympathetic and adrenal activation.[29] The relationship between mortality and glycemic control in hospitalized patients with ACS follows a U-shape curve.[30]

However, several studies have shown that spontaneous hypoglycemia is associated with worse outcomes and mortality than iatrogenic hypoglycemia in hospitalized patients. These results suggest that spontaneous inpatient hypoglycemia may be a marker of disease severity.

INTRODUCTION TO THE MANAGEMENT OF HYPERGLYCEMIA IN THE CCU

The negative impact of hyperglycemia and hypoglycemia in patients admitted to the CCU merits a comprehensive and multidisciplinary management plan. This plan may include dietary modifications, glucose monitoring, personalized glycemic targets to improve hyperglycemia while preventing hypoglycemia, a safe transitioning plan from the CCU to the regular medicine floors and/or home, and proper outpatient follow-up.

GLUCOSE MONITORING IN THE CCU

Given the negative impact of both inpatient hyperglycemia and hypoglycemia, it is necessary to closely monitor the BG levels in all patients admitted to the CCU. Current guidelines recommend glucose monitoring every 1 to 2 hours in critically ill patients. An international consensus meeting recommended against relying solely on the use of capillary BG for monitoring, given the poor reliability in critically ill patients. In patients with permanent vascular access (arterial and/or venous), all samples should be taken from this site following standard safety precautions. Arterial catheters may be preferred in patients with shock, severe peripheral edema, and/or on vasopressor therapy. In patients without arterial or venous catheters, capillary BG can be used. The samples should be analyzed in the blood gas analyzer machines within the intensive care unit (ICU) or CCU, because results can be rapidly available compared to hospitals' central laboratory.[31]

Novel technologies, such as the continuous glucose monitoring (CGM) system, have shown promising results in the area of glucose monitoring in the hospital. Previous studies raised concern for inaccurate BG readings in critically ill patients; however, recent prospective randomized trials have demonstrated better accuracy and safety in patients in the CCU.[32] Closed-loop insulin delivering system is a novel technology that could aid in the management of inpatient and peri-operative hyperglycemia. Closed-loop systems are composed of an insulin pump allowing appropriate insulin doses and a glucose sensor for CGM. Landmark studies in ambulatory patients and a few pilot studies in the hospital have shown that these systems may improve glycemic control, decrease hypoglycemia, and the burden of diabetes care. However, these initial pilot studies are awaiting larger multicenter studies for efficacy and safety validation. Their main limitations at this time are high cost, lack of training among providers and patients, time needed for implementation, and lack of outcome data at this time.[33]

GLYCEMIC TARGETS IN CRITICALLY ILL PATIENTS ADMITTED TO THE CCU

The benefits of a proactive management of inpatient hyperglycemia are well known in the general hospitalized population with or without known diabetes. For critically ill patients, the American Association of Clinical Endocrinologists (AACE) and the ADA recommend starting an IV insulin infusion and frequent glucose monitoring for patients with BG ≥ 180 mg/dL, targeting a BG of 140 to 180 mg/dL, with lower targets of 110 to 140 mg/dL only in selected patients.[11] The Society of Critical Care similarly recommends an insulin infusion for BG > 150 mg/dL and to maintain BG below that target, but absolutely <180 mg/dL.[28]

In patients with ACS, a scientific statement from the American Heart Association Diabetes Committee in 2008, recommended starting intensive insulin therapy in patients with hyperglycemia >180 mg/dL, regardless of their prior history of diabetes. They recommended using a validated and efficient IV insulin protocol with close BG monitoring. Similarly, the European Society of Cardiology in 2012 recommended maintaining BG between 90 and <200 mg/dL in patients with ST segment elevation myocardial infarction, but absolutely avoiding hypoglycemia. Insulin therapy should be decreased and/or adjusted if BG < 70 mg/dL and should be reassessed if BG < 100 mg/dL.[12,34]

For non–critically ill patients, the Endocrine Society and AACE/ADA guidelines recommended a target premeal BG of <140 mg/dL and random BG < 180 mg/dL, with subcutaneous (SQ) basal-bolus regimen preferred.[11]

GLYCEMIC TREATMENT: INSULIN THERAPY IN THE CCU

The LEUVEN study was a landmark study performed by Van den Bergh et al. in Leuven, Belgium in 2001. This study opened an interesting area of investigation in glucose control in surgical critically ill patients and outcomes. Initially, this single-center study showed a mortality benefit in patients treated with insulin to an "intense glycemic target," BG between 80 and 100 mg/dL, compared to a less strict goal of BG between 180 and 200 mg/dL. Notably, there were more severe hypoglycemic episodes in the intervention arm. However, these results were not replicated by several other prospective studies, including the van den Bergh group.[35,36]

The subsequent study by the van der Bergh group in Leuven, including patients in the medical intensive care unit (MICU) this time, showed no difference in mortality. This study also found higher rates of hypoglycemia, presumably because of changes in the nutrition management between the two patient populations, in the intense glycemic group.[37] The largest trial of intense glucose control in the ICU to date is the "Normoglycemia in Intensive Care Evaluation–Survival Using Glucose Algorithm Regulation (NICE-SUGAR)" trial. This trial randomly assigned patients in the MICU and surgical intensive care unit (SICU) to an intensive BG target (BG between 81 and 108 mg/dL) versus a conventional/less strict glucose target (BG < 180 mg/dL). Conversely, this study showed that the intensive glycemic control group had a higher 90-day mortality and incidence of hypoglycemic episodes.[36]

Some small studies have yielded small but significant differences in mortality when goals are less stringent, but comparison is hard and hampered because of the heterogeneity of different studies. The DIGAMI and HI-5 trials are the two landmarks studies of glucose control in the ACS patient population. The first DIGAMI trial studied the effects of intensive in-hospital insulin treatment (insulin-glucose infusion for at least 24 hours followed by multidose SQ insulin regimen) versus usual care in 620 patients with acute myocardial infarction with or without diabetes and an admission glucose of 200 mg/dL. Patients with myocardial infarction were randomized to receive insulin infusion to maintain BG 126 to 180 mg/dL versus standard of care without an insulin infusion. Better glycemic control was achieved in the intensive insulin therapy arm (mean 24-hour posttreatment BG of 173 vs 210 mg/dL in the control group). A significant 28% mortality reduction benefit was seen in the intervention arm after long-term follow up of 3.4 years.[38] The DIGAMI 2 trial attempted to compare three different treatment regimens (acute insulin-glucose infusion followed by insulin-based long-term glucose control; insulin-glucose infusion followed by standard glucose control on discharge; and routine metabolic management in both inpatient and outpatient settings) and found no difference in outcomes between the three regimens.[39] Moreover, the subsequent HI-5 trial was the first randomized trial that included patients with hyperglycemia without a diagnosis of diabetes. Patients were assigned to an intensive insulin infusion arm (BG goal of 72 to 180) and a conventional arm that was treated with their usual diabetes medication including SQ insulin. There was no difference in mortality rates among the groups during hospitalization or at 3 or 6 months. There were, however, significant reductions in post–myocardial infarction HF during the hospitalization (10% absolute risk reduction) and in reinfarction at 3 months.[20]

This brief description of some of the landmark studies regarding hyperglycemia in critically ill patients with ACS was intended to show the conflicting results of intensive glycemic targets in this population. These controversial results may probably be due to heterogeneity in patient characteristics and study protocols. We advise the readers to exercise some caution with extrapolation of the data from general MICU and SICU patients, or combined trials into the CCU practice. Nevertheless, hyperglycemia management targeting less stringent goals has become part of the standard of care in hospitalized patients, as endorsed by several national organizations.[11,12,28,34]

INSULIN INTRAVENOUS INFUSION THERAPY ("DRIP") IN THE CCU

The preferred approach to manage medical or surgical critically ill patients is using an insulin infusion protocol with regular human insulin.[28] There are several validated infusion protocols, some nurse-driven or computer-generated algorithms, that have been validated for their safety and efficacy.[40] Oral hypoglycemic agents are generally not recommended for the critically ill and non–critically ill hospitalized patients, and should be discontinued upon admission to the CCU.[25]

In brief, most insulin infusion protocols include instructions on how much insulin to start infusing based on the initial BG. Then, the insulin rate per hour is adjusted on the basis of the rate of BG change. In addition, the protocol will instruct on how to correct hypoglycemia, and adjust the infusion rate to prevent it again. It has been shown that BG targets are usually achieved within approximately 4 to 8 hours in most patients. The onset of regular insulin after IV administration is within 15 minutes, with a half-life of 9 minutes, a maximal effect within 15 to 30 minutes, and a duration of 30 to 60 minutes. Thus, this safely ensures a

rapid up- or down-titration of the doses in anticipated (ie, rapid decline of BG, use of vasopressors) or unanticipated (ie, acute clinical status deteriorations, hypoglycemia) situations.[28]

Several centers use nurse-driven computer-based algorithms, whereas others use paper-based protocols. The Glucommander is an example of a computer-driven insulin infusion software, developed since 1984. After entering a bedside BG into the system, the Glucommander calculated the initial insulin infusion rate (ie, BG – 60 mg/dL × 0.02 = insulin dose/h). The system will notify the nurse or provider when the next bedside BG is needed. The system continues making adjustment recommendations of the insulin infusion until it is stopped by the provider. The pilot studies by Davidson et al. showed that the system can maintain BG within target range, without significant hypoglycemia, and run by nonspecialized staff.[40]

Peri-operative patients may require additional considerations. Oral hypoglycemic agents and non–insulin injectable agents should be held on the day of the surgery. For patients with DM2 who will be fasting (NPO) for at least 8 hours before surgery, basal insulin should be adjusted to 75% to 100% of the regular home dose the night before surgery, depending on the patient's glycemic curve. Because the patient is fasting, prandial insulin is, by definition, not required. However, correctional sliding-scale insulin every 4 to 6 hours should be used for correction of residual hyperglycemia, while NPO. For patients using neutral protamine Hagedorn (NPH) insulin, because of the increased risk of hypoglycemia compared with basal insulin analogs—glargine or detemir—it is recommended to give about 75% of the usual dose the day before surgery and 50% to 75% on the surgical day. IV insulin infusion protocols can allow for rapid insulin adjustments based on BG in these scenarios of rapid glucose shifts. Close glucose monitoring every 1 to 2 hours is usually recommended for monitoring. For short-duration (approximately <4 hours) and small or simple surgical procedures, SQ insulin can be used. For longer and more complicated procedures (>4 hours) IV insulin infusion is the recommended approach.[41,42]

In our institution, we have created a pathway for management of hyperglycemia in cardiac patients, which is depicted in **Figure 54.4**.[43]

Pathway for the Management of Hyperglycemia in the Cardiac Care Unit

The main goal of this pathway is to provide glycemic control for critically ill patients. Initial assessment of the former group of patients should include history, physical examination, and recording of weight. We have also defined a basic laboratory test panel required for all patients (**Figure 54.5**). We included patients with DKA and patients with hyperosmolar state and provided guidelines for their management (**Figure 54.6**). These patients might not necessarily be treated in the cardiac care unit depending on their associated cardiovascular morbidities. Patients managed in this protocol have a diagnosis of DM. If a patient is not known to have DM, capillary BG determinations every 6 hours will be required. A BG of 180 mg/dL qualifies patients for enrollment into our pathway of insulin infusion protocol (**Figure 54.7**).

Initiation of the insulin infusion is achieved by providing a bolus of 6 units of regular insulin for patients with a BG of 250 mg/dL or more and starting an infusion protocol that is based on weight. If the initial BG value is above 180 but below 250 mg/dL,

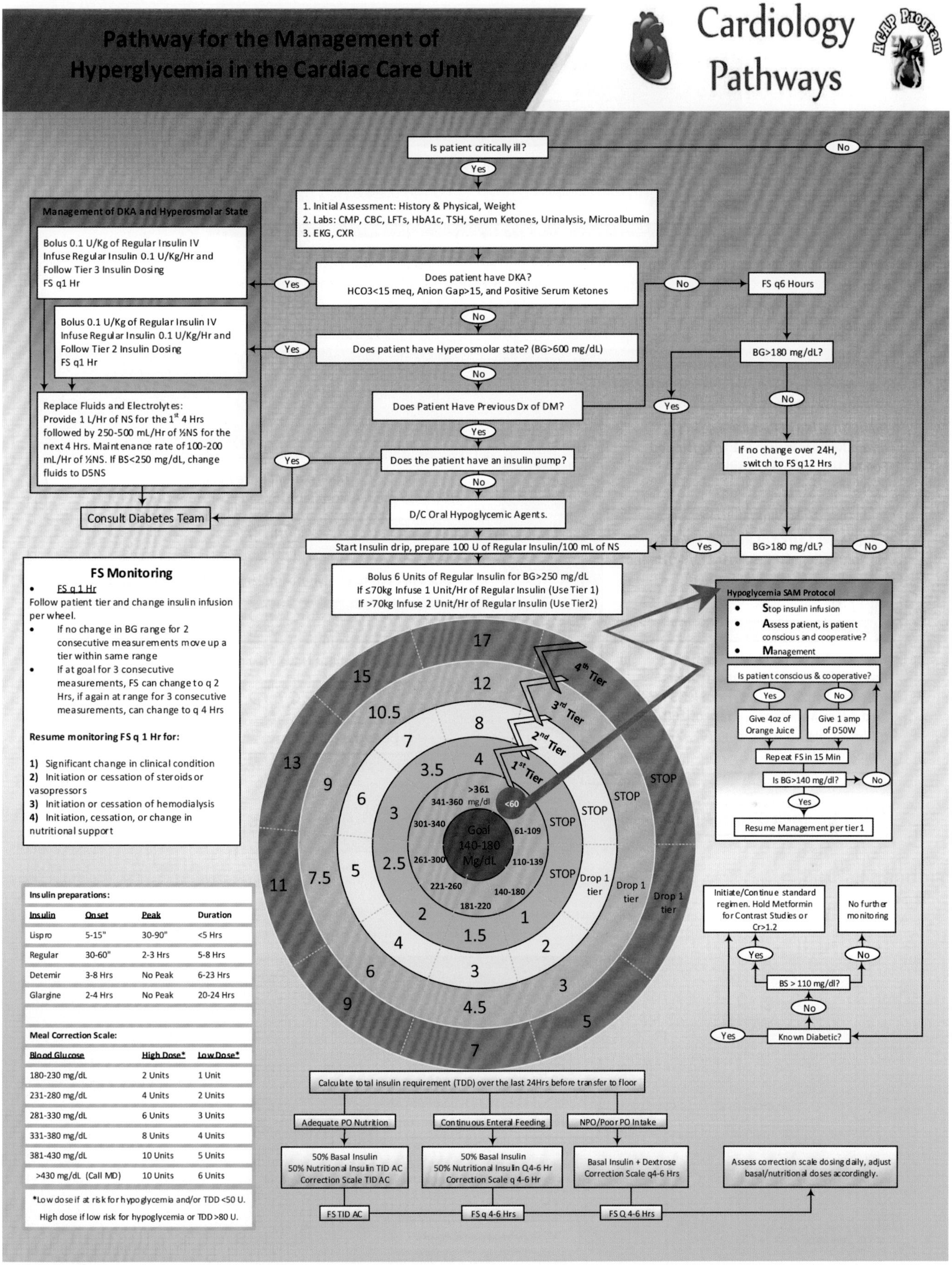

Is patient critically ill? → No

Yes

1. Initial Assessment: History & Physical, Weight
2. Labs: CMP, CBC, LFTs, HbA1c, TSH, Serum Ketones, Urinalysis, Microalbumin
3. EKG, CXR

Management of DKA and Hyperosmolar State

Bolus 0.1 U/Kg of Regular Insulin IV
Infuse Regular Insulin 0.1 U/Kg/Hr and
Follow Tier 3 Insulin Dosing
FS q1 Hr

Does patient have DKA?
HCO3<15 meq, Anion Gap>15, and Positive Serum Ketones → No → FS q6 Hours

No

Bolus 0.1 U/Kg of Regular Insulin IV
Infuse Regular Insulin 0.1 U/Kg/Hr and
Follow Tier 2 Insulin Dosing
FS q1 Hr

Does patient have Hyperosmolar state? (BG>600 mg/dL) → BG>180 mg/dL?

No

Replace Fluids and Electrolytes:
Provide 1 L/Hr of NS for the 1st 4 Hrs
followed by 250-500 mL/Hr of ½NS for the
next 4 Hrs. Maintenance rate of 100-200
mL/Hr of ½NS. If BS<250 mg/dL, change
fluids to D5NS

Does Patient Have Previous Dx of DM? → Yes

Yes → No

If no change over 24H, switch to FS q12 Hrs

Does the patient have an insulin pump? → BG>180 mg/dL?

Consult Diabetes Team

No

D/C Oral Hypoglycemic Agents.

Start Insulin drip, prepare 100 U of Regular Insulin/100 mL of NS → Yes → BG>180 mg/dL? → No

FS Monitoring

- FS q 1 Hr
Follow patient tier and change insulin infusion per wheel.
- If no change in BG range for 2 consecutive measurements move up a tier within same range
- If at goal for 3 consecutive measurements, FS can change to q 2 Hrs, if again at range for 3 consecutive measurements, can change to q 4 Hrs

Bolus 6 Units of Regular Insulin for BG>250 mg/dL
If ≤70kg Infuse 1 Unit/Hr of Regular Insulin (Use Tier 1)
If >70kg Infuse 2 Unit/Hr of Regular Insulin (Use Tier2)

Resume monitoring FS q 1 Hr for:

1) Significant change in clinical condition
2) Initiation or cessation of steroids or vasopressors
3) Initiation or cessation of hemodialysis
4) Initiation, cessation, or change in nutritional support

Hypoglycemia SAM Protocol
- **S**top insulin infusion
- **A**ssess patient, is patient conscious and cooperative?
- **M**anagement

Is patient conscious & cooperative? → Yes / No

Give 4oz of Orange Juice | Give 1 amp of D50W

Repeat FS in 15 Min

Is BG>140 mg/dl? → No

Yes

Resume Management per tier 1

Insulin preparations:

Insulin	Onset	Peak	Duration
Lispro	5-15"	30-90"	<5 Hrs
Regular	30-60"	2-3 Hrs	5-8 Hrs
Detemir	3-8 Hrs	No Peak	6-23 Hrs
Glargine	2-4 Hrs	No Peak	20-24 Hrs

Meal Correction Scale:

Blood Glucose	High Dose*	Low Dose*
180-230 mg/dL	2 Units	1 Unit
231-280 mg/dL	4 Units	2 Units
281-330 mg/dL	6 Units	3 Units
331-380 mg/dL	8 Units	4 Units
381-430 mg/dL	10 Units	5 Units
>430 mg/dL (Call MD)	10 Units	6 Units

*Low dose if at risk for hypoglycemia and/or TDD <50 U.
High dose if low risk for hypoglycemia or TDD >80 U.

(Central wheel diagram — Tiers 1st–4th; Goal 140-180 Mg/dL; glucose ranges: >361, 341-360 mg/dl, 301-340, 261-300, 221-260, 181-220, <60, 61-109, 110-139, 140-180; values 17, 15, 13, 12, 11, 10.5, 9, 8, 7, 7.5, 6, 5, 4, 3.5, 3, 2.5, 2, 1.5, 1, 1.5, 2, 3, 4.5, 5, 4, 6, 9, 7; STOP, Drop 1 tier)

Initiate/Continue standard regimen. Hold Metformin for Contrast Studies or Cr>1.2 → Yes/No

No further monitoring

BS > 110 mg/dl? → No

Yes → Known Diabetic?

Calculate total insulin requirement (TDD) over the last 24Hrs before transfer to floor

Adequate PO Nutrition	Continuous Enteral Feeding	NPO/Poor PO Intake
50% Basal Insulin 50% Nutritional Insulin TID AC Correction Scale TID AC	50% Basal Insulin 50% Nutritional Insulin Q4-6 Hr Correction Scale q 4-6 Hr	Basal Insulin + Dextrose Correction Scale q4-6 Hrs
FS TID AC	FS q 4-6 Hrs	FS Q 4-6 Hrs

Assess correction scale dosing daily, adjust basal/nutritional doses accordingly.

FIGURE 54.4 Pathway for the management of hyperglycemia in the cardiac care unit. BG, blood glucose; CBC, complete blood count; CMP, comprehensive metabolic panel; CXR, chest X-ray; ECG, electrocardiogram; DKA, diabetic ketoacidosis; FS, fasting sugar; LFT, liver function test; NS, normal saline; TDD, total daily dose; TSH, thyroid-stimulating hormone

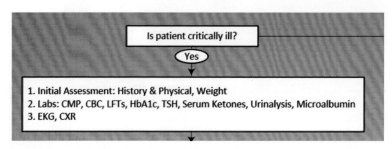

FIGURE 54.5 Initial assessment of patients with hyperglycemia who are screened to a cardiac care unit. CBC, complete blood count; CMP, comprehensive metabolic panel; CXR, chest X-ray; ECG, electrocardiogram; LFT, liver function test; TSH, thyroid-stimulating hormone.

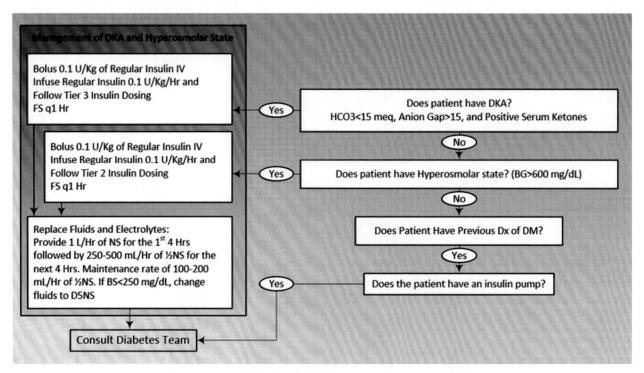

FIGURE 54.6 Management of DKA and hyperosmolar state and activation of diabetes team. DKA, diabetes ketoacidosis; DM, diabetes mellitus; IV, intravenous.

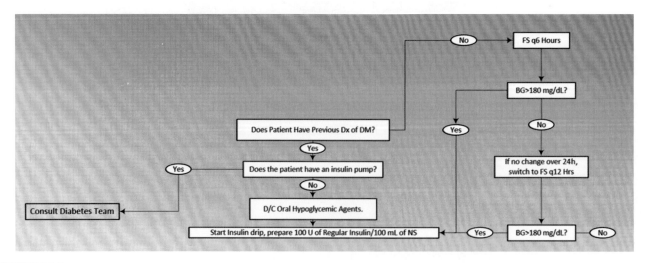

FIGURE 54.7 Blood glucose determination for enrollment into the hyperglycemia pathway. DM, diabetes mellitus ; NS, normal saline.

Bolus 6 units of regular insulin for BG > 250 mg/dL
If ≤ 70 kg Infuse 1 unit/h of regular insulin (use tier 1)
If > 70 kg Infuse 2 unit/h of regular insulin (use tier 2)

FIGURE 54.8 Initiation of insulin infusion protocol. BG, blood glucose; DM, diabetes mellitus; NS, normal saline.

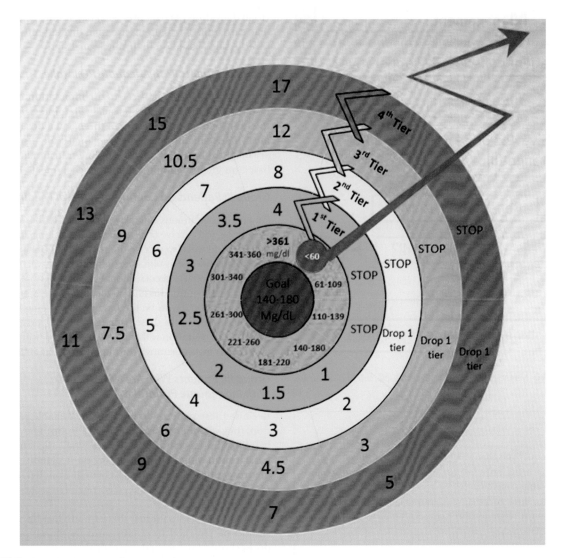

FIGURE 54.9 The "wheel" as a tool for insulin infusion.

the patient will not need the bolus insulin and will be started on weight-based insulin drip only (**Figure 54.8**).

The key element of this pathway is the "wheel" that provides treatment instruction for insulin administration (**Figure 54.9**). This wheel is made up of six circles. The core circle shows the acceptable glycemic range for all the patients and the inner circle represents the measured BG ranges. The four outer circles represent four different rates of insulin infusion, also known as "tiers." For patients who are less than 70 kg, the insulin infusion rate should be calculated on the basis of tier 1. For patients who weigh more than 70 kg, the infusion rate is based on tier 2. BG monitoring is performed every 1 hour. The infusion rate

is then adjusted according to the instructions corresponding to the BG of the same tier: "dialing up and down the wheel within the tier." If there is *no* decrease in BG range for two consecutive measurements, the health care provider moves up a tier at the same glucose range.

A major goal in the management of hyperglycemia is the prevention of hypoglycemia. If a patient is found to be hypoglycemic (defined as BG of 60 mg/dL or less), a protocol for management is provided, as seen in **Figure 54.10**. We named this protocol SAM to reflect the key components of treatment: *S*top insulin infusion, *A*ssess the patient for consciousness and cooperation, and *M*anage the patient (with orange juice or D50%W infusion).

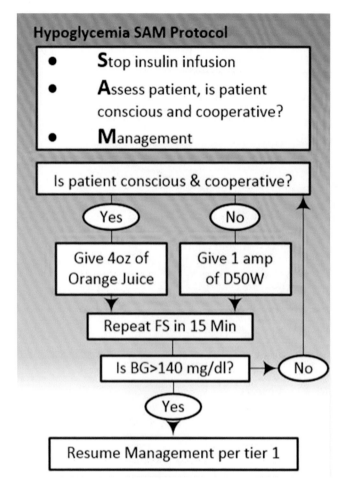

FIGURE 54.10 Management of hypoglycemia. BG, blood glucose; FS, fasting sugar.

FS Monitoring
- FSq 1 h

Follow patient tier and change insulin infusion per wheel.
- If no change in BG range for two consecutive measurements move up a tier within same range
- If at goal for three consecutive measurements, FS can change to q2h, if again at range for three consecutive measurements, can change to q4h

Resume monitoring FS 1 1 h for:
  Significant changes in clinical condition
  Initiation or cessation of steroids or vasopressors
  Initiation or cessation of hemodialysis
  Initiation, cessation, or change in nutritional support

FIGURE 54.11 Guidelines for finger stick monitoring for patients with hyperglycemia. BG, blood glucose; FS, fasting sugar.

If a patient's BG exceeds 140 mg/dL, the management using the "wheel" is resumed with the initial insulin infusion rate based on tier 1 and the corresponding BG.

Instructions for frequency of BG monitoring are provided to the health care provider. Initially, all monitoring is performed every 1 hour. If BG results are at goal for three consecutive readings, then the frequency of monitoring is decreased to every 2 hours and, again, if there is no change for three consecutive readings, it is decreased to every 4 hours. Return to frequent monitoring

(BG every 1 hour) is required for the following conditions: significant change in clinical condition; initiation or cessation of corticosteroids or vasopressors; initiation or cessation of hemodialysis and/or initiation, cessation, or change in nutritional support (**Figure 54.11**).

A protocol was developed to convert from the insulin infusion to SQ insulin injection without sacrificing diabetes control. First, the health care provider calculates the total insulin requirement (total daily dose [TDD]) over the last 24-hour period in the cardiac care unit. The patients are then divided into the following three groups based on their nutritional status.

Group I: Patients With Adequate PO Intake

This group of patients receives a combination of long-acting insulin (50% of the TDD)—usually glargine—at bedtime and the rapid-acting insulin lispro in three equal doses before every meal. They will also receive correctional scale insulin before every meal (to be added to the standing nutritional insulin dose) based on glucose monitoring before each meal (**Figure 54.12**).

Group II: Patients on Continuous Enteral Feeding

Patients on continuous enteral feeding, just like those with adequate PO intake, will receive 50% of their TDD as long-acting insulin at bedtime and will also receive the rest of the TDD in three divided doses of nutritional insulin. The only difference will be in the timing of this nutritional and correctional insulin. Because these patients are receiving continuous enteral feeding, there is no specific meal time during the day to be the base of measurements and administration of insulin. In these patients, both BG measurements and insulin administration will happen every 4 to 6 hours to give them a smoother glycemic range during the day (**Figure 54.12**).

Group III: Patients Who Are NPO or Those With Inadequate PO Intake

Because these patients do not have any reliable source of nutrition, they will not receive nutritional insulin. They will still need basal insulin (specifically if they are type 1 diabetic). To receive basal insulin without hypoglycemia, these patients need to be on dextrose infusion. They will also benefit from BG measurements every 4 to 6 hours and will need correctional scale insulin if these values are high.

In all of these patients, the 24-hour insulin requirements should be checked frequently and the basal and nutritional doses should be adjusted accordingly to minimize the amount of correctional insulin needed (**Figure 54.12**).

Correctional Insulin Scale

We provide two doses for meal correctional insulin in our pathway, the high-dose and the low-dose scale (**Figure 54.13**). The health care provider can also pick the value in between that will represent the medium dose scale of correctional insulin. Use of either of the dosing values is mainly based on clinically estimated risk of hyper- or hypoglycemia.

Medium- or high-dose scale is used mostly in patients who are obese, or have acute, severe illness or infection or those on some medications including steroids, vasopressors, certain antipsychotics, or any other medication that causes a rise in BG level. Low-dose scale is used in patients who are NPO or those who suffer from malnutrition, low body weight, lean type 1 DM, or poor PO intake. This scale is also appropriate to use in those

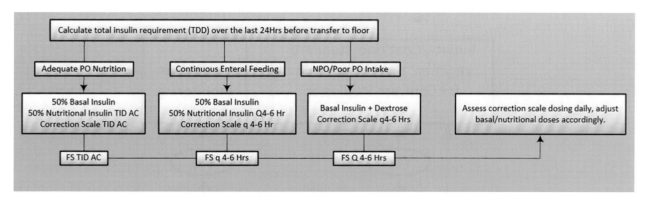

FIGURE 54.12 A protocol for conversion from insulin infusion to subcutaneous insulin injection. FS, fasting sugar; TDD, total daily dose.

Insulin preparations:			
Insulin	**Onset**	**Peak**	**Duration (h)**
Lispro	5–15"	30–90"	<5
Regular	30–60"	2–3 h	5–8
Detemir	3–8 h	No Peak	6–23
Glargine	2–4 h	No Peak	20–24
Meal Correction Scale:			
Blood Glucose		**High Dose* (units)**	**Low Dose* (units)**
180–230 mg/dL		2	1 Unit
231–280 mg/dL		4	2
281–330 mg/dL		6	3
331–380 mg/dL		8	4
381–430 mg/dL		10	5
>430 mg/dL (Call MD)		10	6
*Low dose if at risk for hypoglycemia and/or TDD < 50 U. High dose if low risk for hypoglycemia or TDD> 80 U.			

FIGURE 54.13 Correctional sliding scale and characteristics of different insulin preparations. TDD, total daily dose.

with renal insufficiency, hepatic disease, HF, shock, adrenal failure, burns, alcoholism, malignancy, or those with a history of severe or recurrent hypoglycemia.

Another approach to decide regarding the dosage of the correctional scale is based on patients' total daily insulin intake with low dose used in those with TDD < 50 units, medium dose in those with TDD 51 to 80 units, and high dose in those with TDD > 81 units.

We also provide pharmacologic characteristics of different types of insulin preparation that are used most commonly in the cardiac care unit (**Figure 54.13**).

Non–Critically Ill Patients in the Cardiac Care Unit

Non–critically ill patients will not benefit from aggressive control of their BG using insulin infusion. These patients will need a standard regimen for management of their DM while they are in the hospital. Those with known diabetes who are on established and effective diabetic regimen should be kept on their respective regimens while in the hospital. The only exception will

be to hold the metformin if they are about to undergo contrast studies. Other patients without a history of diabetes who fulfill the criteria for DM diagnosis should be assessed and started on a guideline-based regimen to control their DM. The remainder of the patients who do not fulfill diagnostic criteria of DM will not benefit from frequent BG measurements (**Figure 54.14**).

This comprehensive pathway provides a detailed algorithm for management of hyperglycemia in cardiac care units. It introduces the novel concepts of the "wheel," which is the primary tool permitting rapid restoration of euglycemia and is the focus of this pathway.

TRANSITION OF CARE—FROM THE CCU TO MEDICINE WARD, FROM HOSPITAL WARDS TO HOME

Patients may be transitioned to a SQ insulin regimen once clinically stable, when restarted on oral diet, and/or when transferred out of the CCU. Several factors should be considered during the "transition period," including insulin requirements while on the insulin infusion, current or planned nutrition, and/or concurrent

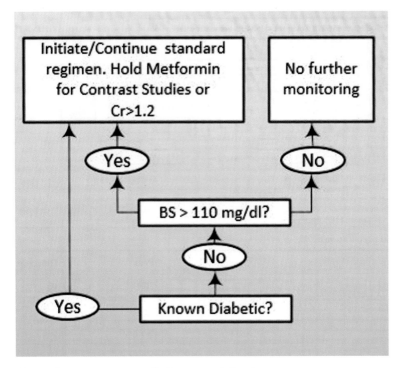

FIGURE 54.14 Management of hyperglycemia in non–critically ill patients. BS, Blood sugar..

infections or medications, such as steroids. Several randomized controlled trials using SQ basal-bolus insulin regimens have reported better glycemic control and reduction of complications compared to sliding-scale insulin in patients with type 2 diabetes.[44] Insulin sliding scales as a sole management approach is strongly discouraged in patients transitioned from the CCU to the general wards. Sliding-scale insulin regimens treat hyperglycemia after it has already occurred, instead of "proactively" preventing the occurrence of hyperglycemia with scheduled insulin doses. This "reactive" approach can lead to rapid changes in BG levels, exacerbating both hyperglycemia and hypoglycemia. The recent Basal-Plus study, a randomized controlled trial consisting of basal insulin plus correctional premeal doses of rapid-acting insulin per sliding scale, showed that this approach may be an alternative in some situations, such as in patients not eating full meals, or with nausea, or with very mild hyperglycemia.[45]

Communication between the multidisciplinary team members, including CCU nurses, diabetes team members, and primary medicine team, is key for a safe transition. The involvement of several members will ensure appropriate glucose monitoring, insulin dose adjustments, and close communication. Before transitioning the patient to the SQ basal-bolus insulin regimen, some clinical characteristics should be evaluated. The patient should have reached clinical stability, have stable glycemic control for several hours, and not continue to require critical medical or nursing care. Some authors suggest a period ranging from 6 to 24 hours of glycemic control with minimal variability in IV insulin rates. Patients should ideally be without vasopressors or inotropic agents and have a stable nutrition plan or should be tolerating PO diet. In patients admitted with DKA, the anion gap and acidosis should have normalized before considering transitioning to SQ insulin. Postoperative stress, pain, variable oral intake, infection, and underlying insulin resistance are all factors that affect insulin requirements. Given the short half-life of IV regular insulin, SQ

insulin should be given before stopping the infusion, to avoid rebound hyperglycemia or acidosis. Consideration should also be given to the time to onset of each type of SQ insulin. For instance, glargine should be given at least 2 hours in advance before stopping the IV insulin.[46]

The insulin infusion requirements are usually high during the first few hours of treatment of patients with DKA or HHS, progressing into a highly variable infusion rate, before finally settling down to a more stable pattern. Similarly, patients with stress hyperglycemia have markedly increased insulin infusion utilization within the first 48 to 72 hours post surgery. Using these variable insulin rates (ie, change greater than two units per hour), especially the initial extremely high rates, in the 24-hour SQ total insulin calculation will yield a result that potentially overestimates the patient's requirements once clinically stable and off the insulin infusion.[46] For this reason, it is recommended to use the hourly insulin rate from a previous period when BG was stable and within target range; in other words, the rate was reasonable and stable for some time. One can then look at the infusion rates during this stable period of time, ideally 6 to 8 hours in duration, to calculate the average insulin rate per hour required. This hourly insulin rate is multiplied by 24 to extrapolate these data to a 24-hour time period and the total 24-hour insulin requirements is calculated. Some authors suggest utilizing 50% to 60% of this 24-hour insulin dose in patients with stress hyperglycemia and no previous diagnosis of diabetes, whereas up to 60% to 80% can be used in patients with DM2 and high insulin requirements. The total insulin dose is then divided into 50% basal and 50% bolus insulin.[46]

In hospital settings, basal insulin analogs, such as glargine or detemir, are generally preferred over NPH or mixed insulin because they have been associated with less glycemic variability and less severe hypoglycemia.[47] Renal dysfunction is common in hospitalized patients, increasing the risk of insulin and non–insulin-related hypoglycemia. Baldwin et al. studied two basal-bolus (glargine-glulisine) insulin-dosing regimens in patients hospitalized with DM and CKD (eGFR < 45 mL/min). The authors found that a weight-based insulin regimen of 0.25 units/kg/d was associated with 50% less hypoglycemia (15.8% vs 30%, $P = 0.08$).[48]

It is important to establish institutional protocol for transition from the inpatient to the outpatient settings. In general, length of stay for patients with diabetes, although longer than for those without, has been gradually decreasing just as for all inpatient stays being on average 5 to 6 days. Therefore, the discharge plan for patients with diabetes has to be set from the admission. In established diabetes, it is important to determine the goals for the patient's level of glycemic control. A recent prospective study recommended using the admission HbA$_{1c}$ to determine the diabetes plan.[49] In patients with stress hyperglycemia, it is important to coordinate appropriate follow-up to assess for the development of diabetes later.

REFERENCES

1. American Diabetes Association: clinical practice recommendations. *Diabetes Care.* 2011;34(suppl 1):S1-S116.

2. Weyer C, Tataranni PA, Bogardus C, Pratley RE. Insulin resistance and insulin secretory dysfunction are independent predictors of worsening of glucose tolerance during each stage of type 2 diabetes development. *Diabetes Care.* 2001;24:89-94.

3. International Association of Diabetes and Pregnancy Study Groups Consensus Panel, Metzger BE, Gabbe SG, Persson B, et al. International association of diabetes and pregnancy study groups recommendations on the diagnosis and classification of hyperglycemia in pregnancy. *Diabetes Care.* 2010;33:676-682.

4. Grundy SM, Cleeman JI, Daniels SR, et al. Diagnosis and management of the metabolic syndrome: an American Heart Association/National Heart, Lung, and Blood Institute Scientific Statement. *Circulation.* 2005;112:2735-2752.

5. Despres JP, Lemieux I. Abdominal obesity and metabolic syndrome. *Nature.* 2006;444:881-887.

6. Grundy SM, Hansen B, Smith SC Jr, Cleeman JI, Kahn RA. Clinical management of metabolic syndrome: report of the American Heart Association/National Heart, Lung, and Blood Institute/American Diabetes Association conference on scientific issues related to management. *Circulation.* 2004;109:551-556.

7. Skyler JS, Bergenstal R, Bonow RO, et al; American Diabetes Association, American College of Cardiology Foundation, American Heart Association. Intensive glycemic control and the prevention of cardiovascular events: implications of the ACCORD, ADVANCE, and VA diabetes trials: a position statement of the American Diabetes Association and a scientific statement of the American College of Cardiology Foundation and the American Heart Association. *Diabetes Care.* 2009;32:187-192.

8. Gaede P, Vedel P, Larsen N, Jensen GV, Parving HH, Pedersen O. Multifactorial intervention and cardiovascular disease in patients with type 2 diabetes. *N Engl J Med.* 2003;348:383-393.

9. Kosiborod M, Deedwania P. An overview of glycemic control in the coronary care unit with recommendations for clinical management. *J Diabetes Sci Technol.* 2009;3(6):1342-1351.

10. Capes SE, Hunt D, Malmberg K, Gerstein HC. Stress hyperglycaemia and increased risk of death after myocardial infarction in patients with and without diabetes: a systematic overview. *Lancet.* 2000;355(9206):773-778.

11. Moghissi ES, Korytkowski MT, DiNardo M, et al. American Association of Clinical Endocrinologists and American Diabetes Association consensus statement on inpatient glycemic control. *Diabetes Care.* 2009;32(6):1119-1131.

12. Deedwania P, Kosiborod M, Barrett E, et al. Hyperglycemia and acute coronary syndrome: a scientific statement from the American Heart Association Diabetes Committee of the Council on Nutrition, Physical Activity, and Metabolism. *Anesthesiology.* 2008;109(1):14-24.

13. Falciglia M, Freyberg RW, Almenoff PL, D'Alessio DA, Render ML. Hyperglycemia-related mortality in critically ill patients varies with admission diagnosis. *Crit Care Med.* 2009;37(12):3001-3009.

14. Goyal A, Mahaffey KW, Garg J, et al. Prognostic significance of the change in glucose level in the first 24 h after acute myocardial infarction: results from the CARDINAL study. *Eur Heart J.* 2006;27(11):1289-1297.

15. Greci LS, Kailasam M, Malkani S, et al. Utility of HbA$_{(1c)}$ levels for diabetes case finding in hospitalized patients with hyperglycemia. *Diabetes Care.* 2003;26(4):1064-1068.

16. Sperling LS, Mechanick JI, Neeland IJ, et al. The cardiometabolic health alliance: working toward a new care model for the metabolic syndrome. *J Am Coll Cardiol.* 2015;66(9):1050-1067.

17. Bhatt DL, Roe MT, Peterson ED, et al. Utilization of early invasive management strategies for high-risk patients with non–ST-segment elevation acute coronary syndromes: results from the CRUSADE Quality Improvement Initiative. *JAMA.* 2004;292(17):2096-2104.

18. Conaway DG, O'Keefe JH, Reid KJ, Spertus J. Frequency of undiagnosed diabetes mellitus in patients with acute coronary syndrome. *Am J Cardiol.* 2005;96(3):363-365.

19. Sarma S, Mentz RJ, Kwasny MJ, et al. Association between diabetes mellitus and post-discharge outcomes in patients hospitalized with heart failure: findings from the EVEREST trial. *Eur J Heart Fail.* 2013;15(2):194-202.

20. Cheung NW, Wong VW, McLean M. The Hyperglycemia: Intensive Insulin Infusion in Infarction (HI-5) study: a randomized controlled trial of insulin infusion therapy for myocardial infarction. *Diabetes Care.* 2006;29(4):765-770.

21. Targher G, Dauriz M, Tavazzi L, et al. Prognostic impact of in-hospital hyperglycemia in hospitalized patients with acute heart failure: results of the IN-HF (Italian Network on Heart Failure) Outcome registry. *Int J Cardiol.* 2016;203:587-593.

22. Rosengren A, Vestberg D, Svensson AM, et al. Long-term excess risk of heart failure in people with type 1 diabetes: a prospective case-control study. *Lancet Diabetes Endocrinol.* 2015;3(11):876-885.

23. Staszewsky L, Cortesi L, Baviera M, et al. Diabetes mellitus as risk factor for atrial fibrillation hospitalization: incidence and outcomes over nine years in a region of Northern Italy. *Diabetes Res Clin Pract.* 2015;109(3):476-484.

24. Gandhi GY, Nuttall GA, Abel MD, et al. Intraoperative hyperglycemia and perioperative outcomes in cardiac surgery patients. *Mayo Clin Proc.* 2005;80(7):862-866.

25. Umpierrez G, Cardona S, Pasquel F, et al. Randomized controlled trial of intensive versus conservative glucose control in patients undergoing coronary artery bypass graft surgery: GLUCO-CABG trial. *Diabetes Care.* 2015;38(9):1665-1672.

26. Lang CC, Beniaminovitz A, Edwards N, Mancini DM. Morbidity and mortality in diabetic patients following cardiac transplantation. *J Heart Lung Transplant.* 2003;22(3):244-249.

27. Galindo RJ, Wallia A. Hyperglycemia and diabetes mellitus following organ transplantation. *Curr Diab Rep.* 2016;16(2):14.

28. Jacobi J, Bircher N, Krinsley J, et al. Guidelines for the use of an insulin infusion for the management of hyperglycemia in critically ill patients. *Crit Care Med.* 2012;40(12):3251-3276.

29. Chow E, Bernjak A, Williams S, et al. Risk of cardiac arrhythmias during hypoglycemia in patients with type 2 diabetes and cardiovascular risk. *Diabetes.* 2014;63(5):1738-1747.

30. Pinto DS, Skolnick AH, Kirtane AJ, et al. U-shaped relationship of blood glucose with adverse outcomes among patients with ST-segment elevation myocardial infarction. *J Am Coll Cardiol.* 2005;46(1):178-180.

31. Finfer S, Wernerman J, Preiser JC, et al. Clinical review: consensus recommendations on measurement of blood glucose and reporting glycemic control in critically ill adults. *Crit Care.* 2013;17(3):229.

32. Kosiborod M, Gottlieb RK, Sekella JA, et al. Performance of the Medtronic Sentrino continuous glucose management (CGM) system in the cardiac intensive care unit. *BMJ Open Diabetes Res Care.* 2014;2(1):e000037.

33. Wallia A, Umpierrez GE, Nasraway SA, Klonoff DC, PRIDE Investigators. Round table discussion on inpatient use of continuous glucose monitoring at the international hospital diabetes meeting. *J Diabetes Sci Technol.* 2016;10(5):1174-1181.

34. Steg PG, James SK, Atar D, et al. ESC Guidelines for the management of acute myocardial infarction in patients presenting with ST-segment elevation. *Eur Heart J.* 2012;33(20):2569-2619.

35. van den Berghe G, Wouters P, Weekers F, et al. Intensive insulin therapy in critically ill patients. *N Engl J Med.* 2001;345(19):1359-1367.

36. Finfer S, Chittock D, Li Y, et al. Intensive versus conventional glucose control in critically ill patients with traumatic brain injury: long-term follow-up of a subgroup of patients from the NICE-SUGAR study. *Intensive Care Med.* 2015;41(6):1037-47.

37. Van den Berghe G, Wilmer A, Hermans G, et al. Intensive insulin therapy in the medical ICU. *N Engl J Med.* 2006;354(5):449-461.

38. Malmberg K, Ryden L, Efendic S, et al. Randomized trial of insulin-glucose infusion followed by subcutaneous insulin treatment in diabetic patients with acute myocardial infarction (DIGAMI study): effects on mortality at 1 year. *J Am Coll Cardiol.* 1995;26(1):57-65.

39. Malmberg K, Ryden L, Wedel H, et al. Intense metabolic control by means of insulin in patients with diabetes mellitus and acute myocardial infarction (DIGAMI 2): effects on mortality and morbidity. *Eur Heart J.* 2005;26(7):650-661.

40. Davidson PC, Steed RD, Bode BW. Glucommander: a computer-directed intravenous insulin system shown to be safe, simple, and effective in 120,618 h of operation. *Diabetes Care.* 2005;28(10):2418-2423.

41. Joshi GP, Chung F, Vann MA, et al. Society for Ambulatory Anesthesia consensus statement on perioperative blood glucose management in diabetic patients undergoing ambulatory surgery. *Anesth Analg.* 2010;111(6):1378-1387.

42. Pichardo-Lowden A, Gabbay RA. Management of hyperglycemia during the perioperative period. *Curr Diab Rep.* 2012;12(1):108-118.

43. Herzog E, Aziz E, Croitor S, et al. Pathway for the management of hyperglycemia in critical care units. *Crit Pathw Cardiol.* 2006;5(2):114-120.

44. Umpierrez GE, Smiley D, Zisman A, et al. Randomized study of basal-bolus insulin therapy in the inpatient management of patients with type 2 diabetes (RABBIT 2 trial). *Diabetes Care.* 2007;30(9):2181-2186.

45. Umpierrez GE, Smiley D, Hermayer K, et al. Randomized study comparing a basal-bolus with a basal plus correction insulin regimen for the hospital management of medical and surgical patients with type 2 diabetes: basal plus trial. *Diabetes Care.* 2013;36(8):2169-2174.

46. Kreider KE, Lien LF. Transitioning safely from intravenous to subcutaneous insulin. *Curr Diab Rep.* 2015;15(5):23.

47. Bueno E, Benitez A, Rufinelli JV, et al. Basal-Bolus regimen with insulin analogues versus human insulin in medical patients with type 2 diabetes: a randomized controlled trial in Latin America. *Endocr Pract.* 2015;21(7):807-813.

48. Baldwin D, Zander J, Munoz C, et al. A randomized trial of two weight-based doses of insulin glargine and glulisine in hospitalized subjects with type 2 diabetes and renal insufficiency. *Diabetes Care.* 2012;35(10):1970-1974.

49. Umpierrez GE, Reyes D, Smiley D, et al. Hospital discharge algorithm based on admission HbA$_{1c}$ for the management of patients with type 2 diabetes. *Diabetes Care.* 2014;37(11):2934-2939.

Patient and Family Information for: DIABETES MELLITUS IN THE CARDIAC CARE UNIT

DIABETES MELLITUS: GENERAL PRINCIPLES

WHAT IS DIABETES MELLITUS AND HOW IS IT DIAGNOSED?

Diabetes Mellitus (DM) is a condition in which the level of glucose or sugar in the blood is higher than normal (also called hyperglycemia). A higher level of glucose in the system over a long period of time leads to injury to different organs in the body, generally affecting the nerves, eyes, and possibly the arteries as well. According to the American Diabetes Association (ADA) criteria, a number of measurements can be used to make the diagnosis of DM, such as the following:

1. Randomly measured levels of glucose in the blood
2. The measurement of glucose while fasting
3. The measurement of blood sugar after a standardized glucose intake is given to the patient orally
4. By measuring the amount of glucose particles attached to blood hemoglobin (A_{1C}), which represents average blood glucose (BG) level over a 3-month period and is a very consistent indicator of risk for diabetes complications

Some of these measurements need to be repeated to confirm the final diagnosis of diabetes.

WHAT CAUSES DIABETES?

DM has various types including type 1, type 2, gestational (associated with pregnancy), or other specified and less common types. Insulin is the hormone mainly responsible for titration of blood sugar level and is secreted from pancreas (an organ in the abdomen that is closely associated with intestinal tract). Type 1 diabetes means that the pancreas is not producing enough, or any, insulin to maintain the blood sugar in the normal range. Type 2 diabetes is not only characterized by resistance to the action of insulin for multiple reasons but also by a relative decrease in the body's ability to secrete insulin (insulin is produced but not in sufficient quantities or in an appropriate pattern to overcome the insulin resistance). Increased resistance to insulin, owing to greater quantities of different hormones in the blood that occur during pregnancy, is the basis for gestational diabetes. The resistance to insulin usually resolves after the patient gives birth but the presence of gestational diabetes constitutes a high-risk factor of developing type 2 diabetes later in the patient's life and therefore these patient's require close follow-up. Other less common types of diabetes could be because of genetic defects affecting insulin's action, pancreatic disease with decreased insulin production, various endocrine dysfunctions, various drugs, rare infections, immune-mediated reactions, and so on. The overall clinical manifestation of these other types are similar to either type 1 or type 2 diabetes.

Type 1 diabetes: Insulin therapy is essential in patients with type 1 diabetes because they do not produce any. DKA is a known complication of type 1 diabetes in patients not receiving insulin injections. This is a very dangerous condition characterized by dehydration, nausea, and vomiting and is so severe that it can lead to coma and even death if left untreated. It is completely reversible with the appropriate administration of insulin and glucose.

Type 2 diabetes: Basically it means a resistance to insulin and the body's inability to compensate by producing more from the pancreas. Type 2 diabetes is always preceded by a condition called prediabetes. Prediabetes is defined by high levels of fasting glucose, unusual rise in blood sugar in response to the higher amounts of glucose intake, and higher levels of A_{1C} but not to the degree seen in full-blown diabetes. A gradual increase in resistance to insulin's action (insulin resistance) occurs with aging, obesity, physical inactivity, and genetic factors. If the insulin resistance is not overcome by producing more insulin then, this will lead to increased glucose in the blood and finally frank DM. It is important to understand that obesity, especially "male-type" abdominal obesity is the central component in developing prediabetes and type 2 diabetes.

Prediabetes can be detected through the same tests as full-blown diabetes. Individuals considered "at risk" should be screened for both prediabetes and type 2 diabetes. Early detection not only allows an early implementation of preventive measures aimed at reducing insulin resistance (weight loss, increased physical activity, etc.) but can also prevent chronic complications and can improve longevity and chances of complication-free survival.

ELEVATED BLOOD GLUCOSE WHILE HOSPITALIZED (INPATIENT HYPERGLYCEMIA)

Sometimes acutely ill patients who are not known to have had diabetes or prediabetes of any kind may develop high BG while admitted to the hospital because the stress on the body from illness causes a state of insulin resistance. This can also happen in patients who have latent diabetes, prediabetes, or just are at risk for diabetes development but are normally glucose tolerant when not sick. It is unclear how frequently this leads to persistent diabetes after hospitalization, but inpatient elevations of BG have been linked to worse outcomes in the critical care units. If the patient survives the critical event but shows signs of impaired glucose tolerance (IGT) (prediabetes), this can be an indication for the future development of diabetes, and it should be addressed by the physician caring for the patient in the outpatient setting.

CLINICAL MANIFESTATION OF DIABETES MELLITUS

Clinical manifestations of DM could be acute (such as diabetic ketoacidosis (DKA) or chronic. The chronic complications may affect the small blood vessels (microvascular) or large blood vessels (macrovascular) in the body. Microvascular complications include worsening vision, nerve dysfunction (neuropathy), and damage to the kidneys. Macrovascular complications include effects on the brain, heart, and other peripheral blood vessels (atherosclerosis and clotting). Other complications include an increased risk of infections and disorders of the skin, joints, and muscles.

TREATING ELEVATED BLOOD GLUCOSE TO ACHIEVE TARGET (OUTPATIENT MANAGEMENT)

Currently it is recommended to aim for tight glucose control early in the course of diabetes. There are several ways to assess glucose control in DM. One can frequently test BG throughout the day with a glucometer (a handheld machine for bedside or home BG measurements), measure A_{1C}, or measure BG continuously through a subcutaneous catheter (inserted under the skin), which is called continuous glucose monitoring. Glucose monitoring is essential for the patients to achieve the glucose targets. A_{1C} reflects mean glucose over a 2- to 3-month period. Beyond the desirable range, it is a marker for risk of complications. The target level of A_{1C} recommended by the ADA is <7% or as close to normal as safely possible to achieve. It should be tested every 6 months if the value is at target or every 3 months when not on target, or when treatment changes. Other glucose targets for tight control have been defined for fasting BG and for glucose checked 2 hours after consumption of a meal (postprandial). The fasting glucose target has been defined by the ADA as 90 to 130 mg/dL, whereas 2-hour postprandial glucose target has been defined as <180 mg/dL peak value. Glucose monitoring is best demonstrated by a diabetes educator, who can also best determine the devices that should be used and how often to test. The glucose should be monitored at least 3 times/day, before each of the main meals, for patients on insulin injections to guide dosing. Those not on insulin could use self-monitoring as a guide to success.

MANAGEMENT OF LOW BLOOD GLUCOSE (HYPOGLYCEMIA)

The correct management of low levels of BG is crucial in all diabetics but especially in those with cardiac disease, vascular disease, or advanced complications. The low BG levels should be correctly evaluated and treated immediately. The severity of low glucose levels is considered mild to moderate when levels of BG range from 50 to 70 mg/dL and/or patients can treat it themselves. It can be treated with simple, and easily absorbable oral sources of carbohydrate such as glucose tablets/gel, orange juice, or soft drinks containing 15 to 20 g glucose. Glucose levels should be checked again in 15 minutes and patients must be educated to carry a source of glucose with them at all times. Extremely low BG levels of <50 mg/dL, when accompanied by altered consciousness and requiring the patients to need assistance, is considered to be very severe. The patient needs to take 20 to 30 g of simple glucose orally if able to or be given glucagon (a hormone produced by the pancreas, which counteracts insulin) by intramuscular injection. If the patient is not responsive to the previous methods, then 911 should be called for IV glucose to be administered. If severe hypoglycemia is consistently present, patients should be referred for a diabetes self-management education workshop, where the use of glucagon injection should be taught to family members or caretakers. In addition, BG goals have to be revised. If patients have frequent episodes of low BG or are unaware of the symptoms that usually accompany these low levels, they need support from family members or friends to prevent them from

harm. These at-risk patients should wear identifying bracelets and it is not recommended that they drive.

IDENTIFYING AND TREATING COMPLICATIONS OF DIABETES

The treatment of chronic complications of diabetes should be conducted according to published standards of care to ensure early diagnosis and to prevent progression. These standards of care are published yearly by the ADA. Retinopathy, nephropathy, and neuropathy are the targeted complications. Retinopathy is one of the eye complications of DM. It can lead to blindness if not treated early with laser or other methods. Diabetes is also a risk factor for the development of cataracts and glaucoma. Patients should have annual dilated eye examinations after 3 years from the onset of type 1 diabetes and immediately at the time of diagnosis for type 2 diabetes. Prevention of retinopathy is through tight control of BG and also by smoking cessation along with control of blood pressure and blood lipids (cholesterol and triglycerides). Diabetic nephropathy (kidney injury) manifests itself as protein leaking into the urine, which eventually can lead to kidney failure requiring dialysis. The amount of protein leaking into the urine should be checked annually with a random spot urine test. Also, the kidney function needs to be monitored at least annually. The prevention of kidney failure should be done through tight glucose and blood pressure control and through administration of agents that lower leakage of protein in the urine. When severe protein leakage is present, there may be swelling of the legs, and the treatment should include dietary protein reduction, blood pressure lowering to <125/75 mm Hg, and revised glucose management goals. Diabetic neuropathy or nerve damage can affect the "peripheral" nerves (those going to the feet and legs, hands, etc.) or the nerves that go to the internal organs. The former can lead to diabetic foot ulcers, damage to the joints, and deformities of the feet with fractures and infections and, ultimately, even amputations. Inspection of the feet should be done at every visit; feet identified to be at high risk should be referred for podiatric care and for orthotics. Patients should have diabetes self-management education including foot care training.

DIABETES MELLITUS IN THE CARDIAC CARE UNIT

HIGH PREVALENCE OF DIABETES MELLITUS AND HYPERGLYCEMIA IN THE ACUTE CORONARY SYNDROME

Patients with type 2 diabetes have a very high incidence of obesity and the so-called metabolic syndrome. Obesity, particularly abdominal obesity, predisposes the body to become more resistant to the effects of insulin. Metabolic syndrome is a constellation of insulin resistance with resultant metabolic derangements that puts the patient at particularly high risk for DM as well as CVD. Other associated metabolic abnormalities of this syndrome that include inflammation, abnormal lipid levels in the blood and a tendency to have blood clots in the vascular system are also associated with acute complications of CVD such as CAD which can lead to coronary syndrome (ACS). or heart attack. Numerous studies have shown that there is a very high prevalence of diabetes in patients admitted to the CCU with acute coronary syndrome (ACS). In addition to being frequently present in ACS, diabetes also predicts unfavorable outcomes in those who have ACS. Patients afflicted with both conditions (diabetes and ACS) have more frequent high blood pressure, high cholesterol, and kidney failure. This is regardless of whether the diabetes is new onset or established. High blood sugar affects ACS outcomes even if diabetes was not present before the event and is diagnosed in the hospital.

STRATEGIES FOR IMPROVING OUTCOMES IN ACUTE CORONARY SYMPTOM COMPLICATED BY DIABETES AND/OR HIGH BLOOD GLUCOSE

To counteract complications from cardiac events in type 2 diabetes, various blood-thinning medications and early strategies to unblock blood vessels are done as early as possible. In addition to these important lifesaving therapies that are similar to those utilized in non–diabetic patients, glucose-lowering therapies and aggressive use of secondary prevention therapies for control of high blood pressure, cholesterol, and inflammation are also utilized. Currently, the consensus is that high BG should be lowered in patients with diabetes and ACS, but the level to be obtained will be dependent on how safe it is to get there without causing hypoglycemia. Both hyperglycemia and hypoglycemia are harmful and should be avoided in the CCU. Many patients with diabetes might need round-the-clock infusions of insulin intravenously to keep their BG level in the appropriate range. The rate at which this infusion enters the body is calculated and adjusted by frequent monitoring of BG levels via glucometers.

TRANSITION TO OUTPATIENT CARE

As soon as the patient's condition is stable and he/she is able to eat, the IV infusion of insulin can be safely switched to SQ (under the skin) injections in preparation for transfer to a general medical floor outside the CCU and eventually home. While in critical conditions, the body's insulin requirements are usually higher and as the acute critical condition improves, the insulin requirements usually go back to their baseline.

OTHER ASPECTS OF DIABETES MANAGEMENT

It is important to assess the goals of diabetes management before the hospital discharge and to follow up with primary care providers outside the hospital to make sure these goals are reached successfully. For anyone with a newly diagnosed DM, essential care also includes diabetes self-management education and nutrition education. If diabetes is diagnosed for the first time while the patient is in hospital, a minimum amount of diabetes education (survival skills) will be taught in the hospital before discharge and patients will be referred to an outpatient, ADA-certified, diabetes self-management education program. Diabetes self-management nutrition education addresses diet and energy balance, weight loss issues if needed, need for carbohydrate (sugar intake) counting in insulin-requiring patients, risk of low BG with decreased calorie intake, increase in physical activity, increase in dietary fiber (14 g/1,000 kcal), and alcohol intake (maximum one drink per day for women and two drinks per day for men).

Physical activity is recommended to be of both aerobic and resistance-type training and should be done in combination. Aerobic activity should be at least 150 minutes per week and it should be of moderate intensity, 50% to 70% of maximum heart rate (220-age). Resistance exercise should be done 3 times a week if there are no contraindications, such as the presence of advanced diabetic retinopathy. Blood pressure targets are lower for diabetics compared to general population (130/80 mm Hg in diabetics and125/75 mm Hg in diabetics with advanced kidney disease). Cholesterol levels also need particular attention in diabetics. Compliance with dietary recommendations and also regular physical activity not only improves the BG but will also significantly improve the cholesterol and triglyceride levels. The doctor might also prescribe cholesterol-lowering medications to help decrease risk of heart and vascular disease. Mood disorders such as depression and anxiety as well as social (family and economic issues) or physical (blindness, amputations, etc.) barriers can affect diabetes management. Inform the doctor about any possible barrier to an optimum diabetes management plan.

In those with inpatient hyperglycemia but without prior history of diabetes, it is important to arrange for regular follow-up after discharge to determine whether the hyperglycemia persists, and if not whether the patient is at risk of developing diabetes.

For more information about diabetes and treatments, visit the ADA website at http://www.diabetes.org/.

Barak Zafrir

55

Lipid Management in the Cardiac Care Unit

LIPIDS, ATHEROSCLEROSIS, AND CARDIOVASCULAR RISK

Elevated plasma lipoproteins are among the most important risk factors for coronary heart disease and are the driving force of atherogenesis. This strong link has been consistently demonstrated over the past decades in pathologic, epidemiologic, genetic, and interventional clinical studies, establishing causality between low-density lipoprotein cholesterol (LDL-C) and atherosclerosis.

Lipoprotein particles accumulate in the intima of arteries in hypercholesterolemic states and undergo oxidative and other modifications that are accelerated during endothelial dysfunction, leading to the uptake of LDL-C by macrophages and generation of foam cells evolving into fatty streaks.[1] This process initiates smooth muscle proliferation and the formation of a fibrous cap, covering the lipid core filled with macrophages. The concept of "response to retention" provides a mechanistic link between accumulation of lipoprotein particles, proinflammatory effects, and the initiation and progression of the atherosclerotic plaque.[2]

Epidemiologic studies have firmly established a direct relationship between serum cholesterol levels and the prevalence of atherosclerotic cardiovascular disease (CVD). Many large randomized controlled trials in the statin era have documented that lowering total cholesterol and LDL-C reduces the risk for both coronary heart disease and stroke, largely irrespective of the initial lipid profile, in a wide range of individuals, including those at relatively low risk for vascular events, and in direct relationship to the intensity of the statin regimen.[3–5] Epidemiologic data have also shown that the concentration of high-density lipoprotein cholesterol (HDL-C) is an independent, inverse predictor for CVD and is important in global risk assessment. However, there is a lack of convincing evidence that raising HDL-C by pharmacologic interventions reduces the risk for CVD, and therefore currently low HDL-C concentration is not a primary target of drug therapy. A renewed interest driven by epidemiologic and genetic data supports triglyceride-rich lipoproteins and their cholesterol content (remnant cholesterol) as an additional contributor to CVD and cardiovascular mortality. However, conclusive evidence as to whether lowering high triglycerides levels reduces the risk of CVD is lacking.

Interindividual variability in blood lipids concentration is derived from both lifestyle and inherited factors. Single-gene mutations in LDL receptor pathway are strongly associated with high cholesterol levels and predispose to familial hypercholesterolemia and premature CVD.[6] In contrast, low cholesterol levels from birth caused by proprotein convertase subtilisin/kexin type 9 (PCSK9) loss-of-function gene mutations confer protection from atherosclerotic disease.[7] Genetic studies further show that genetic variants causing lifetime low LDL-C levels are associated with very low rates of coronary heart disease.[8] Polymorphisms (SNPs) from several genes that are associated with modulation of cholesterol levels were also demonstrated to be an independent risk factor for CVD. In contrast to the causal relationship between LDL-C and CVD, genetic mechanisms that raise plasma HDL-C were not reported to be related to lower risk of myocardial infarction. This challenges the concept that raising plasma HDL-C will uniformly translate into reduction in the risk of coronary heart disease.[9] Research now focuses on assessment of HDL functionality as a marker for atherosclerotic risk and a better target for therapeutic intervention than HDL-C.

PLASMA LIPID PROFILE

Routine lipid profile in most clinical biochemistry laboratories includes direct measurement of total cholesterol, HDL-C, and triglycerides. LDL-C is usually measured indirectly, calculated by the Friedewald equation: LDL-C = Total cholesterol minus HDL-C minus triglycerides/5 (with values in mg/dL). Friedewald equation underestimates LDL-C levels when triglycerides are elevated, and therefore LDL-C is not calculated indirectly when triglycerides are above 300–400 mg/dL, depending on specific institute laboratory. Direct measurement of LDL-C when triglyceride concentrations are high is feasible, but not available routinely at all institutions. Accordingly, calculation of non–HDL-C from standard lipid panel as total cholesterol minus HDL-C is recommended in hypertriglyceridemic states, and expresses the cholesterol content of all atherogenic apolipoprotein B (apoB)–containing particles. Non–HDL-C does not require additional charge, appears to be a more accurate marker of cardiovascular risk than LDL-C, and should be considered an alternative risk marker and a secondary treatment target, especially in hypertriglyceridemic states such as in metabolic syndrome, diabetes, and chronic kidney disease. The specific target for non–HDL-C should be about 30 mg/dL higher than the corresponding LDL-C target. To improve patient compliance with lipid testing, a recent consensus panel advocated the routine use of nonfasting lipid profiles, whereas fasting sampling should be considered when nonfasting triglycerides are signifcantly elevated.[10]

Early studies indicated that cholesterol levels (both LDL-C and HDL-C) start to decline 24 hours after acute myocardial infarction because of an acute-phase response, reach the nadir on approximately day 7, and normalize within 2 months after acute coronary syndrome (ACS). These changes in lipid levels should be taken into account when making clinical decisions in treating hyperlipidemia after ACS, and efforts should be made to take blood samples for lipid profile early in the course of ACS.

LIPOPROTEIN (a)

Lipoprotein(a) [Lp(a)] is a genetic, causal risk factor for CVD, showing an independent and continuous association with cardiovascular risk, including myocardial infarction, stroke, peripheral arterial disease, and calcific aortic valve stenosis.[11,12] Lp(a) is composed of a single molecule of apoB100 covalently linked to apo(a), which contains a unique region that is structurally homologous to plasminogen. It is suggested that Lp(a) induces both prothrombotic activity because of competitively antagonizing plasminogen binding and potential atherogenic effect secondary to arterial deposition of oxidized phospholipids by apoB. Candidates for Lp(a) screening include patients with a strong family history of premature CVD, patients with hypercholesterolemia in which Lp(a) has synergistic effects with elevated LDL-C levels, and patients with ACS and recurrent cardiovascular events despite maximal statin therapy. Niacin is the only medication that has consistently shown a dose-dependent lowering effect on Lp(a), reducing levels up to 30% in clinical trials. Lipoprotein apheresis is an effective therapeutic option reserved for severe cases of progressive coronary disease despite optimal drug therapy.[12] Although Lp(a) is a major causal cardiovascular risk factor in both genetic and population studies, there are no controlled trials that have shown that lowering Lp(a) through pharmacotherapy significantly reduces risk. Novel therapies such as PCSK9 inhibitors reduce 25% to 30% of Lp(a) concentration, and recent promising phase I studies in humans demonstrated a more significant reduction of Lp(a) levels by antisense oligonucleotides (ASOs) that inhibit apo(a) mRNA translation.

ADVANCED LIPOPROTEIN TESTING

Advanced lipoprotein analysis, including testing of lipoprotein subfractions, LDL particle number, and apoB concentration, has been proposed as a more accurate measure to assess the risk attributable to atherogenic lipoproteins and as a potential means to reduce residual cardiovascular risk. The cholesterol content of LDL particles varies substantially between individuals, and subjects with the same LDL-C level may have discordant numbers of LDL particles. Many patients with high cardiometabolic risk or diabetes have relatively normal levels of LDL-C that poorly characterize the excess concentration and risk of small dense LDL particles. The discordance between LDL-C and LDL particle number was shown to impact cardiovascular risk in the Framingham and Multi-Ethnic Study of Atherosclerosis (MESA) studies.[13,14] Therefore, measurements of LDL particle number or apoB rather than the cholesterol content of LDL may be more

adequate to assess the residual risk for coronary disease in high cardiometabolic risk subjects who achieve "optimal" LDL-C levels. However, the clinical utility of advanced lipoprotein analysis is still debated, and this test is not routinely in use in clinical medicine.

FAMILIAL HYPERCHOLESTEROLEMIA

Familial hypercholesterolemia (FH) is a common monogenic disorder of lipoprotein metabolism, associated with high concentrations of LDL-C, predisposing affected individuals and their families to premature coronary heart disease.[6] FH is prevalent globally, reaching 1:300 in the general population in its heterozygous form because of principally autosomal dominant inheritance. Nevertheless, FH is vastly underdiagnosed and undertreated in most countries. Patients with FH are often unrecognized despite typical presentation with premature coronary heart disease and severely elevated LDL-C levels. Cardiovascular risk is driven by the presence of concomitant risk factors and the cumulative LDL-C burden throughout life, which is a function of age of initiation of drug therapy and compliance with treatment. LDL-C $\geq$ 190 mg/dL in adults and $\geq$ 160 mg/dL in children raises the likelihood of the presence of monogenic disorder. However, in the setting of the general population, customary LDL-C cutoffs of 190 mg/dL in children, 220 mg/dL between ages 20 and 29 years, and 240 mg/dL in adults $\geq$30 years are associated with an 80% probability of FH (MEDPED criteria). Secondary causes of severe hypercholesterolemia should be excluded (**Table 55.1**). Family history of hypercholesterolemia and coronary disease at young age in relatives, as well as physical stigmata such as tendon xanthomas and arcus cornea, which are seen in about 30% to 40% of patients and are correlated with severity and duration of hypercholesterolemia, are aditional diagnostic criteria.

Identification of FH patients is important, because early intensive treatment and cascade screening of families may further reduce cardiovascular event rates. Although direct detection of causative gene mutations is available and molecular genetics for screening family relatives is carried out successfully in several countries, genetic testing is still costly and is not systematically feasible in most places. Cardiovascular divisions such as the cardiac care unit may provide ideal locations to promote identification and treatment of high-risk patients with FH.

LIPID MANAGEMENT IN ACS

STATINS

Statins are the cornerstone of pharmacologic therapy in the prevention of atherosclerotic CVD. Statins inhibit HMG-CoA reductase, the rate-limiting step of cholesterol synthesis, subsequently upregulating LDL receptors on the surface of hepatocytes. Statins are targeted mainly for significant reduction of LDL-C levels, up to 55%, but improve, to some extent, all components of the lipid profile. Large-scale, randomized, controlled statin trials of both primary and secondary prevention in humans have shown repeatedly that LDL-C reduction by statins correlates linearly with CVD, reducing myocardial infarction, stroke, and cardiovascular death.[4,5] These trials have demonstrated that the beneficial effects of statins are preserved also in subjects with low baseline LDL-C < 100 mg/dL and in patients with diabetes.

TABLE 55.1	Secondary Causes of Hyperlipidemia
DISORDERS AFFECTING LIPIDS	**MEDICATIONS AFFECTING LIPIDS**
Hypercholesterolemia	Antihypertensives
Nephrotic syndrome	*β-Blockers*
Hypothyroidism	*Thiazides*
Cholestatic liver disease	Steroid hormones
Cushing syndrome	*Combined oral contraceptives*
Anorexia nervosa	*Estrogen replacement therapy*
Pregnancy	*Anabolic steroids (testosterone)*
Autoimmune disorders	*Glucocorticoids*
• Lupus; Rheumatoid arthritis	Antiretroviral therapy
Immunoglobulin excess	*Protease inhibitors*
• Gammopathies	Psychotropic medications
Hypertriglyceridemia	*Clozapine; Olanzapine; Risperidone*
Diabetes mellitus	Antidepressants
Obesity	*Tricyclics; Mirtazapine*
Metabolic syndrome and PCOS[a]	*SSRIs[a] (Sertraline and Paroxetine)*
Hypothyroidism	Retinoic-acid derivatives (isotretinoin)
Chronic kidney disease	Immunosuppressant agents
Pregnancy	*Cyclosporine; Tacrolimus*
Excessive alcohol consumption	Anticonvulsants
Diet high in simple carbohydrates	*Valproic acid*
Lipodystrophies	

[a]PCOS, polycystic ovary syndrome; SSRI, selective serotonin reuptake inhibitors.

Furthermore, intensive lipid lowering with a more potent or higher dose statin resulted in further reduction of both LDL-C levels and major cardiovascular events compared with a less intensive regimen, in both stable and acute coronary artery disease populations. Patients with a history of atherosclerotic vascular disease, including ischemic stroke or peripheral artery disease, are considered coronary heart disease risk equivalents, and, as such, are targeted for high-intensity statin therapy to reduce cardiovascular events.

EFFECTS OF EARLY STATIN TREATMENT ON CLINICAL OUTCOMES AFTER ACS

Early initiation of statin treatment has become a guideline-directed standard of care after ACS because of several landmark randomized prospective trials presented during the years 2001 to 2004. The Myocardial Ischemia Reduction with Aggressive Cholesterol Lowering (MIRACL) study was the first large study investigating the potential clinical benefit of the early use of statins in ACS.[15] Initiation of high-dose atorvastatin (80 mg/d) early (24–96 hours) after ACS reduced cardiovascular adverse events during the first 4 months after starting therapy, especially new hospitalizations for recurrent ischemia. In the A- to -Z trial, patients admitted for ACS and treated with an early intensive statin therapy (simvastatin 40 mg/d for 1 month followed by 80 mg/d) had lower mortality risk compared to less intensive treatment (placebo for 4 months followed by simvastatin 20 mg/d) that was started later.[16] However, the study failed to show an improvement in overall cardiovascular outcomes.

The Pravastatin or Atorvastatin Evaluation and Infection Therapy–Thrombolysis in Myocardial Infarction 22 (PROVE IT–TIMI 22) trial compared a standard statin regime (pravastatin 40 mg/d) to intensive treatment (atorvastatin 80 mg/d), within 10 days of hospital admission for ACS, confirming that high-intensity statin therapy provided greater protection, reducing the rate of cardiovascular adverse events in 16% during a mean follow-up of 24 months, as well as 30-day clinical outcomes.[17] Additional substudy later confirmed the results in the subset of patients who performed percutaneous coronary intervention (PCI) for the acute coronary event, and showed reduced target vessel revascularization in the patients randomized for high-intensity statin.

Although the results of these studies seem to support the protective role of high-intensity statin therapy in the early period after ACS, it should be noted that several meta-analyses summarizing the evidence on early statin therapy for ACS showed favorable but nonsignificant reduction in death or myocardial infarction in the short term, but significant reduction in the occurrence of unstable angina at 4 months following ACS.[18,19] Past ACC/AHA guidelines recommended (Level of Evidence 1A) the use of statin therapy before hospital discharge for all patients with ACS regardless of the baseline LDL-C. The most recent ACC/AHA 2013 guidelines on the treatment of blood cholesterol state that high-intensity statin therapy (atorvastatin 40 to 80 mg or rosuvastatin 20 to 40 mg) should be initiated or continued as first-line therapy in all patients ≤75 years of age that have clinical atherosclerotic CVD but do not relate specifically to the early phase post-ACS.[20]

STATIN-ASSOCIATED BENEFITS IN PATIENTS UNDERGOING PCI

Several studies have reported that short-term preprocedural administration of statins might reduce the incidence of adverse effects after PCI. The Atorvastatin for Reduction of Myocardial Damage during Angioplasty—Acute Coronary Syndromes (ARMYDA-ACS) trial evaluated the loading dose of high-intensity atorvastatin before PCI in NSTEMI ACS, showing a reduced incidence of cardiovascular events in the first month after PCI.[21] A meta-analysis addressing the impact of timing of statin administration given before or after PCI on clinical outcomes reported that administration of statins before PCI reduces the odds of myocardial infarction at 30 days to a greater extent compared with a post-PCI administration, and that the earlier the statin administration, the lower the risk of early major adverse cardiovascular events.[22]

BENEFICIAL MECHANISMS OF EARLY STATIN INITIATION

The mechanisms underlying the protective actions of early statin administration may be independent of LDL-C reduction. Statins have been shown to modulate several mechanisms involved in the pathogenesis of ACS, including inflammation, oxidative stress, and vascular smooth muscle proliferation. Beneficial effects on platelet aggregation and endothelial function were also reported. Intravascular ultrasound (IVUS) studies have shown that statins significantly decrease plaque volume after ACS,[23] and cumulative data support the effectiveness of statin treatment in promoting plaque stabilization and regression, especially after ACS and with the use of high-intensity statins.[24]

STATINS AND THE PREVENTION OF CONTRAST-INDUCED ACUTE KIDNEY INJURY

Patients with ACS have a 3-fold higher risk of developing contrast-induced acute kidney injury, which is associated with prolonged hospitalization and increased morbidity and mortality. The Atorvastatin for Reduction of Myocardial Damage during Angioplasty—Contrast-Induced Nephropathy (ARMYDA-CIN) trial has shown that short-term pretreatment with high-dose atorvastatin decreases the incidence of contrast-induced nephropathy in statin-naïve patients with ACS undergoing early PCI.[25] More recently, the Protective Effect of Rosuvastatin and Antiplatelet Therapy On contrast-induced acute kidney injury and myocardial damage in patients with Acute Coronary Syndrome (PRATO-ACS) study has similarly demonstrated that preprocedural high-dose rosuvastatin given on admission to statin-naïve patients with ACS, who were scheduled for an early invasive procedure, can prevent contrast-induced acute kidney injury and improve short-term clinical outcomes.[26] More effective kidney protection was demonstrated in ACS subjects with higher baseline high-sensitivity C-reactive protein (hs-CRP) levels.

STATIN INTOLERANCE AND ADVERSE EFFECTS

Statin therapy is generally considered to be safe. However, muscular symptoms are common in clinical practice, may reduce patients' adherence to therapy, and can be a barrier in maximizing cardiovascular risk reduction, especially in secondary prevention of CVD, of which high-intensity statins are now indicated. The clinical spectrum of statin-induced myotoxicity includes myalgia (reaching 1%–3% in randomized-controlled trials, but 10%–20% in observational and epidemiologic studies), less commonly myositis with significant elevated creatine kinase levels, and, very rarely, rhabdomyolysis. Asymptomatic rise in creatine kinase concentration is also observed. Factors that increase the risk of statin-induced myopathy include patient-related factors such as advanced-age, female gender, lower weight, excess of alcohol and strenuous exercise, as well as hypothyroidism, vitamin D deficiency, statin–drugs interactions, high statin dose, Asian ancestry, and genetic predisposition. In addition to ruling out possible conditions that may increase the risk of muscle symptoms, the management options include reduction in statin dose, alternate day regimens of statins with longer half-life (atorvastatin and rosuvastatin), transient cessation of therapy, and usage of an alternative statin or other lipid-lowering agent. In cases where muscle symptoms are progressive or creatine kinase is more than X10 the upper limit of normal (ULN), the statin treatment should be stopped. In rare cases of necrotizing autoimmune myopathy, steroids and immunosuppression may be needed. There is no clear evidence that Co-enzyme Q10 treatment is beneficial in statin-induced myotoxicity, because small randomized trials displayed equivocal results.

Mild elevations of hepatocellular liver enzymes are commonly seen in clinical practice. However, liver failure in statin users is rare and is similar to that in the overall population. In cases where hepatic aminotransferase levels are >3 times the ULN values, it is recommended to withhold statin treatment, reassess liver tests, and consider other causes of liver damage. Nevertheless, routine periodic monitoring of liver function tests in patients taking statins is no longer recommended, because it does not appear to be effective for detecting or preventing serious liver injury.

Randomized trials, including recent meta-analyses, have demonstrated a consistent relationship between statins, elevation of blood glucose level, and a modest increase in the risk of incident diabetes.[27] This association seems to be dependent on the dose and potency of the statin. Individuals prone to statin-induced diabetes were shown to have major risk factors for diabetes that were similar to those in the general population, including multiple components of the metabolic syndrome and impaired fasting glucose. The benefits of statins in reducing cardiovascular events outweigh the potential risk for developing new-onset diabetes in patients who are at moderate or high risk for cardiovascular events and in secondary prevention.

Although some patients in observational data and small randomized trials were reported to experience ill-defined memory loss and confusion, recent large meta-analyses and systematic reviews have shown no evidence of increase in the risk of cognitive impairment.

NONSTATIN LIPID-LOWERING THERAPIES

Ezetimibe selectively inhibits cholesterol absorption from the intestine by blocking the transport protein Niemann–Pick C1-Like 1 transporter (NPC1L1) in the brush border of enterocytes, lowering plasma LDL-C levels by 15% to 20%. Ezetimibe is usually used in combination with statins, enhancing LDL-C lowering effect, with a good safety profile. The recently published IMProved Reduction of Outcomes: Vytorin Efficacy International Trial (IMPROVE-IT) showed that when added to simvastatin therapy, ezetimibe resulted in incremental lowering of LDL-C levels and improved cardiovascular outcomes after ACS, demonstrating that lowering LDL-C to levels below previous targets provided additional benefit.[28] This landmark study is the first to show a cardiovascular benefit in adding a nonstatin lipid-modifying agent to statin therapy, reaffirming the LDL hypothesis suggesting that the reduction of LDL-C levels reduces the rate of CVD.

Medications for lowering triglycerides include fibrates, omega-3 polyunsaturated fatty acids (fish oil supplements) in pharmacologic dosages (DHA/EPA 2 to 4 g a day), and niacin. These medications have the ability to reduce 20% to 50% of triglyceride levels in blood and are indicated when levels are above 500 to 1,000 mg/dL in order to prevent acute pancreatitis. However, randomized trials showing the cardiovascular benefit of triglyceride reduction are scarce, and trials assessing fibrates and niacin as an add-on therapy against a background of statin treatment failed to show cardiovascular risk reduction. Therefore, in the statin era the routine use of fibrates and niacin is limited. Nevertheless, subgroup analysis of outcome trials with the major fibrates showed significant relative risk reduction of cardiovascular events in patients with atherogenic dyslipidemia manifested by elevated triglyceride levels (>200 mg/dL) and low HDL-C (<35 mg/dL). Accordingly, fibrates might be considered in high-risk patients with atherogenic dyslipidemia, especially in diabetes and metabolic syndrome, as an add-on treatment to statins in order to reduce the risk for atherosclerotic CVD. Large-scale trials are awaited to provide conclusive evidence as to whether lowering triglycerides reduces the risk of CVD.

PCSK9 inhibitors are a new class of lipid-lowering medications. Binding of PCSK9 to the LDL receptor targets the receptor for lysosomal degradation. The recognition that inhibition of PCSK9 increases LDL receptor activity and the discovery of gene mutations affecting PCSK9 with clinical effects on cardiovascular risk have led to the development of human monoclonal antibodies against PCSK9, self-administered by subcutaneous injections. The PCSK9 inhibitors, approved by the U.S. Food and Drug Administration (FDA) in mid-2015 (evolocumab and alirocumab), when evaluated in numerous phase 3 trials, were found to reduce LDL-C levels up to 65% independent of background statin therapy and with a good safety profile, at least for the short term. However, information on whether PCSK9 inhibitors affect cardiovascular events or mortality is not yet available, and long-term outcome and safety studies are ongoing. Therefore, PCSK9 inhibitors are currently approved for use, in addition to maximally tolerated statin therapy, in patients with FH or clinical atherosclerotic CVD, who require additional lowering of LDL-C to achieve treatment goals.

DIET AND LIFESTYLE INTERVENTIONS

Nonpharmacologic, therapeutic lifestyle interventions are an essential part of the treatment of lipid disorders in both primary and secondary prevention of atherosclerotic CVD. This includes physical activity with an emphasis on aerobic exercise, weight loss, smoking cessation, moderation of alcohol intake, and adjustment of dietary patterns and nutrient intake (discussed separately). Patients with the metabolic syndrome, characterized by central obesity, impaired fasting glucose and insulin resistance, as well as hypertension and atherogenic dyslipidemia (hypertriglyceridemia, low HDL-C and small dense LDL particles), may benefit in particular from lifestyle interventions that were shown to significantly delay conversion to diabetes and its cardiovascular complications. The setting of hospitalization may serve as an ideal opportunity for initial dietary and lifestyle counseling of high-risk patients. In addition, attention should be given to severe hypertriglyceridemia during hospitalization, because it may precipitate acute pancreatitis. Secondary causes of hypertriglyceridemia should be searched for and targeted; these include high carbohydrate intake (especially fructose) and calorie excess, ethanol consumption, central obesity, poor glycemic control, and medications such as systemic glucocorticoids (**Table 55.1**).

GUIDELINES FOR THE TREATMENT OF DYSLIPIDEMIA

Guidelines provide consistency in care, aiming to incorporate new evidence and guide clinical decision making. In 2013, after more than a decade, the American College of Cardiology (ACC) and the American Heart Association (AHA) published a set of guidelines on the control of blood cholesterol to reduce atherosclerotic CVD risk.[20] The AHA/ACC guidelines differed from previous widely adopted national and international guidelines, and thus have been a subject of controversy. Major changes included the abandonment of numerical LDL-C treatment targets, focusing instead on the intensity of statin therapy (**Table 55.2**), and the formation of a newly developed *Pooled Cohort Equations* calculator for estimating 10-year atherosclerotic CVD risk. In addition, in comparison to the previous Adult Treatment Panel III (ATP III) lipid guidelines, the risk threshold for considering statins in the primary prevention setting was lowered to a 10-year absolute atherosclerotic CVD risk of 7.5%. **Table 55.3** compares the similarities and differences in treatment recommendations

TABLE 55.2	Statin Therapy Intensity and LDL-C Reduction		
STATIN INTENSITY	**HIGH INTENSITY**	**MODERATE INTENSITY**	**LOW INTENSITY**
LDL-C lowering (daily dose)	≥50%	30%–50%	<30%
Drugs	Atorvastatin 40–80 mg Rosuvastatin 20–40 mg	Atorvastatin 10–20 mg Rosuvastatin 5–10 mg Simvastatin 20–40 mg Pravastatin 40–80 mg Lovastatin 40 mg Fluvastatin 80 mg Pitavastatin 2–4 mg	Simvastatin 10 mg Pravastatin 10–20 mg Lovastatin 20 mg Fluvastatin 20–40 mg Pitavastatin 1 mg

TABLE 55.3		Comparison Between Lipid Treatment Guidelines	
ACC/AHA (2013) GUIDELINE ON THE TREATMENT OF BLOOD CHOLESTEROL TO REDUCE ASCVD RISK		**ESC/EAS (2011) GUIDELINES FOR THE MANAGEMENT OF DYSLIPIDEMIAS**	
RISK CATEGORIES	**TREATMENT**	**RISK CATEGORIES**	**TREATMENT**
Clinical ASCVD[a]	High-intensity[b] statin Age > 75 or safety concern: Moderate-intensity[b] statin	**Cardiovascular disease**[a]	LDL-C < 70 mg/dL and/or ≥50% reduction.
Diabetes: **Type I or II** **Age 40–75** **LDL-C 70–189 mg/dL**	*High-risk:* (10-y ASCVD risk ≥7.5%): High-intensity statin *Low-risk:* Moderate-intensity statin	**Diabetes (type II or type I with target organ damage) or moderate to severe CKD (GFR ≤ 60 mL/min/1.73 m²)**	LDL-C < 70 mg/dL and/or ≥50% reduction. Second goals: non-HDL-C< 100 mg/dL and apoB < 80 mg/dL.
Primary LDL-C ≥190 mg/dL	High-intensity statin Achieve>50% LDL-C reduction	**Familial dyslipidemia**	LDL-C < 100 mg/dL or maximal reduction with drug combinations and LDL apheresis.
None of the above (primary prevention; age 40–75): **(a) 10-y ASCVD risk ≥ 7.5%** **(b) 10-y ASCVD risk 5%–7.5%** **(risk calculator based on the pooled cohort equations)**	**(a)** Moderate- to high-intensity statin **(b)** Consider moderate-intensity statin	**None of the above:** **10-y risk estimate of First fatal atherosclerotic CV event:** **(a) SCORE > 10%** **(b) SCORE 5%–10%** **(c) SCORE 1%–5%**	**(a)** Very high risk: LDL-C < 70 mg/dL **(b)** High risk: LDL-C < 100 mg/dL **(c)** Moderate risk: LDL-C < 115 mg/dL
If risk-based assessment uncertain, consider: • **Family history premature CVD** • **hsCRP ≥ 2.0 mg/L** • **CAC score ≥ 300 Agatston unit** • **ABI < 0.9** • **LDL-C ≥ 160 mg/dL** • **Lifetime ASCVD risk**		**Additional data modifying risk:** • **Elevated triglycerides** • **Social deprivation** • **Central obesity** • **Familial hypercholesterolemia** • **High lipoprotein (a) levels** • **Subclinical atherosclerosis** • **Chronic kidney disease** • **Family history of premature CVD** • **Low HDL-C**	
Additional recommendations: (a) Encourage lifestyle modifications. (b) Guidelines do not consider data on the use of lipid fractions other than LDL-C. (c) Statins are not routinely recommended for NYHA II–IV heart failure patients and those receiving hemodialysis. (d) Do not routinely measure and monitor ALT or CK, unless symptomatic.		Additional recommendations: **(a)** Encourage lifestyle modifications **(b)** Non-HDL-C and apoB should be considered an alternative risk marker and second treatment target in metabolic syndrome and diabetes (class IIa indication). **(c)** Statins are not indicated in patients with moderate or severe heart failure. Statins are indicated in moderate to severe CKD (LDL-C<70 mg/dL). **(d)** ALT should be measured before treatment, 8 weeks after starting treatment or dose increase, and annually thereafter. CK should be measured before starting treatment, but not necessary for monitoring.	

ABI, ankle-brachial index; ALT, alanine transaminase; ApoB, apolipoprotein B; ASCVD, atherosclerotic cardiovascular disease; CAC, coronary artery calcium; GFR, glomerular filtration rate; HDL-C, high-density lipoprotein cholesterol; hsCRP, high-sensitivity C-reactive protein; CK, creatine kinase; LDL-C, low-density lipoprotein cholesterol.

[a]ACC/AHA clinical ASCVD definition includes acute coronary syndromes, previous myocardial infarction, stable/unstable angina, arterial revascularizations, ischemic stroke or transient ischemic attack, and peripheral arterial disease presumed to be of atherosclerotic origin. ESC/EAS Cardiovascular disease definition includes, in addition, preclinical evidence for atherosclerotic disease on the basis of any imaging modality.

[b]High-intensity statin: daily dose lowers LDL-C by ≥50% (rosuvastatin 20 mg [40 mg]; atorvastatin 40/80 mg). Moderate-intensity: daily dose lowers LDL-C by 30% to 50%.

Initiate high-intensity statin at ACS diagnosis if no contraindication

Blood tests for lipid panel within 24 hours of ACS

If fasting triglycerides >500 mg/dL, consider adding fibrates and in-hospital dietary counselling

Assess characteristics predisposing to statin adverse effects:

comorbidities, impaired renal/hepatic function, hypothyroidism, vitamin D deficiency, history of muscle disorders, drugs affecting statins metabolism, Asian ancestry, >75 years of age

Predischarge counseling on lifestyle modification:

Diet, weight loss, smoking cessation, physical activity, as well as glucose and blood pressure control

Recheck lipid panel 4–6 weeks after ACS

Optimal treatment goal: LDL-C <70 mg/dL

If triglyceride levels >300 mg/dL, use non-HDL-C <100 mg/dL as a therapeutic target

FIGURE 55.1 Algorithm for the management of hyperlipidemia in acute coronary syndrome (ACS). HDL-C, high-density lipoprotein cholesterol; LDL-C, low-density lipoprotein cholesterol.

between the ACC/AHA 2013 guidelines and the most recent European guideline for the management of dyslipidemias.[29] Recently, an ACC expert consensus panel attempted to provide practical guidance for clinicians and patients regarding the use of nonstatin therapies as an add-on to statins, to further reduce CVD risk in situations not covered by the guidelines.[30] An algorithm for the management of lipids in ACS is provided in **Figure 55.1**.

REFERENCES

1. Tabas I, Williams KJ, Boren J. Subendothelial lipoprotein retention as the initiating process in atherosclerosis: update and therapeutic implications. *Circulation.* 2007;116:1832-1844.

2. Libby P, Ridker PM. Inflammation and atherothrombosis: from population biology and bench research to clinical practice. *J Am Coll Cardiol.* 2006;48:A33-A46.

3. Baigent C, Keech A, Kearney PM, et al; Cholesterol Treatment Trialists' (CTT) Collaborators. Efficacy and safety of cholesterol-lowering treatment: prospective meta-analysis of data from 90,056 participants in 14 randomised trials of statins. *Lancet.* 2005;366(9493):1267-1278.

4. Cholesterol Treatment Trialists' (CTT) Collaboration, Baigent C, Blackwell L, Emberson J, et al. Efficacy and safety of more intensive lowering of LDL cholesterol: a meta-analysis of data from 170,000 participants in 26 randomised trials. *Lancet.* 2010;376:1670-1681.

5. Cholesterol Treatment Trialists' (CTT) Collaborators, Mihaylova B, Emberson J, Blackwell L, et al. The effects of lowering LDL cholesterol with statin therapy in people at low risk of vascular disease: meta-analysis of individual data from 27 randomised trials. *Lancet.* 2012;380:581-590.

6. Nordestgaard BG, Chapman MJ, Humphries SJ, et al. Familial hypercholesterolaemia is underdiagnosed and undertreated in the general population: guidance for clinicians to prevent coronary heart disease. Consensus statement of the European Atherosclerosis Society. *Eur Heart J.* 2013;34:3478-3490.

7. Cohen JC, Boerwinkle E, Mosley TH, Hobbs HH. Sequence variations in PCSK9, low LDL, and protection against coronary heart disease. *N Engl J Med.* 2006;354:1264-1272.

8. Ference BA, Yoo W, Alesh I, et al. Effect of long-term exposure to lower low-density lipoprotein cholesterol beginning early in life on the risk of coronary heart disease: a Mendelian randomization analysis. *J Am Coll Cardiol.* 2012;60(25):2631-2639.

9. Voight BF, Peloso GM, Orho-Melander M. Plasma HDL cholesterol and risk of myocardial infarction: a mendelian randomization study. *Lancet.* 2012;380(9841):572-580.

10. Nordestgaard BG, Langsted A, Mora S, et al; European Atherosclerosis Society (EAS) and the European Federation of Clinical Chemistry and Laboratory Medicine (EFLM) Joint Consensus Initiative. Fasting is not routinely required for determination of a lipid profile: clinical and laboratory implications including flagging at desirable concentration cutpoints-a joint consensus statement from the European Atherosclerosis Society and European Federation of Clinical Chemistry and Laboratory Medicine. *Clin Chem.* 2016;62(7):930-946.

11. Kamstrup PR, Tybjaerg-Hansen A, Steffensen R, Nordestgaard BG. Genetically elevated lipoprotein(a) and increased risk of myocardial infarction. *JAMA.* 2009;301(22):2331-2339.

12. Nordestgaard BG, Chapman MJ, Ray K, et al; European Atherosclerosis Society Consensus Panel. Lipoprotein(a) as a cardiovascular risk factor: current status. *Eur Heart J.* 2010;31(23):2844-2853.

13. Cromwell WC, Otvos JD, Keyes MJ, et al. LDL particle number and risk of future cardiovascular disease in the Framingham Offspring Study: implications for LDL management. *J Clin Lipidol.* 2007;1:583-592.

14. Otvos JD, Mora S, Shalaurova I, Greenland P, Mackey RH, Goff DC Jr. Clinical implications of discordance between low-density lipoprotein cholesterol and particle number. *J Clin Lipidol.* 2011;5:105-113.

15. Schwartz GG, Olsson AG, Ezekowitz MD, et al. Effects of atorvastatin on early recurrent ischemic events in acute coronary syndromes: the MIRACL study: a randomized controlled trial. *JAMA.* 2001;285:1711-1718.

16. de Lemos JA, Blazing MA, Wiviott SD, et al. Early intensive vs a delayed conservative simvastatin strategy in patients with acute coronary syndromes: phase Z of the A to Z trial. *JAMA.* 2004;292:1307-1316.

17. Cannon CP, Braunwald E, McCabe CH, et al. Intensive versus moderate lipid lowering with statins after acute coronary syndromes. *N Engl J Med.* 2004;350:1495-1504.

18. Briel M, Vale N, Schwartz GG, et al. Updated evidence on early statin therapy for acute coronary syndromes: meta-analysis of 18 randomized trials involving over 14,000 patients. *Int J Cardiol.* 2012;158:93-100.

19. Vale N, Nordmann AJ, Schwartz GG, et al. Statins for acute coronary syndrome. *Cochrane Database Syst Rev.* 2014;(9):CD006870.

20. Stone NJ, Robinson JG, Lichtenstein AH, et al. 2013 ACC/AHA guideline on the treatment of blood cholesterol to reduce atherosclerotic cardiovascular risk in adults: a report of the American College of Cardiology/American Heart Association Task Force on Practice Guidelines. *Circulation.* 2014;129(25 suppl 2):S1-S45.

21. Patti G, Pasceri V, Colonna G, et al. Atorvastatin pretreatment improves outcomes in patients with acute coronary syndromes undergoing early percutaneous coronary intervention: results of the ARMYDA-ACS randomized trial. *J Am Coll Cardiol.* 2007;49:1272-1278.

22. Navarese EP, Kowalewski M, Andreotti F. Meta-analysis of time-related benefits of statin therapy in patients with acute coronary syndrome undergoing percutaneous coronary intervention. *Am J Cardiol.* 2014;113(10):1753-1764.

23. Okazaki S, Yokoyama T, Miyauchi K, et al. Early statin treatment in patients with acute coronary syndrome: demonstration of the beneficial effect on atherosclerotic lesions by serial volumetric intravascular ultrasound analysis during half a year after coronary event: the ESTABLISH Study. *Circulation.* 2004;110:1061-1068.

24. Nissen SE, Nicholls SJ, Sipahi I, et al; ASTEROID Investigators. Effect of very high intensity statin therapy on regression of coronary atherosclerosis: the ASTEROID trial. *JAMA.* 2006;295(13):1556-1565.

25. Patti G, Ricottini E, Nusca A, et al. Short-term, high-dose Atorvastatin pretreatment to prevent contrast-induced nephropathy in patients with acute coronary syndromes undergoing percutaneous coronary intervention (from the ARMYDA-CIN [atorvastatin for reduction of myocardial damage during angioplasty–contrast-induced nephropathy] trial. *Am J Cardiol.* 2011;108(1):1-7.

26. Leoncini M, Toso A, Maioli M, Tropeano F, Villani S, Bellandi F. Early high-dose rosuvastatin for contrast-induced nephropathy prevention in acute coronary syndrome: Results from the PRATO-ACS Study (Protective Effect of Rosuvastatin and Antiplatelet Therapy On contrast-induced acute kidney injury and myocardial damage in patients with Acute Coronary Syndrome). *J Am Coll Cardiol.* 2014;63(1):71-79.

27. Sattar N, Preiss D, Murray HM, et al. Statins and risk of incident diabetes: a collaborative meta-analysis of randomized statin trials. *Lancet.* 2010;375:735-742.

28. Cannon CP, Blazing MA, Giugliano RP, et al; IMPROVE-IT Investigators. Ezetimibe added to statin therapy after acute coronary syndromes. *N Engl J Med.* 2015;372(25):2387-2397.

29. European Association for Cardiovascular Prevention & Rehabilitation, Reiner Z, Catapano AL, De Backer G, et al; ESC Committee for Practice Guidelines (CPG). ESC/EAS Guidelines for the management of dyslipidemias: the Task Force for the management of dyslipidemias of the European Society of Cardiology (ESC) and the European Atherosclerosis Society (EAS). *Eur Heart J.* 2011;32(14):1769-1818.

30. Lloyd-Jones DM, Morris PB, Ballantyne CM, et al. 2016 ACC expert consensus decision pathway on the role of non-statin therapies for ldl-cholesterol lowering in the management of atherosclerotic cardiovascular disease risk: a report of the American College of Cardiology Task Force on Clinical Expert Consensus Documents. *J Am Coll Cardiol.* 2016;68(1):92-125.

Patient and Family Information for: LIPID MANAGEMENT IN THE CARDIAC CARE UNIT

HYPERLIPIDEMIA

Increased level of lipids (fats) in the blood is termed hyperlipidemia and includes both elevated cholesterol and triglycerides. Hyperlipidemia is a major cause of atherosclerosis, a term that refers to the buildup of fats and other substances in the walls of the arteries in the body, leading to the formation of plaques that can restrict blood flow. Hyperlipidemia significantly increases the risk of developing CVD, damaging the blood vessels supplying the heart, causing coronary artery disease and heart attacks. It may similarly lead to vascular disease in the limbs (peripheral vascular disease) and in the arteries supplying the brain (cerebrovascular disease).

LIPID PROFILE

BLOOD CHOLESTEROL

Cholesterol is a substance found in lipid particles in cells and body fluids, which is important to the cell structure and function and is a precursor to various metabolic pathways. High blood cholesterol is a major risk factor for developing heart disease. Low-density lipoprotein (LDL) particles are the main transporters of cholesterol throughout the body. The retention of LDL cholesterol in the walls of the arteries and the buildup of atherosclerotic plaque may narrow the coronary arteries supplying blood to the heart and cause symptoms such as effort-induced chest pain. Rupture or erosion of plaque in the coronary arteries may precipitate thrombi formation that obstructs the blood vessel and causes heart attack.

Many people are unaware that their cholesterol levels are high. A common genetic disease named "familial hypercholesterolemia" is associated with markedly elevated cholesterol levels and premature heart attack and stroke. Because this genetic disorder may pass to half of first degree relatives, it is important to measure the lipid profile in the blood at a young age in individuals with a family history of high blood cholesterol or premature heart disease, and in everyone at the age of 20. Lowering the cholesterol levels lessens the risk for developing heart disease.

Total Cholesterol Levels

- Desirable: <200 mg/dL
- Borderline high: 200 to 239 mg/dL
- High: ≥ 240 mg/dL

LDL Cholesterol Levels

LDL cholesterol, often called the "bad cholesterol," is directly associated with the risk of developing heart disease, and is therefore the primary target for drug therapy in individuals at risk.

- Optimal: <100 mg/dL
- Mean levels: 100 to 129 mg/dL

- Borderline high: 130 to 159 mg/dL
- High: 160 to 189 mg/dL
- Very high: ≥190 mg/dL

TRIGLYCERIDES

Triglycerides are a form of fat used as an energy source by the body and usually stored in fat cells. High triglyceride levels are often associated with obesity and diabetes and are a risk factor for developing heart disease. Triglyceride-rich lipoprotein particles are broken down by enzymes to smaller particles termed "remnant cholesterol," which are rich in cholesterol and are also atherogenic. Triglycerides should be measured after prolonged fasting of 12 hours.

Triglyceride Levels

- Normal: less than 150 mg/dL
- Borderline high: 150 to 199 mg/dL
- High: 200 to 499 mg/dL
- Very high: 500 mg/dL and above

Triglycerides above 500 mg/dL are a risk factor for developing pancreatitis, which may cause abdominal pain and multiple health complications. Therefore, very high triglyceride levels are an indication for making aggressive lifestyle changes and taking medical treatment.

HDL CHOLESTEROL

HDL cholesterol is the cholesterol carried in particles called high-density lipoproteins (HDL), known as the "good cholesterol," with protective antiatherogenic properties, carrying harmful cholesterol away from the vessel wall back to the liver for metabolism and clearance, a process termed reverse cholesterol transport. Desirable HDL cholesterol levels in blood are above 40 mg/dL in men and 50 mg/dL in women. Low HDL cholesterol is often associated with high triglyceride levels, and both are features of the metabolic syndrome, characterized also by elevated blood pressure, large waist circumference (central obesity), and high glucose levels. Likewise, smoking is associated with reduced HDL cholesterol level and function.

NON-HDL CHOLESTEROL

Non-HDL cholesterol is simply calculated as total cholesterol minus HDL cholesterol. The measurement of non-HDL cholesterol does not require fasting. Non-HDL cholesterol is a good predictor of cardiovascular risk, especially in metabolic syndrome and diabetes. Desirable levels of non-HDL cholesterols and goals for therapy are 30 mg/dL above the LDL cholesterol goals.

CALCULATING RISK FOR DEVELOPING HEART DISEASE

In addition to lipid disorders, major risk factors associated with atherosclerosis and developing heart attack include age, cigarette smoking, high blood pressure, and diabetes. Obesity, physical inactivity, and family history of early heart disease and stroke are also conditions associated with greater risk. Moreover, disorders associated with chronic inflammatory states, such as rheumatoid arthritis and psoriasis, may aggravate atherosclerosis if severe and untreated at an early stage.

Several cardiovascular risk calculators were developed over the years on the basis of large epidemiologic and population studies. These calculators are based on age and common risk factors and aim to predict the 10-year risk for developing atherosclerotic CVD and/or cardiovascular death. The goal of risk calculators is to support clinicians in optimizing individual cardiovascular risk reduction and to make an informed decision about the necessity of drug treatment for prevention of CVD. The most commonly utilized risk calculators are the atherosclerotic cardiovascular disease risk estimator (ASCVD), by American heart societies, and SCORE risk charts, by the European Society of Cardiology. Both risk calculators have a web-based interactive interface available for use online.

MANAGEMENT OF LIPID DISORDERS

WHEN AND WHOM TO TREAT?

The decision to start lipid-lowering treatment is a function of lipid levels, presence of concomitant risk factors, and diagnosis of CVD. Studies have demonstrated that lipid lowering is beneficial in coronary heart disease and significantly reduces the risk of recurrent cardiovascular events. Accordingly, it is common practice today to start cholesterol-lowering medications (ie, statins) in all people with coronary heart disease. Moreover, studies have shown the additional benefit of initiation of high-intensity statin while in the hospital, during the acute coronary event, and preferably before performing cardiac catheterization. In individuals with coronary artery disease, the positive effects of statins are regardless of the baseline LDL cholesterol levels. People with vascular disease of atherosclerotic origin in other arterial blood vessels, such as the carotid arteries and brain (ischemic stroke) and peripheral artery disease, are considered coronary disease equivalent and are therefore eligible for lipid-lowering therapy with statins for secondary prevention of CVD, similar to patients with coronary heart disease. In addition to treating all patients with atherosclerotic CVD with high-intensity statins, international guidelines recommend achieving a target LDL cholesterol level below 100 mg/dL and even less than 70 mg/dL in very high-risk individuals.

In people without a history of CVD, the benefit from lipid-lowering therapy depends on the global risk of developing CVD. People with diabetes or chronic kidney disease are at high risk for heart disease and are entitled to primary prevention therapy with statins. In addition, individuals without diagnosed CVD but with a high predicted risk of developing heart attack according to risk calculators are recommended for initiating statin therapy (eg, a 7.5% risk of developing CVD over 10 years is the threshold suggested for initiating statin therapy for primary prevention in the ASCVD calculator). Additional groups that are recommended for statin therapy regardless of other risk factors are those with very high LDL cholesterol levels, > 190 mg/dL, without apparent secondary reversible cause.

Very high triglyceride levels are also an indication for making aggressive lifestyle changes and taking medical treatment to prevent pancreatitis. Although high triglyceride levels are not the primary treatment target for preventing CVD, in some situations health care providers may recommend specific treatment for this indication, such as in high-risk diabetic patients with increased triglycerides and low HDL cholesterol under statin therapy.

MANAGEMENT OF HIGH CHOLESTEROL

Lifestyle changes are important in the treatment of high cholesterol levels. Losing weight, performing regular physical activity, and diet alterations, including reduction in saturated fats and cholesterol intake, may help reduce blood cholesterol levels. In addition, enrichment of nutrition with soluble dietary fibers is beneficial. Plant stanols and sterols are compounds naturally found in plants and available commercially as food products and dietary supplements, which may further reduce blood cholesterol by 10% to 15%. However, there are no significant data demonstrating a reduced risk of heart disease in people who consume plant sterols and stanols.

Decision making regarding initiation of medications for lowering cholesterol is carried out in accordance with the degree of risk of developing heart attacks or death from heart disease.

Drugs available for cholesterol lowering:

- **Statins:** a powerful group of drugs that are able to reduce LDL cholesterol levels by 30% to 55%. Statins work by inhibiting the production of cholesterol in liver cells and consequently increasing the expression of LDL receptors on the cells' surface, which causes the liver to remove more cholesterol from the blood to disassemble in the liver. Numerous studies in a wide range of populations at various cardiovascular risks have demonstrated over the years the ability of statins to significantly reduce heart attacks, stroke, and cardiovascular death. Accordingly, statins are the drugs of choice in the treatment of high cholesterol levels.

  Some side effects of statins are possible and vary from person to person. The more common side effects include muscle pain or cramps, constipation, and stomach pain. In addition, statin therapy may result in elevation in liver function tests, muscle enzymes, and glucose levels in blood, which are usually mild without clinical implication. Overall, statins have a good safety profile, and serious side effects are very rare.
- **Ezetimibe**: reduces blood cholesterol levels by 15% to 20%, by inhibiting dietary cholesterol absorption in the small intestine. Ezetimibe is most often used in combination with a statin drug.
- **PCSK9 inhibitors**: a novel class of injectable drugs that inhibit PCSK9, an enzyme that is a regulator of the LDL receptor and helps the liver to absorb more cholesterol from the blood when inhibited. Both evolocumab (Repatha) and alirocumab (Praluent) are human monoclonal antibodies against PCSK9 that were recently approved by the FDA for

use in people with very high levels of cholesterol, and in people with a history of coronary disease or who are intolerant to statin therapy and cannot attain lipids treatment goals. These new drugs are very efficient, reducing LDL cholesterol levels by 60% when injected subcutaneously twice a month. Clinical trials with PCSK9 inhibitors are ongoing, to evaluate long-term safety and the ability to improve cardiovascular outcomes.

- **Additional drugs**: bile acid sequestrants, which lower cholesterol indirectly by binding to bile acids, and niacin (nicotinic acid), which has a positive effect on all lipid components, are less commonly used today because they are less potent than statins and have more significant adverse effects.

HDL cholesterol levels are inversely associated with CVD, and low HDL cholesterol is a marker of increased cardiovascular risk. Lifestyle changes may help in raising HDL cholesterol. This includes aerobic exercise most days of the week, smoking cessation, weight loss with maintaining healthy body weight, and diet with alteration of intake of carbohydrates and fats (decreasing refined carbohydrates, avoiding sugary beverages, reducing trans fat, and consuming unsaturated fats). Although some medications such as niacin may increase HDL cholesterol levels, in the statin era, there is no good evidence that raising HDL cholesterol levels pharmacologically on top of statin therapy is beneficial in reducing heart disease.

MANAGEMENT OF HYPERTRIGLYCERIDEMIA

Healthy lifestyle choices have the ability to significantly lower triglycerides:

- **Diet**: dietary changes associated with reduction in triglycerides levels include: (a) reducing saturated fats and trans fats, (b) eating less processed and fast food, (c) increasing fiber intake by consuming more vegetables and whole grains, (d) limiting refined carbohydrates, fruit juices, sugars, and sweets, (e) increasing omega-3 intake, such as in fish like salmon and tuna, and (f) reducing alcohol intake.
- **Exercise**: increasing occupational and leisure-time physical activity; minimum of 150 minutes per week, on most days, preferably aerobic activities.
- **Weight loss**: losing weight by adoption of healthy diet and regular exercise. Even 5% to 7% reduction in weight may significantly improve triglyceride levels and glucose balance.

Drugs available for triglycerides lowering:

Prescription medications aimed at reducing triglyceride levels include fibrates (such as fenofibrate) and niacin. In addition, high-dose fish oil supplements significantly lower triglyceride levels. High blood sugars and uncontrolled diabetes are common precipitators of high triglycerides and should be treated accordingly.

Mary O'Sullivan
Diandra Fortune

Smoking Cessation in the Cardiac Patient

INTRODUCTION

For patients with coronary heart disease, quitting smoking is associated with a 36% reduction in all-cause mortality,[1] yet 1 year post–acute myocardial infarction (AMI), two-thirds of patients given low-intensity counseling have resumed smoking.[2] The decline of cardiovascular mortality in the United States is attributed largely to the reduction in smoking prevalence from about half of US men and a third of US women to 20.5% and 15.3%, respectively.[3,4] Because the benefit is of immediate onset, and because there are effective tools available, smoking cessation for the cardiac patient is an essential component of care.[5] Quitting smoking reduces the risk of coronary events to that of a nonsmoker within 3 years and reduces mortality by half after a heart attack over 3 to 5 years.[6,7] For patients with left ventricular (LV) dysfunction after myocardial infarction (MI), smoking cessation is associated with a 40% lower hazard of all-cause mortality over a median follow-up of 42 months.[8] Smoking post-MI is a powerful independent risk factor for reinfarction and death.[1,9,10] Those who quit have the same risk of sudden death as those who have never smoked.[9] The impact of smoking cessation in this population is therefore of at least the same magnitude as that of angiotensin converting enzyme (ACE) inhibitors (19% relative risk decrease), β-blockers (23% relative risk decrease), and aldosterone antagonists (15% relative risk decrease).[10–12] It is vital that this information be imparted to the Cardiac Care Unit (CCU) patient who has been a smoker.

The effects of smoking on heart rate, blood pressure, cardiovascular blood flow, myocardial oxygen demand, and thrombosis are largely reversible. In this chapter, we review how cigarettes induce cardiac disease, the role of nicotine in this process, the pharmacologic tools available, their safety profile in the cardiac patient, and the basics of behavioral modification for the smoking addiction. Helping patients quit smoking is certainly more challenging than simply ordering a medication. Understanding the biology involved assists us in helping our patients break this notoriously severe addiction.

HOW DOES SMOKING CAUSE HEART DISEASE?

Although the entry portal for cigarette smoke is the lung, where the chemicals present in the smoke are quickly and easily absorbed, the resulting inflammatory cascade has a profound effect that extends well beyond the confines of the lung (**Figure 56.1**). The systemic effects of cigarette smoking include a variety of complicated processes that induce, in the genetically susceptible individual, vascular and hematologic abnormalities that can result in accelerated atherosclerosis as well as the acute events of MI and sudden death.

The main responsible constituents are combustion products that are inhaled and induce (1) oxidative stress, increasing free radicals and lipid peroxidation; (2) systemic inflammation with activation and release of both inflammatory cells and inflammatory mediators; (3) endothelial dysfunction; and (4) abnormalities of coagulation and hemostasis.[13–15]

1. *Oxidative stress.* The particulate (tar) phase of cigarette smoke contains over 10^{17} free radicals/gram, and the gas phase contains over 10^{15} free radicals/puff. Many of the damaging effects of smoking are induced by these molecules. The sustained release of reactive free radicals from the tar and gas phases of smoke imposes an oxidant stress, inducing a variety of chemical injuries, including the formation of proatherogenic oxidized particles, specifically oxidized low-density lipoprotein cholesterol. Also, the inhaled oxidant molecules significantly deplete the body's antioxidant defense system.[13,14]
2. *Systemic inflammation.* Long-term cigarette smoking increases total white blood cell (WBC) counts. There is an increased

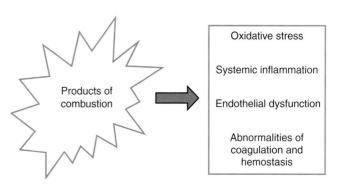

FIGURE 56.1 How smoking causes heart disease.

early bone marrow release of polymorphonuclear leukocytes (PMNs) and platelets into the circulation. These activated inflammatory cells then produce a variety of inflammatory mediators, acute phase proteins, and cytokines, among them C-reactive protein (CRP), fibrinogen, IL-6, and tumor necrosis factor. Some of the inflammatory mediators and hematologic effects of smoking decline rapidly after smoking cessation. However, CRP can remain elevated for 10 to 19 years.[10] These mediators may not be just markers of disease but may be actively involved in the proinflammatory and proatherogenic effects of chronic smoke exposure.

3. *Endothelial dysfunction.* Smoking induces endothelial dysfunction though a variety of biochemical, physiologic, and metabolic factors. Both oxidizing chemicals that are the products of combustion present in cigarette smoke and nicotine appear to be involved. Vasoregulation and changes in endothelial and platelet function affect the microcirculation. Decreased production or availability of NO results in impaired vasodilatory function at the macrovascular level (eg, coronary arteries) as well as at the microvascular level.[16,17] NO is also affected by cigarette smoke via the changes induced on low-density lipoprotein (LDL). In cigarette smokers, LDL gets oxidatively modified by the inhaled oxidant molecules. The modified LDL then interferes with the protective effect of NO on the arterial wall. The result is increased inflammatory cell entry into the arterial wall. The oxidatively modified LDL is taken up by the macrophages that enter the arterial wall; cholesterol esters are deposited and foam cells form.

4. *Abnormalities of coagulation and hemostasis.* Smoking cigarettes induces a hypercoagulable state that is a major factor in acute vascular events in smokers. Viscosity is increased, with increased levels of fibrinogen, lipoproteins, and hematocrit. Antithrombotic and prothrombotic factors and platelet function are affected. There is impaired release of the tissue plasminogen activator (t-PA), the main fibrinolytic activator resulting in impaired fibrinolysis. Hypercoagulability is responsible for 25% to 50% of the link between smoking and coronary artery disease (CAD)[9] and is especially involved in acute cardiac events. This is borne out in multiple clinical situations:

- Smoking increases the risk of MI and sudden death much more than it increases the risk of angina, reflecting the importance of acute thrombus formation.[18]
- Similarly, the prognosis after thrombolysis is better in smokers than in nonsmokers. This reflects the greater part that clots play in the disease process.[19]
- Sudden cardiac death is correlated with the presence of acute thrombosis and not the level of plaque burden.[18]
- Smokers who continue to smoke after thrombolysis or angioplasty have a substantially increased risk of reinfarction or reocclusion.[20,21]
- At least a part of the thrombotic effects of smoking are induced by even passive smoke.[22,23] The remarkable sensitivity of the coagulation system to the effect of cigarette smoke[24] mandates that the cardiac patient must cease all smoking, not just curtail their habit.[25] Patients should be taught the seriousness of this issue.

Although some of the effects of smoking on inflammatory markers may persist for years, a great portion of these effects are reversible by stopping smoking.

WHAT IS THE ROLE OF CO IN THIS PROCESS?

CO acutely poisons the oxygen delivery system, placing the patient at risk for arrhythmia and MI.[18] In patients with CAD, CO induces ischemia at lower levels of work.

HOW DOES NICOTINE PARTICIPATE IN THIS PROCESS?

The major cardiovascular effects of nicotine are mediated through sympathetic neural stimulation as well as the enhanced release of various neurotransmitters. Smoking produces a transient rise in blood pressure and an increase in myocardial work. In patients with coronary disease, smoking constricts epicardial coronary arteries and reduces coronary blood flow.

NICOTINE ADDICTION

After inhalation, nicotine rapidly reaches the nicotinic cholinergic receptors, found in both the peripheral and central nervous systems, resulting in the release of a variety of neurotransmitters, including dopamine, glutamate, γ–aminobutyric acid, norepinephrine, acetylcholine, serotonin, and endorphins, which may contribute to the effects of nicotine on blood vessels but also play an important role in the development of addiction in the susceptible individual. The pleasure derived from the dopamine release contributes to the addictive process.

It is important for the provider to discuss with the patient that nicotine dependence is highly heritable and metabolically driven.[26] Over 50% of the vulnerability to nicotine dependence is in large part a genetically determined phenomenon based on the type of nicotine receptors that the patient has. The type of nicotine receptors the patient has determines its pleasurable effects, its rate of metabolism, its withdrawal syndrome, and the susceptibility to neural plasticity that causes the learned behaviors that become triggers. One of the primary genes involved is the *CYP2A* gene, which is a controller of the rate of metabolism of nicotine, vulnerability to tobacco dependence, and response to smoking treatment and is involved with lung cancer risk. The $\alpha3\beta4$ nicotinic acetylcholine receptor is believed to mediate the cardiovascular effects of nicotine.[27] Thus, depending on the type of nicotine receptors they have, for some patients it is easy to quit, whereas for others it is incredibly difficult. For those who are smoking with known cardiovascular disease, the level of addiction is intense. Understanding that this is a biologically driven process and that, very much like diabetes, it is a chronic illness needing long-term lifestyle modification and medication for support is vitally important. Addressing the interplay of physical addiction and learned behavior is a key feature of therapy (**Figure 56.2**).

With repeated exposure, nicotine tolerance develops via a desensitization of the receptors to the effect of nicotine and an increase in the number of nicotine receptors. Nicotine withdrawal

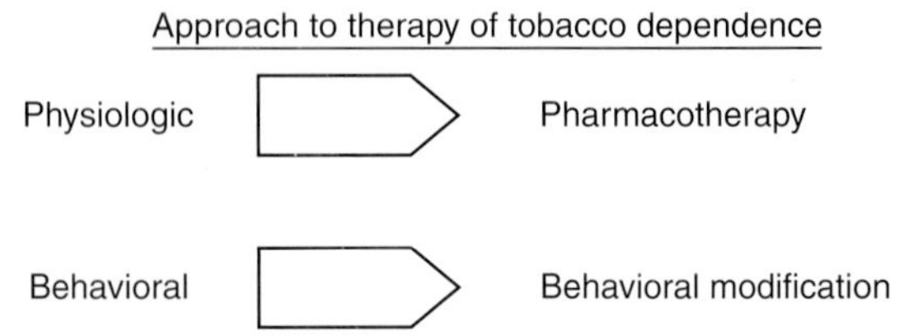

Approach to therapy of tobacco dependence

Physiologic ⟶ Pharmacotherapy

Behavioral ⟶ Behavioral modification

FIGURE 56.2 Approach to therapy of tobacco dependence.

is a complex process, not unlike that of withdrawal from alcohol, cocaine, opiates, and cannabinoids, that results in a state of anxiety, stress, generalized discomfort, inability to concentrate, and depressed mood.[27]

Thus, smokers learn to use the cigarette's nicotine as a modulator of anxiety, concentration, depressive symptoms, and pleasure as a major tool for handling life's stresses. In addition, those who are genetically susceptible to the addiction, after a relatively short period of use, become trapped by an inability to function without the satisfaction of the increased number of less responsive nicotine receptors. Not only does smoking relieve the intense discomfort of withdrawal within 10 seconds, but the relief is also accompanied by significant pleasure and ability to cope.

With time, the smoker associates certain situations with smoking: after a meal, drinks with friends, coffee, stress, etc. This association is learned and contributes significantly to the activity of the nicotine receptors and the expectation of immediate relief. These conditioned responses, also called neural plasticity, play a significant role in maintaining the addiction and become a significant impediment to the process of quitting. These triggers are to be avoided, and understanding the biology elucidates the importance of the behavioral component of smoking cessation.[27] As we will see from the studies on smoking cessation in the cardiac patient, the behavioral component of therapy is as important as the pharmacologic component (**Figure 56.2**). The permanence of the receptors, and the persistence of the learned behavior, makes the incidence of relapse very high; thus the importance of "learning" new sources of pleasure, stress management, concentration, and mood regulation.

WHAT IS THE ROLE OF NICOTINE IN THE DEVELOPMENT OF CARDIOVASCULAR DISEASE?

Sympathetic overactivity is a significant factor by which smoking, and at least in part nicotine, induces cardiovascular disease.[18] Nicotine releases catecholamines, increases heart rate and cardiac contractility, constricts cutaneous and coronary blood vessels, and transiently increases blood pressure.[28] There is an increase in myocardial work and oxygen consumption through an increase in blood pressure, heart rate, and myocardial contractility.[29] Nicotine also reduces sensitivity to insulin and may contribute to endothelial dysfunction.[30,31] How much of the sympathetic overactivity induced by smoking is due to the effect of nicotine in the cigarette is unclear, but this is of obvious concern when we are considering using nicotine replacement therapy (NRT) in the cardiac patient. Interestingly, the effect of nicotine on autonomic ganglia is dose dependent and biphasic. Small doses stimulate all autonomic ganglia. With larger doses, initial stimulation is followed by blockade of catecholamine release and increased splanchnic nerve stimulation, thus resulting in nausea. The dose response curve for the cardiovascular effects, such as heart rate acceleration or the release of catecholamines, is flat, and, consequently, even adding nicotine medication to smoking produces no further effect.[29]

Pharmacologic therapy is strongly recommended. The 2008 U.S. Clinical Practice Guidelines for Treating Tobacco Use and Dependence recommends counseling and medications to help all hospitalized tobacco users maintain abstinence and treat withdrawal symptoms. Three forms of medication are available:

nicotine replacement, bupropion, and varenicline. Each medication has advantages and disadvantages, and the choice should be tailored to the patient's individual clinical profile. Although not widely available now, in the future, identifying slow nicotine metabolizers will predict those who respond best to NRT versus bupropion or varenicline. Resistance to the use of medication is not uncommon but, as we have discussed, for the cardiac patient the stakes are too high to risk failure. Medication use doubles the success rate.

IS THE USE OF NRT SAFE?

After initial concerns regarding the safety of NRT, studies have shown the safety of NRT even as a high-dose patch, with combination NRT and concurrent smoking.[32–34] In a 2010 meta-analysis of adverse events associated with the use of NRT among 177,390 participants, Mills et al.[35] found that NRT is associated with an increased risk of GI complaints and insomnia. There was an observed risk of skin irritation and, with orally administered NRT, oropharyngeal complaints. Although NRT was associated with an increased risk of heart palpitations and chest pain, there was no increased incidence of heart attack or death. Their conclusion was that NRT is associated with adverse effects that may be discomforting for the patient but are not life-threatening. Again, in a more recent meta-analysis that was largely limited to smokers without preexisting heart disease, nicotine replacement therapies had a statistically significant risk of cardiovascular disease events that was driven primarily by less serious effects such as tachycardia. When analysis was limited to major cardiovascular disease events, there was no evidence of harm with NRT.[36] When their review was limited to high-risk patients, the trend toward having an increased risk of overall cardiac events (including tachycardia) remained, but the relative risk decreased and the confidence intervals became wider, not reaching statistical significance.[36]

NICOTINE REPLACEMENT THERAPY

When recommending NRT to a patient, especially one with cardiac disease, multiple questions arise, shown later with responses (**Figure 56.3**).

Nicotine Replacement Comes in a Variety of Delivery Systems

Nicotine Patch

The nicotine patch comes in three strengths—21, 14, and 7 mg—and is equivalent to a full pack a day, half a pack a day, and a third of a pack a day. Variations in the intensity of smoking and differing metabolic rates of nicotine among individuals may necessitate dosing adjustment from these guidelines. If the patch is too strong, the patient experiences nausea, dizziness, and headache. If it is too weak, there are cravings. Adjust the dose to comfort. The patch takes an hour to reach level, which is still well below the level of arterial spike achieved by the cigarette. The gradual delivery allows the body to equilibrate with its effects, contributing to its safety profile. It is applied in the morning and removed at bedtime to avoid potential nightmares. Adjust the dose to comfort. Change the location daily. Some patients are allergic to the adhesive and are unable to use it because they develop blisters.

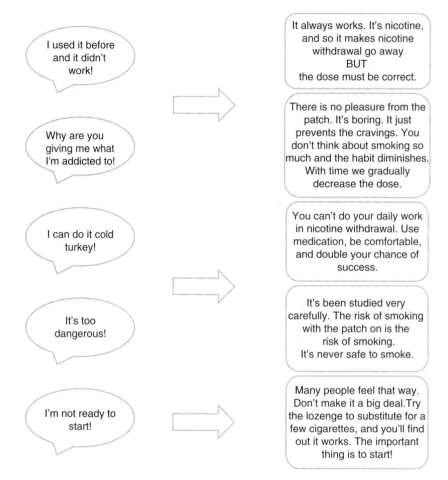

FIGURE 56.3 Common patient concerns regarding use of NRT and answers to these concerns.

Nicotine Gum

The delivery system of the gum is meant to allow a controlled release of nicotine. If it is chewed, it delivers too much nicotine too fast, resulting in nausea, hiccups, and vomiting. Only crack the coating open: it comes in 2- and 4-mg pieces and can be used every hour if needed. The patient can "bite and park," placing it in the cheek and waiting. This is a much faster delivery system compared to the patch, and the patient is aware of a "hit." It is very useful in combination with the patch for craving relief, especially in the morning before the patch has begun to work (**Figure 56.4**).

Nicotine Lozenge

This is similar to the gum in delivery. Allow it to slowly dissolve on the tongue. It can be used alone or in combination with the patch.

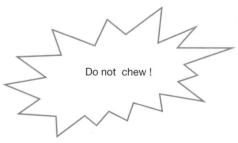

Do not chew!

FIGURE 56.4 Nicotine gum.

Nicotine Inhaler

Puffing on this device delivers straight nicotine to the oral mucosa. It is not meant to be inhaled, but only puffed into the mouth. It can satisfy some of the ritual the smokers may desire. The patient may use six cartridges per day if needed, and each cartridge lasts 30 minutes.

NRT Safety Profile

The use of NRT has presented long-standing safety concerns although the blood level of nicotine achieved with a NRT does not approach the rapid arterial bolus achieved with the cigarette. Multiple studies have shown the safety of NRT even as a high-dose patch, combination patch and gum therapy, and patch and concurrent smoking (10 to 12 Mills and Thornland) (**Figure 56.5**).

In a 2010 meta-analysis of adverse events associated with the use of NRT among 177,390 participants, Mills et al.[35] found that NRT is associated with increased risk of gastrointestinal (GI) complaints, reflecting the previously noted splanchnic nerve stimulation, along with insomnia. There was an observed risk of skin irritation and, with orally administered NRT, oropharyngeal complaints. Although NRT was associated with an increased risk of heart palpitations and chest pain, there was no increased incidence of heart attack or death. Their conclusion was that NRT is associated with adverse effects that may be discomforting for the patient, but are not life-threatening.

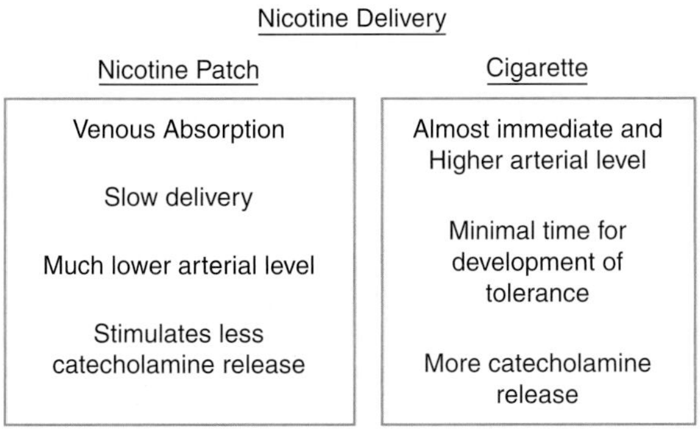

Nicotine Delivery

Nicotine Patch	Cigarette
Venous Absorption	Almost immediate and Higher arterial level
Slow delivery	
Much lower arterial level	Minimal time for development of tolerance
Stimulates less catecholamine release	More catecholamine release

FIGURE 56.5 Nicotine delivery in patch vs. cigarette.

In a more recent meta-analysis that was largely limited to smokers without preexisting heart disease, Mills et al analyzed the data for evidence of cardiac toxicity from NRT. They subdivided the cardiac events into two categories: (1) all cardiac events and (2) major cardiovascular events (MACEs) defined as cardiovascular death, nonfatal MIs, or nonfatal stroke. Although they identified a significant increase in minor events such as tachycardia, there was no increase in MACEs (Mills and Thorlund). This remained true for a subgroup analysis of high-risk patients, although the numbers were small.

IS THE USE OF NRT IN THE CARDIAC PATIENT SAFE?

Early case reports suggested cardiovascular risk associated with use of NRT, especially if the patient smoked while using nicotine replacement. Data are now available[18,32,37–41] from randomized controlled trials, efficacy studies, observational data, and physiologic studies, supporting the safety of NRT used in the stable cardiac patient. There was no increased risk of angina, MI, stroke, arrhythmia, or death. These studies looked at patients with stable cardiovascular disease who had no cardiac event requiring an intervention in the prior 2 weeks.

Although NRT is cautiously prescribed for relief of withdrawal symptoms for cardiac patients in the CCU, there is a lack of randomized evidence to support its safety in the early period after an MI. As previously discussed, nicotine increases heart rate, BP, and myocardial contractility, and has the potential to cause endothelial dysfunction and coronary vasoconstriction. There is only one study[42] that looks at use of NRT among patients who were admitted for acute coronary syndromes (ACS) and who received transdermal NRT during that hospitalization. In this retrospective propensity analysis from Duke University, patients who had undergone a cardiac catheterization for an ACS and received NRT were retrospectively compared with comparable patients from their database. After a propensity-matched analysis, they found no difference in short- or long-term mortality in patients who did or did not receive the patch. There was no significant difference between the groups in the need for undergoing coronary artery bypass graft surgery (CABG) or percutaneous transluminal angioplasty. Nonetheless, nicotine does have hemodynamic effects that could contribute to acute cardiovascular events.

There are two troubling retrospective reports regarding the use of nicotine replacement in critically ill patients. One is among medical intensive care unit patients[43] and the other among patients undergoing CABG.[44] In each study, the use of NRT was associated with an increased mortality. Unfortunately, because of the retrospective nature of the studies and their small size, they could not control for associated comorbidities, thus limiting the weight that we can place on them. However, they most definitely indicate the need for further studies and raise a need for caution.

As far as the e-cigarette is concerned, there is insufficient literature available to address its use in the cardiac patient. There is literature on exposure to both the aerosol and the particulate components that they generate.[45] Using 20 e-cigarette refill solutions from five manufacturers in cultured rat cardiac myoblasts, the aerosols from three solutions were found to be cytotoxic to the cardiac myoblasts. Although tests on e-cigarettes show much lower levels of most toxicants, they do not show reduced levels of particulate matter when compared with that of conventional cigarettes. The distribution of particulate matter generated by the e-cigarette is similar to that of the traditional cigarette. They are small enough to reach deep into the lung and cross into the systemic circulation. Toxicity thresholds are not known, but we know that exposure to ultrafine particles from tobacco smoke or air pollution turns on systemic inflammatory processes and increases the risk of cardiovascular death.[46–48] Overall, although the e-cigarette is likely to be less toxic than the cigarette, the products are unregulated, contain toxic chemicals, and have not been proven as cessation devices. Should the patient insist on e-cigarette use, they should be urged to set a quit date and not plan on using it indefinitely.[45]

Overall, the clinically relevant hemodynamic effects of NRT appear to be very mild, and its use in the stable cardiac patient appears to be quite safe. Clinical trials have not examined the efficacy of NRT in the AMI patient population. However, given the significant health consequences of smoking after MI, and analyzing current data, Benowitz and Prochaska have suggested an approach including, in addition to intensive counseling and follow-up, a personalized prescription of medication that may include NRT to relieve withdrawal symptoms and provide an effective transition from inpatient to outpatient smoking cessation.[49]

BUPROPION FOR SMOKERS WITH CARDIOVASCULAR DISEASE

Bupropion, an atypical antidepressant with a structure related to amphetamine, has, like nicotine replacement, been shown to be an effective smoking cessation tool. After approximately 10 days on treatment, the desire to smoke diminishes significantly. In addition, it prevents the depression that not uncommonly surfaces in patients who stop smoking. The contraindications include a seizure history, alcoholism, bipolar disorder, bulimia nervosa, and panic attacks. The side effects include dry mouth, headache, agitation, and insomnia. Hypertension has been described, especially in patients taking both bupropion and the nicotine replacement. The treatment is usually begun at bupropion 150 mg sustained release (SR) and can subsequently be increased to 150 mg SR twice a day. The side effects are dose dependent, and some patients may obtain an adequate therapeutic benefit with the 150-mg-daily dose. The drug is metabolized in the liver, so dose adjustment is advised with significant liver disease. The drug inhibits the activity of CYP2D6 isoenzyme, which metabolizes β-blockers, antiarrhythmics, certain antidepressants, SSRIs, and antipsychotics.

Bupropion approximately doubles quit rates in otherwise healthy smokers and patients with stable cardiovascular disease.[2] There have been a number of case reports of death and severe adverse cardiovascular reactions occurring in patients taking bupropion,[50] but in the meta-analysis of Mills and Thorlund[35] in a high-risk population (cardiac disease and COPD), bupropion was safe with a MACE relative risk approaching 1. A 2008 clinical practice guideline issued by the U.S. Department of Health and Human Services suggests that bupropion can be safely used in the acute post-MI period.[51]

Although the safety data are encouraging, in the meta-analysis of Mills and Thorlund,[35] efficacy was questioned. Three trials of bupropion therapy that had begun in the CCU did not support significant efficacy at 1 year, with only a 5% improvement in quit rate versus placebo at 1 year.[2,52,53] However, Benowitz and Prochaska point out in their editorial[49] that the 12-month quit rate difference of 5% that was achieved with bupropion over placebo would have a meaningful public health impact for a group at such high risk for ongoing cardiovascular events. There is one randomized trial for smoking cessation comparing bupropion SR 150 mg BID with placebo in outpatients with stable cardiovascular disease,[54] demonstrating improved 1-year quit rates. At 1 year, the quit rates were 27% for the bupropion arm versus 11% for the placebo arm. Safety profile was once again validated.

Duration of therapy with bupropion appears to be a significant factor that needs to be considered in the acute cardiac patient for whom relapse has a particularly high risk. In a five-hospital, double-blind placebo-controlled trial, patients who were admitted with acute cardiovascular disease were randomized to receive either bupropion SR 150 mg BID and intensive counseling or placebo and intensive counseling for 3 months. Bupropion's safety profile was supported for smokers hospitalized with acute cardiovascular disease. The bupropion group did have improved short-term quit rates (37.1% vs 26.8%) but not improved long-term quit rates (25% vs 21.3%) over intensive counseling. After 30 days off the drug, there was a borderline significant increase in cardiac events, and 75% of the subjects were smoking before the event. The patients enrolled in the study were significantly addicted, and 40% of them had been smoking with known CAD before admission, making them a highly addicted group. In addition to supporting the safety of the use of bupropion in the CCU patient, this study raises the question of a need for longer-term therapy with bupropion to help maintain the abstinence advantage seen at 3 months.[53]

In studies of bupropion SR being used as an antidepressant in patients with cardiac disease, few cardiac adverse effects were seen. There was occasional hypertension, but no effect on cardiac conduction or ejection fraction. A black box warning remains on bupropion regarding suicide risk.

Despite the concern raised by case reports, current evidence suggests that bupropion SR is a safe and possibly efficacious treatment for smoking cessation for patients with cardiovascular disease. Full evaluation of bupropion SR in patients with cardiac disease is needed. Bupropion may be used in combination with nicotine replacement. The success rate of this combination has not been shown to be statistically superior[55,56] and has not been evaluated in the cardiac patient. It is suggested that while on combined therapy, blood pressure should be monitored.

WHAT IS THE ROLE OF VARENICLINE FOR THE CARDIAC PATIENT?

Varenicline is a highly effective smoking cessation medication that is both a partial nicotine agonist and an antagonist. After taking this drug for a week, the patient experiences little to no cravings, and if they do smoke they derive no pleasure. Common side effects include insomnia (19%), nausea (16%), abnormal dreams (9%), and constipation (5%). Seizure disorder is a contraindication. Although this drug has had the highest quit rates among healthy individuals, postmarketing data raised concerns regarding the risk of depression, aggressive behavior, suicidal ideation, and suicide. It is well known that depression may surface in patients attempting to quit smoking. Many patients use the nicotine in cigarettes to treat a full-blown or borderline depression, and when they stop smoking, depression may be uncovered. Subsequent studies of varenicline and the risk of depression and suicidal ideation have not substantiated this risk; however, it remains a subject of ongoing research.

More recent studies have validated the use of varenicline in combination with NRT, with a significantly improved quit rate at 24 weeks.[58] In addition, the drug has now been approved for 6 months of therapy. Furthermore, recognizing that gradual reduction may be preferred by some smokers, varenicline has been used in a graduated smoking reduction plan versus placebo with quit rates of 27% versus 9.9% at 1 year.

For the cardiac patient considering use of varenicline, two questions arise. First, is there any excess cardiovascular risk? Second, what is the risk of depression? This is of special concern in this often depressed population.[57]

Theoretically, varenicline should have little to no cardiovascular effects. The sympathomimetic cardiovascular effects of nicotine are mediated primarily by binding to $\alpha 3\beta 4$ nicotinic acetylcholine receptors. Because varenicline binds to a different nicotinic receptor, $\alpha 4\beta 2$, it was theorized not to have cardiovascular effects. In 2010, Rigotti et al.[59] published a multicenter randomized, double-blind placebo-controlled trial comparing the efficacy of 12 weeks of varenicline with counseling versus counseling alone in 714 smokers with stable cardiovascular disease. At the end of a year, the quit rate was 19.2% for the varenicline group versus 7.2% for placebo. Although the trial was small, there was no increase in cardiovascular events or mortality. For this study, patients had to be otherwise well, including no psychiatric history. Mood was not systematically assessed, but there was no difference in spontaneously reported psychiatric symptoms in the varenicline versus placebo group.

Although a meta-analysis by Singh[60] raised concern over the cardiovascular safety of varenicline, other meta-analyses[35,61,62] did not find an increased risk of cardiovascular events. However, in 2011 the FDA issued a safety alert regarding a numerically but not statistically greater rate of adverse cardiovascular events with varenicline compared with placebo. A more recent large retrospective cohort study found no increased risk of cardiovascular events, depression, or self-harm.[63] It appears that varenicline has a small, nonsignificant cardiovascular risk, if any. Similarly, psychiatric concerns have not been supported in the current literature, although the black box warnings persist and change of mood should be taken seriously.

The use of varenicline in the CCU in the acute AMI setting has been studied in the EVITA (Evaluation of Varenicline in Smoking Cessation for Patients Post–Acute Coronary Syndrome) trial, suggesting that 12 weeks of varenicline is both safe and effective in patients with ACS.[64] At 24 weeks, there was a 14.8% absolute difference in point prevalence abstinence for those in the varenicline (47.3%) versus the placebo group (32.5%). Less than a third of those receiving placebo were abstinent at 24 weeks.

Varenicline is our most effective pharmacotherapy for smoking cessation to date. Even though further work is needed to shed more light on the psychiatric risk and to ensure the cardiac safety profile, the risk benefit ratio weighs strongly on the side of this tool. The data provide a strong evidence base to support the safety and effectiveness of varenicline for cardiac patients, both those with stable cardiovascular disease and those in the acute setting of ACS. Questions that need clarification, beyond issues of safety, are the role of more extended courses or even long-term therapy for this chronic severe addiction and the role of integrating intensive behavioral therapy into the varenicline treatment plan.

WHAT IS THE APPROACH TO THE PHARMACOTHERAPY?

In the patient with ACS in the CCU, clinical judgment needs to guide the approach. Given the significant health consequences of smoking after MI, and based on the available current data, Benowitz and Prochaska have emphasized the importance of a personalized plan including behavioral modification along with the prescription of medication to relieve withdrawal symptoms and provide an effective transition from inpatient to outpatient smoking cessation.[49] NRT has no safety data in the acute setting but abundant safety data for the stable cardiac patient. It has the advantage of immediate relief of withdrawal symptoms. The disadvantage of the delayed onset of action of both bupropion and varenicline is counterbalanced by substantial safety data in the acute setting. The improved effectiveness of varenicline along with its safety data gives support to its use in this group of patients. The ongoing, although decreasing, concern regarding psychiatric comorbidities remains. Until we have better randomized long-term control trials, the approach needs to be guided by informed clinical judgment.

Even when we have devised a plan, some patients may be unwilling to stop abruptly. Recent investigations have shown that gradual reduction may be effective, although in the cardiac patient this is not ideal.[65]

BEHAVIORAL MODIFICATION

Although 30% to 45% of smokers who suffer an initial cardiac event stop smoking,[66] 60% to 70% of them relapse within a year. No matter which pharmacologic therapy one uses to stop smoking, there is a 50% relapse rate. The problem is that nicotine addiction is permanent. The patient who smokes immediately on waking or who is uncomfortable in places where they cannot smoke for any length of time is very addicted. The faster and stronger the craving, the more addicted the patient. Other patients are able to wait hours before their first cigarette. They are less affected by the decreased nicotine level that occurs over a night without smoking. They have fewer or no cravings. They have a larger behavioral component to their habit and are less in need of medication to quit.

As previously noted, patients who are highly addicted need more than medication to have sustained success. They need to learn behavioral techniques to allow them to remain smoke free through a lifetime. We know that smoking cessation programs that do not include postdischarge counseling and that do not provide follow-up for more than a month are ineffective.[67–70]

Follow-up of at least 3 months is indicated.[50,71] Cardiologists should attend to these simple techniques and the importance of lifestyle modification on an ongoing basis.[72,73]

WHAT ARE THE PRINCIPLES INVOLVED?

- Most importantly, convince the patient that he or she can succeed and that you are confident that they will. Put the patient on a positive footing. Identify areas of accomplishment. A cardiac patient who is smoking is often tremendously guilt-ridden. You, as their health care provider, will support them through the process. Medications and behavioral techniques will help control the withdrawal and the cravings.
- Allow them to lead the conversation regarding what aspect of smoking is of concern to them. Address their concerns, whether they are financial, social, or health related, to get the conversation going. Identify why they use the cigarette: for pleasure, relief of depression, boredom, anxiety, or stress; improved concentration, relief from cravings, or all of these? Together, consider alternative approaches to each of those problems, which requires identifying other pleasures, as well as addressing depression,[43] stress and anger management techniques, exercise, being otherwise occupied, and avoiding the situations that lead to the urge to smoke.
- Have the patient make a concrete plan for what he or she will do to cope with cravings (eg, gum, water, or deep breathing).
- Identify and plan for avoidance of triggers such as coffee, alcohol, friends who smoke.
- Identify substitutes that the patient likes and can look forward to, for example, movies, museums, friends who do not smoke, or magazines.
- Encourage the patient to be as busy as possible, especially immediately after meals.
- Most importantly, discuss with the patient the permanence of the addiction and the need to be on guard even years later, especially in situations of stress. Unfortunately, the thought of picking up another cigarette recurs for a very long time, and one puff can lead to full relapse.
- Patients should never allow others to smoke around them or endanger their sobriety. As their cardiologist, you are giving them the license to be an inconvenience to others who want to smoke around them, because of their cardiac health. Their success is so important that nothing should be allowed to endanger it.
- Web-based interventions are available. The http://www.smokefree.gov website of the National Cancer Institute (NCI) combines evidence-based guidelines tailored to readiness to quit with available professional assistance via instant messaging and quitline (1-877-44U-QUIT).
- Texting interventions show borderline results.
- Social media (Twitter and Facebook) have potential benefit, utilizing buddy groups.
- Monetary incentives have shown only short-term benefit.

Smoking cessation in the cardiac patient covers a spectrum of therapy from simple behavioral modification to complex decisions involving pharmacotherapeutic options. We have ample data indicating that the approach must be a combination of techniques, with months of ongoing support. Still, the relapse rate remains unacceptably high. As we have reviewed, the risks of ongoing smoking are high, as are the benefits from quitting. Clearly, we need more physician participation in this process, and who could be more effective in guiding the patient to success than their own cardiologist?

REFERENCES

1. Critchley JA, Capewell S. WITHDRAWN: smoking cessation for the secondary prevention of coronary heart disease. *Cochrane Database Syst Rev.* 2012;(2):CD003041.

2. Eisenberg MJ, Grandi SM, Gervais A, et al. Bupropion for smoking cessation in patients hospitalized with acute myocardial infarction: a randomized, placebo-controlled trial. *J Am Coll Cardiol.* 2013;61(5):524-532.

3. U.S. Department of Health and Human Services. The Health Consequences of Smoking: 50 years of progress. A Report of the Surgeon General. Atlanta, GA: U.S. Department of Health and Human Services, Centers for Disease Control and Prevention, National Center for Chronic Disease Prevention and Health Promotion, Office on Smoking and Health, 2014.

4. Jamal A, King BA, Neff LJ, Whitmill J, Babb SD, Graffunder CM. Current cigarette smoking among adults—United States, 2005–2015. *MMWR Morb Mortal Wkly Rep.* 2016;65(44):1205-1211.

5. Thomson CC, Rigotti NA. Hospital- and clinic-based smoking cessation interventions for smokers with cardiovascular disease. *Prog Cardiovasc Dis.* 2003;45(6):459-479.

6. Critchley J, Capewell S. Smoking cessation for the secondary prevention of coronary heart disease. *Cochrane Database Syst Rev.* 2003;(4):CD003041.

7. Gerber Y, Rosen LJ, Goldbourt U, Benyamini Y, Drory Y. Smoking status and long-term survival after first acute myocardial infarction a population-based cohort study. *J Am Coll Cardiol.* 2009;54(25):2382-2387.

8. Shah AM, Pfeffer MA, Hartley LH, et al. Risk of all-cause mortality, recurrent myocardial infarction, and heart failure hospitalization associated with smoking status following myocardial infarction with left ventricular dysfunction. *Am J Cardiol.* 2010;106(7):911-916.

9. Goldenberg I, Jonas M, Tenenbaum A, et al. Current smoking, smoking cessation, and the risk of sudden cardiac death in patients with coronary artery disease. *Arch Intern Med.* 2003;163(19):2301-2305.

10. Pfeffer MA, Braunwald E, Moyé LA, et al. Effect of captopril on mortality and morbidity in patients with left ventricular dysfunction after myocardial infarction. Results of the survival and ventricular enlargement trial. The SAVE Investigators. *N Engl J Med.* 1992;327(10):669-677.

11. Yusuf S, Hawken S, Ounpuu S, et al. Effect of potentially modifiable risk factors associated with myocardial infarction in 52 countries (the INTERHEART study): case-control study. *Lancet.* 2004;364(9438):937-952.

12. Conroy RM, Pyörälä K, Fitzgerald AP, et al. Estimation of ten-year risk of fatal cardiovascular disease in Europe: the SCORE project. *Eur Heart J.* 2003;24(11):987-1003.

13. Yanbaeva DG, Dentener MA, Creutzberg EC, Wesseling G, Wouters EF. Systemic effects of smoking. *Chest.* 2007;131(5):1557-1566.

14. Pasupathi P, Rao Y. Effect of cigarette smoking on lipids and oxidative stress biomarkers in patients with acute myocardial infarction. *Res J Med Med Sci.* 2009;4(2):151-159.

15. Wannamethee SG, Lowe GD, Shaper AG, Rumley A, Lennon L, Whincup PH. Associations between cigarette smoking, pipe/cigar smoking, and smoking cessation, and haemostatic and inflammatory markers for cardiovascular disease. *Eur Heart J.* 2005;26(17):1765-1773.

16. Pryor W, Stone K. Oxidants in cigarette smoke radicals, hydrogen peroxides, peroxynitrate and peroxynitrite. *Ann N Y Acad Sci.* 1993;686(1):12-27.

17. Ludwig PW, Hoidal JR. Alterations in leukocyte oxidative metabolism in cigarette smokers. *Am Rev Respir Dis.* 1982;126:977-980.

18. Benowitz NL, Gourlay SG. Cardiovascular toxicity of nicotine: implications for nicotine replacement therapy. *J Am Coll Cardiol.* 1997;29:1422-1431.

19. Barbash GI, Reiner J, White HD, Wilcox RG, Armstrong PW, Sadowski Z, Morris D, Aylward P, Woodlief LH, Topol EJ. Evaluation of paradoxic beneficial effects of smoking in patients receiving thrombolytic therapy for acute myocardial infarction: mechanism of the "smoker's paradox" from the GUSTO-I trial, with angiographic insights. Global Utilization of Streptokinase and Tissue-Plasminogen Activator for Occluded Coronary Arteries. *J Am Coll Cardiol.* 1995;26(5):1222-1229.

20. Rivers JT, White HD, Cross DB, Williams BF, Norris RM. Reinfarction after thrombolytic therapy for acute myocardial infarction followed by conservative management: incidence and effect of smoking. *J Am Coll Cardiol.* 1990;16(2):340-348.

21. Galan KM, Deligonul U, Kern MJ, Chaitman BR, Vandormael MG. Increased frequency of restenosis in patients continuing to smoke cigarettes after percutaneous transluminal coronary angioplasty. *Am J Cardiol.* 1988;61(4):260-263.

22. Glantz SA, Parmley WW. Passive smoking and heart disease: mechanisms and risk. *JAMA.* 1995;273:1047-1053.

23. Barnoya J, Glantz SA. Cardiovascular effects of secondhand smoke: nearly as large as smoking. *Circulation.* 2005;111(20):2684-2698.

24. Ambrose JA, Barua RS. The pathophysiology of cigarette smoking and cardiovascular disease, an update. *J Am Coll Cardiol.* 2004;43:1731-1737.

25. Godtfredsen NS, Osler M, Vestbo J, et al. Smoking reduction, smoking cessation, and incidence of fatal and non-fatal myocardial infarction in Denmark 1976–1998: a pooled cohort study. *J Epidemiol Community Health.* 2003;57:412-416.

26. Lerman C, Schnoll RA, Hawk LW, et al. Use of the nicotine metabolite ratio as a genetically informed biomarker of response to nicotine patch or varenicline for smoking cessation: a randomised, double-blind placebo-controlled trial. *Lancet Respir Med.* 2015;3(2):131-138.

27. Benowitz NL. Pharmacology of nicotine: addiction, smoking-induced disease, and therapeutics. *Ann Rev Pharmacol Toxicol.* 2009;49:57-71.

28. Benowitz NL. Cigarette smoking and cardiovascular disease: pathophysiology and implications for treatment. *Prog Cardivasc Dis.* 2003;46:91-111.

29. Najem B, Houssiere A, Pathak A, et al. Acute cardiovascular and sympathetic effects of nicotine replacement therapy. *Hypertension.* 2006;47:1162-1167.

30. Eliasson B. Cigarette smoking and diabetes. *Prog Cardiovasc Dis.* 2003;45:405-413.

31. Puranik R, Celermajer DS. Smoking and endothelial function. *Prog Cardiovasc Dis.* 2003;45:443-458.

32. Joseph AM, Norman SM, Ferry LH, et al. The safety of transdermal nicotine as an aid to smoking cessation in patients with cardiac disease. *N Engl J Med.* 1996;335(24):1792-1798.

33. Haustein KO, Krause J, Haustein H, Rasmussen T, Cort N. Comparison of the effects of combined nicotine replacement therapy vs. cigarette smoking in males. *Nicotine Tob Res.* 2003;5:195-203.

34. Zevin S, Jacob P 3rd. Dose-related cardiovascular and endocrine effects of transdermal nicotine. *Clin Pharmacol Ther.* 1998;64:87-95.

35. Mills EJ, Wu P, Lockhart I, Wilson K, Ebbert JO. Adverse events associated with nicotine replacement therapy (NRT) for smoking cessation. A systematic review and meta-analysis of one hundred and twenty studies involving 177,390 individuals. *Tob Induc Dis.* 2010;8:8.

36. Mills E, Thorlund K, Eapen S, Wu P, Prochaska JJ. Cardiovascular events associated with smoking cessation pharm acotherapies A network meta-analysis. *Circulation.* 2014;129(1):28-41.

37. Ludvig J, Miner B, Eisenberg MJ. Smoking cessation in patients with coronary artery disease. *Am Heart J.* 2005;149:565-572.

38. Ford CL, Zlabek JA. Nicotine replacement therapy and cardiovascular disease. *Mayo Clin Proc.* 2005;80:652-656.

39. Hubbard R, Lewis S, Smith C, et al. Use of nicotine replacement therapy and the risk of acute myocardial infarction, stroke, and death. *Tob Control.* 2005;14:416-421.

40. Fishbein L, O'Brien P, Hutson A, Theriague D, Stacpoole PW, Flotte T. Pharmacokinetics and pharmacodynamic effects of nicotine nasal spray devices on cardiovascular and pulmonary function. *J Investig Med.* 2000;48:435-440.

41. Tzivoni D, Keren A, Meyler S, Khoury Z, Lerer T, Brunel P. Cardiovascular safety of transdermal nicotine patches in patients with coronary artery disease who try to quit smoking. *Cardiovasc Drugs Ther.* 1998;12(3):239-244.

42. Meine TJ, Patel MR, Washam JB, Pappas PA, Jollis JG. Safety and effectiveness of transdermal nicotine patch in smokers admitted with acute coronary syndromes. *Am J Cardiol.* 2005;95(8):976-978.

43. Lee A, Alessa B The association of nicotine replacement therapy with mortality in a medical intensive care unit. *Crit Care Med.* 2007;35:1517-1521.

44. Paciullo C, Short M, Steinke DT, Jennings HR. Impact of nicotine replacement therapy on postoperative mortality following coronary artery bypass graft surgery. *Ann Pharmacother.* 2009;43:1197-1202.

45. Grana R, Benowitz N, Glantz SA. e-Cigarettes a scientific review. *Circulation.* 2014;129:1972-1986.

46. Brook RD, Rajagopalan S, Pope CA 3rd, et al. Particulate matter air pollution and cardiovascular disease: an update to the scientific statement from the American Heart Association. *Circulation.* 2010;121:2331-2378.

47. Pope CA 3rd, Burnett RT, Krewski D, et al. Cardiovascular mortality and exposure to airborne fine particulate matter and cigarette smoke: shape of the exposure-response relationship. *Circulation.* 2009;120:941-948.

48. Mehta S, Shin H. Ambient particulate air pollution and acute lower respiratory infections: a systematic review and implications for estimating the global burden of disease. *Air Qual Atmos Health.* 2013:1-15.

49. Benowitz N, Prochaska J. Smoking cessation after acute myocardial infarction. *J Am Coll Cardiol.* 2013;61(5):533-535.

50. Treating tobacco use and dependence: 2008 update U.S. Public Health Service Clinical Practice Guideline executive summary. *Respir Care.* 2008;53(9):1217-1222.

51. Joseph AM, Fu SS. Safety issues in pharmacotherapy for smoking in patients with cardiovascular disease. *Prog Cardiovasc Dis.* 2003;45(6):429-441.

52. Planer D, Lev I, Elitzur Y, et al. Bupropion for smoking cessation in patients with acute coronary syndrome. *Arch Intern Med.* 2011;171(12):1055-1060.

53. Rigotti N, Thorndike A, Regan S, et al. Bupropion for smokers hospitalized with acute cardiovascular disease. *Am J Med.* 2006;119:1080-1087.

54. Tonstad S, Farsang C, Klaene G, et al. Bupropion SR for smoking cessation in smokers with cardiovascular disease: a multicentre, randomized study. *Eur Heart J.* 2003;24:946-955.

55. Jorenby D, Leischow S, Nides M, et al: A controlled trial of sustained-release bupropion, a nicotine patch, or both for smoking cessation. *N Engl J Med.* 1999;340:685-691.

56. Simon J, Duncan C, Carmody T, Hudes E. Bupropion for smoking cessation. *Arch Intern Med.* 2004;164:1797-1803.

57. Thorndike AN, Rigotti NA. A tragic triad: coronary artery disease, nicotine addiction and depression. *Curr Opin Cardiol.* 2009;24:447-453.

58. Koegelenberg CF, Noor F, Bateman ED, et al. Efficacy of Varenicline combined with Nicotine Replacement Therapy vs Varenicline alone for Smoking Cessation. *JAMA.* 2014;312(2):155-161.

59. Rigotti NA, Pipe A, Benowitz NL, Arteaga C, Garza D, Tonstad S. Efficacy and safety of varenicline for smoking cessation in patients with cardiovascular disease. *Circulation.* 2010;121:221-229.

60. Singh S, Loke YK, Spangler JG, Furberg CD. Risk of serious adverse cardiovascular events associated with varenicline: a systematic review and meta-analysis. *CMAJ.* 2011;183(12):1359-1366.

61. Prochaska JJ, Hilton JF. Risk of cardiovascular serious adverse events associated with varenicline use for tobacco cessation: systematic review and meta-analysis. *BMJ.* 2012;344:e2856.

62. Ware JH, Vetrovec GW, Miller AB, et al. Cardiovascular safety of varenicline: patient-level meta-analysis of randomized, blinded, placebo-controlled trials. *Am J Ther.* 2013;20:235-246.

63. Kotz D, Viechtbauer W, Simpson C, Van schayck OC, West R, Sheikh A. Cardiovascular and neuropsychiatric risks of varenicline: a retrospective cohort study. *Lancet Respir Med.* 2015;3(10):761-768.

64. Eisenberg M, Windle S, Roy N, et al. Varenicline for smoking cessation in hospitalized patients with acute coronary syndrome. *Circulation.* 2016;133:21-23.

65. Lindson-Hawley N, Aveyard P, Hughes JR. Reduction versus abrupt cessation in smokers who want to quit. *Cochrane Database Syst Rev.* 2010;11:CD008033.

66. Rigotti NA, Singer DE, Mulley AG, Thibault GE. Smoking cessation following admission to a coronary care unit. *J Gen Intern Med.* 1991;6(4):305-311.

67. Aziz O, Skapinakis P, Rahman S, et al. Behavioural interventions for smoking cessation in patients hospitalised for a major cardiovascular event. *Int J Cardiol.* 2008;137:171-174.

68. Quist-Paulsen, Gallefoss P. Randomised controlled trial of smoking cessation intervention after admission for coronary heart disease. *BMJ.* 2003;327:1254-1257.

69. Rigotti NA, Munafo MR, Stead LF. Smoking cessation interventions for hospitalized smokers: a systematic review. *Arch Intern Med.* 2008;168(18):1950-1960.

70. Smith P, Burgess E. Smoking cessation initiated during hospital stay for patients with coronary artery disease: a randomized controlled trial. *CMAJ.* 2009;180(13):1297-1303.

71. Mohiuddin S, Mooss AN, Hunter CB, et al. Intensive smoking cessation intervention reduces mortality in high-risk smokers with cardiovascular disease. *Chest.* 2007;131:446-452.

72. Chow C, Jolly S, Rao-Melacini P, Fox KA, Anand SS, Yusuf S. Association of diet, exercise, and smoking modification with risk of early cardiovascular events after acute coronary syndromes. *Circulation.* 2010;121:750-758.

73. Bullen C. Impact of tobacco smoking and smoking cessation on cardiovascular risk and disease. *Expert Rev Cardiovasc Ther.* 2008;6(6):883-895.

Patient and Family Information for: SMOKING CESSATION FOR THE CARDIAC PATIENT

As a cardiac patient who smokes, you have an urgent need to understand not only how much cigarettes endanger your survival, but also how rapidly and thoroughly stopping smoking will improve your health and outcome. For patients with coronary heart disease, quitting smoking produces a 36% reduction in death from any cause. As you well know, cigarette addiction can be very intense for many people. But despite the intensity of this addiction, with your own determination and a little help from medication and behavioral techniques, you really will succeed.

HOW DOES IT BEGIN?

You most likely began smoking as a teenager, when you were very vulnerable to the addictive properties of nicotine. You tried a cigarette and found that it gave you a certain degree of confidence and pleasure. That feeling came from a substance called dopamine, which the nicotine in cigarette smoke causes to be released in the brain. Quickly, as you developed tolerance to nicotine, you found that in order to get the same effect you needed two cigarettes. Eventually, you found that you needed a cigarette to get going in the morning. Nowadays, it is hard to function without that morning cigarette and maybe a cup of coffee. The discomfort before that first cigarette in the morning is called withdrawal, and when you first felt it you were hooked.

WHY CAN SOME PEOPLE STOP "COLD TURKEY" AND I CANNOT?

The level of addiction varies from person to person. It is determined genetically, by how your body handles nicotine, the addicting substance in the cigarette. Some people can be "social" smokers and just have an occasional cigarette. They experience the harmful effects of the cigarette, but they are not addicted. Their bodies handle nicotine differently. They do not have the genetic makeup that causes them to be susceptible to the addictive properties of nicotine. Why is this important to understand? Accepting that your smoking is an addiction is a heavy burden, but it is important for you and your loved ones to understand it, accept it, and look forward to getting you the help that you need to quit.

HOW DO YOU KNOW IF YOU ARE ADDICTED?

The easiest way to know if you are addicted to cigarettes is to ask yourself how soon after you wake up you have your first cigarette. If it is within minutes, you are very addicted and quitting may be tough for you. We therefore suggest that for you, quitting will be most successful if you combine medication with behavioral changes. Participating in a program with ongoing support, such as a smoking cessation clinic, is likely to be a major help.

WHAT IS NICOTINE WITHDRAWAL?

Nicotine withdrawal is a real physical brain dysfunction. You cannot do your day's work. You get irritable, unable to concentrate. And what makes cigarettes so addicting is that within 10 seconds of smoking, not only is that uncomfortable feeling gone, but you experience real pleasure.

IS IT TOO LATE TO QUIT?

Absolutely not! Much of the effect of smoking on the heart and circulation is reversible and, within 3 years of quitting, the risk of recurrent coronary events becomes that of someone who never smoked. The benefits begin immediately. Within hours of quitting smoking, the carbon monoxide that poisons your oxygen delivery system and the chemically induced tightening of your blood vessels dissipate.

An important part of what happens when a person has a heart attack is caused by the development of clots in the coronary arteries. That is why your doctor is giving you medicines like aspirin and other anticoagulants to thin your blood. Smoking, however, causes your blood to clot, and that effect is not blocked by aspirin. The clotting system is so sensitive to the effect of smoking that even one cigarette causes it to be disrupted. It is therefore very important to understand that it is not enough to cut down on your smoking. You must quit entirely. Even one cigarette endangers your survival. The good news is that your clotting system renews itself very well and fairly rapidly, so the benefits of quitting begin almost immediately.

Smoking also contributes to vascular damage over the years; damage not just to your coronary arteries, but to all the vessels in your body. If you are also diabetic, this effect is further enhanced with an increased risk of blindness, kidney damage, stroke, and loss of limb.

HOW DO I STOP?

There are two parts to this process: medication, for the physical withdrawal, and behavioral change for the habit. You may be disturbed by the idea of taking another medication and believe that you can do this without pharmacologic support. The truth is, if you are addicted, you double your chance of success with treatment, and stopping smoking is as important for your cardiac health as taking some of your cardiac medications, ACE inhibitors, or β-blockers.

MEDICATION

Your doctor will speak with you about using medication to help with nicotine withdrawal. It may be a nicotine patch or gum or even an inhaler, a medication called bupropion, which can be used with or without nicotine replacement or varenicline, which is used alone.

If you have been a heavy smoker and are using nicotine replacement therapy, you will need higher doses of nicotine replacement or possibly a combination of medications such as the patch and gum. If you used nicotine replacement before and felt that it did not help, be aware that the dose must be just right for you. Also, it may seem strange to take nicotine to quit smoking when it is nicotine that you are trying to get away from. The reason this works is that the patch satisfies your need for nicotine without giving you any pleasure. It also breaks the ritual of the smoking habit, doubling your chance of success. As you become comfortable not smoking, the dose of nicotine is gradually reduced and finally stopped.

Your doctor may prescribe bupropion, which helps with the desire to smoke, cravings, as well as with depression. If you have been depressed, it is important to let your doctor know, because bupropion may be very helpful.

There is also a newer, highly effective medicine for stopping smoking called varenicline. It may cause nausea and strange dreams, but after taking it for 7 days you will not feel like smoking. You continue to take varenicline for several months. Unfortunately, some people can become very depressed and even suicidal while taking it. Your doctor may ask a family member to be aware of this and monitor you for any change of mood. If you do experience any change of mood, you need to stop varenicline immediately and speak with your doctor. Although warnings of mood change and depression are concerning, the effectiveness of this drug is very real. You and your doctor need to discuss this option in light of previous quit attempts, level of addiction, and the vulnerability of your cardiac status.

No matter which pharmacotherapy you use, a year later the relapse rate is the same. Something more is needed to remain smoke free, and this is called behavioral therapy: learning new life skills to cope with the issues that made you want to smoke in the first place.

WHAT IS THE BEHAVIORAL PART OF MY TREATMENT?

In addition to dealing with the nicotine withdrawal, you must have a plan for handling the behavioral part of your addiction. Do you use cigarettes for stress, boredom, anger, pleasure, socializing? It is important to look at the reasons for your smoking in order to plan a lifetime change, not just while you are taking medication, but a whole new approach to handling those situations that make you want to smoke.

Develop a clear plan for limiting your stress, avoiding situations that upset you. Exercise regularly, giving yourself real rewards. Put relaxation into your day. Develop hobbies that you can substitute for the pleasure that you derived from cigarettes. Bring a magazine to work for what used to be your smoking break. Have a game on your cell phone to play when you are waiting for the bus. Music, reading, meditation, yoga, sketching, deep breathing, whatever gives you pleasure.

Some tips:
- Develop a list of activities that you can use to keep yourself busy, happy, and relaxed.
- Do not let anyone interfere with or endanger your success. No one can smoke around you!
- Avoid alcohol: it is the strongest trigger.
- For some, coffee is a trigger. Get a substitute, tea or juice or chocolate, at least for the first few days, to change your routine and make it easier to quit.
- Purchase healthy snacks and keep them on hand to relieve the cravings and avoid weight gain.

Pick a quit day and have all your tools ready to go. Choose a busy, nonstressful day; have no cigarettes in the house; throw out all your ashtrays. Keep very busy and go to bed early. If this thought is overwhelming, you are not alone. Some need to begin in a more stepwise fashion. Try using the nicotine lozenge to substitute for a few cigarettes for a few days to get started. Discuss this with your doctor. For the cardiac patient, this is not ideal because all cigarettes are dangerous, but the important message is to start.

Cigarette addiction can be overcome, but it never goes away completely, even as your body becomes much healthier. If you do have a relapse, get back to your plan immediately. Relapse is very common, but it is best to think of it as a learning opportunity—how you could handle that situation differently in the future. It is all part of the process of becoming smoke free.

May Bakir
Eyal Herzog

57

Women's Heart Disease in the Cardiac Care Setting

Case Presentation

A 44-year-old woman presents to the emergency room complaining of chest pain. The patient began to experience chest discomfort during lunch and initially thought it was heartburn. The patient was awoken from recurrent chest pain later that evening around 4 pm and called emergency medical services. In the emergency room, the patient was found to have <1 mm ST elevations in leads aVR, V1, and V2. The patient's initial troponin level was 0.12 ng/mL. Blood pressure and heart rate were within normal limits. Bedside echocardiogram demonstrated left ventricular ejection fraction (LVEF) of 50% and no overt segmental wall motion abnormalities. The patient was admitted to the telemetry floor.

The following morning, the patient's troponin level was <0.03 ng/mL, and the patient was scheduled to have a stress echocardiography. During the stress test, the patient began to experience chest pain and had ST elevations in leads aVR, V1, and V2. Echocardiogram showed new segmental wall motion abnormalities during stress in the basal anterior, anteroseptal, and septal regions. Chest pain and ST elevations resolved quickly with the termination of the stress test. The patient was transferred to the cardiac intensive care unit. She remained hemodynamically stable and was scheduled for cardiac angiography that evening.

Cardiac catheterization was completed and did not demonstrate significant angiographic stenosis. Nitrate medication was initiated, and the patient was scheduled to follow up with a cardiologist as an outpatient.

This case broaches the question "why were there ST elevations and normal coronary anatomy?"

INTRODUCTION

Women with signs and symptoms of cardiac ischemia will undergo cardiac angiography. Many of these patients are found to have normal-appearing coronary arteries. Several studies have demonstrated that up to 40% of patients who undergo cardiac catheterization will not have angiographically significant coronary stenosis.[1] Historically, these patients were said to have cardiac syndrome X. Cardiovascular disease accounts for about 1 in 3 female deaths. For women presenting for evaluation of suspected ischemic symptoms, a diagnosis of normal coronary arteries is 5 times more common than for men.[2] A substantial percentage of these patients have coronary microvascular dysfunction (CMD). In the past two decades, in part because the National Heart, Lung and Blood Institute initiated the Women's Ischemia Syndrome Evaluation in 1996, an extensive amount of research has focused on coronary microvasculature. CMD is now acknowledged as a cause of cardiac ischemia and can occur alone or along with macrovascular coronary artery disease (CAD). Patients with CMD have a significantly higher rate of hospitalization, heart failure, sudden cardiac death, and myocardial infarction (MI).[3] CMD can affect the cardiac vasculature in a number of ways that essentially disrupt the coronary arteries' vasodilatory ability and therefore hinders coronary blood flow (CBF), causing ischemia.[4]

MYOCARDIAL ISCHEMIA IN WOMEN IN THE CRITICAL CARE SETTING

All patients with acute coronary syndrome (ACS) are evaluated for placement in the cardiac care unit (CCU). Patients who are believed to have high-risk lesions, such as left main coronary disease, will be appropriately monitored in the CCU until further diagnostic procedures can be obtained. As with the patient in the case presentation, because of the ST elevations in leads aVR, V1, and V2 and concordant echocardiographically demonstrated wall motion abnormalities during exercise stress, it was thought that there was a high likelihood of left main coronary disease. Optimal medical therapy for women experiencing ACS does not differ from that for men. In the absence of absolute contraindications, aggressive therapy should be initiated with antiplatelet therapy with aspirin, a platelet $P2Y_{12}$ receptor blocker, anticoagulation therapy, β-blockade, and lipid-lowering medication. Cardiac angiography would be the next diagnostic approach to assess the coronary arteries. It is well known that about 50% of patients who undergo clinically indicated coronary angiography will not have obstructive CAD. Of the patients without obstructive CAD, more than half are believed to have CMD. The importance of the diagnosis of CMD lies in its poor prognosis.

PROGNOSIS

In women who present with ACS, it is not uncommon for the angiogram to demonstrate nonobstructive CAD. National data have shown that the odds for obstructive CAD in the ACS setting are 50% lower in women when compared with men.[5] However, in the setting of ACS, nonobstructive coronary anatomy does not carry a benign prognosis. Studies have shown that women with signs and symptoms of ischemia and no obstructive CAD have elevated major adverse cardiac event (MACE) rates, including MI and cardiac death. In some patients, the worse prognosis is attributed to advanced age and comorbidities, but younger women in particular do worse. This may be due to underutilization of lifesaving therapies and medications.[6] CMD can occur secondary to either endothelial-dependent or non–endothelial-dependent regulatory systems. Endothelial-dependent CMD is defined as impaired vasomotor response to acetylcholine. Endothelial-dependent CMD has been shown to be an independent risk factor for MACE.[7] Non–endothelial-dependent CMD is diagnosed when there is reduced coronary flow reserve (<2.36), and it is significantly associated with MACE in 5-year follow-up from initial diagnosis.[3]

TAKOTSUBO CARDIOMYOPATHY

Stress cardiomyopathy, also known as Takotsubo cardiomyopathy or broken heart syndrome, is a syndrome characterized by regional systolic dysfunction of the left ventricle (LV) where the presentation mimics troponin-positive ACS or ST-elevation MI, but lacking obstructive disease on cardiac angiography.[8] There are several forms of Takotsubo cardiomyopathy, the most common presentation being apical ballooning of LV apex, with hypokinesis of the mid-and apical segments and hyperkinesis of the basal segments of the LV[9] (**Figure 57.1**). This syndrome is more common in women, and the pathogenesis, although not fully understood, is postulated to be secondary to catecholamine release, coronary spasm, or microvascular dysfunction. These patients, although lacking obstructive CAD, demonstrate abnormal myocardial perfusion.[10] Several findings argue that Takotsubo cardiomyopathy is consistent with CMD, including abnormal coronary flow reserve (CFR) measured by echocardiography and improvement of LV function with the administration of adenosine.[11,12]

DIAGNOSIS

STRESS TESTING

Exercise stress testing is commonly used to assess CAD. However, stress testing is not very sensitive or specific in detecting heart disease in women. Currently, there are no methods to directly visualize the coronary microvasculature. Indirect assessment of the coronary microvasculature is made through functional testing. CFR is one method that provides vasodilator response to adenosine. CFR is calculated as the ratio of the CBF at maximal dilation to the CBF at rest and can be obtained through various imaging modalities. There is not an absolute cutoff for the CFR in defining CMD; however, most are considered to have CMD if the CFR is <1.5.[13]

POSITRON EMISSION TOMOGRAPHY

Cardiac positron emission tomography (PET) scanning is used for myocardial perfusion scanning as a technique to identify perfusion defects, which in turn reflect CAD. In nonobstructive CAD, perfusion defects reflect microvascular ischemia along distribution of the three main coronary arteries.[14]

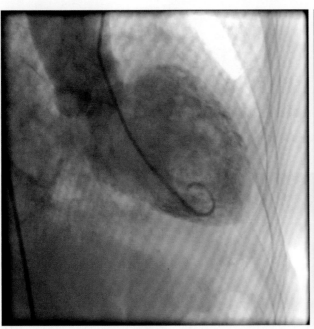
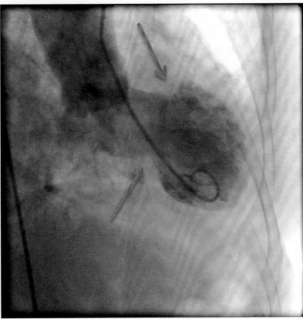

FIGURE 57.1 Takotsubo cardiomyopathy on cardiac angiography. Arrows indicate the hinge points between hyperdynamic basal segments and akinetic mid- and apical segments.

CONTRAST ECHOCARDIOGRAPHY

Assessing the coronary arteries with cardiac angiography can be challenging in a critically ill patient. Contrast echocardiography can be safely used at the bedside.[15] Features of ACS are commonly seen in critically ill patients, including ECG changes, troponin elevation, and angina. These features of ACS are frequently seen in conditions other than obstructive CAD, such as Takotsubo cardiomyopathy and CMD. Cardiac microvasculature in the endocardial regional has the lowest flow reserve and is more susceptible to ischemia than the epicardium possibly because of the larger epicardially placed coronary arteries.[16] Therefore, in CMD there may be a reduction in the blood flow in the endocardial myocardium to a greater extent than in the epicardial myocardium (**Figure 57.2**), which can be seen with reduced perfusion during contrast echocardiography.[15]

CARDIAC MAGNETIC RESONANCE IMAGING

Myocardial scar can be detected by cardiac magnetic resonance imaging (CMRI) late gadolinium enhancement (LGE) and is a known predictor of MACE. Women with signs and symptoms of ischemia and no obstructive CAD have been shown to have a prevalence of myocardial scar detected by CMRI LGE, with a predominant traditional MI pattern (**Figure 57.3**) indicative of CMD. The amount of ischemia can be assessed on the basis of the intensity of gadolinium that is perfused in the myocardium.[17] The use of CMRI has confirmed that many of these women can have irreversible myocardial injury, which appears to be clinically underdiagnosed.[18]

CORONARY REACTIVITY TESTING

The gold standard for diagnosing CMD is through coronary reactivity testing. This is done while the patient is having a cardiac angiography. Adenosine is used to assess endothelial-independent dysfunction, and acetylcholine is used to assess endothelial-dependent dysfunction. Coronary flow is quantified before the adenosine injection and again after administration. In non–endothelial-dependent dysfunction, the CFR, in response to adenosine, will be ≤2.5.[19] Endothelial-dependent dysfunction is seen when there is less than 50% increase in coronary blood flow after the bolus of acetylcholine.[20] Coronary spasm can also be assessed with acetylcholine if the patient has chest pain in addition to ECG changes and if the change in the coronary artery diameter is less than 90%.[21]

TREATMENT

Currently, there are no guidelines to treat CMD. Treating CMD begins with risk factor control and lifestyle modification.

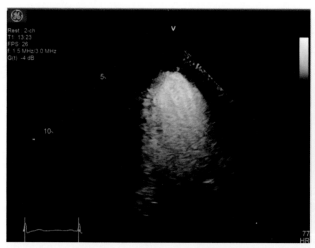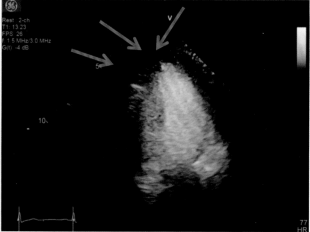

FIGURE 57.2 Contrast echocardiography demonstrating decreased circulation at the apical segment (arrows).

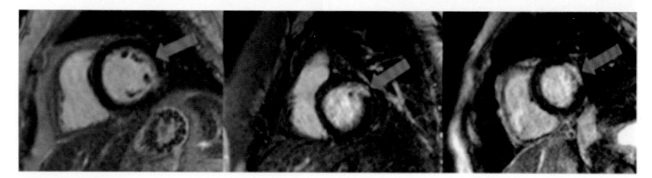

FIGURE 57.3 Cardiac magnetic resonance imaging with late gadolinium enhancement (arrows): Typical infarction pattern along the coronary arteries seen in coronary microvascular dysfunction.

Treatment should be aimed at reducing ischemic disease to reduce the risk of adverse cardiac events, ameliorating symptoms to improve quality of life and to decrease the morbidity from unnecessary and repeated cardiac catheterization.

Patients with endothelial dysfunction should be counseled on smoking cessation, which is known to improve endothelial dysfunction and therefore CMD.[22] Adrenergic modulation seems to play an important role, and therefore exercise should also be encouraged in this population. Angiotensin-converting enzyme inhibitors and statin medications improve endothelial dysfunction and should be used as first-line therapy. Statins lower cholesterol and have anti-inflammatory properties that have been shown to increase CFR.[23]

Patients with non–endothelial-dependent CMD benefit from β-blocker and nitrate medications. Nitrates help with angina by decreasing preload with venous dilation. β-Blockers are beneficial in that they decrease myocardial oxygen demand and increase diastolic filling time.

Ranolazine is a medication that is used to treat angina with varying results. Ranolazine inhibits the late sodium channels and reduces intracellular calcium, leading to improved ventricular relaxation.[24] Patients who have refractory angina despite being on maximal medical therapy should have a trial of Ranolazine to see if their symptoms improve.

CONCLUSION

Myocardial ischemia has specific sex differences. Despite having a lower prevalence of obstructive CAD, women have a higher prevalence of symptoms, ischemia, and mortality relative to men. Diagnostic testing can be used to accurately assess for myocardial ischemia in symptomatic women, in addition to providing important prognostic information. Women who are critically ill because of unstable angina or ACS and who do not have obstructive CAD should not be dismissed from care without further workup. Many of these women have been shown to have CMD that has been proven to be associated with high mortality, and, therefore, CMD is important to consider when diagnosing and treating these patients.

REFERENCES

1. Patel MR, Peterson ED, Dai D, et al. Low diagnostic yield of elective coronary angiography. *N Engl J Med.* 2010;362:886-895.
2. Sullivan AK, Holdright DR, Wright CA, Sparrow JL, Cunningham D, Fox KM. Chest pain in women: Clinical, investigative, and prognostic features. *BMJ.* 1994;308:883-886.
3. Pepine CJ, Anderson RD, Sharaf BL, et al. Coronary microvascular reactivity to adenosine predicts adverse outcome in women evaluated for suspected ischemia: results from the national heart, lung and blood institute wise (women's ischemia syndrome evaluation) study. *J Am Coll Cardiol.* 2010;55:2825-2832.
4. Camici PG, Crea F. Coronary microvascular dysfunction. *N Engl J Med.* 2007;356:830-840.
5. Shaw LJ, Shaw RE, Merz CNB, et al. Impact of ethnicity and gender differences on angiographic coronary artery disease prevalence and in-hospital mortality in the American College of Cardiology–National Cardiovascular Data Registry. *Circulation.* 2008;117:1787-1801.
6. Vaccarino V, Parsons L, Every NR, Barron HV, Krumholz HM. Sex-based differences in early mortality after myocardial infarction. *N Engl J Med.* 1999;341:217-225.
7. Gulati M, Cooper-DeHoff RM, McClure C, et al. Adverse cardiovascular outcomes in women with nonobstructive coronary artery disease: a report from the Women's Ischemia Syndrome Evaluation Study and the St James Women Take Heart Project. *Arch Intern Med.* 2009;169:843-850.
8. Sato H, Tateishi H, Uchida T. Takotsubo-type cardiomyopathy due to multivessel spasm. In: Kodama K, Haze K, Hon M, eds. *Clinical Aspect of Myocardial Injury: From Ischemia to Heart Failure.* Tokyo, Japan: Kagakuhyouronsha, 1990:56-64.
9. Abe Y, Kondo M, Matsuoka R, Araki M, Dohyama K, Tanio H. Assessment of clinical features in transient left ventricular apical ballooning. *J Am Coll Cardiol.* 2003;41:737-742.
10. Elesber A, Lerman A, Bybee KA, et al. Myocardial perfusion in apical ballooning syndrome: correlate of myocardial injury. *Am Heart J.* 2006;152:469.e9-469.e413.
11. Rigo F, Sicari R, Citro R, Ossena G, Buja P, Picano E. Diffuse, marked, reversible impairment in coronary microcirculation in stress cardiomyopathy: a doppler transthoracic echo study. *Ann Med.* 2009;41:462-470.
12. Galiuto L, De Caterina AR, Porfidia A, et al. Reversible coronary microvascular dysfunction: a common pathogenetic mechanism in apical ballooning or tako-tsubo syndrome. *Eur Heart J.* 2010;31:1319-1327.
13. Löffler AI, Bourque JM. Coronary microvascular dysfunction, microvascular angina, and management. *Curr Cardiol Rep.* 2016;18:1-7.
14. Marroquin OC, Holubkov R, Edmundowicz D, et al. Heterogeneity of microvascular dysfunction in women with chest pain not attributable to coronary artery disease: implications for clinical practice. *Am Heart J.* 2003;145:628-635.
15. Orde S, McLean A. Bedside myocardial perfusion assessment with contrast echocardiography. *Crit Care.* 2016;20:1.
16. Linka AZ, Sklenar J, Wei K, Jayaweera AR, Skyba DM, Kaul S. Assessment of transmural distribution of myocardial perfusion with contrast echocardiography. *Circulation.* 1998;98:1912-1920.
17. Cullen J, Horsfield M, Reek C, Cherryman G, Barnett D, Samani N. A myocardial perfusion reserve index in humans using first-pass contrast-enhanced magnetic resonance imaging. *J Am Coll Cardiol.* 1999;33:1386-1394.
18. Bakir M, Wei J, Thomson L, et al. Prevalence of myocardial scar in women with signs and symptoms of ischemia but no obstructive coronary artery disease: a report from the Women's Ischemia Syndrome Evaluation. *J Am Coll Cardiol.* 2015;65(10):A1580.
19. Murray KJ. Cyclic AMP and mechanisms of vasodilation. *Pharmacol Ther.* 1990;47:329-345.
20. Blaise G, Stewart D, Guerard M. Acetylcholine stimulates release of endothelium-derived relaxing factor in coronary arteries of human organ donors. *Can J Cardiol.* 1993;9:813-820.
21. Chen C, Wei J, AlBadri A, Zarrini P, Merz CNB. Coronary microvascular dysfunction—epidemiology, pathogenesis, prognosis, diagnosis, risk factors and therapy. *Circ J.* 2016;81:3-11.
22. Lim TK, Choy AJ, Khan F, Belch JJ, Struthers AD, Lang CC. Therapeutic development in cardiac syndrome X: a need to target the underlying pathophysiology. *Cardiovasc Ther.* 2009;27:49-58.
23. Zhang X, Li Q, Zhao J, et al. Effects of combination of statin and calcium channel blocker in patients with cardiac syndrome X. *Coron Artery Dis.* 2014;25:40-44.
24. Hasenfuss G, Maier L. Mechanism of action of the new anti-ischemia drug ranolazine. *Clin Res Cardiol.* 2008;97:222-226.

Patient and Family Information for: WOMEN'S HEART DISEASE IN THE CARDIAC CARE SETTING

Coronary microvascular disease (CMD) is a disease that affects the small vessels of the heart that branch off from the larger coronary arteries. Patients often have signs and symptoms that are consistent with a blockage of the larger coronary arteries, but after cardiac angiography are not seen to have blockage. CMD is defined as damage to the inner walls of the blood vessels that can lead to spasms and decreased blood flow to the heart muscle. CMD affects more women than men. Despite not having obstructive disease of the large vessels of the heart, patients with CMD have a high risk of recurrent hospitalization, chronic chest pain, heart attack, and sudden cardiac death.

Stress-induced cardiomyopathy, also known as Takotsubo cardiomyopathy, is thought to be partially secondary to CMD. Patients who have experienced stressful situations, which could include anything from the loss of a family member to an illness or any general life hardship, can be affected by this type of cardiomyopathy. The pump function of the heart decreases in stress-induced cardiomyopathy because the apex of the heart will not contract as it should. Most often, this cardiomyopathy is reversible if treated properly.

The diagnosis of CMD has been evolving over the past two decades. There are noninvasive imaging modalities that can be used, such as positron emission tomography, echocardiography, and cardiac magnetic resonance imaging. Invasive testing can be done during cardiac angiography to see how the small vessels respond to certain medications to determine if there is a dysfunction within the lining of the blood vessels.

There are no specific guidelines on the treatment of CMD. All patients with CMD should undergo risk adjustment with lifestyle modification. Smoking cessation is essential because cigarette smoke affects the lining of the small blood vessels and exacerbates the symptoms of CMD. Exercise should be encouraged because it increases blood flow throughout the body, including to the small vessels. Medications that increase blood flow to the small vessels should be considered. These include angiotensin receptor blockers, β-blockers, nitrates, and Ranolazine, each having their respective mechanism of action. Cholesterol-lowering medications should be started because they both lower cholesterol and have anti-inflammatory properties, which are thought to aid in the treatment of symptomatology.

To conclude, women with chest pain should have a thorough workup done by a cardiologist. Women who have been admitted to the hospital for an acute coronary syndrome but have not been found to have obstructive coronary disease of the large vessels should not go without follow-up because if they do have CMD and go undiagnosed and untreated, the prognosis is often poor.

Alan Rozanski
Randy Cohen

Lifestyle Management after the Diagnosis of Heart Disease

As the 20th century approached, pneumonia, tuberculosis, and diarrhea/enteritis were the leading causes of death in the United States. However, marked advances in our understanding of the determinants and transmission of diseases were beginning to reduce the mortality risk from acute illnesses. These included such measures as sanitation, chlorination, the introduction of measures to ensure a safer food supply, and the development of vaccines against acute illnesses, which by 1900 included vaccines against cholera, tetanus, typhoid fever, and bubonic plague. By the 1920s, chronic diseases were replacing acute illnesses as the major causes of mortality, with cardiovascular disease (CVD) as the leading cause of death. Thus, a "war" against CVD was initiated by the American medical community.

Initial success was slow because of a limited understanding of the disease and its risk factors. CVD increased in epidemic proportion before peaking in its incidence in the late 1960s. Since then, the reversal of disease has been remarkable. In the late 1960s, heart disease dwarfed cancer as a cause of death, and strokes were all too common. Since 1970, however, the mortality rates from cardiac disease and stroke have fallen by 70%, and the death rates from heart disease and cancer are now comparable (**Figure 58.1**).[1]

Two broad factors have accounted for this success: remarkable improvements in the treatments for heart disease and important advances in CVD prevention. Each of these factors is estimated to account for approximately 50% of the decline in heart disease.[2]

The medical advances have been broad based, including the initiation of cardiac care units, introduction of stress testing, development of cardiac bypass surgery and percutaneous coronary interventions, echocardiography, radionuclide stress testing, defibrillators, pacemakers, ablation procedures for arrhythmias, cardiac transplant, and the development of many effective classes of cardiac medications. The increasing sophistication of treatment has led to the development of many cardiac subspecialties, such as in cardiac imaging, electrophysiology, interventional cardiology, heart failure, and preventive cardiology. In each of these arenas, there have been continual advances that have improved care and survival. For instance, in the early introduction of angioplasty, reocclusion was a common problem. Improvement came with the development of bare metal stents, but in-stent restenosis remained a problem. The subsequent introduction of drug-eluting stents reduced the incidence of in-stent stenosis and

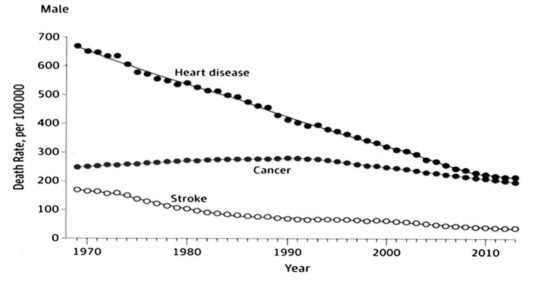

FIGURE 58.1 Temporal decline in death rates from heart disease, cancer, and stroke since 1969. (From Ma J, Ward EM, Siegel RL, Jemal A. Temporal trends in mortality in the United States, 1969–2013. *JAMA*. 2015;314:1731-1739.)

allowed the performance of more complex procedures. Now fully bioabsorbable stents have been approved for use and will be tested for their added efficacy. Similarly, the treatment of heart failure has been revolutionized by ever safer ventricular assist devices and resynchronization devices. Cardiac imaging has expanded to include cardiac MRI, coronary artery calcium scanning and coronary CT angiography, as well as continued advances in echo and nuclear cardiology. Other important recent advances include the expanding use of trans-aortic valvular replacement (TAVR), hypothermia for cardiac arrest, and many new drug therapies, such as those used to treat diabetes, the introduction of PCSK 9 inhibitors for hyperlipidemia, and novel anticoagulants.

The improvements in CVD prevention have also been broad based and impressive. An important advance in this regard was the initiation of the famous Framingham Study in 1948, which was dedicated to determining what risk factors accounted for heart disease in the town of Framingham, Massachusetts. By the early 1960s, the study had revealed that high cholesterol, hypertension, smoking, and diabetes were all important risk factors for CVD. At that time, nearly 45% of Americans smoked, often with great frequency, and many others were subject to secondhand smoke. The greatest single advance in cardiac prevention that has occurred since that time has been the dramatic drop in smoking rates (**Figure 58.2**),[3] aided by societal measures to prevent individuals from being exposed to sec-ondhand smoking. Second, dietary guidelines and change in eating habits, such as the reduction in animal lard use and trans fats, have helped reduce serum cholesterol levels (which began even before the statin era) (**Figure 58.3**).[4] In addition, the advent of statins to treat dyslipidemia and powerful medications to control hypertension and diabetes has markedly improved our ability to prevent CVD.

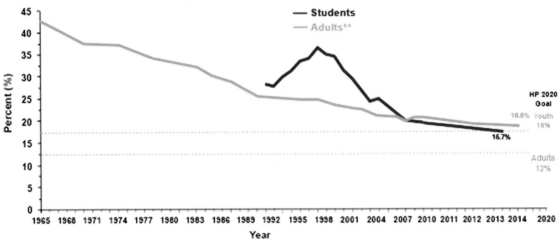

FIGURE 58.2 Temporal decline in the prevalence of smoking in the United States since 1965 for adults (green line) and students (blue line). (From Trends in current cigarette smoking among high school students and adults, United States, 1965–2014. Atlanta, GA: Office on Smoking and Health, National Center for Chronic Disease Prevention and Health Promotion; March 2016.)

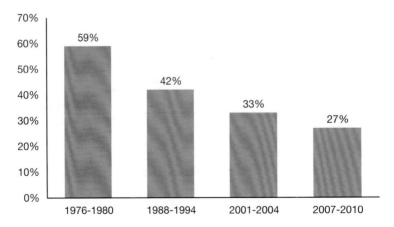

FIGURE 58.3 Temporal decline in the prevalence of high LDL cholesterol levels in the United States as assessed over four temporal periods. (From Kuklina EV, Carroll MD, Shaw KM, Hirsch R. Trends in high LDL cholesterol, cholesterol-lowering medication use, and dietary saturated-fat intake: United States, 1976–2010. Atlanta, GA: National Center for Health Statistics Brief No. 117; March 2013.)

Because of these remarkable advances in prevention, there has been a marked decline in sudden cardiac death, and both the frequency and magnitude of myocardial infarction have declined.[5,6] So too has the incidence of peripheral vascular disease.[7] There has also been a marked decline in the frequency of inducible myocardial ischemia among patients presenting to stress labs for the workup of suspected CVD (**Figure 58.4**).[8] In sum, heart disease today is not only less frequent but also milder than yesteryear.

Nevertheless, despite all of this progress, CVD remains the number one cause of death in the United States, among both men and women.[9] Further progress will depend on addressing two interrelated problems. First, although the medical advances cited earlier have remarkably altered the course of CVD, they have also markedly increased the cost of cardiovascular health care, which has been projected to triple between 2010 and 2030 (**Figure 58.5**).[9] Thus, efforts to reduce CVD costs have become an important driving force in health care policy. Second, although some risk factors for CVD have declined, three important risk factors have increased in frequency: obesity, sedentary behavior, and diabetes.

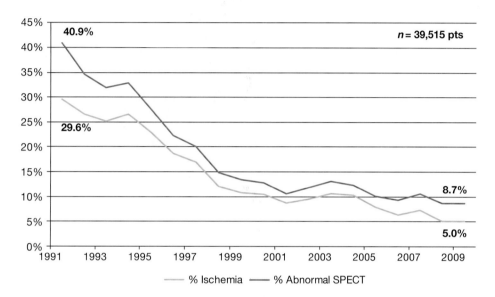

FIGURE 58.4 Temporal decline in the frequency of abnormal stress-rest myocardial perfusion SPECT studies (red line) and frequency of inducible ischemia (green line) between 1991 and 2009 among 39,515 patients referred for testing at a single medical center because of suspected CAD. (From Rozanski A, Gransar H, Hayes SW, et al. Temporal trends in the frequency of inducible myocardial ischemia during cardiac stress testing: 1991 to 2009. *J Am Coll Cardiol.* 2013;61:1054-1065.)

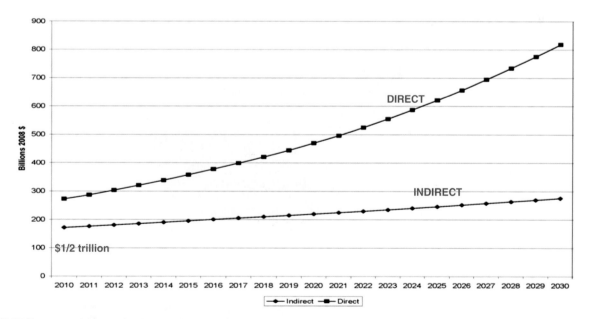

FIGURE 58.5 Projected direct and indirect medical costs for cardiovascular care in the United States between 2010 and 2030, according to an American Heart Association analysis. (From Heidenreich PA, Trogdon IG, Khaugov OA, et al. Forecasting the future of cardiovascular disease in the United States. A policy statement from the American Heart Association. *Circulation.* 2011;123:933-944.)

Since the 1980s, obesity has increased around the world in epidemic fashion. To exemplify the problem, the Centers for Disease Control and Prevention (CDC) maps the prevalence of obesity by state on a yearly basis. For instance, **Figures 58.6** and **58.7** show the U.S. obesity maps for 1990 and 2010. In 1990, not one state had a prevalence of obesity that was >15%.[10] By contrast, in 2010, a mere 20 years later, approximately one-quarter of states had obesity rates >30%. Today, approximately 30% of Americans are overweight and >30% are obese. It is widely recognized that this sudden rise in obesity is not due to genetic change, but rather to societal and environmental changes that have occurred since the 1980s, including such factors as eating more refined grains, changes in how food is processed, advertising of unhealthy foods, increasingly sedentary behavior, growth of

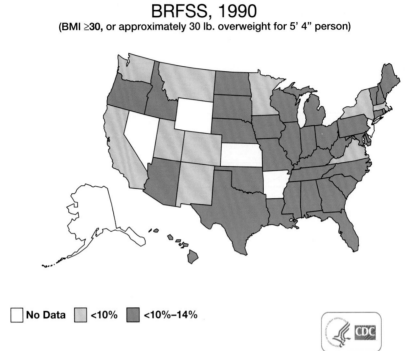

FIGURE 58.6 Prevalence of obesity in the United States, by state, according to a Behavioral Risk Factor Surveillance System (BRFSS) analysis in 1990. As shown on the color maps, no state exceeded a 15% prevalence of obesity.

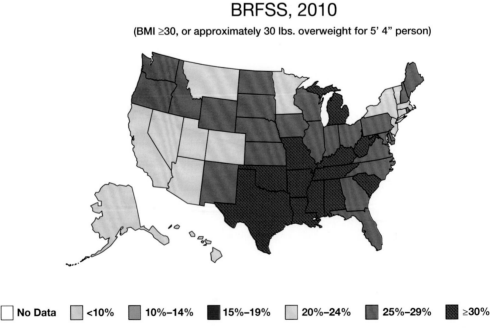

FIGURE 58.7 Prevalence of obesity in the United States, by state, according to a Behavioral Risk Factor Surveillance System (BRFSS) analysis in 2010. As shown on the color maps, 12 states exceeded a 29% prevalence of obesity.

convenience stores, increasing size of food portions, and decreasing sleep patterns. The poor diet of Americans is a large part of this story. The American Heart Association has identified seven components of "ideal" cardiovascular health, on the basis of diet, physical activity, body mass index, abstinence from tobacco use, blood pressure, cholesterol, and blood glucose levels.[11] Of these factors, Americans' poor diet is a particularly challenging one, with the vast majority of Americans scoring poorly on their diet metric.

Sedentary behavior has become normative in our society and may be increasing because of various societal trends. Excessive TV watching, increasing screen time, sedentary pastimes (eg, video games), a shift to more sedentary jobs,[12] convenience devices

that have led to less physical activity at home (**Figure 58.8**),[13] less maternal time spent engaged in physical activity (**Figure 58.9**),[13] and a drop in physical activity among teenagers (**Figure 58.10**),[14] a time when physical activity habits are being set, are among the reasons for too little physical activity in today's society. Today's society has also become more fast paced and time pressed, resulting in greater difficulty for finding time to exercise among many people.

The result of poor nutritional habits, the rise of obesity, and the decline in physical activity have fueled an epidemic rise in diabetes (**Figure 58.11**), which now affects nearly 30 million Americans (approximately 9.3% of the population), and nearly 85 million Americans over the age of 20 are also considered prediabetic.[15] The presence of these three risk factors has helped

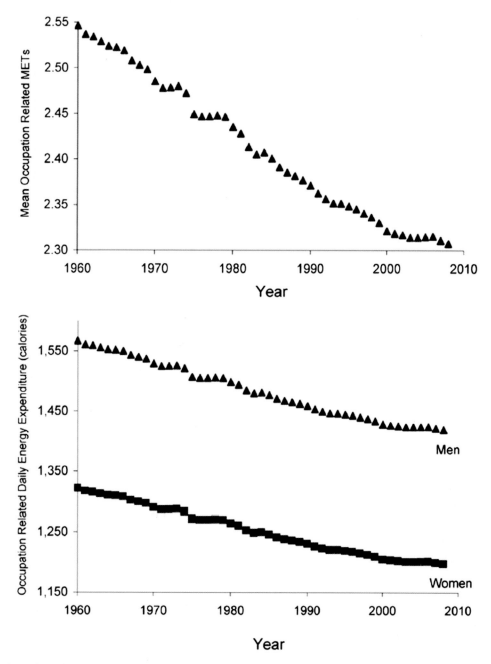

FIGURE 58.8 Decline in household levels of energy expenditure over a 45-year period. (From Archer E, Lavie CJ, McDonald SM, et al. Maternal inactivity: 45-year trends in mothers' use of time. *Mayo Clin Proc.* 2013;88[12]:1368-1377.)

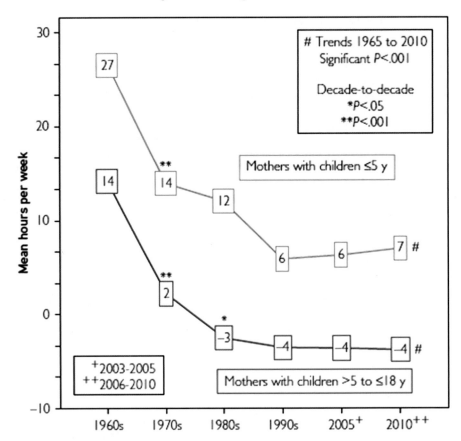

FIGURE 58.9 Time reallocation (mean hours per week spent in physically active behaviors minus hours per week spent in sedentary behaviors; numbers rounded to the nearest whole number) in US mothers, 1965–2010. Negative values denote more time spent in sedentary than in physically active behaviors. (From Archer E, Lavie CJ, McDonald SM, et al. Maternal inactivity 45-year trends in mothers' use of time. *Mayo Clin Proc.* 2013;88[12]:136-1377.)

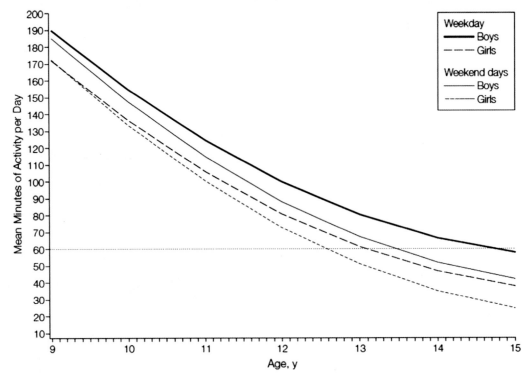

FIGURE 58.10 Daily minutes of physical activity for children between the ages of 9 and 15, for boys and girls, including weekdays and weekends. Note the marked decline in physical activity during the teenage years. (From Nader PR, Bradley RH, Houts RM, McRitchie SL, O'Brien M. Moderate-to-vigorous physical activity from ages 9 to 15 years. *JAMA.* 2008;300[3]:295-305.)

Number and Percentage of U.S. Population with Diagnosed Diabetes, 1958-2013

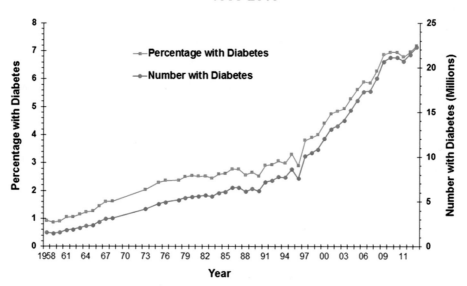

FIGURE 58.11 The number (blue) and percentage (gold) of Americans with diagnosed diabetes between 1958 and 2013. (From Centers for Disease Control and Prevention. National diabetes statistics report: estimates of diabetes and its burden in the U.S., 2014. Atlanta, GA: U.S. Department of Health and Human Services; 2014.)

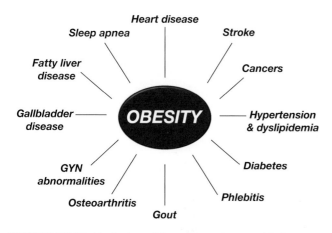

FIGURE 58.12 Medical conditions that are increased in frequency because of obesity.

to sustain our continued high rate of CVD, and these risk factors also lead to many other chronic medical conditions, as shown for obesity in **Figure 58.12**. It is estimated that the majority of chronic diseases could be obviated if people would adopt healthy lifestyle habits.[16,17] For this reason, increasing emphasis now needs to be placed on the promotion of healthy nutrition, exercise, and successful weight management.

However, changing negative health habits is not simple. Even adherence to medication change is often difficult for patients. Thus, a new field of behavioral cardiology has emerged, which is dedicated to studying the behavioral and psychosocial determinants of cardiac disease and the behavioral approaches to modifying negative health habits.[18,19] This field has made rapid strides in recent decades.[20] The field is based on a psychosocial model of health that recognizes that psychosocial factors both contribute

to negative health habits and help cause disease directly through various pathophysiologic mechanisms. The field is also dedicated to the application of psychological principles for aiding patients to change their negative lifestyle behaviors.

To illustrate the development of behavioral cardiology and its application to patients following myocardial infarction, we present the story of David, a patient recovering from myocardial infarction, in the next three chapters. The first chapter deals with David's dietary management based on a new body of scientific literature that has identified which foods and dietary patterns are associated with better health and a reduced risk of CVD.[21] The second chapter focuses on the growing science of exercise physiology and epidemiology and how it might apply to a patient like David.[22] The third chapter focuses on a dramatic growth in the field of behavioral cardiology: identification of the psychosocial risk factors that help contribute to the development of CVD and the increasing application of psychological principles for the management of negative health habits and psychosocial risk factors for CVD.[23] Together, these three chapters provide growing insights into the application of behavioral cardiology for the betterment of patients' lifestyles following the occurrence of cardiac events.

REFERENCES

1. Ma J, Ward EM, Siegel RL, Jemal A. Temporal trends in mortality in the United States, 1969–2013. *JAMA.* 2015;314:1731-1739.

2. Ford ES, Ajani UA, Croft JB, et al. Explaining the decrease in U.S. deaths from coronary disease, 1980-2000. *N Engl J Med.* 2007;356:2388-2398.

3. Trends in current cigarette smoking among high school students and adults, United States, 1965–2014. Office on smoking and health, National Center for Chronic Disease Prevention and Health Promotion. March 2016.

4. Kuklina EV, Carroll MD, Shaw KM, Hirsch R. Trends in high LDL cholesterol, cholesterol-lowering medication use, and dietary saturated-fat intake: United States, 1976–2010. National Center for Health Statistics Brief No. 117, March 2013.

5. Yeh RW, Sidney S, Chandra M, Sorel M, Selby JV, Go AS. Population trends in the incidence and outcomes of acute myocardial infarction. *N Engl J Med*. 2010;362:2155-2165.

6. Myerson M, Coady S, Taylor H, Rosamond WD, Goff DC Jr; ARIC Investigators. Declining severity of myocardial infarction from 1987 to 2002: the Atherosclerosis Risk in Communities (ARIC) Study. *Circulation*. 2009;119:503-514.

7. Murabito JM, Evans JC, D'Agostino RB Sr, Wilson PW, Kannel WB. Temporal trends in the incidence of intermittent claudication from 1950 to 1999. *Am J Epidemiol*. 2005;162:430-437.

8. Rozanski A, Gransar H, Hayes SW, et al. Temporal trends in the frequency of inducible myocardial ischemia during cardiac stress testing: 1991 to 2009. *J Am Coll Cardiol*. 2013;61:1054-1065.

9. Heidenreich PA, Trogdon IG, Khaugov OA, et al. Forecasting the future of cardiovascular disease in the United States. A policy statement from the American Heart Association. *Circulation*. 2011;123:933-944.

10. Prevalence of self-reported obesity among U.S. adults by state and territory, Behavioral Risk Factor Surveillance System. Division of Nutrition, Physical Activity, and Obesity, National Center for Chronic Disease Prevention and Health Promotion, September 2016.

11. Lloyd-Jones DM, Hong Y, Labarthe D, et al. Defining and setting National Goals for Cardiovascular Health Promotion and Disease Reduction: the American Heart Association's Strategic Impact Goal Through 2020 and beyond. *Circulation*. 2010;121(4):586-613.

12. Church TS, Thomas DM, Tudor-Locke C, et al. Trends over 5 decades in U.S. occupation-related physical activity and their associations with obesity. *PLoS One*. 2011;6(5):e19657.

13. Archer E, Lavie CJ, McDonald SM, et al. Maternal inactivity: 45-year trends in mothers' use of time. *Mayo Clin Proc*. 2013;88(12):1368-1377.

14. Nader PR, Bradley RH, Houts RM, McRitchie SL, O'Brien M. Moderate-to-vigorous physical activity from ages 9 to 15 years. *JAMA*. 2008;300(3):295-305.

15. Centers for Disease Control and Prevention. National diabetes statistics report: estimates of diabetes and its burden in the U.S., 2014. Atlanta, GA: U.S. Department of Health and Human Services; 2014.

16. Stampfer MJ, Hu FB, Manson JE, et al. Primary prevention of coronary heart disease in women through diet and lifestyle. *N Engl J Med*. 2000;343(1):16-22.

17. Akesson A, Larsson SC, Discacciati A, Wolk A. Low-risk diet and lifestyle habits in the primary prevention of myocardial infarction in men: a population-based prospective cohort study. *J Am Coll Cardiol*. 2014;64(13):1299-1306.

18. Rozanski A, Blumenthal JA, Kaplan J. Impact of psychological factors on the pathogenesis of cardiovascular disease and implications for therapy. *Circulation*. 1999;99:2192-2217.

19. Rozanski A, Blumenthal JA, Davidson KW, Saab PG, Kubzansky L. The epidemiology, pathophysiology, and management of psychosocial risk factors in cardiac practice: the emerging field of Behavioral Cardiology. *J Am Coll Cardiol*. 2005;45:637-651.

20. Rozanski A. Behavioral cardiology: current advances and future directions. *J Am Coll Cardiol*. 2014;64:100-110.

21. Cohen R, Rozanski A. Nutrition and weight management in cardiac patients. In Herzog's CCU Book-Chapter 59.

22. Cohen R, Rozanski A. Exercise and physical activity in cardiac patients. In Herzog's CCU Book-Chapter 60.

23. Rozanski A, Cohen R. Applying psychological principles for the lifestyle management of cardiac patients. In Herzog's CCU Book-Chapter 61.

59

Randy Cohen
Alan Rozanski

Nutrition and Weight Management in Cardiac Patients

David is a 52-year-old male who until recently felt well. One day, however, he developed sudden chest pain, prompting him to go to the local hospital. Much to his surprise, he was diagnosed with a heart attack and needed a coronary stent placed to open up a blocked artery. Although David had been told by his doctor for years to lose weight, change his diet, and start exercising in order to avoid developing medical conditions that can predispose to heart disease, he just didn't have the necessary time to commit to these lifestyle changes. Having three teenage children and a working wife, David had a very demanding job that required long hours, a long commute, and expectations to work from home. In David's mind, it was more important to work hard and provide for his family than to tend to these lifestyle changes, which he mentally thought of as something one does after retirement.

David's heart attack was real and life changing. As he sat recuperating in his hospital bed, he thought about all the things he could have done differently to avoid this major medical event that, for better or worse, has now affected his life and put a burden on his family, coworkers, and friends. Thankfully, David's hospitalization was unremarkable, and he was given an excellent prognosis. As he was being discharged to his home, David felt a deep sense of responsibility to himself and his family to make all the important lifestyle changes necessary to regain his sense of health and vitality. The only problem was he didn't know where to start. As a first step, he established care with a local cardiologist and began asking questions: "How can I change my diet and poor eating habits? What is the most safe and effective way to lose weight? How do I initiate an exercise program? What is the best way to manage the stress in my life?"

David's first visit with the cardiologist started out with a general assessment of his health. Although he felt well, during the hospitalization David found out that he had mild hypertension and high cholesterol, both of which required medical therapy for adequate control. He was also told that he was overweight with a body mass index of 28 and was prediabetic with a fasting blood glucose of 110 mg/dL and a HbA1C of 6.2%. His blood pressure was controlled on medication, and his physical exam and ECG were unremarkable. David expressed his reluctance to take medications and asked if he could manage his heart condition with only diet and exercise. His cardiologist explained that the medications were essential to stabilizing his condition after the heart attack and preventing recurrent problems from developing in the future. In fact, research indicates that many of the medications David was taking can lower his risk of a recurrent heart event by 20% to 30%. That being said, however, his cardiologist went on to explain that medications can only do so much and that changing his lifestyle would be the only way to achieve and maintain health and vitality.

After a prolonged discussion, David and his cardiologist agreed to focus first on diet and nutrition. He was referred to a local dietitian, who sent him a primer on nutrition before his first visit, with copies of articles that had been extracted for those who wanted to delve more closely into nutrition.

THE DIET CONUNDRUM

David took on his nutrition packet as a homework assignment. He quickly became aware of how vast the topic of nutrition is and how much information is out there. In an age when dietary advice is dispensed through so many sources, it should be easy for patients to know what constitutes a good diet. However, the easy access to information is also often a hindrance: much contradictory information is often provided. For years, diet information was based on scant data or poorly designed nutritional studies. But over the last 15 to 20 years, a new evidence-based science of nutrition has emerged. In addition, an evidence-based set of principles have also emerged that help guide patients on the psychological barriers and approaches that can be used to implement a new diet.

WHY FOCUS ON NUTRITION?

At the beginning of his first session with the dietitian, she asked David why he was interested in meeting with her. David told her he had been frightened by his heart attack and wanted to do everything he could to improve his health. To reinforce the issue, the dietitian asked David what the potential health benefits of a good diet were. David answered that they included rising good cholesterol, decreasing bad cholesterol, preventing heart disease, and preventing obesity.

"Very good" responded the dietitian. "That is all correct. But the effects of diet on our physiology are actually even more extensive than that." She then showed him a diagram (**Figure 59.1**) that revealed the many ways in which the food we eat can affect our physiology. Besides the factors that David mentioned, these include effects upon our blood pressure, increase or decrease in systemic microinflammation, endothelial health of our blood vessels, and many other factors. She explained that people do not sufficiently realize that so much of what we can eat can affect our health either for the better or for the worse. Over time, the effects can be powerful. Intrigued, David asked her to explain more.

UNDERSTANDING THE BASICS OF NUTRITION

The dietitian then asked David if she could review with him some basic facts about nutrition. She understood that David did not have a science background, but there were a few central principles that she thought David and everyone should understand. She first discussed the concept of calories. She explained that our body requires a certain amount of energy each day to perform all of its basic functions—eating, working, playing, and even breathing. Energy for these basic activities is expressed in the form of "calories." She told David that in his case, on the basis of his age, height, and weight, he required about 2,000 calories per day in

order to maintain his weight. If he consumed more than this (ie, more energy than his body needs to perform his daily activities), this would place him in "positive energy balance" and he would gain weight. If he consumed less than this (ie, less energy than his body needs to perform his daily activities), he would be in "negative energy balance" and would begin to lose weight. She explained that food (in any form) represents energy (calories).

UNDERSTANDING THE MAJOR DIETARY COMPONENTS

She then introduced the topic of major dietary components, or what we term *macronutrients* and *micronutrients*. She explained that most people go straight to asking what diet or dietary pattern they should be on, but she felt understanding this first was essential.

There are three main macronutrients: fat, carbohydrate, and protein. The "typical" American diet is comprised of about 20% protein, 30% to 35% fat, and 45% to 50% carbohydrate. Of note, whereas the protein content of various diets remains relatively fixed, the fat and carbohydrate content can fluctuate greatly. In fact, it is the variation in fat and carbohydrate that often differentiates various popular diet patterns, as shown in **Table 59.1**. The dietitian then began to explain these macronutrients in more detail, beginning with fats.

DIETARY FATS

The dietitian explained that there are three basic types of fat, which can be distinguished biochemically, according to the number of carbon–carbon double bonds that are present in their chemical structure. Saturated fats have zero double bonds, monounsaturated fats have one double bond, and polyunsaturated fats have two or more double bonds. Polyunsaturated fats are broadly categorized as either omega-6 or omega-3 fatty acids. Another type of fat, trans fat, is formed by taking a polyunsaturated fat and converting it through a process called hydrogenation into hydrogenated fat.

All fats contain 9 calories of energy per gram of fat consumed. By comparison, carbohydrates and proteins contain only 4 calories of energy per gram. Thus, fat represents the most energy-dense form of food.

The dietitian then showed David a chart that contained examples of saturated, monounsaturated, and polyunsaturated fats (**Table 59.2**).

With this knowledge in hand, the dietitian then explained that on the basis of considerable scientific study, we now make a distinction between fats that are healthy, neutral, and

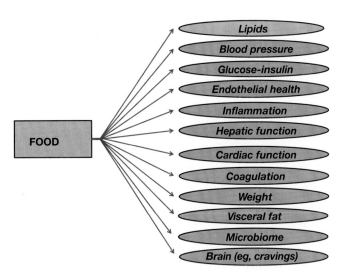

FIGURE 59.1 Illustration of how the food we eat impacts diverse bodily functions.

TABLE 59.1	Types of Diets		
	LOW-/VERY LOW–FAT DIETS (eg, ORNISH)	**MODERATE-FAT DIETS (eg, MEDITERRANEAN, DASH)**	**HIGH-FAT DIETS (eg, ATKINS)**
Fat	11%–19%	20%–40%	50%–55%
Carbohydrate	>65%	55%–60%	<25%
Protein	10%–20%	15%–20%	25%–30%

TABLE 59.2	Types of Fat	
SATURATED FATS	**MONOUNSATURATED FATS**	**POLYUNSATURATED FATS**
Palmitic (palm oil, meat)	Oleic and palmitoleic (nuts, olives, avocado)	**Omega-6** Linoleic (soybean, corn, and safflower oils)
Myristic (dairy foods)		Arachidonic (meats)
Lauric (coconut oil, palm kernel oil)		**Omega-3** Alpha linolenic (soybean and canola oils, nuts, and flaxseed)
Stearic (meat, cocoa butter)		DHA/EPA (fatty cold water fish—trout, herring, salmon, sardines)

unhealthy. The healthiest fats are polyunsaturated fats. Lipids have been most studied over the years for their effect on serum lipid values (low-density lipoprotein [LDL], high-density lipoprotein [HDL], and triglycerides), but the analysis of lipids is only one important effect of lipids. For example, not only do foods high in polyunsaturated fats lower LDL cholesterol and triglycerides and raise HDL, but they can also lead to improvement in blood pressure and endothelial function and reduce inflammatory biomarkers in the body. Monounsaturated fats also have beneficial effects on health. These fats have a neutral or even lowering effect upon total and LDL cholesterol, while having a lowering effect on triglycerides and a raising effect on HDL. At the other end of the spectrum are the trans fats, which are particularly atherogenic. Trans fats are known to raise total and LDL cholesterol as well as promote oxidation of lipids, a key step in atherosclerosis. These fats have strong and consistent associations with cardiovascular disease (CVD). Although recently banned by the Food and Drug Administration (FDA), trans fats have historically been present in packaged and processed foods including frozen pizza, pastries, deep-fried foods, and stick margarine.

After asking David if he had any further questions about fat, the dietitian then turned to the second major macronutrient: carbohydrates.

CARBOHYDRATES

Carbohydrates in their most basic form are sugars. Carbohydrates come in various forms ranging from simple sugars such as sucrose (table sugar), lactose (milk sugar), and fructose (fruit sugar), to more complex forms such as starch and fiber. As with fats, the quality of carbohydrates in one's diet is related to one's overall health. A complete understanding of what constitutes healthy carbohydrates centers around a variety of factors, including the glycemic response to digestion, the degree to which the carbohydrate is processed, and its fiber content.

The Glycemic Response to Digestion

The ease with which carbohydrates are broken down by the body into simple sugars often determines how it will affect blood sugar levels. For example, refined starches (eg, white bread, white rice, potatoes) can be quickly broken down to sugar, which can lead to spikes in blood sugar levels. Alternatively, unrefined carbohydrates rich in fiber (eg, whole-grain breads, brown/multigrain

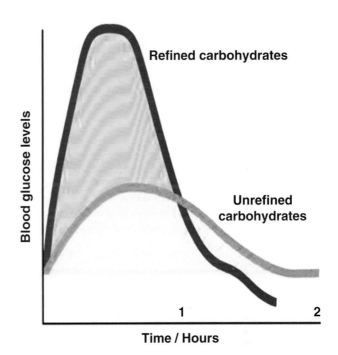

FIGURE 59.2 Impact of carbohydrate quality on blood glucose levels. Highly refined carbohydrates cause large spikes in blood glucose levels over a short period of time, often leading to periods of relative hypoglycemia. Unrefined carbohydrates, however, cause a slow and steady rise of blood glucose levels followed by a gradual decline to baseline. GI, glycemic index.

rice) take much longer to break down, thus leading to a slow and steady rise in blood sugar (**Figure 59.2**).

Among the dietary sugars, it is important to distinguish between those sugars consumed in their natural form, such as lactose or fructose, and those that are added to food during cooking, processing, or packaging. Sugars such as lactose and fructose, in moderation, can be a healthy part of one's diet. Milk contains not only lactose, but also protein, calcium, and vitamin D. Similarly, fruits contains not only fructose, but also important vitamins, minerals, and fiber. On the other hand, added sugars, which are sugars that are added to foods to enhance flavor (eg, pastries, candy, soda, fruit juice, or other sugary drinks), have been consistently linked to weight gain, diabetes, and even CVD.

The Degree to Which the Carbohydrate is Processed

Similar to the differences between added sugars and natural sugars, there are important differences in how grains are prepared for consumption. Although wheat is among the more popular types of grains, there are, in fact, many other types of grains (**Table 59.3**). In its most basic, natural form, a grain of wheat is composed of the bran, endosperm, and germ (**Figure 59.3**).

Diets containing excessive refined grains have been linked to diabetes, high triglycerides, metabolic syndrome, weight gain, and CVD.

When a food product contains whole-grain wheat, for example, it refers to the entire grain (bran, endosperm, and germ). Food products containing whole grains (unrefined grains) are always preferred because they contain fiber (bran), starch (endosperm), and vitamins, protein, and fat (germ). Unfortunately, over the years whole grains have undergone extensive processing to promote mass production and prolonged shelf life. During the refinement process, whole grains are often stripped of the fiber-rich bran, and sometimes the germ, bleached to achieve a more visually appealing white color, and enriched with artificial forms of fiber, vitamins, and minerals. These refined grains are very easily digested, often leading to spikes in blood sugar.

Fiber Content

Diets rich in fiber can help lower cholesterol, blood sugar, and blood pressure, while helping increase satiety. It is recommended that most individuals consume diets with at least 25 g of fiber per day. Unfortunately, the "typical" American diet falls quite short of this recommendation. Good sources of fiber include (but are not limited to) whole grains such as whole wheat, brown/multigrain rice and quinoa, vegetables, fruit with the skin, nuts, and legumes.

In summary, although there is no single parameter that best characterizes carbohydrate content, attempting to minimize refined grains, added sugars, and starchy foods, such as russet or white potatoes, is highly recommended. Each of these foods produces a sharp rise in blood glucose and insulin, leading to multiple adverse effects, including a craving for more food.

Another useful index of carbohydrate quality is the total carbohydrate-to-fiber ratio (gram/serving). The lower the ratio, the healthier the carbohydrate. Generally, a ratio of <10:1 is preferable. **Figure 59.4** illustrates the important differences in fiber content (and the carbohydrate-to-fiber ratio) between two similar honey-flavored cereals.

PROTEIN

Protein is an essential component of our diets, required for normal growth, development, and metabolism. In broad terms, protein can originate from either plant or animal sources, as shown in **Table 59.4**. Although animal meat is a good source of protein, important differences in health outcomes exist. For example, poultry has a relatively health-neutral effect, whereas processed meats are consistently associated with negative cardiovascular outcomes. Unprocessed red meat, however, is more controversial. Some studies have found similar health-damaging effects as processed meat (albeit less damaging), whereas other studies have found relatively neutral effects.

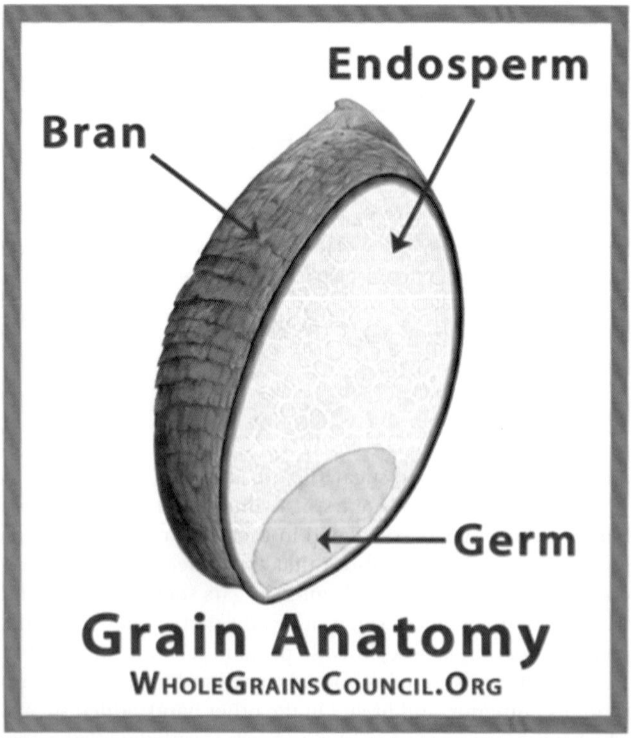

MINOR DIETARY COMPONENTS: MICRONUTRIENTS

After this discussion, David felt like he had a basic understanding of macronutrients. He then asked, "What about things like salt, vitamins, and minerals, and where do they fit in?" To save time, the dietitian focused only on a few key points in response to David's question. She stated that vitamins, minerals, and trace elements are considered minor dietary elements (ie, micronutrients), which are essential components of any diet, but present in small quantities. Among them, sodium is a mineral of considerable importance because it is required for normal cellular function throughout the body. Abundant in the food supply, sodium is found mainly in the form of sodium chloride (salt). According to national surveys, the average American consumes about 3,400 mg of sodium each day. By contrast, the American Heart Association recommends consuming 1,500 mg of sodium each day. Although most people think of salt as a seasoning, which is sprinkled on to foods after cooking to enhance flavor, by far the more common source of salt is in prepacked and processed foods, as well as fast food and chain restaurant foods. Although there is some controversy in the medical literature as to whether or not too much dietary salt can cause high blood pressure, there is universal agreement that the typical American diet contains excessive salt. Among individuals with high blood pressure, or other cardiac conditions, excessive dietary salt can lead to elevations in blood pressure, retention of water, and even congestive heart failure.

FIGURE 59.3 Anatomy of a grain with an outer coating of bran, a middle endosperm, and the germ at the core.

Nutrition Facts

Serving Size 3/4 Cup (32g)

Amount Per Serving

Calories 120   Calories from Fat 15

% **Daily Value***

Total Fat 1.5g	**2%**
Saturated Fat 0g	**0%**
Trans Fat 0g	
Polyunsaturated Fat 0.5g	
Monounsaturated Fat 0.5g	
Cholesterol 0mg	**0%**
Sodium 85mg	**4%**
Potassium 90mg	**3%**
Total Carbohydrate 26g	**9%**
Dietary Fiber 4g	**15%**
Soluble Fiber less than 1g	
Insoluble Fiber 3g	
Sugars 5g	
Protein 3g	

Vitamin A 0%	•	Vitamin C 0%
Calcium 0%	•	Iron 4%

* Percent Daily Values are based on a 2,000 calorie diet. Your daily values may be higher or lower depending on your calorie needs:

		Calories	2,000	2,500
Total Fat	Less than		65g	80g
Sat. Fat	Less than		20g	25g
Cholesterol	Less than		300mg	300mg
Sodium	Less than		2,400mg	2,400mg
Potassium			3,500mg	3,500mg
Total Carbohydrate			300g	375g
Dietary Fiber			25g	30g

Nutrition Facts

Serving Size: 3/4 cup (28g)

Amount Per Serving

Calories 110   Calories from Fat 14

% **Daily Value***

Total Fat 1.5 g	**2%**
Saturated Fat 0 g	**0%**
Trans Fat 0 g	
Cholesterol 0 mg	**0%**
Sodium 190.12 mg	**8%**
Potassium 115.08 mg	**3%**
Total Carbohydrate 21.65 g	**7%**
Dietary Fiber 1.99 g	**8%**
Sugars 9 g	
Sugar Alcohols	
Protein 3 g	
Vitamin A 500.08 IU	10%
Vitamin C 5.99 mg	10%
Calcium 99.96 mg	10%
Iron 4.5 mg	25%

FIGURE 59.4 Nutrition fact sheets for two different brands of honey-flavored cereal. Although very similar products, note the differences in carbohydrate quality as demonstrated by the varying fiber content and the total carbohydrate-to-fiber ratio.

TABLE 59.3	Examples of Whole Grains
Barley	Quinoa
Buckwheat	Rye
Corn	Spelt
Farro	Wheat
Millet	Wild rice
Oats	

TABLE 59.4	Sources of Protein	
PLANT SOURCES	**ANIMAL**	
Nuts	Meat (eg, beef, poultry, pork)	
Whole grains	Dairy (eg, cheese, milk, yogurt)	
Legumes	Fish	
	Eggs	

Besides her comments on salt, the dietitian raised the issue of supplements. These represent a broad category of substances that are taken to enhance one's usual dietary intake and promote health and wellness. Examples include vitamins, minerals, trace elements, herbs, and other substances. In general, it is always better to consume vitamins, minerals, and trace elements as a part of a healthy balanced diet, rather than supplements. Should additional supplementation be necessary for medical reasons, a health care professional should be consulted. If one is interested in taking supplements to promote health and wellness, it is still useful to consult with a health care professional first to ensure it is appropriate and will not interact with other medications.

A HISTORIC CHANGE IN OUR UNDERSTANDING OF NUTRITION

After completing their session, the dietitian told David to review his notes before the next session and come back with any questions. She said she would ask him to summarize his understanding at the beginning of the next session. When they next met, David remarked that not only he, but also his family and friends had presumed that too much fat was not good. In fact, many of his friends were currently on a high-carbohydrate/low-fat diet. Why were the recommendations so different now?

The dietitian explained. In the 1940s and 1950s, researchers working with the Framingham Heart Study discovered an association between various health conditions and heart disease. Among these "risk factors" were conditions such as high blood pressure, smoking, and high blood cholesterol. Later in the 1960s, work by Drs. Keys and Hegsted established a link between dietary saturated fat and high blood cholesterol. Subsequent to this, there were a number of large-population studies that confirmed the relationship between dietary saturated fat, high blood cholesterol, and heart disease–related events. It was this groundbreaking series of work that led to large-population–level public health campaigns against diets high in total and saturated fat.

Over the next 30 to 40 years, dietary fat became a major target for the primary and secondary prevention of CVD. In response to public and private sector efforts to promote lower-fat diets, the U.S. population effectively lowered its consumption of total and saturated fat. The lower U.S. consumption of fat was balanced by an increased consumption of carbohydrates (**Figure 59.5**). Over the same general period that the U.S. population was lowering their consumption of saturated fat and increasing their consumption of carbohydrates, epidemiologic studies indicated a rising prevalence of obesity (**Figure 59.6**) and diabetes mellitus. Further examination of these trends revealed a higher consumption of refined grains and lower consumption of fiber (**Figure 59.7**).

Thus, in our efforts to lower our collective risk of heart disease by reducing our intake of dietary saturated fat, we increased our consumption of highly processed, refined (poor-quality) grains, with the net effect of higher rates of obesity, diabetes mellitus, and the metabolic syndrome.

Subsequently, more authoritative studies revealed that there was no significant association between saturated fat and important health outcomes.[1] In related work,[2] investigators examined not only the CV effects of a reduced saturated fat diet, but also what macronutrient was being substituted for the fat. This was amplified by a study examining over 120,000 patients over 24 years, in which CVD risk was assessed according to the macronutrient that was being substituted for dietary fat.[3] The studies were concordant for observing the following:

- When dietary saturated fat was replaced with refined grains, CVD risk either remained similar to or was increased compared with that of saturated fat.
- If dietary saturated fat was replaced with whole grains or high-quality fats (ie, polyunsaturated fat), CVD risk was reduced.

Thus, simply reducing the saturated fat content of our diets is not sufficient, the dietitian said. Rather, we must replace this fat with higher quality fats and/or higher quality carbohydrates to effectively reduce our risk of CVD.

At this point, the dietitian introduced a diagram summarizing what she had covered with David (**Figure 59.8**). Foods can be categorized as healthy to unhealthy on the basis of hard scientific evidence finding consumption of individual foods to cause heart disease, diabetes, stroke, and other adverse outcomes. The healthiest foods include fruits, vegetables, whole grains, and legumes. The unhealthiest foods include processed meat, refined grains, and added sugars. The neutral zone foods are to be consumed in moderation. These include milk, cheese, eggs, poultry, butter, and red meat (unprocessed).

FOCUSING ON DIETARY PATTERNS RATHER THAN SPECIFIC NUTRIENTS

At this point, the dietitian felt ready to establish a specific diet plan with David. She had just covered with him what foods are known to increase and decrease health risk. However, her training had taught her that most individuals follow a dietary pattern rather than focusing on any particular food group. She now decided to broach this subject with David.

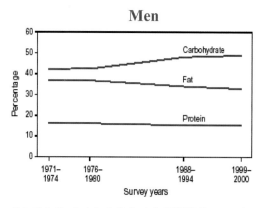
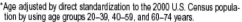
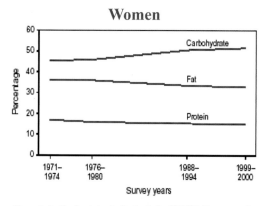

FIGURE 59.5 Survey data illustrating how the average fat content of the U.S. population declined over time, however, at the expense of a greater proportion of carbohydrates.

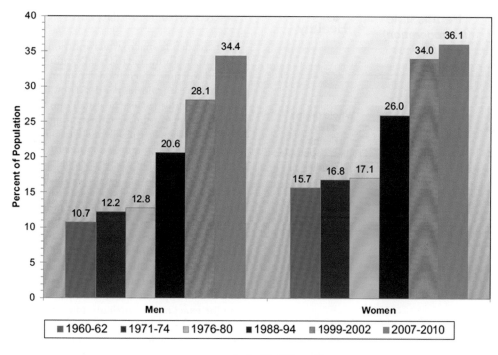

Adult Obesity

FIGURE 59.6 Survey data illustrating how the U.S. population has become more obese over time.

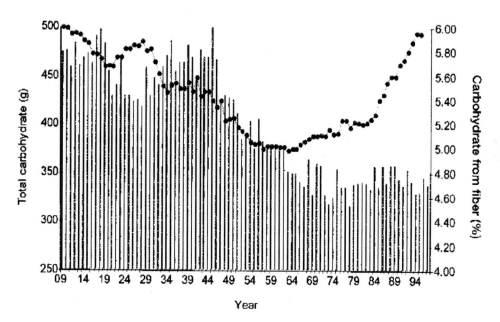

FIGURE 59.7 Survey data illustrating how the carbohydrate quality of the U.S. diet has changed over time. Although carbohydrate consumption was high in the early 1900s, most of it was high-quality carbohydrates rich in fiber. From the 1960s to 1990s, carbohydrate consumption was on the rise, but fiber consumption remained low, indicating that Americans were consuming poorer quality carbohydrates.

She explained to David that the study of what constitutes healthy diet patterns has been an important breakthrough in nutritional science. Important insights have come from the use of food questionnaires, which inquire about the frequency and quantity of different foods (anywhere from 50 to 150 different foods) consumed over the prior week to month. Using a statistical method called principal components analysis, investigators

have been able to ascertain which foods are consumed in high versus low quantities by a given population of subjects. This then allows for different dietary patterns that can be extrapolated and correlated with various clinical outcomes (eg, biomarkers, CVD, mortality).

The consistent finding from these epidemiologic cohort studies is that diets rich in fruits, vegetables, whole grains, legumes, high

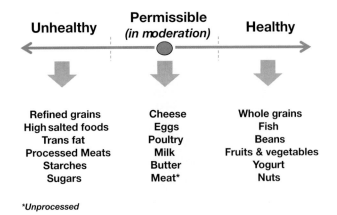

FIGURE 59.8 Illustration of how the food we eat lies along a spectrum from unhealthy to healthy. Dietary intake should be focused on those foods at the far right, with moderate consumption of foods in the middle and little consumption of foods at the far left.

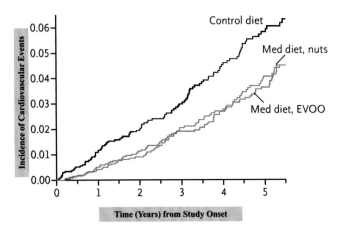

FIGURE 59.9 The PREDIMED study was a landmark clinical trial that demonstrated how consuming a Mediterranean diet (Med diet + nuts or Med diet with extra-virgin olive oil) was associated with a significant reduction in cardiovascular events relative to a low-fat diet. EVOO, extra virgin olive oil.

fiber, fish, lean meats, moderate alcohol, and low-fat dairy are consistently associated with a reduced risk for CVD.

Conversely, diets high in red and processed meat, refined grains, processed foods, soda, and other added sugars are associated with an increased risk for CVD.

Further study revealed that the "heart healthy" dietary pattern previously noted is most consistent with the diet consumed in most parts of the Mediterranean region—hence the term *Mediterranean diet.*

Importantly, a number of studies have since confirmed the beneficial effects of a Mediterranean-style diet, including a lower risk of heart disease, diabetes, cancer, and all-cause mortality.[4–6] **Figure 59.9** is an example of one of the landmark studies showing the reduction in cardiovascular events with a Mediterranean diet. As a result of this consistent body of literature, the FDA now recommends a similar (Mediterranean-style) diet pattern in the 2015 Dietary Guidelines for Americans.[7] It is important to remember, however, that these recommendations are only a guide, the foundation of which can be applied to individual tastes as well as cultural, ethnic, and religious preferences.

EATING AND SHOPPING HABITS

After discussing macro/micronutrients and diet patterns, the dietitian briefly turned to David's eating habits. In particular, she wanted to know which foods he liked and disliked, how much he liked to eat (calories per day), how he usually ate (distracted, mindless eating), where he usually ate (in front of the television or computer), why he ate (stress eating, social eating, food addictions), and when he typically ate (late-night meals, skipping meals). Furthermore, she inquired about participation in food shopping and meal preparation. Each one of these factors plays a crucial role in shaping one's dietary habits. On the basis of David's responses, she recommended that David take on a Mediterranean-style diet, focusing on foods that are rich in mono- and polyunsaturated fats, high-quality carbohydrates rich in fiber (found in whole grains), lean sources of protein (eg, fish, poultry), nuts, low-fat dairy, fruits, vegetables, legumes, and olive oil.

In conjunction with this recommendation, the dietitian wanted to make sure that David was sufficiently savvy in reading food labels. She explained that almost all foods have labels outlining the exact macronutrients, micronutrients, and ingredients they contain and that he could use this information to make more informed decisions about his food purchases. Much like reading a menu at a restaurant, it is important to read food labels to gain a deeper understanding of what is in the food (ie, key ingredients) and the nutritional value of the food. Some time ago, the FDA required labeling of all food products sold in stores and many chain restaurants. This has allowed consumers to become more aware of the nutritional value of individual foods, compare foods within similar categories, and make more informed decisions. Two examples of a nutrition fact sheet are shown in Figure 59.4. Although both foods are honey-flavored cereals, there are important differences in the nutritional content.

Of similar importance to reading nutrition fact sheets is reading ingredient lists for foods. Gaining a deeper understanding of the actual ingredients that make up the food is a necessary step to making better food choices. In most instances, the ingredient in highest proportion appears first, with the remaining ingredients in descending order of proportion. Examples of two ingredient lists are shown in **Figure 59.10**. Although both products are bread, important differences exist.

The dietitian suggested that David go food shopping this coming week, analyze food labels, and come into their next scheduled session with any questions that he experienced while reviewing the labels. David was very excited by the idea.

At their next session, David and the dietitian reviewed his success in following his new Mediterranean-style diet, his trip to the grocery store, and his questions about food labels. David was pleased that he was now able to incorporate foods into his diet, such as eggs and cheese, that he had previously thought he had to avoid as a heart patient.

The dietitian concluded by imparting some additional advice on the basis of her previous screening of David's eating habits. Her suggestions included eating smaller, more frequent meals during the day, avoiding late-night meals or meal skipping, as well as adopting healthy mealtime habits—for example, eating to satiety and nondistracted, mindful eating. David thanked the dietitian for her counsel and left enthused with his newly acquired knowledge base and commitment to eating according to a healthy dietary plan.

Whole Wheat Flour, **Unbleached Enriched Wheat Flour** (Flour, Malted Barley Flour, Reduced Iron, Niacin, Thiamin Mononitrate [Vitamin B_1], Riboflavin [Vitamin B_2], Folic Acid), Water, Sugar, Sunflower Seeds, Wheat Gluten, Wheat, Rye, Cellulose Fiber, Oats, Yeast, Soybean Oil, Ground Corn, Salt, Molasses, Buckwheat, Brown Rice, Calcium Propionate (Preservative), Monoglycerides, Triticale, Barley, Flaxseed, Millet, Calcium Sulfate, Datem, Grain Vinegar, Calcium Carbonate, Citric Acid, Soy Lecithin, Nuts (Walnuts and/or Hazelnuts and/or Almonds), Whey, Soy Flour, Nonfat Milk.

Whole Wheat Flour, Water, **High Fructose Corn Syrup**, Wheat Gluten, Sugar, Yeast, Contains 2% or less of each of the following: Soybean Oil, Calcium Sulfate, Salt, Dough Conditioners (May Contain One or More of the Following: Mono- and Diglycerides, Ethoxylated Mono- and Diglycerides, Sodium Stearoyl Lactylate, Calcium Peroxide, Datem, Ascorbic Acid, Azodicarbonamide, Enzymes), Wheat Bran, Guar Gum, Distilled Vinegar, Calcium Propionate (Preservative), Yeast Nutrients (Monocalcium Phosphate, Calcium Phosphate, Ammonium Phosphate), Corn Starch, Vitamin D3, Soy Lecithin, Milk, Soy Flour.

FIGURE 59.10 Examples of ingredient lists from two types of commercial breads. Although the products appear similar, important differences in wheat quality and sugar exist.

WEIGHT LOSS AND WEIGHT MANAGEMENT

David had a follow-up visit with his cardiologist 2 weeks later. At this point, David was maintaining his new diet, but he had not lost any weight. The cardiologist had not set weight loss as an initial goal because he first wanted David to get on a healthy diet plan. He now explained to David that while specific foods and diet patterns have been shown to favorably impact blood pressure, cholesterol, and blood glucose levels, modest weight loss has also been associated with favorable changes in these risk factors. For example, he explains, in the Look AHEAD (Action for Health in Diabetes) study that involved over 5,000 men and women with a mean baseline weight of 100 ± 19 kg, weight loss of 5% to 10% was associated with significant improvements in blood glucose, blood pressure, high-density cholesterol (HDL), and triglyceride levels at 1 year.[8] Encouraged by this research, David asked for specific suggestions to modify his diet program to achieve weight loss. Although he was encouraged to follow up with the dietitian for more specifics, he was offered the following explanation by his physician.

A number of diet strategies exist to facilitate weight loss and weight maintenance, including fad diets (eg, Paleo), commercial weight-loss programs (eg, Weight Watchers), variable macronutrient composition diets (eg, low-fat diets), and dietary patterns (eg, Mediterranean diet). Although considerable public opinion exists as to which diet strategy is superior for achieving and maintaining weight loss, research suggests that calorie restriction is the common underlying mechanism responsible for the success of these diet programs rather than any particular food, macronutrient, or diet pattern. In a landmark study by Williamson et al., 811 overweight adults were randomized to one of four diet plans varying in macronutrient composition.[9] On 2-year follow-up, there was no significant difference in achieved weight loss among the different macronutrient composition diets. Participants in all four diet programs achieved similar weight loss, which averaged 4 kg at 2 years. Of note, successful weight loss was also associated with greater participation in group counseling sessions.

His cardiologist emphasized that a gradual reduction in weight should be sought, with a goal of losing 2 to 4 pounds per month. To this end, he suggested that David attempt to reduce his daily caloric intake by about 250 to 500 calories per day, if possible. Both agreed that he should see the dietitian for further follow-up

concerning his weight-loss goals. His physician also recommended that David begin an exercise program, both for overall health promotion and for facilitating his pursuit of successful weight loss and maintenance of weight loss. This program is the subject of the next chapter.

CONCLUSION

Reflecting on his journey over the past few months, David admits to undergoing a significant transformation. What started out as years of denial and misinformation has now evolved to a deep understanding of health and wellness. He has committed not only to obtaining the necessary information to make informed decisions about his health, but also to the process of lifestyle modification as it relates to diet, nutrition, and successful weight loss. David notes that his sense of self-esteem and vitality have both increased since he started his diet. While his initial heart attack was frightening to him, he now realizes that this event was a blessing in disguise. David now feels far more energetic than he did before his heart attack, as well as knowing that he is on a path to better health.

WHAT PATIENTS AND FAMILY NEED TO KNOW

1. Learn to become an educated consumer of food.
   - Read food labels and nutrition fact sheets on food products.
   - Participate in food shopping and meal preparation to promote healthier eating.
   - Consider taking a healthy cooking class or subscribing to healthy eating magazines.

2. If you are overweight or obese, or have known or suspected heart disease, consider consulting with a dietitian to gain a deeper understanding of your dietary habits and how to make healthier choices to promote better health.

3. Consider adopting a Mediterranean-style diet as this type of dietary pattern has been consistently shown to be associated with a reduced risk of heart disease, diabetes, and cancer and improved longevity.

4. Foods with saturated fats can be eaten in moderation.

5. Sugars, refined grains, processed meats, and high-sodium foods should be avoided because of their harmful health effects.

6. As discussed later in the chapter on exercise, regular physical activity is an important part of lifestyle modification for high blood pressure, high blood cholesterol, and high blood sugar, as well as effective weight loss and weight maintenance.

REFERENCES

1. Siri-Tarino PW, Sun Q, Hu FB, Krauss RM. Meta-analysis of prospective cohort studies evaluating the association of saturated fat with cardiovascular disease. *Am J Clin Nutr.* 2010;91:535-546.

2. Jakobsen MU, Dethlefsen C, Joensen AM, et al. Intake of carbohydrates compared with intake of saturated fatty acids and risk of myocardial infarction: importance of the glycemic index. *Am J Clin Nutr.* 2010;91:1764-1768.

3. Li Y, Hruby A, Bernstein AM, et al. Saturated fats compared with unsaturated fats and sources of carbohydrates in relation to risk of coronary heart disease: a prospective cohort study. *J Am Coll Cardiol.* 2015;66:1538-1548.

4. Trichopoulou A, Costacou T, Bamia C, Trichopoulos D. Adherence to a Mediterranean diet and survival in a Greek population. *N Engl J Med.* 2003;348:2599-2608.

5. Estruch R, Ros E, Salas-Salvado J, et al. Primary prevention of cardiovascular disease with a Mediterranean diet. *N Engl J Med.* 2013;368:1279-1290.

6. Salas-Salvado J, Bullo M, Babio N, et al. Reduction in the incidence of type 2 diabetes with the Mediterranean diet. Results of the PREDIMED-Reus nutrition intervention randomized trial. *Diabetes Care.* 2011;34:14-19.

7. U.S. Department of Health and Human Services and U.S. Department of Agriculture. 2015-2020 Dietary Guidelines for Americans. 8th edition. December 2015.

8. Wing RR, Lang W, Wadden TA, et al. Benefits of modest weight loss in improving cardiovascular risk factors in overweight and obese individuals with type 2 diabetes. *Diabetes Care.* 2011;34:1481-1486.

9. Sacks FM, Bray GA, Carey VJ, et al. Comparison of weight-loss diets with different compositions of fat, protein, and carbohydrates. *N Engl J Med.* 2009;360:859-873.

Randy Cohen
Alan Rozanski

60

Exercise and Physical Activity in Cardiac Patients

Six months after the initial hospitalization for a heart attack, David visited his cardiologist for a routine follow-up visit. David had not experienced any chest pain since his initial event, and reported success in maintaining a Mediterranean-style diet after his visits to a dietician. This had resulted in a nearly 10-pound weight loss, which David was proud of. All of David's laboratory work and his blood pressure, on medications, were now within normal limits. However, David had not taken up his physician's request to initiate an exercise program, citing the heavy workload at his job.

David's cardiologist, however, had gotten to know David well by now and felt that he was ready to add exercise to his routine. He suspected that David was not yet sufficiently motivated to start exercising because he did not realize the medical importance of being physically active. Further, David could probably benefit from formal instruction and supervision as to how to exercise. The cardiologist's institution offered two options for patients like David. One was a formal cardiac rehabilitation program that people like David could join. The other was a hybrid gym-based program, which involved initial supervision by a physical therapist who worked with their Rehabilitation unit. The Rehab facility offered an introductory lecture given by a physiatrist that met monthly. The next lecture was taking place in a few days. David's cardiologist suggested that David attend this introductory lecture and then either call him or make an appointment for a follow-up visit a week afterward. David was more than eager to do so.

At the start of the lecture, the physiatrist asked each participant to write down on a piece of paper their daily work and physical activity routine, with as much detail as possible. David wrote that he did not currently engage in any planned physical activity. Although he had tried to engage in regular physical activity at various points over his life, he always seemed to find excuses not to go to the gym. In fact, David wrote, he found himself becoming increasingly sedentary with each passing year. David described his daily routine as one characterized by a great deal of sitting time with long periods of inactivity. Specifically, David spent an hour commuting to work each day, then worked at a desk job, sitting at his computer for most of the time during his 8 to 10 hour workday, and then commuting another hour back home. Once at home, David sat to eat dinner with his family and then either worked

further using his home computer or relaxed, watching TV with his wife and children. As he wrote this down, David was surprised to realize just how much time he sat during the day. He decided he was going to pay keen attention to the lecture.

THE BIRTH OF EXERCISE EPIDEMIOLOGY

The physiatrist first remarked that the modern study of exercise was spurred, in part, by a landmark study conducted by Morris and colleagues in the 1950s.[1] In a classic study, these investigators followed drivers and conductors of double-decker buses among London's Transport Workers, comparing bus drivers (sedentary occupation) with conductors (active occupation). The bus drivers had a classically sedentary job, whereas the conductors were constantly standing, going between the first and second levels of the bus. During the follow-up period, the conductors were observed to have a significantly lower incidence of cardiac events. In subsequent work, these investigators also followed sedentary clerical workers versus postmen in the British civil service. Again, the more active group (ie, the postmen) developed less heart disease during follow-up.

Many subsequent epidemiologic studies have shown how important leisure-time physical activity is. For instance, in 1986 Paffenbarger et al. published their findings on the assessment of leisure-time physical activity levels in over 16,000 Harvard alumni who had been followed for 16 years (**Figure 60.1**).[2] As a result of the groundbreaking work by Morris, and those who followed, the field of exercise science was born.

ASSESSING EXERCISE ABILITY IN THE STRESS LABORATORY

The physiatrist then noted that at first, cardiologists had no formal ability to quantify an individual's exercise capacity in their offices. The first formalized approach was developed by Dr. Arthur Masters in the 1920s. His initial approach involved having patients step up and down two steps as fast as they could for 90 seconds (later extended to 3 minutes). The longer it took,

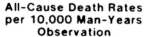

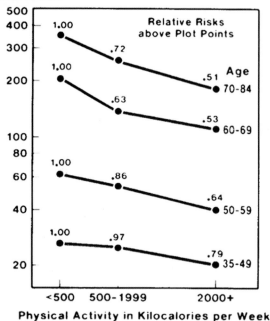

All-Cause Death Rates
per 10,000 Man-Years
Observation

FIGURE 60.1 Decline in all-cause mortality with increasing physical activity, stratified by age groups.

the greater was the patient's risk of heart disease. Initially, this task was performed without electrocardiographic monitoring, but as this technology developed, postexercise ECG and then, eventually, ECG monitoring both during and following exercise were added to the evolving stress test.

A major advance was the development of the motorized treadmill, which allowed the performance of progressively higher levels of exercise while patients were electrocardiographically monitored. In 1963, Dr. Robert Bruce validated what has subsequently been called the Bruce protocol: a progressive graded exercise test, increased by two degrees of incline and by increasing speed during each 3 minutes of exercise.[3] Today, the Bruce treadmill exercise protocol is still the standard for performing exercise ECG testing in cardiac practice.

Exercise electrocardiography permits the assessment of ischemia (how much ST-segment deviation is elicited during exercise), patients' clinical response to exercise (ie, whether chest pain was elicited during stress testing), and the assessment of patients' overall exercise functional capacity (eg, how many minutes patients were able to exercise). Hundreds of outcome studies have shown that all three of these parameters are prognostically useful, but the most potent parameter is patients' functional exercise capacity. For example, Myers et al. followed 6,213 individuals for 6.2 years after exercise ECG testing, including a group with and without known cardiovascular disease (CVD).[4] In both groups, after adjusting for age, the mean exercise capacity, measured in metabolic equivalents (METs), was the strongest predictor of outcome. For each 1-MET increase in exercise capacity, there was a 12% improvement in survival.

In another particularly large study, Gupta et al. reported on the follow-up of 66,371 individuals without preexisting heart disease who underwent exercise ECG testing as part of the

Cooper Center Longitudinal Study between 1970 and 2006. All subjects were followed for CVD mortality.[5] The presence of traditional risk factors, such as hypertension, diabetes, and smoking, was associated with an increased risk of CVD events during follow-up (**Figure 60.2**). However, consideration of exercise capacity was quite important. After adjusting for the presence of these risk factors, each quintile of increasing exercise fitness was associated with a progressively greater decrease in the risk of CVD mortality.

THE PHYSIOLOGIC BENEFITS OF EXERCISE

The physiatrist then turned his attention to the principal mechanisms by which physical activity and exercise promote better health. The beneficial physiologic effects are shown in **Table 60.1**. Among these is a favorable reduction in blood pressure. Although acute bouts of exercise cause transient elevations in heart rate and blood pressure, the hours immediately following exercise are characterized by consistently lower systolic and diastolic blood pressure readings and a lower pulse. In a review of 14 studies by Thompson et al., the mean change in systolic and diastolic blood pressure after acute dynamic exercise was −2.1 mm Hg and −0.3 mm Hg, respectively.[6] In contrast, regular physical activity and cardiorespiratory fitness have been consistently associated with −3.4 to −10.5 mm Hg and −2.4 to −7.6 mm Hg reductions in systolic and diastolic blood pressure, respectively.[7] Although these reductions in blood pressure may not seem clinically important, epidemiologic data inform us that a 2-mm Hg reduction in systolic and diastolic blood pressure translate into a 14% and 17% reduction in stroke, and a 9% and 6% reduction in coronary artery disease.[8]

Another favorable effect of exercise is its influence on serum lipids, including a rise in serum high-density lipoprotein (HDL) cholesterol, and reduction in serum triglycerides. But extensive research has shown that even chronic, high-intensity aerobic exercise leads to only modest improvements in total and low-density lipoprotein (LDL) cholesterol. Thus, exercise is not a primary tool used to lower serum LDL cholesterol.

Exercise has many other effects, including an enhancement in glucose metabolism and insulin sensitivity; decrease in negative inflammatory markers; better autonomic function (ie, increased vagal tone); increased endurance and muscle strength; and greater bone strength and joint health.

In addition, exercise helps promote better vascular health through a number of mechanisms. Vascular function, which is a measure of how well the arteries expand and contract in response to every heartbeat, is known to be significantly better among individuals with versus without cardiorespiratory fitness. The mechanism behind improved vascular function is thought to be related to exercise-induced reduction in oxidative stress and chronic inflammation, as well as enhanced production of nitric oxide, a potent vasodilator. In addition, exercise promotes favorable vascular remodeling, including enlargement of the coronary vessels, and it improves the endothelial function of blood vessels, thus making them less susceptible to negative pathophysiologic changes, such as the buildup of plaque.

Regular physical activity is also an important component of weight loss as well as the prevention of weight gain after successful weight loss. Even among obese individuals unable to successfully achieve meaningful weight loss, regular physical activity and

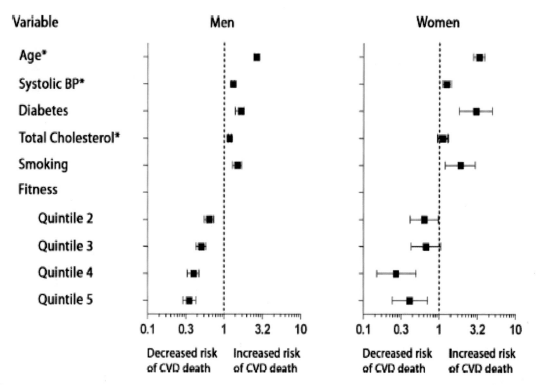

FIGURE 60.2 Lower risk of cardiovascular death (CVD) with increasing quintiles of cardiorespiratory fitness. Even in the lowest quintile (Q2) of fitness, there is a reduced risk of cardiovascular death.

*Hazard ratios are per 1 SD (per 10 years for age, per 14 mm Hg for systolic blood pressure and per 40 mg/dL for total cholesterol).

TABLE 60.1	Beneficial Physiologic Effects of Exercise

- Reduced blood pressure
- Increases serum high-density lipoprotein level; minimal lowering of serum low-density lipoprotein levels
- Lowering of triglyceride levels
- Improved glucose metabolism
- Increased insulin sensitivity
- Decrease in inflammatory markers
- Improved autonomic function
- Enhanced endurance and muscle strength
- Promotes bone and joint health
- Promotes positive vascular remodeling
- Improves endothelial function
- Aids weight management
- Promotes cognitive function and reduces dementia risk
- Promotes better moods

cardiorespiratory fitness are important goals to achieve. As shown by Barry et al. in a meta-analysis of 10 studies, all-cause mortality rates were similar among those individuals demonstrating cardiorespiratory fitness, regardless of their body mass index (normal weight or obese).[9]

Finally, exercise has important psychological benefits. Exercise can help reduce feelings of stress, anxiety, and depression. In fact, randomized controlled studies have found exercise to be comparable to antidepressant medications for reducing depression symptoms in those studies.[10]

THE RELATIONSHIP BETWEEN PHYSICAL ACTIVITY AND CHRONIC DISEASE

After reviewing the physiologic benefits of exercise, the physiatrist reviewed the particular benefits of exercise with respect to disease prevention. He pointed out that given the diverse benefits of regular physical activity on various bodily functions (eg, cardiovascular, metabolic, bone health) that he had just discussed, it is not surprising that physical activity has been found to significantly reduce the risk of many chronic diseases. For example, in a large prospective cohort study, Wen et al. assessed leisure-time physical activity in over 400,000 individuals and then followed them for an average of 8 years.[11] Relative to the inactive group, those in the low, medium, high, or very high activity levels had significant reductions in all-cause as well as cancer- and cardiovascular-related mortality (**Figure 60.3**). Of note, even among those able to engage in only 15 minutes of leisure-time physical activity per day, a 14% reduction in all-cause mortality and a 3-year longer life expectancy was observed. In related work, Blair and colleagues examined how changes in fitness over time impacted mortality.[12] As expected, those who were found to be fit by treadmill testing at both baseline and follow-up visits had the lowest all-cause and cardiovascular mortality. However, among those who improved their fitness level (unfit at baseline → fit on follow-up), a 44% reduction in mortality was observed. This association was maintained even after correcting for age, health status, and other factors associated with premature mortality. These findings underscore the importance of establishing a regular physical activity program, even if one is not healthy or fit at baseline.

In related work, Moore et al. examined the association between leisure-time physical activity and 26 different types of cancer in over 1.4 million subjects.[13] After 15+ years of follow-up, regular

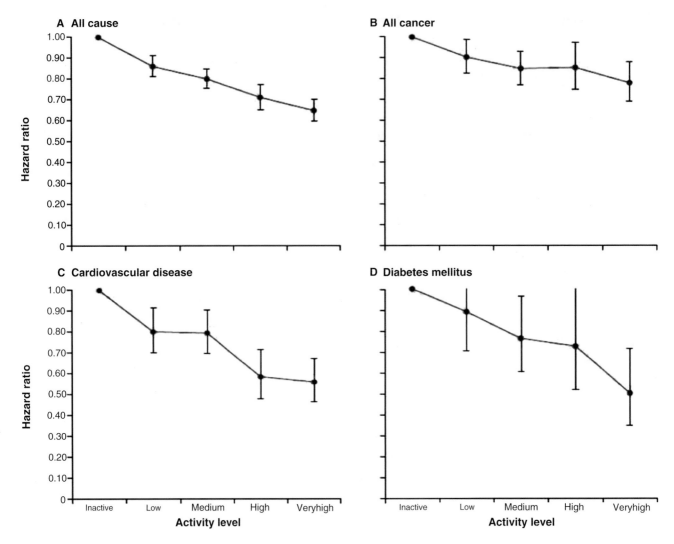

FIGURE 60.3 Decline in all-cause mortality, cancer, cardiovascular disease, and diabetes with increasing levels of leisure-time physical activity.

leisure-time physical activity was associated with substantial reductions in many cancers, including lung, kidney, endometrial, colon, rectal, myeloid leukemia, and bladder.

Regular physical activity, as well as physical activity that is part of a comprehensive lifestyle modification program, has also been shown to substantially reduce the risk of developing diabetes mellitus. In a review of 10 studies involving over 300,000 participants, brisk walking (≥2.5 hours/week) was associated with a 30% reduction in new onset diabetes mellitus.[14] In the landmark Diabetes Prevention Program trial, involving over 3,000 patients, regular physical activity along with healthy eating and modest weight loss reduced the incidence of diabetes mellitus by 58%.[15]

Another beneficial effect of exercise is its role in maintaining bone health and muscle strength during the aging process. For instance, regular physical activity has been shown to be of critical importance in preventing osteoporosis and frailty. In a review by Hendricks et al., regular exercise reduced the risk of developing osteoporosis and subsequent injuries by promoting bone strength as well as strengthening muscle groups that contribute to balance, coordination, and gait stability.[16] In recent years, frailty

has emerged as an important threat to successful aging and has been associated with a number of poor health outcomes.[17,18] Specifically, frailty is defined as a clinical syndrome involving any three of the following characteristics: unintentional weight loss, low physical activity, weakness, fatigue or exercise intolerance, and slowed motor performance.[19] In a recent review by de Labra et al., exercise was found to be an effective intervention for older adults exhibiting signs of frailty, although the exact type and duration of exercise remain unclear.[20]

Another important and exciting area of exercise science relates to cognitive function. In a recent review by Bherer et al., regular physical activity was shown to have a significant and positive impact on cognitive function among a variety of individuals, ranging from asymptomatic elderly adults to those with established cognitive impairment.[21] In related work, Erickson and colleagues concluded that physical activity can induce important, dynamic changes in cognitive function that can slow or delay the onset of cognitive decline.[22] In particular, physical activity can promote brain plasticity and enhance the growth of the prefrontal and hippocampal regions, which are involved in memory function.

THE CURRENT RISE OF PHYSICAL INACTIVITY

At this point of his presentation, the physiatrist paused to summarize the physiologic and medical benefits of exercise. He then moved on to an interesting aspect of his presentation: how societal trends were leading to decreasing, rather than increasing, levels of physical activity. He began this section by citing many recent studies that have documented population-level declines in physical activity. For example, Church et al. identified a significant decline in occupational physical activity over a 50-year time frame (**Figure 60.4**).[23] Similar declines in physical activity have been observed across the globe (**Figure 60.5**),[24] as well as in different demographic groups.[25]

Another trend causing concern is the amount of screen time (TV, computer/tablets, phone) individuals engage in each day. According to the U.S. Bureau of Labor Statistic's Time Use Survey for 2015, at least 56% of all daily leisure-time activity involves screen time (**Figure 60.6**). This has had a particularly detrimental effect on youth, and significant declines in leisure-time physical activity have been documented in children and adolescents.[26,27]

Relatedly, there has been increasing research into the health detriments posed by excessive sitting. Although often necessary for occupational, transportation, and recreational needs, excessive sitting time (often related to excessive screen time—computers, TV, video games) has now been linked to a variety of negative health outcomes, including obesity, diabetes, CVD, cancer, and all-cause mortality (**Figure 60.7**).[28–31] Although initial studies linking sitting time with health outcomes were often based on subjective questionnaires, more recent studies involving objectively measured sitting time using accelerometers yielded similar results. A recent study involving over 5,000 individuals examined the interaction between objectively measured (via accelerometer) sedentary time and moderate to vigorous physical activity (MVPA).[32] Although both outcomes (sedentary time and MVPA) were independently associated with all-cause mortality, interestingly, among those above the median level of MVPA, sedentary time was no longer associated with mortality. What this suggests is that, among those who are perhaps committed to prolonged sitting time (eg, occupational or transportation-related sitting), those who are able to engage in MVPA are somewhat protected from the deleterious effects of excessive sitting. To combat excessive sitting, health professionals recommend standing/walking breaks every 30 to 60 minutes. In fact, pointed out the physiatrist, a recent study found that standing > 2 hours per day (vs < 2 hours per day) was associated with a 10% reduction in all-cause mortality.[33]

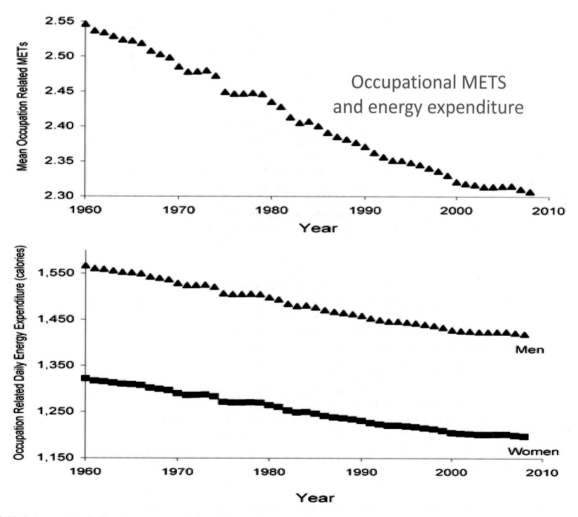

FIGURE 60.4 Progressive decline in occupational physical activity (METs) and energy expenditure (calories) over a 50-year period.

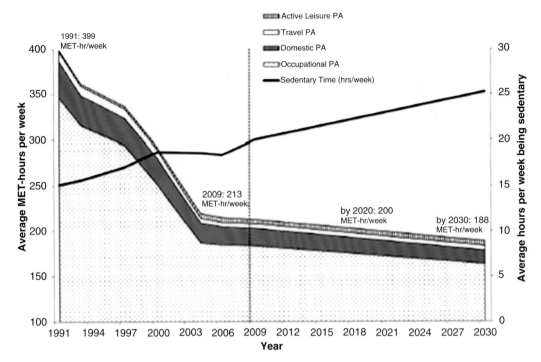

FIGURE 60.5 Progressive decline in all types of physical activity, and increasing sedentary time, over a 25-year period in China.

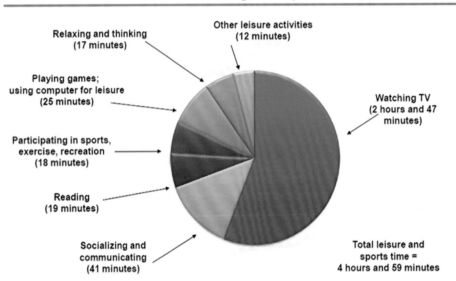

FIGURE 60.6 Time spent in various leisure-time activities, according to the U.S. Bureau of Labor Statistics. Note the significant amount of time per day spent on screen-related activities (eg, computers, video games, television).

EXERCISE ACTIVITIES

At this point, the physiatrist turned his attention toward a general discussion of exercise activities. Aware that many individuals in the audience were people like David, with different forms of cardiac conditions, the physiatrist emphasized that the initiation of exercise among cardiac patients should be done only under medical supervision. He thus said that although he would cover general points about exercise, patients should check with their doctors before initiating a specific exercise program. The physiatrist covered three general forms of activity:

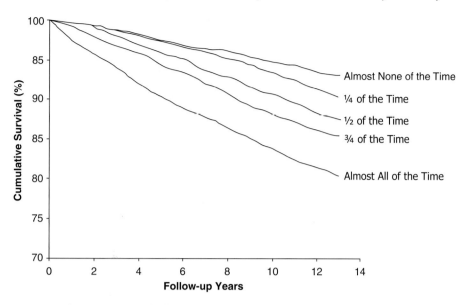

FIGURE 60.7 Daily sitting time and its association with all-cause mortality, cardiovascular disease, and cancer.

TABLE 60.2	Examples of Moderate- and Vigorous-Intensity Physical Activities
MODERATE INTENSITY (3.0–5.9 METs)	**VIGOROUS INTENSITY (≥ 6.0 METs)**
Brisk walking	Running or jogging (10-min mile or faster)
Bicycle riding on level ground	Bicycle riding at brisk pace/up hills
Doubles tennis	Singles tennis
Mowing the lawn (push mower)	Shoveling/carrying heavy loads
Washing windows/vacuuming/mopping	Basketball
Water aerobics	Lap swimming
Ballroom dancing	Soccer
	Aerobic classes (Zumba, spinning, etc.)

AEROBIC EXERCISE

According to the U.S. physical activity guidelines,[34] adults should work toward achieving 150 minutes of moderate-intensity aerobic exercise per week. Alternatively, individuals can engage in 75 minutes of vigorous-intensity exercise per week for similar health benefits. Examples of moderate and vigorous exercise activities are listed in **Table 60.2**. It should be emphasized that although substantial health benefits are achieved with these levels of physical activity, research indicates that any amount of regular physical activity can promote cardiovascular health and wellness. As for patients, many of whom have been completely sedentary, transitioning from sedentary behavior to aerobic physical activity can be quite daunting, and should be taken up with a graduated program that minimizes the risk of physical injury.

One tool that has been shown to be effective in promoting the initiation and maintenance of exercise activities is pedometers. These portable electronic devices are capable of monitoring one's daily steps, thus tracking physical activity. More advanced devices are even able to track sitting time and issue alarms when the user has exceeded a predetermined amount of sitting (eg, 1 hour). Pedometers have become so prevalent and technologically advanced that most smartphones and smart watches now have them built in. A useful way to start using a pedometer is to simply wear the device (from first thing in the morning till bedtime) every day for 1 week. Do not worry about monitoring step counts, sitting time, etc.; just wear the device and carry on with your usual weekly activities. At the end of 1 week, review the recorded data for total daily step count and calculate the average number of steps per day (eg, 3,000 steps/day). This will now serve as your baseline level of physical activity from which you can start to add steps.

It is worth noting that time recommendations can be achieved in a variety of ways. For example, for moderate-intensity activities, 30 minutes/day, 5 days/week will fulfill the 150-minute/week goal. The 30 minutes/day can even be divided into three 10-minute bouts of activity throughout the day.

TABLE 60.3	Examples of Strength (Resistance) Training Exercises
Light free or machine weights	
Push-ups/sit-ups/pull-ups	
Yoga	
Pilates	
Fitness bands	

TABLE 60.4	Examples of Activities for Promoting Balance
Walking backward	
Walking sideways	
Walking on heels	
Walking on toes	
Repeated standing from sitting position	
Tai chi	

STRENGTH (RESISTANCE) TRAINING

Although not well known, strength training is an equally important component of any exercise routine, and should be performed at least 2 times/week (in addition to the aerobic exercise recommendations). As noted earlier, strength training is important for maintaining muscle tone and strength, which are essential for successful aging and the prevention of injuries. Examples of strength (resistance) training exercises are listed in **Table 60.3**. In general, strength training can include the use of weights or, alternatively, resistance from body weight (eg, push-ups) or elastic bands. For optimal results, strength training should include as many large muscle groups as possible, including hips, back, legs, arms, chest, abdomen, and shoulders. Although no fixed rule exists, in general, strength (resistance) training exercises should be performed in 1 to 3 sets of 8 to 12 repetitions each.

BALANCE TRAINING

Older adults, and those at increased risk for falls, should engage in balance training in addition to aerobic and strength exercises. Numerous studies have noted benefits from balance training relating to overall strength, coordination, and prevention of falls and fall-related injuries among older adults. Established balance exercises include backward and sideways walking, heel walking, toe walking, and repeated standing from a sitting position (**Table 60.4**). Tai chi is also an accepted form of balance training, many exercises of which can also be used for strength training.

THE QUESTION-AND-ANSWER SESSION

After completing his general presentation, the physiatrist asked the audience to write down any questions they had and to hand

them to his assistant. He briefly reviewed these questions and then chose the following questions to discuss with the entire audience:

HOW DO I KNOW IF I AM GETTING ENOUGH EXERCISE?

The official recommendations for leisure-time physical activity are 150 minutes of moderate-intensity exercise each week or, alternatively, 75 minutes of vigorous-intensity exercise each week. This time requirement, regardless of whether it is moderate or vigorous, can be divided into different blocks throughout the day or week. For example, one can engage in 30 minutes of moderate-intensity exercise daily for 5 days, 25 minutes of vigorous-intensity exercise daily for 3 days, or any combination of moderate and/or vigorous activity to achieve the weekly recommendation. However, for those individuals just starting with exercise activities, these recommendations may be too demanding to achieve at first. Rather, one should start by committing to walking or another similar activity for a few minutes per day. After achieving some degree of success, and developing a new habit of regular exercise, one can work toward achieving progressively higher levels of exercise activity.

WHAT ARE METs AND VO$_2$ MAX, AND DO I NEED TO KNOW THESE TO START MY EXERCISE PROGRAM?

METs are metabolic equivalents and represent energy expenditure by the body during various physical activities. 1 MET is the amount of energy expended by the body at rest. Thus, various physical activities represent multiples of the baseline energy expenditure. For example, if resting quietly is equal to 1 MET, a brisk walk might be 3 to 4 METs, and jogging might be 6 to 7 METs.

VO$_2$ max represents the maximal amount of oxygen an individual can use during high-intensity exercise. Although typically used to help train high-level athletes, it is also used to guide the evaluation and management of patients with advanced heart and lung disease.

If the goal is to initiate and maintain a physical activity program for the purposes of health and wellness, it is not necessary to learn and use METs or VO$_2$ max. Rather, it would be more useful to understand which activities are generally classified as being of moderate versus vigorous intensity to help identify the types of activities and the time duration needed to meet official recommendations (Table 60.2).

WHAT IS THE DIFFERENCE BETWEEN PHYSICAL ACTIVITY AND PHYSICAL FITNESS?

Physical activity simply refers to the act of engaging in coordinated movements of the body for the purpose of achieving health (eg, walking, jogging, sports). Fitness, on the other hand, refers to the ability of the heart and lungs to adequately supply oxygen to the muscles during regular sustained exercise activity. Cardiorespiratory fitness is a more specific form of fitness that integrates not only physical and aerobic capacity, but other factors as well, including age, gender, and ethnicity. Thus, it is no surprise that cardiorespiratory fitness is the most potent measure of fitness and correlates the most with various health outcomes. In fact, cardiorespiratory fitness has been found to be as strong a predictor of all-cause mortality as other commonly accepted risk factors, including smoking, diabetes mellitus, high blood pressure, and high cholesterol. In general, cardiorespiratory fitness levels < 5 METs are associated with a higher risk of mortality, whereas levels > 8 METs are associated with increased survival.[35] Another important distinction is that physical activity, and even fitness, can be assessed by detailed questionnaires, whereas cardiorespiratory fitness can be assessed only by actual exercise testing.

IS THERE SUCH A THING AS TOO MUCH EXERCISE?

One can think of exercise in terms of both volume (duration of time spent) and intensity (low or moderate or vigorous). In terms of volume, as we noted earlier in this chapter, even the lowest level of activity (eg, standing for > 2 hours per day vs < 2 hours per day) is associated with better health outcomes. As shown by Powell et al., progressively larger volumes of exercise are associated with greater reductions in CVD, with no apparent upper limit beyond which benefit is lost (**Figure 60.8**).[36] Of note, the greatest reductions in cardiovascular risk appear to be when transitioning from sedentary to low or moderate activity. With respect to exercise intensity, no upper limit of low- or moderate-intensity exercise exists beyond which benefit is lost. In terms of vigorous-intensity exercise, some data suggest an upper limit of benefit (11 MET-hours/week); however, there is no consistent evidence of actual harm.[37]

THE PHYSIATRIST'S SUMMARY

The physiatrist concluded by reiterating the value of making regular physical activity an important part of one's daily routine. He reminded the audience that there is now an overwhelming amount of scientific research that associates physical activity with a reduced likelihood of many chronic diseases. Furthermore, physical activity can even be used as a successful treatment of various diseases and in some cases lead to the regression of disease (eg, type II diabetes mellitus). Another compelling reason to engage in regular physical activity is to promote one's sense of wellness and vitality. He told the audience that as the U.S. population ages, those who are hitting social security age (age 65) can expect to now live, on average, another 20 years. Unfortunately, too many elderly adults find themselves living with chronic debilitating diseases (eg, arthritis, obesity) in older age. This can greatly impair one's sense of wellness and vitality, decreasing one's ability to enjoy and contribute to all that life has to offer. The goal, therefore, should be to defer chronic disease and disability to the last *few years* of one's life, not the last *few decades*. This concept is referred to as the "compression of morbidity" and is tightly linked to maintaining health, wellness, and a sense of vitality for as many years as possible before illness and disability set in.[38]

If deferring illness and disability to the latter years of one's life is not sufficient reason to engage in physical activity, perhaps saving money will be another, as shown by a recent study in which higher fitness in middle age was associated with less health costs in later life (**Figure 60.9**).[39] As we learned earlier in this presentation, said the physiatrist, physical inactivity has been directly associated with an increased risk of obesity, diabetes mellitus, cardiovascular disease, and cancer, and can greatly impair cognitive function and promote musculoskeletal dysfunction and injury, as well as overall unsuccessful aging. At an economic level, physical inactivity has been estimated to contribute to over $53 billion in worldwide health care costs, creating a substantial economic burden on the public and private sectors, as well as individual households.[40] In the United States alone, physical inactivity has been estimated to contribute to approximately 11% of aggregate health care expenditures.[41]

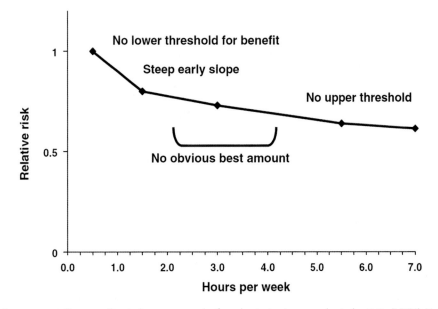

FIGURE 60.8 Risk of all-cause mortality according to hours per week of moderate to vigorous physical activity (MVPA). Note the lack of an upper or lower threshold above or below which benefit of MVPA is lost.

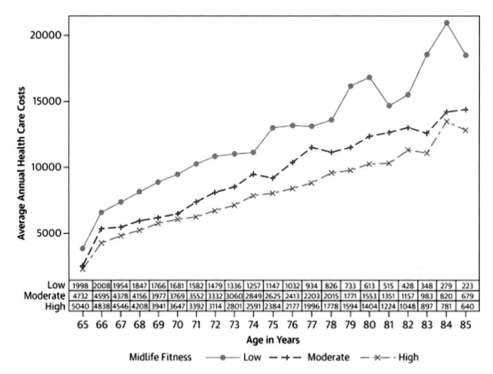

	65	66	67	68	69	70	71	72	73	74	75	76	77	78	79	80	81	82	83	84	85
Low	1998	2008	1954	1847	1766	1681	1582	1479	1336	1257	1147	1032	934	826	733	613	515	428	348	279	223
Moderate	4732	4595	4378	4156	3977	3769	3552	3332	3060	2849	2625	2413	2203	2015	1771	1553	1351	1157	983	820	679
High	5040	4838	4546	4208	3941	3647	3392	3114	2801	2591	2384	2177	1996	1778	1594	1404	1224	1048	897	781	640

FIGURE 60.9 Health care–associated costs later in life according to cardiorespiratory fitness level in middle age.

David's Follow-Up Visit With His Cardiologist

David scheduled a return visit to his cardiologist, as suggested, a week after the lecture. It was clear that David had been very inspired by the lecture and was motivated to start adding an exercise program to his health regimen. Knowing that inspiration is fleeting, his cardiologist decided to get David to commit to a specific exercise plan before he left the office. He first suggested a formal cardiac rehabilitation program that David was eligible for, which involved group exercise under medical supervision, including electrocardiographic monitoring. However, the Rehabilitation Center was located 40 minutes away from David's work, and he was afraid the time involved in traveling would make the program prohibitive. However, the cardiologist was aware of this type of problem and knew of alternative options within the community. He suggested that David join a general gym that also sponsored a cardiac patient program three nights per week between 6 and 7 PM and that was also conducted by members of the Hospital's Rehabilitation team. David indicated that option would work fine. The cardiologist wrote down the name of the gym and the contact person for David and asked him when he would make the call to join. David promised to do so that very afternoon.

His cardiologist then suggested that David also purchase a pedometer and gave him a sheet with various options.

Finally, he asked David if there was anything else he planned to do. David mentioned that he was particularly impressed about the discussion regarding the hazards of sitting and that he had already gone ahead and ordered a standing desk. His cardiologist was very impressed. He saw that David had not only been inspired to be more physically active, but had now taken important steps to anchor this motivation into a plan that would promote David's health for years to come.

REFERENCES

1. Morris JN, Heady JA, Raffle PAB, Roberts CG, Parks JW. Coronary heart disease and physical activity at work. *Lancet.* 1953;265:1053-1057.

2. Paffenberger RS Jr, Hyde RT, Wing AL, Hsieh CC. Physical activity, all-cause mortality and longevity of college alumni. *N Engl J Med.* 1986;314:605-613.

3. Bruce RA, Blackmon JR, Jones JW, Strait G. Exercise testing in adult normal subjects and cardiac patients. *Pediatrics.* 1963;32(4):742-756.

4. Myers J, Prakash M, Froelicher V, Do D, Partington S, Atwood JE. Exercise capacity and mortality among men referred for exercise testing. *N Engl J Med.* 2002;346:793-801.

5. Gupta S, Rohatgi A, Ayers CR, et al. Cardiorespiratory fitness and classification of risk of cardiovascular disease mortality. *Circulation.* 2011;123:1377-1383.

6. Thompson PD, Crouse SF, Goodpaster B, Kelley D, Moyna N, Pescatello L. The acute versus chronic response to exercise. *Med Sci Sports Exerc.* 2001;33(6):S438-S445.

7. Kokkinos P, Myers J. Exercise and physical activity: clinical outcomes and applications. *Circulation.* 2010;122:1637-1648.

8. Pescatello LS, Franklin BA, Fagard R, Farquhar WB, Kelley GA, Ray CA. American College of Sports Medicine position stand. Exercise and hypertension. *Med Sci Sports Exerc.* 2004;36:533-553.

9. Barry VW, Baruth M, Beets MW, Durstine JL, Liu J, Blair S. Fitness vs. fatness on all-cause mortality: a meta-analysis. *Prog Cardiovasc Dis.* 2014;56:382-390.

10. Blumenthal JA. Exercise and pharmacological treatment of depressive symptoms in patients with coronary heart disease: results from the UPBEAT (Understanding the Prognostic Benefits of Exercise and Antidepressant Therapy) study. *J Am Coll Cardiol.* 2012;60:1053-1063.

11. Wen CP, Wai JPM, Tsai MK, et al. Minimum amount of physical activity for reduced mortality and extended life expectancy: a prospective cohort study. *Lancet.* 2011;378:1244-1253.

12. Blair SN, Kohl HW 3rd, Barlow CE, Paffenbarger RS Jr, Gibbons LW, Macera CA. Changes in physical fitness and all-cause mortality. A prospective study of healthy and unhealthy men. *JAMA.* 1995;273:1093-1098.

13. Moore SC, Lee I-M, Weiderpass E, et al. Association of leisure-time physical activity with risk of 26 types of cancer in 1.44 million adults. *JAMA Intern Med.* 2016;176(6):816-825.

14. Jeon CY, Lokken RP, Hu FB, van Dam RM. Physical activity of moderate intensity and risk of type 2 diabetes: a systematic review. *Diabetes Care.* 2007;30(3):744-752.

15. Knowler WC, Barrett-Connor E, Fowler SE, et al. Diabetes Prevention Program Study Group. Reduction in the incidence of type 2 diabetes with lifestyle intervention or metformin. *N Engl J Med.* 2002;346:393-403.

16. Hendricks NK, White CP, Eisman JA. The roles of exercise and fall risk reduction in the prevention of osteoporosis. *Endocrinol Metab Clin North Am.* 1998;27(2):369-387.

17. Bartley MM, Geda YE, Christianson TJ, Pankratz VS, Roberts RO, Petersen RC. Frailty and mortality outcomes in cognitively normal older people: sex differences in a population-based survey. *J Am Geriatr Soc.* 2016;64(1):132-137.

18. Sergi G, Veronese N, Fontana L, et al. Pre-frailty and risk of cardiovascular disease in elderly men and women. The Pro. V.A. Study. *J Am Coll Cardiol.* 2015;65(10):976-983.

19. Fried LP, Tangen CM, Walston J, et al. Frailty in older adults: evidence for a phenotype. *J Gerontol A Biol Sci Med Sci.* 2001;56(3):M146-M156.

20. De Labra C, Guimaraes-Pinheiro C, Maseda A, Lorenzo T, Millán-Calenti JC. Effects of physical exercise interventions in frail older adults: a systematic review of randomized controlled trials. *BMC Geriatr.* 2015;15:154.

21. Bherer L, Erickson KI, Liu-Ambrose T. A review of the effects of physical activity and exercise on cognitive and brain functions in older adults. *J Aging Res.* 2013;2013:657508.

22. Erickson KI, Weinstein AM, Lopez OL. Physical activity, brain plasticity, and Alzheimer's disease. *Arch Med Res.* 2012;43(8):615-621.

23. Church TS, Thomas DM, Tudor-Locke C, et al. (2011) Trends over 5 decades in U.S. occupation-related physical activity and their associations with obesity. *PLoS One.* 2011;6(5):e19657.

24. Ng SW, Popkin B. Time Use and physical activity: a shift away from movement across the globe. *Obes Rev.* 2012;13(8):659-680.

25. Archer E, Lavie CJ, McDonald SM, et al. Maternal inactivity: 45-year trends in mothers' use of time. *Mayo Clin Proc.* 2013;88:1368-1377.

26. Kimm SYS, Glynn NW, Kriska AM, et al. Decline in physical activity in black girls and white girls during adolescence. *N Engl J Med.* 2002;347:709-715.

27. Nader PR, Bradley RH, Houts RM, McRitchie SL, O'Brien M. Moderate-to-vigorous physical activity from ages 9 to 15 years. *JAMA.* 2008;300:295-305.

28. Hu FB, Li TY, Colditz GA, Willett WC, Manson JE. Television watching and other sedentary behaviors in relation to risk of obesity and type 2 diabetes mellitus in women. *JAMA.* 2003;289:1785-1791.

29. Petersen CB, Bauman A, Grønbæk M, Helge JW, Thygesen LC, Tolstrup JS. Total sitting time and risk of myocardial infarction, coronary heart disease and all-cause mortality in a prospective cohort of Danish adults. *Int J Behav Nutr Phys Act.* 2014;11:13.

30. Patel AV, Hildebrand JS, Campbell PT, et al. Leisure-time spent sitting and site-specific cancer incidence in a large U.S. cohort. *Cancer Epidemiol Biomarkers Prev.* 2015;24:1350-1359.

31. Chau JY, Grunseit AC, Chey T, et al. Daily sitting time and all-cause mortality: a meta-analysis. *PLoS One.* 2013;8:e80000.

32. Loprinzi PD, Loenneke JP, Ahmed HM, Blaha MJ. Joint effects of objectively-measured sedentary time and physical activity on all-cause mortality. *Prev Med.* 2016;90:47-51.

33. van der Ploeg HP, Chey T, Ding D, Chau J, Stamatakis E, Bauman AE. Standing time and all-cause mortality in a large cohort of Australian adults. *Prev Med.* 2014;69:187-191.

34. Physical activity guidelines advisory committee. Physical activity guidelines advisory committee report, 2008. Washington, DC: U.S. Department of Health and Human Services; 2008.

35. Sedentary behavior and cardiovascular morbidity and mortality. A science advisory from the American Heart Association. *Circulation.* 2016;134:e262-e279.

36. Powell KE, Paluch AE, Blair SN. Physical activity for health: what kind? How much? How intense? On top of what? *Annu Rev Public Health.* 2011;32:349-365.

37. Eijsvogels TMH, Molossi S, Lee D-C, Emery MS, Thompson PD. Exercise at the extremes: the amount of exercise to reduce cardiovascular events. *J Am Coll Cardiol.* 2016;67(3):316-329.

38. Fries JF. Aging, natural death, and the compression of morbidity. *N Engl J Med.* 1980;303:130-135.

39. Bachmann JM, DeFina LF, Franzini L, et al. Cardiorespiratory fitness in middle age and health care costs in later life. *J Am Coll Cardiol.* 2015;66:1876-1885.

40. Ding D, Lawson KD, Kolbe-Alexander TL, et al. The economic burden of physical inactivity: a global analysis of major non-communicable diseases. *Lancet.* 2016;388:1311-1324.

41. Carlson SA, Fulton JE, Pratt M, Yang Z, Adams EK. Inadequate physical activity and health care expenditures in the United States. *Prog Cardiovasc Dis.* 2015;57:315-323.

Alan Rozanski
Randy Cohen

61

Applying Psychological Principles for the Lifestyle Management of Cardiac Patients

Fifteen months after sustaining his heart attack, David is scheduled for a routine follow-up with his cardiologist. Now 53 years old, David's preexisting hypertension and high cholesterol are presently well controlled on his current medical regimen and dietary changes. David had also been noted to have a high HgbA$_{1C}$ after his heart attack (6.2%), signaling a prediabetic state, but this value has now decreased to 5.7%. At his 3, 6, and 9-month follow-up visits, David had sustained his new health habits, including a strict adherence to a restricted-calorie (1,800 calories) Mediterranean diet, and an exercise regimen that he had adopted after his three-month visit, including joining a health club, which he attended for 45 to 60 minutes 3 times/week. During this time, he had also bought a standing desk and purchased a pedometer, which he wore every day.

However, 5 months before his current visit, David began to experience more stress at his law firm, which had recently expanded its operations. As one of the senior associates, David was traveling more and cutting back on some of his sleep. Feeling quite time pressed, he decided he would defer his exercise program for a week or 2, and he allowed himself permission to eat an extra snack or 2 during the day. Without thinking about it, David had resumed a prior pattern of night eating, and once he stopped exercising, he did not restart his exercise program. By the time he saw his cardiologist, he had regained 8 of the 14 lb he had previously lost during the first 9 months following his heart attack. David was pleased that his risk factors were under control, but he was quite discouraged by his failure to maintain his new health habits.

However, David's cardiologist was not perturbed by the setback. Instead, he praised David for his initial success and said that this proved he could do it again. He then mentioned to David that he knew a health psychologist, Dr. Jones, who helped coach patients who were having trouble adopting new health behaviors and maintaining them for the long term. He mentioned that Dr. Jones gave a monthly lecture on stress and heart disease at the hospital and suggested that David attend the lecture.

David was very eager to do so. At the lecture, Dr. Jones explained that his presentation was divided into three parts. First, he would discuss the scope of psychological factors that are related to heart disease. Second, he would describe psychological principles related

to the management of health behaviors and stress management. Third, he would provide the participants with a self-reflective exercise that could guide their future self-management of their health goals.

PSYCHOSOCIAL RISK FACTORS FOR HEART DISEASE

Dr. Jones began the first portion of his lecture by showing a slide that listed the psychological domains that he would discuss (**Table 61.1**). He then spent a few minutes discussing the following essentials regarding each psychological domain that was listed on the slide.

DEPRESSION

Depression is a common psychological symptom that can range from very mild symptoms to those that are very severe. Severe or "major depression" is said to be present when patients experience a markedly depressed mood or the lack of interest in nearly all of their activities in life for at least 2 consecutive weeks, in conjunction with other psychological symptoms, including either loss or increase in appetite, insomnia, fatigue, difficulty concentrating, and feelings of guilt.

The systemic pathophysiologic effects of depression are profound. When depression is chronic, it can result in persistent activation of the hypothalamic pituitary adrenal axis and dysregulation of the sympathetic nervous system, leading to a rise in serum cortisol levels and elevated norepinephrine levels. This in turn can lead to profound systemic effects affecting many physiologic functions and organ systems, as shown in **Figure 61.1**.[1] For instance, people suffering from depression have a higher frequency of insulin resistance and elevated risk for diabetes. They are also more prone to develop abdominal obesity and elevation in inflammatory proteins, as well as pathology in the inner lining of blood vessels ("endothelial dysfunction"). Depression also leads to platelet abnormalities in the blood. All of these changes combine to accelerate the development and progression of atherosclerosis in the coronary vessels.

Secondly, depression also has an important negative effect on the health habits of individuals. People who are depressed are more likely to eat poorly, be sedentary, smoke, and be less proactive about their health in general. Moreover, once depression sets in, people find it harder to comply with recommended behavioral changes, such as suggestions for exercise, or even with their prescription medications.

TABLE 61.1	Psychosocial Risk Factors for Cardiovascular Disease

1. Depression
2. Anxiety syndromes
   • Elevated anxiety symptoms
   • Phobias
   • Generalized anxiety disorder
   • Posttraumatic stress disorder
3. Pessimism
4. Hostility/anger
5. Loneliness and poor social support
6. Lack of life purpose
7. Chronic stress
   • Work stress
   • Marital stress
   • Caregiver stress
   • Effects of trauma and abuse
   • Chronic illness
8. Fatigue states
   • Vital exhaustion
   • Burnout
   • Lack of sleep

Epidemiologic study indicates that chronic depression is a particularly potent factor for promoting heart disease. In a large meta-analysis of 54 epidemiologic studies, the adjusted risk for developing adverse cardiac events among individuals who were depressed was increased nearly 2-fold among depressed versus nondepressed subjects in both community cohorts as well as in patients with prior cardiovascular disease (CVD) (**Figure 61.2**).[2]

Investigators have also found a graded relationship between the degree of depressive symptoms and the likelihood of adverse cardiac events. For example, Lesperance et al.[3] conducted a follow-up study in 896 patients who had sustained a myocardial infarction. All patients filled out a questionnaire (the Beck Depression Inventory) to assess their degree of depressive symptoms at baseline, and were then followed for 5 years (**Figure 61.3**). The risk of cardiac mortality during the follow-up period increased in direct proportion to the magnitude of depressive symptoms. Notably, even mild depressive symptoms increased risk somewhat in comparison with patients who had no signs of depressive symptoms.

Notably, the prevalence of depression is substantial among cardiac patients. The 1-month community-based prevalence of major depression is approximately 4% to 5%. By contrast, this prevalence is approximately 2-fold higher in cardiac populations.[4] In addition, depressive symptoms of a milder degree than major depression are found in another 15% of cardiac patients.[4] The high prevalence typifies a reciprocal relationship: depression is a risk factor for heart disease, but in addition, the development of heart disease can lead to depressive symptoms in some patients.

ANXIETY

Anxiety symptoms are also common in society and increase in prevalence among patients with heart disease and other chronic medical symptoms. As with depression, symptoms may range from

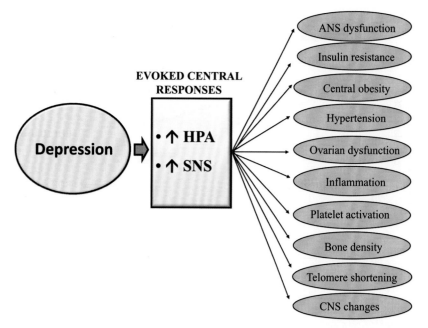

FIGURE 61.1 In the presence of chronic depression, there is persistent stimulation of the sympathetic nervous system and the hypothalamic pituitary axis (HPA). The result is diverse pathophysiologic effects, as shown. ANS, autonomic nervous system. (Modified from Rozanski A, Blumenthal JA, Davidson KW, Saab PG, Kubzansky L. The epidemiology, pathophysiology, and management of psychosocial risk factors in cardiac practice: the emerging field of behavioral cardiology. *J Am Coll Cardiol.* 2005;45:637-651.)

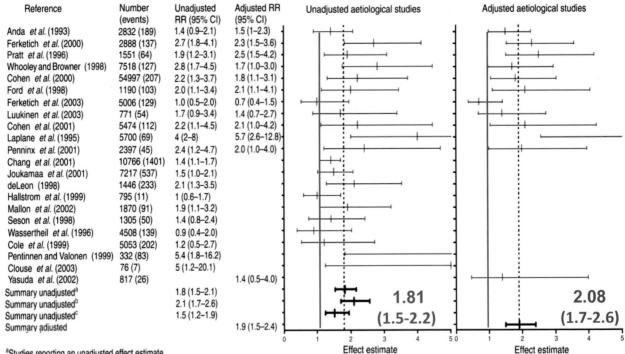

FIGURE 61.2 Relative risks (RR) are shown for the occurrence of coronary disease events (cardiac death or myocardial infarction) in association with depression among community cohorts, according to both unadjusted and adjusted data. A substantial elevation in risk is noted. RR, risk ratio; CHD, coronary heart disease; CI, confidence interval. (From Nicholson A, Kuper H, Hemingway H. Depression as an aetiologic and prognostic factor in coronary heart disease: a meta-analysis of 6,362 events among 146,538 participants in 54 observational studies. *Eur Heart J.* 2006;27:2763-2774.)

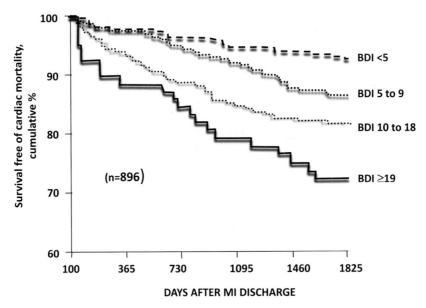

FIGURE 61.3 A 5-year follow-up of 896 post–myocardial infarction (MI) patients who were assessed according to their degree of depressive symptoms according to the Beck Depression Inventory (BDI), ranging from no depressive symptoms (BDI < 5) to moderate to severe depressive symptoms (BDI ≥ 19). There was a gradient relationship between the magnitude of depressive symptoms and the frequency of subsequent deaths. (From Lesperance F, Frasure-Smith N, Talajiv M, Bourassa MG. Five-year risk of cardiac mortality in relation to initial severity and one-year changes in depression symptoms after myocardial infarction. *Circulation.* 2002;105:1049-1053.)

mild symptoms to severe psychiatric conditions, including phobias, panic disorder, generalized anxiety disorder, and posttraumatic stress disorder (PTSD). The relationship between anxiety and cardiac disease was recently assessed in a very large meta-analysis of 46 studies, involving 2,017,276 participants and 222,253 subjects with anxiety.[5] Anxiety was associated with a moderately elevated risk for cardiac disease, cardiac death, stroke, and heart failure, as shown in **Figures 61.4 and 61.5.**

Psychiatric-level anxiety syndromes are associated with even further cardiac risk.[6–9] For instance, an interesting study concerning PTSD was conducted in 562 twins in whom only one of the two twins had suffered from PTSD. The twins were followed for

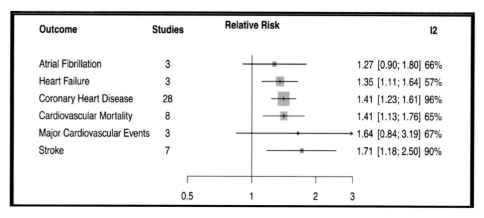

FIGURE 61.4 The relative risk posed by anxiety in association with various cardiac conditions. (From Emdin CA, Odutayo A, Wong CX, et al. Meta-analysis of anxiety as a risk factor for cardiovascular disease. *Am J Cardiol.* 2016;118:511-519.)

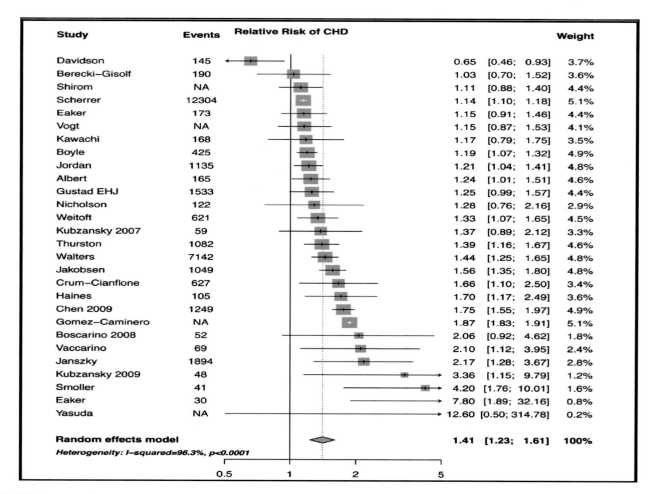

FIGURE 61.5 The relative risk of developing coronary heart disease (CHD) is shown for each of 28 studies included in this meta-analysis. (From Emdin CA, Odutayo A, Wong CX, et al. Meta-analysis of anxiety as a risk factor for cardiovascular disease. *Am J Cardiol.* 2016;118:511-519.)

a mean of 13 years.[10] The presence of PTSD in one of the twins was associated with a more than 2-fold increase in cardiac disease.

PESSIMISM

It has been demonstrated that optimism is a general life asset, associated with greater likelihood of successful goal achievement in life and an enhanced sense of resilience. Pessimism, by contrast, can diminish coping skills and self-confidence, and it is associated with an increased risk of depression. Studies on the specific effects of pessimism versus optimism as a cardiac risk factor, however, have only been recent.

Pessimism is generally characterized as a personality disposition toward expecting negative outcomes in the future. Optimists, on the other hand, tend toward expecting positive outcomes. Another way psychologists have assessed optimism versus pessimism in the past is by examining people's "explanatory style." Pessimists tend to evoke an explanatory style of self-blame when negative events occur, and they tend to expect that these events will be persistent and affect many aspects of their lives. Optimists, on the other hand, tend to avoid self-blame for negative events, and view these events as transient and limited in scope.

Both dispositional and explanatory pessimism have been linked to negative health outcomes. The results, in fact, have been quite consistent. Pessimism is associated with reduced longevity and increased risk of cardiovascular events and stroke.[11–15] Optimism has the opposite effect. As with most psychological risk factors, a graded relationship has been noted between the level of pessimism or optimism and the occurrence of these negative events. Recent data from the Nurses' Health Study (NHS) have also demonstrated important effects of optimism on reduction of other health outcomes, including cancer, respiratory disease, and infection.[16]

As with other psychological risk factors, the impact of optimism versus pessimism on health appears to be related to both biologic and behavioral mechanisms. Biologic mechanisms include a positive effect of optimism on immune function, better autonomic function, and, pending further study, potentially slower rates of telomere shortening over time. In addition, optimists tend to exhibit a higher likelihood of engaging in exercise, eating a healthy diet, and a lower likelihood of smoking and other negative behaviors.

HOSTILITY

Hostility is a broad construct that encompasses the traits of anger, cynicism, and mistrust. The study of hostility has been an outgrowth of initial work by Friedman and Rosenman to study a personality complex that they termed "Type A behavior pattern," based on three features: the presence of easily provoked hostility, a competitive drive, and a sense of time urgency and impatience. Over time, epidemiologic data did not confirm initial positive findings concerning Type A behavior pattern as a cardiac risk factor, but the hostility component has been shown to demonstrate a modest relationship to heart disease. This construct is hard to study because many patients with hostility tend to have some degree of self-denial or lack of self-awareness about their anger and hostility. Nevertheless, a large meta-analysis found that individuals with a pattern of anger/hostility have about a 20% to 25% elevated risk for heart disease compared to individuals without hostility.[17]

LONELINESS AND POOR SOCIAL SUPPORT

Individuals have a basic need to be socially connected to others. Here, we can make a distinction between being alone and feeling lonely. People vary in the depth of their need for connectivity to others, but unmet social needs and/or a feeling of loneliness is not only painful, but often health damaging. One of the first studies to examine the relationship between social factors and adverse outcomes was the "Alameda County study."[18] This study asked individuals to characterize how many people were in their social network and then followed them for a number of years. The investigators found that as the size of one's "social network" decreased, the risk of all-cause mortality increased (**Figure 61.6**). Since then, this finding has been reproduced in many studies. Similarly, other studies have demonstrated that a variety of social factors are related to health, including the size, structure, and

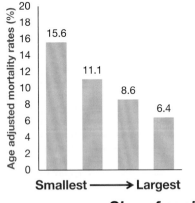
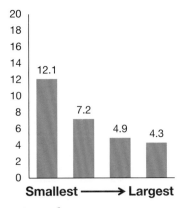

Size of social networks

FIGURE 61.6 The age-adjusted mortality results are shown for men and women who were characterized at baseline according to the size of their social network size in the Alameda County study. Mortality rates were highest in those with small social networks and lowest in those with high social networks. (From Berkman LF, Syme SL. Social networks, host resistance, and mortality: a nine-year follow-up study of Alameda county residents. *Am J Epidemiol*. 1979;109:186-204.)

frequency of contacts within one's social network, and the quality of either functional and/or emotional support that one receives from others. A recent meta-analysis of 148 studies found that individuals who scored high on a measure of social integration had an approximately 2-fold increase in survival compared to individuals who were less socially integrated.[19] Such an increase in survival is a substantial health benefit when compared to other clinical parameters that can affect health.

PURPOSE IN LIFE

Living with intentionality and goal directedness provides individuals with a strong sense of life purpose. By contrast, a lack of life purpose is associated with boredom and increases the risk of future depression. Over the last decade, a series of studies have studied the relationship between one's sense of life purpose and important clinical outcomes, such as heart disease, dementia, and longevity. In one recent meta-analysis of 10 prospective studies that involved over 136,000 subjects, investigators found that a high sense of life purpose was associated with a reduced risk ratio for cardiac events and for all-cause mortality (**Figure 61.7**).[20] The results were highly consistent among the individual studies constituting this meta-analysis. A higher sense of purpose has also been linked to a reduced risk of stroke, future physical disability, and dementia. Prospective study is needed to study the mechanisms by which this occurs, but preliminary data suggest that people who live with a high sense of life purpose tend to maintain more positive health behaviors and have a greater sense of psychological well-being.

In addition, purpose in life may be associated with greater resilience, as suggested by a meta-analysis of 70 studies that found that purpose in life was associated with a greater sense of competence, stronger social integration, and more positive affect.[21]

CHRONIC STRESS

Another psychological factor associated with heart disease is chronic stress. More distinctively, it is "toxic" stress, or a chronic sense of distress, that seems to be associated with adverse medical outcomes. That is, not all stress is bad. Rather, individuals, as part of their desire to live a life of purpose, like to take on life challenges. Successful coping with life stress can provide both life satisfaction and an increased sense of self-esteem.

As with depression, chronic distress can lead to stimulation of the hypothalamic–pituitary–adrenocortical axis and the sympathetic nervous system, leading to many similar effects on physiologic functions and organ systems. Of note, people under chronic distress are also more likely to become physiologic "hyper-reactors," meaning that there is a tendency for heart rate and blood pressure responses to rise higher and recover more slowly following acute stimulations compared to people who are not under distress. Other studies indicate that chronic distress can lead to signs of accelerated aging, as measured by DNA evidence.[1,22] Finally, chronic distress can result in adverse changes in the brain's plasticity, including increase in the size of the amygdala, which is the brain's fear center, and reduction in the size of the hippocampus and prefrontal cortex.[23]

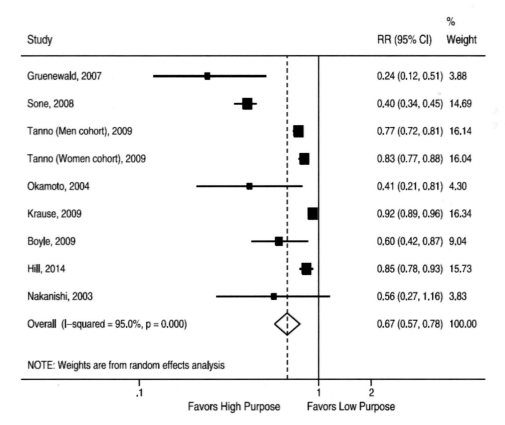

FIGURE 61.7 Meta-analysis of the risk ratio for having adverse cardiac outcomes according to the presence of having a high versus low sense of life purpose. The presence of high purpose was associated with a diminished risk of cardiac events. CI, confidence interval; RR, risk ratio. (From Cohen R, Bavishi C, Rozanski A. Purpose in life and its relationship to all-cause mortality and cardiovascular events: a meta-analysis. *Psychosom Med.* 2016;78:122-133.)

There are various types of distress that have been linked to a higher risk of heart disease, including work stress and marital strain. In addition, acute and chronic illnesses can also produce a stress response among some patients. For instance, Edmonsdon et al.[24] found that among patients presenting with acute coronary syndrome (ACS) patients, 12% developed symptoms of PTSD. Other common negative chronic stressors include caregiving strain and the enduring effects of childhood abuse or trauma. For instance, in the NHS II, involving a 16-year follow-up of 66,798 women, a history of childhood abuse was associated with an approximately 1.5-fold increase in the onset of cardiovascular events by middle age.[25] The investigators found that adult risk factors such as smoking, diabetes, and increased body mass index, as well as the presence of other psychosocial factors, such as depression, accounted for the majority of this elevated risk.

NEGATIVE FATIGUE STATES

Another negative psychological risk factor is the presence of negatively charged fatigue states (ie, a feeling of tiredness that is intermixed with negative emotions or a sense of tension). This is in contrast to calm-tiredness, which may occur after a long day of satisfying work. The latter is regenerative, whereas a state of "tense-tiredness" can induce negative moods and a need for quick fix behaviors.[26,27] When individuals are in sync in terms of physical health, social well-being, and a sense of purpose, they have a greater sense of vitality. The presence of vitality promotes an overall sense of well-being and provides people with energy for successful coping and emotional regulation. On the other end of the spectrum is the presence of "vital exhaustion," a condition of excessive fatigue, feelings of demoralization, and increased irritability, which has been postulated to be a result of prolonged distress.[28] Epidemiologic study has consistently linked vital exhaustion to an increased risk of cardiac events and/or all-cause mortality. For instance, vital exhaustion was recently compared to other CVD risk factors in a follow-up of 8,882 individuals who were initially free from CVD in the Copenhagen City Heart Study.[29] Vital exhaustion was found to be a strong independent risk factor for the development of CVD in both genders, with manifestation of a strong risk-adjusted gradient relationship. Another negative fatigue state is the presence of burnout, which is characterized by a sense of exhaustion, depersonalization, and diminished efficacy at work. Preliminary study also suggests that burnout can increase the risk for heart disease.[30-31] In addition, chronic poor sleep, including insomnia, represents another risk factor for heart disease.[32,33]

"CLUSTERING" OF PSYCHOSOCIAL RISK FACTORS

Although psychosocial stresses are often studied in isolation, in life they often tend to cluster together. For example, people with poor social support are also more likely to feel life stress. When such negative psychosocial risk factors cluster, they tend to magnify the potential pathophysiologic effects of these factors. For example, in a study of post–MI patients, the presence of high levels of life stress and social isolation were both found to be associated with an approximately 2-fold increase in subsequent clinical events.[34] But overall clinical risk was increased 4-fold among post–MI patients reporting both social isolation and life stress. Similarly, clinical risk is magnified among patients who report both anxiety and depression.[35] Notably, psychosocial factors also interact synergistically with physical risk factors to increase overall clinical risk. For example, depressed patients who are physically inactive are at increased risk for future cardiac events (**Figure 61.8**).[36] Such data emphasize the need to treat any and all risk factors as best as one can to reduce the overall clinical risk among patients.

MANAGING HEALTH BEHAVIORS AND LIFE STRESS

After providing the audience with this overview, Dr. Jones asked if there were any questions and then began the second portion of his lecture. He mentioned that any health goal, like goals in

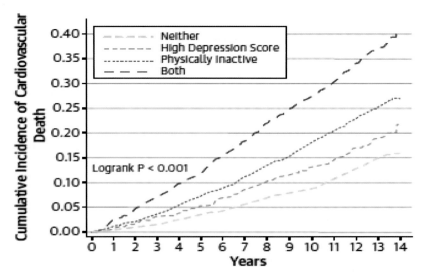

FIGURE 61.8 The cumulative incidence of cardiovascular death among patients divided into four groups according to being physically active or inactive and according to having a high versus low depression score in the Cardiovascular Health Study. (From Win S, Parakh K, Eze-Nliam CM, et al. Depressive symptoms, physical inactivity and risk of cardiovascular mortality in older adults: the Cardiovascular Health Study. *Heart.* 2011;97:500-505.)

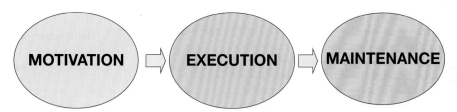

FIGURE 61.9   The pursuit of goals can be divided into three components, as shown. Techniques that can be used to foster motivation, execution, and maintenance in each group are shown. (From Rozanski A. Behavioral cardiology: current advances and future directions. *J Am Coll Cardiol.* 2014;64:100-110.)

general, could be broken down into three phases, as illustrated in another slide he showed them (**Figure 61.9**). These three phases included: (1) motivation; (2) goal execution; and (3) goal maintenance. Under each category, Dr. Jones listed a number of representative tools and techniques that could be used by individuals to foster that phase of goal pursuit. To save time, Dr. Jones chose to address just a few of these tools in his lecture, as follows:

AUTONOMY

Motivation can be classified as either "intrinsic" or "extrinsic" in origin. Examples of extrinsic motivation include warning, provision of incentives, or the provision of case managers. When motivation comes from within, this is termed internal motivation. Patients, as with all people, are more likely to stick with a goal that is derived from internal motivation. The desire to choose a goal based on your own volition rather than being told by someone else what to do is termed "autonomy." For instance, whereas physicians can provide patients with compelling health reasons for exercise, diet, and so forth, a schooled physician will also look for other angles by which to foster internal motivation in patients. For instance, a patient may want to start a diet to feel good or to please a spouse or merely to please his or her physician. The more compelling the personal reason is, the more likely the patient will follow through. In addition, merely asking patients to verbalize their own personal reasons helps patients to take more ownership of their health goals. Various studies have found that when patients leave their doctors' office with a sense of autonomy regarding a suggested health goal, they are more likely to adhere to their health goals over time.

SELF-EFFICACY

The setting of unrealistic goals is a prescription for failure. By contrast, the more someone believes that a certain goal can be accomplished (ie, the greater the sense of "self-efficacy"), the more the person will be willing to try. For instance, health organizations recommend that individuals get at least 20 to 30 minutes of moderate physical exercise on most days of the week. Although this is a reasonable goal for people who are generally fit, this is generally

too hard for a completely sedentary person. It is more important that sedentary people first establish a goal that is compatible with their individual sense of "self-efficacy," even if this means a very minimal goal at first, such as walking 5 to 10 minutes/day. Once patients have tasted some success in a new health domain, goals can then be increased incrementally.

SPECIFIC ACTION PLANS

Vague action plans are another prescription for failure. Rather, the more specific the action plan, the greater the likelihood of patient adherence. For instance, establishing a goal to get more exercise is a vague goal. Deciding to join a gym is more specific. Even better is committing to which days of the week one may go to the gym and for how long. Writing down one's goals helps build one's sense of commitment.

SELF-MONITORING

Self-monitoring helps to anchor health goals by providing a mechanism for daily self-awareness and personal feedback. The most obvious example of self-monitoring is using a scale to weigh oneself daily. Studies indicate that overweight individuals who weigh themselves daily are more successful in maintaining weight loss compared to individuals who do not. More recently, the use of pedometers as a means of self-monitoring one's physical activity has become increasingly promulgated. For example, a review of medical studies found that the use of pedometers was associated with a 27% increase in physical activity compared to physical activity before initiating pedometer use.[37] The use of pedometers has a number of potential advantages: it is a way of becoming more cognizant of one's physical activity; it can be motivational for some to monitor their steps and try to increase them; and the information can also represent a form of feedback to patients as they learn to monitor and track their daily steps.

There are different potential walking goals that can be established with the use of a pedometer. Some providers have popularized a goal of achieving 10,000 steps/day, but caution needs to be employed, because such a goal may not be practical initially for many older adults, those with chronic illnesses, or those who are significantly deconditioned. Rather, an incremental approach in terms of increasing pedometer steps based on one's baseline level of activity is preferred for those who are initially sedentary. For instance, after determining baseline step counts based on a week of observation, patients may begin by seeking to increase their physical activity by a mere 100 to 200 steps/day, with progressive increases according to an individual's sense of self-efficacy during subsequent weeks.

IMPLEMENTATION INTENTIONS

When a patient commits to a new health goal, the new practice is highly vulnerable because of the pressures of daily life. A new practice must be repeated continually before it becomes a habit. To strengthen habit formation, a group of investigators, Gollwitzer and colleagues, have developed a technique called "implementation intentions."[38] An implementation intention involves the use of an external stimulus to cue a specific behavior ("X"), followed by a specific action ("Y") that will be initiated when that cue occurs. The cue can be a stimulus in time, place, or situation. Gollwitzer et al. suggest that the formulation should always be stated as follows:

> **"When it is X, I will do Y," where "X" is the cue, and "Y" is the behavior.**

Although this technique might seem simple, a large meta-analysis of many studies involving the use of implementation intentions has found that implementation intentions are associated with a moderate to large effect in stimulating successful goal achievement.[39] One such example comes from a study of women who were being encouraged to perform breast self-examination (BSE) to promote early detection of breast cancer.[40] In the study, all women received a lecture on the importance of BSE, but half of the women were also asked to perform an implementation intention around how and when they would perform this task (eg, *"On the first evening of each new month, I will perform my breast self-examination."*). Notably, the women who were asked to form an implementation intention concerning BSE manifested a substantially higher rate of adherence to this health practice during follow-up.[40] Similar findings were noted in a study concerning implementation intentions and physical activity (**Figure 61.10**).[41]

CONTINGENCY PLANS

Developing contingency plans around new goals is an important step in fostering long-term goal maintenance. Stressful life events, boredom, new competing priorities, and many other factors frequently intervene to challenge a patient's ability to stick with a new health goal. The key thing during such times is to not let the desired goal activity go down to zero, since the complete cessation of activity increases the risk that the health goal will not be reinstituted. A contingency plan represents a certain floor of minimal activity that will be maintained during times of stress. For example, if a patient has committed to exercising at the gym five times per week, the contingency plan may be a temporary reduction to exercising only 2 times/week.

SOCIAL SUPPORT

Having social support can provide both renewable motivation and coping help to maintain new health goals. Medical studies

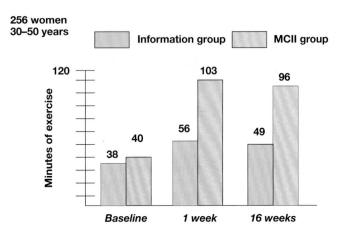

FIGURE 61.10 Minutes of moderate to vigorous physical activity per week among two groups of women, randomized to either an information group about exercise or to a group that were also asked to perform mental contrasting and make an implementation intention about exercise (MCII). The MCII group had nearly double the amount of physical activity at both one week and four months. (From Stadler G, Oettingen G, Gollwitzer PM. Physical activity in women: effects of a self-regulation intervention. *Am J Prev Med.* 2009;36:29-34.).

reveal that when social support is lacking, patients are less likely to adhere to their physicians' health recommendations.[42] Building appropriate social support is highly personal and depends on many factors, such as one's personal need for social support, the availability of friends, social opportunities in one's community, and time constraints.

FEEDBACK

Feedback represents a specific form of tangible support, combining components of the aforementioned tools. Knowing that feedback will be provided by one's health provider tends to increase one's sense of accountability. Feedback may also help people gain insights into the natural blind spots that they experience when pursuing difficult goals. Feedback also provides a sense of social support and a sense of teamwork—"we're in this thing together."

STRESS MANAGEMENT

One of the common reasons why patients fail to maintain new health habits over the long term is their difficulty in balancing this new commitment with other life priorities. Many patients can benefit from enhanced stress management skills. One useful approach that may be particularly relevant for cardiac patients is to consider stress from the perspective of one's sense of energy and sense of tension. This was the focus of research by Dr. Robert Thayer years ago.[26,27] Through his work, he developed his model of tension and energy, as shown in **Figure 61.11**. He observed that when people are both tense and tired, they tend to be more moody and more likely to resort to "quick fix" behaviors that will reduce their tension or increase their energy. Very often, these quick fixes are counterproductive and health damaging, such as the use of cigarette smoking to reduce tension or frequent ingestion of candy bars to mollify stress or increase energy.

Either increasing energy and/or reducing stress can be used to decrease the frequency of tense-tiredness that a person may feel. The best way to reduce chronic stress is to reduce the source

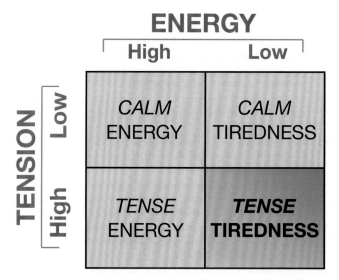

FIGURE 61.11 Per work developed by Thayer et al., personal states can be characterized by one's level of energy and tension, as shown. Periods of tense-tiredness tend to be characterized by a higher frequency of low moods and quick-fix behaviors.

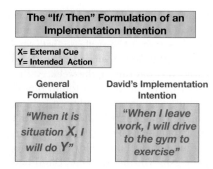

FIGURE 61.12 General formulation of an Implementation Intention and the specific Implementation Intention formulated by David. "X" is the external cue, which may be a specific time, place, or situational cue. "Y" is the intended action.

of the tension. However, even when this is not possible, the breakup of continuous tension can be quite beneficial. Tension-busters include breathing exercises, guided meditation exercises, engaging in interests that one finds stimulating or relaxing, and social diversions. In addition, individuals may turn to specific forms of stress-reducing physical activities such as yoga and tai-chi.

Alternatively, individuals can attempt to reduce tense-tiredness by taking steps to increase their general energy level. Importantly, research shows that people tolerate their stress better when they feel energetic. Taking on positive health behaviors, such as exercise, adequate sleep, and a healthy diet plan all help in this regard. In addition, if a person realizes that there is a point in the day at which they are particularly prone to feeling tired, they can build an energy plan around that, such as taking a short nap, or developing the habit of taking out a 10- to 15-minute physical or mental breather that is restorative of energy during energetically low points of the day.

When one feels that their stress is unmanageable, seeking the advice of trained coaches may be useful for isolated problems, such as poor time management skills, and/or the consideration of mental health counseling, particularly if there is also an overlay of anxiety, depressive symptoms, increasing pessimism, sleeping problems, an inability to relax physically or mentally, or feelings of social alienation.

AN EXERCISE IN LIFESTYLE MANAGEMENT

After completing the second phase of his lecture, Dr. Jones explained that life stress and psychological challenges are commonplace, and can frequently be exaggerated by acute or chronic illnesses. He then mentioned that there is no specific formula for dealing with life stress, because of the highly varied differences in individuals' "life settings" (eg, income, social circumstances), personalities, coping skills, level of conflicting priorities, and many other factors, intrinsic talents, upbringing to them. To illustrate some of the points of his lecture, Dr. Jones gave the audience participants the following assignment:

First, he asked the people to identify all negative health habits and psychological problems that were relevant to them on the basis of his lecture presentation. David thought about this. He certainly did not feel depressed, unduly anxious, or hostile toward anyone. He was quite dissatisfied with his failure to exercise and to maintain his new diet. In addition, he recognized that he was overdoing it at work and that he had to work on his time management skills He was also not getting enough sleep. David realized that he had a lot on his plate.

Dr. Jones then asked each individual to identify one problem that they would like to work on over the next 3 months. This did not preclude working on other problems, but he explained that strong success in one area often breeds energy to succeed in other arenas. David was fascinated by the question. He decided to take on the issue of restarting an exercise program. He recalled how good he had felt when he was getting more physically fit and how that had helped him to maintain his health diet during that time.

Dr. Jones then asked each participant to form a specific health goal to address a chosen problem, with the greatest specificity possible. David realized that the only time he was likely to exercise was when he left work. He got to work too early to consider exercise, and exercising during the day was not an option. Once he got home at night, he was either too distracted or tired to go out to the gym again. Thus, the only practical option was to exercise after leaving the office, before he got home. As to the frequency, David figured he would try to exercise daily after work, so that he could make this more habitual. He further decided to devote a total of 1 hour at the gym per session, which would include time to change into and out of his gym gear and a 30-minute workout.

Dr. Jones then asked the audience to form an implementation intention around their new health goal. David had really enjoyed that part of the lecture and he quickly formulated his intention (**Figure 61.12**):

"When I leave the office on Monday through Friday, I will drive directly to the gym to work out for 30 minutes."

Leaving work was David's cue to engage in his health behavior. Working out at the gym was the specific behavior.

Finally, Dr. Jones suggested that each individual formulate a contingency plan for their new goal. For David, this amounted to going to the gym on Fridays, for one half-hour of exercise, with a second makeup session on the weekends.

Dr. Jones then asked the participants to write down their implementation intention and share it with someone who could hold them accountable. He also suggested that the participants calendar their intended program, if possible, in their daily planners.

David left the lecture feeling very pleased with what he learned. Over the course of the next 3 months, David found himself exercising nearly every day during the week. At first, it was very difficult. As he drove to the gym, he found himself having all sorts of complaints, such as "I am too tired tonight" or "I have too much to do" or "I am hungry." But he stuck with the plan and was now realizing that the goal was taking root as a new habit. In fact, he was beginning to feel uncomfortable on the days that he did not go to the gym. During this time, David had also begun to eat better again and had lost 4 lb. He was excited to make his next follow-up meeting with his cardiologist. David shared with him his success, the life skills he felt he had learned in the process, and his overall sense of feeling quite energetic. At the end of the visit, David thanked his physician for being attuned to the psychological dimensions of health care and left the office with a sense of confidence about his health and his future.

REFERENCES

1. Rozanski A, Blumenthal JA, Davidson KW, Saab PG, Kubzansky L. The epidemiology, pathophysiology, and management of psychosocial risk factors in cardiac practice: the emerging field of behavioral cardiology. *J Am Coll Cardiol.* 2005;45:637-651.

2. Nicholson A, Kuper H, Hemingway H. Depression as an aetiologic and prognostic factor in coronary heart disease: a meta-analysis of 6362 events among 146 538 participants in 54 observational studies. *Eur Heart J.* 2006; 27:2763-2774.

3. Lesperance F, Frasure-Smith N, Talajiv M, Bourassa MG. Five-year risk of cardiac mortality in relation to initial severity and one-year changes in depression symptoms after myocardial infarction. *Circulation.* 2002;105:1049-1053.

4. Rozanski A, Blumenthal JA, Kaplan J. Impact of psychological factors on the pathogenesis of cardiovascular disease and implications for therapy. *Circulation.* 1999;99:2192-2217.

5. Emdin CA, Odutayo A, Wong CX, Tran J, Hsiao AJ, Hunn BH. Meta-analysis of anxiety as a risk factor for cardiovascular disease. *Am J Cardiol.* 2016;118:511-519.

6. Roest AM, Zuidersma M, de Jonge P. Myocardial infarction and generalised anxiety disorder: 10-year follow-up. *Br J Psychiatry.* 2012;200:324-329.

7. Roest AM, Martens EJ, Denollet J, de Jonge P. Prognostic association of anxiety post myocardial infarction with mortality and new cardiac events: a meta-analysis. *Psychosom Med.* 2010;72:563-569.

8. Tully PJ, Turnbull DA, Beltrame J, et al. Panic disorder and incident coronary heart disease: a systematic review and meta-regression in 1131612 persons and 58111 cardiac events. *Psychol Med.* 2015;45:2909-2920.

9. Edmondson D, Kronish IM, Shaffer JA, Falzon L, Burg MM. Posttraumatic stress disorder and risk for coronary heart disease: a meta-analytic review. *Am Heart J.* 2013;166:806-814.

10. Vaccarino V, Goldberg J, Rooks C, et al. Post-traumatic stress disorder and incidence of coronary heart disease: a twin study. *J Am Coll Cardiol.* 2013;62:970-978.

11. Kubzansky LD, Sparrow D, Vokonas P, Kawachi I. Is the glass half empty of half full? A prospective study of optimism and coronary heart disease in the normative aging study. *Psychosom Med.* 2001;63:910-916.

12. Tindle HA, Chang YF, Kuller LH, et al. Optimism, cynical hostility, and incident coronary heart disease and mortality in the women's health initiative. *Circulation.* 2009; 120: 656-662.

13. Giltay EJ, Kamphuis MH, Kalmijn S, Zitman FG, Kromhout D. Dispositional optimism and the risk of cardiovascular death: the Zutphen Elderly Study. *Arch Intern Med.* 2006;166:431-436.

14. Nabi H, Koskenvuo M, Singh-Manoux A, et al. Low pessimism protects against stroke: the Health and Social Support (HeSSup) prospective cohort study. *Stroke.* 2010;41:187-190.

15. Kim ES, Park N, Peterson C. Dispositional optimism protects older adults from stroke: the Health and Retirement Study. *Stroke.* 2011;42:2855-2859.

16. Kim ES, Hagan KA, Grodstein F, DeMeo DL, De Vivo I, Kubzansky L. Optimism and cause-specific mortality: a prospective cohort study. *Am J Epidemiol.* 2017;185:21-29.

17. Chida Y, Steptoe A. The association of anger and hostility with future coronary heart disease: a meta-analytic review of prospective evidence. *J Am Coll Cardiol.* 2009;53:936-946.

18. Berkman LF, Syme SL. Social networks, host resistance, and mortality: a nine-year follow-up study of Alameda county residents. *Am J Epidemiol.* 1979;109:186-204.

19. Holt-Lunstad J, Smith TB, Layton JB. Social relationships and mortality risk: a meta-analytic review. *PLoS Med.* 2010;7:e1000316.

20. Cohen R, Bavishi C, Rozanski A. Purpose in life and its relationship to all-cause mortality and cardiovascular events: a meta-analysis. *Psychosom Med.* 2016;78:122-133.

21. Pinquart M. Creating and maintaining purpose in life in old age: a meta analysis. *Aging Int.* 2002;27:90-114.

22. Rozanski A. Behavioral cardiology: current advances and future directions. *J Am Coll Cardiol.* 2014;64:100-110.

23. McEwen BS. Physiology and neurobiology of stress and adaptation: central role of the brain. *Physiol Rev.* 2007;87:873-904.

24. Edmondson D, Richardson S, Falzon L, Davidson KW, Mills MA, Neria Y. Posttraumatic stress disorder prevalence and risk of recurrence in acute coronary syndrome patients: a meta-analytic review. *PLos One.* 2012;7:e38915.

25. Rich-Edwards JW, Mason S, Rexrode K, et al. Physical and sexual abuse in childhood as predictors of early-onset cardiovascular events in women. *Circulation.* 2012;126:920-927.

26. Thayer RE. Energy, tiredness, and tension effects of a sugar snack versus moderate exercise. *J Pers Soc Psychol.* 1987;52:119-125.

27. Thayer RE. *The Biopsychology of Mood and Arousal.* New York, NY: Oxford University Press; 1991.

28. Appels A, Happener P, Mulder P. A questionnaire to assess pre-monitoring symptoms of myocardial infarction. *Int J Cardiol.* 1987;17:15-24.

29. Schnohr P, Marott JL, Kristensen TS, et al. Ranking of psychosocial and traditional risk factors by importance for coronary heart disease: the Copenhagen City Heart Study. *Eur Heart J.* 2015;36:1385-1393.

30. Ahola K, Vaaananen A, Kskinen A, Kouvonen A, Shirom A. Burnout as a predictor of all-cause mortality among industrial employees: a 10-year prospective register-linkage study. *J Psychosom Res.* 2010;69:51-57.

31. Toker S, Melamed D, Berliner S, Zeltser D, Shapira I. Burnout and risk of coronary heart disease: a prospective study of 8,838 employees. *Psychosom Med.* 2012;74:840-847.

32. Cappuccio FP, Cooper D, D'Elia L, Strazzullo P, Miller MA. Sleep duration predicts cardiovascular outcomes: a systematic review and meta-analysis of prospective studies. *Eur Heart J.* 2011;32:1484-1492.

33. Sofi F, Cesari F, Casini A, Macchi C, Abbate R, Gensini GF. Insomnia and risk of cardiovascular disease: a meta-analysis. *Eur J Prev Cardiol.* 2014;21(1):57-64.

34. Ruberman W, Weinblatt E, Goldberg JD, Chaudhary BS. Psychosocial influences on mortality after myocardial infarction. *N Engl J Med.* 1984;311:552-529.

35. Watkins LL, Koch GG, Sherwood A, et al. Association of anxiety and depression with all-cause mortality in individuals with coronary heart disease. *J Am Heart Assoc.* 2013;2:e000068.

36. Win S, Parakh K, Eze-Nliam CM, Gottdiener JS, Kop WJ, Ziegelstein RC. Depressive symptoms, physical inactivity and risk of cardiovascular mortality in older adults: the Cardiovascular Health Study. *Heart.* 2011;97:500-505.

37. Bravata DM, Smith-Spangler C, Sundaram V, et al. Using pedometers to increase physical activity and improve health. *JAMA.* 2007;298(19):2296-2304.

38. Gollwitzer PM. Implementation intentions: strong effects of simple plans. *Am Psychol.* 1999;54:493-503.

39. Gollwitzer PM, Sheeran P. Implementation Intentions and goal achievement: a meta-analysis of effects of processes. *Adv Exp Soc Psychol.* 2006;38:69-119.

40. Orbell S, Hodgkins S, Sheeran P. Implementation intentions and the theory of planned behavior. *Pers Soc Psych Bull.* 1997;23:945-954.

41. Stadler G, Oettingen G, Gollwitzer PM. Physical activity in women: effects of a self-regulation intervention. *Am J Prev Med.* 2009;36:29-34.

42. Dimatteo MR. Social support and patient adherence to medication treatment: a meta-analysis. *Health Psychol.* 2004;23:207-218.

Index

Page numbers followed by "*f*" and "*t*" denotes figures and tables respectively